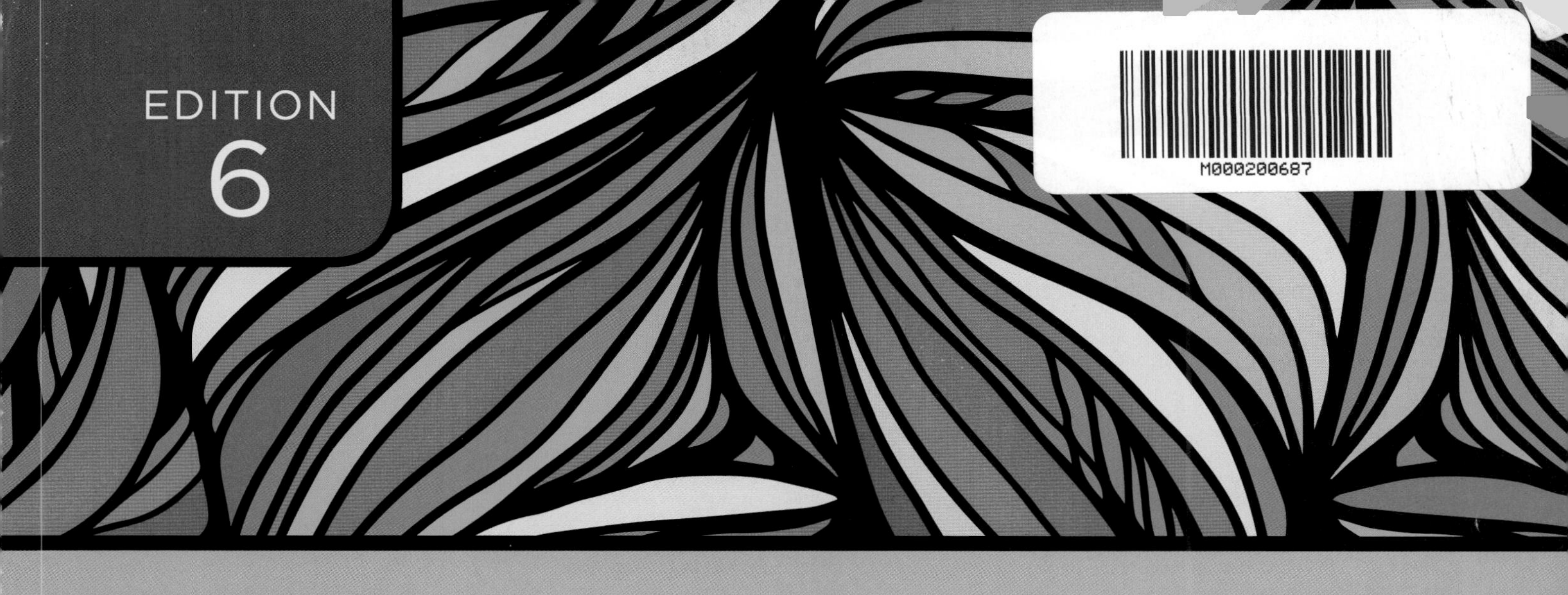

ESSENTIALS OF Dental Assisting

DEBBIE S. ROBINSON, CDA, MS
Research Associate and Project Manager
Gillings School of Global Public Health
University of North Carolina
Chapel Hill, North Carolina

DONI L. BIRD, CDA, RDA, RDH, MA
Dental Education Consultant
DB Bird Management;
Former Director, Allied Dental Education Program
Instructor, Continuing Education
Santa Rosa Junior College
Santa Rosa, CA

ELSEVIER

ELSEVIER

3251 Riverport Lane
St. Louis, Missouri 63043

ESSENTIALS OF DENTAL ASSISTING, SIXTH EDITION ISBN: 978-0-323-40064-0

International Standard Book Number: 978-0-323-40064-0

Senior Content Strategist: Kristin Wilhelm
Content Development Manager: Luke Held
Content Development Specialist: Kelly Skelton
Publishing Services Manager: Julie Eddy
Project Manager: Michael Sheets
Design Direction: Renee Duenow

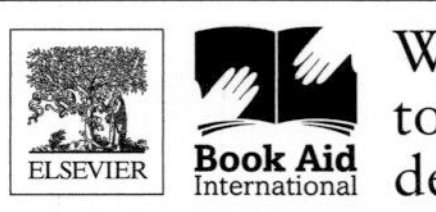

Printed in China

Last digit is the print number: 9 8 7 6 5 4 3 2 1

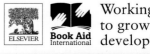

About the Authors

DEBBIE S. ROBINSON is currently a Research Associate Professor at the University of North Carolina, where she is involved in clinical research within the Gillings School of Global Public Health. Her educational background includes an associate degree in Dental Assisting from Broward Community College, a bachelor's degree in Health Administration from Florida Atlantic University, and a master's degree in Dental Auxiliary Teachers Education from the University of North Carolina. Her clinical experience includes practicing as a clinical chairside assistant for 7 years in a pediatric dental office, as well as in the dental research center and the special patient care clinic at the University of North Carolina (UNC) Dental School. With more than 20 years of teaching, Debbie has held teaching positions at community college settings in Florida and North Carolina. She has served as Clinical Assistant Professor and Director of the Dental Assisting Program and Dental Assisting Specialty Program at UNC School of Dentistry. She has presented continuing education for practicing dental assistants at local, state, and international meetings. She has served as a member of the Dental Assisting National Board (DANB) test construction committee for two terms and has authored and coauthored journal articles for *The Dental Assistant.* Additional endeavors include consulting with community colleges and proprietary schools on the development of new dental assisting programs across the country.

DONI L. BIRD is the former Director of the Allied Dental Education Programs at Santa Rosa Junior College in Santa Rosa, California. She has taught dental assisting at City College of San Francisco, College of Marin, and the University of New Mexico. Before becoming a dental assisting educator, she practiced as a dental assistant in private practice and as a supervisor of the Dental Clinic at Mount Zion Hospital and Medical Center in San Francisco. Doni holds a bachelor's degree in Education and a master's degree in Education from San Francisco State University and a degree in dental hygiene from the University of New Mexico in Albuquerque. She has served as a member and Chairman of the board of directors of the Organization for Safety, Asepsis, and Prevention (OSAP). She is a member of the American Dental Assistants Association (ADAA) and has served as President of the Northern California Dental Assistants Association and as a board member and Chairman of the Dental Assisting National Board (DANB). She served as a consultant to the Registered Dental Assisting Test Construction Committee in California and on the board of directors of the California Association of Dental Assisting Teachers (CADAT). She has also served as a consultant in dental assisting education to the Commission on Dental Accreditation (CODA) of the American Dental Association (ADA). Additional endeavors include consulting with private dental practices, community colleges, and proprietary schools on the development of new dental assisting programs across the country.

Preface

Welcome to the sixth edition of *Essentials of Dental Assisting*. Our goal for this edition was to design a textbook along with ancillaries that meet the needs of specific groups in the population of dental assisting professionals, that is, individuals who are gaining general background knowledge and skills, those who are in entry-level positions in a clinical setting, and those on-the-job–trained dental assistants who are preparing to take the Dental Assisting National Board certification examinations.

Many of the chapters in this edition have been revised and enhanced to include the most up-to-date knowledge and skills that are being taught in dentistry and practiced in clinical settings. The book is divided into 10 parts, beginning with historical information, legal and ethical issues, and scientific background, leading into preclinical and clinical areas, and finishing with preparation for employment and national board examinations. Each chapter provides specific objectives for the reader to achieve, terms for the reader to review to ensure comprehension of the content, specific figures and tables that are designed to assist the reader in grasping the material, and, finally, procedures that provide detail and exercises designed to test comprehension.

The role of the dental assistant in today's dental practice requires an individual who is well informed and skilled from the very basic level of patient care and continuing to the performance of advanced intraoral procedures. To be an efficient and competent member of the dental team, the clinical assistant of today must have critical-thinking abilities when solving problems, as well as knowledge and understanding when making legal and ethical decisions.

A career as a dental assistant can be challenging and rewarding. Becoming a well-educated and clinically competent dental assistant will require dedication, determination, and desire. This may sound like quite a challenge, but you can do it!

The Learning Package

The sixth edition of *Essentials of Dental Assisting* is designed as a comprehensive learning package.

The student package includes:

- Textbook
- Evolve Resources
- Student Workbook (sold separately)

The faculty package includes all student resources plus:

- Test bank
- TEACH Instructor Resources

Textbook

Specific updated guidelines and recommendations are integrated into this edition, which provides:

- Comprehensive coverage that spans the entire dental assisting curriculum
- Cutting-edge content in an approachable writing style
- Expert authorship
- Top-notch artwork
- Step-by-step procedures for basic and expanded functions identified by icons
- The most recent CDC Guidelines for Infection Control in Dentistry to promote adherence to the most advanced infection control procedures for patients and dental professionals
- Intraoral, panoramic, and digital radiographic techniques used in dentistry today
- Standards that apply to performing CPR
- HIPAA requirements that address patient confidentiality as ensured by the health care system
- Nutritional guidelines as determined by the Food and Nutrition Board of the National Academy of Sciences
- Anesthesia color coding system designed by the American Dental Association Council on Scientific Affairs
- Excellent clinical photographs

The following tools guide the reader:

- **Key Terms** are introduced throughout the chapter. Each chapter features two different types of highlighted terms: terms that appear in bold and blue and terms that appear in bold and black. The terms appearing in bold and blue are key terms and appear in the Key Terms list at the beginning of each chapter. The terms that appear in bold and black are important to the material being discussed in the chapter (and are therefore emphasized) but were first introduced in an earlier chapter. All terms are also included in a comprehensive Glossary at the back of the book, which provides chapter cross-references. The definitions reinforce these new terms.
- **Learning Objectives** are introduced at the beginning of each chapter so that readers will know what is expected of them at both the theoretical and the performance levels.
- **Ethical Implications** boxes will help readers focus on ethical and legal behaviors that they must know to protect themselves, dental patients, and dental practices.
- **Multiple-Choice Questions** are found at the end of each chapter for readers to use to test their immediate knowledge. Answers are available to instructors in the *Instructor's Resource Manual* on the Evolve Web site.

- **Apply Your Knowledge** allows readers to analyze and initiate discussions in the classroom setting or with the dental team.
- **Procedures** are presented in a step-by-step sequence with illustrations, lists of equipment and supplies that the dental assistant will need, and the rationale behind each step. Procedural icons are included to remind the reader of the preparation and precautions that are needed. Examples of how the procedure might be entered in the patient's chart are provided at the end of many procedures.

It should be noted that there may be more than one way to perform a procedure correctly. Some dental assistants may perform a procedure one way, whereas others may choose to perform the same procedure using a slightly different technique. We have chosen to feature the methods used by most dental assisting programs.

Evolve Resources

Elsevier has created a Web site to support this learning package at http://evolve.elsevier.com/Robinson/essentials/. This Evolve site includes both student and instructor resources.

Student Resources

- Chapter quizzes in instant-feedback format
- Competency skill sheets for all procedures in the text
- Multiple-choice practice examination (250 questions)
- Content updates
- Procedural videos (more information follows)

Videos

Visual presentation is vital for learning clinical skills. The student Evolve Resources provide 65 video clips of specific skills that the dental assistant may perform in the clinical setting; they are organized into the following categories:

- Oral Health and Prevention of Disease
- Infection Prevention in Dentistry
- Occupational Health and Safety
- Patient Information and Assessment
- Clinical Dentistry
- Dental Imaging
- Dental Materials
- Comprehensive Dental Care

Emphasis in these videos is placed on the expanded functions delegated to the credentialed dental assistant. Again, it should be noted that there may be more than one way to perform any technique correctly. We have chosen to feature the techniques used by most dental assisting programs.

The videos also feature:

- Interactive review questions at the end of each skill
- Optional English and Spanish closed-captioning
- Animations that showcase common medical emergency conditions
- The collection in a downloadable format
- Scripts in English and Spanish

Instructor Resources

- Access to all student resources
- Image collection
- Instructor-specific content updates
- Test bank with 1,000 questions and answers, rationales for all choices, page number references for remediation, cognitive level, Certified Dental Assistant (CDA) examination blueprint category, and chapter objectives to which the question maps, available in ExamView.
- TEACH Instructor Resources (more information follows)

TEACH Instructor Resources

TEACH for *Essentials of Dental Assisting* is an all-in-one resource designed to save educators time and take the guesswork out of classroom planning and preparation. TEACH includes detailed lesson plans with chapter teaching focus, pretests, background assessments, and related class discussions and activities, all designed to fit into 50-minute classroom increments to ease the work involved in classroom preparation. These lesson plans are centered on mapping textbook and ancillary content (by page number) to specific chapter learning and performance outcomes. Answers to the chapter exercises and the student workbook questions and exercises are also available with TEACH. In addition, lecture outlines provide detailed PowerPoint presentations with teaching notes or talking points as a ready-to-use classroom resource for educators.

Note: If you are unable to access TEACH on the Evolve Web site, contact your Elsevier Education Solutions Consultant.

Student Workbook

The student workbook is a supplement to the learning process. The workbook includes review exercises for all chapters, competency skills sheets for all procedures in the textbook, and 42 flashcards as a bonus study aid.

Acknowledgments

The authors would like to recognize and thank many people whose contributions were instrumental in the completion of this project.

Thank you to our publishing family at Elsevier: Kristin Wilhelm, Senior Content Strategist; Kelly Skelton, Content Development Specialist; Julie Eddy, Publishing Services Manager; Mike Sheets, Project Manager; Traci Cahill, Marketing Manager; and Renee Duenow, Designer. In addition, a huge thank you to the sales associates nationwide who really do the legwork to get "EDA" to instructors and programs. We truly appreciate everyone's support, advice, contributions, and collaboration in creating such a comprehensive learning package.

We sincerely appreciate and thank the reviewers who took the time to evaluate our work carefully and to provide constructive suggestions and recommendations.

Finally, a special thank you to our family, friends, and colleagues for their ongoing patience, adjustments to their schedules, and support that go hand in hand with working in the publishing world.

Debbie and Doni

How to Use *Essentials of Dental Assisting*

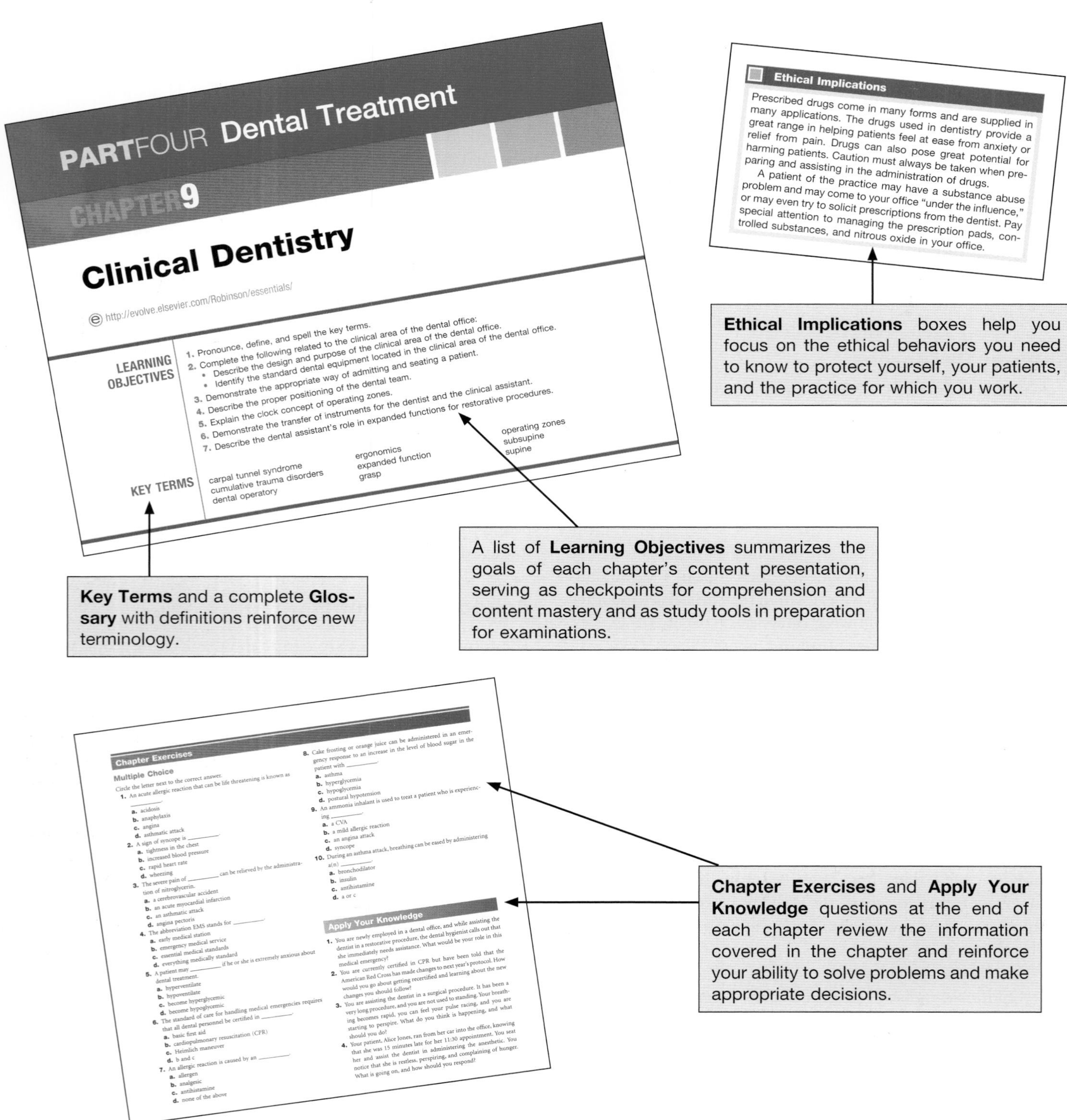

PARTFOUR Dental Treatment
CHAPTER 9
Clinical Dentistry
http://evolve.elsevier.com/Robinson/essentials/
LEARNING OBJECTIVES
1. Pronounce, define, and spell the key terms.
2. Complete the following related to the clinical area of the dental office:
• Describe the design and purpose of the clinical area of the dental office.
• Identify the standard dental equipment located in the clinical area of the dental office.
3. Demonstrate the appropriate way of admitting and seating a patient.
4. Describe the proper positioning of the dental team.
5. Explain the clock concept of operating zones.
6. Demonstrate the transfer of instruments for the dentist and the clinical assistant.
7. Describe the dental assistant's role in expanded functions for restorative procedures.
KEY TERMS
carpal tunnel syndrome
cumulative trauma disorders
dental operatory
ergonomics
expanded function
grasp
operating zones
subsupine
supine
Ethical Implications
Prescribed drugs come in many forms and are supplied in many applications. The drugs used in dentistry provide a great range in helping patients feel at ease from anxiety or relief from pain. Drugs can also pose great potential for harming patients. Caution must always be taken when preparing and assisting in the administration of drugs.
A patient of the practice may have a substance abuse problem and may come to your office "under the influence," or may even try to solicit prescriptions from the dentist. Pay special attention to managing the prescription pads, controlled substances, and nitrous oxide in your office.
Ethical Implications boxes help you focus on the ethical behaviors you need to know to protect yourself, your patients, and the practice for which you work.
A list of Learning Objectives summarizes the goals of each chapter's content presentation, serving as checkpoints for comprehension and content mastery and as study tools in preparation for examinations.
Key Terms and a complete Glossary with definitions reinforce new terminology.
Chapter Exercises
Multiple Choice
Apply Your Knowledge
Chapter Exercises and Apply Your Knowledge questions at the end of each chapter review the information covered in the chapter and reinforce your ability to solve problems and make appropriate decisions.

Step-by-step procedures in the textbook include illustrations, the equipment and supplies you will need, icons, and the rationale behind certain steps. An example of how you might enter the procedure in the patient's chart is provided at the end of many procedures.

Procedural icons are located with each procedure to remind you at a glance of those important precautions that are required during the performance of a procedure.

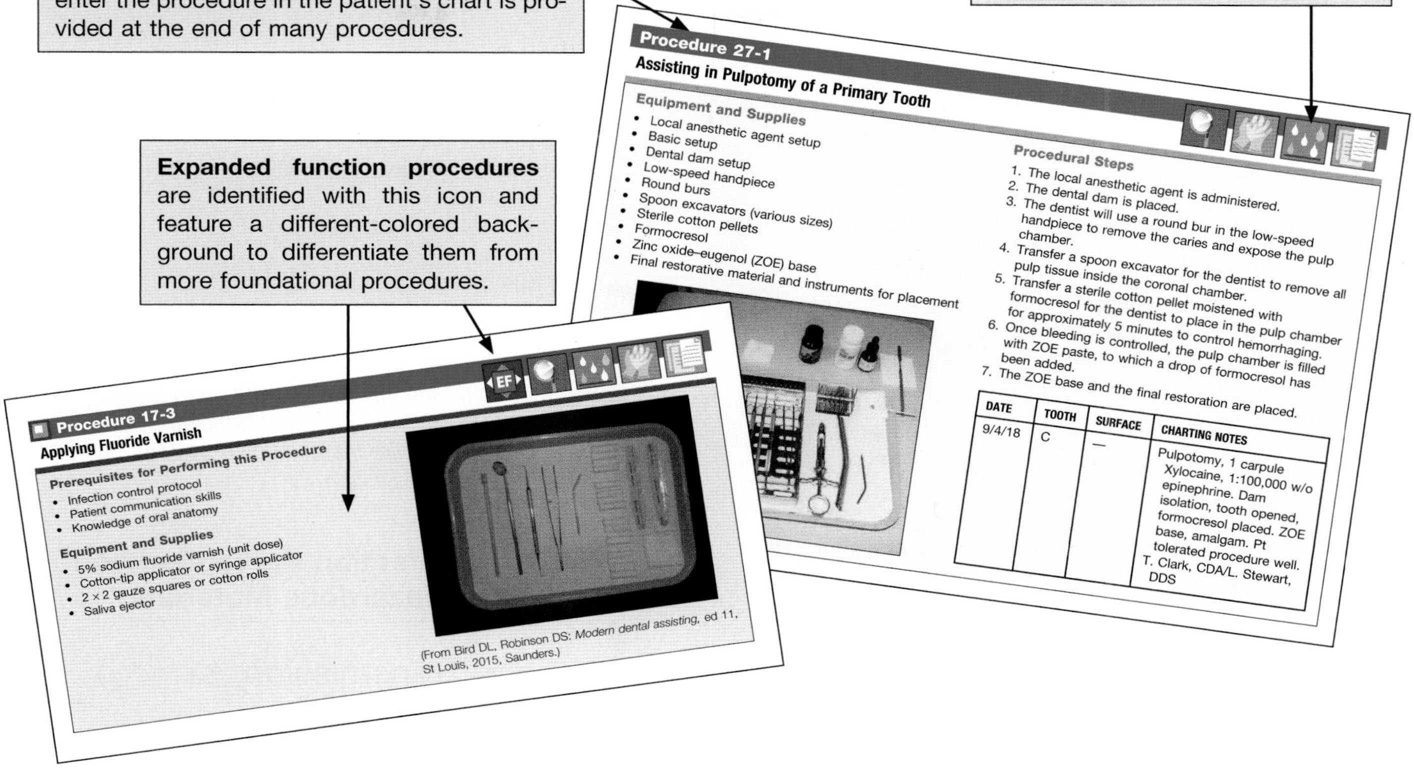

Procedure 27-1

Assisting in Pulpotomy of a Primary Tooth

Equipment and Supplies

- Local anesthetic agent setup
- Basic setup
- Dental dam setup
- Low-speed handpiece
- Round burs
- Spoon excavators (various sizes)
- Sterile cotton pellets
- Formocresol
- Zinc oxide–eugenol (ZOE) base
- Final restorative material and instruments for placement

Procedural Steps

1. The local anesthetic agent is administered.
2. The dental dam is placed.
3. The dentist will use a round bur in the low-speed handpiece to remove the caries and expose the pulp chamber.
4. Transfer a spoon excavator for the dentist to remove all pulp tissue inside the coronal chamber.
5. Transfer a sterile cotton pellet moistened with formocresol for the dentist to place in the pulp chamber for approximately 5 minutes to control hemorrhaging.
6. Once bleeding is controlled, the pulp chamber is filled with ZOE paste, to which a drop of formocresol has been added.
7. The ZOE base and the final restoration are placed.

DATE	TOOTH	SURFACE	CHARTING NOTES
9/4/18	C	—	Pulpotomy, 1 carpule Xylocaine, 1:100,000 w/o epinephrine. Dam isolation, tooth opened, formocresol placed. ZOE base, amalgam. Pt tolerated procedure well. T. Clark, CDA/L. Stewart, DDS

Expanded function procedures are identified with this icon and feature a different-colored background to differentiate them from more foundational procedures.

Procedure 17-3

Applying Fluoride Varnish

Prerequisites for Performing this Procedure

- Infection control protocol
- Patient communication skills
- Knowledge of oral anatomy

Equipment and Supplies

- 5% sodium fluoride varnish (unit dose)
- Cotton-tip applicator or syringe applicator
- 2 × 2 gauze squares or cotton rolls
- Saliva ejector

(From Bird DL, Robinson DS: Modern dental assisting, ed 11, St Louis, 2015, Saunders.)

Icon Key

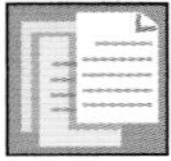

The procedure should be documented in the patient record.

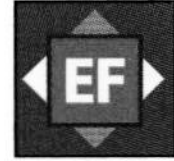

In some states, the procedure is considered an expanded function if it is delegated to the dental assistant. Always review the regulations in the Dental Practice Act of your state.

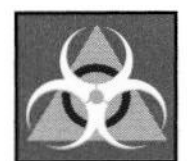

The procedure involves contact with materials that are considered hazardous. Review the safety data sheet (SDS) on this procedure. Special handling, labeling, or disposal techniques may be required.

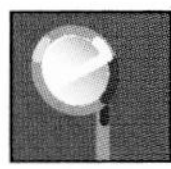

The student should be able to identify the instruments required for the stated procedure and to recognize their use.

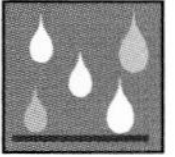

The procedure is sensitive to moisture contamination. Special precautions such as cotton roll placement, oral evacuation, and the use of a dental dam must be applied to avoid moisture in the oral cavity.

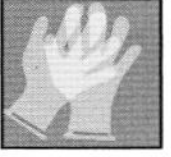

The procedure involves exposure to potentially infectious materials and requires the use of appropriate personal protective equipment (PPE), such as protective clothing, mask, eyewear, and gloves.

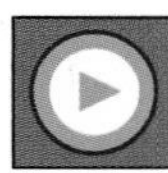

The procedure is featured in a video on the Evolve Resources Web site.

Contents

PART SIX Dental Imaging

PART SEVEN Preventive Dentistry

CHAPTER 1

Introduction to Dental Assisting

http://evolve.elsevier.com/Robinson/essentials/

LEARNING OBJECTIVES

1. Pronounce, define, and spell the key terms.
2. Describe the highlights in the history of dental assisting and dentistry, including but not limited to the following:
   - Name the individual who discovered x-rays.
   - Name the first dentist to employ a dental assistant.
   - Name the first African American to receive the Doctor of Medical Dentistry degree from Harvard University.
   - Name the first African-American woman to receive a dental degree in the United States.
   - Name the first Native American Indian to receive a dental degree in the United States.
- Name the first Native-American Indian woman to receive a dental degree in the United States.
3. Complete the following related to the members of the healthcare team:
   - Name each member of the dental team, and explain the role of each.
   - List and describe each of the specialties of dentistry.
   - Describe the various roles of the dental assistant.
4. Identify and describe the areas of a dental office.

KEY TERMS

C. Edmund Kells
certified dental technician (CDT)
Commission on Dental Accreditation (CODA) of the American Dental Association (ADA)
dental assistant
dental health care team
dental laboratory technician
dental public health
dental specialties
dentist
Doctor of Dental Surgery (DDS)
Doctor of Medical Dentistry (DMD)
endodontics
expanded-functions dental assistant (EFDA)
George Blue Spruce, Jr.
Ida Gray-Rollins
Jessica A. Rickert
oral and maxillofacial radiology
oral and maxillofacial surgery
oral pathology
orthodontics
pediatric dentistry
prosthodontics
radiographs
registered dental hygienist (RDH)
Robert Tanner Freeman
Wilhelm Conrad Roentgen

Dental assistants are important members of the **dental health care team**. A dental assistant career is exciting, challenging, and very rewarding. Many opportunities are available for young people who are deciding on a career and individuals who may be older and wish to return to school to begin a new career.

This chapter takes you through the highlights in the history of dentistry, including how the **Lady in Attendance** evolved into the highly skilled dental health professional recognized today as the dental assistant. You will learn the roles and responsibilities of each member of the dental health team, as well as how the members interact to provide patients with quality dental care. You will also learn about the specialty areas of dentistry.

History of Dentistry

Dentistry has a long and fascinating history. From the earliest times, humans have suffered from dental pain and have sought a variety of means to treat it. From the earliest times, humans also cleaned and cared for their teeth. Early toothbrushes ranged from wooden sticks with frayed ends to ivory-handled brushes with animal-hair bristles for cleaning the teeth. Today, many people think of "cosmetic dentistry" as a relatively new field, but skulls of ninth-century Mayans have numerous inlays of decorative jade and turquoise on the front teeth. Skulls of the Incas discovered in Ecuador have gold pounded into prepared holes in the teeth, similar to modern gold inlay restorations. As B.W. Weinberger noted in *Dentistry: An Illustrated History*, a profession that is ignorant of its past experiences has lost a valuable asset because "it has missed its best guide to the future." Table 1-1 lists the major highlights in the history of dentistry.

Wilhelm Conrad Roentgen (rent-ken) (1845-1923) was a Bavarian physicist who discovered the x-ray beam in 1895 (Figure 1-1). His discovery revolutionized diagnostic capabilities and forever changed the practice of medicine and dentistry. The images produced by x-ray beams on film are known as **radiographs**.

C. Edmund Kells (1856-1928), a New Orleans dentist, is usually credited with employing the first dental assistant (Figure 1-2). In 1885 the first "lady assistant" was actually a "lady in attendance" who made it respectable for an unaccompanied woman patient to visit a dental office. The assistant helped with office duties, and Dr. Kells was working with both a chairside dental assistant and a secretarial assistant by the year 1900. Soon other dentists saw the value of dental assistants and began to train dental assistants in their own offices.

Today, the dental assistant is a key member of the dental health team, performing a wide variety of duties.

African Americans in Dental History

African Americans were not accepted for training at any dental schools until 1867, when Harvard University initiated its first dental class and accepted **Robert Tanner Freeman** as its first black student. Since then, African Americans have been appointed deans and faculty members at a number of American dental schools. **Ida Gray-Rollins** (1867-1953) was the first African-American woman in the United States to earn a dental

TABLE 1-1
Highlights in the History of Dentistry

Date	Group/Individual	Event
3000-2151 BC	Egyptians	Hesi-Re is the earliest dentist known by name.
900-300 BC	Mayans	Teeth receive attention for religious reasons or self-adornment.
460-322 BC	Greeks	Hippocrates and Aristotle write about tooth decay.
166-201 AD	Romans	Decayed teeth are restored with gold crowns.
570-950	Muslims	Siwak is used as a primitive toothbrush
1510-1590	Ambroise Paré	Writes extensively about dentistry, including extractions.
1678-1761	Pierre Fauchard	Becomes the "Father of Modern Dentistry."
1728-1793	John Hunter	Performs the first scientific study of teeth.
1844	Horace Wells	Uses nitrous oxide for the relief of dental pain.
1859		The American Dental Association is founded.
1885	C. Edmund Kells	Employs the first dental assistant.
1895	G.V. Black	Becomes the "Grand Old Man of Dentistry" and perfects amalgam.
1895	W.C. Roentgen	Discovers the x-ray beam.
1908	Frederick McKay	Discovers that fluoride is associated with the prevention of dental caries.
1913	Alfred C. Fones	Establishes the first dental hygiene school in Bridgeport, Connecticut.
1924		The American Dental Assistants Association is founded.
1947		The Dental Assisting National Board is founded.
1970	Congress	Creates the Occupational Safety and Health Administration.
1978	*Journal of the American Dental Association*	Publishes a report on infection control for dental offices.
1982		The first hepatitis B vaccine becomes commercially available.
2000		*Oral Health in America: A Report of the Surgeon General* is released.
2003	Centers for Disease Control and Prevention	Releases *Guidelines for Infection Control in Dental Health-Care Settings—2003.*

degree. She practiced dentistry in Chicago until she retired in 1928 (Table 1-2).

Native Americans in Dental History

Dr. George Blue Spruce, Jr. is the first Native-American dentist in the United States. He graduated Dental School from Creighton University in 1956, where he was the only Native American on campus (Figure 1-3). He began treating patients on Native American reservations and later became an Assistant Surgeon General in the United States Public Health Service. He is currently the Assistant Dean for American Indian Affairs at the Arizona School of Dentistry and Oral Health.

"... Never be afraid to go after your dream. You, too, can meet and beat the challenges that come your way. Sometimes simply discovering and sharing your dreams can be a big step forward" (Dr. George Blue Spruce, Jr.).

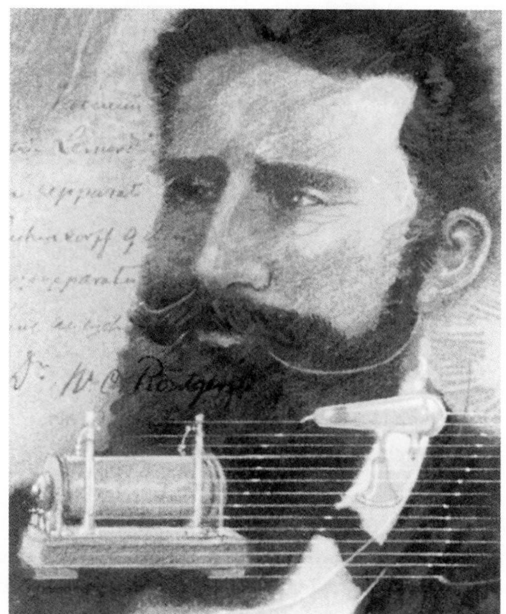

FIGURE 1-1 Wilhelm Conrad Roentgen discovered the early potential of the x-ray beam in 1895.

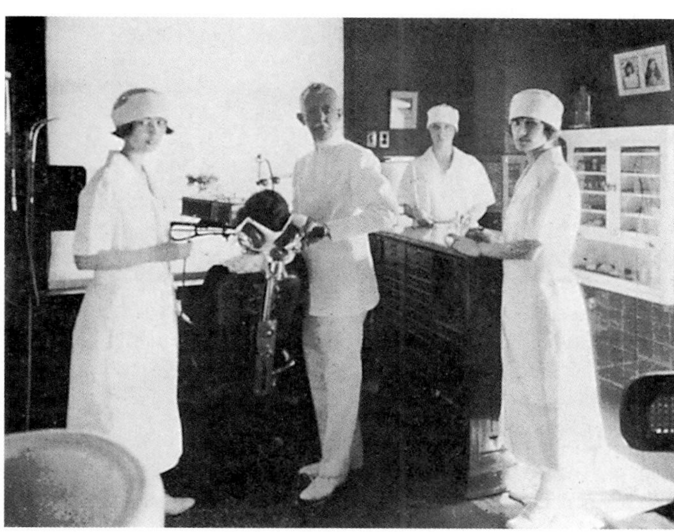

FIGURE 1-2 Dr. C. Edmund Kells and his "working unit."

TABLE 1-2
Highlights of African Americans in Dentistry

Date	Group/Individual	Event
1765	Peter Hawkins	A native-born, itinerant preacher in Richmond, Virginia, performs extractions for parishioners.
1851	John S. Rock	Is awarded a silver medal for making artificial teeth. Examples of his work were exhibited by the Benjamin Franklin Institute.
1869	Robert Tanner Freeman	Is the first African-American dentist to receive the Doctor of Medical Dentistry (DMD) degree from Harvard University.
1963	Andrew Z. Kellar	Publishes "The epidemiology of lip, oral and pharyngeal cancers" in the *American Journal of Public Health*.
1967	Van E. Collins	Is the first African-American dentist in regular military service to be promoted to the rank of colonel.
1973	Konneta Putman	Is installed as the president of the American Dental Hygienists Association.
1975	Jeanne C. Sinkford	Is the first African-American female dean of a United States dental school.
1989	Raymond J. Fonseca	Is appointed dental dean at the University of Pennsylvania.
1994	Juliann Bluitt	Is the first woman dentist elected president of the American College of Dentists.
1994	Caswell A. Evans	Is the first African-American dentist elected president of the American Public Health Association.
1994	Eugenia Mobley	Is the first African-American woman dentist to earn a degree in public health and the second female dean of a United States dental school.
1994	Clifton O. Dummett	Is the distinguished professor emeritus of the University of Southern California School of Dentistry and author and historian for the National Dental Association.

From Bird DL, Robinson DS: *Modern dental assisting,* ed 11, St. Louis, 2015, Elsevier.

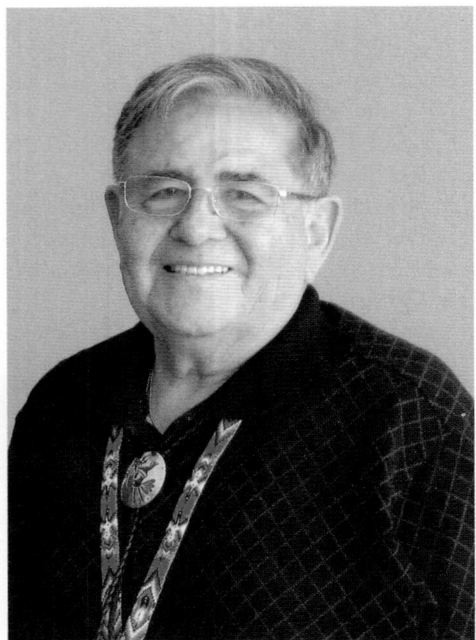

FIGURE 1-3 Dr. George Blue Spruce, Jr., the first American Indian dentist. (Courtesy Dr. George Blue Spruce, Jr.)

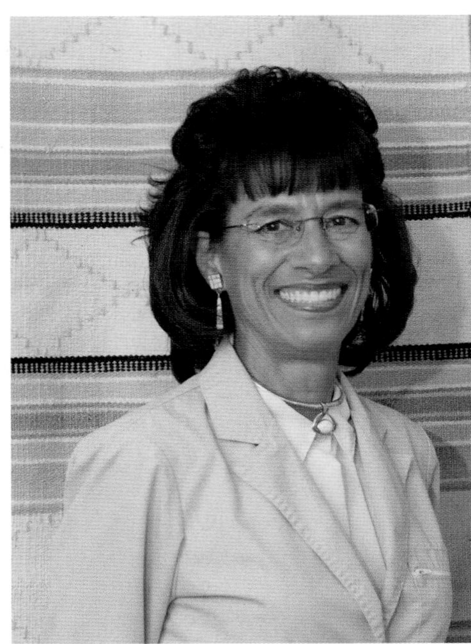

FIGURE 1-4 Dr. Jessica A. Rickert. The first Native-American female Indian dentist. (Courtesy Dr. Jessica Rickert.)

In 1975, **Jessica A. Rickert** became the first recognized Native-American female dentist. She attended the University of Michigan School of Dentistry, and she was the only Native American in a class of approximately 150 students. Also, during this time, there were very few female dentists or female dental students. Jessica Rickert received the 2005 Access Recognition Award from the American Dental Association (ADA) for leadership in helping people in need gain access to dental care. In particular, she was nominated for her work in educating Native Americans on dental care and encouraging them to pursue careers in the field. In 2009 she was honored for her work by being inducted into the Michigan Women's Hall of Fame (Figure 1-4).

Members of the Dental Health Care Team

The members of the dental health care team strive to provide quality oral care for patients in the practice. Although each member of the team plays an important role, the most important person in the dental office is always the **patient.** The roles and responsibilities of each team member are listed in Box 1-1. The dental health care team consists of the following members:

1. Dentist (general dentist or specialist)
2. Dental assistant (clinical, expanded functions, business)
3. Dental hygienist
4. Dental laboratory technician

Dentist

The **dentist** is the individual who is legally and ultimately responsible for the care of patients and for the supervision of all other members of the team. The dentist is often referred to as the leader of the team. The dentist trained in the United States must graduate from a dental university approved by the **Commission on Dental Accreditation (CODA) of the American Dental Association (ADA)**. Most dentists also have an undergraduate degree before being admitted to a dental university. Dental education programs usually last 4 academic years. When dentists graduate from a dental university, they are awarded either the **Doctor of Dental Surgery (DDS)** or the **Doctor of Medical Dentistry**, depending on which dental school they attended. Before going into practice, all dentists must pass a **written** national board examination. Dentists are then required to take a **clinical** board examination for licensure in the state in which they choose to practice. Dentists have a variety of practice options available to them. Some will choose to practice alone, some may choose to have a practice partner, and others may choose to join a large group practice. Other career options for dentists include the military, public health, community clinics, research, teaching, or returning to school for specialty training. Although a general dentist is trained and legally permitted to perform all dental functions, many dentists prefer to refer more difficult cases to specialists who have advanced training in certain areas. Most dentists are members of their professional organization, the ADA.

Dental Specialists

All licensed dentists have received basic education in all areas of dentistry. However, many choose to pursue advanced education and training in a specialty area. The ADA recognizes nine **dental specialties**. Depending on the type of specialty, the time to complete additional education to become a specialist varies from 2 to 6 years. Most dentists who are specialists will belong to a professional organization for their specialty, in addition to membership in the ADA. The nine dental specialties recognized by the ADA are listed in Box 1-2.

BOX 1-1 Roles and Responsibilities of Dental Health Care Team Members

Dentist or Dental Specialist

- Is legally responsible for the care of the patient
- Assesses the patient's oral health needs as related to physical and emotional well-being
- Uses up-to-date diagnostic skills
- Uses current techniques and skills in all aspects of patient care
- Provides legally required supervision for dental auxiliaries

Chairside Dental Assistant (Clinical Assistant, Circulating Assistant)

- Seats and prepares patients
- Maintains and prepares treatment rooms and instruments
- Assists dentist at chairside during patient treatment
- Prepares and delivers dental materials
- Provides postoperative patient instructions
- Manages infection control program
- Performs radiographic procedures
- Performs basic laboratory procedures (e.g., pouring impressions to create diagnostic casts)
- Provides assurance and support for the patient

Expanded-Functions Dental Assistant (EFDA)

- Performs only those intraoral (inside-mouth) procedures that are legal in the state in which the EFDA practices
- Check with your state board of dentistry for a current listing of dental assistant duties

Registered Dental Hygienist

- Assesses the periodontal status of patients; measures the depth of periodontal pockets and the condition of oral tissues.
- Performs dental prophylaxis (e.g., removal of plaque from crowns and root surfaces).
- Performs scaling and root-planing procedures.
- Exposes, processes, and evaluates the quality of radiographs.
- Performs additional procedures, such as administration of local anesthetic and administration of nitrous oxide if allowed by the state.

Business Assistant (Administrative Assistant, Secretarial Assistant, Receptionist)

- Greets patients and answers the telephone.
- Makes and confirms appointments.
- Manages patient records, payroll, insurance billing, and financial arrangements.
- Ensures that patient privacy measures are in place and are followed.
- Oversees patient relations.

Dental Laboratory Technician

- Performs laboratory work only under the prescription of a licensed dentist.
- Constructs and repairs prosthetic devices (e.g., full and partial dentures).
- Constructs restorations (e.g., crowns, bridges, inlays, veneers).

BOX 1-2 Dental Specialties Recognized by the American Dental Association

Dental public health involves developing policies at the county, state, and national levels for programs to control and prevent disease. Examples include dental public health professionals involved with fluoridation issues, community oral health education, and Head Start programs. Dental public health also includes dental screenings within a community to assess the needs of the community. In dental public health, the community rather than the individual is the patient.

Endodontics involves the causes, diagnosis, prevention, and treatment of diseases and injuries of the pulp and associated structures. The common term for most of the treatment is *root canal.* The specialist is an endodontist.

Oral and maxillofacial radiology became the first new dental specialty in 36 years when it was granted recognition by the ADA in 1999. The dental radiologist uses new and sophisticated imaging techniques to locate tumors and infectious diseases of the jaws, head, and neck and assists in the diagnosis of patients with trauma and temporomandibular disorders.

Oral and maxillofacial surgery involves the diagnosis and surgical treatment of diseases, injuries, and defects of the oral and maxillofacial regions. It involves significantly more than tooth extractions. The specialist is an oral and maxillofacial surgeon.

Oral pathology involves the nature of diseases affecting the oral cavity and adjacent structures. The specialist is an oral pathologist. A major function of an oral pathologist is to perform biopsies and to work closely with oral surgeons to provide a diagnosis.

Orthodontics involves the diagnosis, treatment, and prevention of malocclusions of the teeth and associated structures. This specialty entails significantly more than the fitting of braces. The specialist is an orthodontist.

Pediatric dentistry involves the oral health care of children from birth to adolescence. The pediatric dentist often treats children with emotional and behavioral problems.

Periodontics involves the diagnosis and treatment of diseases of the oral tissues supporting and surrounding the teeth. The specialist is a periodontist.

Prosthodontics involves the restoration and replacement of natural teeth with artificial constructs, such as crowns, bridges, and dentures. The specialist is a prosthodontist.

Registered Dental Hygienist

Generally, a **registered dental hygienist** (RDH) removes deposits on the teeth (calculus), exposes radiographs, places topical fluoride and dental sealants, and provides patients with home care instructions (Figure 1-5). The duties delegated to the dental hygienist vary from state to state. In many states, dental hygienists are allowed to administer local anesthesia. A thorough understanding of the laws of the state in which they practice is important for dental hygienists. Employment opportunities for dental hygienists are available in private and specialty dental offices, health clinics, school systems, research facilities, public health departments, educational programs, and marketing and sales of dental products.

The minimal education required for a dental hygienist is 2 academic years of college study and an associate's degree in an ADA-accredited dental hygiene program. Dental hygiene is also offered in bachelor's and master's degree programs. The RDH must pass both written national or regional board examinations and clinical state board examinations to be licensed by the state in which he or she plans to practice. In most states, the RDH is required to work under the supervision of a licensed dentist.

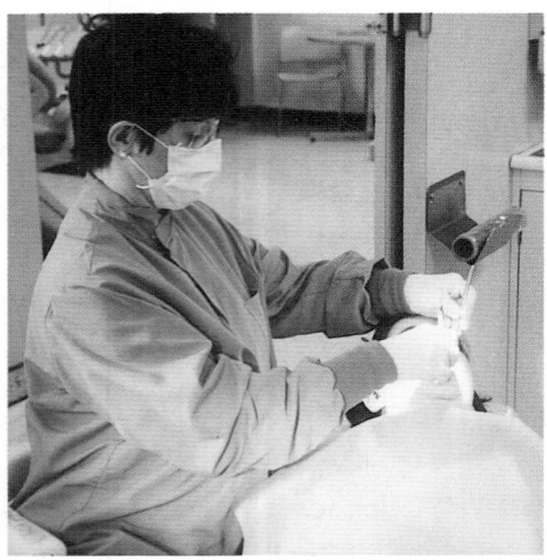

FIGURE 1-5 Registered dental hygienist performing an oral prophylaxis. (Courtesy Nordent Manufacturing, Inc., Elk Grove Village, Illinois.)

Dental hygienists may be members of their professional organization, the **American Dental Hygienists Association (ADHA)**. For additional information on dental hygiene, visit the Web site at http://www.adha.org.

Dental Assistant

An educationally qualified **dental assistant** will be able to assume many activities that do not require the professional skill and judgment of a licensed dentist. However, the responsibilities assigned to a dental assistant are limited by the regulations of the Dental Practice Act of the state in which he or she practices (see Chapter 2). Advancements in technology are changing the practice of dentistry and include changes in the role of the dental assistant. Today, computerized patient charting is replacing paper charts, digital imaging is replacing x-ray film. The Cone Beam 3D Imaging System produces three-dimensional images of the head and neck (Figure 1-6). Intraoral scanners are beginning to replace conventional dental impressions for many procedures. Dental implants are replacing missing or extracted teeth.

The dental assistant has many important responsibilities in the dental office of tomorrow. Each dental practice is unique and has specific needs, and the educationally qualified dental assistant is quick to adapt to new situations as needs arise.

Several states have created their own titles to recognize dental assistants who have had additional training and are legally allowed to perform specific procedures within that particular state.

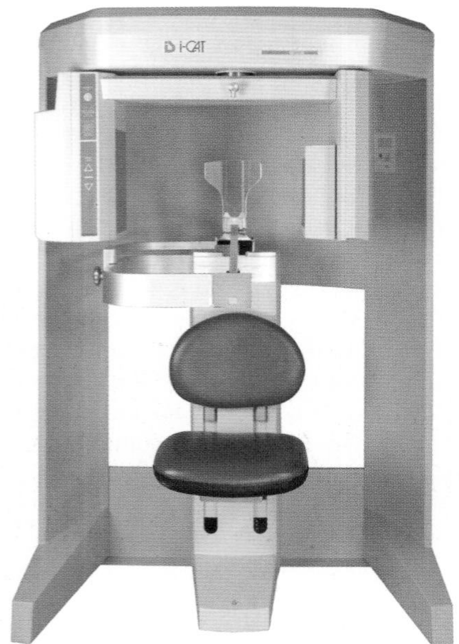

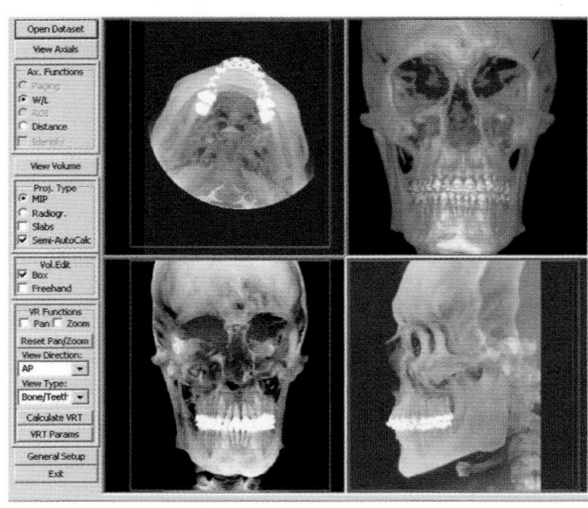

FIGURE 1-6 Cone Beam 3D Imaging System. (Courtesy Air Techniques, Inc., Melville, New York.)

Although not all states require formal education for dental assistants, CODA has established minimal standards for their accreditation. CODA Standards require a program of approximately 1 academic year in length, conducted at a post–high school educational institution. The curriculum must include didactic, laboratory, and clinical content. Dental assistants may also receive training at vocational schools or proprietary schools accredited through the state's board of dentistry.

This chapter provides an introduction to the basic dental assisting skills.

Chairside Dental Assistant

The chairside dental assistant is directly involved in patient care. The duties include charting, placing and removing the rubber dam, passing instruments, mixing and passing dental materials, suctioning, and reassuring the nervous patient, among other duties (Figure 1-7).

The **circulating assistant** serves as an extra pair of hands when needed throughout the clinical areas of the practice and is referred to as **six-handed dentistry** (Figure 1-8). In many practices, the circulating assistant is responsible for seating and dismissing patients and for preparing and caring for instruments and treatment rooms.

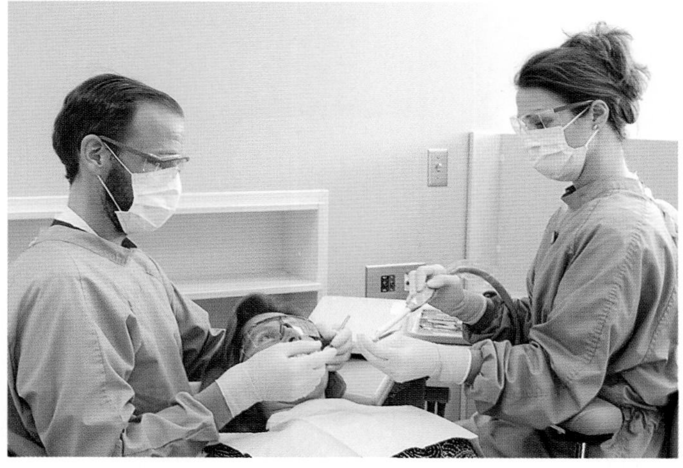

FIGURE 1-7 Dentist and chairside dental assistant working together.

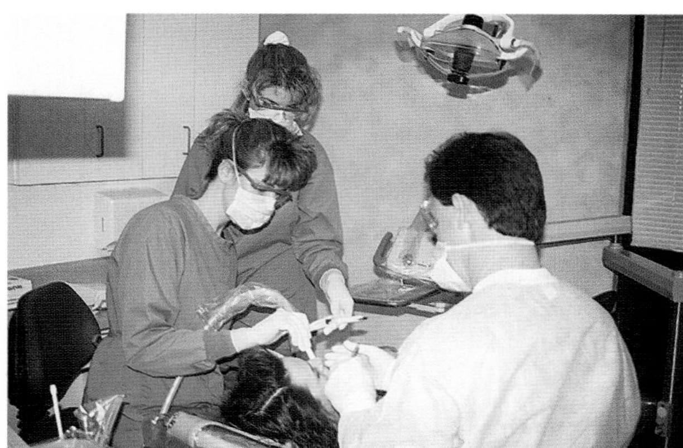

FIGURE 1-8 Chairside dental assistant is supported by a circulating assistant (six-handed dentistry).

Sterilization Assistant

In many offices, the responsibility for sterilization procedures is delegated to a specific individual. In other offices, all dental assistants share this important responsibility. The **sterilization assistant** efficiently and safely processes all instruments and manages biohazardous waste. Other responsibilities include weekly monitoring of sterilizers and maintaining sterilization monitoring reports (Figure 1-9). The sterilization assistant is often responsible for the selection of infection control products and for performing quality assurance procedures (see Chapters 7 and 8).

State-Specific Categories

Many states have created special categories and titles for dental assistants. The titles and allowable duties are specific to a state and vary according to the Dental Practice Act in each state.

Dental assistants in a special category have received additional training and are legally permitted to provide certain intraoral patient care procedures beyond the duties traditionally performed by a dental assistant (Figure 1-10). Knowing which functions are legal in a state and performing **only** those functions are important for dental assistants (see Chapter 2).

Business Assistant

Business assistants, also known as **administrative assistants**, **secretarial assistants**, and **receptionists**, are primarily responsible for the smooth and efficient operation of the business office (Figure 1-11). Two or more assistants may work in the business area of a dental office. The duties of a business assistant include controlling appointments, communicating on the telephone, coordinating financial arrangements with patients, and handling dental insurance claims. It is not uncommon for a chairside dental assistant to move into a business office position. It is very helpful when the individual at the desk has an excellent understanding of how the clinical practice functions.

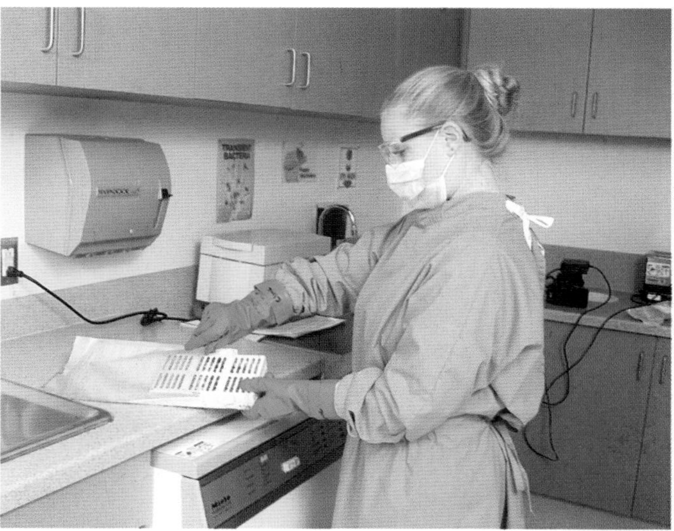

FIGURE 1-9 A sterilization assistant is an important member of the dental team.

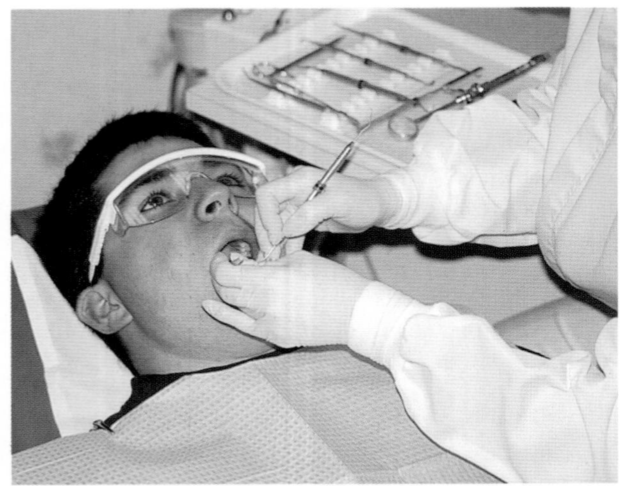

FIGURE 1-10 **Expanded-functions dental assistant (EFDA)** removes excess cement.

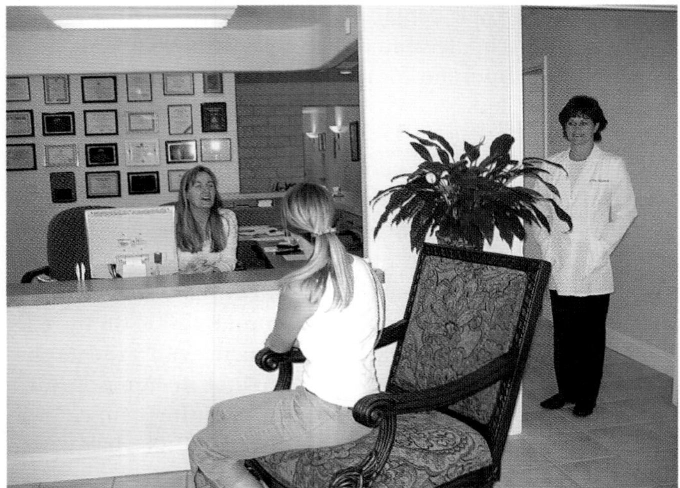

FIGURE 1-11 A patient is greeted by the business assistant before meeting the dental hygienist. (Courtesy Cr. Peter Pang, Sonoma, California.)

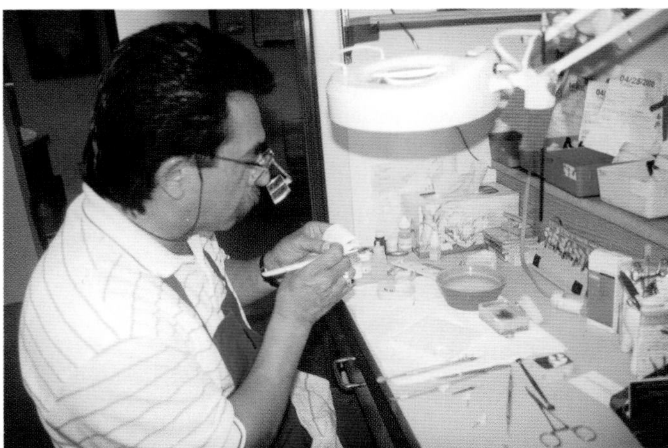

FIGURE 1-12 Dental laboratory technician fabricates a crown.

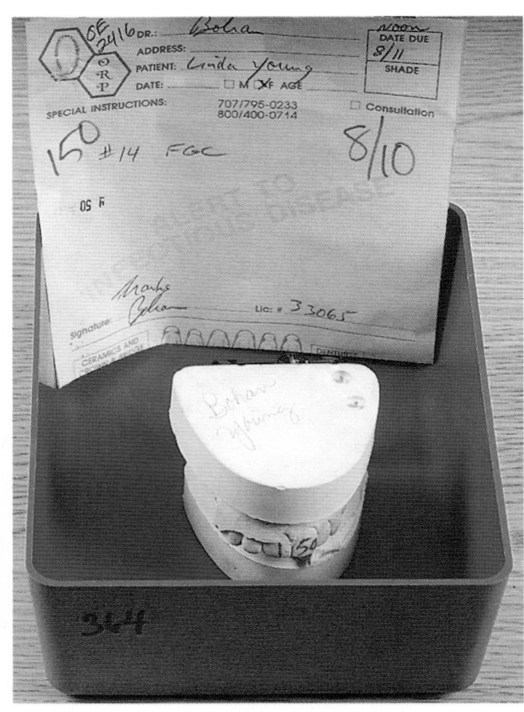

FIGURE 1-13 Laboratory case and prescription (Rx).

Dental Laboratory Technician

Although some dental offices have "in-house" laboratories, the **dental laboratory technician** usually does not work in the dental office with the other team members. Many dental technicians choose to be employed in private laboratories, and others choose to own and operate their own laboratory (Figure 1-12). In either case, the dental laboratory technician may legally perform only those tasks specified by the **written prescription** of the dentist (Figure 1-13). Dental technicians make crowns, bridges, and dentures from impressions taken by the dentist and sent to the dental laboratory. The dental assistant often communicates with the dental laboratory technician to discuss the length of time needed to return a case or to relay special instructions from the dentist about a case. Maintaining a good working relationship with the dental laboratory is important for the dental assistant.

Dental laboratory technicians can receive their training through apprenticeship, commercial schools, or CODA-accredited programs. Many have received their training in CODA-accredited programs that are 2 years in length. Dental laboratory technicians have extensive knowledge of dental anatomy and materials and excellent manual dexterity.

To become a **certified dental technician (CDT)**, the dental laboratory technician must pass a written examination. Dental technicians may be members of their professional organization, the **American Dental Laboratory Technician Association (ADLTA)**.

Overview of the Dental Office

The types and sizes of dental offices vary greatly, and the interior design and decor usually reflect the dentist's personal style.

However, certain areas are found in every dental office; these include the reception area, the business office, nonclinical areas, an instrument-processing area, the dental laboratory, and treatment rooms.

Reception Area

The reception area is where patients are received, pleasantly greeted, and made to feel welcome. The reception area should not be a "waiting room"; with proper scheduling, patients can be seen on time for their appointments.

Patients often judge the quality of their care by the appearance of the office. Therefore the reception area and all areas of the dental office must be kept neat and clean at all times (Figure 1-14).

Business Office

The business office is the hub for the management of the business aspect of the dental practice, and it includes a **scheduling area,** where patients can make future appointments; an area where patients can make **financial arrangements**; and an area for **record storage**, where patient records can be safeguarded and privacy maintained. It is not uncommon for a dental office to have two or more staff members working in this important area.

Nonclinical Areas

The dentist will usually have a **private office** for his or her personal use. Other staff members should respect the privacy of this area.

The dentist discusses the proposed treatment plans with patients in the **consultation room.** When no consultation area is available, the dentist's private office is used for this purpose.

The **staff lounge** is an area where the staff may rest, eat, and hold meetings. Contaminated clothing or items must not be brought into this area. Staff members are responsible for keeping this area clean and neat at all times.

FIGURE 1-14 Reception area of a modern dental office. (Courtesy of Dr. Peter Pang, Sonoma, California.)

Instrument-Processing Area

The instrument-processing area is where contaminated instruments are cleaned, packaged, sterilized, and stored for reuse (Figure 1-15; see Chapters 7 and 8).

Dental Laboratory

The dental laboratory in the dental office is used by the staff to pour impressions, prepare study models, and polish removable items, such as dentures or space maintainers. Wearing safety goggles is important for staff when using laboratory equipment. In addition, the entire laboratory must be kept clean and neat at all times. Food or drink should never be present in the laboratory area because it is considered an area of potential contamination.

Major equipment in the dental laboratory usually includes the following:

1. **Laboratory handpiece** for tasks such as trimming custom trays or temporary restorations
2. **Laboratory work pans** for storing together all the parts of individual cases
3. **Model trimmer** for use when trimming diagnostic casts and study models (Figure 1-16)

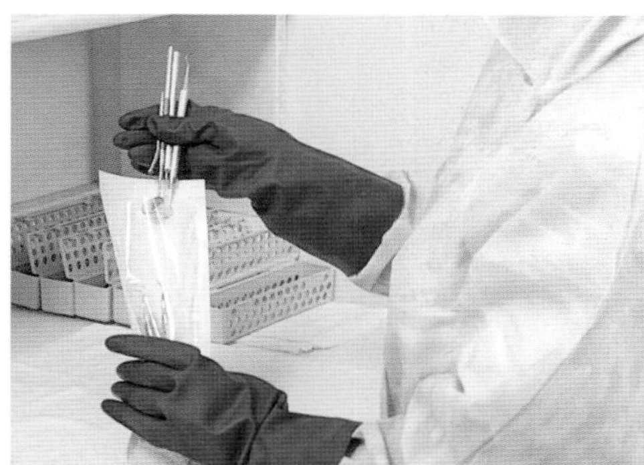

FIGURE 1-15 Instruments are cleaned and packaged in preparation for sterilization.

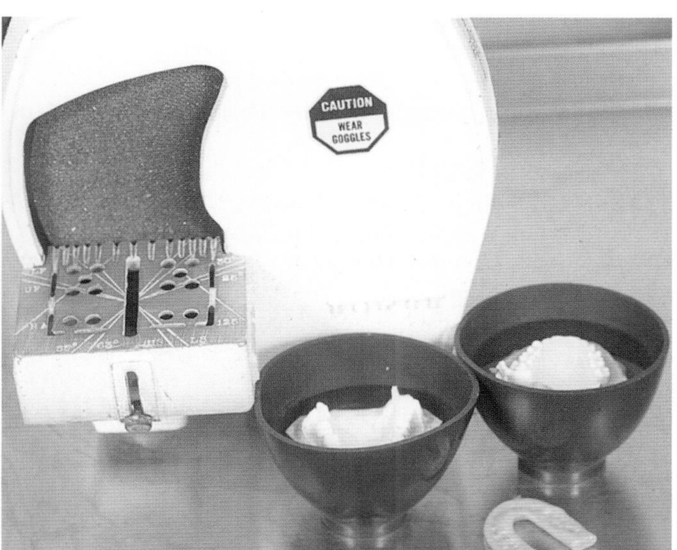

FIGURE 1-16 Model Trimmer. (From Boyd LRB: *Dental instruments: A pocket guide,* ed 5, St. Louis, 2015, Saunders.)

4. **Vacuum former** used to create custom trays, bleaching trays, and mouth guards
5. **Dental lathe** to grind metals and polish dentures and precious metal crowns

Treatment Rooms

Dental treatment rooms, also known as operatories, are the heart of the clinical area of the dental practice. Patients receive treatment in the treatment rooms. Most practices have several treatment rooms.

Usually, at least one treatment room is for the dental hygienist. In some practices, separate treatment rooms serve as an extra room for emergencies or short procedures, such as a checkup after surgery.

Ethical Implications

Dental assisting is a wonderful career. It offers you pride and professional opportunities. You may decide to pursue a career in general dentistry, specialty practices, public health clinics, or dental schools. Someday, you may even choose to become a dental assisting educator.

Always remember to maintain an attitude of professionalism and cooperative teamwork with other staff members, and never forget that the patient is the most important person in the office.

Chapter Exercises

Multiple Choice

Circle the letter next to the correct answer.

1. The dental specialty in which the patient is the entire community is __________.
- **a.** periodontics
- **b.** orthodontics
- **c.** public health dentistry
- **d.** pediatric dentistry

2. A patient who needs a root canal treatment might be referred to a(n) __________.
- **a.** periodontist
- **b.** oral surgeon
- **c.** endodontist
- **d.** oral pathologist

3. The MOST important person in the dental practice is the __________.
- **a.** dentist
- **b.** dental hygienist
- **c.** dental assistant
- **d.** patient

4. Contaminated dental instruments should be returned to the __________.
- **a.** dental laboratory
- **b.** clean area of the sterilization center
- **c.** contaminated area of the sterilization center
- **d.** operatories

5. The newest dental specialty is __________.
- **a.** oral and maxillofacial surgery
- **b.** oral and maxillofacial radiology
- **c.** dental public health
- **d.** endodontics

6. The member of the dental health team who is licensed to scale and polish teeth is the __________.
- **a.** dental hygienist
- **b.** dental assistant
- **c.** dental laboratory technician
- **d.** all of the above

7. Model trimmers and dental lathes are found in the __________.
- **a.** business office area
- **b.** staff lounge
- **c.** dental laboratory
- **d.** operatories

8. The dentist explains the treatment plan to the patient in the __________ of the practice.
- **a.** staff lounge
- **b.** business office
- **c.** consultation room
- **d.** dental laboratory

9. The leader of the dental health care team is the __________.
- **a.** dentist
- **b.** dental hygienist
- **c.** dental assistant
- **d.** patient

10. The dentist recognized as having used the first dental assistant was __________.
- **a.** Dr. C. Edmund Kells
- **b.** Dr. Louis Pasteur
- **c.** Dr. W.C. Roentgen
- **d.** Dr. G.V. Black

Apply Your Knowledge

1. Visit the Web page of your state's Dental Board to learn what functions a dental assistant in your state may legally perform. Are there any special credentialing or licensing requirements for dental assistants in your state?

2. Visit a dental office in your area, and explain to the dentist that you are a dental assisting student and would like to observe the various members of the dental health team at work. Be prepared to ask questions that are of interest to you.

CHAPTER 2

Professional and Legal Aspects of Dental Assisting

http://evolve.elsevier.com/Robinson/essentials/

LEARNING OBJECTIVES

1. Pronounce, define, and spell the key terms.
2. Complete the following related to characteristics of a professional dental assistant:
   - Discuss the concept of professionalism.
   - Discuss the characteristics of a professional dental assistant.
   - Demonstrate the personal qualities of a professional dental assistant.
3. Explain the differences between ethics and law, as well as discuss the different types of law.
4. Explain the purpose of a state's Dental Practice Act and discuss the legal aspects of dentistry.
5. Describe the levels of dental auxiliary supervision.
6. Explain the differences between certified dental assistants and registered dental assistants.
7. Discuss risk management, including the steps necessary to help avoid malpractice suits.
8. Discuss the guidelines for informed consent, patient records, and how to report child abuse and neglect.
9. Complete the following related to regulatory and professional organizations:
   - Name the professional organizations for dentists, dental assistants, and dental hygienists.
   - Give the full names and identify the roles of the following agencies: OSHA, CDC, OSAP, EPA, and FDA.

KEY TERMS

act of commission
act of omission
breach of contract
certified dental assistant (CDA)
civil law
contract law
dental auxiliary
direct supervision
ethics
general supervision
implied consent
indirect supervision
informed consent
legal
licensure
patient of record
professionalism
reciprocity
registered dental assistant (RDA)
res gestae
risk management
tort law

You chose an exciting and challenging career when you decided to become a professional dental assistant. A career in dental assisting offers variety, job satisfaction, opportunity for service, and financial reward. Dental assisting is a career that requires dedication, personal responsibility, integrity, and a commitment to continuing education.

A highly skilled dental assistant is a vital member of the dental health care team. Reducing patient anxiety, making decisions, simplifying treatment procedures, and improving the quality of patient care are all part of a dental assistant's day (Figure 2-1).

Characteristics of a Professional Dental Assistant

Becoming a dental assistant involves more than acquiring the knowledge and developing the skills necessary to perform a variety of duties. Becoming a dental assistant is about becoming a **professional.**

Professionalism is an attitude that is apparent in everything you do and say, in and out of the dental office. Professionalism is what distinguishes people who "have a job" from those who "pursue a career." The public's expectations of health care

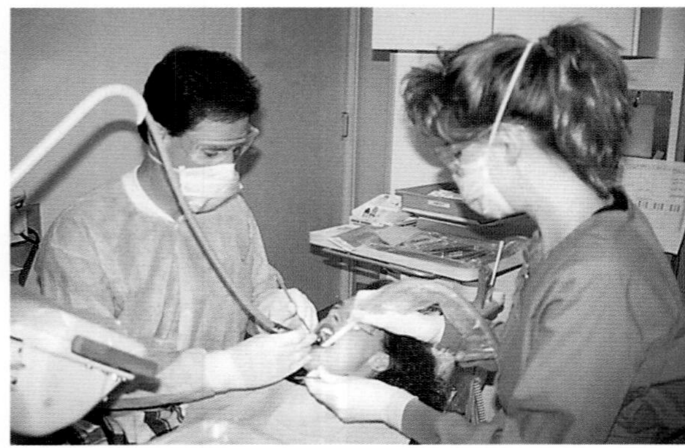

FIGURE 2-1 The dental assistant is an important member of the dental health care team.

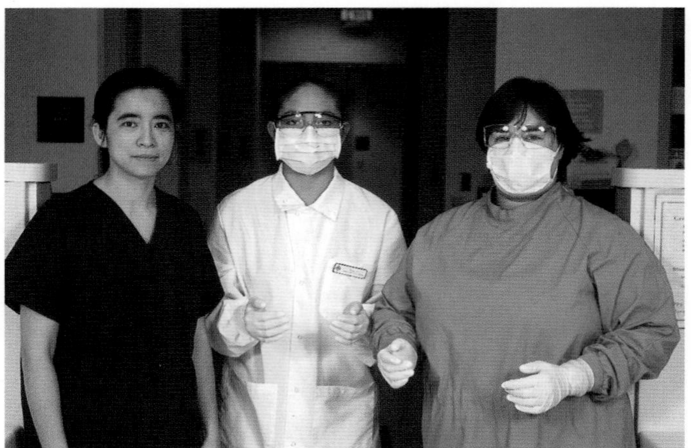

FIGURE 2-2 The attire of a professional dental assistant may vary, depending on the duties performed. *Left,* Scrubs are acceptable at times. *Center,* Full personal protective wear is indicated for chairside procedures. *Right,* Surgical gowns may be indicated for surgery or hospital dentistry.

workers are higher than the expectations of individuals in other occupations. The dental assistant must demonstrate patience and compassion when communicating with patients and other team members. When you demonstrate professionalism, you earn respect and acknowledgment from your colleagues and patients as a valued member of the dental health care team.

Professional Appearance

The dental assistant who has a professional appearance promotes the patient's confidence in the entire office and improves his or her dental experience. Essential aspects of a professional appearance include (1) good health, (2) good grooming, and (3) appropriate dress.

Good health requires getting an adequate amount of rest, eating well-balanced meals, and exercising enough to keep fit. Dental assisting is a physically demanding profession.

For **good grooming,** your hair should be neat and away from your face. Your fingernails should be clean and not extend beyond your finger. Long nails can cause cuts in the fingertips of your gloves. Avoid the use of artificial fingernails; they harbor bacteria.

Personal cleanliness involves taking a daily bath or shower, using a deodorant, and practicing good oral hygiene. Perfume or cologne should not be used. You are working in very close personal proximity to coworkers and patients who may be allergic to or irritated by some scents. Avoid the use of tobacco products because the odor lingers on your hair and clothing and is offensive, especially in a professional setting.

Appropriate dress involves wearing clothing appropriate for the type of position in which you are working. Regardless of the type of professional wear, it must be clean, wrinkle-free, and worn over appropriate undergarments (Figure 2-2). Personal protective clothing is discussed in greater detail in Chapter 6. In any position in a dental office, excessive makeup and jewelry are not considered appropriate for a professional appearance. Infection control requirements must also be considered when clinical clothing and jewelry are selected (see Chapters 7 and 8).

Teamwork

Teamwork is extremely important in a dental office. Think of the letters in the word **team,** "**T**ogether, **E**veryone **A**ccomplishes **M**ore." Dental assistants should step in to do the work of an absent colleague and be willing to help coworkers when other tasks are completed. When several assistants are in an office, each should be able and willing to substitute for the others in an emergency.

Attitude

Patients, employers, and coworkers appreciate the dental assistant who has a good attitude. Showing a willingness to get along by avoiding criticism of others, showing appreciation for what others have done, and being willing to pitch in and help are important. The dental office can be a stressful place for patients and staff, so maintaining a positive attitude is important. Using your cell phone in a dental office for personal use sends a message to your patients and coworkers that you are more interested in your personal life than in your professional life.

Dedication

Professional dental assistants are dedicated to their dental practice, their patients, and the profession of dental assisting. Dedication is possible only if the assistant truly cares for people, is empathetic to their needs, and maintains a positive attitude.

Remember. ... Patients don't care how much you know until they know how much you care.

Responsibility and Initiative

The dental assistant can demonstrate work responsibility by (1) arriving on time, (2) staying for the full shift, (3) being a cooperative team member, and (4) not asking to leave early. Assistants should understand what is expected in their regular job and, if time permits, should be willing to help others who may be overworked.

You can show a willingness to learn additional skills by asking questions and observing others. Finding tasks to perform without being asked shows initiative. Calling the office when you are ill or unavoidably late shows responsibility. Personal problems should never be discussed in the dental office with your patients or with other staff members.

Confidentiality

Everything that is said or done in the dental office must remain confidential. Dental assistants have access to a vast amount of personal and financial information about their patients. Such information must be held in strict confidence and must not be discussed with others (Figure 2-3). Breaches of confidentiality can result in lawsuits against all parties involved.

You cannot reveal the identity of a patient or any information from his or her records without the patient's written consent. You must never discuss patients with anyone outside the dental office. You will learn more about the legal requirements associated with record keeping in Chapter 11.

Personal Qualities

Most people do not enjoy a visit to the dentist, and many are stressed or intimidated. The dental assistant must (1) demonstrate sensitivity to the patient's needs, (2) show empathy, (3) say "the right thing at the right time," and (4) **be sincere** (Box 2-1).

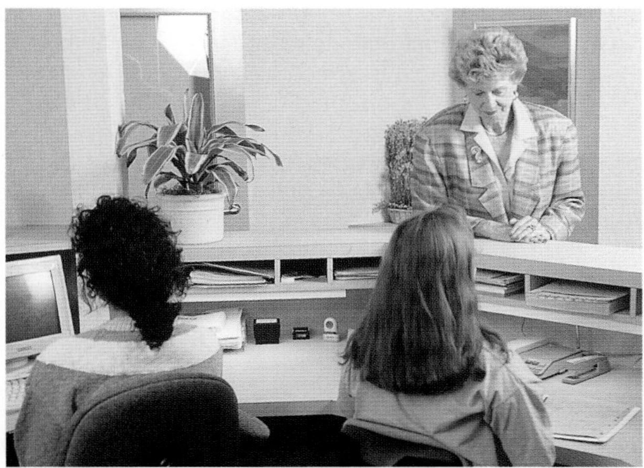

FIGURE 2-3 Patients have the right to expect confidentiality of their conversations in a dental office.

BOX 2-1 Check Your Qualities as a Dental Assistant

How Do I Interact with Patients?

- Am I friendly? Do I have a pleasant attitude?
- Do I listen more than I speak?
- Am I courteous?
- Am I considerate, respectful, and kind?
- Do I control my temper?
- Do I try to see the other person's point of view?

Am I Responsible?

- Am I dependable?
- Am I attentive to details?
- Am I calm in an emergency?
- Am I responsible for my own actions?
- Do I tend to blame others or find fault with others?
- Do I offer to help others without being asked?
- Do I avoid office gossip?

By learning to be a good listener, you will develop sensitivity for the opinions and concerns of others. Building **rapport** (good relations) with the patients in your office is nearly impossible if they do not trust you. Nonverbal signals such as a reassuring smile or a pat on the arm can be very comforting to a nervous patient.

Ethics and Law

In today's society, we have laws that enforce certain standards of behavior. In addition to the law, each of us has our own personal values, morals, and standards of behavior. Throughout life, our values and morals may be modified as a result of increased knowledge, improved understanding, and life experiences.

Laws are written to indicate the *minimum standard* of required behavior. Ethics are voluntary and are higher standards.

Difference Between Ethics and Law

Ethics deals with moral conduct—right and wrong behavior, "good" and "evil." Ethics includes values, high standards of conduct, and personal obligations in our interactions with other professionals and patients. Very few absolutes and many gray areas exist regarding ethics. Ethical issues are subject to individual interpretation as to the right or wrong of particular situations. A behavior can be unethical and still be legal, but it cannot be illegal and still be ethical.

Ethics refers to what you *should* do, not what you must do. The law deals with what you *must* do.

All major professions have a written code of ethics. The code of ethics states the ideal behavior, which is always higher than the minimum standard set forth by the law (Box 2-2). Ethical behavior is important to dental health care professionals as they provide dental care and privacy to their patients (Boxes 2-3 and 2-4).

Types of Law

Law can be divided into **criminal law** and civil law. Criminal law involves crimes against society. In criminal law, a governmental agency, such as law enforcement or the board of dentistry, begins the legal action. For example, a dental assistant who performs a procedure that is not legal is in violation of criminal law. Insurance fraud is another example of a criminal offense that may be committed in a dental office. Civil law involves crimes against an individual with another individual initiating legal action (i.e., lawsuit). For example, a patient sues a dentist because he or she is dissatisfied with the treatment or has been injured during treatment. A civil action against a dentist may involve either contract law or tort law (Boxes 2-5 and 2-6).

Legal Aspects of Dentistry

Regulations regarding **dental assistants** vary greatly from state to state. Having a clear understanding of the law in your state is important, as it relates to dental assisting and the practice of dentistry. You must always practice within the laws of your state.

BOX 2-2 ADAA: Principles of Ethics and Code of Professional Conduct

- Abide by the bylaws of the Association.
- Maintain loyalty to the Association.
- Pursue the objectives of the Association.
- Hold in confidence the information entrusted to you by the Association.
- Maintain respect for the members and employees of the Association.
- Serve all members of the Association in an impartial manner.
- Recognize and follow all laws and regulations related to activities of the Association.
- Exercise and insist on sound business principles in the conduct of affairs of the Association.
- Use **legal** and ethical means to influence legislation or regulation affecting members of the Association.
- Issue no false or misleading statements to fellow members or the public.
- Refrain from disseminating malicious information concerning the Association or any member or employee of the Association.
- Maintain high standards of personal conduct and integrity.
- Do not imply Association endorsement of personal opinions or positions.
- Cooperate in a reasonable and proper manner with staff and members.
- Accept no personal compensation from fellow members, except as approved by the Association.
- Promote and maintain the highest standards of performance in service to the Association.
- Assure public confidence in the integrity and service of the Association.

ADAA, American Dental Assistants Association.

State Dental Practice Act

Each state has a right to regulate the practice of dentistry within that state. To protect the public from incompetent dental health care providers, each state has established a **Dental Practice Act**. The Dental Practice Act specifies the legal requirements for the practice of dentistry within each state. It may be a single law or a compilation of laws that regulate the practice of dentistry. The Dental Practice Act defines the duties a dental assistant may perform in that state. Each state's Dental Practice Act is now accessible on the Internet. You will find links to each state's Dental Practice Act at http://www.ada.org.

State Board of Dentistry

An agency, usually called the state board of dentistry or the dental board, is responsible for enforcing the state's Dental Practice Act within that state. The members of the state board of dentistry are appointed by the governor of the state. In addition to licensed dentists, some state boards have members that are dental assistants, dental hygienists, and public members. The state board of dentistry has the authority to not only issue licenses but also **revoke**, **suspend**, or **deny renewal** of a license. Most states will take action if the licensed person has a felony conviction or a misdemeanor involving drug addiction, moral corruptness, incompetence, or mental or physical disability that may cause harm to patients.

BOX 2-3 Dentist's Duty of Care to the Patient

- Be properly licensed.
- Use reasonable skill, care, and judgment.
- Use standard drugs, materials, and techniques.
- Use Standard Precautions in the treatment of all patients.
- Maintain confidentiality of all information.
- Obtain and update patients' medical-dental health histories.
- Make appropriate referrals, and request consultation when indicated.
- Maintain a level of knowledge and competence in keeping up with advances in the dental profession.
- Do not exceed the scope of practice or allow assistants under your general supervision to perform unlawful acts.
- Complete patients' care in a timely manner.
- Do not use experimental procedures.
- Obtain informed consent from the patient or guardian before beginning an examination or treatment.
- Arrange for patients' care during a temporary absence.
- Give adequate instructions to patients.
- Achieve reasonable treatment results.

BOX 2-4 Patient's Responsibility to the Dentist

- Pay a reasonable and agreed-on fee for service.
- Follow instructions and cooperate in the treatment.

BOX 2-5 Requirements for Contract Law to Apply

Legally Competent

Both parties must be legally competent. If a minor or a mentally incompetent individual signed a contract, then that contract would not be valid.

Legal Service

A contract cannot be written for an illegal service or act.

Payment

Payment must be made. If something is being given away free with no money or services in exchange, then there can be no contract.

Note: **Breach of contract** lawsuits occur when either party fails to meet his or her end of a written or verbal contract.

Licensure

Licensure is having a license to practice in a specific state. Licensure is one method of supervising individuals who

BOX 2-6 Requirements for Tort Law to Apply

Legal Duty

Once the dentist accepts a patient, the dentist then has specific professional and legal duties to the patient.

Breach of Duty

The dentist must have failed to perform a legal duty.

Damage or Harm

The patient must have suffered some type of harm or injury.

Cause of Damage or Harm

The dentist's wrongful act directly caused the damage or harm.

Note: All four elements must exist before a lawsuit claiming a tort is valid.

practice in the state. The purpose of licensure is to protect the public from unqualified or incompetent practitioners. The requirements for licensure vary from state to state, but dentists and dental hygienists, and, in some states, dental assistants must be licensed or registered by the state in which they practice.

An increasing number of states are requiring either licensing or registration for dental assistants. Some states have assigned various titles to dental assistants that allow them to perform specific functions. Understanding the requirements for practice in a state is essential. In every state, any person who practices dentistry without a license is guilty of an illegal act.

Some states have a reciprocity agreement with another state. **Reciprocity** is an agreement between two or more states that allows a dentist or a dental hygienist who is licensed in one state to receive, usually without further examination, a license to practice in any of the other states in the reciprocity agreement. Reciprocity agreements are usually made between states with adjoining borders and similar testing requirements. States without reciprocity agreements require dentists and dental hygienists licensed in another state to take their state board examination.

Levels of Dental Auxiliary Supervision

In states that allow the dentist to delegate intraoral functions to a **dental auxiliary** (dental assistant or dental hygienist), the rules in the state's Dental Practice Act are usually specific regarding the types of auxiliary supervision that the dentist must provide. The following terms are used often in Dental Practice Acts:

A **patient of record** is an individual who has been examined and diagnosed by a licensed dentist and has had his or her treatment planned by the dentist.

Direct supervision generally means that the dentist has delegated a specific procedure to be performed for a patient of record by a legally qualified dental auxiliary, who meets the requirements of the state board of dentistry. The dentist must examine the patient before delegating the procedure and again when the procedure is complete. *The dentist must be physically present in the office at the time the procedure is performed.*

BOX 2-7 DANB National Certifications

The Dental Assisting National Board (DANB) offers five national certifications:

- National Entry Level Dental Assistant (NELDA)
- Certified Dental Assistant (CDA)
- Certified Orthodontic Assistant (COA)
- Certified Preventive Functions Dental Assistant (CPFDA)
- Certified Restorative Functions Assistant (CRFDA)

Contact DANB at www.danb.org.

General supervision (indirect supervision) generally means that the dentist has authorized and delegated specific procedures that may be performed by a legally qualified dental auxiliary for a patient of record. Exposing radiographs and recementing a temporary crown that has become dislodged are examples of functions that are often delegated under general supervision.

Unlicensed Practice of Dentistry

As a dental assistant, you may legally perform only those functions that have been delegated to you under the Dental Practice Act of the state in which you practice. Performing procedures that are not legal is the same as practicing dentistry without a license, which is a **criminal act**. Ignorance of the Dental Practice Act is no excuse for illegally practicing dentistry. *If the dentist asks you to perform an expanded function that is not legal in your state and you choose to do so, then you are committing a criminal act.*

Credentialing of Dental Assistants

Certified Dental Assistants

A **certified dental assistant (CDA)** is an individual who has taken and passed a *national examination* administered by the Dental Assisting National Board (DANB). To remain currently certified, the CDA must complete a specified number of continuing education hours and must pay a renewal fee each year. Some states require a dental assistant to be a CDA to perform certain expanded functions. Additional information regarding certification can be obtained by or visiting the DANB Web site at www.danb.org (Box 2-7).

Registered Dental Assistant

A **registered dental assistant (RDA)** is an individual who has taken and passed an examination required by a specific state to perform functions allowed only in that state. States that require registration usually require periodic (annual or biannual) renewal through the payment of a fee and a specified number of clock hours of continuing education credits. Registration of dental assistants is not available in all states.

Risk Management

Risk management refers to concepts and techniques that members of the dental team can use to help prevent malpractice lawsuits. The major areas of risk management (prevention of malpractice lawsuits) involve (1) maintaining accurate and complete records, (2) obtaining **informed consent**, and (3) doing everything possible to maintain the highest standards of clinical excellence. Most patients who sue are angry and believe they have been wronged. When patients become angry or frustrated and believe they are not being heard, they are more likely to file a lawsuit.

The primary factor in avoiding legal entanglements with patients is maintaining good rapport and open communication with all patients.

Avoiding Malpractice Lawsuits

Prevention and good communication with the patient are the best defenses against malpractice (Figure 2-4). Patients are less likely to initiate a lawsuit when they have a clear understanding of the following:

- Planned treatment
- Reasonable treatment results
- Potential treatment complications
- Financial obligations

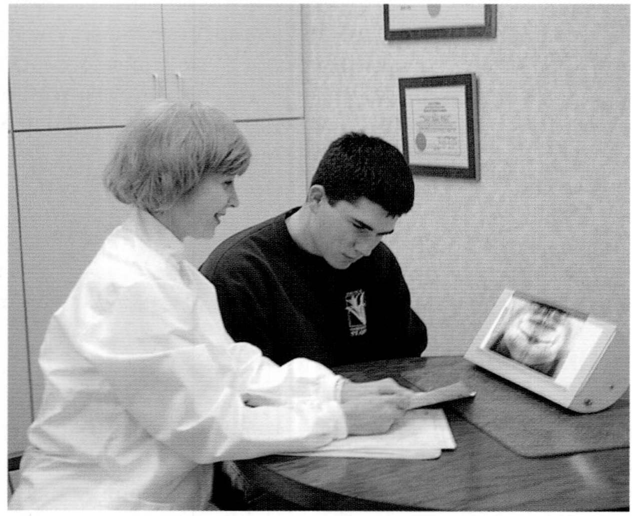

FIGURE 2-4 An important role of the dental assistant is to help maintain good communication with the patient.

The dental assistant plays an important role in the prevention of malpractice litigation by being aware of the signs of patient dissatisfaction and alerting the dentist.

"Silence Is Golden"

The dental assistant must never make critical remarks about dental treatment rendered by an employer or another dentist. The dental assistant should never discuss other patients and should avoid discussing the dentist's professional liability insurance.

Under the concept of **res gestae** ("part of the action"), statements spontaneously made by anyone (including the dental assistant) at the time of an alleged negligent act are admissible as evidence and may be damaging to the dentist and the dental assistant in a court of law. Comments such as "whoops" or "uh-oh" may unnecessarily frighten the patient and should be avoided.

Guidelines for Informed Consent

The concept of informed consent is based on the idea that the patient is the one who must pay the bill, as well as endure the pain and suffering that may result from treatment. Therefore the patient has the right to know all important facts about the proposed treatment.

Informed Patient Consent

Two things must occur for the patient to give informed consent: (1) **being informed** and (2) **giving consent**. This means that the dentist must give the patient enough information about his or her condition and explain all available treatment options. The patient and the dentist must first discuss these options, and then the patient chooses the most suitable treatment alternative.

When a patient enters a dentist's office, the patient gives **implied consent**, at least for the dental examination. Provided the patient is capable, implied consent is given when the patient agrees to treatment or at least does not object to treatment. In a court of law, implied consent is a less reliable form of consent in a malpractice suit. **Written consent** is the preferred means of obtaining and documenting the patient's consent and understanding of the procedure.

Informed Refusal

If a patient refuses the proposed treatment, then the dentist must inform the patient about the likely consequences and must obtain the patient's informed refusal.

However, obtaining the patient's informed refusal does not release the dentist from the responsibility of providing the standard of care. A patient may not consent to substandard care, and the dentist may not legally or ethically agree to provide such care. For example, if a patient refuses radiographs, then the dentist may refer the patient to another provider because the dentist believes radiographs are a necessary standard of care. Another dentist, however, may be willing to treat the patient without radiograph images and may request that the patient sign a written and dated informed refusal for radiographs. This statement is then filed with the patient's record.

Informed Consent for Minors

The parent, custodial parent, or legal guardian must give consent for treating minor children. When parents live separately, the child's personal information form should indicate which parent is the custodial parent. When separated parents share custody, the child's record should contain letters from each parent providing consent and authorization to treat. Asking in advance for a parent's or a custodial parent's *blanket* consent for emergency treatment avoids confusion and delays should the child require emergency care when a parent or guardian is not present.

Documenting Informed Consent

Most states do not require a specific means for documenting discussions on informed consent. At minimum, the patient's record should indicate that the patient received information about the risks, benefits, and alternatives and consented to or refused the proposed treatment.

When the treatment is extensive, invasive, or risky, a written informed consent document is recommended. The patient, the dentist, and a witness should sign the written consent form. The patient should receive a copy of the form, and the original should be kept with the patient's chart.

Patient Records

Records regarding patient care are referred to as the **dental chart** or **patient record.** These records are important legal documents that must be protected and handled with care. All examination records, diagnoses, radiographs, consent forms, updated medical histories, copies of medical and laboratory prescriptions, and correspondence to or about a patient are filed together in the patient's folder. Financial information is not included with the patient chart.

Patient records are acceptable in court and clearly show the dates and the details of services rendered for each patient. Nothing should be left to memory. Incomplete or unclear records are damaging evidence in a malpractice case. Every entry in a chart should be made as if the chart will be seen in a court of law.

Ownership of Dental Records and Radiographs

The dentist technically "owns" all patient records and radiographs. According to most state laws, patients have the right to **access** (review) and **retrieve** (remove) their records and radiographs.

Original records and radiographs are not allowed to leave the practice without the dentist's permission. In most situations, duplicate radiographs and a photocopy of the record will satisfy the patient's needs. If a disagreement with the patient arises on this subject, then the dental assistant should not attempt to make a decision but should immediately refer the matter to the dentist (see Chapter 11).

Reporting Child Abuse and Neglect

Cases of child abuse and neglect are increasingly reported throughout the United States. Approximately 65% of child abuse injuries involve the head, neck, or mouth area (Figure 2-5). Therefore dental personnel are appropriate health care providers to identify signs of abuse in their pediatric patients. In many states, dental professionals are required by law to report known or suspected cases of child abuse.

The primary intent of reporting abuse is to protect the child. Providing help for the parents is equally important. Parents may be unable to ask for help directly, and child abuse may be a means of revealing family problems. The report of abuse may lead to changes in the home and lower the risk of further abuse.

Child abuse is legally defined as any act of omission or act of commission that endangers or impairs a child's physical or emotional health and development. These acts include (1) physical abuse and corporal punishment resulting in injury, (2) emotional abuse, (3) emotional deprivation, (4) physical neglect or inadequate supervision, and (5) sexual abuse or exploitation.

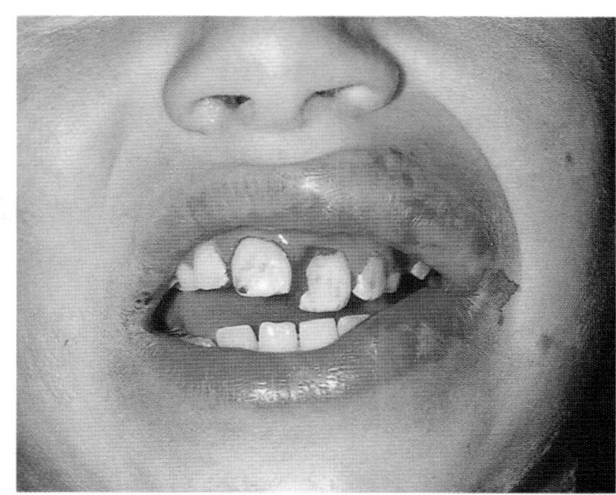

FIGURE 2-5 This boy is a victim of child abuse.

In states that identify dental professionals as **mandated reporters**, dental assistants must report suspected child abuse if they observe signs of abuse or if they have reasonable suspicion of abuse. The report may be made to a child protection agency, such as a county welfare or probation department or to the police or sheriff's department.

Immunity

In states that legally mandate the reporting of child abuse, immunity is granted from criminal or civil liability for reporting as required. This immunity means that the dental assistant cannot be sued for reporting suspicions in an attempt to protect the child.

Regulatory and Professional Organizations

Recognizing and understanding the roles of the government agencies and professional organizations that have a direct influence on the practice of dentistry are important for the dental assistant (Table 2-1). When you are in practice as a dental assistant, these agencies are excellent resources for information for you, and they are easily accessed on the Internet.

Ethical Implications

Having a clear understanding of the Dental Practice Act in your state, especially as it relates to the duties assigned to the dental assistant, is very important. If you move to another state, be certain to check with the state board of dentistry regarding the laws of that state before you begin to practice there. Remember that your personal and professional ethics are the basis of your dental assisting career.

TABLE 2-1
Functions of Professional Organizations and Government Agencies in Dentistry

Professional Organization	Function
American Dental Association (ADA)	Professional organization for dentists The ADA does not regulate or mandate guidelines; it sets standards of practice for dentists. Dental schools and dental assisting, dental hygiene, and dental laboratory technology programs are accredited by the Commission on Dental Accreditation through the ADA.
American Dental Assistants Association (ADAA)	Professional organization for dental assistants ADAA membership gives the dental assistant a voice in national affairs.
American Dental Hygienists Association (ADHA)	Professional organization for dental hygienists
Dental Assisting National Board (DANB)	Independent organization DANB administers the Dental Assisting Board Examination and issues the credential of Certified Dental Assistant (CDA).
Organization for Safety, Asepsis and Prevention (OSAP)	Dentistry's resource for infection control and safety information The OSAP is a nonprofit organization made up of all members of the dental health team, dental manufacturers, researchers, and dental consultants and educators. Its mission is to promote infection control and related health and safety policies and practices.
Government Agencies	**Function**
Occupational Safety & Health Administration (OSHA)	Division of the U.S. Department of Labor OSHA issues and enforces regulations pertaining to employee safety in the workplace.
Centers for Disease Control and Prevention (CDC)	The recognized expert in matters concerning public health The primary mission of the CDC is to track, investigate, and report the spread, virulence (strength), and incidence of specific diseases affecting the U.S. population. The CDC publishes treatment guidelines and provides information on disease prevention and education.
U.S. Environmental Protection Agency (EPA)	The EPA deals with issues of concern for the environment or public safety that involve air and water pollution and waste management. The EPA is also responsible for the registration of chemical disinfectants.
U.S. Food and Drug Administration (FDA)	The FDA issues clearance for all medical and dental devices marketed in the United States. The FDA regulates sterilization technology, which can include equipment and liquid chemical sterilants, to ensure that they are consistent with the claims on their labels.

Chapter Exercises

Multiple Choice

Circle the letter next to the correct answer.

1. The aspect of dentistry that deals with codes of behavior, values, and morals is __________.
   a. ethics
   b. legal
2. A violation of licensing regulations or an inappropriate use of drugs would be regulated under __________.
   a. civil law
   b. criminal law
   c. tort law
   d. contract law
3. The agency in each state that is responsible for regulating the practice of dentistry is the __________.
   a. American Dental Association
   b. state dental association
   c. state board of dentistry
   d. none of the above
4. Reciprocity occurs when __________.
   a. the fees are the same in two dental offices
   b. one state recognizes the dental license of an individual from another state
   c. a dental assistant practices dentistry without a license
   d. all patients are treated equally
5. The type of supervision that requires the dentist to be in the office while the dental auxiliary performs certain functions is __________.
   a. direct supervision
   b. general supervision
6. The credential of a certified dental assistant (CDA) is awarded by the __________.
   a. American Dental Assistants Association
   b. Dental Assisting National Board
   c. state board of dentistry
   d. American Dental Association
7. The methods of preventing lawsuits in a dental office are called __________.
   a. tort law
   b. risk management
   c. liability prevention
   d. risk assessment
8. Another term for malpractice is __________.
   a. professional negligence
   b. risk management
   c. liability
   d. none of the above
9. When a dentist fails to recognize a dental disease and the patient's condition worsens, this scenario is known as __________.
   a. an act of commission
   b. reciprocity
   c. an act of omission
   d. risk management
10. When a patient is given specific information about a dental procedure and any possible risks involved and then signs a form that states that he or she understands the risks and agrees to the dental procedure about to be performed, this process is called __________.
    a. implied consent
    b. informed consent
    c. general consent

Apply Your Knowledge

1. You are a new dental assisting graduate beginning your first job in a beautiful new office with an excellent salary and benefits. Dr. Morris is very nice and is quite impressed with your clinical skills and is anxious to have you use them. On a very busy morning, Dr. Morris asks you to place a retraction cord around a crown preparation while he treats a patient in an emergency situation. Although you know that placing a retraction cord is not a legal function for dental assistants in your state, you have seen it done many times and are certain that you can safely do it. What should you do? You definitely do not want to lose this job.
2. Mrs. Weirs has called your office and has asked you to send her records to another dentist because she is unhappy with the treatment she received in your office. When you check her clinical record, you notice that the last entry is not as complete as it should be. However, you remember that appointment very well and could "adjust" the record to make the entry more complete. What should you do?
3. Your patient is a 78-year-old gentleman who does not speak English very well. You are explaining the reasons he should have a crown on one of his molars. You think he understands you because he is smiling and nodding his head. Do you think this is informed consent? Why or why not? What would you do?

PART TWO The Sciences

CHAPTER 3

Anatomy and Physiology

http://evolve.elsevier.com/Robinson/essentials/

LEARNING OBJECTIVES

1. Pronounce, define, and spell the key terms.
2. Name and describe the terms used to designate directions in the body, as well as the planes and sections of the body.
3. List and describe the organizational levels of the human body.
4. Name each body system, and identify its major function.
5. Discuss the structures of the head and neck, and explain why a dental assistant should be familiar with these structures.
6. Identify the major muscles of mastication and facial expression, and state the function of each.
7. Name and locate the landmarks of the face and oral cavity.

KEY TERMS

ala of the nose
alveolar socket
anatomy
angle of the mandible
anterior
anterior naris
attached gingivae
buccal
canthus
cells
distal
frontal plane
glabella
inferior
innervation
lateral
lingual
mandibular
masticatory mucosa
maxillary
medial
mental protuberance
midsagittal plane
mucogingival junction
mucous membrane
nasion
organs
palate
philtrum
physiology
posterior
proximal
sagittal plane
septum
superior
tissues
tragus
transverse plane
trigeminal nerve
zygomatic arch

The human body is an incredible living creation. It has 11 body systems that function together more smoothly than the world's greatest computers. Having a basic understanding of the study of **anatomy** (study of the structure of the human body) and **physiology** (study of how the human body functions) is important for the dental assistant. This knowledge will also help you keep your own body healthy, communicate with medical personnel, and understand treatments or medications that may be prescribed for you. This chapter also introduces you to the basic terms and definitions that you need to communicate effectively as a dental health care professional.

Directions and Body Planes

Directions in the Body

Directional terms are used to describe the relative position of one part of the body to another. Note that the pairs of directional terms in Table 3-1 are opposites (e.g., left and right, up and down, forward and back).

Planes and Sections of the Body

Three imaginary planes are used to help visualize the spatial relationships of internal body parts. These planes are

TABLE 3-1
Directional Terms for the Body

Term	Example	Term	Example
Anterior Toward the front of the body	The heart is anterior to the spinal column.	**Posterior** Toward the back of the body	The ear is posterior to the nose.
Medial Toward, or nearer to, the midline of the body	The nose is medial to the ears.	**Lateral** Toward the side; away from the midline	The ears are lateral to the nose.
Proximal Part closer to the trunk of the body or point of attachment	The elbow is proximal to the wrist.	**Distal** Part farther away from the midline of the body	The fingers are distal to the wrist. In dentistry, the surface of a tooth that is farthest from the midline is the distal surface.
Superior Above or higher	The nose is superior to the mouth.	**Inferior** Below or under	The nose is inferior to the eyes.

used to describe the location of an organ or a problem (Figure 3-1).

1. The **sagittal plane** refers to a lengthwise cut that divides the body into right and left portions. If the cut passes through the midline of the body, then it is called a **midsagittal plane**.
2. The **transverse plane**, also known as the horizontal plane, is any vertical plane at right angles to the sagittal plane that horizontally cuts across the body, dividing the body into **anterior** (front) and **posterior** (back) portions. This type of view is sometimes called a cross section.
3. The **frontal plane** divides the body into anterior and posterior sections and is perpendicular to both the sagittal plane and the transverse plane. The frontal plane is sometimes called a coronal plane.

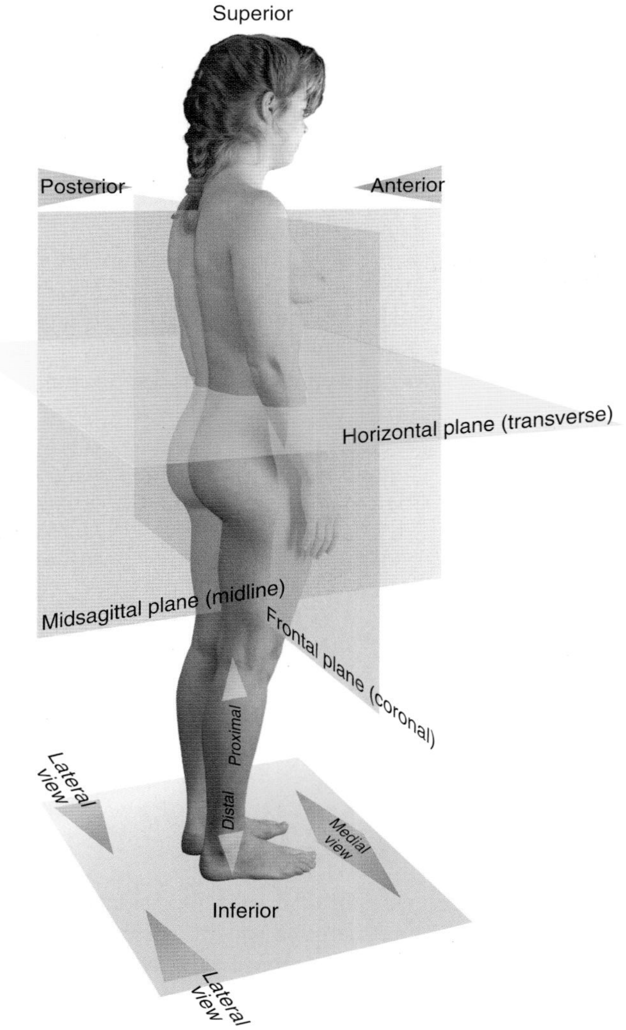

FIGURE 3-1 Body in anatomic position. (Modified from Abrahams PH, Boon J, Spratt J: *McMinn's clinical atlas of human anatomy*, ed 6, St. Louis, 2008, Mosby.)

Organizational Levels of the Body

The human body has four organizational levels or units. From the simplest to the most complex, they include **cells**, **tissues**, **organs**, and body systems (Figure 3-2).

Cells

Cells are the smallest units in the human body. A variety of cell types are known, and each type has its own special functions. The structure of a particular cell is based on the function of that cell. For example, blood cells have a very different function from heart cells. Cells do not function alone. Approximately 75 to 100 trillion cells join together to form special groups known as *tissues.*

Tissues

Four primary types of tissues are found in the human body: **epithelial**, **connective**, **muscle**, and **nervous.** Similar to cells, each type of tissue is designed to perform a specific function (Table 3-2). Related tissue types join together to form organs. For example, heart muscles function together to keep the heart beating.

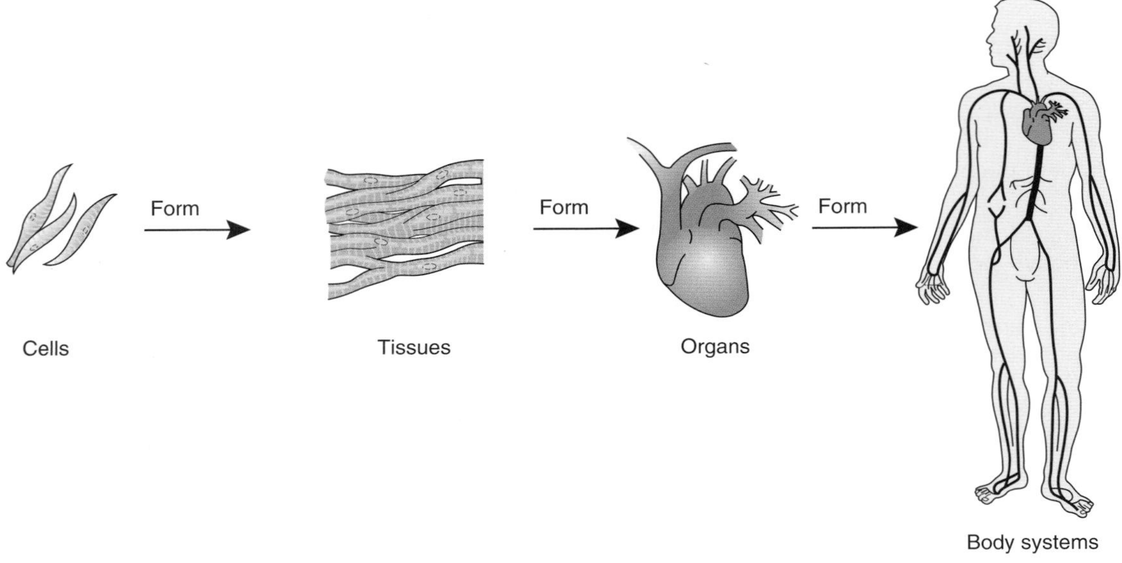

FIGURE 3-2 Organizational levels of the body.

TABLE 3-2
Tissue Types and Functions

Tissue	Function	Examples
Epithelial	Forms the covering of all body surfaces, and lines body cavities and hollow organs.	Skin, intestines, lungs, tubes of the reproductive system, and lining of the oral cavity
Connective	Binds structures together. Forms the framework and support for organs and the entire body. Stores fat, transports substances, and helps repair tissue damage.	Fat, tendons and ligaments, cartilage, blood, and bone
Muscle	Produces movement of body parts.	Body movements, pumping action of the heart, food movement through the digestive process, and urine movement through the bladder
Nervous	Is found in the brain, spinal cord, and nerves. Coordinates and controls many body activities.	Stimulates muscle contraction. Creates awareness of the environment. Plays a major role in emotions, memory, and reasoning.

Organs

Organs work together as a team to keep each body system functioning. The heart, skin, ear, stomach, and liver are examples of organs.

Body Systems

Body systems are made up of organs. Occasionally, the same organ belongs to more than one system. For example, ovaries and testes clearly belong to the reproductive system, but because one of their functions is to produce hormones, they are also part of the endocrine system. Body systems do not function independently. For example, when you exercise hard, your muscular system needs extra oxygen. Your respiratory system meets this need by supplying additional oxygen.

Systems of the Body

Eleven major systems are present in the human body (Figure 3-3). Although each system has its own specific functions, all systems work together as a team to support life (Table 3-3).

Digestive System

The digestive system is composed of the **mouth**, **teeth**, **tongue**, **pharynx**, **esophagus**, **stomach**, **intestines**, and **glands** such as the **salivary glands**, **pancreas**, and **liver**. The functions of the digestive system are to ingest food, process it into molecules that can be used by the body, and then eliminate the residue.

Nervous System

The nervous system causes muscles to contract, stimulates glands to secrete, and regulates many other systems of the body.

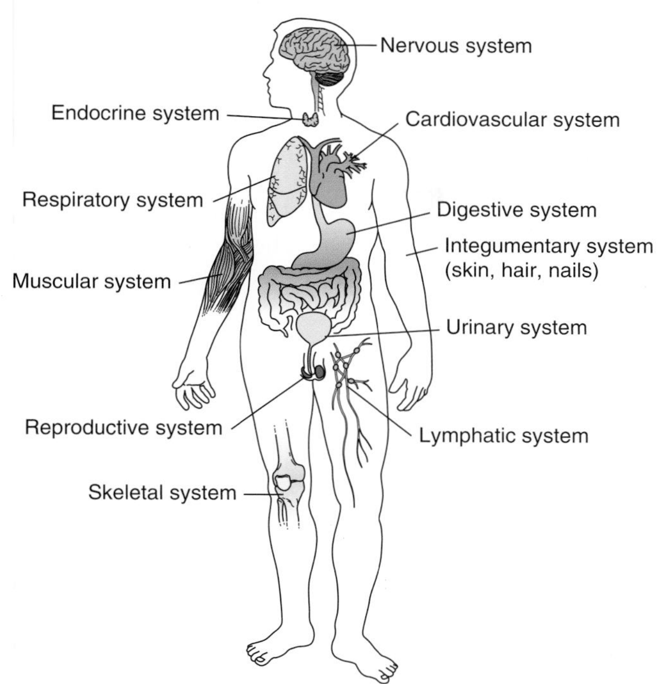

FIGURE 3-3 The eleven body systems.

The nervous system also allows sensations such as pain, pressure, and touch to be perceived. The two primary divisions of the nervous system are the **central nervous system**, which consists of the spinal cord and brain, and the **peripheral nervous system**, which consists of the cranial and spinal nerves.

Cardiovascular System

The cardiovascular system includes the heart, blood vessels, and blood. The functions of the cardiovascular system are to circulate blood, carry oxygen and nutrients to all areas of the body, and filter and eliminate wastes. The two major subdivisions of this system are the pulmonary circulation and the systemic circulation. **Pulmonary circulation** includes the flow of blood from the heart, through the lungs (where it receives oxygen), and back to the heart. **Systemic circulation** includes blood flow to all parts of the body except to the lungs.

Endocrine System

The endocrine system consists of glands that produce hormones that regulate the rate of metabolism, growth, and sexual development and functioning. Hormones are directly secreted into the bloodstream (not through a duct). The endocrine glands include the **thyroid** and **parathyroid glands**, **ovaries**, **testes**, **pituitary gland**, **pancreas**, and **adrenal medulla**.

Respiratory System

The respiratory system is responsible for carrying oxygen from the air to the bloodstream and for expelling the waste product

TABLE 3-3
Major Body Systems

Body System	Components	Major Functions
Skeletal	206 bones	Protection, support, and shape; hematopoietic; storage of certain minerals
Muscular	Striated, smooth, and cardiac muscle	Holding body erect, locomotion, movement of body fluids, production of body heat, communication
Cardiovascular	Heart, arteries, veins, and blood	Respiratory, nutritive, excretory
Lymphatic and immune	White blood cells; lymph fluid, vessels, and nodes; spleen and tonsils	Defense against disease, conservation of plasma proteins and fluid, lipid absorption
Nervous	Central and peripheral nervous systems, special sense organs	Reception of stimuli, transmission of messages, coordinating mechanism
Respiratory	Nose, paranasal sinuses, pharynx, epiglottis, larynx, trachea, bronchi, and lungs	Transportation of oxygen to cells, excretion of carbon dioxide and some water wastes
Digestive system	Mouth, pharynx, esophagus, stomach, intestines, and accessory organs	Digestion of food, absorption of nutrients, elimination of solid wastes
Urinary system	Kidneys, ureters, bladder, and urethra	Formation and elimination of urine, maintenance of homeostasis
Integumentary system	Skin, hair, nails, sweat glands, and sebaceous glands	Protection of body, regulation of body temperature
Endocrine system	Adrenals, gonads, pancreas, parathyroids, pineal, pituitary, thymus, and thyroid	Integration of body functions, control of growth, maintenance of homeostasis
Reproductive system	Male: testes and penis Female: ovaries, fallopian tubes, uterus, and vagina	Production of new life

carbon dioxide. The respiratory system comprises the **nose**, **paranasal sinuses**, **pharynx**, **epiglottis**, **larynx**, **trachea**, **alveoli**, and **lungs**.

Lymphatic System

The lymphatic system is part of the immune system and plays important roles in the defense of the body against infection and disease and also in the absorption of fats from the intestine. The lymphatic system includes the **thymus**, **spleen**, **tonsils**, **lymph vessels**, **lymph nodes**, and **lymphatic nodules** located in the digestive system.

Muscular System

The muscular system consists of three basic types of muscles: **striated** (striped), **smooth**, and **cardiac**. These types of muscle are described according to their appearance and function (Figure 3-4).

Types of Muscle

Striated muscles are known as the skeletal or voluntary muscles. Skeletal muscles attach to the bones of the skeleton and make bodily motions possible.

Smooth muscle fibers move the internal organs, such as the digestive tract, blood vessels, and secretory ducts leading from the glands.

Cardiac muscle forms most of the wall of the heart and is the contraction of the muscle that causes the heart to beat.

Skeletal System

The skeletal system consists of 206 bones. It provides the framework for the attached muscles and plays an indispensable role in movement and in supporting the brain and spinal cord, which are encased in the skull and spine.

Urinary System

The urinary system consists of the **kidneys**, in which urine is formed to carry away waste materials from the blood; the **ureters**, which transport urine from the kidney; the **bladder**, where the urine is stored until it can be disposed; and the **urethra**, through which the bladder is emptied to the outside through the process of urination. The kidneys require a large blood supply and are close to the primary artery of the body—the aorta. More than 2 pints of blood pass through the kidneys every minute.

Integumentary or Skin System

The integumentary (skin) system has many important functions. It helps regulate body temperature, keeps bacteria from entering the body, excretes liquids and salts, and provides sensitivity to touch. The skin also absorbs ultraviolet rays from the sun and uses them to convert chemicals into vitamin D, which is necessary for the absorption of calcium.

Reproductive System

The female reproductive system consists of the **ovaries**, **fallopian tubes**, **uterus**, and **vagina**. Fertility begins at puberty (the onset of menstruation) and ceases at the time of menopause. The male reproductive system includes the **testes**, **prostate**, and **seminal vesicles**.

Structures of the Head and Neck

As a dental assistant, your knowledge and understanding of the structures of the head and neck will be useful for almost every task you perform. (See Procedure 3-1: Identify the Major Landmarks and Structures of the Face.)

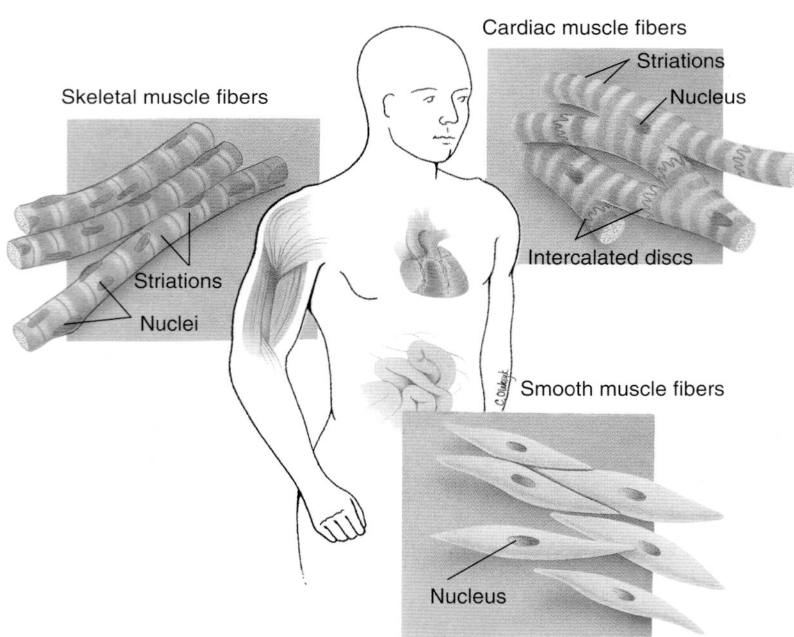

FIGURE 3-4 Types of muscle. (From Thibodeau GA, Patton KT: *The human body in health and disease*, ed 5, St. Louis, 2010, Mosby.)

Types of Bone

Bone is the hard connective tissue that makes up most of the human skeleton. There are two types of bone (Figure 3-5).

Compact bone, also known as cortical bone, is hard, dense, and very strong. It forms the outer layer of bones where it is needed for strength. For example, the outer layer of the mandible (lower jaw) is made of compact bone (Figure 3-6, **A**).

Cancellous bone, also known as **spongy bone,** is found in the interior of bones and is lighter in weight and not as strong as compact bone. For example, the inner layer of the maxillary bones (upper jaw) is made of cancellous bone (Figure 3-6, **B**).

The **periosteum** is the specialized connective tissue covering of all bones in the body.

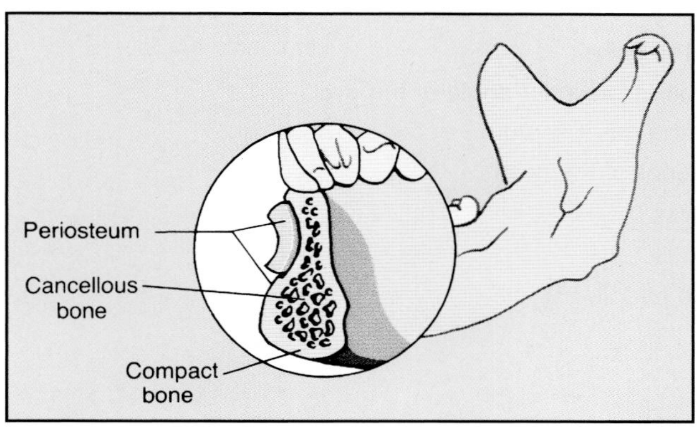

FIGURE 3-5 Structure of bone.

Anatomy of the Skull

The human skull is made up of the bones of the cranium and the face. (The **cranium** forms the bony protection for the brain.) The bones of the skull are summarized in Table 3-4.

The dental assistant should know the anatomic landmarks of the skull. These landmarks are illustrated in Figures 3-7 through 3-13.

Paranasal Sinuses

The paranasal sinuses are spaces that contain air within the bones of the skull. Their functions include providing mucus, making the bones of the skull lighter, and helping to produce sound (Figure 3-14). These sinuses are named for the bones in which they are located (Table 3-5).

Temporomandibular Joint

A joint is the junction between two or more bones. The temporomandibular joint (TMJ) is located on each side of the head where the temporal bone and the mandible join (Figure 3-15). The TMJ makes it possible for the lower jaw to move so that we can speak and chew. A patient may have a disorder with one or both of their TMJs. The dental professional must have an understanding of the anatomy of the TMJ, the normal movements of the joint, and any possible disorders of the joint (Figure 3-16).

Capsular Ligament

The capsular ligament is a dense fibrous capsule that completely surrounds the TMJ. It is attached to the neck of the condyle and

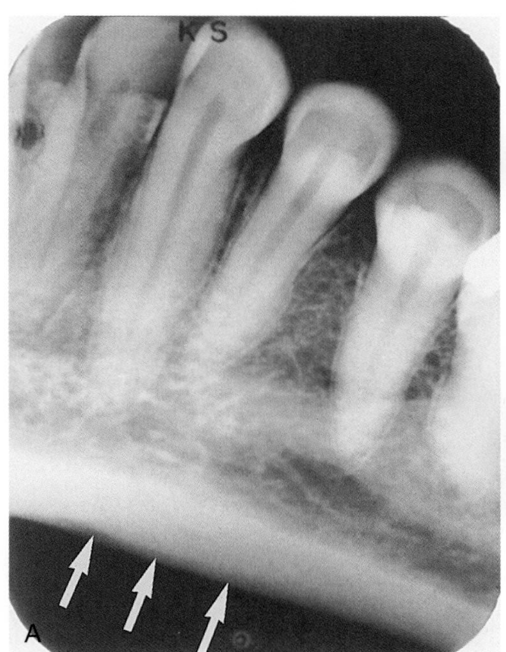

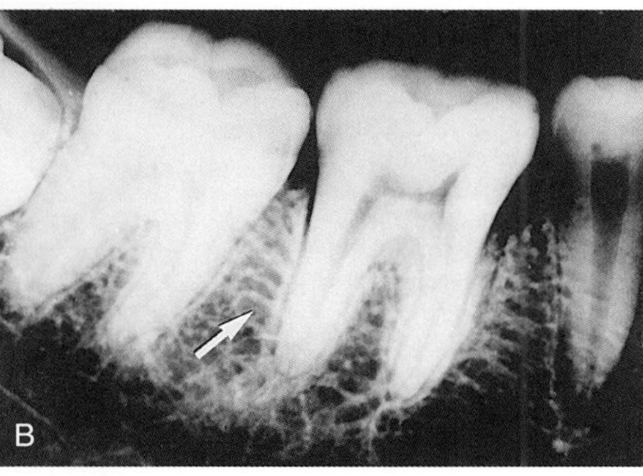

FIGURE 3-6 **A,** Cortical bone appears hard and dense. **B,** Cancellous bone appears spongy. (From Haring JI, Lind LJ: *Radiographic interpretation for the dental hygienist,* Philadelphia, 1993, Saunders.)

TABLE 3-4
Bones of the Skull

Bone	Number	Location
Eight Bones of the Cranium		
Frontal	1	Forms the forehead, most of the orbital roof, and the anterior cranial floor.
Parietal	2	Form most of the roof and upper sides of the cranium.
Occipital	1	Forms the back and base of the cranium.
Temporal	2	Form the sides and base of the cranium.
Sphenoid	1	Forms part of the anterior base of the skull and part of the walls of the orbit.
Ethmoid	1	Forms part of the orbit and the floor of the cranium.
Fourteen Bones of the Face		
Zygomatic	2	Form the prominence of the cheeks and part of the orbit.
Maxillary	2	Form the upper jaw.
Palatine	2	Form the posterior part of the hard palate and the floor of the nose.
Nasal	2	Form the bridge of the nose.
Lacrimal	2	Form part of the orbit at the inner angle of the eye.
Vomer	1	Forms the base for the nasal septum.
Inferior conchae	2	Form part of the interior of the nose.
Mandible	1	Forms the lower jaw.
Six Auditory Ossicles		
Malleus, incus, stapes	6	Are the bones of the middle ear.

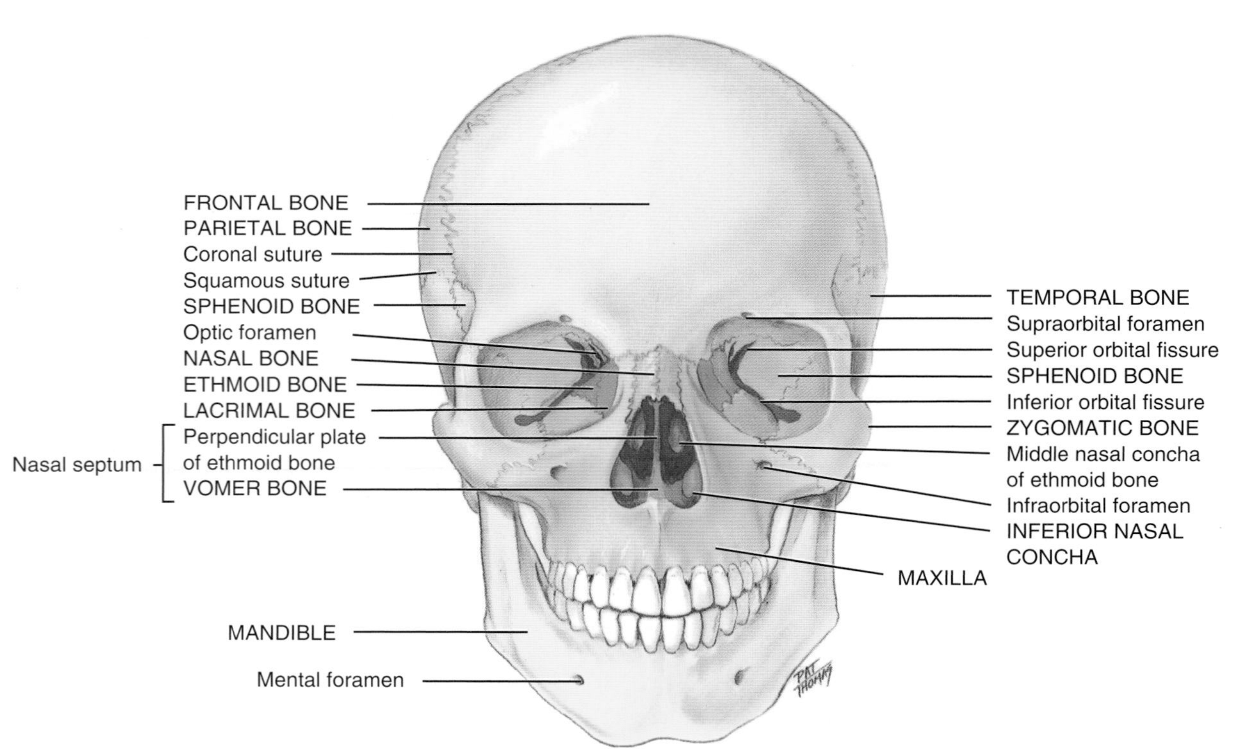

FIGURE 3-7 Frontal view of the skull. (From Applegate E: *The anatomy and physiology learning system*, ed 4, St. Louis, 2011, Saunders.)

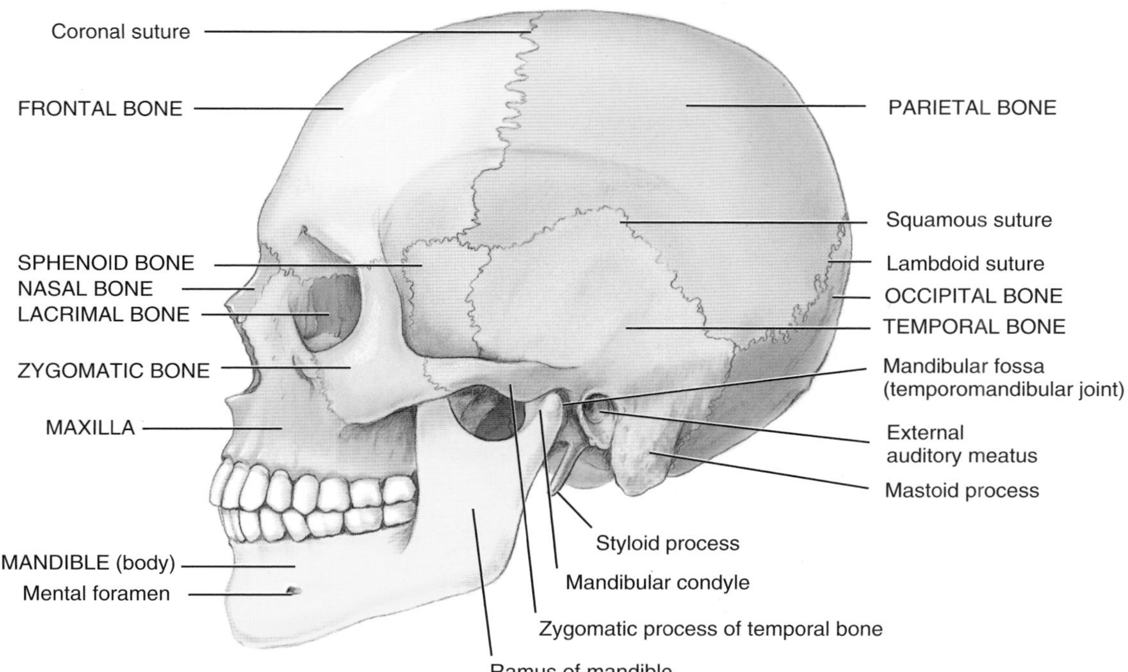

FIGURE 3-8 Lateral view of the skull. (From Applegate E: *The anatomy and physiology learning system*, ed 4, St. Louis, 2011, Saunders.)

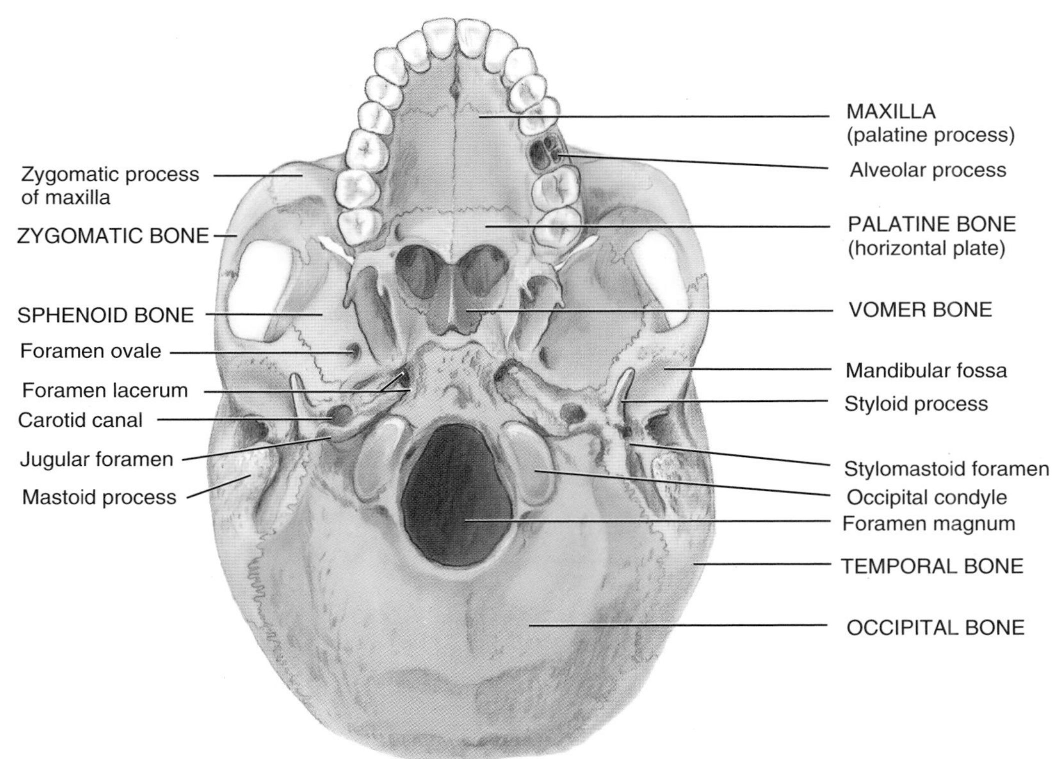

FIGURE 3-9 Base of the skull. (From Applegate E: *The anatomy and physiology learning system*, ed 4, St. Louis, 2011, Saunders.)

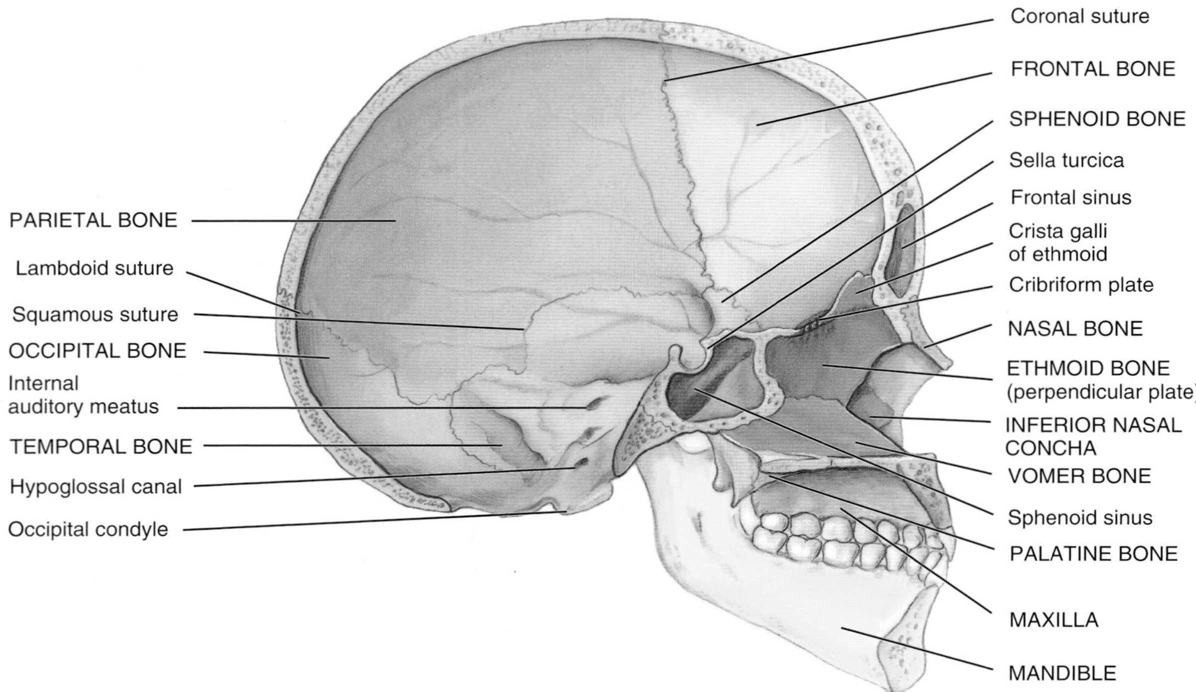

FIGURE 3-10 Midsagittal view of the skull. (From Applegate E: *The anatomy and physiology learning system*, ed 4, St. Louis, 2011, Saunders.)

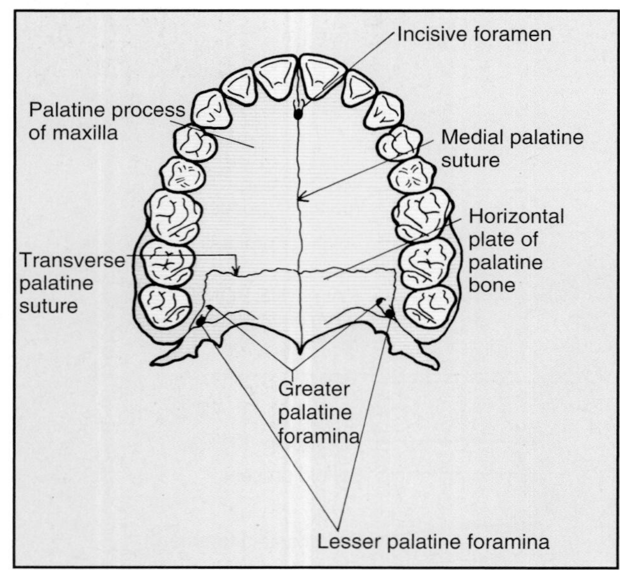

FIGURE 3-11 Bones and landmarks of the hard palate.

to the nearby surfaces of the temporal bone. The ligaments of the TMJ attach the mandible to the cranium (Figure 3-17).

Articular Space

The articular space is the area between the capsular ligament and the surfaces of the glenoid fossa and the condyle. The **articular disc**, also known as the meniscus, is a cushion of dense connective tissue that divides the articular space into fluid-filled upper and lower compartments. The structure of these compartments and the presence of fluid make smooth movement of the joint possible.

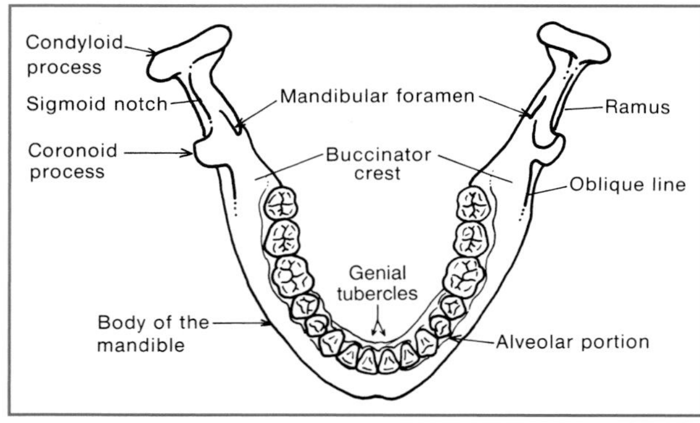

FIGURE 3-12 Topical view of the mandible.

Movements of the Temporomandibular Joint

The TMJs are constructed for specialized hinge-and-glide movements, which allow the mouth to open and close (Figure 3-18).

Hinge Action

The hinge action is the first phase in opening the mouth. During this movement, the body of the mandible drops downward and backward.

Gliding Action

Gliding action is the second phase in opening the mouth. This phase consists of a gliding movement by the condyle and articular disc forward and downward along the articular eminence. This movement occurs during the forward movement

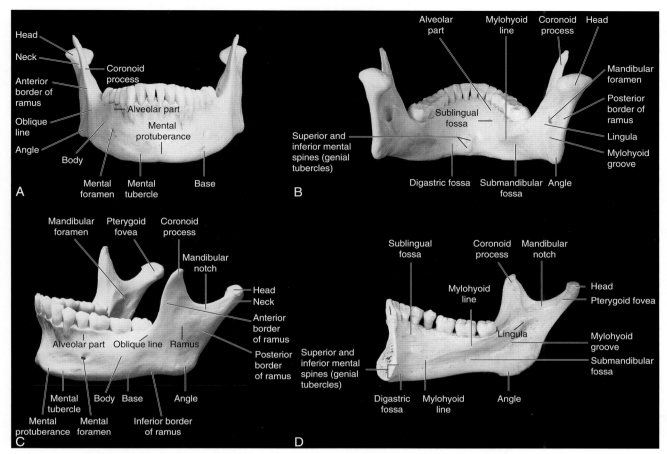

FIGURE 3-13 Views of the mandible. **A,** From the front. **B,** From behind and above. **C,** From the left and front. **D,** Internal view from the left. (From Malamed SF: *Handbook of local anesthesia,* ed 6, St. Louis, 2013, Mosby. Data from Abrahams PH, Boon J, Spratt J: *McMinn's clinical atlas of human anatomy,* ed 6, St. Louis, 2008, Mosby.)

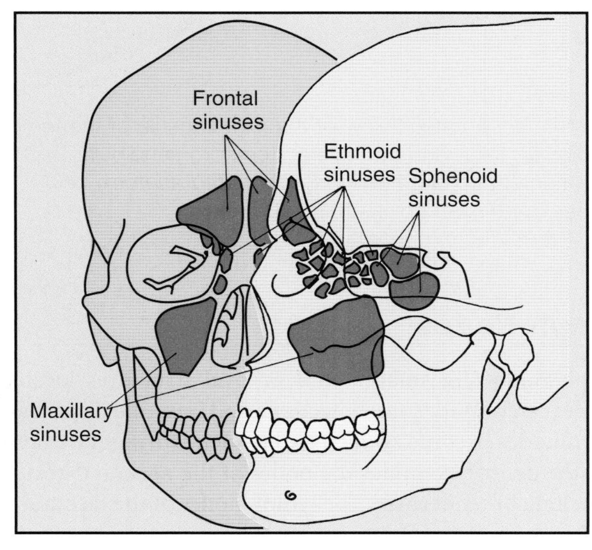

FIGURE 3-14 The paranasal sinuses.

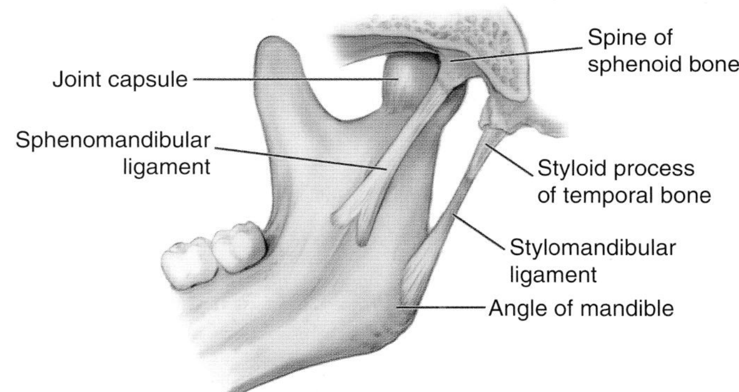

FIGURE 3-15 Lateral view of the skull showing the mandible and the temporomandibular joint. (From Fehrenbach M, Herring S: *Illustrated anatomy of the head and neck,* ed 4, St. Louis, 2012, Saunders.)

TABLE 3-5
The Paranasal Sinuses

Sinuses	Location	Significance of Sinuses
Maxillary	Are located in the maxillary bones and are the largest sinuses.	Infection in any of the maxillary sinuses may cause pain in the maxillary teeth. The symptoms of sinusitis (inflamed sinuses) are headache, foul-smelling discharge, fever, and weakness. Infection in one sinus can travel through the nasal cavity to the other sinuses, leading to serious complications for the patient.
Frontal	Are located in the frontal bone, within the forehead, just above the eyes.	
Ethmoid	Are located in the ethmoid bone and are irregularly shaped air cells separated from the orbital (eye) cavity by a very thin layer of bone.	
Sphenoid sinuses	Are located in the sphenoid and close to the optic nerves.	Infection in these sinuses may damage vision or the brain or both.

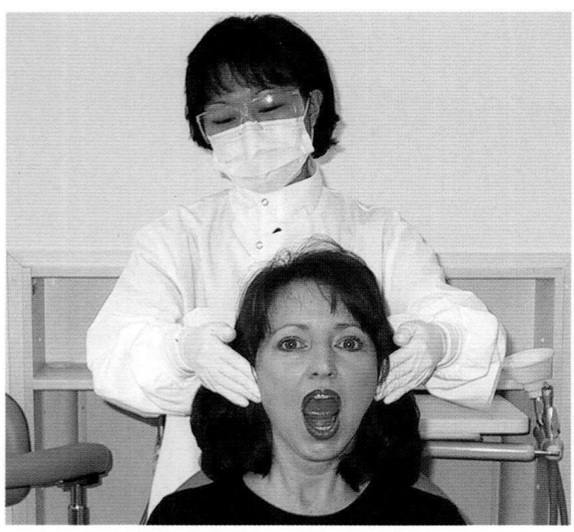

FIGURE 3-16 Palpation of the patient during movements of both temporomandibular joints.

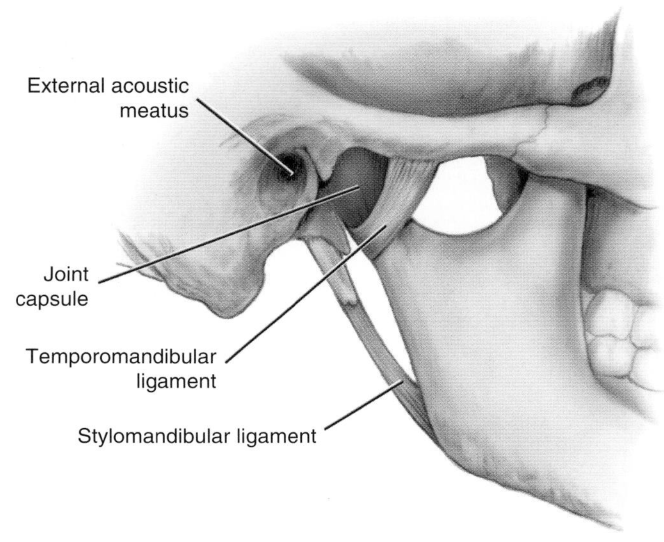

FIGURE 3-17 Lateral view of the joint capsule of the temporomandibular joint and its lateral temporomandibular ligament. (From Fehrenbach M, Herring S: *Illustrated anatomy of the head and neck,* ed 4, St. Louis, 2012, Saunders.)

(protrusion) of the mandible. The backward movement is called *retrusion.*

Major Muscles of Mastication and Facial Expression

The muscles of mastication are responsible for closing the jaws, bringing the lower jaw forward and backward, and shifting the lower jaw from side to side. The muscles of mastication work with the TMJ to accomplish these movements (Table 3-6).

Blood Supply to the Face and Mouth

Arteries carry oxygenated blood away from the heart to all parts of the body with a pulsing motion. Veins carry blood back to the heart. The major arteries and veins of the face and mouth are shown in Figure 3-19 and listed in Table 3-7.

Lymph Nodes

Lymph nodes are small round or oval structures located in lymph vessels. With some infections and immune disorders, the lymph nodes become swollen and tender. During the examination, the dentist examines the nodes of the neck to detect signs of swelling or tenderness. The lymph nodes of the face and neck are shown in Figure 3-20.

Nerve Supply to the Mouth

The **trigeminal nerve**, which is a branch of the fifth cranial nerve, is the primary source of the nerve supply for the mouth.

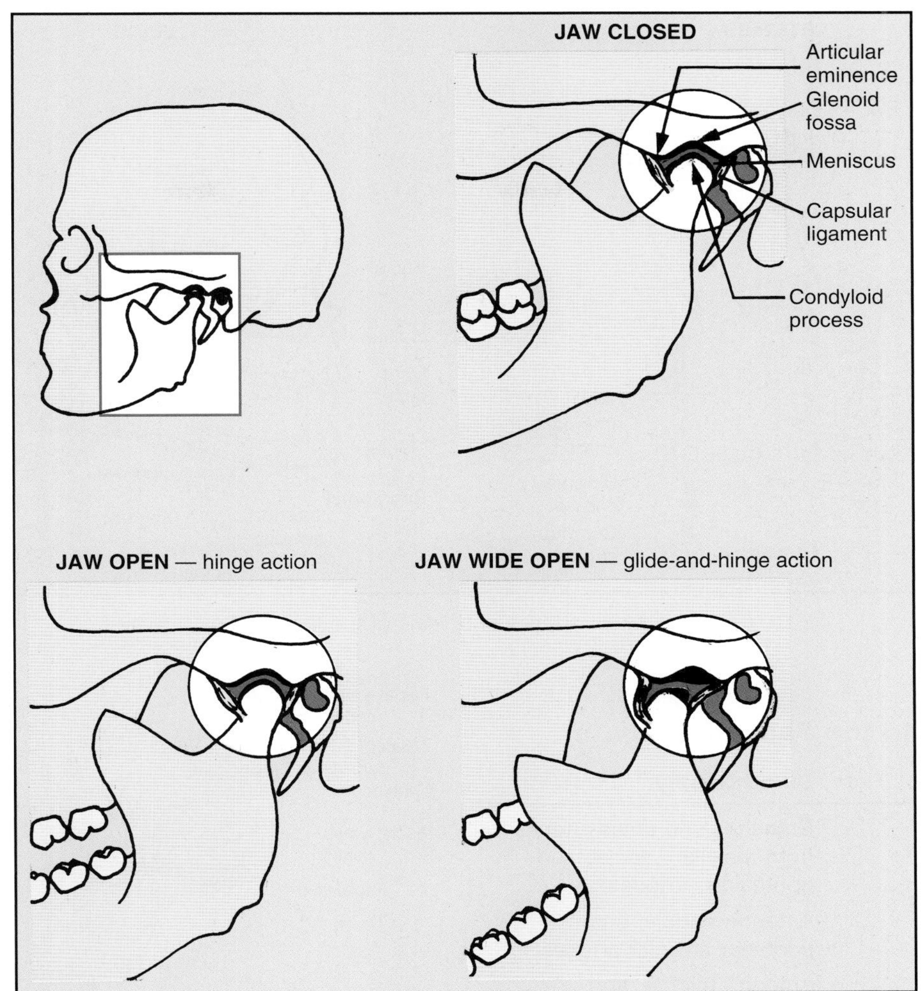

FIGURE 3-18 Hinge-and-gliding actions of the temporomandibular joint.

TABLE 3-6
Muscles of Mastication and Facial Expression

Muscle	Function
Buccinator	Compresses the cheeks and holds food in contact with the teeth.
External (lateral) pterygoid	Depresses, protrudes, and moves the mandible from side to side.
Internal (medial) pterygoid	Closes and aids in sideways movement.
Masseter	Raises the mandible, closes the jaws, and occludes the teeth.
Mentalis	Raises and wrinkles the skin of the chin and pushes up the lower lip.
Orbicularis oris	Closes and puckers the lips and aids in chewing by pushing the food against the teeth.
Temporal	Raises the mandible, closes the jaw, and occludes the teeth.
Zygomatic major	Draws the angles of the mouth upward and backward, as in laughing.

Innervation is another term for nerve supply. The trigeminal nerve divides into **maxillary** and **mandibular** branches to serve the mouth (Figures 3-21 and 3-22).

Maxillary Innervation

The maxillary division of the trigeminal nerve supplies the maxillary (upper) teeth, periosteum, mucous membrane, maxillary sinuses, and soft **palate**. The **mucous membrane** is the specialized tissue that lines the inside of the mouth.

The maxillary division further subdivides to provide the following routes of the nerve supply:

- The **nasopalatine nerve**, which passes through the incisive foramen, supplies the tissue palatal to the maxillary anterior teeth. (Anterior means *toward the front*. A **foramen** is an

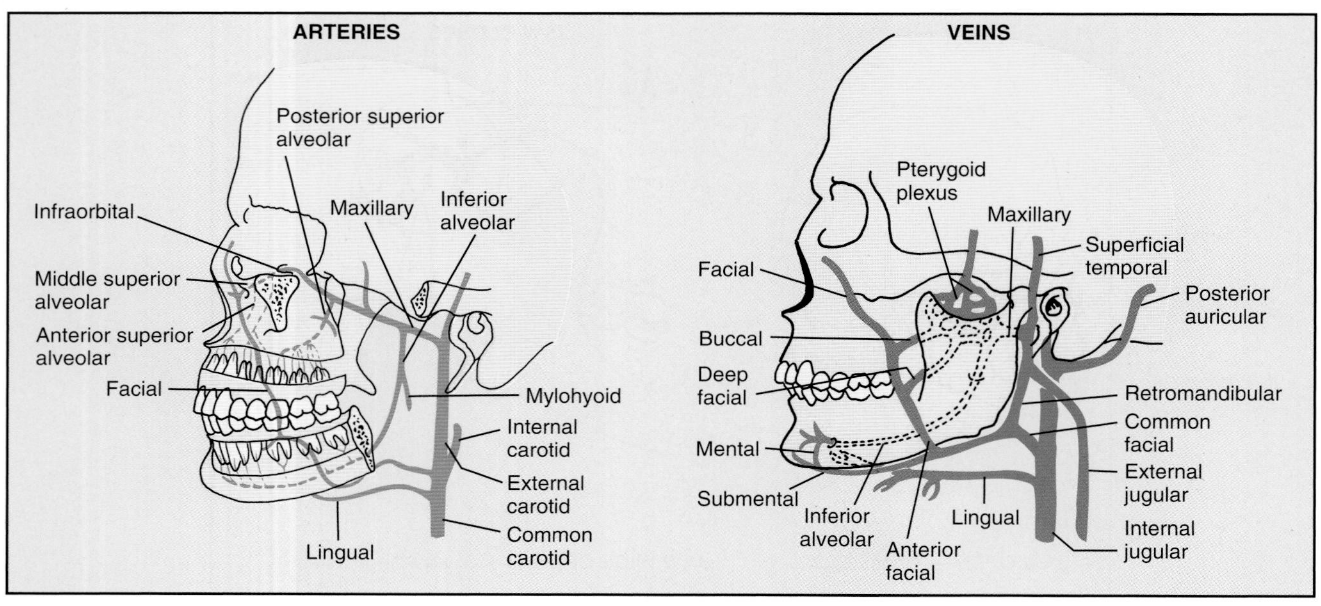

FIGURE 3-19 Major arteries and veins of the face and oral cavity.

TABLE 3-7
Major Arteries to the Face and Mouth

Structure	Blood Supply
Muscles of facial expression	Branches and small arteries from maxillary, facial, and ophthalmic arteries
Maxilla	Anterior, middle, and posterior alveolar arteries
Maxillary teeth	Anterior, middle, and posterior alveolar arteries
Mandible	Inferior alveolar arteries
Mandibular teeth	Inferior alveolar arteries
Tongue	Lingual artery
Muscles of mastication	Facial arteries

opening in a bone through which blood vessels, nerves, and ligaments pass.)

- The anterior palatine nerve, which passes through the posterior palatine foramen and forward over the palate, supplies the **mucoperiosteum** (mucoperiosteum is periosteum that has a mucous membrane surface).

The anterior superior alveolar nerve supplies the maxillary central, lateral, and cuspid teeth plus their periodontal membrane and gingivae. This nerve also supplies the maxillary sinus.

- The middle superior alveolar nerve supplies the maxillary first and second premolars, the mesiobuccal root of the maxillary first molar, and the maxillary sinus.
- The posterior superior alveolar nerve supplies the other roots of the maxillary first molar and the maxillary second and third molars. This nerve also branches forward to serve the lateral wall of the maxillary sinus.
- The buccal nerve supplies branches to the buccal mucous membrane and to the mucoperiosteum of the maxillary and

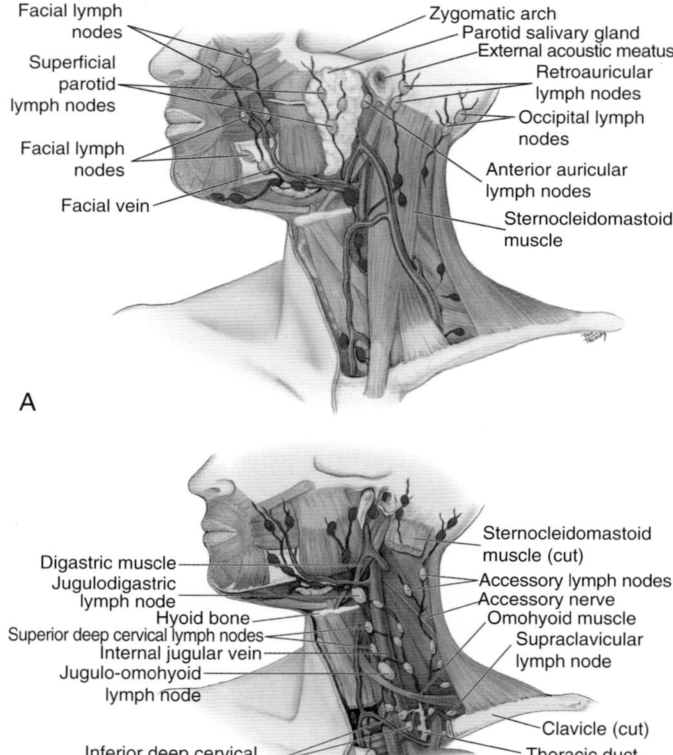

FIGURE 3-20 **A,** Superficial lymph nodes of the head and associated structures. **B,** Deep cervical lymph nodes and associated structures. (From Fehrenbach M, Herring S: *Illustrated anatomy of the head and neck,* ed 4, St. Louis, 2012, Saunders.)

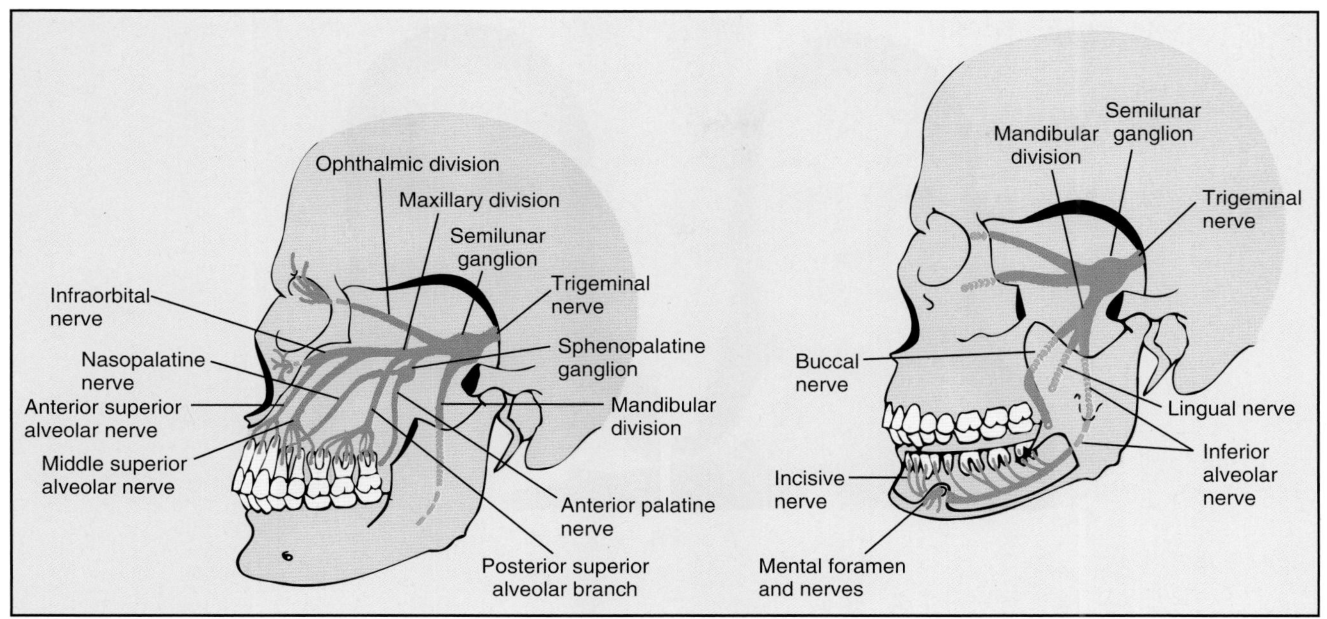

FIGURE 3-21 Maxillary and mandibular innervation.

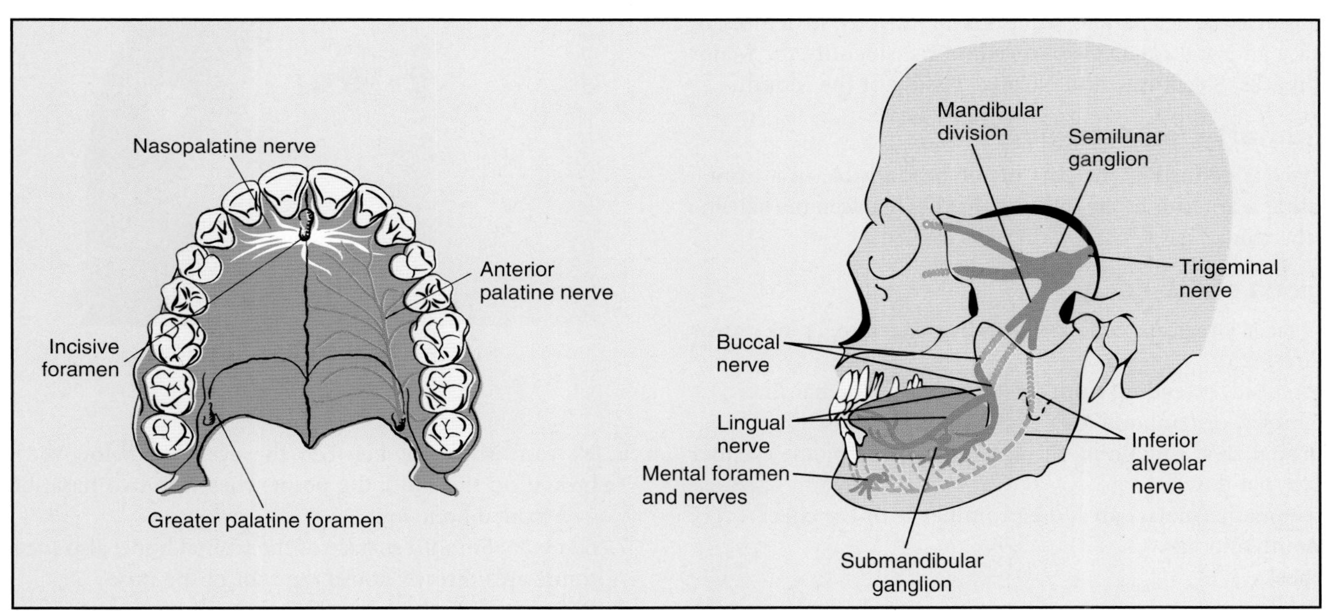

FIGURE 3-22 Palatal, lingual, and buccal innervation.

mandibular molar teeth. (**Buccal** means *pertaining to* or *directed toward the cheek.*)

Mandibular Innervation

The mandibular division of the trigeminal nerve subdivides into the buccal, **lingual**, and **inferior** alveolar nerves.

- The buccal nerve supplies branches to the buccal mucous membrane and to the mucoperiosteum of the maxillary and mandibular molar teeth.
- The lingual nerve supplies the anterior two thirds of the tongue and gives off branches to supply the lingual mucous membrane and mucoperiosteum. (Lingual means of, or pertaining to, the tongue.)
- The inferior alveolar nerve subdivides into the following:
- The mylohyoid nerve supplies the mylohyoid muscles and the anterior belly of the digastric muscle.
- The small dental nerves supply the molar teeth and premolar teeth, alveolar process, and periosteum of the mandible.
- The mental nerve moves outward through the mental foramen and supplies the chin and mucous membrane of the lower lip.
- The incisive nerve continues interiorly and gives off small branches to supply the cuspid, lateral, and central teeth.

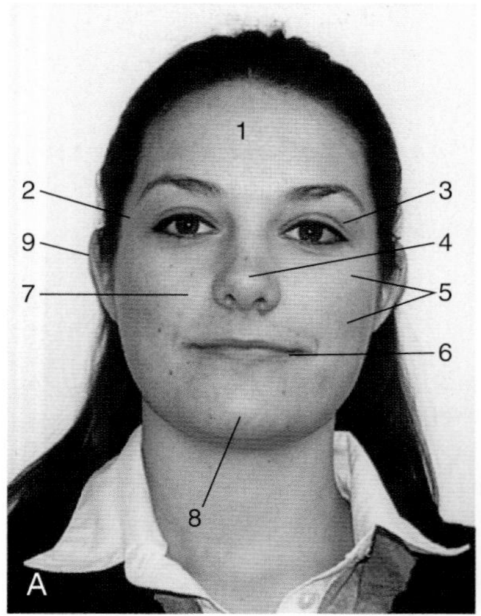

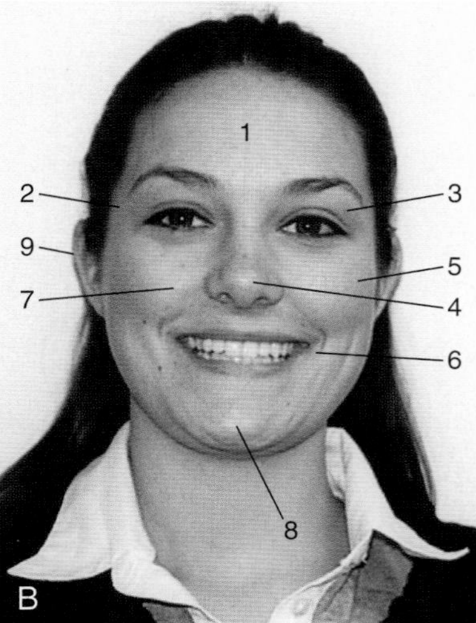

FIGURE 3-23 **A** and **B,** Regions of the face.

Structures of the Face and Oral Cavity

Before beginning more advanced procedures, such as exposing dental radiographs or assisting with intraoral procedures, you must learn the terms and locations of various structures of the face and oral cavity. See Procedure 3-2: Identify the Major Landmarks, Structures, and Normal Tissues of the Mouth.

Landmarks of the Face

The face is defined as the part of the head visible in a frontal view that is anterior to the ears and that lies between the hairline and the chin.

Regions of the Face

The facial region can be subdivided into nine areas (Figure 3-23):

1. Forehead, extending from the eyebrows to the hairline
2. Temples, or temporal area posterior to the eyes
3. Orbital area, containing the eye and covered by the eyelids
4. External nose
5. Zygomatic (malar) area, the prominence of the cheek
6. Mouth and lips
7. Cheeks
8. Chin
9. External ear

Features of the Face

The dental assistant should be able to identify the following important facial landmarks (Figure 3-24):

1. Outer **canthus** of the eye: Fold of tissue at the outer corner of the eyelids
2. Inner canthus of the eye: Fold of tissue at the inner corner of the eyelids
3. **Ala of the nose**: Winglike tip on the outer side of each nostril
4. **Philtrum**: Rectangular area between the two ridges running from under the nose to the midline of the upper lip
5. **Tragus** of the ear: Cartilaginous projection anterior to the external opening of the ear

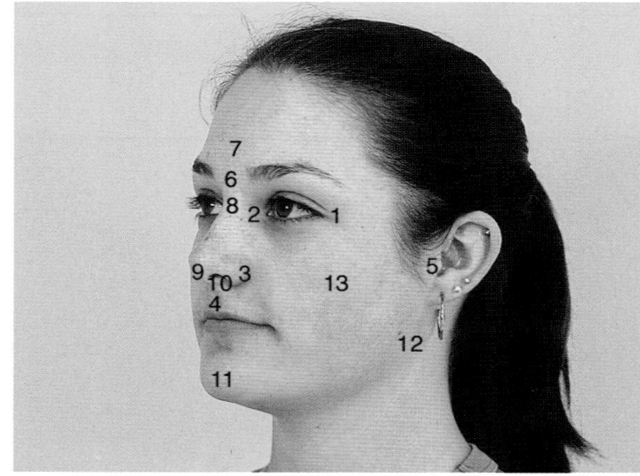

FIGURE 3-24 Features of the face.

6. **Nasion**: Midpoint between the eyes just below the eyebrows; on the skull, the point where the two nasal bones and frontal bone join
7. **Glabella**: Smooth surface of the frontal bone; also the anatomic area directly above the root of the nose
8. Root: Commonly called the *bridge* of the nose
9. **Septum**: Tissue that divides the nasal cavity into two nasal fossae
10. **Anterior naris**: Nostril
11. **Mental protuberance**: Part of the mandible that forms the chin
12. **Angle of the mandible**: Lower posterior of the ramus
13. **Zygomatic arch**: Prominence of the cheek

Oral Cavity

The entire oral cavity is lined with mucous membrane tissue. This type of tissue is moist and is adapted to meet the needs of the area it covers.

The oral cavity consists of the following two areas:

1. Vestibule: Space between the teeth and the inner mucosal lining of the lips and cheeks

2. Oral cavity proper: Space on the tongue side within the upper and lower dental arches

Tongue

The tongue is primarily made up of muscles. It is covered on top with a thick layer of mucous membrane and thousands of tiny projections called *papillae.* Inside the papillae are the sensory organs and the nerves for both taste and touch. On a healthy tongue, the papillae are usually pinkish-white and velvety smooth.

The tongue is one of the body's most versatile organs and is responsible for a number of functions: (1) speaking, (2) positioning food while eating, (3) tasting and tactile sensations, (4) swallowing, and (5) cleansing the oral cavity. After eating, notice how your tongue moves from crevice to crevice, seeking out and removing bits of retained food in your mouth.

The anterior two thirds of the tongue, called the *body,* is found in the oral cavity. The root of the tongue is the posterior part that turns vertically downward to the pharynx. The dorsum consists of the superior (upper) and posterior roughened aspects of the tongue and is covered with small papillae of various shapes and colors (Figure 3-25).

The sublingual surface of the tongue is covered with thin, smooth, transparent mucosa through which many underlying vessels can be seen (Figure 3-26). Two small papillae are present on either side of the lingual frenulum (frenum) just behind the central incisors. Through these papillae into the mouth are the openings of the submandibular ducts. The saliva enters the oral cavity through these ducts. On either side of the lingual surface are two smaller fimbriated folds. The lingual frenum is the thin fold of mucous membrane that extends from the floor of the mouth to the underside of the tongue.

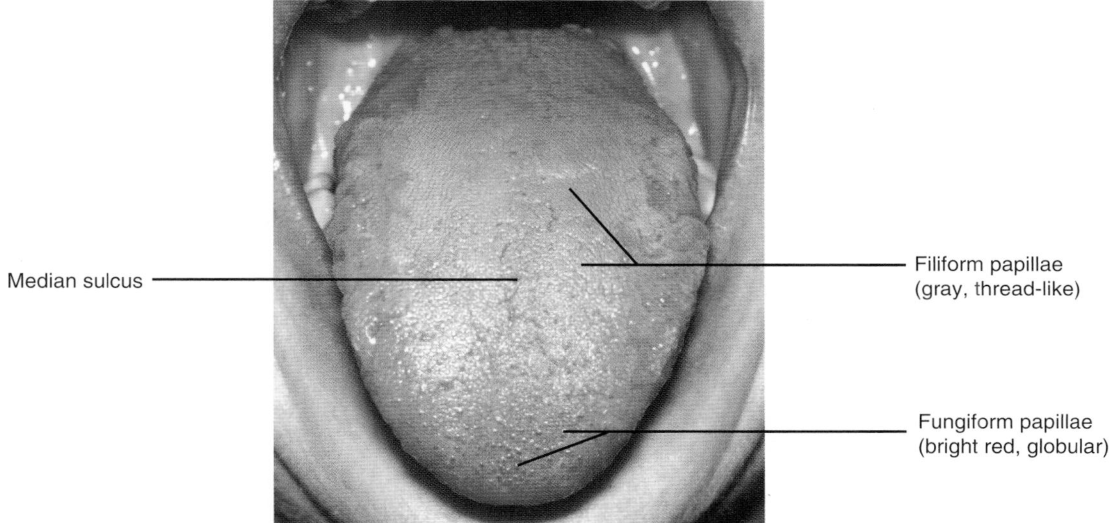

FIGURE 3-25 Dorsum of the tongue. (From Liebgott B: *The anatomical basis of dentistry,* ed 3, St. Louis, 2010, Mosby.)

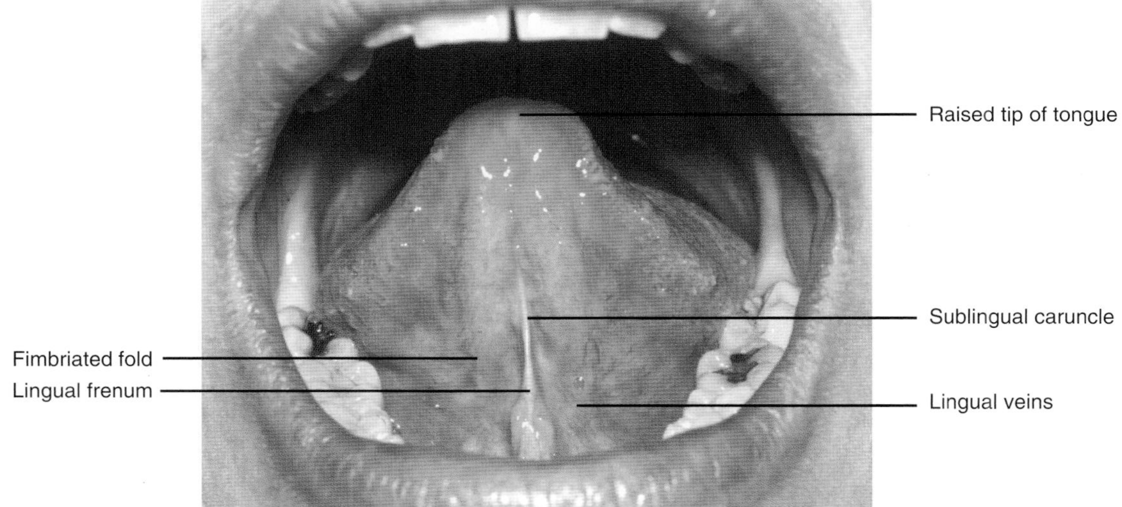

FIGURE 3-26 Sublingual aspect of the tongue. (From Liebgott B: *The anatomical basis of dentistry,* ed 3, St. Louis, 2010, Mosby.)

Frenum

A frenum is a narrow band of tissue that connects two structures. The maxillary labial frenum passes from the oral mucosa at the midline of the maxillary arch to the midline of the inner surface of the upper lip. The mandibular labial frenum passes from the oral mucosa at the midline of the mandibular arch to the midline of the inner surface of the lower lip (Figure 3-27).

In the area of the first maxillary permanent molar, the buccal frenum passes from the oral mucosa of the outer surface of the maxillary arch to the inner surface of the cheek. The lingual frenum passes from the floor of the mouth to the midline of the ventral border of the tongue.

Salivary Glands

The salivary glands produce saliva that lubricates and cleans the oral cavity and helps with digestion. The nervous system controls these glands. The salivary glands have ducts (openings) to help drain the saliva directly into the oral cavity where the saliva is used. The salivary glands may become enlarged, tender, and possibly firm as the result of various disease processes. Certain medications or disease processes may result in decreased or increased production of saliva by these glands (Table 3-8 and Figure 3-28).

Hard and Soft Palates

The hard and soft palates serve as the roof of the mouth, and they separate the mouth from the nasal cavity (Table 3-9 and Figure 3-29).

Gag Reflex

The gag reflex is an involuntary protective mechanism located in the posterior region of the mouth. This very sensitive area includes the soft palate, the uvula, the surrounding tissue, and the posterior portion of the tongue.

Contact of a foreign body with the membranes of this area causes gagging, retching, or vomiting when placing impression

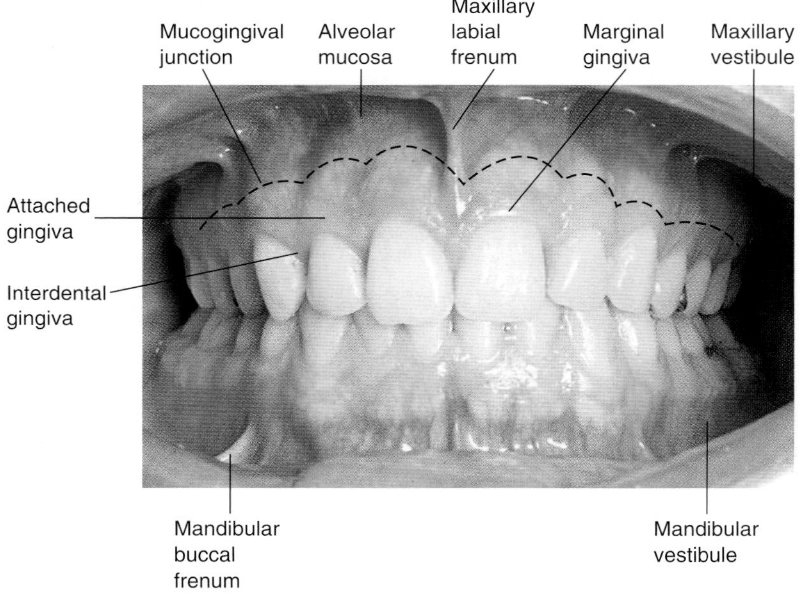

FIGURE 3-27 View of the gingivae and associated anatomic structures.

TABLE 3-8
Three Pairs of Salivary Glands and Ducts

Gland	Location	Associated Duct
Parotid	Is the largest pair of glands; located under the skin just in front of and below each ear. The parotid glands can be felt by gently touching that area.	Saliva enters through Stensen duct, located in the cheek opposite the maxillary second molar.
Sublingual	This gland is present on each side underneath the tongue.	Saliva enters through the sublingual duct through the sublingual caruncle.
Submandibular	Is the second largest pair of salivary glands; they lie beneath the mandible in the submandibular fossa, posterior to the sublingual salivary gland.	Saliva enters through Wharton duct.

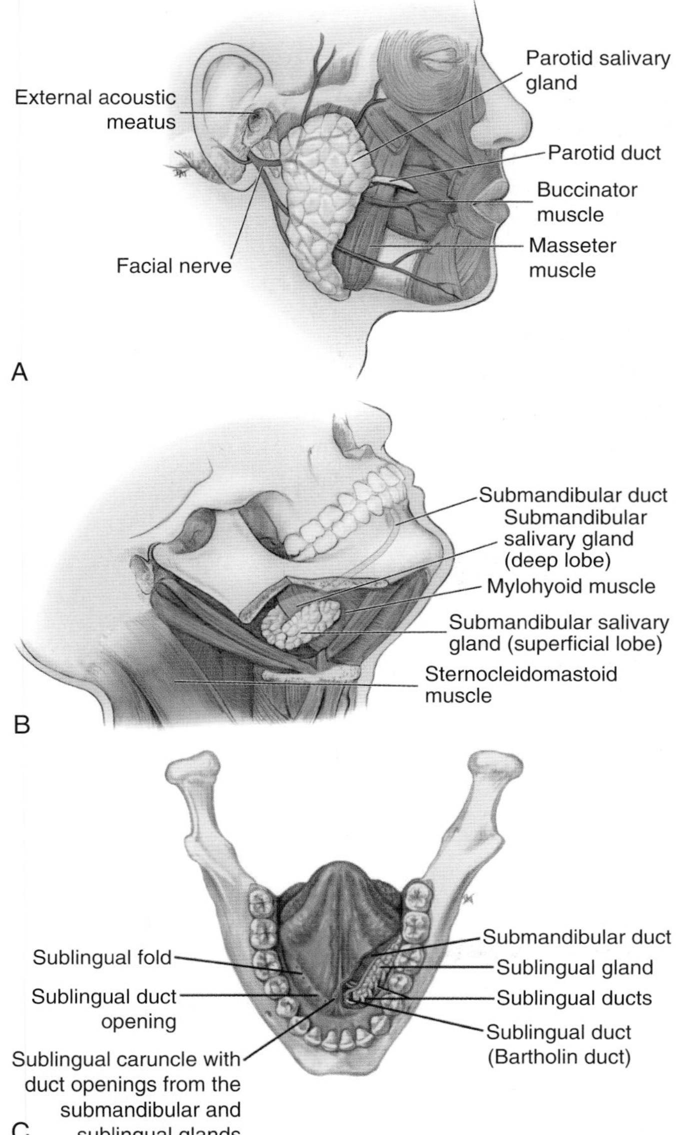

FIGURE 3-28 Major salivary glands. **A,** Parotid salivary glands. **B,** Submandibular salivary gland. **C,** Sublingual salivary gland. Note the elevated tongue and the tissues sectioned in the highlighted area. (From Fehrenbach M, Herring S: *Illustrated anatomy of the head and neck,* ed 4, St. Louis, 2012, Saunders.)

trays or working in the mouth. It is extremely important to avoid stimulating the gag reflex.

Alveolar Process

The alveolar process is the extension of the bones that form the mandible and the maxilla. The teeth are firmly held in place within the bone of the alveolar process.

Cortical Plate

The cortical plate, also known as the *cribriform plate,* is the dense outer layer of bone covering the alveolar process that provides strength and protection. The cortical plate of the mandible is dense with few openings. The cortical plate of the maxilla is not as dense.

TABLE 3-9
Structures of the Hard and Soft Palates

Structure	Location
Hard palate	Bony anterior portion covered with masticatory mucosa
Palatine rugae	Irregular ridges or folds in the mucosa on the palate just behind the maxillary central incisors
Incisive papilla (a small or nipple-shaped pad of tissue)	Pear-shaped pad of tissue located directly behind the maxillary central incisors
Soft palate	Flexible posterior portion of the palate that can be lifted upward and backward to block the entrance to the throat during swallowing and speech The uvula hangs from the posterior soft palate.

The Alveolar Crest

The alveolar crest is the highest point of the alveolar ridge. In an unhealthy mouth, the alveolar crest can be destroyed.

Alveolar Socket

The alveolar socket is the space within the alveolar process in which the root of a tooth is held in place by the periodontal ligament (Figure 3-30).

Oral Mucosa

The entire mouth is lined with mucous membrane tissue (Figure 3-31). Two types of oral mucosa are known as:

- The **lining mucosa**, which covers the inside of the cheeks, vestibule, lips, ventral surface of the tongue, and soft palate, is delicate, thin, and easily injured.
- The masticatory mucosa, which covers the gingivae (gums), hard palate, and dorsum of the tongue, is firmly attached to the bone, is very dense, and designed to withstand the vigorous activity of chewing and swallowing food.

Gingivae

The gingivae are the tissues that surround the teeth (Table 3-10 and see Figure 3-27).

The gingiva (plural, *gingivae*), commonly referred to as the *gums,* is masticatory mucosa that covers the alveolar processes of the jaws and surrounds the necks of the teeth.

Epithelial Attachment

Healthy gingivae cover the alveolar bone and attach to the teeth on the enamel surface just above the neck of the tooth. This structure is known as the *epithelial attachment.*

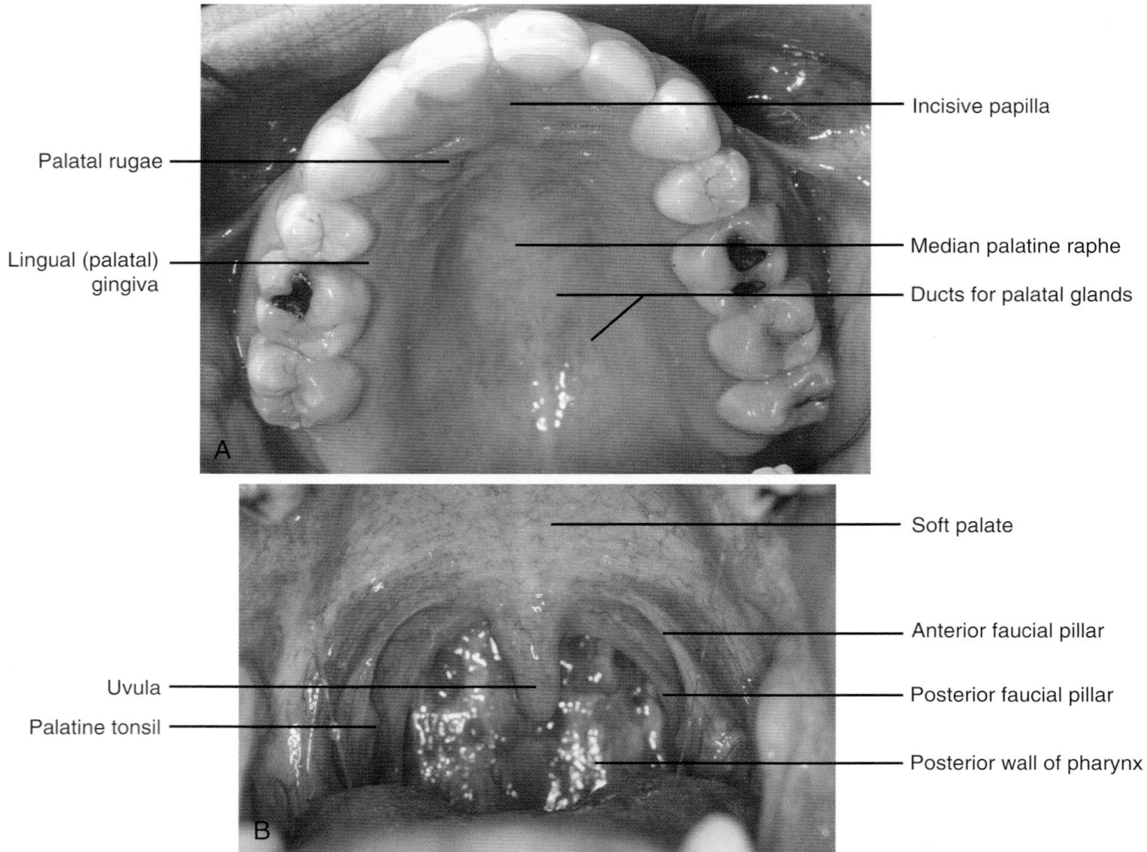

FIGURE 3-29 **A,** Surface features of the hard palate. **B,** Surface features of the soft palate. (From Liebgott B: *The anatomical basis of dentistry,* ed 3, St. Louis, 2010, Mosby.)

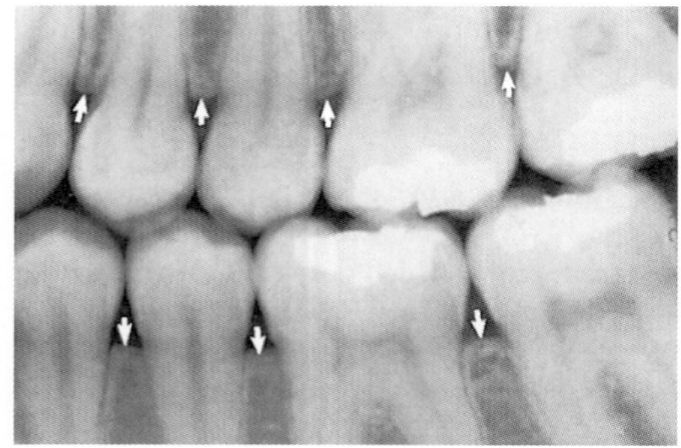

FIGURE 3-30 The alveolar crest *(arrows)* as it appears on a radiograph. (From Haring JI, Lind LJ: *Radiographic interpretation for the dental hygienist,* Philadelphia, 1993, Saunders.)

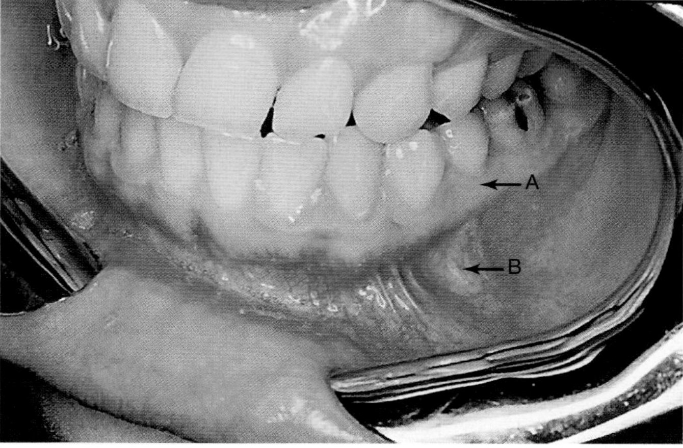

FIGURE 3-31 **A,** Dense masticatory mucosa makes up the gingiva. **B,** Delicate lining mucosa covers the vestibule.

Free Gingivae

The free gingivae are the parts of the gingiva that extend higher than the epithelial attachment. They are made up of tissue from the gingival margin to the base of the gingival sulcus and are normally light pink and coral in color in light-skinned people. The gingival sulcus is the space between the free gingivae and the tooth.

Teeth

The types of teeth, their structures, and their tissues are discussed in Chapter 4.

TABLE 3-10
Gingivae

Structure	Location
Epithelial attachment	The epithelial attachment is healthy gingiva that covers the alveolar bone and attaches to the teeth on the enamel surface just above the neck of the tooth.
Free gingiva	The free gingiva extends from the base of the gingival sulcus to the gingival margin. It is not attached to the surface of the tooth.
Gingival sulcus	The gingival sulcus is the space between the free gingiva and the tooth. A normal, healthy gingival sulcus is 3 mm or less in depth.
Gingival margin	The gingival margin is the upper edge of the gingiva. Its shape follows the curvatures of the cervical line of the tooth.
Free gingival groove	The free gingival groove is a shallow groove that extends from the base of the sulcus to the mucogingival junction. It is a stippled, dense tissue that is firmly bound to the underlying bone.
Attached gingivae	The attached gingivae extend from the base of the sulcus to the mucogingival junction.
Mucogingival junction	The mucogingival junction is the line that separates the attached gingivae from the alveolar mucosa.

Procedure 3-1

Identify the Major Landmarks and Structures of the Face

Goal

To identify the major landmarks and structures of the face correctly.

1. Ala of the nose.
2. Inner canthus and outer canthus of the eye.
3. Commissure of the lips.
4. Location of the frontal sinuses.
5. Location of the maxillary sinuses.
6. Location of the parotid glands.
7. Philtrum.
8. Tragus of the ear.
9. Vermilion border.
10. Zygomatic arch.

Procedure 3-2

Identify the Major Landmarks, Structures, and Normal Tissues of the Mouth

Goal

To identify and locate correctly the major landmarks, structures, and normal tissues of the mouth.

1. Locate the dorsum of the tongue.
2. Locate the area of the gag reflex.
3. Identify the hard and soft palates.
4. Identify the gingival margin.
5. Locate the incisive papilla.
6. Identify the mandibular labial frenum.
7. Identify the maxillary labial frenum.
8. Locate the sublingual frenum.
9. Identify the vestibule of the mouth.
10. Locate Wharton duct.

Chapter Exercises

Multiple Choice

Circle the letter next to the correct answer.

1. The simplest organizational level in the human body is the __________.

a. cell
b. organ
c. tissue
d. body system

2. The body system that causes muscles to contract and stimulates glands to secrete is the __________ system.

a. digestive
b. nervous
c. cardiovascular
d. endocrine

3. The thymus, spleen, and tonsils are components of the __________ system.

a. respiratory
b. muscular
c. lymphatic
d. nervous

4. The type of movements made by the TMJ is __________.

a. hinge
b. glide
c. hinge and glide

5. The nerve that supplies the maxillary first and second premolars and the mesiobuccal root of the maxillary first molar is the __________ nerve.

a. anterior superior alveolar
b. middle superior alveolar
c. posterior superior alveolar
d. buccal

6. The structures that carry blood back to the heart are the __________.

a. arteries
b. lymph nodes
c. veins
d. trigeminal nerve

7. The top of the tongue is called the __________ surface.

a. lateral
b. ventral
c. dorsal
d. facial

8. Which of the following is(are) functions of the salivary glands?

a. Provide lubrication.
b. Clean the oral cavity.
c. Aid in digestion.
d. All of the above are functions.

9. Which type of oral mucosa covers the inside of the cheeks, vestibules, lips, and ventral surface of the tongue?

a. Lining mucosa
b. Masticatory mucosa
c. Gingiva
d. Epithelial attachment

10. The __________ is the cavity within the alveolar process that holds the tooth.

a. alveolar crest
b. alveolar socket
c. cortical plate
d. periodontal ligament

Apply Your Knowledge

1. A patient comes into your office complaining that when he bit into a hot piece of pizza, he "burned the bump of skin in the front part" of the roof of his mouth. Which oral landmark was most likely injured?

2. The dentist asks you to place a cotton roll over the Stensen duct to help control the flow of saliva. Where would you place the cotton roll?

3. To perform a restorative procedure on the mandibular teeth, which nerve must be anesthetized?

4. When placing x-ray film in the maxillary posterior regions of the mouth, care must be taken to avoid stimulating a certain response from the patient. What is this involuntary response?

CHAPTER 4

Dental Anatomy

http://evolve.elsevier.com/Robinson/essentials/

LEARNING OBJECTIVES

1. Pronounce, define, and spell the key terms.
2. Discuss the anatomic parts of the tooth and explain the composition of each of the tissues of a tooth.
3. Complete the following related to describing the teeth and associated structures:
   - Identify the different types of teeth.
   - Discuss the two dental arches.
   - Describe the difference between anterior and posterior teeth.
   - Use the correct terminology when describing the teeth.
4. Identify the locations of all surfaces of the teeth, name the tooth surfaces, and describe the anatomic features of the teeth.
5. Complete the following related to dentition:
   - Identify the number of teeth in the primary dentition.
   - Discuss mixed dentition.
   - Identify the number of teeth in the permanent dentition.
6. Use the Universal National System, International Standards Organization System, or Palmer Notation System to designate and name the surfaces of each tooth, as well as identify the correct location of each permanent tooth.

KEY TERMS

anatomic crown
apex
apical
bifurcation
cementoenamel junction
cementum
clinical crown
contact point
cusp
dentin
dentinal fiber
dentinal tubules
embrasure
enamel
enamel prisms
exfoliation
Federation Dentaire Internationale (FDI) System
fossae
International Standards Organization (ISO) System
mixed dentition
numbering systems
Palmer Notation System
periapical
periodontal ligament
periodontium
permanent dentition
primary dentition
pulp
trifurcation
Universal National System

In this chapter, you will learn the anatomic parts of the tooth and the names and locations of the various types of teeth in the human dentition. You will also learn their functions and features. In preparation for learning dental charting, you will learn the common systems of tooth numbering.

Anatomic Parts of the Tooth

Each tooth consists of a crown and one or more roots. The size and shape of the crown and the size and number of roots vary according to the type of the tooth (Figure 4-1).

Crown

Anatomic Crown

The **anatomic crown** is the portion of the tooth covered with enamel (Figure 4-2). The size of the anatomic crown remains the same throughout the life of the tooth, regardless of the position of the gingiva (see Figure 4-2).

Clinical Crown

The **clinical crown** is the portion of the tooth that is visible in the mouth. The length of the clinical crown varies during the

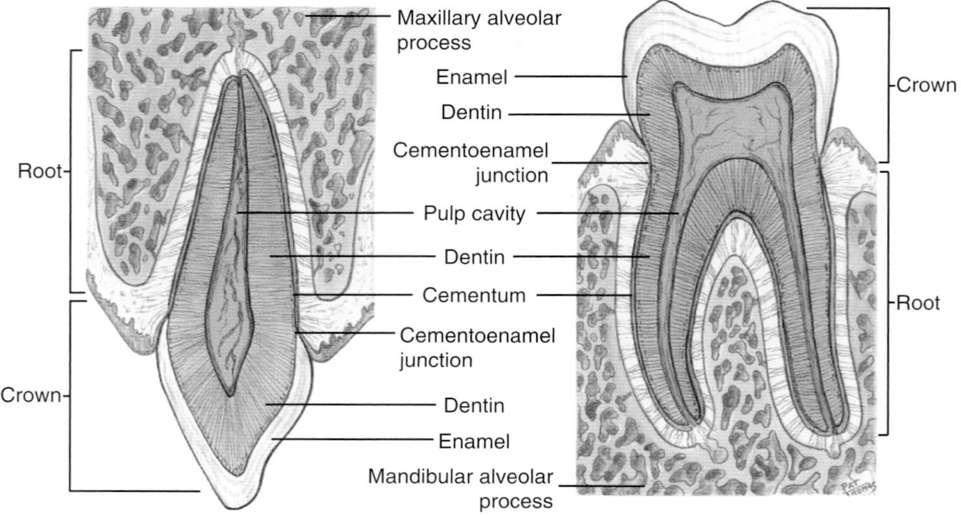

FIGURE 4-1 Tissues of the tooth and surrounding structures. (From Fehrenbach MJ, Herring SW: *Illustrated anatomy of the head and neck*, ed 4, St. Louis, 2012, Saunders.)

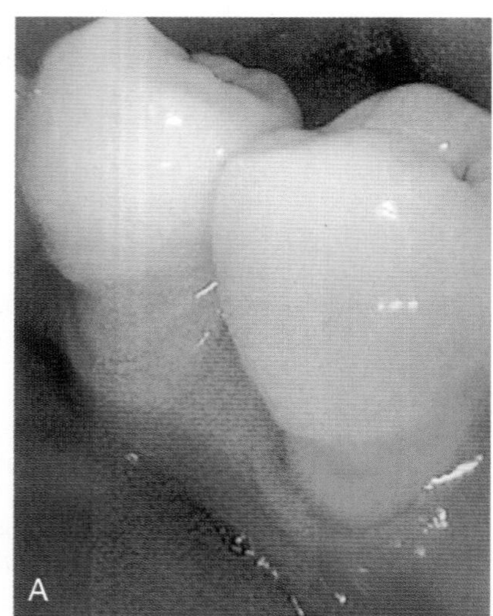

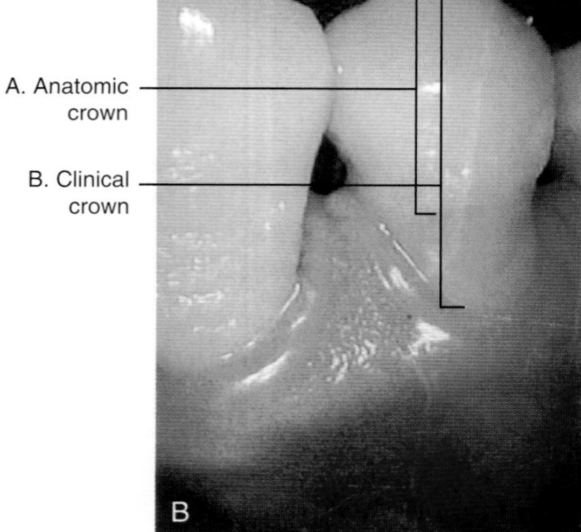

FIGURE 4-2 **A**, The anatomic crown, the portion of the tooth covered with enamel, remains the same. **B**, The clinical crown, the portion of the tooth visible in the mouth, may vary as changes occur in the position of the gingiva.

life cycle of the tooth, depending on the level of the gingiva. The clinical crown is shortest when the tooth erupts into position and becomes longer as the surrounding gingiva recedes.

Root

The root is the portion of the tooth that is normally embedded in the alveolar process and is covered with cementum.

Depending on the type of tooth, one, two, or three roots may be present. **Bifurcation** means division into two roots, and **trifurcation** means division into three roots.

The tapered end of each root tip is known as the **apex**. Anything that is located at the apex is referred to as **apical**, and anything surrounding the apex is said to be **periapical**.

Cervix

The cervix is the narrow area of the tooth where the crown and the root meet. (**Cervix** means *neck*.)

The **cementoenamel junction** is formed by the enamel of the crown and the cementum of the root. This area is also known as the *cervical line* or the *cementoenamel junction (CEJ)*.

Tissues of the Tooth

Enamel

Enamel, which makes up the anatomic crown of the tooth, is the hardest material of the body. This hardness is important because enamel forms the protective covering for the softer underlying dentin. It also provides a strong surface for tearing, crushing, grinding, and chewing food.

Enamel is translucent and ranges in color from yellow-white to gray-white. (*Translucent* means that the substance allows some light to pass through it.)

Enamel is similar to bone in its hardness and mineral content. Unlike bone, mature enamel does not contain cells that are capable of repairing themselves. However, some remineralization is possible (see Chapter 17). Enamel is composed of millions of calcified enamel prisms, which are also known as *enamel rods*. These extend from the surface of the tooth to the dentinoenamel junction.

The enamel prisms tend to be grouped into rows that follow a course that is approximately perpendicular to the surface of the tooth.

Dentin

Dentin makes up the primary portion of the tooth structure and extends almost the entire length of the tooth. It is covered by enamel on the crown and by cementum on the root.

In the primary teeth, dentin is very light yellow. In the permanent teeth, it is light yellow and somewhat transparent. The color of the dentin tends to darken as we age.

Structure of Dentin

Dentin is a mineralized tissue that is harder than bone and cementum but not as hard as enamel. Although hard, dentin is a very porous tissue made up of microscopic canals called dentinal tubules that extend from the exterior surface, where the dentin joins the enamel or cementum, to the interior surface, which forms the pulp chamber. If the dentin is not protected by enamel, then these tubules form a direct passage for invading bacteria into the pulp.

Each tubule contains a dentinal fiber that transmits pain into the pulp. Dentin is a very sensitive living tissue; therefore it must be protected against dehydration (excessive drying) and thermal shock (sudden temperature changes) during dental treatment.

Because dentin is capable of some repair, the dentist can use materials that will help encourage the repair process when placing a restoration.

Pulp

The inner aspect of the dentin forms the boundaries of the pulp chamber (Figure 4-3). Similar to the dentin surrounding it, the contours of the pulp chamber follow the contours of the exterior surface of the tooth.

At the time of eruption, the pulp chamber is large. However, because of the continuous deposition of dentin, it becomes smaller with age.

The portion of the pulp that lies within the crown portion of the tooth is called the *coronal pulp;* this includes the pulp horns, which are extensions of the pulp that project toward the cusp tips and incisal edges.

The other portion of the pulp is more apically located and is referred to as *radicular* or *root pulp.* The radicular pulp of each root is continuous with the tissues of the periapical area via an apical foramen.

In young teeth, the apical foramen is not yet fully formed, and this opening is wide. With increasing age, the pulp chamber becomes smaller.

Structure of the Pulp

The pulp is made up of blood vessels and nerves that enter the pulp chamber through the apical foramen. The blood supply is derived from branches of the dental arteries and from the periodontal ligament.

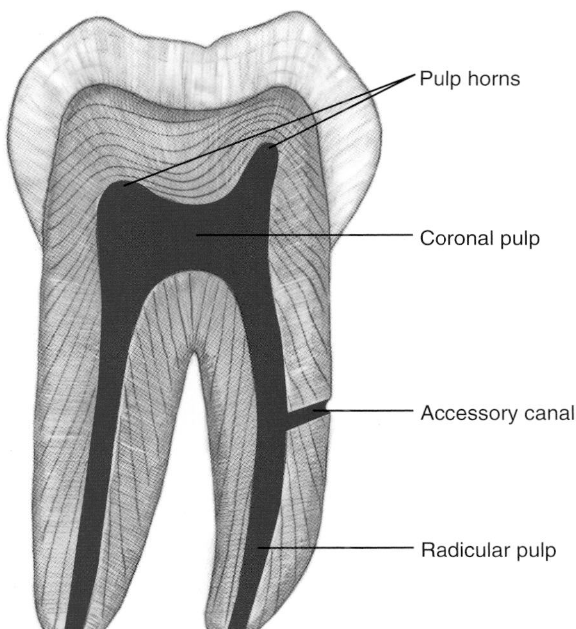

FIGURE 4-3 The dental pulp. (From Fehrenbach MJ, Popowics T: *Illustrated dental embryology, histology, and anatomy*, ed 4, St. Louis, 2016, Saunders.)

The nerves in the pulp receive and transmit pain stimuli. When the stimulus is weak, the response by the pulpal system is weak, and the interaction goes unnoticed. However, when the stimulus is great, the reaction is greater, and the patient feels pain.

Cementum

Cementum, which is not as hard as either enamel or dentin, protects the root of the tooth and joins the enamel at the CEJ. Cementum is of a light yellow shade that is somewhat lighter than the color of dentin and darker than enamel. Cementum also lacks the luster and translucent qualities of enamel.

Normally, cementum is covered by bone and gingival tissue. If it is exposed because of gingival recession and bone loss, then cementum is very sensitive and susceptible to decay.

Periodontium

The periodontium supports the teeth in the alveolar bone and consists of cementum, alveolar bone, and the periodontal ligaments. These tissues also protect and nourish the teeth.

Periodontal Ligament

The periodontal ligament is dense connective tissue organized into groups of fibers that connect the cementum covering the root of the tooth with the alveolar bone of the socket wall. At one end, the fibers are embedded in cementum; at the other end, they are embedded in bone. These embedded portions become mineralized and are known as *Sharpey fibers.* The periodontal ligament ranges in width from 0.1 to 0.38 mm, with the thinnest portion around the middle third of the root. As we age, a gradual progressive decrease in the width of these fibers occurs (Figure 4-4).

Types of Teeth

Humans eat a diet that includes meats, vegetables, grains, and fruit. To accommodate this variety in our diet, our teeth are designed for cutting, shearing or incising, tearing, and grinding different types of food (Table 4-1).

Dental Arches

Two dental arches—the maxillary and the mandibular—are found in the human mouth. The lay person may refer to the maxillary arch as the upper jaw and the mandibular arch as the lower jaw (Figure 4-5). The **mandibular arch** is capable of movement through the action of the temporomandibular joint. The **maxillary arch,** which is actually part of the skull, is fixed and not capable of movement (see Chapter 3).

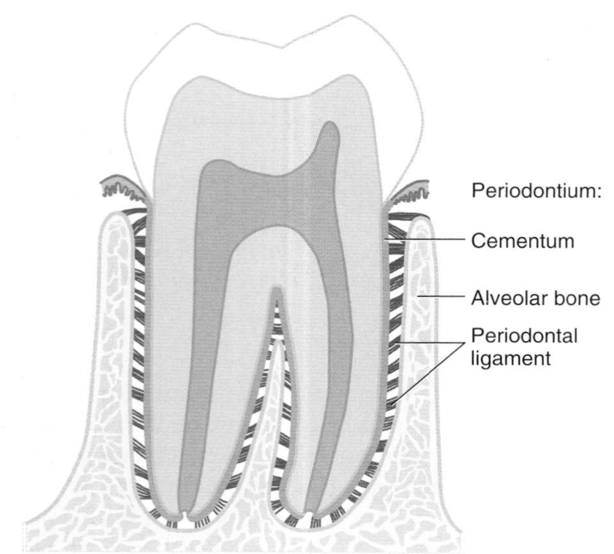

FIGURE 4-4 Periodontium of the tooth. (From Fehrenbach MJ, Popowics T: *Illustrated dental embryology, histology, and anatomy,* ed 4, St. Louis, 2016, Saunders.)

Quadrants and Sextants

An imaginary midline divides each dental arch into mirror halves. The two arches, each divided into halves, create four sections, which are called **quadrants** (Figure 4-6).

Quadrants

When the maxillary and mandibular arches are each divided into halves, the following four sections, called *quadrants*, result:

Maxillary right quadrant
Maxillary left quadrant
Mandibular left quadrant
Mandibular right quadrant

Each quadrant of permanent dentition contains eight permanent teeth ($4 \times 8 = 32$), and a quadrant of primary dentition contains five teeth ($4 \times 5 = 20$).

As the dental assistant looks into the patient's oral cavity, the directions are reversed. This concept is the same as it is when two people face each other and shake hands.

Sextants

Each arch can also be divided into sextants rather than quadrants. A sextant is one sixth of the dentition. There are three sextants in each arch. The dental arch is divided as follows (Figure 4-7):

1. Maxillary right posterior sextant
2. Maxillary anterior sextant
3. Maxillary left posterior sextant
4. Mandibular right posterior sextant
5. Mandibular anterior sextant
6. Mandibular left posterior sextant

TABLE 4-1
Types of Teeth

Types of Teeth	Characteristics	Functions
Incisors	Incisors are single-rooted teeth with a relatively sharp and thin edge; they are located at the front of the mouth.	Are designed to cut food without heavy force.
Canines	Also known as *cuspids,* canines are located at the "corner" of the dental arch. The crown is thick, with one well-developed pointed cusp. Because of their long root, canines are the most stable teeth in the mouth and are usually the last teeth to be lost.	Are designed for cutting and tearing of food that requires the application of force.
Premolars	Also known as *bicuspids,* premolars are similar to canines in that they have points and cusps but have a broader chewing surface. There are no premolars in the primary dentition.	Are designed for grasping and tearing; they also have a broad surface for chewing.
Molars	Molars have more cusps than the other teeth in the dentition. The shorter, blunter cusps provide a chewing surface.	Are designed for chewing and grinding solid masses of food that require the application of heavy forces.

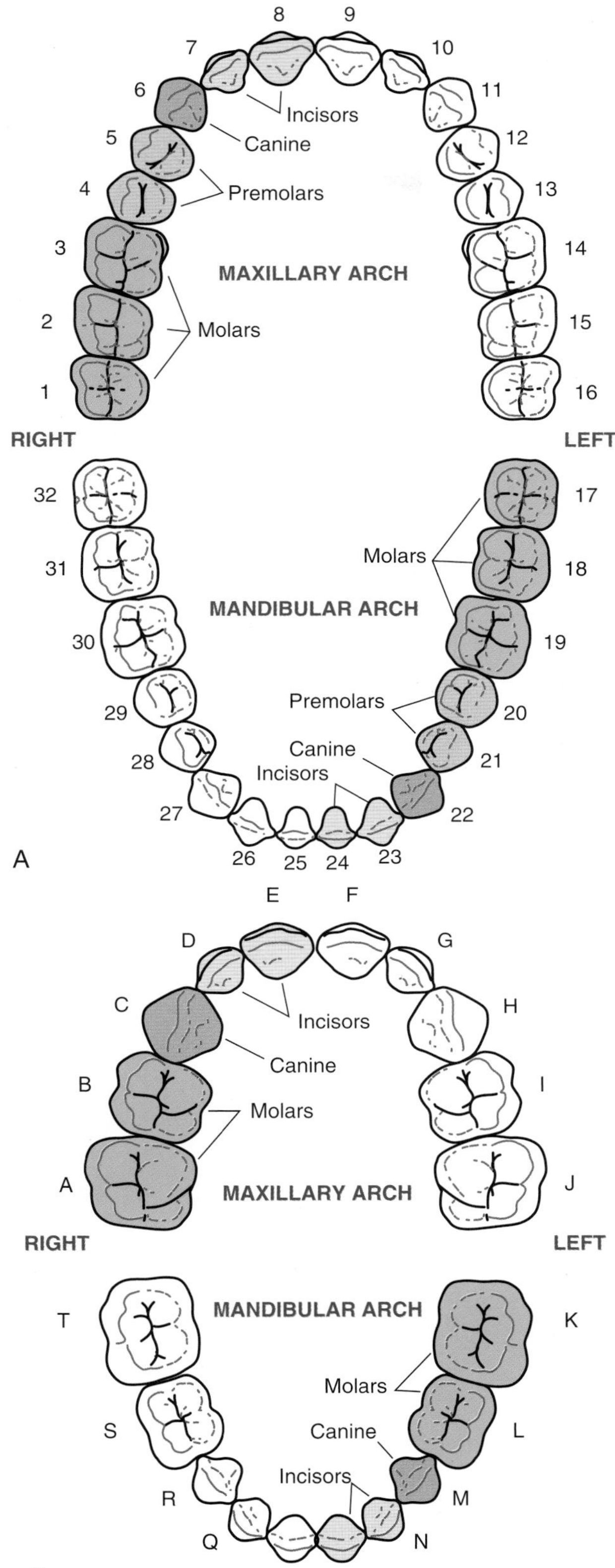

FIGURE 4-5 **A**, Occlusal view of the permanent dentition. The types of teeth are identified using the Universal National System. **B**, Occlusal view of the primary dentition. (From Fehrenbach MJ, Popowics T: *Illustrated dental embryology, histology, and anatomy*, ed 4, St. Louis, 2016, Saunders.)

TABLE 4-2
Surfaces of the Teeth

Name of Surface	Description
Facial surface	Is the surface closest to the face. The facial surfaces closest to the lips are also termed *labial surfaces.* The facial surfaces close to the inner cheek are also termed *buccal surfaces.*
Lingual surface	Is the surface closest to the tongue.
Masticatory surfaces	
Incisal surface or edge	Is the surface on the anterior teeth.
Occlusal surface	Is the surface on the posterior teeth.
Mesial surface	Is the surface closest to the midline.
Distal surface	Is the surface farthest away from the midline.
Palatal surface	Is the surface closest to the palate.

Anterior and Posterior Teeth

To assist in describing their locations and functions, the teeth are classified as being **anterior** (toward the front) or **posterior** (toward the back). In Figure 4-8, the anterior teeth are not shaded, and the posterior teeth are shaded.

The anterior teeth are the incisors and canines and are usually visible when people smile. The anterior teeth are aligned in a gentle curve. The posterior teeth are the premolars and molars and are aligned with little or no curvature; they appear to be in an almost straight line. Remembering how these teeth are aligned in the dental arch will be important when you begin exposing radiographs.

Tooth Surfaces

Each tooth has five surfaces: facial, lingual, masticatory, mesial, and distal. The surfaces and their subdivisions are described in Table 4-2.

See Procedure 4-1: Identify the Teeth and Name the Tooth Surfaces.

Anatomic Features of the Teeth

The anatomic features of the teeth—contours, contacts, and embrasures—help maintain the positions of the teeth in the dental arch and protect the tissues during chewing.

Contours

All teeth have a curved surface except when the tooth is fractured or worn. Some surfaces are convex (curved outward); others are concave (curved inward). Although the general contours vary, the general principle that the crown of the tooth narrows toward the cervical line is true for all types of teeth.

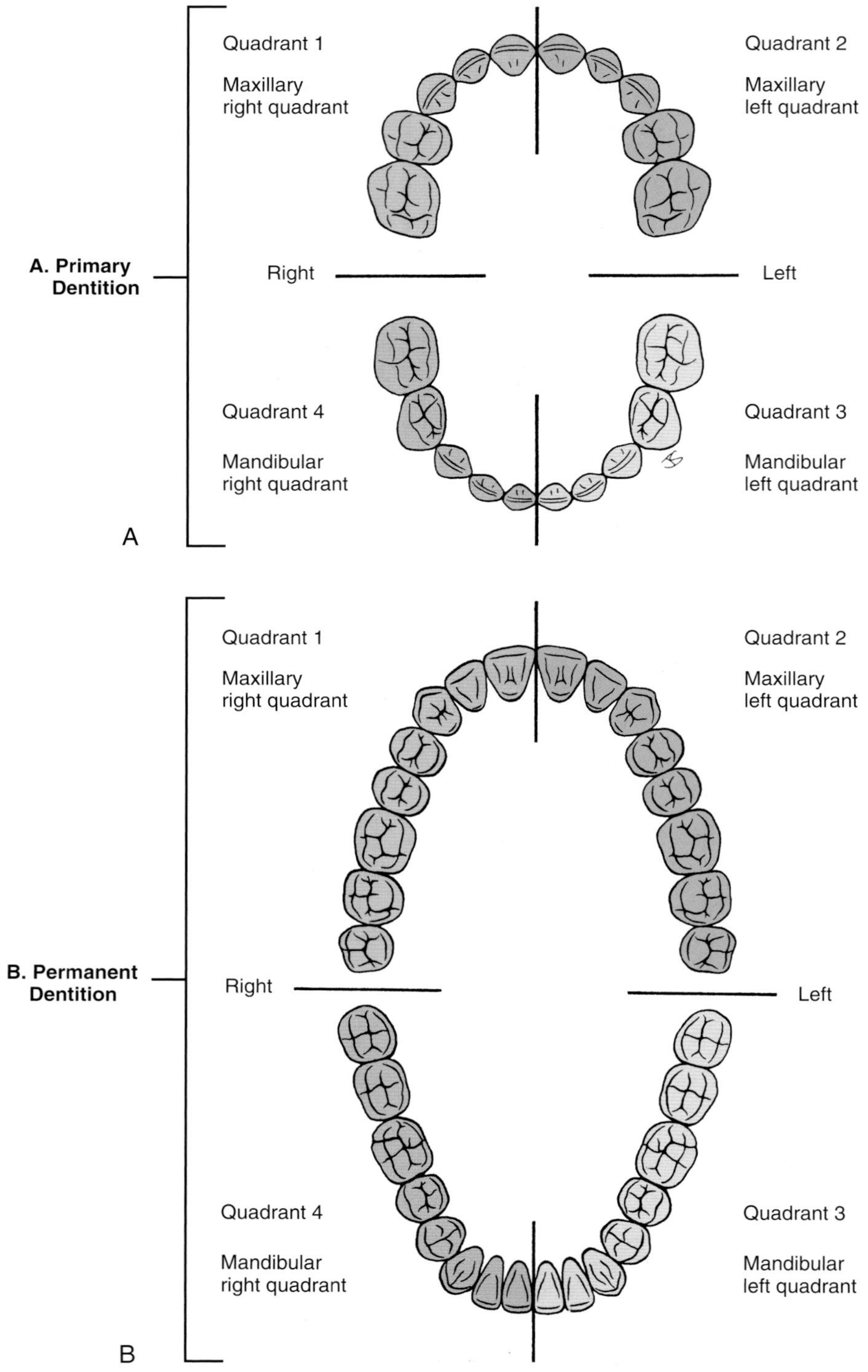

FIGURE 4-6 **A**, Primary dentition separated into quadrants. **B**, Permanent dentition separated into quadrants. (From Finkbeiner B, Johnson C: *Comprehensive dental assisting*, St. Louis, 1995, Mosby.)

Facial and Lingual Contours

The curvatures found on the facial and lingual surfaces provide natural passageways for food. This action protects the gingiva from the impact of foods during mastication. The normal contour of a tooth provides the gingiva with adequate stimulation for health and still protects it from being damaged by food (Figure 4-9, **A**).

When a tooth is restored, returning it to a normal contour is important. With inadequate contour, the gingiva may be traumatized by food pushing against it (Figure 4-9, **B**). With

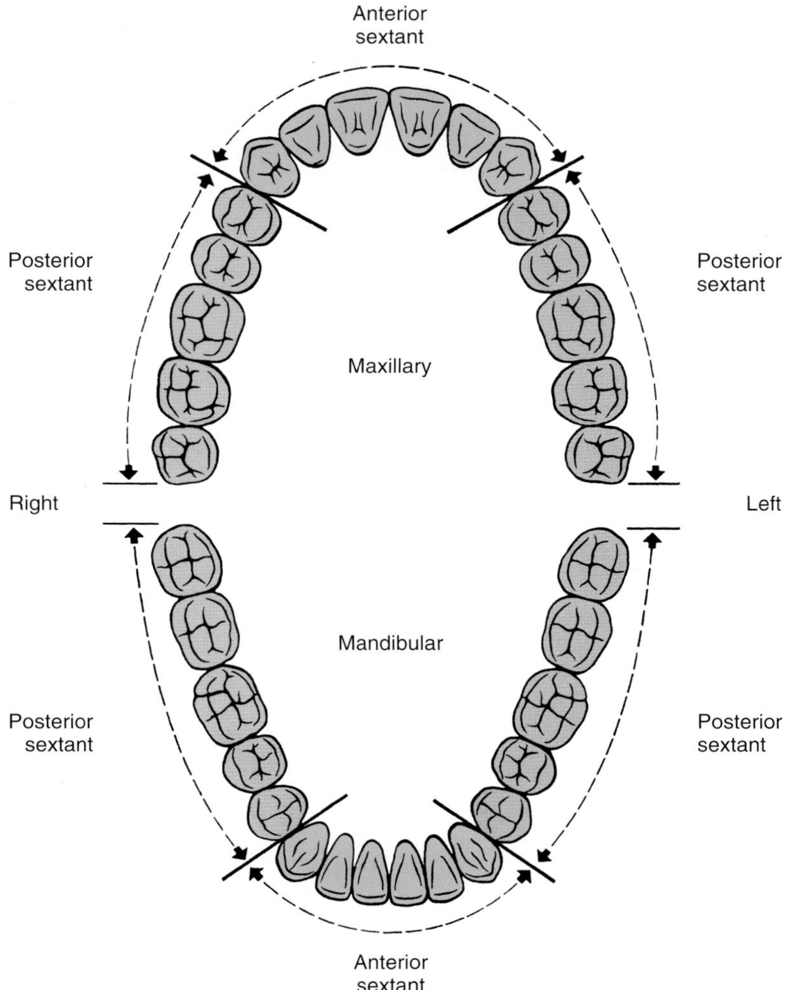

FIGURE 4-7 Permanent dentition separated into sextants. (From Finkbeiner B, Johnson C: *Comprehensive dental assisting*, St. Louis, 1995, Mosby.)

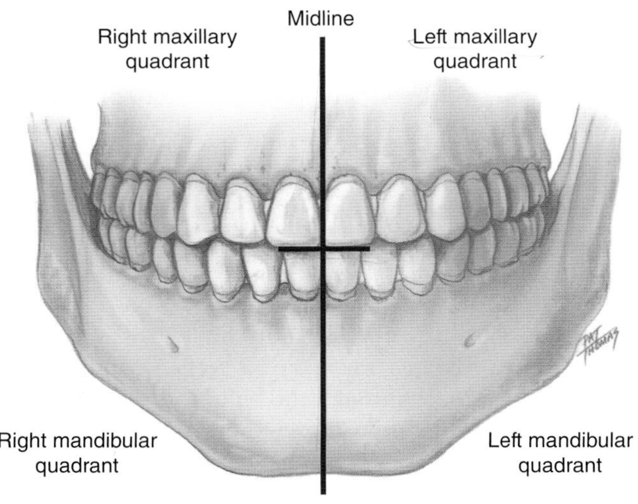

FIGURE 4-8 Oral cavity with the permanent teeth. The midline, quadrants, and anterior and posterior teeth are identified. (From Fehrenbach MJ, Popowics T: *Illustrated dental embryology, histology, and anatomy*, ed 4, St. Louis, 2016, Saunders.)

overcontouring, the gingiva will lack adequate stimulation and will be difficult to clean (Figure 4-9, **C**).

Contacts

The contact area of the mesial or distal surface of a tooth is the area that touches the adjacent tooth in the same arch. The **contact point** is the exact spot at which the teeth actually touch each other. The terms *contact* and *contact area* are frequently used interchangeably to refer to the contact point.

The crown of each tooth in the dental arches should be in contact with its adjacent tooth or teeth. A proper contact relationship between adjacent teeth serves the following three purposes:

1. Prevents food from being trapped between the teeth.
2. Stabilizes the dental arches by holding the teeth in either arch in positive contact with each other.
3. Protects the interproximal gingival tissue from trauma during mastication.

Embrasures

An **embrasure** is a triangular space near the gingiva between the proximal surfaces of two adjoining teeth. Embrasures are

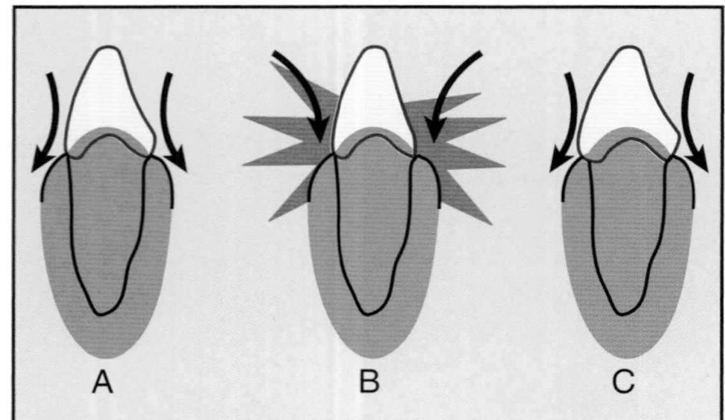

FIGURE 4-9 Tooth contours. **A**, Normal contour. **B**, Inadequate contour. **C**, Overcontouring.

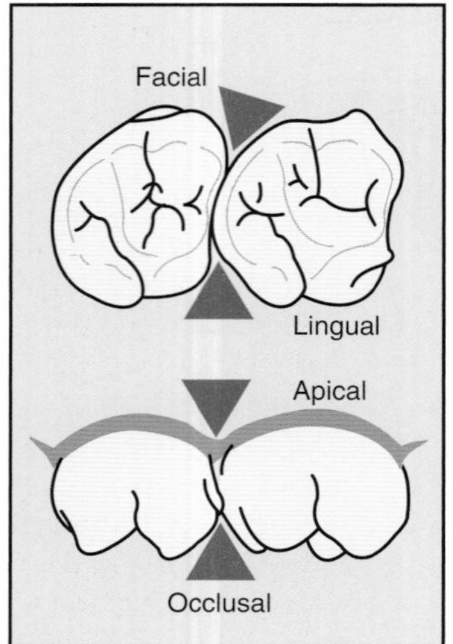

FIGURE 4-10 Embrasures may diverge facially, lingually, apically, or occlusally.

continuous with the interproximal spaces between the teeth. All tooth contours, including contact areas and embrasures, are important in the function and health of the oral tissue (Figure 4-10).

Occlusion

Occlusion is the contact between the maxillary and mandibular teeth in all mandibular positions and movements. The occlusal surfaces consist of cusps (raised areas) and fossae (indentations or grooves). The cusps of the teeth in one arch fit into the fossae of the teeth in the opposing arch, which produces a very effective grinding action for chewing food.

Dentition

The term *dentition* refers to the natural teeth in the dental arches. The term *edentulous* means without natural teeth and is used to describe the condition when the permanent teeth have been lost.

The normal human has two complete sets of teeth in a lifetime: primary dentition and permanent dentition. The transition from one dentition state to the other is known as the mixed dentition. During this period, both primary teeth and permanent teeth are in the mouth.

TABLE 4-3
Primary Dentition in Order of Eruption

Dentition	Date of Eruption (in months)	Date of Exfoliation (in years)
Maxillary Teeth		
Central incisor	6-10	6-7
Lateral incisor	9-12	7-8
First molar	12-18	9-11
Canine	16-22	10-12
Second molar	24-32	10-12
Mandibular Teeth		
Central incisor	6-10	6-7
Lateral incisor	7-10	7-8
First molar	12-18	9-11
Canine	16-22	9-12
Second molar	20-32	10-12

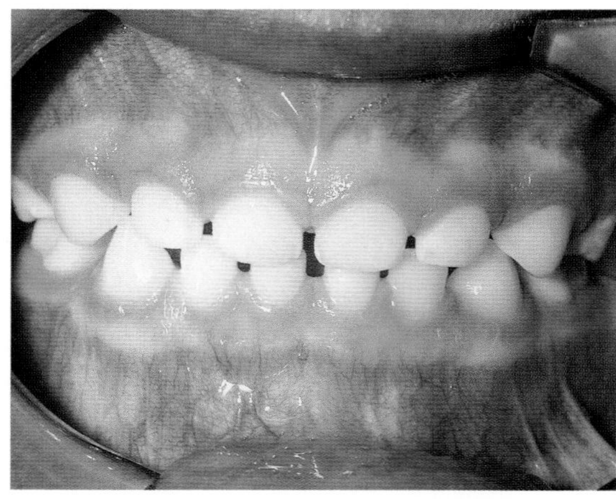

FIGURE 4-11 Facial and buccal view of a primary dentition.

Primary Dentition

All 20 teeth of the **primary dentition** should have erupted and be in place shortly after the age of 2 years. (**Eruption** is the movement of a tooth through the bone and gingival tissue.) Each quadrant of the primary dentition contains one central incisor, one lateral incisor, one canine, one first molar, and one second molar.

All of the primary teeth, also known as *deciduous teeth,* are exfoliated to make way for their replacements. (Exfoliation is the normal process by which primary teeth are shed.) During this process, the root of the primary teeth is **resorbed** (removed by a normal body process). Table 4-3 shows average ages at eruption and exfoliation of the primary dentition (Figure 4-11).

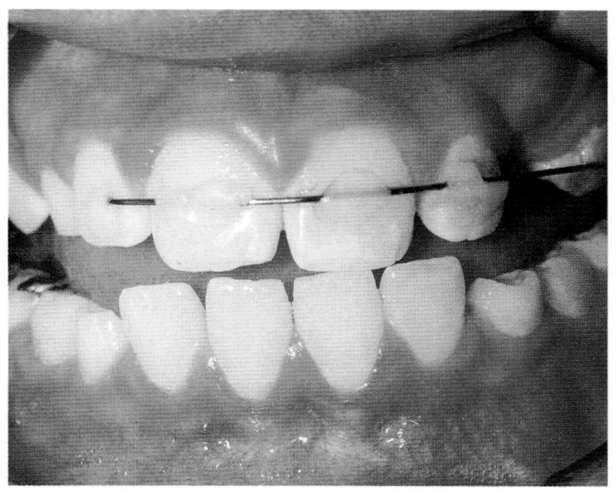

FIGURE 4-12 Facial and buccal view of a mixed dentition.

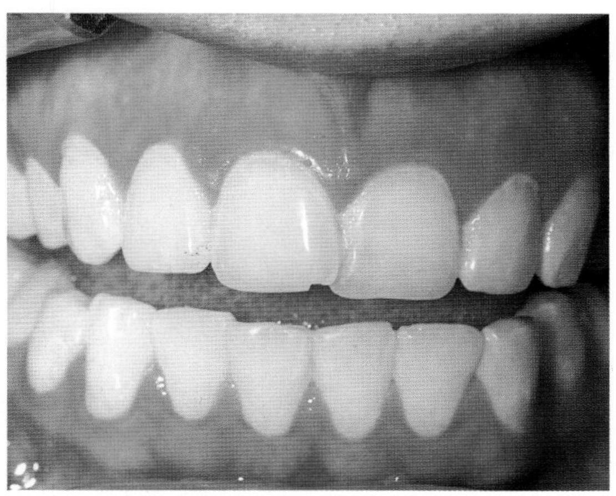

FIGURE 4-13 Facial and buccal view of a permanent dentition.

Mixed Dentition

When primary teeth no longer meet the needs of the growing child, they are lost and replaced by the permanent teeth, which are larger, stronger, and more numerous.

The exfoliation, or shedding process, of the primary teeth takes place between the ages of 5 and 12 years. During the time of this **mixed dentition**, the child has some permanent and some primary teeth (Figure 4-12).

Permanent Dentition

The **permanent dentition** period begins when the last primary tooth is shed, after approximately 12 years of age, and includes the eruption of all 32 of the permanent teeth (Figure 4-13). The jaws have nearly completed their growth when the stages of puberty pass.

Tooth Numbering Systems

Numbering systems are used as a simplified means of identifying the teeth for charting and descriptive purposes (Table 4-4).

See Procedure 4-2: Identify the Primary and Permanent Dentition Using the Universal National System, the Federation Dentaire Internationale System, and the Palmer Notation System.

Universal National System

The Universal National System, which is approved by the American Dental Association, is used throughout the United States. In the Universal National System, the permanent teeth are numbered from 1 to 32. Numbering begins with the upper-right third molar (tooth #1), works around to the upper-left third molar (tooth #16), drops to the lower-left third molar (tooth #17), and works around to the lower-right third molar (tooth #32) (see Figure 4-5, **A**).

TABLE 4-4
Tooth Designation Systems

Tooth Name	Universal National System	ISO/FDI System	Palmer Notation System
Permanent Dentition			
Maxillary Teeth			
Right third molar	1	18	8
Right second molar	2	17	7
Right first molar	3	16	6
Right second premolar	4	15	5
Right first premolar	5	14	4
Right canine	6	13	3
Right lateral incisor	7	12	2
Right central incisor	8	11	1
Left central incisor	9	21	1
Left lateral incisor	10	22	2
Left canine	11	23	3

Continued

TABLE 4-4
Tooth Designation Systems—cont'd

Tooth Name	Universal National System	ISO/FDI System	Palmer Notation System
Left first premolar	12	24	4
Left second premolar	13	25	5
Left first molar	14	26	6
Left second molar	15	27	7
Left third molar	16	28	8
Mandibular Teeth			
Left third molar	17	38	8
Left second molar	18	37	7
Left first molar	19	36	6
Left second premolar	20	35	5
Left first premolar	21	34	4
Left canine	22	33	3
Left lateral incisor	23	32	2
Left central incisor	24	31	1
Right central incisor	25	41	1
Right lateral incisor	26	42	2
Right canine	27	43	3
Right first premolar	28	44	4
Right second premolar	29	45	5
Right first molar	30	46	6
Right second molar	31	47	7
Right third molar	32	48	8
Primary Dentition			
Maxillary Teeth			
Right second molar	A	55	E
Right first molar	B	54	D
Right canine	C	53	C
Right lateral incisor	D	52	B
Right central incisor	E	51	A
Left central incisor	F	61	A
Left lateral incisor	G	62	B
Left canine	H	63	C
Left first molar	I	64	D
Left second molar	J	65	E
Mandibular Teeth			
Left second molar	K	75	E
Left first molar	L	74	D
Left canine	M	73	C
Left lateral incisor	N	72	B
Left central incisor	O	71	A
Right central incisor	P	81	A
Right lateral incisor	Q	82	B
Right canine	R	83	C
Right first molar	S	84	D
Right second molar	T	85	E

FDI, Federation Dentaire Internationale; *ISO,* International Standards Organization.
From Bath-Balogh M, Fehrenbach MJ: *Illustrated dental embryology, histology, and anatomy,* ed 2, St. Louis, 2005, Saunders.

The primary teeth are lettered with capital letters from A to T. Lettering begins with the upper-right second primary molar (tooth A), works around to the upper-left second primary molar (tooth J), drops to the lower-left second primary molar (tooth K), and works around to the lower-right second primary molar (tooth T; see Figure 4-5, **B**).

International Standards Organization System

The **International Standards Organization (ISO) System** is based on the **Federation Dentaire Internationale (FDI) System** and is used in most other countries.

The ISO/FDI System uses a two-digit, tooth-recording system. The first digit indicates the quadrant, and the second digit indicates the tooth within the quadrant, with numbering from the midline toward the posterior. The permanent teeth are numbered as follows:

1. Maxillary right quadrant is digit 1 and contains teeth #11 to #18.
2. Maxillary left quadrant is digit 2 and contains teeth #21 to #28.
3. Mandibular left quadrant is digit 3 and contains teeth #31 to #38.
4. Mandibular right quadrant is digit 4 and contains teeth #41 to #48.

The primary teeth are numbered as follows:

1. Maxillary right quadrant is digit 5 and contains teeth #51 to #55.
2. Maxillary left quadrant is digit 6 and contains teeth #61 to #65.
3. Mandibular left quadrant is digit 7 and contains teeth #71 to #75.
4. Mandibular right quadrant is digit 8 and contains teeth #81 to #85.

The digits should be separately pronounced. For example, the permanent canines are teeth #1-3 ("number one-three"), #2-3 ("number two-three"), #3-3 ("number three-three"), and #4-3 ("number four-three").

To avoid miscommunication internationally, the ISO/FDI System also provides designation of areas in the oral cavity (see Table 4-4). A two-digit number designates these, and at least one of the two digits is zero (0). In this system, for example, 00 ("zero-zero") designates the whole oral cavity, and 01 ("zero-one") indicates the maxillary area only.

Palmer Notation System

In the **Palmer Notation System**, each of the four quadrants is given its own tooth bracket made up of a vertical line and a horizontal line (Figure 4-14). The Palmer method is a shorthand diagram of the teeth as if the patient's teeth are viewed from the outside. The teeth in the right quadrant would have the vertical midline bracket to the right of the tooth numbers or letters, as when looking at the patient. The midline is to the right of the teeth in the right quadrant.

For example, if the tooth is a maxillary tooth, the number or letter should be written above the horizontal line of the bracket, thus indicating an upper tooth. Conversely, a mandibular tooth symbol should be placed below the line, indicating a lower tooth.

The number or letter assigned to each tooth depends on its position relative to the midline. For example, central incisors, the teeth closest to the midline, have the lowest number 1 for permanent teeth and the letter A for primary teeth. All central incisors, maxillary and mandibular, are given the number 1. All lateral incisors are given the number 2, canines are given the number 3, premolars are numbers 4 and 5, molars are 6 and 7, and third molars are number 8.

The Palmer Notation System for Permanent Teeth

Maxillary Right	Maxillary Left
8 7 6 5 4 3 2 1	1 2 3 4 5 6 7 8
8 7 6 5 4 3 2 1	1 2 3 4 5 6 7 8
Mandibular Right	Mandibular Left

Tooth Numbers	
Central incisors	#1
Lateral incisors	#2
Canines	#3
1st premolar	#4
2nd premolar	#5
1st molar	#6
2nd molar	#7
3rd molar	#8

Examples of Charting

- 1 Maxillary right central incisor
- 2 Mandibular right lateral incisor
- 4 Maxillary left first premolar
- 8 Mandibular left third molar

The Palmer Notation System for Primary Teeth

Maxillary Right	Maxillary Left
E D C B A	A B C D E
E D C B A	A B C D E
Mandibular Right	Mandibular Left

Examples of Charting

- A Maxillary right central incisor
- B Mandibular right lateral incisor
- C Maxillary left canine
- D Mandibular left first primary molar

Tooth Letters	
Central incisors	A
Lateral incisors	B
Canines	C
1st primary molar	D
2nd primary molar	E

FIGURE 4-14 Palmer Notation System.

Tooth Diagrams

The diagrams used for dental charting have the teeth in the right quadrants arranged on the left side of the page and the teeth in the left quadrants arranged on the right side of the page. The purpose of this layout is to simulate looking into the patient's mouth. The skills you have learned in this chapter will be used when you study dental charting in detail in Chapter 12.

Ethical Implications

Your understanding of dental terminology and dental anatomy is fundamental to a variety of clinical procedures you will be performing every day in the dental setting. In addition, your ability to use the proper terminology when communicating with patients and other dental professionals demonstrates your level of training and education and enhances your image as a dental professional.

Procedure 4-1

Identify the Teeth and Name the Tooth Surfaces

Goal

To identify the teeth and name the tooth surfaces correctly.

Equipment and Supplies

- Study model or typodont

Procedural Steps

Identify each of the following:

1. Maxillary central incisors
2. Mandibular central incisors
3. Maxillary lateral incisors
4. Mandibular lateral incisors
5. Maxillary canines
6. Mandibular canines
7. Maxillary premolars
8. Mandibular premolars
9. Maxillary molars
10. Mandibular molars
11. Occlusal surfaces
12. Incisal surfaces
13. Lingual surfaces
14. Facial surfaces
15. Mesial surface of the maxillary central incisors
16. Distal surface of the mandibular central incisors

Procedure 4-2

Identify the Primary and Permanent Dentitions Using the Universal National System, the Federation Dentaire Internationale System, and the Palmer Notation System

Goal

To identify the teeth correctly using each numbering system.

Equipment and Supplies

- Study model or typodont
- Worksheet from student workbook or Evolve (or create your own worksheet by dividing a piece of paper into three columns labeled with the three numbering systems and a row to fill in the name of each tooth)

Procedural Steps

Identify each of the following:

1. Primary teeth in each arch using the Universal National System.
2. Primary teeth in each arch using the Federation Dentaire Internationale System.
3. Primary teeth in each arch using the Palmer Notation System.
4. Permanent teeth in each arch using the Universal National System.
5. Permanent teeth in each arch using the Federation Dentaire Internationale System.
6. Permanent teeth in each arch using the Palmer Notation System.

Chapter Exercises

Multiple Choice

Circle the letter next to the correct answer.

1. The chewing surfaces of the posterior teeth are called __________ surfaces.
   - **a.** incisal
   - **b.** lingual
   - **c.** buccal
   - **d.** occlusal
2. How many teeth are included in the permanent dentition?
   - **a.** 28
   - **b.** 32
   - **c.** 16
   - **d.** 20
3. In the Universal National System, tooth #9 is the __________.
   - **a.** maxillary left central incisor
   - **b.** maxillary right central incisor
   - **c.** mandibular left central incisor
   - **d.** mandibular right central incisor
4. In the FDI System, tooth #11 is the __________.
   - **a.** maxillary right third molar
   - **b.** maxillary right central incisor
   - **c.** maxillary left central incisor
   - **d.** maxillary left canine
5. The surfaces of the teeth that are nearest to the tongue are the __________ surfaces.
   - **a.** buccal
   - **b.** lingual
   - **c.** occlusal
   - **d.** incisal
6. *Occlusion* refers to the __________.
   - **a.** contact area on the proximal surfaces of the teeth
   - **b.** contact area between the maxillary and mandibular arches
   - **c.** space between the proximal surfaces of the teeth
   - **d.** contact area of the teeth
7. When the arches are divided into six parts, each part is called a(n) __________.
   - **a.** quadrant
   - **b.** sextant
   - **c.** arch
   - **d.** embrasure
8. The primary dentition contains four premolars.
   - **a.** True
   - **b.** False
9. The teeth that are sometimes called the "corner" of the arch are the __________.
   - **a.** lateral incisors
   - **b.** premolars
   - **c.** canines
   - **d.** first permanent molars
10. The proximal surface that is located farthest away from the midline is the __________ surface.
    - **a.** distal
    - **b.** mesial
    - **c.** facial
    - **d.** lingual

Apply Your Knowledge

1. Provide the professional terminology for each of the following lay terms: front tooth, back tooth, top teeth, bottom teeth, and chewing surfaces.
2. If the dentist asked you to take a radiograph of tooth #19, in what area would you place the film?
3. The parent of a 3-year-old asks you to tell her about the process of her daughter losing her "baby" teeth and wants to know when she will get her permanent teeth. How would you reply?

PART THREE Infection Prevention and Hazardous Materials

CHAPTER 5

Disease Transmission

http://evolve.elsevier.com/Robinson/essentials/

LEARNING OBJECTIVES

1. Pronounce, define, and spell the key terms.
2. Compare and contrast the types of pathogens, as well as provide examples of each.
3. Explain the concept of the chain of infection.
4. Explain the differences among acute, chronic, latent, and opportunistic infections.
5. Identify the various modes in which disease transmission can occur in the dental office setting.
6. Name and describe the viral diseases that are of major concern to dental health care professionals.
7. Name and describe the bacterial diseases that are of major concern to dental health care professionals.

KEY TERMS

acute infection
aerosols
bacteria
bacterial endocarditis
bloodborne diseases
chronic infection
cross-contamination
direct transmission
fungi
hepatitis A
hepatitis B
hepatitis C
hepatitis D
HIV
host
host susceptibility
indirect transmission
infectious disease
latent infection
mists
opportunistic infection
parenteral transmission
pathogen
portal of entry
spores
tuberculosis
virulence
viruses

The dental assistant is at risk of exposure to infectious diseases through occupational exposure. In this chapter, you will learn about the organisms that cause infectious diseases and how to recognize the diseases that are of particular concern to dental professionals. You will learn how these diseases can spread in the dental office and the steps you can take to protect yourself, other staff members, and patients from disease transmission in the dental office.

Pathogens

A **pathogen** is a microorganism that is capable of causing disease. These microorganisms are so small that they can be seen only under a microscope.

Bacteria

Bacteria (singular bacterium) are a large group of one-celled microorganisms that vary in size, shape, and arrangement of cells. Most bacteria are capable of living independently under favorable environmental conditions. Pathogenic bacteria usually grow best at 98.6° F (37° C) in a moist, dark environment.

A bacterial infection can be spread by many means of transmission. Humans **host** a variety of bacteria at all times. The skin, respiratory tract, and gastrointestinal tract are inhabited by a great variety of harmless bacteria, called normal flora. They are beneficial and protect the human host by aiding in metabolism and preventing entrance of harmful bacteria. An infection occurs when bacteria occurring naturally in one

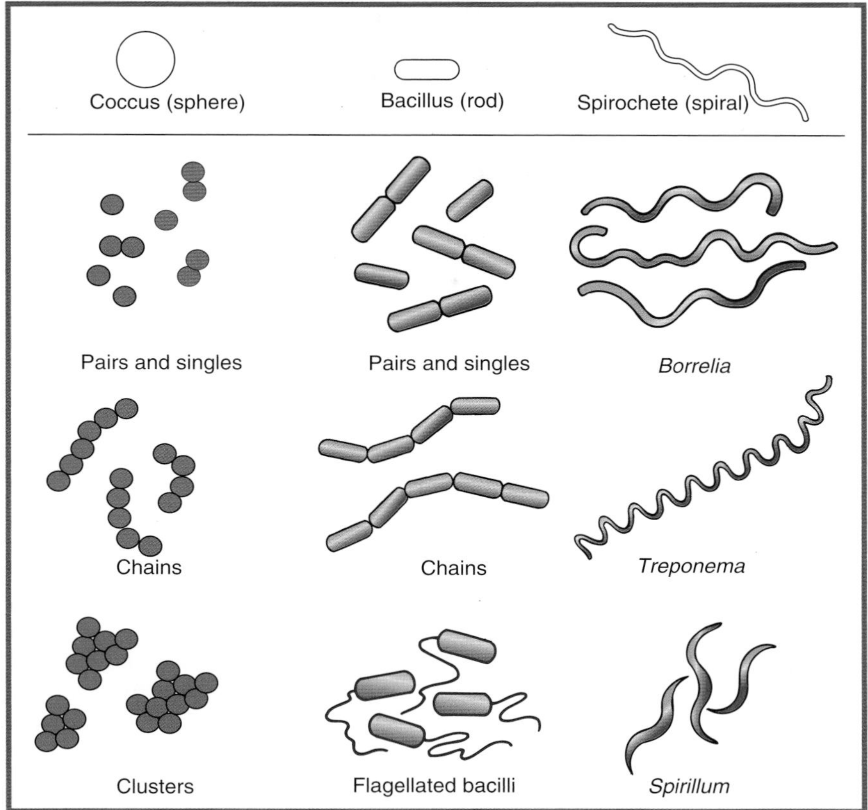

FIGURE 5-1 Three basic shapes of bacteria.

TABLE 5-1
Shapes of Bacteria and Diseases in Which They Occur

Shape	Name	Disease
Spherical	Streptococci	"Strep" throat, pneumonia, tonsillitis
	Staphylococci	Boils, skin infections, pneumonia
Rod-shaped	Bacilli	Tuberculosis
Spiral-shaped	Spirochetes	Syphilis, Lyme disease

part of the body invade another part of the body and become harmful. Most bacterial infections are treated with antibiotic medications.

When viewed under a microscope, bacteria have three shapes: spherical, rod shaped, and spiral (Figure 5-1 and Table 5-1).

Spores

Under unfavorable conditions, some bacteria change into a highly resistant form called **spores**. Tetanus is an example of a disease caused by a spore-forming bacillus.

Bacteria remain alive in the spore form but are inactive. In the spore state, they cannot reproduce or cause disease. When conditions are again favorable, the bacteria become active and are capable of causing disease.

Spores represent the most resistant form of life known. They can survive extremes of heat and dryness, as well as the presence of disinfectants and radiation. Because of this incredible resistance, harmless spores are used to test the effectiveness of techniques designed to sterilize dental instruments (see Chapter 8).

Viruses

Viruses are significantly smaller than bacteria. Despite their tiny size, many viruses cause fatal diseases. New and increasingly destructive viruses are being discovered and have resulted in the creation of a special area within microbiology called *virology* (the study of viruses and their effects).

Viruses can live and multiply only inside an appropriate host cell. Host cells may be human, animal, plant, or bacteria.

A virus invades a host cell, replicates (produces copies of itself), and then destroys the host cell, releasing the viruses into the body. The various forms of viral hepatitis and the human immunodeficiency virus (**HIV**) are discussed in greater detail later in this chapter.

Latency

Some viruses establish a latent (dormant) state in host cells. A latent virus can be reactivated in the future and can produce more infective viral particles, followed by signs and symptoms of the disease.

Stress, infection with another virus, and exposure to ultraviolet light can reactivate a virus. Some patients with the HIV infection have experienced prolonged periods of latency and have remained in good health for many years. For example, hepatitis C is known to have a latency period of 15 to 25 years.

Treatment of Viral Diseases

Viruses cause many clinically significant diseases in humans. Unfortunately, most viral diseases can only be symptomatically treated, that is, by treating the symptom, not the infective cause.

General antibiotic medications are ineffective in preventing or curtailing viral infections. Even the few drugs that are effective against specific viruses have limitations because viruses often produce different types of infection, have different host cells, or can cause serious side effects.

Viruses are also capable of mutation (changing). Viruses can change to become better suited to survive current conditions and to resist efforts to kill them. Developing vaccines against viruses is very difficult because of their ability to change their genetic code.

Fungi

Fungi are plants such as mushrooms, yeasts, and molds that lack chlorophyll. (Chlorophyll is the substance that makes plants green.) Athlete's foot, ringworm (which is not a worm), and candidiasis are examples of diseases caused by fungi.

Oral candidiasis is caused by the yeast *Candida albicans.* All forms of candidiasis are considered to be opportunistic infections, especially affecting the very young, very old, and patients who are very ill. Infants and patients who are terminally ill are also at risk. Candidiasis is common under the dentures in patients with HIV infection.

Oral candidiasis is characterized by white membranes on the surface of the oral mucosa, on the tongue, and elsewhere in the oral cavity. The lesions may resemble thin cottage cheese; wiping reveals a raw, red, and sometimes bleeding base (Figure 5-2). Candidiasis is treated with topical antifungal preparations such as nystatin in the form of lozenges.

Chain of Infection

To understand how infections can occur, imagine a chain that has six links. Each link is a condition that *must be present* before infection or disease can occur. Infection control practices are designed to break one or more of the links. The links in the chain of infection include: (1) infectious agent, (2) reservoir, (3) portal of exit (4) method of transmission, (5) portal of entry, and (6) susceptible host (Figure 5-3).

An **infectious agent** is a pathogen (e.g., bacterium, virus, fungus) and must be present in sufficient numbers to cause infection. In addition to the numbers, the organism must be **virulent**. Virulence means the degree, or the strength, of an organism's ability to cause disease. If an organism is not very virulent, then it may not be capable of causing disease.

Reservoir is a place where the organisms normally live and reproduce. Examples of reservoirs include humans, animals, water, food, contaminated surfaces, and bioburden. *Bioburden* refers to organic materials such as blood and saliva. Handwashing and cleaning contaminated surfaces will minimize reservoirs for microorganisms.

Portal of exit refers to the method the pathogen uses to leave the reservoir. It could be from contaminated hands, surfaces or instruments, or body fluids such as a sneeze.

Transmission is the mechanism the pathogen uses to spread from one host to another.

Portal of entry refers to the method by which the pathogen enters the body. The portals of entry for airborne pathogens are through the mouth and nose. Bloodborne pathogens must have access to the blood supply as a means of entry into the body. The portal of entry into the blood supply can occur through a break in the skin caused by a needlestick, a cut, or even a human bite. It can also occur through the mucous membranes of the nose and oral cavity (Table 5-2).

Host susceptibility is the ability of the human body (host) to resist a pathogen. The healthier you are, the better your resistance to disease. Low resistance can result from fatigue, physical or emotional strain, poor nutrition, injury, surgery, or the presence of other diseases.

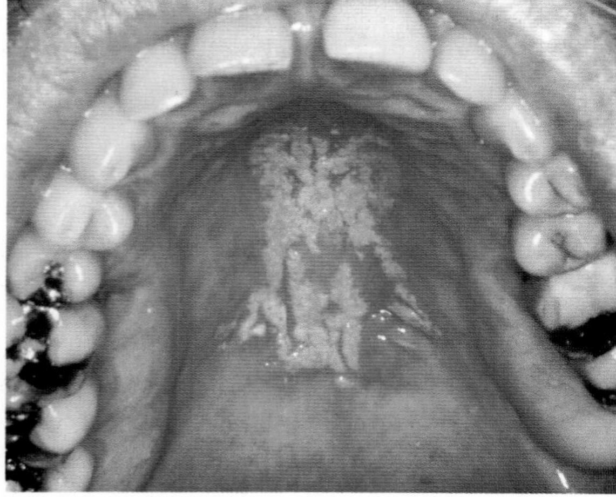

FIGURE 5-2 Pseudomembranous candidiasis. (From Ibsen OAC, Phelan JA: *Oral pathology for the dental hygienist*, ed 6, St. Louis, 2014, Saunders.)

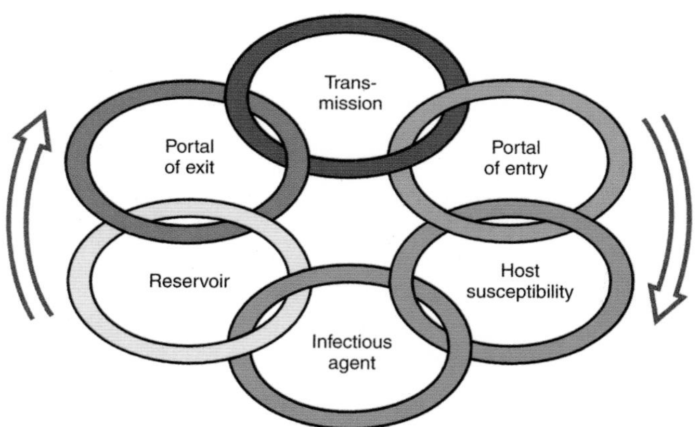

FIGURE 5-3 At least one link must be removed to break the chain of infection. (From Potter PA, Perry AG, Stockert P, et al: *Mosby's basic nursing*, ed 7, St. Louis, 2013, Mosby.)

TABLE 5-2
Portals of Entry for Disease Transmission

Portal	Examples	Means of Prevention
Inhalation	Breathing aerosols generated from handpieces or the air-water syringe or from uncovered ultrasonic cleaning devices	Wear face masks during chairside procedures and when processing contaminated instruments and surfaces. Note: Face shields protect against splatter but not against inhalation.
Ingestion	Swallowing droplets of blood or saliva spattered into the mouth Bare hands coming into contact with contaminated surfaces or items and the hands then handling food items	Wear face masks, frequently wash hands, and keep surfaces free from contamination by using barriers or surface disinfectants.
Mucous membrane	Droplets of blood or saliva spattering into the eyes, nose, or mouth	Wear face masks and safety glasses with side and bottom shields during chairside procedures and when processing contaminated instruments and surfaces.
Breaks in skin	Cuts or sticks from contaminated sharps Instrument punctures Cuts or cracks on ungloved hands or torn gloves	Develop and practice safe work habits. Replace torn or punctured gloves as soon as possible. Protect hands from becoming chapped or cracked.

BOX 5-1 Factors Affecting Resistance to Infection

- Patient's immune status
- Patient's age
- Patient's nutritional status
- Medications
- Allergies
- Alcohol consumption
- Psychologic condition

Infection control efforts are aimed at preventing the transmission of disease and reducing the number of pathogens that are present (Box 5-1).

Numbers refers to the concentration of pathogens that are present. The more pathogens that are present, the better their chances of overwhelming the host and producing disease.

Types of Infections

An infection occurs when a pathogenic microbe is able to multiply in the tissue within which it is lodged. An **infectious disease** is one that is communicable or contagious. This term means that the disease can be transmitted (spread) in some way from one host to another.

Acute Infection

In an **acute infection**, symptoms are often severe and usually appear soon after the initial infection occurs. Acute infections are short in duration. For example, with a viral infection, such as the common cold, the body's defense mechanisms usually eliminate the virus within 2 to 3 weeks.

Chronic Infection

A **chronic infection** is one during which the microorganism is present for a long duration; in some chronic infections, microorganisms may persist for life. The person may be asymptomatic (not showing symptoms of the disease) but may still be a carrier of the disease, as with hepatitis B virus (HBV), hepatitis C virus (HCV), or HIV infection.

Latent Infection

A **latent infection** is a persistent infection during which the symptoms "come and go." Cold sores (oral herpes simplex) and genital herpes are latent viral infections.

The virus first enters the body and causes the original lesion. It then lies dormant away from the surface in a nerve cell until certain conditions, such as illness with fever, sunburn, or stress, cause the virus to leave the nerve cell and again seek the surface. Once the virus reaches the surface, it becomes detectable for a short time and causes another outbreak at that site.

Opportunistic Infection

An **opportunistic infection** is normally caused by nonpathogenic organisms and occurs in individuals whose resistance is decreased or compromised. For example, an individual recovering from influenza may develop pneumonia or an ear infection. Opportunistic infections are common in patients with autoimmune disease or diabetes and in older adults.

Modes of Disease Transmission

Before you can prevent disease transmission in the dental office, you must first understand how **infectious diseases** are spread (Figure 5-4 and Table 5-3).

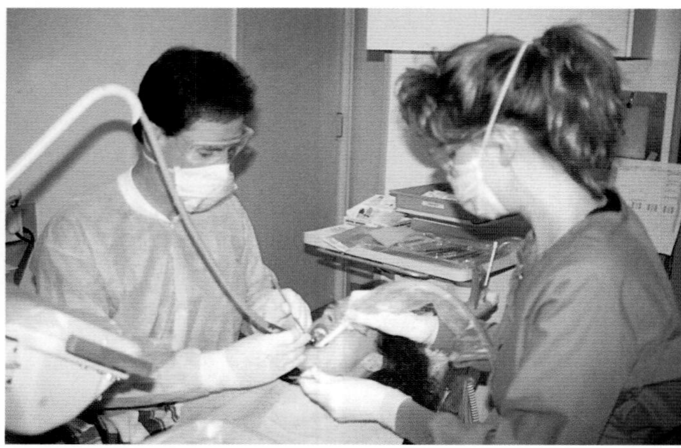

FIGURE 5-4 Pathogens can be transferred from staff member to patient, from patient to staff member, and from patient to patient through contaminated equipment.

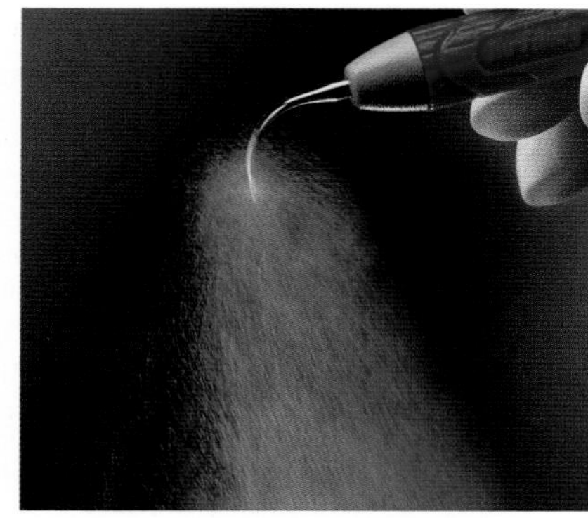

FIGURE 5-5 Aerosol from an ultrasonic scaler. (Courtesy Hu-Friedy Manufacturing. Company, Chicago, Illinois.)

TABLE 5-3
Modes of Disease Transmission in the Dental Office

Mode	Description
Direct	Contact with infectious lesions or infected blood and/or saliva
Indirect	Contact with a contaminated object, such as an instrument, any surface, or dental equipment
Splash or spatter	Contact of blood, saliva, or other body fluids onto broken or nonintact skin or mucosa
Airborne	Transfer of microorganisms via sprays, mists, or aerosols
Dental unit water lines	Ingestion or inhalation of water containing pathogenic microorganisms released from the biofilm within dental unit water lines

Direct Transmission

Pathogens can be transferred through **direct transmission** by coming into direct contact with an infectious lesion or infected body fluids, including blood, saliva, semen, and vaginal secretions. Many viruses and pathogenic bacteria are directly transmitted and cause hepatitis, herpes infection, HIV infection, and tuberculosis.

Exposure to blood and saliva is of particular concern for dental professionals during dental treatment. Although blood may not be visible in the saliva, it is often present.

Indirect Transmission

Indirect transfer of organisms to a susceptible person can occur by handling contaminated instruments or by touching contaminated surfaces and then touching the face, eyes, or mouth. Frequently washing your hands to avoid indirect transmission of microorganisms is important. **Indirect transmission** is also known as **cross-contamination**.

In the dental office, diseases may be indirectly transmitted via soiled hands and towels, contaminated instruments, and even dust. In addition, anything that is touched during patient care—faucet handles, switches, handpieces, instrument drawer handles, dental materials, the patient's chart, protective eyewear, and even the pen used to make the chart entry—is considered contaminated and potentially capable of spreading disease.

Splash or Spatter

Blood, saliva, or nasopharyngeal (nasal) secretions can be sprayed or spattered during dental procedures. Diseases can be transmitted during a dental procedure by splashing the mucosa (mouth or eyes) or nonintact skin with blood or blood-contaminated saliva.

Intact skin, which is not broken in any way, acts as a natural protective barrier. Nonintact skin, in which a cut, scrape, or needlestick injury has occurred, provides an entrance for pathogens to enter the body.

Airborne Transmission

Airborne transmission, also known as **droplet infection**, is the spread of disease through droplets of moisture containing bacteria or viruses. Most of the contagious respiratory diseases are caused by pathogens carried in droplets of moisture. Some of these pathogens are carried long distances through the air and ventilation systems. Airborne transmission can also occur when someone coughs or sneezes.

Aerosols containing saliva, blood, and microorganisms are created with the use of the high-speed handpiece, air-water syringe, and ultrasonic scaler during dental procedures (Figure 5-5). Inhaling bacteria and debris in the aerosol (without the protection of a face mask) is comparable with having someone sneeze in your face twice a minute at a distance of 1 foot.

Mists are droplet particles larger than those generated by the aerosol spray. Mists, such as those from coughing, can transmit respiratory infections. However, mists do not appear to transmit HBV or HIV infection, despite being inhaled.

Spatter consists of large droplet particles contaminated with blood, saliva, and other debris. Spatter is created during all restorative and hygiene procedures involving rotary and ultrasonic dental instruments. The use of the air-water syringe may also produce spatter.

Spatter droplets travel farther than the aerosol mist and tend to land on the upper surfaces of the wrist and forearms, upper arms, and chest. Droplets may also reach the necktie or collar area of the dentist, assistant, or hygienist.

Parenteral Transmission

Parenteral means through the skin, as with cuts or punctures. **Parenteral transmission** of bloodborne pathogens (disease-causing organisms transferred through contact with blood or other bodily fluids) can occur through needlestick injuries, human bites, cuts, abrasions, or any break in the skin.

Bloodborne Transmission

Certain pathogens, referred to as *bloodborne,* are carried in the blood and body fluids of infected individuals and can be transmitted to others. Bloodborne transmission occurs through direct or indirect contact with blood and other body fluids. Saliva is of particular concern during dental treatment because it is frequently contaminated with blood. Remember, although blood is not visible in the saliva, it may be present.

Improperly sterilized instruments and equipment can transfer all **bloodborne diseases**. Individuals who share needles while using illegal drugs easily transmit these diseases to each other. Unprotected sex is another common method of transmitting a bloodborne disease.

Common bloodborne microorganisms of concern in dentistry include HCV, HBV, and HIV. Because dental treatment often involves contact with blood and always with saliva, bloodborne diseases are of major concern in the dental office.

Food and Water Transmission

Many diseases are transmitted by contaminated food that has not been properly cooked or refrigerated and by water that has been contaminated with human or animal fecal material. For example, contaminated food or water spread tuberculosis, botulism, and staphylococcal and streptococcal infections.

Fecal-Oral Transmission

Many pathogens are present in fecal matter. If proper sanitation procedures, such as handwashing after using the toilet, are not followed, then these pathogens may be directly transmitted by touching another person or may be indirectly transmitted by contact with contaminated surfaces or food.

Fecal-oral transmission occurs most often among health care and daycare workers (who frequently change diapers) and in careless food handlers.

Transient Bacteremia

Bacteria entering the bloodstream and causing the temporary presence of bacteria in the blood is called *transient bacteremia.* (**Transient** means *temporary* or *moving*, and **bacteremia** means the *presence of bacteria in the blood.*)

For most healthy patients, transient bacteremia is not a problem because the body is able to destroy the bacteria quickly. However, even the temporary presence of bacteria in the blood is dangerous for high-risk patients, such as those with a history of congenital heart disease, rheumatic fever, or open heart surgery; those with certain forms of heart disease; those wearing pacemakers; and those with an artificial joint, such as a hip replacement.

For high-risk patients, the danger of **bacterial endocarditis** (bacterial infection of the lining of the heart) or a bacterial infection at the site of the implant exists. The administration of prophylactic (preventive) antibiotic medications for these patients is discussed in Chapter 11.

Viral Diseases of Major Concern to Dental Health Care Workers

Viral Hepatitis

There are at least five types of viral hepatitis, each of which is caused by a different virus: **hepatitis A** virus (HAV), **hepatitis B** virus (HBV), **hepatitis C** virus (HCV), **hepatitis D** virus (HDV), and hepatitis E virus (HEV) (Table 5-4).

Hepatitis A

HAV can affect anyone. It is spread from person to person by putting something in the mouth that has been contaminated with the stool of a person with HAV. This type of transmission is called *fecal-oral.* Good personal hygiene and proper sanitation can help prevent HAV. Always wash your hands after changing a diaper or using the bathroom. HAV is the least serious form of viral hepatitis. A vaccine is available that provides long-term prevention in persons older than 2 years.

TABLE 5-4
Primary Types of Hepatitis

	A	B	C	D	E
Source of the virus	Fecal-oral	Blood and body fluids	Blood and body fluids	Blood and body fluids	Fecal-oral
Route of transmission	Fecal-oral	Percutaneous and mucosal tissues	Percutaneous and mucosal tissues	Percutaneous and mucosal tissues	Fecal-oral
Chronic infection	No	Yes	Yes	Yes	No
Prevention	Vaccine	Immunization	Perform blood donor screening; modify risky behavior	Hepatitis B vaccine	Ensure safe drinking water

From Bird D, Robinson D: *Modern dental assisting*, ed 11, St. Louis, 2015, Elsevier.

Hepatitis B

HBV causes a very serious disease that may result in prolonged illness, liver cancer, cirrhosis of the liver, liver failure, and even death. HBV is a bloodborne disease that may also be transmitted by other body fluids, including saliva.

Anyone who has ever had HBV and some who have been exposed but have not actually been ill may be carriers of HBV, which means that patients who appear to be healthy and have no history of the disease may actually be spreading the infection to others. HBV is responsible for 34% of all types of acute viral hepatitis, which presents a high risk for dental personnel because dental treatment brings them into contact with saliva and blood. In addition, dental personnel may unknowingly be carriers of the disease. In this situation, the risk of transmitting the infection to the patient during treatment is always present.

Hepatitis B immunization A highly effective vaccine is available to prevent HBV. All dental personnel with a chance of occupational exposure should be vaccinated against HBV. The Occupational Safety & Health Administration (OSHA) Bloodborne Pathogens (BBP) Standard (see Chapter 6) requires that an employer offer the HBV vaccination at no cost to an employee within 10 days of initial assignment to a position in which the chance of occupational exposure to blood and/or other body fluids exists. The employee has the right to refuse the offer of vaccination; however, that employee must sign a release form indicating that the employer offered the vaccine and that the employee understands the potential risks of contracting HBV.

Postvaccination testing is recommended 1 to 6 months after the third injection to ensure that the individual has developed the antibodies necessary for immunity. Should antibodies not be present, the three-dose series should be repeated. The HBV vaccine is considered safe for pregnant women.

Hepatitis C

HCV is most efficiently transmitted through a blood transfusion or percutaneous exposure to blood. *Percutaneous* means performed through the skin and can occur from an accidental needlestick to an employee in a dental office, from sharing contaminated needles among injection drug users, or from contaminated tattoo needles. The carrier rate associated with HCV is higher than that associated with HBV. Unfortunately, no vaccine against HCV exists, nor has a cure for the disease been found. The U.S. Food and Drug Administration approved two new direct-acting antiviral drugs to treat chronic HCV infection. The primary concern of occupational exposure to HCV is needlesticks or other percutaneous injuries.

Hepatitis D

HHDV is a defective virus that cannot replicate itself without the presence of HBV. Therefore, infection with HDV may occur only simultaneously as a co-infection with HBV or may occur in an HBV carrier. Persons with co-infection of HBV and HDV often have more severe acute disease and a higher risk of death compared with those infected with HBV alone. Vaccination against HBV will also prevent infection with HDV.

Hepatitis E

HEV is not transmitted through bloodborne contact and is most frequently transmitted via the fecal-oral route through contaminated food or water. The disease is most frequently seen in the form of an epidemic in developing countries, and transmission is not a major concern in a standard dental setting.

Human Immunodeficiency Virus

The **HIV** infection is a bloodborne viral disease. The virus attacks and weakens or destroys the immune system. A blood test can be used to determine the presence of antibodies to HIV before symptoms appear.

A **positive test**, also known as a *seropositive result,* indicates that the individual is infected with the HIV, is a carrier, and is capable of transmitting the virus to others. (As used here, *sero-* refers to serum, which is the liquid portion of blood.)

A **negative test**, also known as *seronegative result,* means that no infection was present at the time of the test. However, this result does not suggest immunity to the virus.

A person with the HIV infection may remain healthy for many years. People who are HIV positive develop acquired immunodeficiency syndrome (AIDS) when they become sick with serious illnesses and infections that can occur with the HIV infection. Several oral conditions are frequently associated with the HIV infection.

Routes of Human Immunodeficiency Virus Transmission

The HIV infection is spread by sexual contact with an infected person of by needle sharing among drug users. Before blood donor screening for HIV, the virus was also transmitted by blood transfusions. Now that blood is screened for HIV antibodies, the blood supply in this country is safe. Babies born to HIV-infected mothers may become infected before or during birth or through breastfeeding after birth.

In (nondental) health care settings, workers have been infected with HIV by being stuck with needles containing HIV-infected blood or, less frequently, after infected blood gets into the worker's bloodstream through an open cut or splashes into a mucous membrane (e.g., eyes, inside of the nose).

Transmission of HIV, itself, is a concern but is not a major threat in the dental setting. However, patients who are HIV positive often have other diseases that can be transmitted more easily through dental treatment. Transmission of these diseases, particularly tuberculosis and HBV, poses a threat to dental personnel (Table 5-5).

Herpesviruses

Four major herpesviruses may affect humans (Table 5-6):

Herpes simplex virus (HSV) is divided into two types: HSV type 1 (HSV-1), which causes primarily oral lesions, and HSV type 2 (HSV-2), which primarily causes genital lesions.

Herpes zoster virus (HZV) or varicella-zoster virus causes herpes zoster, shingles, and chickenpox.

Cytomegalovirus (CMV) is normally latent (does not produce disease) but may become active when the immune

TABLE 5-5
Routes of Human Transmission of the Human Immunodeficiency Virus (HIV)

Routes of Transmission	Comments
Sexual contact	Is most easily transmitted through blood, semen, and vaginal secretions during sexual intercourse. Women are 10 times more likely than men to become infected in this manner.
Shared needles	Is transmitted through exposure to shared needles during illegal drug use and through tattoo needles.
Exposure to blood	Is transmitted through accidental exposure to blood that occurs in the health care setting.
Organ donation Blood or blood product transfusions	Transmission can also occur in rituals during which commingling of blood occurs, such as becoming "blood brothers."
During birth During breastfeeding	An infected mother can transmit the HIV infection to her child.

TABLE 5-6
Types of Human Herpesviruses

Herpes simplex virus (HSV)	
HSV-1	Primarily causes oral lesions.
HSV-2	Primarily causes genital lesions.
Herpes zoster virus (HZV)	Causes herpes zoster, shingles, and chickenpox.
Cytomegalovirus (CMV)	Is normally latent (does not cause disease) but may become active when the immune system is damaged. Once active, CMV is highly contagious and transmitted through most body fluids.
Epstein-Barr virus (EBV)	Causes infectious mononucleosis and Burkitt lymphoma, which is a malignancy of the lymph tissues.

For more information about these conditions, visit www.cdc.gov/ and search for the specific condition.

system is damaged; once active, CMV is highly contagious and transmitted by most body fluids.

The Epstein-Barr virus (EBV) causes infectious mononucleosis and Burkitt lymphoma, which is a malignant neoplasm involving lymphatic tissue.

Herpes Simplex Virus Type 1

HSV-1 is a viral infection that causes recurrent sores on lips. Because these sores frequently develop when the patient has a cold or fever of another origin, the disease has become commonly known as *fever blisters* or *cold sores.*

Primary Herpes

Primary herpes, which is highly contagious, makes its first appearance in very young children (1 to 3 years of age) and is known as *primary herpes.*

The child may have a slight fever, pain in the mouth, increased salivation, bad breath, and a general feeling of illness. The inside of the mouth becomes swollen, and the gingivae are inflamed.

Natural healing begins within 3 days, and the illness is usually over in 7 to 14 days. During this time, supportive measures can be taken to make the child more comfortable, to relieve the pain, and to prevent secondary infection.

Recurrent Herpes Labialis

After an initial herpes labialis infection during childhood, the HSV lies dormant and reappears later in life as the familiar recurring fever blister or cold sore (Figure 5-6).

Recurrences tend to take place when the patient's general resistance is lowered as a result of stress, fever, illness, injury, and exposure to the sun. Use of sunscreen with a sun protection factor (SPF) of 15 helps prevent sun-induced recurrences of herpes.

Attacks may recur as infrequently as once a year or as often as weekly or even daily. As in the case of primary herpes, recurrent herpes labialis sores heal by themselves in 7 to 10 days, leaving no scar.

Herpes Simplex Virus Type 2

HSV-2, also known as *genital herpes,* is one of the most common sexually transmitted diseases (STDs) in the United States. Initial symptoms, which generally appear 2 to 10 days after infection, include tingling, itching, and a burning sensation during urination.

Once a person is infected with HSV-2, outbreaks will recur. The disease can be transmitted only during these recurrences.

A mother with active vaginal or cervical herpetic lesions at the time of delivery can pass HSV-2 to her newborn. Approximately 50% of such newborns will be infected as they pass through the birth canal. At least 85% of infected infants will be severely damaged or killed by the virus.

Herpes Zoster Virus

HZV (human herpesvirus type 3) causes both varicella (chickenpox) and herpes zoster (shingles). Although these are two different diseases, both are caused by the identical organism. Chickenpox is the primary infection, and herpes zoster is the reactivation of illness. HZV is a highly contagious infection in individuals who have not been previously exposed to the virus. Transmission occurs by direct contact with skin lesions or by droplet infection from infectious saliva.

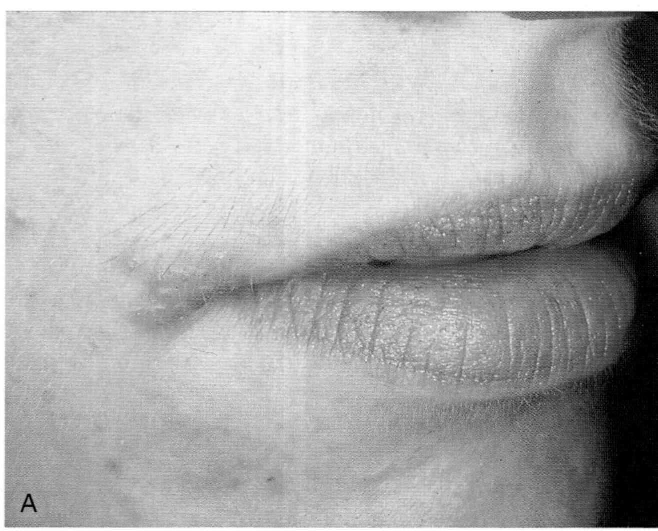

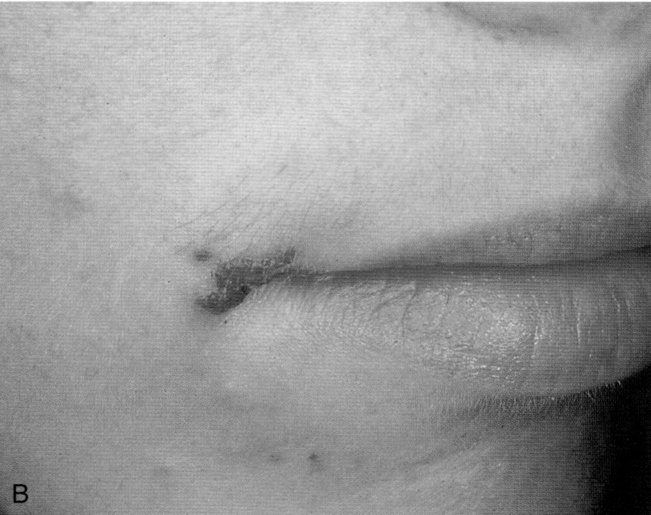

FIGURE 5-6 Herpes labialis. **A,** Twelve hours after onset. **B,** Forty-eight hours after onset. (From Ibsen OAC, Phelan JA: *Oral pathology for the dental hygienist*, ed 6, St. Louis, 2014, Saunders.)

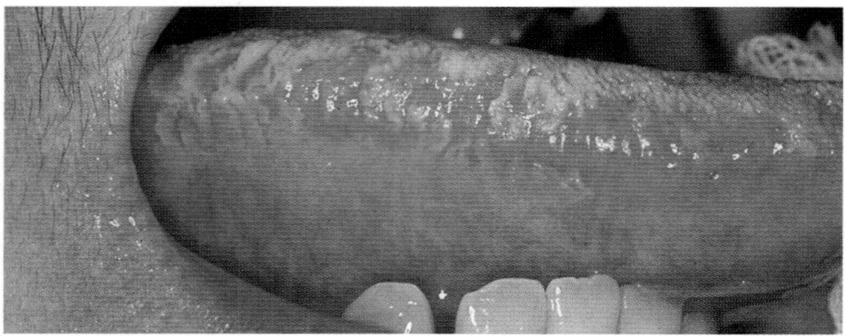

FIGURE 5-7 Hairy leukoplakia. (From Ibsen OAC, Phelan JA: *Oral pathology for the dental hygienist*, ed 6, St. Louis, 2014, Saunders.)

Cytomegalovirus

CMV (human herpesvirus type 5) rarely causes disease unless other factors, such as a compromised immune system, are present. However, CMV can infect the fetus during pregnancy. In some cases, infants will be born deaf or will suffer mental retardation. The route of transmission of CMV is unclear.

Epstein-Barr Virus

EBV (human herpesvirus type 4) is responsible for a number of infections, including infectious mononucleosis, nasopharyngeal cancer, lymphoma, and oral hairy leukoplakia (a condition commonly seen in patients with HIV) (Figure 5-7). Infectious mononucleosis is an acute infectious disease that primarily affects people between 15 and 20 years of age. EBV is present in the saliva and is transmitted by kissing, hence it is often called the "kissing disease."

Herpes Transmission

The major transmission route for the herpesvirus is through direct contact with lesions or with infectious saliva. When oral lesions are present, the patient may be asked to reschedule his or her appointment for a time after the lesions have healed. Even when no active lesions are present, viral transmission through saliva or through the aerosol spray from the dental handpiece is still a possibility.

Because no preventive vaccine is available to protect against herpes, taking precautions to prevent exposure is essential.

Protective eyewear for the dental professional is particularly important because a herpes infection in the eye may cause blindness. Gloves protect the dental professional against infection through lesions or abrasions on the hands.

Measles

Measles, which can be prevented by the administration of a vaccine, is a potentially serious viral disease and is easily transmitted via airborne transmission. It has an incubation period of 10 to 12 days. Measles is characterized by a rash, but the first symptoms are a cough and fever.

Bacterial Diseases of Major Concern to Dental Health Care Workers

Tuberculosis

Tuberculosis, which is caused by the bacterium *Mycobacterium tuberculosis,* is the leading cause of death worldwide from infectious diseases (Box 5-2).

BOX 5-2 Signs of Tuberculosis

1. Productive cough lasting longer than 3 weeks (Sputum comes up into the mouth in a productive cough. Sputum is thick mucus from the lungs that is ejected through the mouth.)
2. Unexplained fever, fatigue, or night sweats
3. Unexplained weight loss and anorexia (loss of appetite)
4. Member of a high-risk group

Because patients infected with the HIV have a weakened immune system, they are highly susceptible to tuberculosis;

therefore, HIV and tuberculosis are often present together. Of the two, tuberculosis presents a greater health risk for health care workers. One reason for this is that the rod-shaped tubercle bacillus is able to withstand disinfectants that kill many other bacteria. Surface disinfectants are further discussed in Chapter 7.

Transmission of Tuberculosis

Infection with active disease A patient who is diagnosed with the signs described in Box 5-2 is in the active stage. This patient may easily spread the disease through prolonged close contact. Tuberculosis is primarily spread when the individual coughs and the tubercle bacilli, which are present in the sputum, are expelled through the mouth. These bacteria are inhaled by others and carried to their lungs. A healthy individual is usually able to fight off the infection; however, someone who is already weakened with other illnesses may become infected.

Transmission of the disease can also occur through the consumption of contaminated milk and through contact with infected cattle.

Infection without active disease Of all people who are exposed to tuberculosis, 90% are infected without active disease; that is, they carry the disease but never have active symptoms. Although they do not transmit the disease at this stage, if resistance is weakened, then the tubercle bacilli may become active.

After a patient has had the active disease and seems to be well, he or she will always be a carrier for the disease.

Legionnaires' Disease

The *Legionella pneumophila* bacterium (named after an epidemic of this disease during an American Legion convention in Philadelphia) is responsible for two acute bacterial diseases: Pontiac fever and legionnaires' disease. Bacteria are transmitted through aerosolization and aspiration of contaminated water (see Chapter 7 for a discussion on dental unit water lines).

No person-to-person transmission occurs. *L. pneumophila* bacteria have been found to thrive in lakes, creeks, hot tubs, spas, air-conditioning systems, shower heads, water distillation systems, and the biofilm found in dental unit water lines (Figure 5-8). Dental personnel have higher antibodies against *L. pneumophila* than the general public, indicating occupational exposure and a resistance to this organism.

Pontiac fever is the least serious form of infection, causing acute flulike symptoms with headache, high fever, dry cough, chills, diarrhea, chest pain, and abdominal pain.

Legionnaires' disease is the more serious form of infection, causing very severe pneumonia. In those who are immunocompromised or in older adults, the disease can be fatal.

Tetanus

Tetanus, which is also known as *lockjaw,* is an extremely dangerous and often fatal disease that is caused by a spore-forming bacillus found in soil, dust, or animal or human feces. This microbe is usually introduced into the body through a wound or break in the skin (as in a puncture wound from a soiled instrument).

The organism causing tetanus produces the severe muscle spasms and rigidity that give the disease its popular name of lockjaw. The disease can be prevented by the administration of a vaccine; however, immunity must be kept current through booster doses. (It is important that dental personnel keep all immunizations current.)

Syphilis

Syphilis, an STD, is caused by *Treponema pallidum* spirochetes. Although these bacteria are fragile outside of the body, the danger of direct cross-infection exists in the dental operatory through contact with oral lesions.

The first stage of syphilis involves the presence of a painless ulcerating sore, known as a *chancre,* which is infectious on contact. When it occurs on the lip, it may resemble herpes, but the crusting is darker (Figure 5-9).

The second stage of syphilis is also infectious, and immediate infection may occur through contact with an open sore (Box 5-3). The third stage, known as *latent syphilis,* is usually fatal and may occur after the disease has been dormant for 20 years.

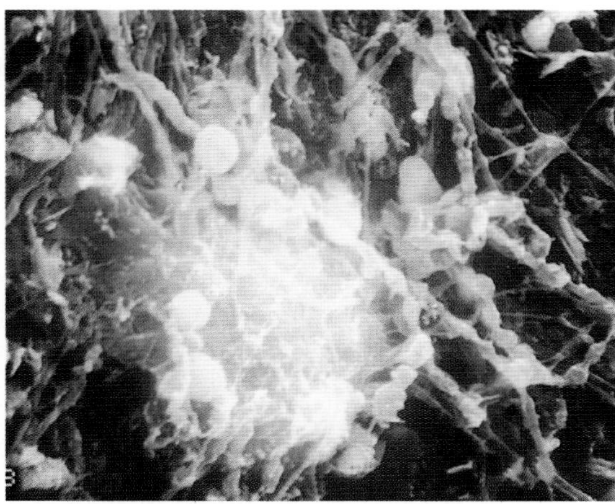

FIGURE 5-8 Bacteria in biofilm taken from dental unit water lines. (Courtesy Dr. Shannon Mills.)

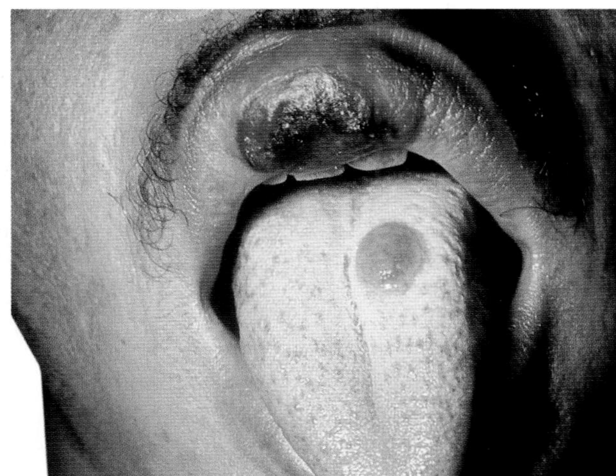

FIGURE 5-9 Chancres on the tongue and lip seen in a person with primary syphilis. (From Schachner LA, Hansen RC, eds: *Pediatric Dermatology,* ed 4, London, 2011, Mosby.)

BOX 5-3 Oral Signs of Syphilis of Special Interest to Dental Personnel

1. Split papules at the corners of the mouth
2. Grayish-white, moist mucous patches on the tongue, roof of mouth, tonsils, or inner surfaces of the lips (These patches are highly infectious.)
3. Generalized rash resembling a measles rash, poxlike pustules, oozing sores, and hair falling out of the scalp

Ethical Implications

Regardless of whether your state has established minimum standards for infection control in the dental setting, doing everything possible to prevent the transmission of disease to patients, to other staff members, and to yourself is your ethical responsibility.

Chapter Exercises

Multiple Choice

Circle the letter next to the correct answer.

1. A microorganism that can cause disease is called a(n) __________.
- **a.** pathogen
- **b.** host
- **c.** virulence
- **d.** autogenous

2. A large group of one-celled microorganisms that are capable of causing disease are ________.
- **a.** pathogens
- **b.** bacteria
- **c.** viruses
- **d.** all of the above

3. Forms of life that are most resistant to extremes of heat and dryness are __________.
- **a.** bacteria
- **b.** viruses
- **c.** fungi
- **d.** spores
- **e.** all of the above

4. Another term for the disease often called *lockjaw* is __________.
- **a.** hepatitis
- **b.** Pontiac fever
- **c.** tetanus
- **d.** bacterial endocarditis

5. The serious disease that can be transmitted from contaminated dental water in dental lines is __________.
- **a.** hepatitis
- **b.** tuberculosis
- **c.** legionnaires' disease
- **d.** herpes

6. The sexually transmitted form of herpes is __________.
- **a.** HSV-1
- **b.** HSV-2
- **c.** HZV
- **d.** EBV

7. The virus that enters the human body and attacks the immune system is __________.
- **a.** HBV
- **b.** HCV
- **c.** HZV
- **d.** HIV

8. Which of the following types of hepatitis is *NOT* a bloodborne disease?
- **a.** HAV
- **b.** HBV
- **c.** HCV
- **d.** HDV

9. Which of the following types of hepatitis is *NOT* capable of replicating itself?
- **a.** HAV
- **b.** HBV
- **c.** HCV
- **d.** HDV

10. An infection resulting from bacteria that are normally present in the patient's mouth is called ______.
- **a.** co-infection
- **b.** autogenous infection
- **c.** transient bacteremia
- **d.** carrier transmission

Apply Your Knowledge

1. Mr. Jerry Davis informs you that he tested positive on a tuberculosis test, but he thinks the results are a mistake because he feels very healthy and has no symptoms of tuberculosis. What would you do?

2. Mrs. Quock brings her 7-year-old son, Stanley, for a fluoride treatment. Stanley shows you several yellowish-colored sores inside his mouth. What could these sores be, and what should you do?

3. Mrs. Robinson accompanies her 87-year-old mother (who resides in a nursing home) for her dental visit. The older woman appears weak and is coughing into a handkerchief. What concerns might you have about the potential medical condition of this patient?

4. A newly hired dental assistant in your office confides in you that she is afraid of shots. Because of her fear, she does not think she will get the hepatitis B vaccine, and she asks you for your opinion. How would you advise her?

CHAPTER 6

Infection Control and Management of Hazardous Materials

http://evolve.elsevier.com/Robinson/essentials/

LEARNING OBJECTIVES

1. Pronounce, define, and spell the key terms.
2. Provide an overview of the roles and responsibilities of the Centers for Disease Control and Occupational Safety & Health Administration when it comes to workplace safety and infection control in dentistry.
3. Complete the following related to OSHA's Bloodborne Pathogens Standard (BBP).
   - Explain the components of the OSHA BBP Standard.
   - Name the components of an exposure control plan.
   - Explain the difference between Universal Precautions and Standard Precautions.
   - Categorize tasks and procedures according to occupational exposure risks.
   - Discuss employee training in relation to the BBP Standard.
   - Describe the indications for the hepatitis B vaccine.
   - Discuss the storage of employee medical records.
   - Describe and demonstrate the proper disposal of contaminated sharps.
   - State how to prevent needle sticks.
   - Describe postexposure management, as well as how to provide first aid after an exposure incident.
4. Describe and demonstrate the proper technique of handwashing.
5. Describe and demonstrate the appropriate use of alcohol-based hand rubs.
6. Explain the requirements for personal protective equipment, including the steps to putting on personal protective equipment and removing personal protective equipment.
7. Describe the types of dental waste and the management of each.
8. Identify and discuss the five components of the Occupational Safety & Health Administration Hazard Communication Standard.

KEY TERMS

alcohol-based hand rubs
Bloodborne Pathogens (BBP) standard
Centers for Disease Control and Prevention (CDC)
Globally Harmonized System (GHS) of Classification and Labeling of Chemicals
hazard class
Hazard Communication Standard (HCS)
hazard statement
hazardous waste
infectious waste
occupational exposure
Occupational Safety & Health Administration (OSHA)
percutaneous
permucosal
personal protective equipment (PPE)
pictogram
regulated waste
safety data sheets (SDSs)
sharps
signal word
Standard Precautions
Universal Precautions

Roles and Responsibilities of the CDC and OSHA

Both the **Centers for Disease Control and Prevention (CDC)** and the **Occupational Safety & Health Administration (OSHA)** federal agencies play very important roles in workplace safety and infection control for dentistry.

The CDC is not a regulatory agency. Its role is to issue specific recommendations based on sound scientific evidence on health-related matters. Although not law, the CDC Guidelines for Infection Control in Dental Health Care Settings are now the standard of care (Figure 6-1 and Box 6-1).

OSHA is a regulatory agency. Its role is to issue specific regulations, also called *standards,* to protect the health of employees in the United States. Failure to comply with OSHA requirements can have serious consequences, including heavy fines. As a dental assistant, following all of the guidelines and recommendations is important.

This chapter discusses the basic concepts and the step-by-step procedures you will need to prevent the transmission of disease and to manage hazardous material safely in the dental office.

OSHA's Bloodborne Pathogens Standard

OSHA's **Bloodborne Pathogens (BBP) Standard** is the most important infection control law in dentistry. It is designed to protect employees against occupational exposure to bloodborne, disease-causing organisms, such as the hepatitis B virus (HBV), hepatitis C virus (HCV), and human immunodeficiency virus (HIV).

The BBP Standard requires employers to protect their employees from exposure to blood and other potentially infectious material (OPIM) in the workplace and to provide proper care to the employee if an exposure should occur. The Standard applies to any type of facility in which employees might be exposed to blood and other body fluids, including dental and medical offices, hospitals, funeral homes, emergency medical services, and nursing homes.

OSHA requires that a copy of the BBP Standard be present in every dental office and clinic. A copy of the OSHA BBP Standard may be obtained by visiting http://www.osha.gov and searching for "Bloodborne Pathogens Standard."

Exposure Control Plan

Each dental office must have a written exposure control plan that clearly describes how that office complies with the BBP Standard. The exposure control plan must be reviewed and updated at least annually. A copy must be accessible to all employees (Box 6-2).

Standard and Universal Precautions

The term **Universal Precautions** is still referred to in OSHA's BBP Standard. Universal Precautions is based on the concept that all human blood and certain body fluids (including saliva)

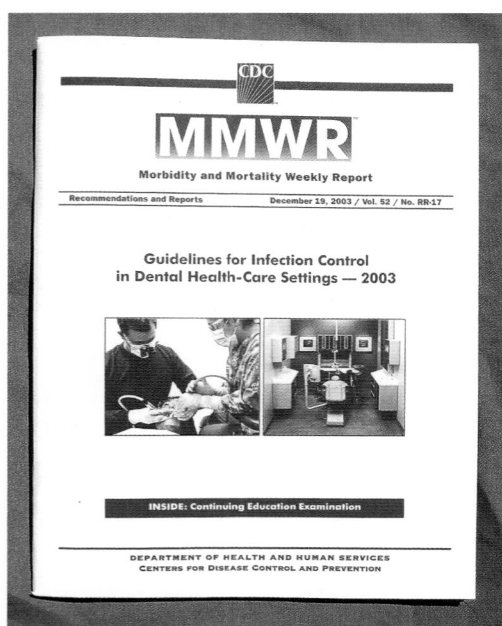

FIGURE 6-1 The December 19, 2003, issue of *Morbidity and Mortality Weekly Report* includes the Centers for Disease Control and Prevention (CDC) Guidelines for Infection Control in Dental Health-Care Settings—2003. NOTE: Although the date on these Guidelines is 2003, the CDC has regularly reviewed them since then and has not found changes necessary, thus the date of 2003 remains in the current title.

BOX 6-1 Overview of CDC Guidelines for Infection Control in Dental Health-Care Settings—2003

- Use of Standard Precautions rather than Universal Precautions
- Work restrictions for health care personnel infected with infectious diseases
- Postexposure management of occupational exposure to bloodborne pathogens (HBV, HIV, HCV)
- Selection of devices with features to prevent sharps injuries
- Hand hygiene products and surgical hand asepsis
- Contact dermatitis and latex hypersensitivity
- Sterilization of unwrapped instruments
- Dental unit water line concerns
- Dental radiology infection control
- Aseptic technique for injectable medications
- Preprocedural mouth rinses for patients
- Oral surgical procedures
- Laser and electrosurgery plumes
- Tuberculosis
- Creutzfeldt-Jakob disease and other prion-related diseases
- Evaluation of infection control program
- Research considerations

Modified from CDC Guidelines for Infection Control in Dental Health-Care Settings—2003. *NOTE: Although these Guidelines were adopted in 2003, they have been continually reviewed, and no updates have been issued.* Copies of these guidelines may be requested at oralhealth@cdc.gov, or by telephone at (770) 488-6054 or by fax at (770) 488-6080.

CDC, Centers for Disease Control and Prevention; *HBV,* hepatitis B virus; *HCV,* hepatitis C virus; *HIV,* human immunodeficiency virus.

BOX 6-2 Written Exposure Control Plan Required by OSHA

General policy of implementing the Centers for Disease Control and Prevention Guidelines and the American Dental Association Infection Control Recommendations

- Use of Universal Precautions
- Required use of personal protective equipment
- Standardized housekeeping
- Laundering of contaminated protective clothing
- Standardized policy on cleaning and disinfecting
- Policy on general waste disposal
- Labeling procedure (secondary labeling)
- Policy on sterilization (including monitoring) and disinfection
- Use of sharps containers and disposal system
- Standardized handwashing protocol
- HBV vaccination
- Postexposure evaluation and medical follow-up

OSHA, Occupational Safety & Health Administration.

are to be treated as if known to be infected with the bloodborne diseases such as HBV, HCV, or HIV infection. The rationale for this concept is that identifying those individuals who are infectious is not possible; therefore Universal Precautions are to be used for all health care personnel and their patients.

The CDC later expanded the concept and changed the term to **Standard Precautions**. Standard Precautions apply not only to contact with blood but also contact with (1) all body fluids, secretions, and excretions (except sweat), regardless of whether they contain blood; (2) nonintact skin; and (3) mucous membranes. Saliva has always been considered a potentially infectious material in dental infection control; therefore there is no difference in clinical dental practice between Universal Precautions and Standard Precautions. Standard Precautions apply to contact with:

- Blood
- All body fluids, secretions, and excretions except sweat, regardless of whether they contain blood
- Nonintact skin
- Mucous membranes

Categories of Employees

OSHA's BBP Standard requires employers to categorize tasks and procedures during which an employee might have an occupational exposure (Table 6-1).

The BBP Standard defines an **occupational exposure** as "any reasonably anticipated skin, eye, [or] mucous membrane contact, or percutaneous injury, with blood or any other potentially infectious materials." **Percutaneous** (through the skin, such as needlesticks, cuts, and human bites) and **permucosal** (contact with mucous membranes, such as the eyes or mouth) exposures to blood, saliva, and other body fluids pose the greatest risk for the transmission of HIV, HBV, and HCV.

Employee Training

The BBP Standard requires the dentist and/or employer to provide training in infection control and safety issues to all personnel who may come in contact with blood, saliva, or contaminated instruments or surfaces. The employer must keep records of all training sessions. The record of each training session must include the date of the session, the name of the presenter, the topic, and the names of all employees who attended (Box 6-3).

TABLE 6-1
Occupational Exposure Determination

Category	Definition	Examples
I	Routinely exposed to blood, saliva, or both	Dentist, dental hygienist, dental assistant, sterilization assistant, dental laboratory technician
II	May, on occasion, be exposed to blood, saliva, or both	Receptionist or office manager who may, on occasion, clean a treatment room or handle instruments or impressions
III	Never exposed to blood, saliva, or both	Financial manager, insurance clerk, computer operator

BOX 6-3 OSHA's Bloodborne Pathogens Standard Training Requirements

Employee training is required in each of the following areas:

- Epidemiology, modes of transmission, and prevention of HBV and HIV
- Possible risks to the fetus from HIV and HBV
- Location and proper use of all protective equipment
- Proper work practices using Universal Precautions
- Meaning of color codes, biohazard symbol, and precautions to follow in handling infectious waste
- Procedures to be followed if a needlestick or other exposure incident occurs

Employee training must be provided at the time of initial assignment to tasks during which occupational exposure may occur. Annual training is required within 12 months of the previous training. The training shall be tailored to the education and language level of the employee and offered during the normal work shift.

HBV, Hepatitis B virus; *HIV,* human immunodeficiency virus; *OSHA,* Occupational Safety & Health Administration.

Hepatitis B Immunization

The BBP Standard requires the dentist and/or employer to offer the HBV vaccination series to all employees whose assignments include category I and II tasks. The vaccine must be offered within 10 days of assignment to an occupational exposure category I or II task. To document compliance, the dentist or employer must obtain proof from the physician who administered the vaccination to the employee.

The employee has the right to refuse the HBV vaccine for any reason. The employee is then required to sign an informed refusal form that is kept on file in the dental office. Although the employee originally signed the refusal form, he or she always has the right to reverse the decision and to receive the vaccine at a later date at no charge.

Need for an HBV Booster Vaccine

The CDC *does not* recommend routine booster doses of the HBV vaccine, nor does it recommend routine blood testing to monitor the HBV antibody level in individuals who have already had the vaccine, assuming that the individual was tested after receiving the vaccine and was known to have initially developed antibodies. An exception is the immunized individual who has a documented exposure incident and for whom the attending physician orders a booster dose.

Employee Medical Records

The dentist or employer must keep a confidential medical record for each employee. The employer must store these records in a locked file for the duration of employment plus 30 years (Box 6-4).

Managing Contaminated Sharps

Contaminated needles and other disposable sharps, such as scalpel blades, orthodontic wires, and broken glass, must be placed into a sharps container. The sharps container must be puncture resistant, closable, leakproof, and color-coded or labeled with the biohazard symbol (Figure 6-2).

Sharps containers must be located as close as possible to the place of immediate disposal. Needles should not be cut, bent, or broken before disposal, and a needle should never be removed from a disposable-type device.

Preventing Needlesticks

Some needles on the market have safety guards to prevent accidental needlesticks (Figure 6-3). The single-handed scoop technique or some type of safety device (Figure 6-4) should always be used.

Postexposure Management

Despite efforts to prevent occupational exposure incidents, accidents happen. Therefore before an accident occurs, the BBP

BOX 6-4 Requirements for Employee Medical Records

- Employee's name and Social Security number
- Proof of employee's hepatitis B virus (HBV) vaccination or signed refusal
- Circumstances of any exposure incident (e.g., needlestick) involving the employee and the name of the source individual (patient whose blood or bodily fluid is involved in the incident)
- Copy of the postexposure follow-up procedures for any injuries sustained by that employee

These records must be retained by the dentist or employer for the duration of employment plus 30 years.

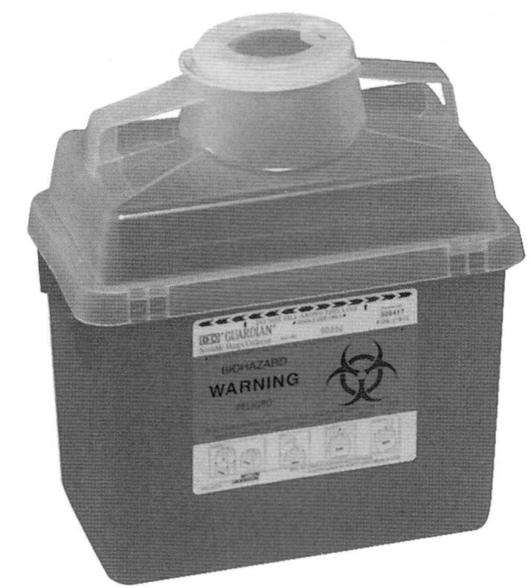

FIGURE 6-2 A puncture-resistant sharps disposal container should be located as close as possible to the area where the disposal of sharps takes place.

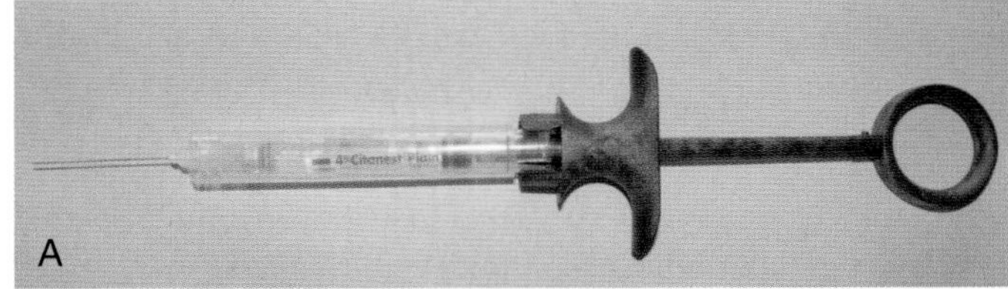

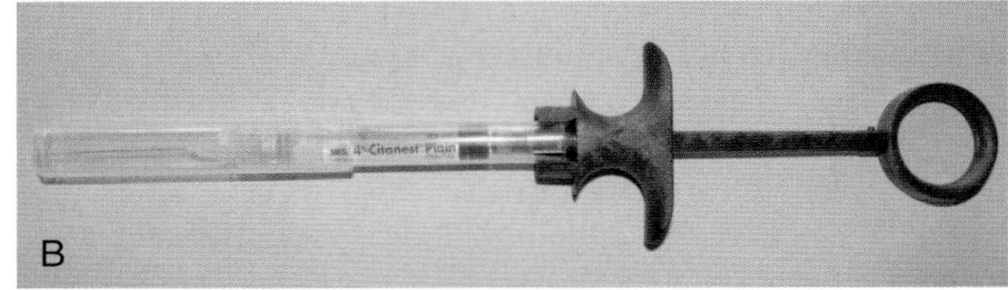

FIGURE 6-3 Ultra Safety Plus XL aspirating syringe. **A,** Ready for injection. **B,** Needle sheathed to prevent a needlestick injury. (From Logothesis DD: *Local anesthesia for the dental hygienist,* St. Louis, 2012, Mosby.)

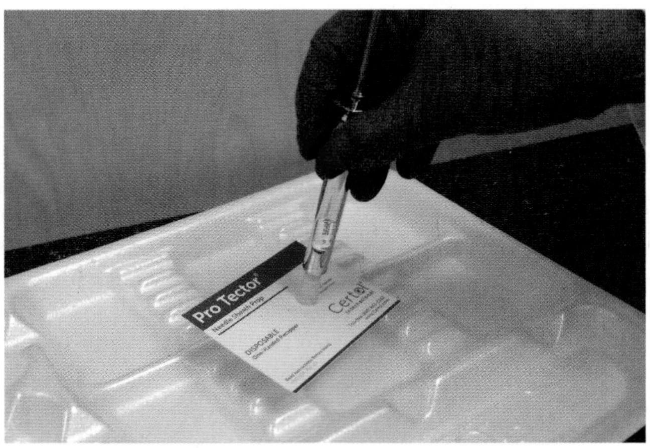

FIGURE 6-4 ProTector® disposable needle guard. (ProTector® Needle Sheath Prop, Courtesy Certol International, Commerce City, Colorado.)

BOX 6-5 Postexposure Follow-Up for an Exposed Worker

The following services must be offered to the employee without charge:

- Confidential medical counseling
- HIV test series (immediately and at 6-week, 12-week, and 6-month intervals)
- HBV immunoglobulin (if the employee has not been vaccinated for HBV)
- Tetanus booster
- Documentation of the incident on the appropriate OSHA form

An employee has the right to refuse testing, and no adverse actions can be taken against him or her. However, the employee will be required to sign an informed refusal form.

HBV, Hepatitis B virus; *HIV,* human immunodeficiency virus; *OSHA,* Occupational Safety & Health Administration.

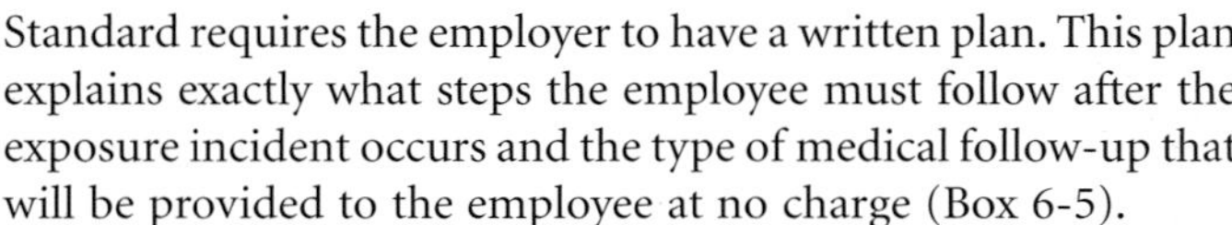

Standard requires the employer to have a written plan. This plan explains exactly what steps the employee must follow after the exposure incident occurs and the type of medical follow-up that will be provided to the employee at no charge (Box 6-5).

The employer must provide training to employees on the proper response to an exposure incident. Procedure 6-1 reviews first-aid steps after an exposure incident.

Handwashing and Hand Care

Handwashing

You must wash your hands before you put on gloves (Procedure 6-2) and immediately after you remove gloves. Washing your hands after you remove your gloves is important because the growth of bacteria on your skin will increase as a result of the warm, moist environment under the glove. Washing before gloving reduces the number of microorganisms to begin with, and washing after glove removal reduces the number of organisms that have increased.

Handwashing is also required if you inadvertently touch contaminated objects or surfaces while barehanded. You should always use liquid soap during handwashing. Bar soap should never be used because it may transmit contamination. In addition, you should not "top off" containers of soap or lotion. Bacteria can grow in liquid soaps and lotions. The container should be used until empty, then washed and dried and then refilled. An alternative is to use disposable containers that can be recycled.

To minimize cross-contamination, treatment room sinks equipped with *hands-free* faucets that are electronically activated or are activated with foot pedals are preferable (Figure 6-5).

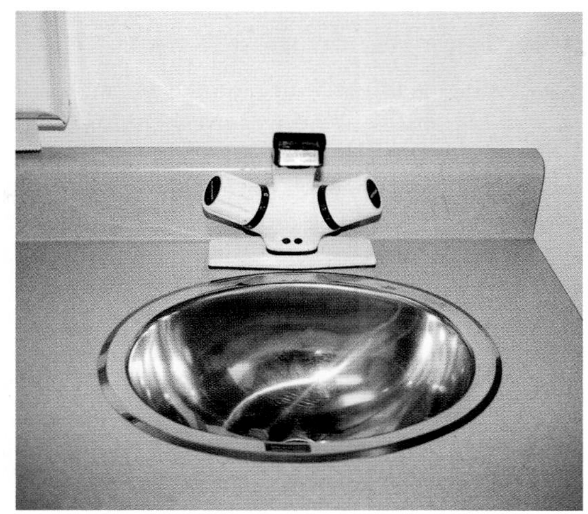

FIGURE 6-5 Sensing device automatically turns the water on and off with hands-free operation.

Alcohol-Based Hand Rubs

Waterless antiseptic agents are alcohol-based products that are available in gels, foams, or rinses (Figure 6-6). They do not require the use of water. The product is simply applied to the hands, which are then rubbed together to cover all surfaces.

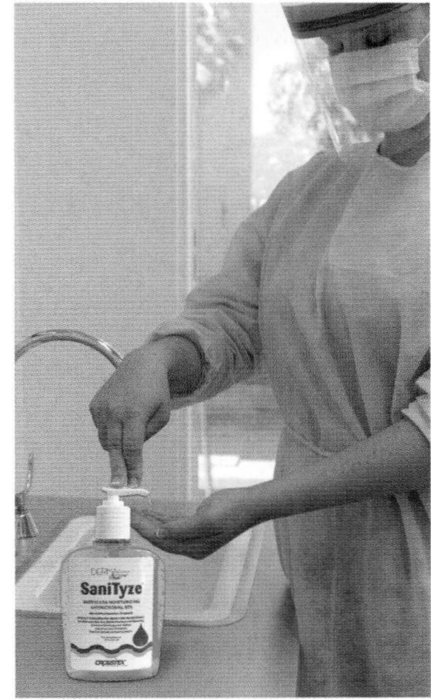

FIGURE 6-6 Alcohol-based hand rub agents are available for refillable wall-mounted containers, in counter size, and in purse size. (Courtesy Crosstex International, Inc., Hauppauge, New York.)

These products are more effective at reducing microbial flora than plain soap or even an antimicrobial hand wash. Concentrations of 60% to 95% are the most effective. In addition, these products are actually good for your skin. They contain emollients that reduce the incidence of chapping, irritation, and drying of the skin.

Alcohol-based hand rubs are NOT indicated if your hands are visibly soiled or are contaminated with organic matter, such as blood or saliva. In this case, your hands need to first be washed with soap and water and then followed with the alcohol-based product.

See Procedure 6-3: Applying Alcohol-Based Hand Rubs.

Hand-Hygiene Recommendations

Healthy skin is better able to withstand the damaging effects of repeated washing and of wearing gloves. Drying your hands well is important before donning gloves.

Dental personnel with open sores or weeping dermatitis must avoid activities involving direct patient contact and handling contaminated instruments or equipment until the condition on the hands is healed.

Because rings and long fingernails can harbor pathogens and damage gloves, nails should be kept short and well manicured. Rings, long nails, and artificial nails are likely to puncture examination gloves. In addition, microorganisms can enter the body through any break in the skin. CDC guidelines recommend that rings, fingernail polish, and artificial nails not be worn at work.

Lotions

You can use lotions to prevent skin dryness caused by frequent handwashing. However, you must use caution in selecting a product. Lotions with a base of petroleum, lanolin, mineral oil, palm oil, or coconut oil have a negative effect on latex gloves. Use these products only at the end of the workday. You can use lotions containing aloe vera, glycerin, vitamin E, or vitamin A.

Personal Protective Equipment

OSHA's BBP Standard requires the employer to provide employees with appropriate **personal protective equipment (PPE)** (Figure 6-7) without charge to the employee. Examples of PPE include protective clothing, surgical masks, face shields, protective eyewear, disposable patient treatment gloves, and heavy-duty utility gloves.

Because the dental assistant is likely to come in contact with blood and saliva, you must wear PPE whenever you are performing tasks that could produce contact with body fluids.

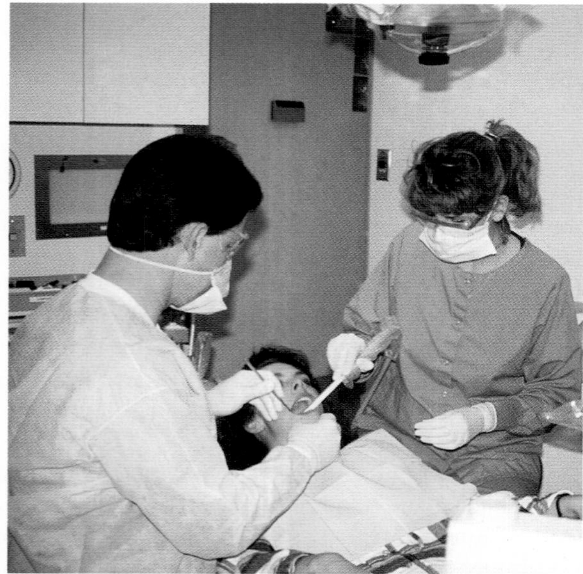

FIGURE 6-7 Appropriate personal protective equipment (PPE) at chairside includes long-sleeved gowns, gloves, and eyewear.

See Procedure 6-4: Putting on Personal Protective Equipment (PPE) and Procedure 6-5: Removing Personal Protective Equipment.

You must also wear appropriate PPE when you perform other clinical activities that require handling items contaminated with patient secretions. Examples include processing dental radiographs and handling laboratory cases, dentures, and other prosthetic appliances or contaminated equipment and surfaces.

Protective Clothing

The purpose of protective clothing is to protect the skin and underclothing from exposure to saliva, blood, aerosol, and other contaminated materials. Types of protective clothing can include smocks, pants, skirts, laboratory coats, surgical scrubs (hospital surgical unit clothing), scrub (surgical) hats, and shoe covers. Technically, clinic shoes and hosiery are also part of PPE.

The decision as to the type of protective clothing you should wear is based on the degree of anticipated exposure to infectious materials. For example, assisting with the high-speed handpiece during a cavity preparation carries a high risk of exposure to contaminated aerosol. Charting during an oral examination, on the other hand, carries a low risk of exposure because it does not involve use of the handpiece or air-water syringe, which creates contaminated aerosol (Figure 6-8).

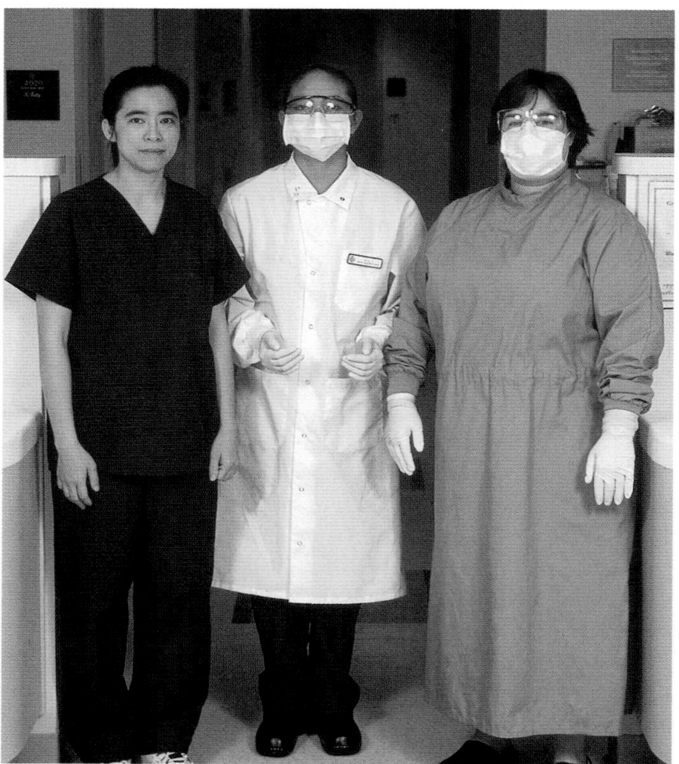

FIGURE 6-8 Depending on the task, the dental assistant's attire might be scrubs, laboratory coats, or surgical gowns. *Left,* Dental assistant in scrubs. *Center,* Dental assistant in a laboratory coat. *Right,* Dental assistant in surgical gown.

Protective Clothing Requirements

Protective clothing should be made of fluid-resistant material. Cotton, cotton-polyester mix, or disposable jackets or gowns are usually satisfactory for routine dental procedures.

To minimize the amount of uncovered skin, clothing should have long sleeves and a high neckline. The design of the sleeve should allow the cuff to be tucked inside the band of the glove.

During high-risk procedures, protective clothing must cover dental personnel at least to the knees when seated.

Buttons, trim, zippers, and other ornamentation (which may harbor pathogens) should be kept to a minimum.

Note: The type and characteristics of protective clothing depend on the anticipated degree of exposure (Box 6-6).

Handling Contaminated Laundry

The BBP Standard prohibits an employee from taking protective clothing home to be laundered. Laundering contaminated protective clothing is the responsibility of the employer, and many offices have a laundry service that will pick up contaminated laundry from the dental office. Some dental offices have chosen to install washers and dryers for PPE within the office. In this situation, any employee responsible for laundering contaminated PPE must be trained in the proper handling of contaminated PPE and must wear PPE when handling contaminated items.

Contaminated linens that are removed from the office for laundering should be in a leakproof bag with a biohazard label or an appropriately color-coded label (Figure 6-9). Disposable gowns must be discarded daily and more often if visibly soiled.

Protective Masks

A surgical mask is worn over the nose and mouth to protect the person from inhaling infectious organisms spread by the aerosol spray of the handpiece or air-water syringe and by accidental splashes. A mask with at least 95% filtration efficiency for particles 3 to 5 micrometers (μm) in diameter should be worn whenever splash or spatter is likely. Surgical masks do not provide a perfect seal around the edges; therefore unfiltered air can pass through the edges. For this reason, selecting a mask that fits your face well is important. Masks should be changed between patients or during patient treatment if the mask becomes wet.

BOX 6-6 Guidelines for Wearing Protective Clothing

- Protective clothing should not be worn out of the office for any reason; it can spread contamination.
- Protective clothing should be changed at least daily or more often if it becomes visibly soiled.
- Protective clothing should be IMMEDIATELY changed if it becomes soiled or saturated with body fluids or chemicals.
- Protective clothing must NEVER be worn in the staff lounge areas or when coworkers are eating or consuming beverages.

The two most common types of masks are the dome-shaped and flat types. Some operators prefer the dome-shaped type, particularly during lengthy procedures, because it conforms or "molds" more effectively to the face and creates an air space between the mask and the wearer (Figures 6-10 and 6-11 and Box 6-7).

When not in use, face masks should never be worn below the nose or on the chin. Remember, the outer surface of the mask is highly contaminated (Figure 6-12).

Protective Eyewear

Eyewear is worn to protect the eyes against damage from aerosolized pathogens, such as herpes simplex viruses and staphylococci, and from flying debris, such as scrap amalgam and tooth fragments. Protective eyewear also prevents injury from splattered solutions and caustic chemicals. Such damage may be irreparable and may lead to permanent visual impairment or blindness.

The BBP Standard requires the use of eyewear with both front and side protection (solid side shields) for use during exposure-prone procedures. If you wear prescription glasses, you must add protective side and bottom shields. Protective eyewear that can be worn over prescription glasses is also available. If you wear contact lenses, then you must also wear protective eyewear with side shields or a face shield.

The CDC guidelines recommend that you clean your eyewear with soap and water or, if visibly soiled, clean and disinfect reusable facial protective wear between patients.

The two types of protective eyewear used during patient care are (1) glasses with protective side shields and (2) clear face shields.

Face Shields

A chin-length plastic face shield may be worn as an alternative to protective eyewear. However, a shield cannot replace a face

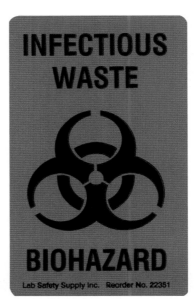

FIGURE 6-9 Containers of contaminated laundry must be labeled with the universal biohazard symbol.

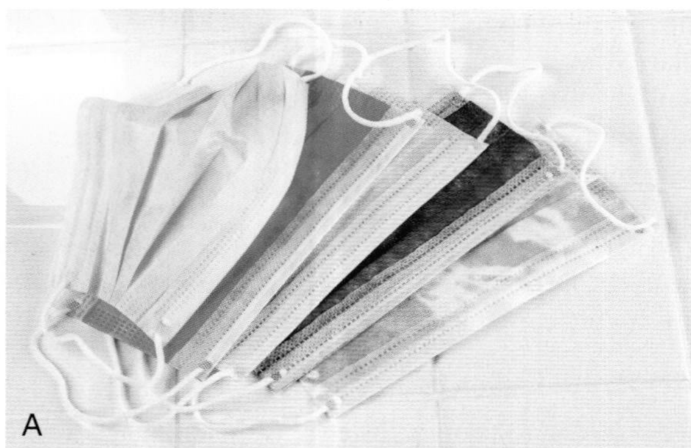

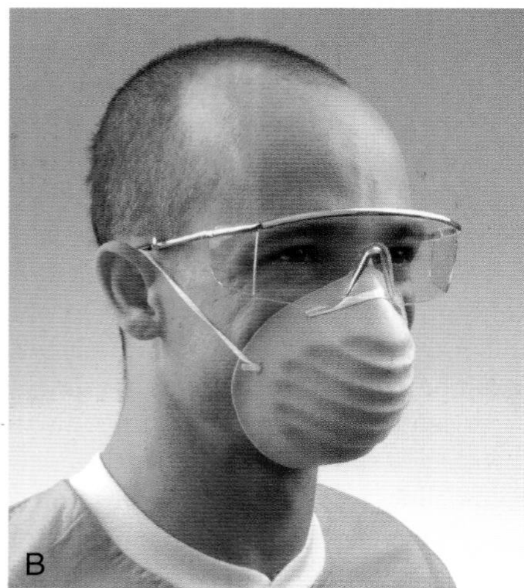

FIGURE 6-10 Types of face mask. **A,** Flat. **B,** Dome-shaped or molded. (**A,** Courtesy Practicon Dental, Greenville, North Carolina. **B,** Courtesy Crosstex International, Inc., Hauppauge, New York.)

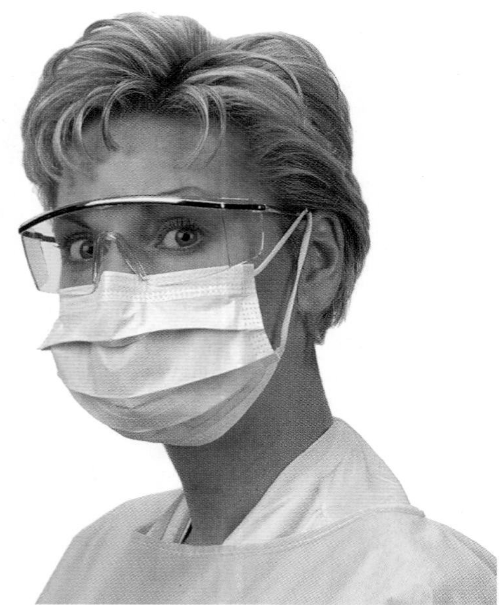

FIGURE 6-11 Face mask and safety glasses. (Courtesy Crosstex International, Inc., Hauppauge, New York.)

BOX 6-7 Guidelines for Using Protective Masks

- Change masks for every patient or more often, particularly if heavy spatter is generated during treatment or if the mask becomes damp.
- Handle masks ONLY by touching the side edges, and avoid contact with the more heavily contaminated body of the mask.
- Conform the mask to your face.
- Do not allow the mask to contact your mouth when being worn. The moisture will reduce the mask filtration efficiency. A damp or wet mask is not an efficient mask.
- Change your mask approximately once each hour during a long procedure.
- Remember, a face shield is not a substitute for a mask because it provides no protection from aerosols.
- Never wear your face mask below your nose or on your chin. The outer surface of the mask is highly contaminated.

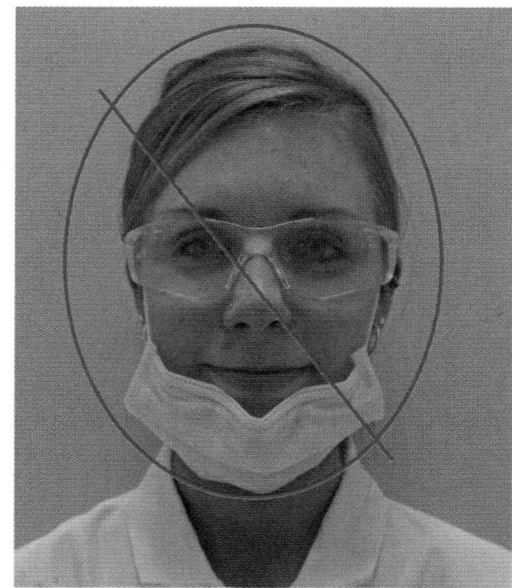

FIGURE 6-12 Face masks should never be worn below the nose or on the chin. (From Bird DL, Robinson DS: *Modern dental assisting*, ed 11, St. Louis, 2015, Saunders.)

mask because the shield does not protect against the inhalation of contaminated aerosols (Figure 6-13).

When splashing or spattering of blood or other body fluids is likely during a procedure such as surgery, a face shield is often worn in addition to a protective mask.

Patient Eyewear

Patients should be provided with protective eyewear because they may also be subject to eye damage from (1) handpiece spatter; (2) spilled or splashed dental materials, including caustic chemical agents; and (3) airborne bits of acrylic or tooth fragments (Figure 6-14).

When laser treatments are performed, patients must be supplied with special filtered-lens glasses.

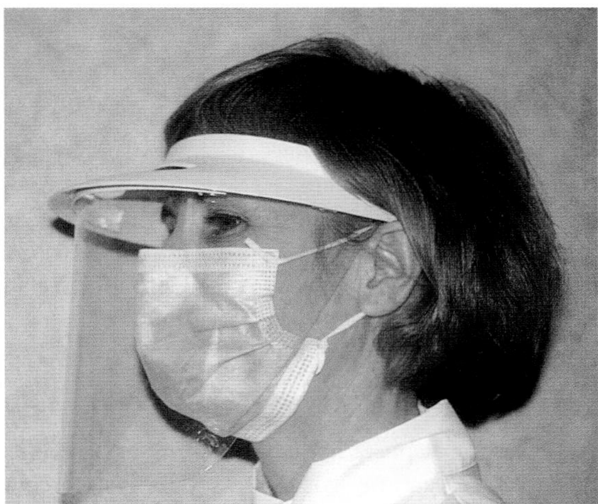

FIGURE 6-13 Face shields provide adequate eye protection, but a face mask is still required when assisting with aerosol-generating procedures.

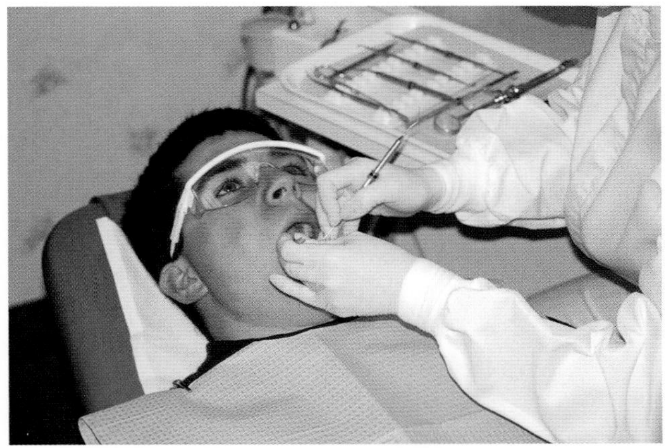

FIGURE 6-14 Protective eyewear should be provided to patients.

Gloves

The types of gloves used in a dental practice vary by the various types of procedures that are performed in the practice (Box 6-8).

Examination Gloves

Medical examination gloves are usually latex or vinyl and are often referred to as *exam gloves* or *procedure gloves.* These gloves are most frequently worn by dental personnel during patient care (Figure 6-15).

Examination gloves are inexpensive, available in a range of sizes from extra-small to extra-large, and fit either hand. These gloves are nonsterile and strictly serve as a protective barrier for the wearer.

Gloves Damaged during Treatment

Gloves are effective only when they are intact (not damaged, torn, ripped, or punctured). If gloves are damaged during treatment, then immediately change them and wash your hands before regloving. The procedure for regloving in this situation is as follows:

1. Excuse yourself, and leave the chairside.
2. Remove and discard the damaged gloves.
3. Thoroughly wash your hands.
4. Reglove before returning to the chairside to resume the dental procedure.

BOX 6-8 Types of Gloves in Dentistry

Patient Care Gloves

- Sterile latex surgical gloves
- Sterile neoprene surgical gloves*
- Sterile styrene surgical gloves*
- Sterile synthetic copolymer gloves*
- Sterile reduced-protein latex surgeon's gloves
- Latex examination gloves
- Vinyl examination gloves*
- Synthetic copolymer examination gloves*
- Nitrile examination gloves*
- Styrene-butadiene examination gloves*
- Polyurethane gloves*
- Powderless gloves
- Flavored gloves
- Low-protein gloves

Utility Gloves

- Heavy latex gloves
- Heavy nitrile gloves
- Thin copolymer gloves
- Thin plastic (food handler) gloves

Other Gloves

- Heat-resistant gloves
- Dermal (cotton) gloves

From Miller CH: *Infection control and management of hazardous materials for the dental team,* ed 5, St. Louis, 2014, Mosby.

*One should review the labeling or check with the manufacturer to confirm that these are latex-free gloves.

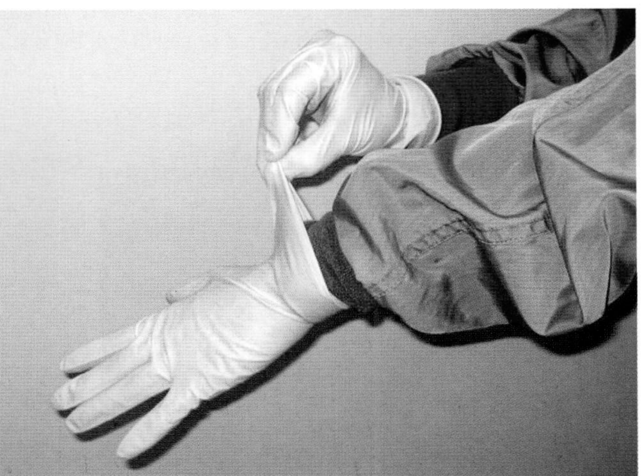

FIGURE 6-15 Nonsterile examination gloves. (Courtesy Crosstex International, Inc., Hauppauge, New York.)

If you leave the chairside for any reason during the treatment of a patient, then overgloves should be used. You must remove your contaminated examination gloves and wash your hands before you leave the chairside. When you return, you should wash and dry your hands and use fresh examination gloves.

Overgloves

Overgloves, also known as *food handler gloves*, are made of lightweight, inexpensive, clear plastic. They may be worn over contaminated treatment gloves (overgloving) to prevent contamination of clean objects handled during treatment (Figure 6-16).

Sterile Surgical Gloves

Sterile gloves, which are the type used in hospital surgical units, should be worn for invasive procedures involving the cutting of bone or significant amounts of blood or saliva, such as oral surgery or periodontal treatment.

Sterile gloves are supplied in prepackaged units to maintain sterility before use. They are provided in specific sizes and are fitted to the left or right hand.

Utility Gloves

Utility gloves are not used for direct patient care. Utility gloves are worn (1) when the treatment room is cleaned and disinfected between patients, (2) where contaminated instruments are being cleaned or handled, and (3) for surface cleaning and disinfecting (Figure 6-17). Utility gloves may be washed, disinfected, or sterilized and reused. Utility gloves must be discarded, however, when they become worn and no longer have the ability to provide barrier protection. After use, utility gloves must be considered contaminated and must be appropriately handled until they have been properly disinfected or sterilized. Each staff member responsible for cleanup procedures must have his or her own designated pair of utility gloves.

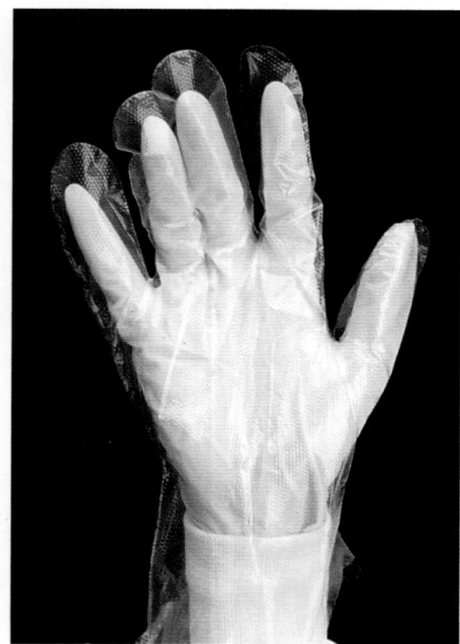

FIGURE 6-16 Overglove worn over a latex examination glove.

Non–Latex-Containing Gloves

Occasionally, health care providers or patients may experience serious allergic reactions to latex. The person who is sensitive to latex can wear gloves made from vinyl, nitrile, and other non–latex-containing materials (Figure 6-18). If you think you may be developing an allergy to latex, you should have a blood test to confirm the diagnosis.

Medical Waste Management

All waste must be disposed of according to applicable federal, state, and local regulations. Although the term **medical waste** is commonly used, more accurate terms are **contaminated waste** and **infectious waste** or **regulated waste**.

Classifications of Waste

Handling, storing, labeling, and disposing waste depend entirely on the type of waste. For example, when reprocessing a

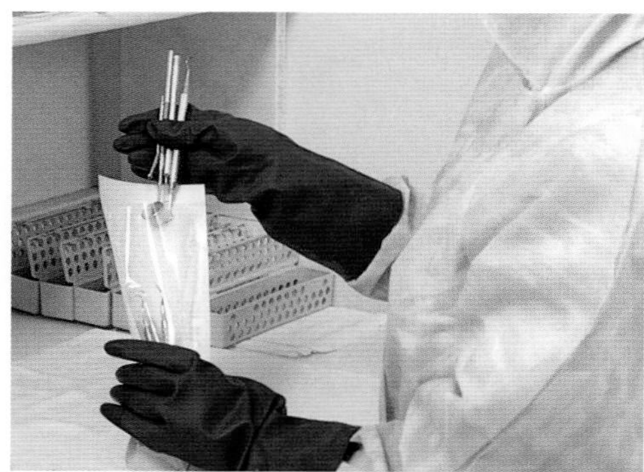

FIGURE 6-17 Utility gloves are used when preparing instruments for sterilization.

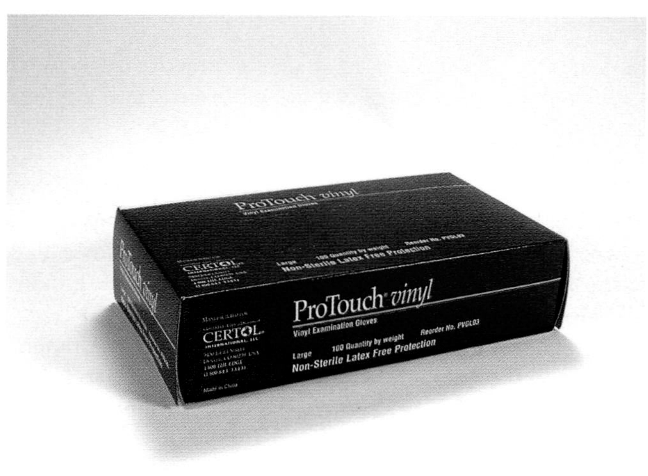

FIGURE 6-18 Latex-free vinyl gloves. (Courtesy Certol International, Commerce City, Colorado.)

TABLE 6-2
Classification of Waste

Type	Examples	Handling Requirements
General waste	Paper towels, paper mixing pads, empty food containers	Discard in covered containers made of durable materials, such as plastic or metal.
Hazardous waste	Waste that presents a danger to humans or the environment (e.g., toxic chemicals)	Follow your specific state and local regulations.
Contaminated waste	Waste that has been in contact with blood or other body fluids (e.g., used barriers, patient napkins)	In most states, contaminated waste is disposed of with the general waste.
Infectious or regulated waste (biohazard)	Waste that is capable of transmitting an infectious disease	Follow your specific state and local regulations. Containers for all three types of infectious waste must be labeled with the biohazard label.
1. Blood and blood-soaked materials	Blood or saliva that can be squeezed out, or dried blood that may flake off of an item	Follow your specific state and local regulations.
2. Pathologic waste	Soft tissue and extracted teeth	Follow your specific state and local regulations. Never dispose of extracted teeth with amalgam restorations with waste that will be incinerated.
3. Sharps	Contaminated needles, scalpel blades, orthodontic wires, endodontic instruments (e.g., reamers files)	Containers should be closeable, leakproof, and puncture resistant. Containers should be color coded red and marked with the biohazard symbol. Sharps containers should be located as close as possible to the work area.

treatment room, the waste should be separated into different containers. You must understand the types of waste to know what goes into which container (Table 6-2).

OSHA's Hazard Communication Standard

OSHA issued the Hazard Communication Standard (HCS) to require employers to inform their employees about the identity and hazards of chemicals that they use in the workplace. The HCS, also known as the "Employee Right-to-Know Law," requires employers to implement a hazard communication program.

Revision of the Hazard Communication Standard

In 2012, OSHA revised the HCS and adopted the Globally Harmonized System (GHS) of Classification and Labeling of Chemicals (Figure 6-19). Although most of the standard remains unchanged, some modifications to the terminology have been made. For example, the term *hazard determination* has been changed to hazard classification, and *material safety data sheet* has been changed to safety data sheet.

Under the new international system, each chemical will be classified and labeled the same, regardless of where in the global market the chemical is manufactured or used, thus ending confusion and eliminating the need for different labels.

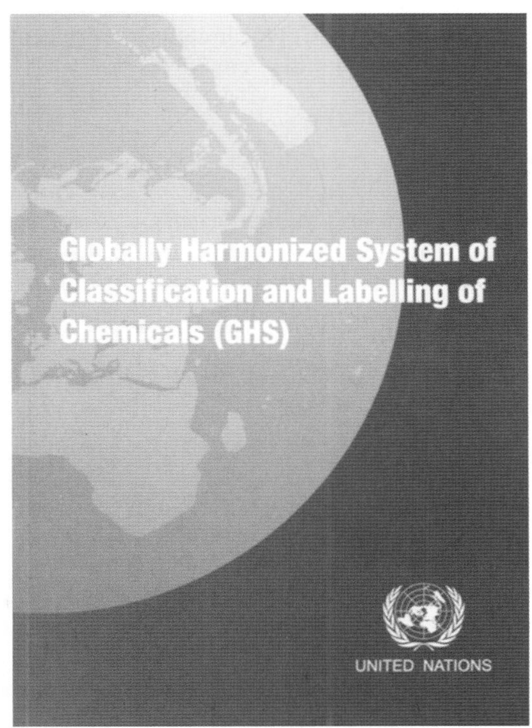

FIGURE 6-19 Globally Harmonized System of Classification and Labeling of Chemicals. (From https://www.osha.gov/dsg/hazcom/global.html. Accessed April 26, 2013.)

The three major areas of change are in **hazard classification**, **labels**, and safety data sheets (SDSs).

The revised HCS will still require chemical manufacturers and importers to evaluate the chemicals they produce or import and provide hazard information to employers and workers by applying specific labels on containers and preparing SDSs. The new system is being implemented throughout the world by countries including Canada, the European Union, China, Australia, and Japan.

Hazard Communication Standard

The hazard communication program has the following five parts:

1. Written program
2. Chemical inventory
3. Safety data sheets (SDSs)
4. Labeling
5. Employee training

Written Program

The written program must identify, by name, all employees in the office who are exposed to hazardous chemicals. It must also identify the individual who is responsible for the program. The program describes (1) staff training; (2) how chemicals are handled in the office, including all labeling and safety measures; and (3) how to respond to chemical emergencies, such as spills or exposures.

If several dentists are working in one clinic or practice, then all employers must be aware of the hazards and protective measures so that they can train their employees.

Chemical Inventory

The chemical inventory is a list of every product used in the office that contains chemicals and includes amalgam, composites, bonding materials, etching agents, disinfectants, and impression materials, among others. Each time a new product containing any chemical is brought into the office, it must be added to the chemical inventory list. The dentist will often appoint the dental assistant to be the program coordinator and to be responsible for maintaining the chemical inventory and updating the SDS file.

Safety Data Sheet

In the revised HCS, **SDSs** have replaced Material Safety Data Sheets (MSDSs). The SDSs contain health and safety information about every product in the office that contains chemicals. The SDSs provide comprehensive technical information and are a resource for employees working with chemicals. They describe the physical and chemical properties of a chemical, its health hazards, routes of exposure, and precautions for safe handling and use, as well as emergency and first-aid procedures and spill control measures.

The manufacturer of a product that contains chemicals is required to supply the dental office with an SDS for the product. However, the program coordinator for dental office is responsible for ensuring that the office has an SDS for every chemical used. An SDS is often enclosed in the package with the product. SDSs should be organized in binders, providing employees ready access to be able to locate a particular SDS easily. The SDS now has a specified 16-section format (Table 6-3).

Labeling

As of June 1, 2015, all labels will be required to have a harmonized signal word, pictogram, and hazard statement for each hazard class and category (Figure 6-20).

When a chemical is transferred to a different container, the new container must also be labeled. For example, when a concentrated chemical disinfectant is mixed fresh and placed into a spray bottle or tub (secondary containers), the spray bottle or tub must be labeled. Other examples of secondary containers that hold chemicals and require labeling are automatic x-ray film processors and manual processing tanks, ultrasonic cleaning tanks, and chemical vapor sterilizers.

Hazard Classification

Specific criteria for hazards have been developed, and chemicals are classified into categories that compare hazard severity within a hazard class. Once a chemical is classified, warnings are automatically assigned so that each chemical in the same category will have the same label requirements and language. This consistency will help ensure that evaluations of the hazardous effects are consistent for all manufacturers and that labels and SDSs are also consistent.

The two most important considerations are that (1) OSHA HCS labels are used, and (2) all employees are properly trained to understand and read the label.

Employee Training

Employee training is essential for a successful hazard communication program. Staff training is required (1) when a new employee is hired, (2) when a new chemical product is added to the office, and (3) once a year for all continuing employees. Records of each training session must be kept on file for at least 5 years.

Although the dentist is responsible for providing the training, the dental assistant is responsible for routinely following safety precautions.

Outline for Hazard Communication Training Program*

1. Requirements of the Hazard Communication Standard (HCS)
2. Written communication plan for the office (e.g., location, use)
3. Understanding of the hazards of the chemicals with which the employees work
4. Ability to interpret warning labels and safety data sheets (SDSs)

*On completion, employees are asked to sign a training record that will remain in the personnel file.

TABLE 6-3
Sections of Hazard Communication Safety Data Sheets

The Hazard Communication Standard (HCS) requires chemical manufacturers, distributors, or importers to provide Safety Data Sheets (SDSs) (formerly known as Material Safety Data Sheets or MSDSs) to communicate the hazards of hazardous chemical products. As of June 1, 2015, the HCS will require all new SDSs to be in a uniform format and include the section numbers, the headings, and associated information under the headings below:

Section	Description	Explanation
1	Identification	Includes product identifier; manufacturer or distributor name, address, and telephone number; emergency telephone number; recommended use; and restrictions on use.
2	Hazard(s) identification	Includes all hazards regarding the chemical and required label elements.
3	Composition and information on ingredients	Includes information on chemical ingredients and trade secret claims.
4	First-aid measures	Includes important symptoms and effects, acute and delayed effects, and required treatment(s).
5	Fire-fighting measures	Lists suitable extinguishing techniques and equipment and chemical hazards from fire.
6	Accidental release measures	Lists emergency procedures, protective equipment, and proper methods of containment and cleanup.
7	Handling and storage	Lists precautions for safe handling and storage, including incompatibilities.
8	Exposure controls and personal protection	Lists OSHA's permissible exposure limits (PELs), threshold limit values (TLVs), appropriate engineering controls, and personal protective equipment (PPE).
9	Physical and chemical properties	Lists the chemical's characteristics.
10	Stability and reactivity	Lists chemical stability and possibility of hazardous reactions.
11	Toxicologic information	Includes routes of exposure; related symptoms and acute and chronic effects; and numerical measures of toxicity.
12	Ecologic information*	
13	Disposal considerations*	
14	Transport information*	
15	Regulatory information*	
16	Other information	Includes the date of preparation or the date of the last revision.

*Since other agencies regulate this information, OSHA will not be enforcing Sections 12 through 15(29 CFR 1910.1200(g)(2)).
For more information: www.osha.gov; (800) 321-OSHA (6742); U.S. Department of Labor.

Responsibilities of the Dental Assistant as Coordinator of the Hazard Communication Program

- Read and understand OSHA's Hazard Communication Standard (HCS).
- Implement the written hazard communication program.
- Compile a list (chemical inventory) of products in the office that contain hazardous chemicals.
- Obtain safety data sheets (SDSs).
- Update the SDS file as new products are added to the office inventory.
- Inform other employees of the location of the SDSs.
- Label appropriate containers.
- Provide training to other employees.

OSHA, Occupational Safety & Health Administration.

Exemptions to Labeling Requirements

Certain chemicals are exempted from the standard, including tobacco and tobacco products, wood and wood products, food, drugs, cosmetics, and alcoholic beverages sold and packaged for consumer use. Drugs dispensed by a pharmacy to a health care provider for direct administration to a patient also are exempt from the labeling requirement, as are over-the-counter drugs, such as aspirin and first-aid supplies, and drugs intended for personal consumption by employees while in the workplace.

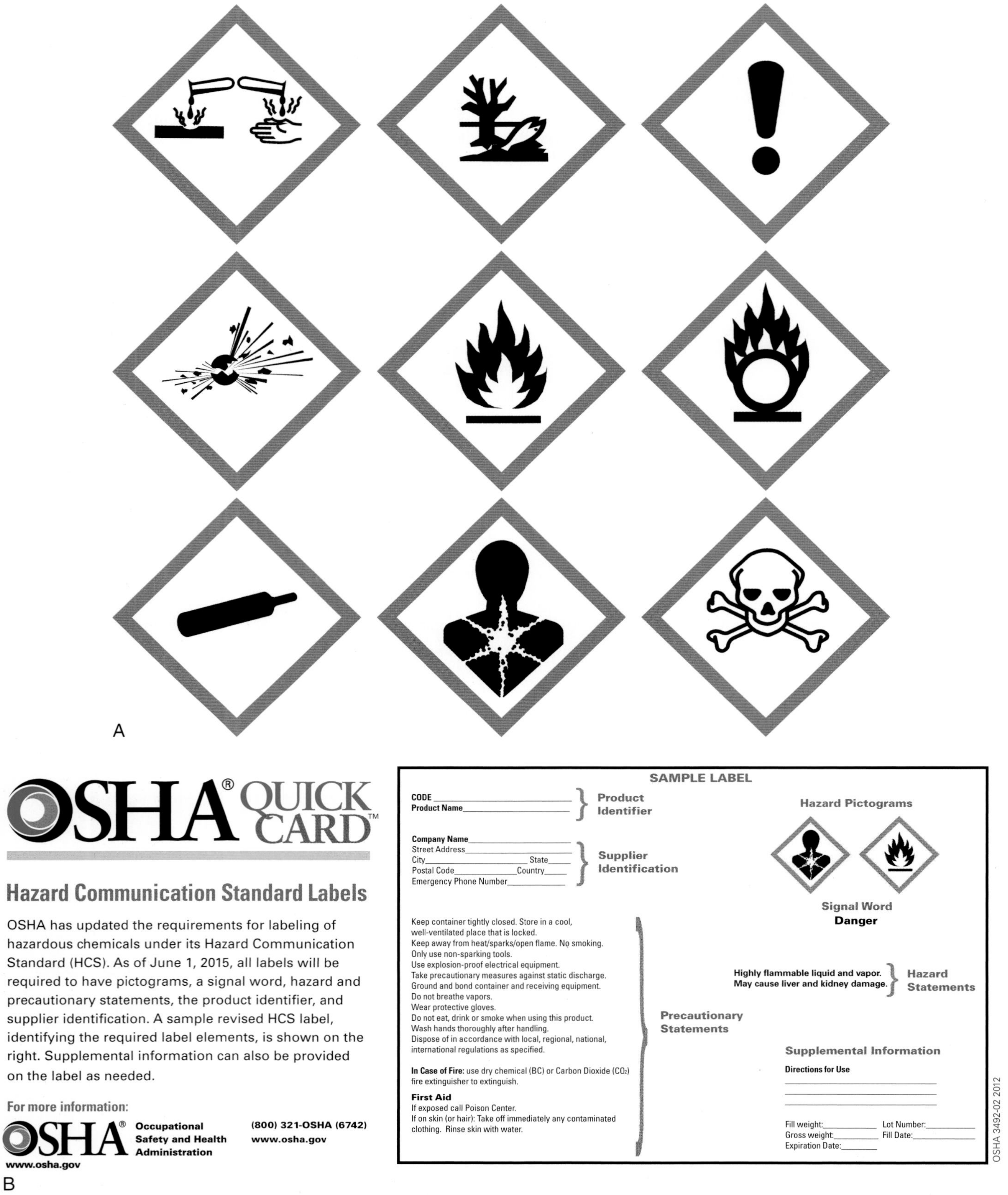

A

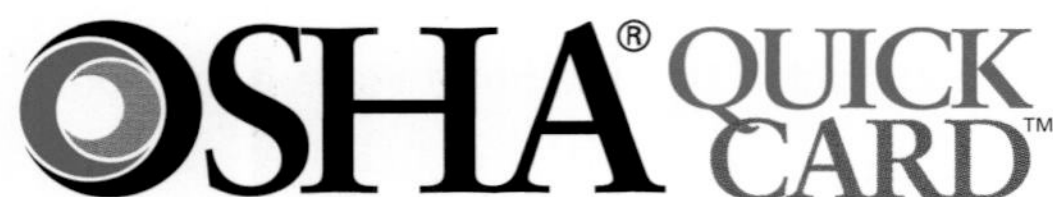

Hazard Communication Standard Labels

OSHA has updated the requirements for labeling of hazardous chemicals under its Hazard Communication Standard (HCS). As of June 1, 2015, all labels will be required to have pictograms, a signal word, hazard and precautionary statements, the product identifier, and supplier identification. A sample revised HCS label, identifying the required label elements, is shown on the right. Supplemental information can also be provided on the label as needed.

For more information:

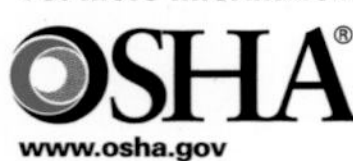

Occupational Safety and Health Administration

(800) 321-OSHA (6742)
www.osha.gov

SAMPLE LABEL

CODE________________
Product Name________________ } **Product Identifier**

Company Name________________
Street Address________________
City________________ State____
Postal Code________________ Country____
Emergency Phone Number________________ } **Supplier Identification**

Hazard Pictograms

Signal Word
Danger

Highly flammable liquid and vapor.
May cause liver and kidney damage. } **Hazard Statements**

Keep container tightly closed. Store in a cool, well-ventilated place that is locked.
Keep away from heat/sparks/open flame. No smoking.
Only use non-sparking tools.
Use explosion-proof electrical equipment.
Take precautionary measures against static discharge.
Ground and bond container and receiving equipment.
Do not breathe vapors.
Wear protective gloves.
Do not eat, drink or smoke when using this product.
Wash hands thoroughly after handling.
Dispose of in accordance with local, regional, national, international regulations as specified.

In Case of Fire: use dry chemical (BC) or Carbon Dioxide (CO_2) fire extinguisher to extinguish.

First Aid
If exposed call Poison Center.
If on skin (or hair): Take off immediately any contaminated clothing. Rinse skin with water. } **Precautionary Statements**

Supplemental Information

Directions for Use

____
____
____

Fill weight:________ Lot Number:________
Gross weight:________ Fill Date:________
Expiration Date:________

OSHA 3492-02 2012

B

FIGURE 6-20 **A,** Hazard Communication Standard (HCS) pictograms. **B,** Sample label. (From http://www.osha.gov/dsg/hazcom/standards.html. Accessed April 26, 2013.)

Guidelines for Minimizing Exposure to Chemical Hazards in the Dental Office

- Keep a minimum of hazardous chemicals in the office.
- Read the labels, and use only as directed.
- Store each chemical according to the manufacturer's directions.
- Keep containers tightly covered.
- Avoid mixing chemicals unless consequences are known.
- Wear appropriate personal protective equipment (PPE) when handling hazardous substances.
- Immediately wash hands after removing gloves.
- Avoid skin contact with chemicals; immediately wash skin that has come in contact with chemicals.
- Maintain good ventilation.
- Do not eat, drink, smoke, apply lip balm, or insert contact lenses in areas in which chemicals are used.
- Keep chemicals away from open flames and heat sources.
- Always have an operational fire extinguisher on hand.
- Know and use proper cleanup procedures.
- Keep neutralizing agents available for strong acid and alkaline solutions.
- Dispose of all hazardous chemicals according to safety data sheet (SDS) instructions.

Ethical Implications

Infection control and management of **hazardous waste** can present legal and ethical issues for dental assistants. Taking shortcuts can lead to the transmission of disease or accidents. Always following proper infection control and chemical management procedures is a matter of personal commitment and integrity.

Patients should have absolute confidence that infection control procedures followed in the office are never compromised. This confidence is as important for the protection of the dental team as it is for the patient.

Procedure 6-1

First Aid After an Exposure Incident

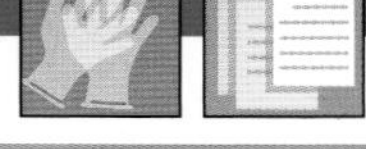

Goal

To perform appropriate first aid after an exposure incident

Equipment and Supplies

- Soap and water
- Paper towels
- Antiseptic cream or ointment
- Adhesive bandage
- Exposure incident report form

Procedural Steps

Immediately stop operations.

1. Remove your gloves.
2. Thoroughly wash your hands using antimicrobial soap and warm water.
3. Dry your hands.
4. Apply a small amount of antiseptic to the affected area.

Note: Do not apply caustic agents, such as bleach or disinfectant solutions, to the wound.

5. Apply an adhesive bandage to the area.
6. Complete applicable postexposure follow-up paperwork.

Note: The employer should be immediately notified of the injury after initial first aid is provided.

Procedure 6-2

Handwashing Before Gloving

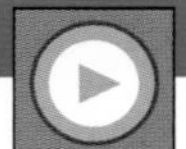

Goal

To wash hands properly before gloving

Equipment and Supplies

- Sink with running water
- Liquid soap in a dispenser
- Nailbrush or orange stick
- Paper towels in a dispenser

Procedural Steps

1. Remove all jewelry, including watch and rings.

Purpose: Jewelry is difficult to clean, can harbor microbes, and can puncture the gloves.

2. Use the foot or electronic control to regulate water flow. If this is not available, then use a paper towel to grasp the faucets to turn them on and off. Discard the towel after use. Allow your hands to become wet.

Purpose: Faucets may have been contaminated by being touched with soiled or contaminated hands.

3. Apply soap; lather using a circular motion with friction while holding your fingertips downward. Rub well between your fingers. If this is the first handwashing of the day, then use a nailbrush or an orange stick. Inspect and clean under every fingernail during this step.

Purpose: Friction removes soil and contaminants from your hands and wrists.

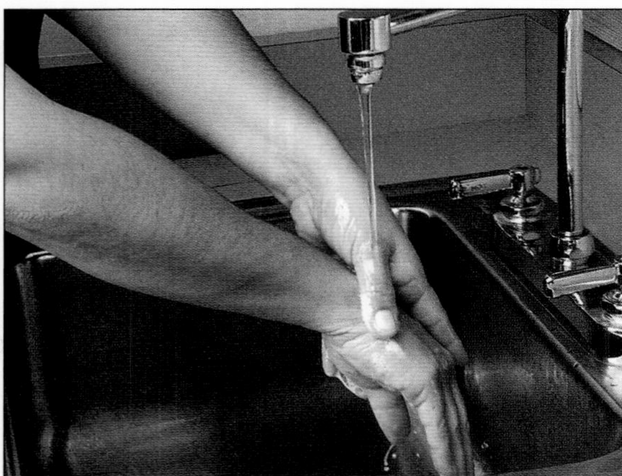

4. Vigorously rub the lathered hands together under a stream of water to remove surface debris.

Purpose: Scrubbing the first time removes gross debris.

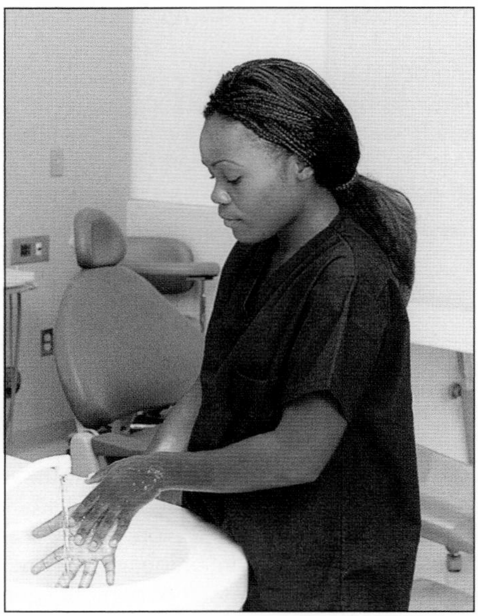

5. Apply more soap, and vigorously rub the lathered hands together for a minimum of 10 seconds under a stream of water.

Purpose: Secondary scrubbing removes residual debris and tenacious microorganisms, which thrive under the free edges of the fingernails.

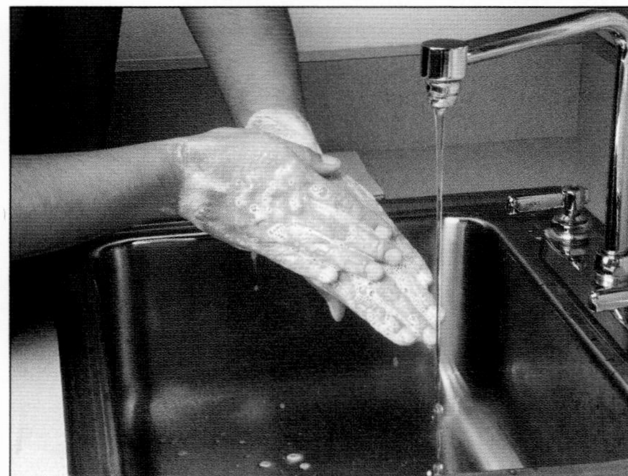

Procedure 6-2

Handwashing Before Gloving—cont'd

6. Rinse the hands with cool water.

Purpose: Cool water closes the pores.

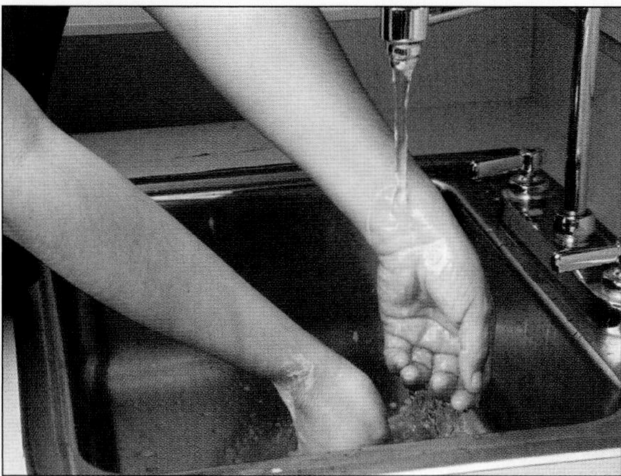

7. Use a paper towel to dry the hands thoroughly, and then dry the forearms.

Purpose: Reusable cloth towels remain moist, contribute to microbial growth, and spread contamination.

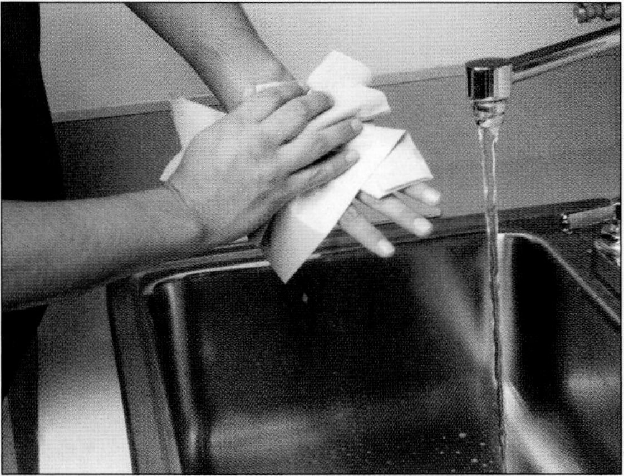

8. If water faucets are not foot operated, turn off the faucet with a clean paper towel.

Purpose: The faucet is dirty and will contaminate your clean hands.

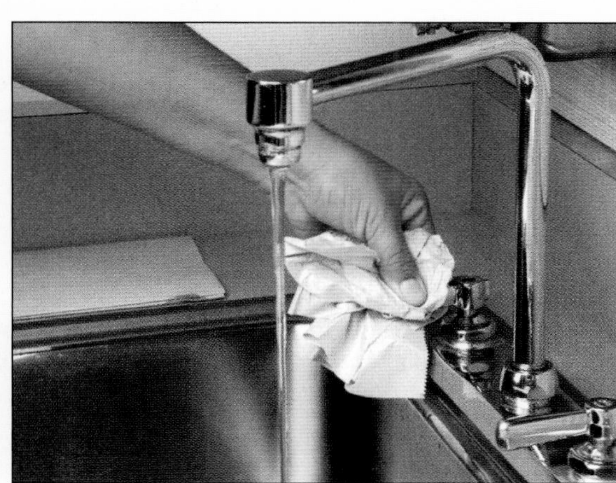

Illustrations from Proctor DB, Adams AP: *Kinn's the medical assistant: an applied learning approach*, ed 12, St. Louis, 2014, Saunders.

Procedure 6-3

Applying Alcohol-Based Hand Rubs

Goal

To apply an alcohol-based hand rub

Equipment and Supplies

- Alcohol-based hand rub (60% to 95% concentration)

Procedural Steps

1. Check your hands to be sure they are not visibly soiled or contaminated with organic matter, such as blood or saliva. If necessary, wash your hands with soap and water and dry them thoroughly.

Purpose: Alcohol-based hand rubs are not effective in the presence of organic matter.

2. Carefully read directions to determine the proper amount to dispense.

Purpose: These products are dose sensitive. If you use a smaller amount than is recommended, then their effectiveness will be seriously decreased.

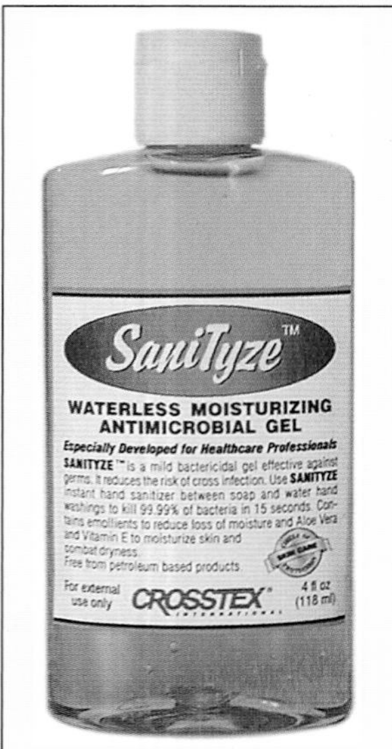

(Courtesy Crosstex International, Inc., Hauppauge, New York.)

3. Dispense the proper amount of the product into the palm of one hand.

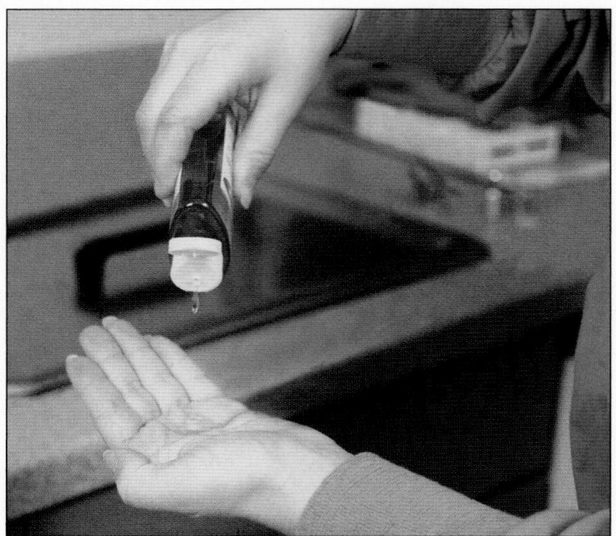

4. Rub the palms of your hands together.

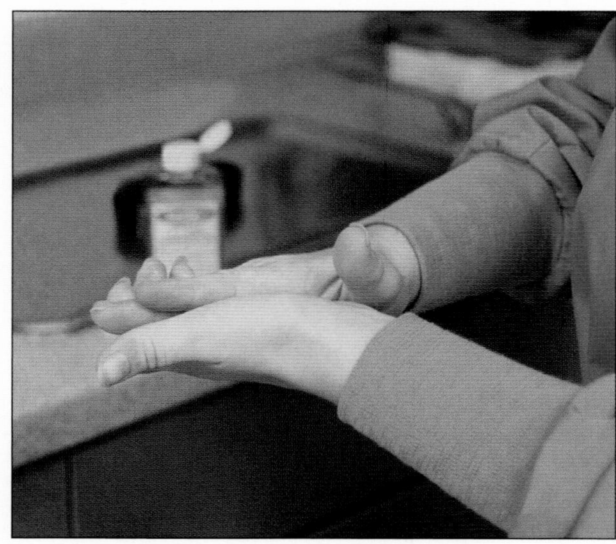

Procedure 6-3

Applying Alcohol-Based Hand Rubs—cont'd

5. Rub the product between your fingers.

Purpose: Thoroughly covering both of your hands is important.

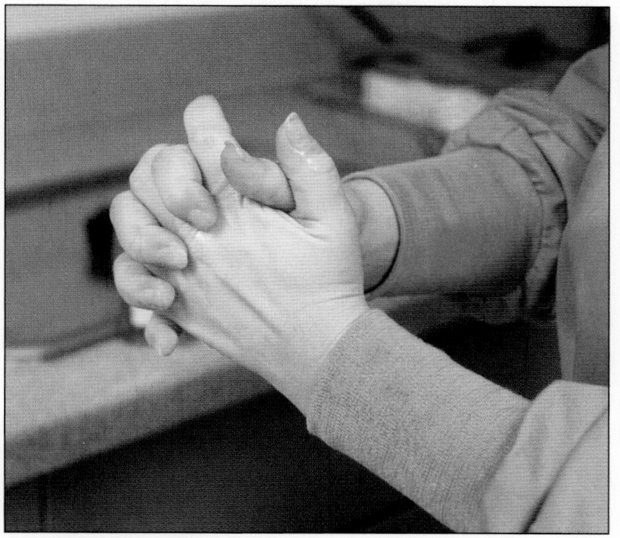

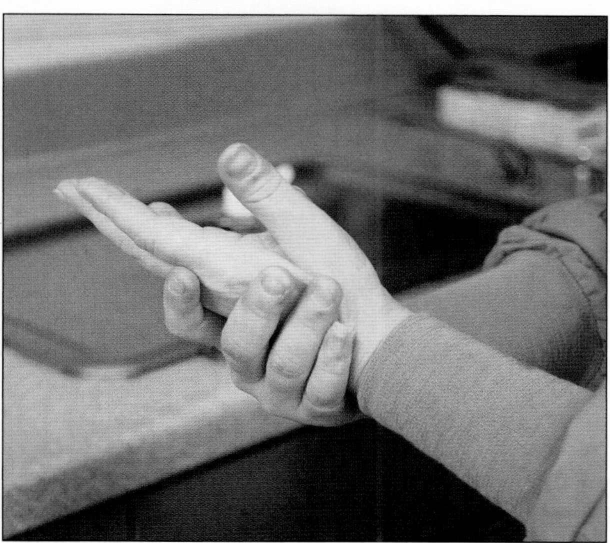

6. Rub the product over the backs of your hands.

Procedure 6-4

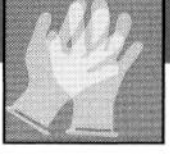

Putting on Personal Protective Equipment (PPE)

Goal

To put on PPE before patient care

Equipment and Supplies

- Protective clothing
- Surgical mask
- Protective eyewear
- Gloves

Procedural Steps

1. Put your protective clothing over your uniform, street clothes, or scrubs.

Note: Protective clothing can be long-sleeved laboratory coats, clinic jackets, or gowns.

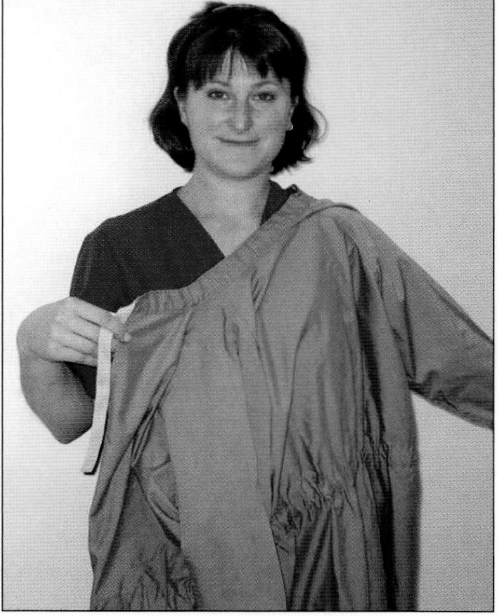

Continued

Procedure 6-4

Putting on Personal Protective Equipment (PPE)—cont'd

2. Put on your surgical mask, and adjust the fit.

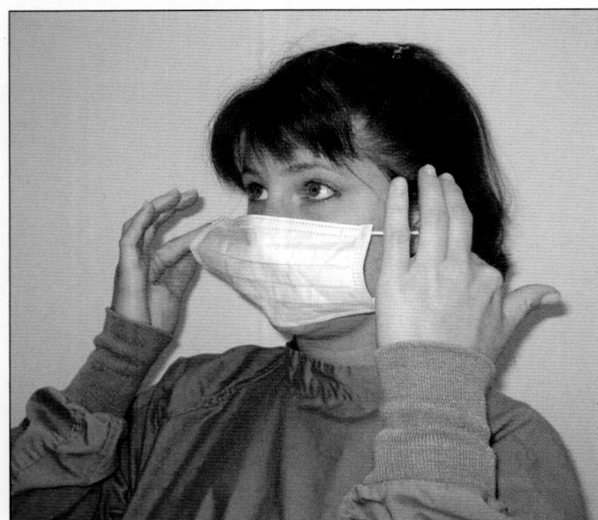

3. Put on your protective eyewear.

Note: Eyewear should be impact resistant and have side protection. Goggles or face shields are also acceptable.

4. Thoroughly wash and dry your hands.

Note: If your hands are not visibly soiled, then you may use an alcohol-based hand rub.

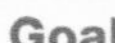

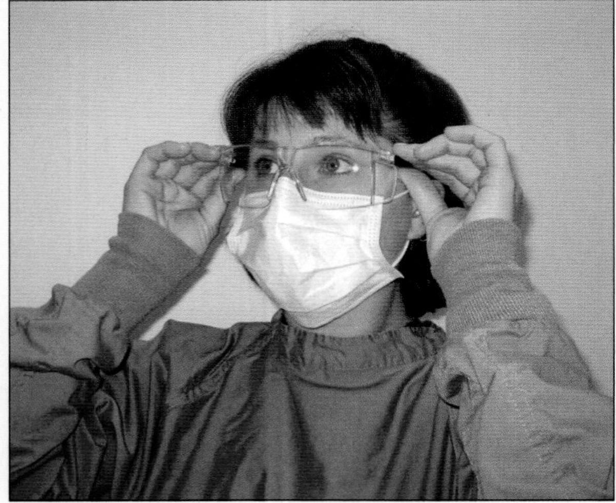

5. Hold one glove at the cuff, place your opposite hand inside the glove, and pull it onto your hand. Repeat with a new glove for your other hand.

Important Note: Regarding the sequence of putting on PPE, putting on the gloves last to avoid contaminating them before your hands are placed in the patient's mouth is the most important step.

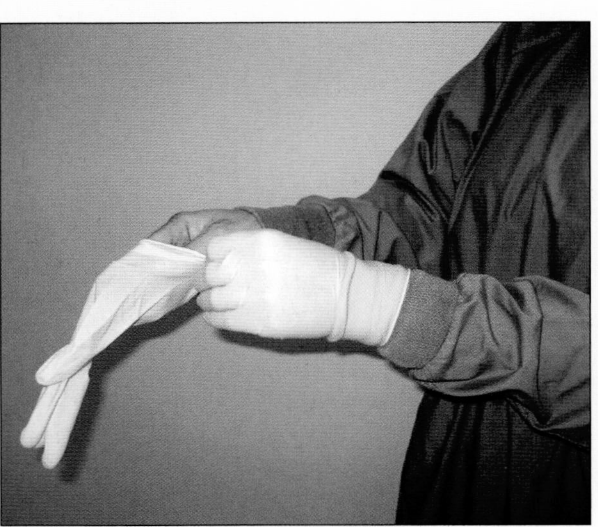

Modified from Organization for Safety Asepsis and Prevention: *Policy to practice: OSAP's guide to the guidelines*, Annapolis, Md, 2004, OSAP.

Procedure 6-5

Removing Personal Protective Equipment

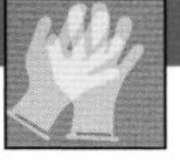

Goal

To remove personal protective wear

Equipment and Supplies

- Protective clothing
- Surgical mask
- Protective eyewear
- Gloves

Procedural Steps

1. Use your gloved hand to grasp the other glove at the outside cuff. Pull downward, turning the glove inside out as it pulls away from your hand.
2. For the other hand, use your ungloved fingers to grasp the inside (uncontaminated area) of the cuff of the remaining glove. Pull downward to remove the glove, turning it inside out. Discard the gloves into the waste receptacle.

Procedure 6-5

Removing Personal Protective Equipment—cont'd

3. Wash and thoroughly dry your hands.

Note: **If no visible contamination exists and if the gloves have not been torn or punctured during the procedure, then you may use an alcohol-based hand rub in place of handwashing. However, if your hands are damp from perspiration or have glove powder, then you may prefer to wash them with antimicrobial soap and water.**

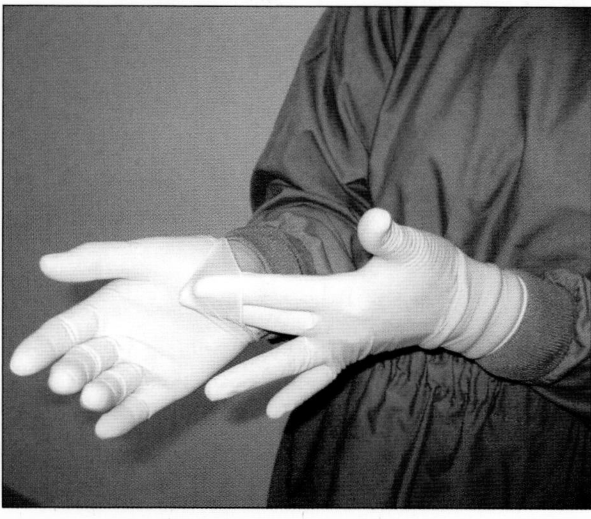

Eyewear

1. Remove eyewear by touching it only on the ear rests (which are not contaminated).
2. Place the eyewear on a disposable towel until it can be properly cleaned and disinfected.

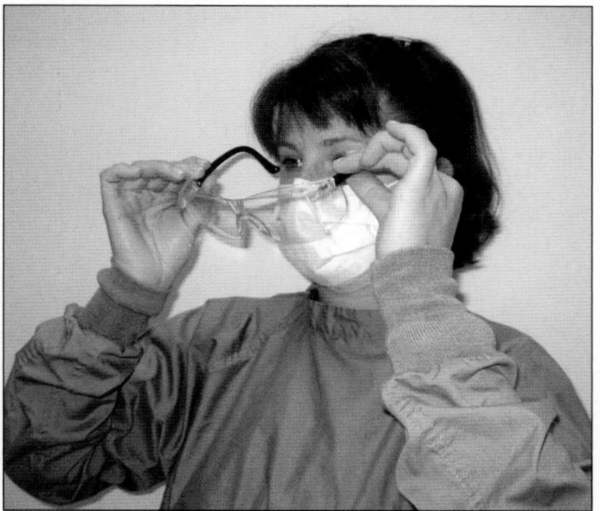

Masks

1. Slide the fingers of each hand under the elastic strap in front of your ears, and remove the mask. Discard the mask into the waste receptacle.

Note: **Be sure your fingers contact only the mask's ties or elastic strap.**

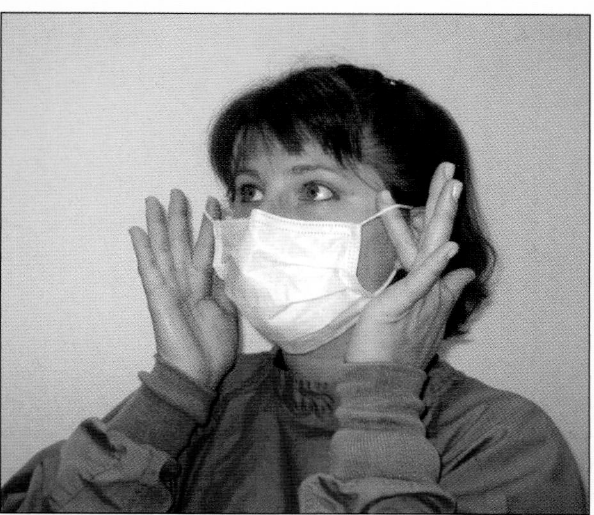

Protective Clothing

1. Pull the gown off, turning it inside out as it comes off.

Note: **Be careful not to allow the gown to touch underlying clothes or skin.**

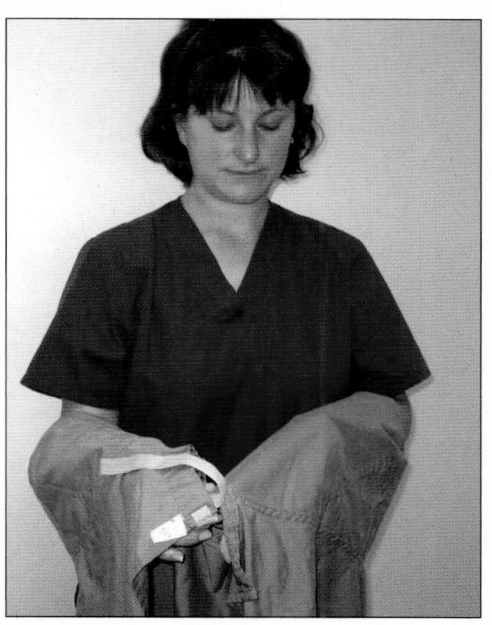

Modified from Organization for Safety Asepsis and Prevention: *Policy to practice: OSAP's guide to the guidelines*, Annapolis, Md, 2004, OSAP.

Chapter Exercises

Multiple Choice

Circle the letter next to the correct answer.

1. The goal of an infection control program is to prevent disease transmission to the __________.
   a. patient from the staff
   b. staff from the patient
   c. patient from another patient
   d. a, b, and c

2. Which of the following could result in a percutaneous injury?
   a. Splash to the eyes
   b. Cut from an instrument
   c. Splash to the mouth
   d. Needlestick
   e. b and d

3. As a dental assistant, when should you wash your hands?
   a. Before you glove
   b. After you remove your gloves
   c. Both before and after wearing your gloves

4. Which of the following are considered PPE?
   a. Protective clothing
   b. Mask
   c. Eyewear or chin-length face shield
   d. Disposable gloves
   e. All of the above

5. Which of the following statements is *NOT* true regarding the use of face masks?
   a. They should be changed between patients.
   b. They should be changed if they become damp.
   c. The inside of the mask should contact your mouth while being worn.
   d. The mask should conform to your face.

6. Which type of glove should be used when cleaning and disinfecting the treatment room?
   a. Latex examination gloves
   b. Vinyl overgloves
   c. Sterile surgical gloves
   d. Utility gloves

7. Safety data sheets (SDSs) should be supplied by the __________.
   a. manufacturer of the material
   b. sales person
   c. delivery person
   d. all of the above

8. Which of the following items are exempt from the chemical labeling laws?
   a. Tobacco and tobacco products
   b. Foods
   c. Cosmetics and drugs for employees' personal use in the workplace
   d. All of the above

9. Wearing jewelry under latex gloves is considered a safe practice.
   a. True
   b. False

10. Waste that presents a danger to humans or the environment (e.g., toxic chemicals) is classified as __________ waste.
   a. general
   b. hazardous
   c. contaminated
   d. pathologic

Apply Your Knowledge

1. While preparing instruments for sterilization, you accidentally stick the palm of your hand with a contaminated surgical instrument. What would you do for postexposure follow-up?

2. During Miss Parish's first visit to your office, she asks you why everyone is wearing such "elaborate garb" as masks and gloves. She seems annoyed and tells you that her previous dentist knew she did not have any disease and that he did not feel that gloves were necessary. How do you handle this situation?

3. Pamela Leong is a new employee hired to work at the front desk and, on occasion, clean up an operatory or process instruments. However, Pamela has not had formal dental assisting training. According to the OSHA BBP Standard, what would be her category of risk?

4. If you are working as a dental assistant and accidentally spill a chemical used for cleaning instruments, where would you be able to find information on how to clean up and dispose of that chemical?

CHAPTER 7

Surface Disinfection and Treatment Room Preparation

http://evolve.elsevier.com/Robinson/essentials/

LEARNING OBJECTIVES

1. Pronounce, define, and spell the key terms.
2. Discuss surface barriers, as well as demonstrate placing and removing surface barriers.
3. Complete the following related to precleaning and disinfection:
   - Perform treatment room cleaning and disinfection.
   - Describe the process of precleaning.
   - Discuss disinfection and list the levels, characteristics, and types of disinfectants.
   - Name the governmental agency that is responsible for registering disinfectants and sterilants.
   - Discuss several considerations when selecting a surface disinfectant.
4. Describe the classifications of instruments, equipment, and surfaces that are used to determine the type of posttreatment processing.
5. Discuss additional aseptic techniques that can be used to reduce the spread of microorganisms in the dental office.
6. Demonstrate cleaning and disinfection of the laboratory area, including how to disinfect an alginate impression.
7. Discuss cleaning and disinfection of the radiology area.

KEY TERMS

alcohol
antiseptic
bioburden
biofilm
chlorine dioxide
critical instruments
disinfection
glutaraldehyde
iodophors
noncritical instruments
ortho-phthalaldehyde (OPA)
precleaning
semicritical instruments
sodium hypochlorite
surface barriers
synthetic phenol

During patient treatment, the equipment and treatment room surfaces become contaminated with saliva or by aerosol containing blood and/or saliva. A primary source of contamination occurs when a member of the dental team touches surfaces with contaminated gloves. Although no cases of cross-infection have been linked to dental treatment room surfaces, cleaning and disinfecting these surfaces are important components in an effective infection control program. In addition, the Occupational Safety & Health Administration (OSHA) Bloodborne Pathogens (BBP) Standard requires that contaminated work surfaces be disinfected between patient visits. Two methods are used to deal with surface contamination. One method is to prevent the surface from becoming contaminated by using a surface barrier. The second method is to preclean and disinfect the surface between patients. Advantages and disadvantages of both methods are known, and most dental offices use a combination of the two methods (Table 7-1).

Surface Barriers

Surface barriers are used to prevent contamination on the surface and will not need to be cleaned and disinfected between patients.

Types of Surface Barriers

A wide variety of surface barriers are available today. All should be resistant to fluids to keep microorganisms in saliva, blood, and other liquids from soaking through to contact the surface

TABLE 7-1
Comparison of Surface Barriers versus Precleaning and Disinfection

	Advantages	Disadvantages
Surface barrier	Protects surfaces that are not easily cleaned and disinfected. Prevents contamination when properly placed. Is less time-consuming. Reduces handling and storage of chemicals. Provides patient with visual assurance of cleanliness. Does not damage equipment or surfaces.	Adds plastics to the environment after disposal. May be more expensive than precleaning and disinfecting. Requires a variety of sizes and shapes. May become dislodged during treatment.
Precleaning and disinfecting	May be less expensive than surface barriers. Does not add plastic to the environment. Some dentists do not like the appearance of plastic barriers.	Requires more time; therefore cleaning and disinfecting are sometimes not properly performed. Not all surfaces can be adequately precleaned. Over time, some chemicals are destructive to dental equipment surfaces. Chemical containers must be properly labeled, and safety data sheets must be on file in the office. No method is available to determine whether the microbes have been removed or killed. Some disinfectants must be prepared fresh daily. Chemicals are added to the environment upon disposal.

underneath. Some plastic bags are especially designed to fit the shape of items, such as the dental chair, an air-water syringe, hoses, pens, and light handles, among other items. Plastic barrier sticky tape is frequently used to protect smooth electrical surfaces, such as touch pads on equipment or electrical switches on chairs or x-ray equipment. Aluminum foil can also be used because it is easily formed around any shape (Figures 7-1 to 7-3).

See Procedure 7-1: Placing and Removing Surface Barriers.

Precleaning and Disinfection

Precleaning and disinfecting techniques are most effective when used on smooth and easily accessible contaminated treatment room surfaces (Figure 7-4). Always wear your utility gloves, mask, protective eyewear, and protective clothing when precleaning and disinfecting.

See Procedure 7-2: Performing Treatment Room Cleaning and Disinfection.

Surfaces Typically Protected With Barriers*

Headrest on dental chair
Control button on dental chair
Light handles
Light switches
Evacuator hoses and controls
X-ray control switches
Air-water syringe handles
Dental unit control touch pads
Patient mirror handles
Handle on light-curing device
Switch on amalgamators or other automatic mixing devices
Drawer handles
Adjustment handles on operator and assistant stools
Bracket table

Always Single-Use-Only Items

Prophy cups and brushes
Sterilization pouches
Irrigating syringes
Patient napkins
Surface barriers
Face masks
Examination and surgical gloves
Syringe needles
Suture needles
Plastic orthodontic brackets
Sharps containers (dispose of when fill-to line is reached; *never* empty and reuse)

Either Disposable or Reusable Items

Air-water syringe tips
High-volume evacuator tips
Impression trays
Mirrors
Prophy angles
Dental diamond burs
Vacuum line traps

*If surface cannot be easily and thoroughly cleaned and disinfected, it should have barrier protection.

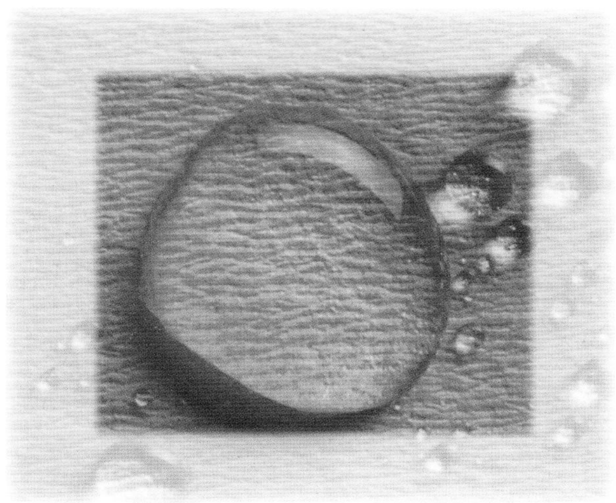

FIGURE 7-1 An example of water on a fluid-resistant material. (Courtesy Crosstex International, Inc., Hauppauge, New York.)

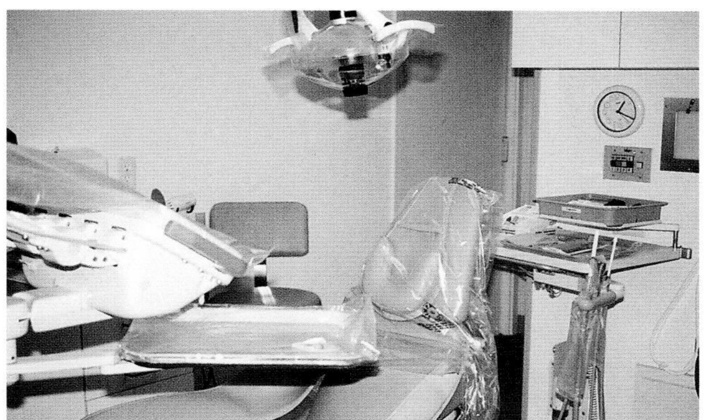

FIGURE 7-2 Surfaces touched during patient care should be covered with protective barriers. If not protected, then the surfaces should be cleaned and disinfected.

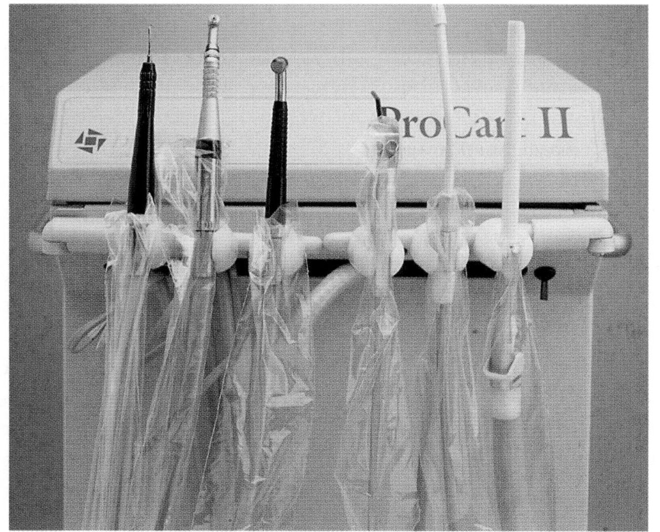

FIGURE 7-3 Tube socks provide barrier protection for difficult-to-clean areas. (Courtesy Certol International, Commerce City, Colorado.)

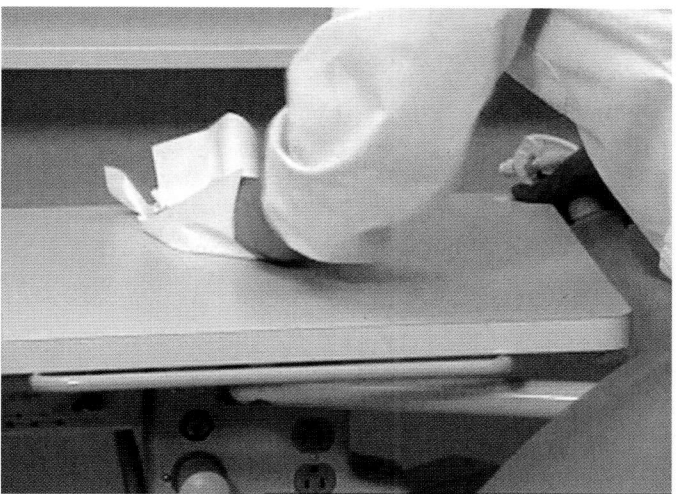

FIGURE 7-4 Smooth surfaces are easily sprayed and wiped.

Precleaning

Precleaning means to clean before disinfecting. All contaminated surfaces **must** be precleaned before they can be disinfected. This sequence reduces the number of microbes and removes the blood and/or saliva (also called bioburden). Not all types of disinfectants contain a precleaning agent.

Regular soap and water may be used for precleaning, but selecting a disinfectant that contains detergents for both the precleaning step and the disinfecting steps is more efficient. Remember—if a surface is not clean, it cannot be disinfected.

Disinfection

Disinfection is intended to kill disease-producing microorganisms that remain on the surface after precleaning. Spores are *not killed* during disinfection procedures. Do not confuse disinfection with sterilization. **Sterilization** is the process during which all forms of life are destroyed. Sterilization techniques are discussed in Chapter 8.

The term **disinfectant** is used for chemicals that are applied to inanimate surfaces, such as countertops and dental equipment, and the term antiseptic is used for antimicrobial agents that are applied to living tissue. Disinfectants and antiseptics should never be interchangeably used because tissue toxicity and damage to equipment can result.

Levels of Disinfectants

The **U.S. Environmental Protection Agency (EPA)** registers and regulates disinfectants and chemical sterilants and places them in categories (Table 7-2). In dentistry, only those products that are registered with the EPA as hospital disinfectants with tuberculocidal claims (kills the organism *Mycobacterium tuberculosis*) should be used to disinfect dental treatment areas. *M. tuberculosis* is highly resistant to disinfectants (Figure 7-5).

Characteristics of Disinfectants

Ideally, the perfect disinfectant would be one that rapidly kills all types of pathogenic organisms and is odorless, gentle to dental equipment surfaces, nontoxic, and economical to use.

TABLE 7-2
Chemical Classification

Level of Disinfection	EPA Classification	Use
High level	High-level disinfectant with a relatively short contact time and a sterilant when used with a prolonged contact time Monitoring not possible for sterilization	Semicritical items that cannot tolerate heat sterilization
Intermediate level	Hospital disinfectant with tuberculocidal activity	Noncritical items or surfaces that have been contaminated with blood or saliva
Low level	Nontuberculocidal activity	Surfaces not contaminated with blood

EPA, U.S. Environmental Protection Agency.

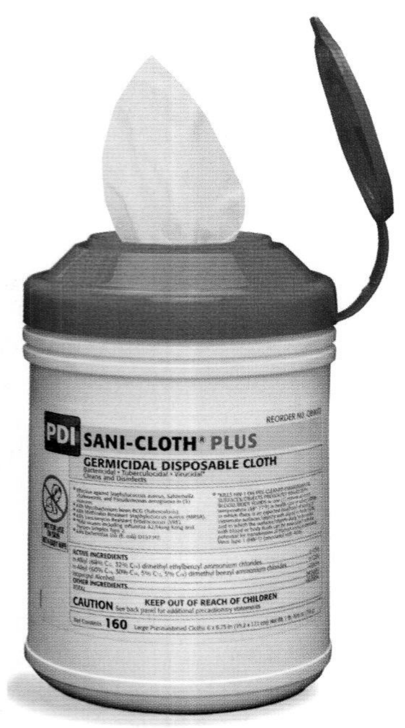

FIGURE 7-5 Disposable premoistened wipes with tuberculocidal activity. (Courtesy Crosstex International, Inc., Hauppauge, New York.)

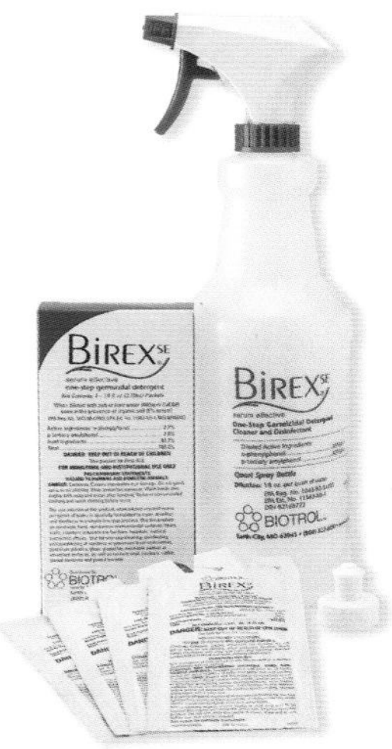

FIGURE 7-6 Intermediate-level surface disinfectant. (Courtesy Biotrol, Earth City, Missouri.)

Unfortunately, no perfect surface disinfectant is available; informed choices must be made. Nevertheless, several classes of disinfecting chemicals are available for use in dentistry (Table 7-3).

Many manufacturers of dental equipment will recommend specific surface disinfectants that are most appropriate for their dental chairs and unit accessories.

Types of Chemical Disinfectants

Iodophors Iodophors are EPA-registered, intermediate-level hospital disinfectants with tuberculocidal action. Iodophors are recommended for disinfecting surfaces that have been soiled with potentially infectious patient material. When used according to the manufacturer's instructions, iodophors are usually effective within 5 to 10 minutes. Iodophors are inactivated by hard water; consequently, they must be mixed with soft or distilled water. Because they contain iodine, iodophors may corrode or discolor certain metals or may temporarily cause red or yellow stains on clothing and other surfaces.

Synthetic phenol compounds Synthetic phenol compounds are EPA-registered, intermediate-level hospital disinfectants with broad-spectrum activity, meaning that they can kill a wide range of microbes. When properly diluted, phenols are used for surface disinfection, provided the surface has first been thoroughly cleaned.

Phenols can be used on metal, glass, rubber, or plastic. They also can be used as a holding solution for instruments; however, phenols leave a residual film on treated surfaces. A synthetic phenol compound is prepared daily. Phenols may also be used to disinfect impressions; however, always check with the manufacturer of the impression material.

Sodium hypochlorite Sodium hypochlorite is classified as an intermediate-level disinfectant and the primary active ingredient is ortho-phenylphenol (Figure 7-6). Sodium hypochlorite is a fast-acting, economical, and broad-spectrum disinfectant. Under the 1993 CDC guidelines, it was a recommended disinfectant. However, under the more recent CDC guidelines, household bleach, alone, is no longer a recommended product for use in dental settings as a disinfectant because it is not an EPA-registered disinfectant (Box 7-1).

TABLE 7-3
EPA-Registered Surface Disinfectants for Dentistry

Category and Active Ingredient	Pros	Cons
Chlorines: Sodium hypochlorite diluted in-office, chlorine dioxide, and commercial preparations of sodium hypochlorite with added surfactants	Economical Rapid, broad-spectrum activity Tuberculocidal action Effective in diluted solutions	Diluted solutions must be prepared daily; they cannot be reused. Are corrosive to some metals and may destroy fabrics. May irritate skin and other tissue. Chlorine dioxide is a poor cleaner.
Complex phenols: Synthetic phenols containing multiple phenolic agents	Broad-spectrum activity Residual activity Effective cleaner and disinfectant Tuberculocidal action Compatible with metal, glass, rubber, and plastic	Extended exposure may degrade some plastics or leave etchings on glass. Many preparations are limited to 1 day of use. May leave a residual film on treated surfaces.
Dual and synergized quaternary ammonium compounds: Alcohol and multiple quaternary ammonium compounds	Broad-spectrum activity Tuberculocidal action Hydrophilic virus claims Low toxicity Contains detergent for cleaning	Are readily inactivated by anionic detergents and organic matter. Can damage some materials.
Iodophors: Iodine, combined with a surfactant	Broad-spectrum activity Tuberculocidal action Relatively nontoxic Effective cleaner and disinfectant Residual biocidal action	Are unstable at higher temperatures; may discolor some surfaces. Inactivated by alcohol and hard water. Must be prepared daily. Dilution and contact times are critical.
Phenol-alcohol combinations: Phenolic agent in an alcohol base	Tuberculocidal action Fast-acting Residual activity Some inhibit the growth of mold, mildew, and other fungi	May cause porous surfaces to dry and crack. Have poor cleaning capabilities.
Other halogens: Sodium bromide and chlorine	Fast-acting Tuberculocidal action Supplied in tablet form for simple dilution Requires minimal storage space	Are for use on hard surfaces only. Have a chlorine smell.

From Organization for Safety, Asepsis and Prevention: *Infection control in practice,* vol 1, no 3, Annapolis, Md, 2002, OSAP.
EPA, U.S. Environmental Protection Agency.
Note: Glutaraldehydes and simple quaternary ammonium compounds should not be used for surface disinfection in dentistry. High-concentration alcohols (ethyl alcohol or isopropyl alcohol of at least 70%) should be used on precleaned surfaces.
Note: Always follow manufacturer's recommendations regarding surface contact time.

BOX 7-1 Disadvantages of Sodium Hypochlorite

- Unstable, and needs daily preparation.
- Has a strong odor, and is corrosive to some metals.
- Is destructive to fabrics, and eventually may cause plastic chair covers to crack.
- Is irritating to the eyes and skin.

EPA-approved disinfectant products that contain sodium hypochlorite or other chlorine compounds are available on the market. Always check the product label for the EPA registration number.

Alcohol Ethyl alcohol and isopropyl alcohol have been used over the years as skin antiseptics and surface disinfectants. However, alcohols are not effective in the presence of bioburden, such as blood and saliva, and the rapid rate of evaporation limits the antimicrobial activity of the alcohol. In addition, alcohols are damaging to certain materials, such as plastics and vinyl, which are prevalent in the dental environment.

The American Dental Association (ADA), the CDC, and the Organization for Safety and Asepsis Procedures (OSAP) do not recommend alcohol as an environmental surface disinfectant.

Liquid chemical sterilants and high-level disinfectants Liquid chemical sterilants are chemicals on the market that are classified for use as a sterilant or high-level disinfection. When used as sterilants, they destroy all microbial life, including bacterial endospores. Depending on the type of sterilant, the time for sterilization can range from 6 hours to 30 hours. At weaker dilutions or at shorter contact times, these chemicals provide high-level disinfection, which inactivates all microorganisms except endospores (Table 7-4). However, in the dental office, monitoring for microbial kill is not possible, as it is with

TABLE 7-4
FDA-Cleared Instrument Immersion Disinfectants for Dentistry

Category and Active Ingredient	Classification
Glutaraldehyde 2.4%-3.4% alkaline and acidic formulations*	Sterilant High-level disinfectant
Hydrogen peroxide, 7.3%	Sterilant High-level disinfectant
Ortho-phthalaldehyde, 0.55%	High-level disinfectant
Synergistic Solutions	
1.12% glutaraldehyde and 1.93% phenol/phenate	Sterilant High-level disinfectant
7.35% hydrogen peroxide and 0.23% peracetic acid	Sterilant High-level disinfectant

From Organization for Safety, Asepsis and Prevention: *Infection control in practice,* vol 1, no 3, Annapolis, Md, 2002, OSAP.
FDA, U.S. Food and Drug Administration.
Note: Glutaraldehydes and simple quaternary ammonium compounds should not be used for surface disinfection in dentistry. High-concentration alcohols (ethyl alcohol or isopropyl alcohol of at least 70%) should be used on precleaned surfaces.
Note: Always follow manufacturer's recommendations regarding surface contact time.
*Varies by active ingredient or disinfectant brand.

heat sterilization. Spore tests for biologic monitoring have not yet been developed for office testing.

Most of these chemicals are toxic and can irritate the eyes, skin, and lungs. Personal protective equipment (PPE) must always be worn when using these chemicals. They are to be used for immersion (soaking) of heat-sensitive items and should never be used as surface disinfectants.

Always keep the container lid closed to minimize fumes.

Glutaraldehyde Glutaraldehyde is classified as a high-level disinfectant and sterilant. It can be used as a liquid sterilant when the immersion time is greatly increased (see Chapter 8). Times for disinfection range from 10 to 90 minutes; always read the manufacturer's recommendations. Glutaraldehyde products are useful for plastics or other items that cannot withstand heat sterilization. Some glutaraldehyde products are effective for only 28 days after activation.

Glutaraldehyde is very toxic and should be carefully handled to avoid the fumes. Glutaraldehyde-treated instruments should never be used on patients unless the items have been thoroughly rinsed with water. Prolonged contact of certain types of instruments with glutaraldehyde solutions can lead to discoloration and corrosion of instrument surfaces and cutting edges.

Chlorine dioxide Chlorine dioxide is classified as a high-level disinfectant and sterilant. Products containing chlorine dioxide can be used as effective, rapid-acting, environmental surface disinfectants (3 minutes) or as chemical sterilants (6 hours). However, chlorine dioxide products do not readily penetrate organic debris and must be used with a separate cleaner.

Other disadvantages of chlorine dioxide include the following: (1) it must be prepared fresh daily, (2) it must be used with good ventilation, and (3) it is corrosive to aluminum containers.

Ortho-phthalaldehyde Ortho-phthalaldehyde (OPA) is a chemical used in high-level disinfectant and is effective in achieving high-level disinfection within 12 minutes at room temperature. OPA is more expensive than glutaraldehyde solutions, but it may be a good alternative for health care workers with sensitivity to glutaraldehyde. OPA has very little odor and does not require activation or mixing.

Disadvantages of an OPA solution include: (1) high cost, (2) can only be used half as long as most glutaraldehyde products in dentistry, (3) may stain skin and fabrics, (4) turns plastics a blue-green color where proteins have not been removed, and (5) does not have a sterilization claim.

Classifications of Instruments, Equipment, and Surfaces

Instruments, equipment, and surfaces used during patient care are divided into three classifications: critical, semicritical, and noncritical items. These classifications are used to determine the type of posttreatment processing (Table 7-5).

Critical Instruments

Critical items *must be* **heat sterilized.** Critical instruments are items used to penetrate soft tissue or bone. They have the greatest risk of transmitting infection and must be sterilized by heat. Examples of critical instruments include forceps, scalpels, bone chisels, scalers, and burs.

Semicritical Instruments

Semicritical items *should be* **heat sterilized.** Semicritical instruments touch mucous membranes or nonintact skin and have a lower risk of transmission. Most semicritical items in dentistry are heat tolerant and should be sterilized. If the item will be damaged by heat, then it should receive, at a minimum, high-level disinfection (see Chapter 8).

Examples of semicritical items include plastic-handled brushes, high-volume evacuator (HVE) tips, rubber dam forceps, x-ray film holders, and amalgam carriers. Items manufactured for single use should be disposed, not disinfected.

In dental offices today, most items used intraorally are capable of withstanding the heat of sterilization. A fundamental rule of infection control states, "If an item can be heat sterilized, it should be heat sterilized."

Noncritical Instruments

Noncritical instruments pose the least risk of transmission of infection because they contact only intact skin, which is an effective barrier to microorganisms. These items should be cleaned and processed with an EPA-registered, intermediate-level or low-level disinfectant after each patient use.

Noncritical clinical devices include the position indicator device (PID) of the x-ray unit tube head, the lead apron, and the curing light that comes into contact only with intact skin.

TABLE 7-5
CDC Classification of Instruments and Procedures

Category	Functions and Examples	Intraoral Use	Risk of Disease Transmission	Procedure
Critical	**Function:** To touch bone or to penetrate soft tissue **Examples:** Surgical and other instruments used to penetrate soft tissue or bone, including forceps, scalpels, bone chisels, scalers, and burs	Yes	Very high	Sterilization
Semicritical	**Function:** To touch mucous membranes but will not touch bone or penetrate soft tissue **Examples:** Mouth mirrors and amalgam condensers	Yes	Moderate	Sterilization or high-level disinfection
Noncritical	**Function:** Contact only with intact skin **Examples:** External dental x-ray head	No	Very low or none	Intermediate-to low-level disinfection or basic cleaning

CDC, Centers for Disease Control and Prevention.
Note: Always follow manufacturer's recommendations regarding surface contact time.

BOX 7-2 Steps to Reduce the Spread of Microorganisms

- Avoid unnecessary touching of surfaces.
- Use high-volume evacuation.
- Use the rubber dam.
- Use preprocedure mouth rinses.
- Use disposable items.
- Reduce dental unit water line contamination.

Additional Aseptic Techniques

In addition to precleaning and disinfecting equipment and surfaces, several additional steps can be taken to reduce the spread of microorganisms in the dental office (Box 7-2).

Unnecessary Touching of Surfaces

During patient care procedures, gloves become contaminated with blood and saliva, and that contamination is easily transferred when members of the dental team touch items or surfaces with their gloved hands. Plan ahead to have all needed items present at chairside before the procedure begins, which will reduce the need for leaving chairside or reaching into drawers with contaminated gloves. If you must leave chairside, then use an overglove to reach for necessary items. Remember not to touch or rub your eyes, nose, or skin, or touch your hair with gloved hands.

High-Volume Evacuation

The use and proper placement of the HVE greatly reduce the quantity of salivary aerosols and spatter emitted from the patient's mouth. The HVE system should be cleaned at the end of the day by evacuating a detergent or a water-based detergent-disinfectant through the system. In addition, the disposable trap should be periodically replaced. Remember to always wear masks, protective eyewear, and protective clothing when cleaning the HVE system or replacing traps.

Rubber Dam

Using a rubber dam with simultaneous use of the HVE provides the best approach to minimize dental aerosols and spatter emitted from the patient's mouth.

Preprocedure Mouth Rinse

Some dentists have their patients rinse with an antimicrobial mouth rinse before dental procedures are begun. This procedure is intended to reduce the number of microorganisms released in the form of aerosol or spatter. In addition, preprocedural mouth rinsing can decrease the number of microorganisms introduced into the patient's bloodstream during invasive dental procedures. Preprocedural mouth rinses are especially useful before procedures during which a rubber dam cannot be used (e.g., ultrasonic scaler).

Use of Disposables

Disposable items, usually made of plastic and not heat tolerant, are made for a single use. A disposable item must be properly disposed after use, and you *should not attempt* to preclean and disinfect or sterilize it for reuse on another patient.

Dental Unit Water Line Contamination

The water in a dental unit is commonly contaminated with microorganisms (Figure 7-7). The municipal water entering the dental office contains a few waterborne bacteria and a small quantity of nutrients that may support the growth of bacteria. As water stands in narrow dental unit water lines, some of the bacteria attach to and accumulate on the inside walls of the lines, forming a **biofilm** (Figures 7-8 and 7-9). (Bacteria in dental plaque serve as an excellent example of biofilm formation.) When bacteria are embedded in the protective biofilm, they are extremely difficult to remove. As water flows through

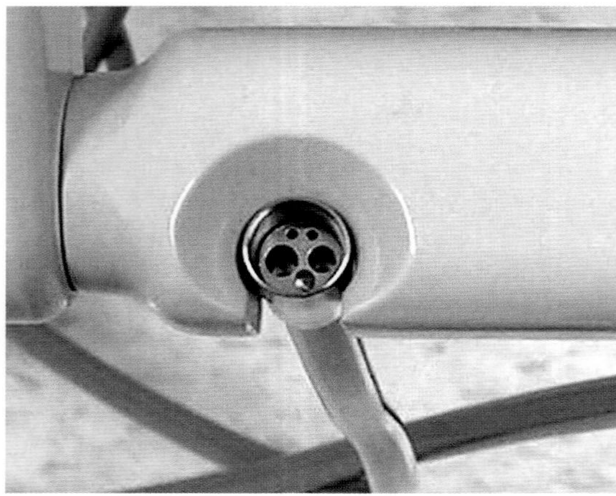

FIGURE 7-7 Close-up of dental tube opening.

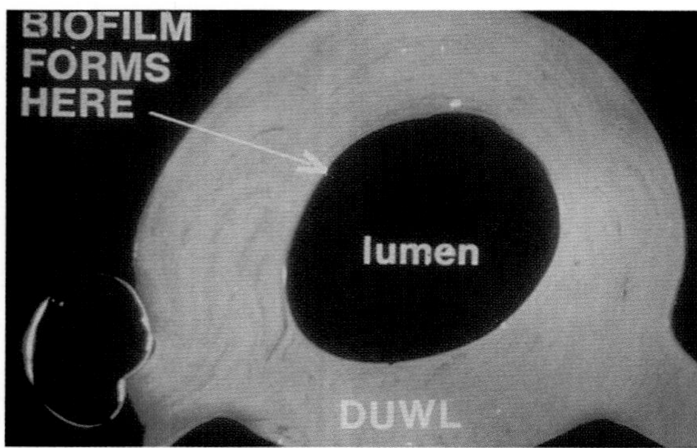

FIGURE 7-8 Cross-section of a dental unit water line (DUWL) illustrating the formation of biofilm on the inside wall of a dental tube. (Courtesy United States Air Force [USAF].)

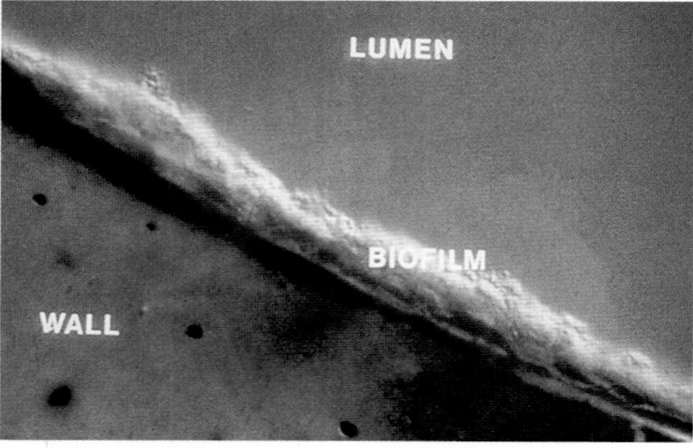

FIGURE 7-9 Magnification of a cross section of a dental unit water line showing biofilm formation.

the lines, bacteria from the biofilm may be released into the water and sprayed into the patient's mouth during the use of the high-speed handpiece and air-water syringe.

Bacteria in dental unit water not only potentially contaminate patients, but they can also contaminate the dental team through aerosols and spatter generated by the use of the high-speed handpiece, ultrasonic scalers, and air-water syringes.

BOX 7-3 Methods to Reduce Bacterial Contamination of Dental Unit Water Lines

1. Flush water lines for several minutes at the beginning of the day and longer after weekends.

Note: Biofilms cannot be removed by flushing alone. Flushing 20 to 30 seconds between patients is recommended to eliminate material retracted from the previous patient.

2. Use a self-contained water reservoir system.
3. Use a self-contained water reservoir system combined with periodic or continuous application of chemical germicides as recommended by the equipment manufacturer.
4. Use a separate (sterile water) system for surgical procedures.
5. Purge the water from the dental lines, and dry the lines with air at the end of each day.
6. Use microfiltration cartridges in the water lines.
7. Stay current with new techniques and manufacturing technology for dental unit water lines.
8. Follow the recommendations for monitoring water quality provided by the manufacturer of the dental unit or water line treatment product.

Although eliminating biofilm from dental unit water lines is not yet entirely possible, methods have been found to greatly reduce the level of bacterial contamination (Box 7-3).

Cleaning and Disinfection of the Laboratory Area

In contrast to the dental treatment room, the laboratory area in the dental office is often overlooked when infection control practices are implemented. Steps should be taken to prevent cross-contamination between patients and dental team members or to other patients. Standard precautions should be observed in the dental laboratory at all times.

The counter surfaces should be covered with impervious paper or cleaned and disinfected on a regular basis. All case pans should be cleaned and disinfected before they are used for another case. You should not eat, drink, smoke, apply cosmetics or lip balm, handle contact lenses, or store food in the laboratory area because it is an area of contamination.

Impressions

After removal from the patient's mouth, the impression is contaminated with saliva and possibly blood. Some viral and bacterial pathogens can exist for long periods outside the human body. Although the risk of disease transmission from an impression is low, the risk is real. Gloves, protective eyewear, and outerwear must be worn whenever contaminated impressions are handled.

A wide variety of impression materials are available on the market, and the chemicals and techniques recommended for disinfection also vary. Always check the manufacturer's

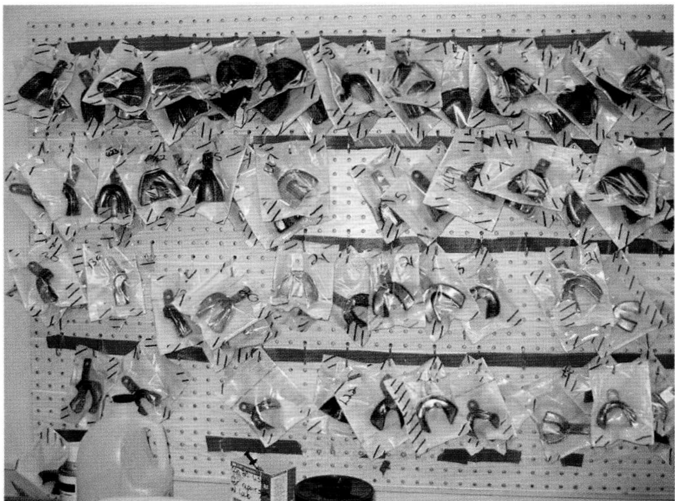

FIGURE 7-10 Impression trays are heat sterilized in individual bags.

recommendations for the disinfectant best suited for the impression material.

See Procedure 7-3: Disinfecting an Alginate Impression.

Disinfection of Casts

Casts are the most difficult prosthodontic items to disinfect without causing damage. Disinfecting the impression so that the resulting cast, itself, will not have to be disinfected is preferable. However, accidental contamination may make disinfection necessary. Casts should be set on their ends to allow drainage and should be sprayed with an iodophor or chlorine product, rinsed, and allowed to dry.

Disinfection of Other Materials

Articulators, case pans, and face bow components can be cleaned and disinfected with an intermediate-level disinfectant. The pumice for the polishing lathe should be dispensed using the unit dose concept (just enough for one patient). All brushes, rag wheels, and other laboratory tools should be sterilized or disinfected between patients (Figure 7-10).

Cleaning and Disinfecting the Radiology Area

Multiple opportunities for cross-contamination occur during an oral radiographic procedure.

The surfaces that the operator touches while producing radiographs are considered noncritical and must be cleaned and disinfected with an intermediate-level or a low-level disinfectant after the patient is dismissed. A very desirable alternative to surface disinfection is to cover the noncritical surfaces with removable plastic barriers.

Plastic wrap and plastic bags are most commonly used as barriers. Barriers should be placed over the chair headrest, countertops, extension arm, tube head, PID of the x-ray machine, control panel, and exposure button (Figure 7-11).

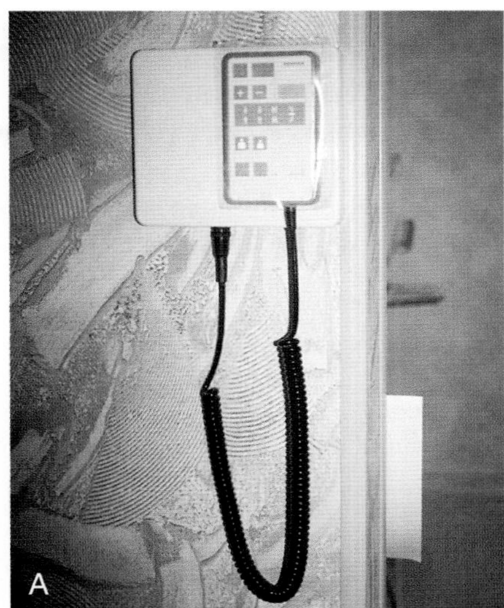

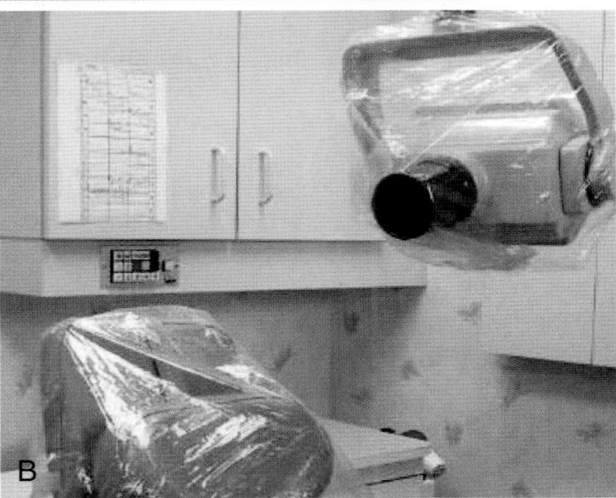

FIGURE 7-11 **A,** Exposure control protected with barrier. **B,** Radiography operatory with barriers in place.

Ethical Implications

As a dental assistant, you play a very important role in organizing, managing, and implementing the infection control program in the office. Infection control is a rapidly expanding and changing area within dentistry. New diseases continue to emerge, and familiar pathogens have become resistant to antibiotics. Your employer, fellow staff members, and your patients depend on you to have a solid understanding of the basic concepts of infection control and the ability to perform step-by-step procedures.

Today, more than at any other time in history, patients are concerned about the risk of disease transmission in the dental office. From a legal and ethical aspect, malpractice lawsuits have occurred as a result of disease transmission to patients caused by improper infection control techniques. Everyone in the dental office must understand the importance of good infection control and must follow all infection control procedures.

Procedure 7-1

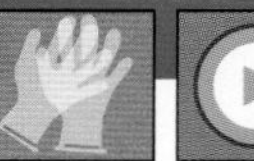

Placing and Removing Surface Barriers

Goal

To place surface barriers before patient treatment and to remove the barriers at the end of the procedure

Equipment and Supplies

- Liquid antimicrobial hand soap
- Utility gloves
- Plastic surface barriers
- Noncontaminated surfaces in dental treatment room

Procedural Steps

1. Wash and dry hands.
2. Select the appropriate surface barrier to be placed over the clean surface.

Note: If the surfaces to be covered have been previously contaminated, then put on utility gloves and preclean and disinfect the surface. Then wash, disinfect, and remove your utility gloves. Wash and dry your hands before applying the surface barriers.

3. Place each barrier over the entire surface to be protected. Check to ensure that the barrier is secure and will not come off.

Purpose: If the barrier slips out of position, then the underlying surface will become contaminated and will require precleaning and disinfecting, negating the barrier's purpose.

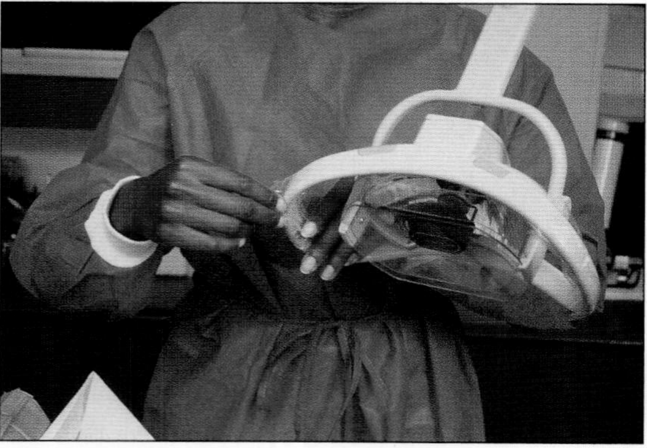

4. Wear utility gloves to remove contaminated surface barriers after dental treatment.

Purpose: Utility gloves protect the skin from contamination.

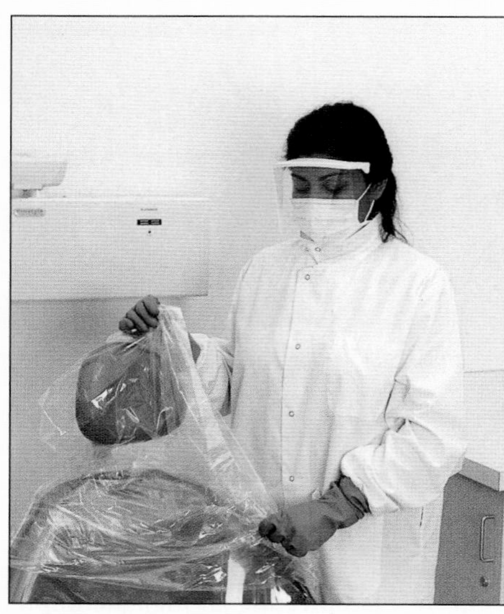

5. Very carefully remove each cover without touching the underlying surface with either the utility glove or the contaminated outside surface of the barrier.

Purpose: If a surface is accidentally touched during removal of the cover, then the surface must be precleaned and disinfected.

6. Discard the used covers in the regular waste trash. (Check disposal laws in your state.)

Purpose: Most states do not consider barriers to be regulated waste (requiring special disposal) unless an item is soaked or caked with blood or saliva that would be released if the item were to be compressed.

7. Wash, disinfect, and remove your utility gloves. Wash and dry your hands, then apply fresh surface covers for the next patient.

Purpose: Your utility gloves are contaminated from handling the used barriers. By washing, drying, and disinfecting your utility gloves, you will know they are ready for their next use.

Procedure 7-2

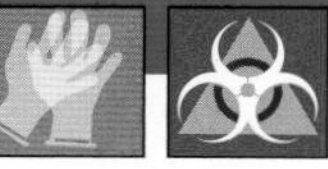

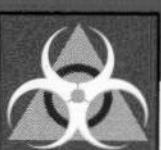

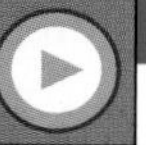

Performing Treatment Room Cleaning and Disinfection

Goal

To clean and disinfect dental treatment rooms effectively

Equipment and Supplies

- Personal protective equipment (PPE), including utility gloves, goggles, and mask
- Intermediate-level surface cleaner and/or disinfectant
- Paper towels

Procedural Steps

1. Put on utility gloves, protective eyewear, and protective clothing.

Purpose: To prevent contact with contaminated surfaces and chemicals.

Note: The latex examination gloves used in patient care should not be used for precleaning and disinfecting procedures. The chemicals will degrade the latex glove

Procedure 7-2

Performing Treatment Room Cleaning and Disinfection—cont'd

and allow chemicals and contaminants to penetrate to the skin.

2. Make sure that the precleaning and/or disinfecting products have been correctly prepared and are fresh. Always read and follow the manufacturer's instructions.

Purpose: Some products are concentrated and must be diluted for use. In addition, some products must be prepared daily.

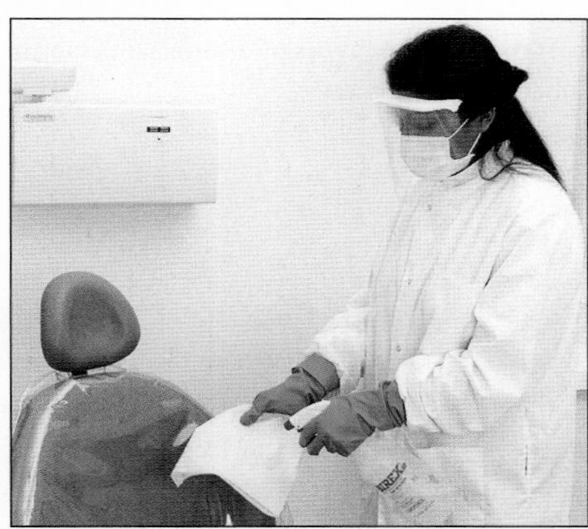

3. To preclean, spray the paper towel or gauze pad with the product and vigorously wipe the surface. You may use a small brush for surfaces that do not become visibly clean from wiping. If you are cleaning a large area, then use several towels or gauze pads.

Purpose: Overspray is reduced by spraying the product onto the towel or gauze pad. Large areas require more towels or pads to avoid spreading bioburden instead of removing it.

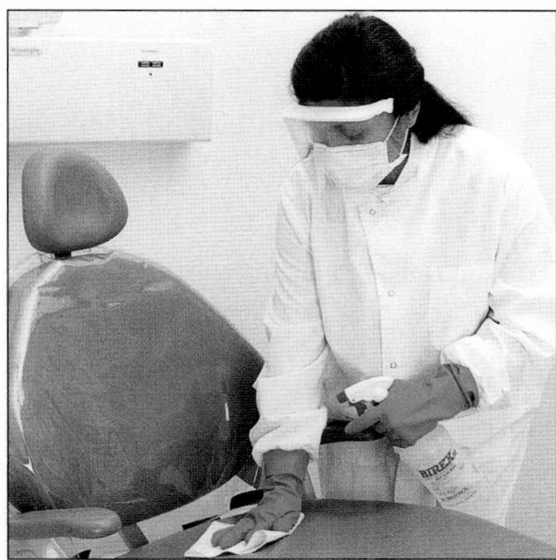

4. To disinfect, spray a fresh paper towel or gauze pad with the product. Let the surface remain moist for the manufacturer's recommended time for tuberculocidal action (usually 10 minutes).
5. If the surface is still moist after the kill time and you are ready to seat another patient, then you may wipe the surface dry. Use water to rinse any residual disinfectant from surfaces that will come in contact with the patient's skin or mouth.

Purpose: The chemicals used for precleaning and disinfecting may irritate the patient's skin or damage the patient's clothing.

Procedure 7-3

Disinfecting an Alginate Impression

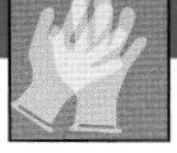
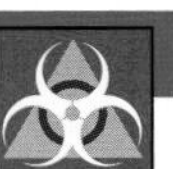

Goal

To disinfect an alginate impression

Equipment and Supplies

- Protective clothing
- Surgical mask
- Protective eyewear
- Chemical-resistant utility gloves
- Disinfectant solution

Procedural Steps

1. Rinse the impression under running tap water to clean it. If necessary, use a soft, camel-hair brush to remove debris.

Purpose: To remove any blood and/or saliva.

2. Disinfect the impression using an intermediate-level hospital disinfectant for the contact time recommended on the germicide's label.

Note: Immersion or spraying is recommended for disinfecting impressions. Spraying uses less solution, and often you can use the same disinfectant that you use for the operatory. However, sprayed disinfectants may pool, which may prevent some surfaces from being adequately exposed to the germicide. Some organizations encourage immersion disinfection of all dental impressions.

3. If spraying is used, then thoroughly spray the impression and wrap it with well-moistened paper towels. Unwrap the impression after the manufacturer's recommended contact time has elapsed.
4. If immersion is used, then remove the impression after the manufacturer's recommended contact time has elapsed.
5. Rinse the disinfected impression under tap water to remove any residual germicide.
6. After a thorough rinse, gently shake the impression within the sink basin to remove the remaining water with minimal spatter.

Note: Always check the recommendations of the impression manufacturer as to the stability of the impression material during disinfection.

Modified from Organization for Safety, Asepsis and Prevention: *Policy to practice: OSAP's guide to the guidelines,* Annapolis, Md, 2004, OSAP.

Chapter Exercises

Multiple Choice

Circle the letter next to the correct answer.

1. A mouth mirror is an example of a __________ instrument.
- **a.** critical
- **b.** semicritical
- **c.** noncritical

2. A dental bur is an example of a __________ instrument.
- **a.** critical
- **b.** semicritical
- **c.** noncritical

3. Which of the following PPE should NOT be worn while precleaning and disinfecting a treatment room?
- **a.** Mask
- **b.** Eyewear
- **c.** Gown
- **d.** Latex examination gloves

4. Surface barriers are NOT necessary on surfaces that are __________.
- **a.** electrical connections
- **b.** smooth and easily cleaned
- **c.** irregular

5. The best way to manage surface asepsis is with the use of __________.
- **a.** surface disinfectants only
- **b.** surface barriers only
- **c.** a combination of surface barriers and surface disinfectants

6. Laboratory items such as rag wheels should be changed __________.
- **a.** daily
- **b.** weekly
- **c.** after each patient use

7. Which of the following items can produce contaminated dental unit water?
- **a.** High-speed handpieces
- **b.** Air-water syringes
- **c.** Ultrasonic handpieces
- **d.** All of the above

8. When placing surface barriers on a surface that has already been cleaned and disinfected, you should use __________.
- **a.** clean bare hands
- **b.** latex examination gloves
- **c.** utility gloves

9. __________ instruments must be heat sterilized between patients.
- **a.** Semicritical
- **b.** Critical
- **c.** Noncritical
- **d.** All of the above

10. Which of the following types of disinfectants may not necessarily have tuberculocidal action?
- **a.** High level
- **b.** Intermediate level
- **c.** Low level

Apply Your Knowledge

1. While in the process of preparing a dental treatment room for the next patient, you notice that the surface barrier on the light handle has become dislodged and is barely hanging on. Although you do not see any visible contamination on the light handle, you realize that the barrier must have slipped sometime during the previous procedure. How would you deal with this as you prepare the room for the next patient?

2. A very nice patient has baked some cookies for everyone in your dental office. As she enters the hallway en route to the treatment room, she offers to put the cookies in the laboratory for you so you can enjoy them later. What would you do?

3. After seeing a recent television program about acquired immunodeficiency syndrome (AIDS), a patient expresses his concern about the possibility of disease transmission in your dental office. How would you reassure this patient?

4. Imagine you are preparing a dental treatment room. Where would you place surface barriers and why?

CHAPTER 8

Instrument Processing

http://evolve.elsevier.com/Robinson/essentials/

LEARNING OBJECTIVES

1. Pronounce, define, and spell the key terms.
2. Describe the seven steps of processing dental instruments.
3. Describe the "ideal" instrument-processing area.
4. Complete the following related to precleaning and packaging instruments:
   - List and describe the three ways to preclean instruments.
   - Operate an ultrasonic cleaner.
   - Describe packaging instruments.
   - Discuss the various types of packaging materials used for sterilization.
5. Complete the following related to methods of sterilization:
   - Identify the three most commonly used methods of heat sterilization, and describe the advantages and disadvantages of each.
   - Describe the process of using an autoclave.
   - Sterilize instruments with chemical vapor, dry heat, and chemical liquid.
6. Complete the following related to sterilization monitoring:
   - Identify the three forms of sterilization monitoring that are currently used.
   - Explain the differences between process indicators and process integrators.
7. Describe the purpose of, as well as perform, biologic monitoring.
8. Identify the reasons for sterilization failure.

KEY TERMS

autoclave
biologic monitoring
chemical vapor sterilization
clean areas
contaminated area
dry heat sterilization
forced air sterilizer
holding solution
instrument processing
process indicators
process integrators
static air sterilizer
ultrasonic cleaner

One of the most important responsibilities of the dental assistant is to process contaminated instruments and other patient care items for reuse.

Instrument processing involves much more than sterilization. Proper processing of contaminated dental instruments is actually a seven-step process (Table 8-1). Although the seven steps are not difficult to learn, having a clear understanding of how and why each step is performed is very important. To prevent disease agents from a previous patient from being transferred to you, to another member of the dental team, or to the next patient, instrument-processing procedures must be performed in a consistent and disciplined manner.

Processing reusable instruments begins at the chairside at the completion of the patient visit and ends with procedures that ensure the quality of the entire reprocessing procedure.

First, the dental assistant puts on utility gloves and discards disposable needles, scalpels, and other contaminated sharp items into a puncture-resistant sharps disposal container. Other waste, such as used cotton rolls and gauze squares, is disposed (Figure 8-1). The contaminated instruments are then taken to the sterilization center (processing area). To prevent injury, the instruments should be transported in a rigid, leakproof, and covered container (Box 8-1).

Sterilization Center

The instrument-processing area, or sterilization area, should be centrally located in the office to allow easy access from all patient care areas. This centralized location minimizes the need to carry contaminated items through **clean areas** of the office,

TABLE 8-1
Seven Steps for Instrument Processing

Step	Technique
Transport	Transport contaminated instruments to the processing area in a manner that minimizes the risk of exposure to persons and the environment. Use appropriate PPE and a rigid, leakproof container.
Cleaning	Clean instruments using a hands-free, mechanical process, such as an ultrasonic cleaner or instrument washer. If instruments cannot be immediately cleaned, then use a holding solution.
Packaging	In the clean area, wrap and/or package instruments in appropriate types of materials. Place a chemical indicator inside the package next to the instruments. If an indicator is not visible on the outside of the package, then place an external process indicator on the package.
Sterilization	Load the sterilizer according to the manufacturer's instructions. Label the packages. Do not overload the sterilizer. Place the packages on their edges in single layers or on racks to increase circulation of the sterilizing agent around the instruments. Operate the sterilizer according to the manufacturer's instructions. Allow packages to cool before removing them from the sterilizer. Allow packages to cool before handling.
Storage	Store instruments in a clean, dry environment in a manner that maintains the integrity of the package. Rotate packages so that those with the oldest sterilization dates will be used first.
Delivery	Deliver packages to the point of use in a manner that maintains sterility of the instruments until they are used. Inspect each package for damage. Aseptically open each package.
Quality assurance program	An effective quality assurance program should incorporate training, record keeping, maintenance, and the use of biologic indicators.

Modified from the Organization for Safety, Asepsis and Prevention (OSAP).
PPE, Personal protective equipment.

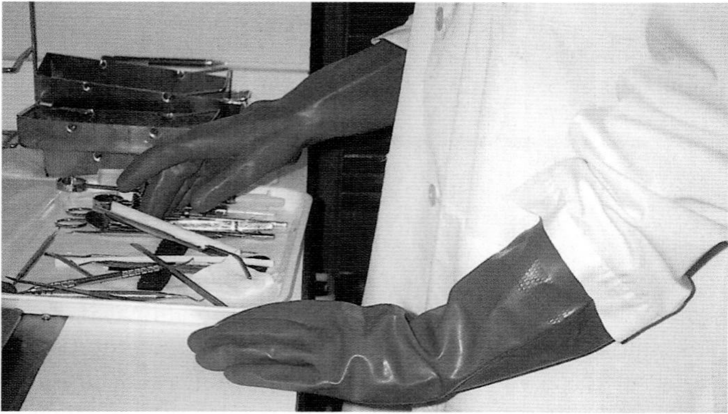

FIGURE 8-1 Personal protective equipment (PPE) must be worn while preparing instruments for sterilization.

BOX 8-1 Requirements for Personal Protective Equipment During Instrument Processing

- Nitrile utility gloves, protective clothing, and protective eyewear must be worn when soiled instruments are handled.
- A mask must be worn if the cleaning method generates splash, spatter, or aerosols, such as hand scrubbing of instruments or rinsing of instruments.
- Examination gloves are worn when reassembling preset trays of wrapped sterile instruments.

where sterilized instruments, fresh disposable supplies, and prepared trays are stored.

The ideal instrument-processing area should (1) be dedicated only to instrument processing, (2) be physically separated from the operatories and the dental laboratory, and (3) not be a part of a common walkway. The size of the area should accommodate all the equipment and supplies necessary for instrument processing, with multiple outlets and proper lighting, water, and an airline and vacuum line for flushing high-speed handpieces.

A deep sink should have hands-free controls for instrument rinsing and (if space permits) a foot-operated or other hands-free trash receptacle. The flooring should be an uncarpeted, seamless, and hard surface. The size, shape, and accessories of the instrument-processing area vary among dental offices.

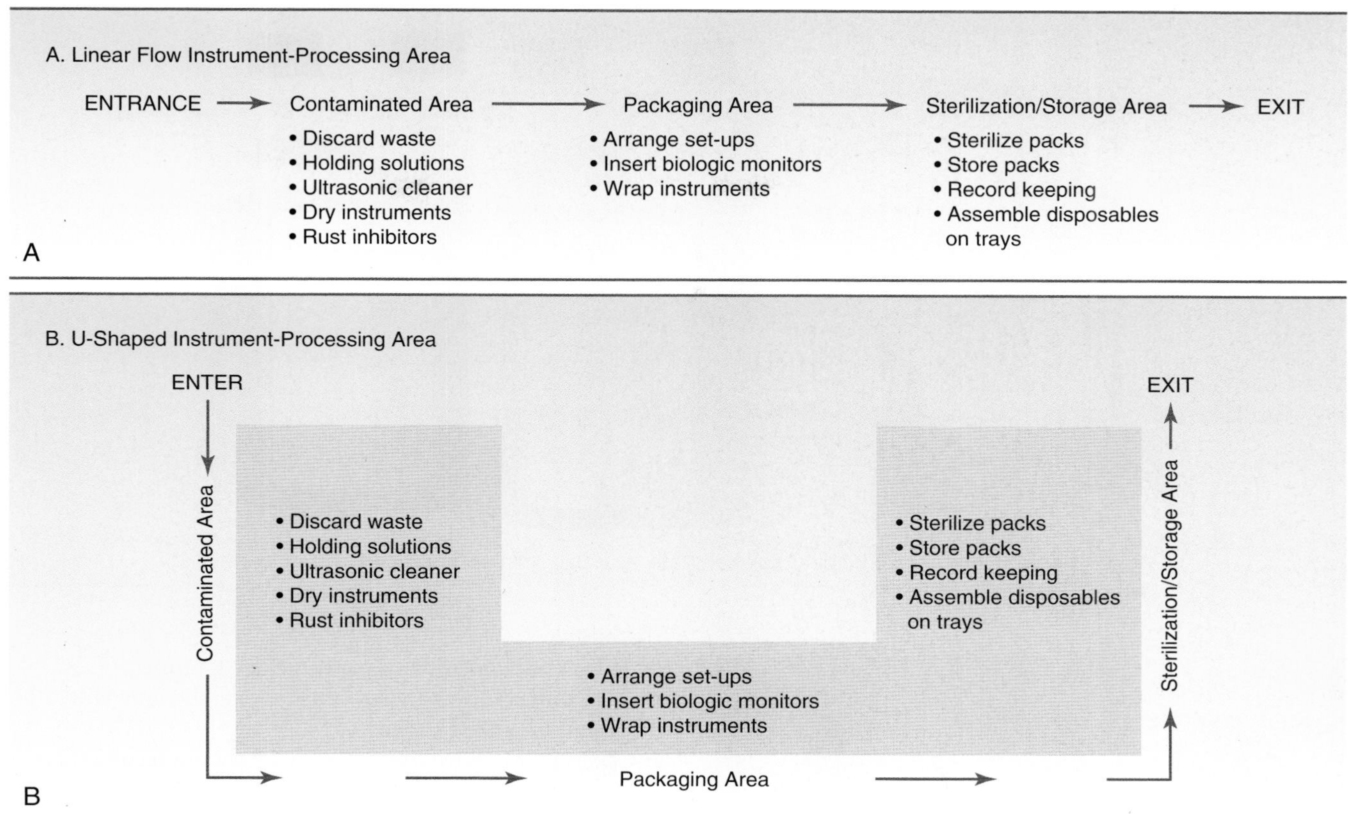

FIGURE 8-2 Instrument processing area. **A,** Linear. **B,** U-shaped.

Workflow Pattern

Regardless of the size or shape of the instrument-processing area, four basic areas govern the pattern of workflow. Instruments that are being processed should proceed in a single loop—from dirty to clean to sterile to storage—without ever *doubling back* (Figure 8-2).

If the instrument-processing area is small, then signs can be used that read, "Contaminated items only," "Precleaning area," "Cleaned items only," "Sterile items only," or "Sterilization area" to separate contaminated areas from clean areas. This method works well to prevent mixing contaminated and sterile items in a small sterilization area.

Contaminated Area

All soiled instruments are brought into the **contaminated area**, the initial receiving area where they are held for processing. Any disposable items not already discarded in the treatment room are removed from the instrument tray and disposed of as contaminated waste.

The contaminated area contains clean protective eyewear and utility gloves, counter space, a sink, a waste disposal container, a **holding solution**, an **ultrasonic cleaner**, an eyewash station, and supplies for wrapping instruments before sterilization.

Note: Soiled and clean instruments are never stored in the same cabinet.

Holding Solution

If the instruments cannot be immediately cleaned after the procedure, then they should be placed in a holding solution to prevent blood and debris from drying on the instruments.

The holding solution may be any noncorrosive liquid. A commercial enzymatic solution that partially dissolves organic debris may be used (Figure 8-3). Dishwasher detergent also makes a good holding solution because it is low cost, low foaming, and readily available. Using a disinfectant alone as a holding solution is neither cost-effective nor desirable. The dental professional should read and follow the manufacturer's instructions on the ultrasonic unit when choosing a solution.

The container must have a lid and must be labeled with both a biohazard label (because of the contaminated instruments) and a chemical label (because of the cleaner and/or detergent). The holding solution should be changed at least twice daily and more frequently if it becomes clouded.

Remember, a holding solution is necessary only when contaminated instruments cannot be immediately processed.

Clean Area

In the clean area, cleaned instruments and other dental supplies should be inspected, assembled into sets or trays, and wrapped or placed in packages for sterilization (Figure 8-4).

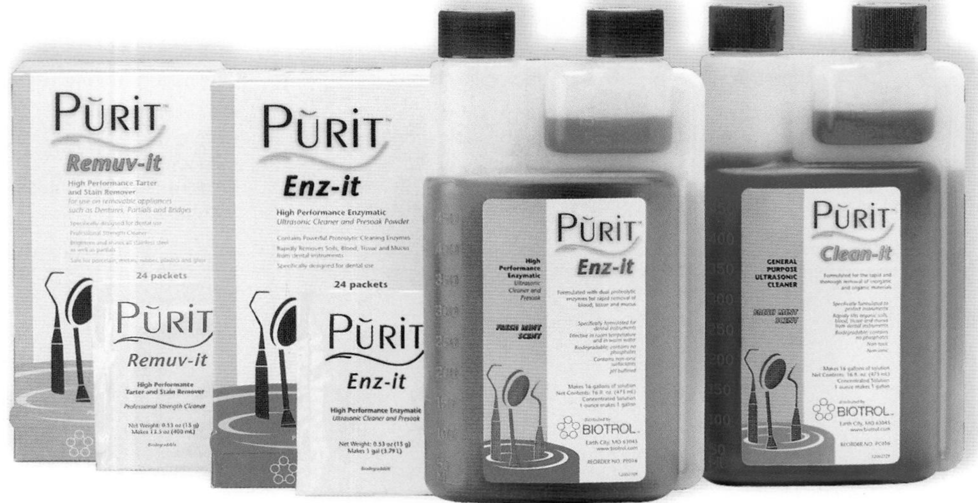

FIGURE 8-3 Commercial holding solutions are available for use in precleaning. (Courtesy Biotrol, Earth City, Missouri.)

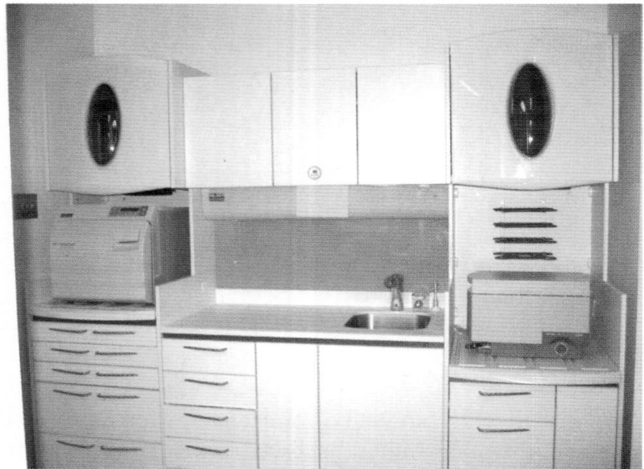

FIGURE 8-4 The clean area includes the sterilizer and space to store prepared trays. (Courtesy Sterilizers.com.)

Clean instruments *are not* sterile and can still harbor pathogens. Instruments must be packaged and sterilized before being used on a patient.

Precleaning and Packaging Instruments

Instruments may be precleaned in one of three ways: (1) hand scrubbing, (2) ultrasonic cleaning, and (3) instrument washing machines.

Hand Scrubbing

Hand scrubbing is the LEAST desirable method of cleaning instruments because it requires direct hand contact with the contaminated instrument. If you absolutely must hand-scrub instruments, then adhere to the following precautions:

- Wear goggle-type eyewear, puncture-resistant gloves, and protective clothing.
- Clean only one or two instruments at a time.
- Use only a long-handled brush, preferably one with a hand guard or a wide surface.
- Keep items above the water line; fully immersing them in a basin of soapy water interferes with the ability to see sharp ends.
- Allow the instruments to air dry, or carefully pat them with thick toweling. Never rub or roll the instruments inside the towel because of the risk of accidental injury.

Note: Some states have specific infection control guidelines or Occupational Safety & Health Administration (OSHA) plans that prohibit hand scrubbing of instruments. In these states, an ultrasonic cleaner or machine cleaning must be used.

Ultrasonic Cleaning

Ultrasonic cleaners are used to loosen and remove debris from instruments. These cleaners also reduce the risk of hand injuries from cuts and punctures during the cleaning process.

See Procedure 8-1: Operating the Ultrasonic Cleaner.

Puncture-resistant utility gloves, a mask, protective eyewear, and a protective gown should always be worn when the ultrasonic cleaner is used. To further limit contact with contaminated instruments, keep a set of tongs near the ultrasonic unit for removing instruments after the cleaning cycle (Figure 8-5).

The ultrasonic cleaner works by producing sound waves beyond the range of human hearing. These sound waves, which can travel through metal and glass containers, cause cavitation (formation of bubbles in liquid). The bubbles, which are too small to be seen, burst by implosion (bursting inward, the opposite of an explosion). The mechanical cleaning action of the bursting bubbles combined with the chemical action of the ultrasonic solution removes the debris from the instruments.

Instruments should be processed in the ultrasonic cleaner until they are visibly clean. The time may vary from 5 to 15 minutes, depending on the amount and type of material on the instruments and the efficiency of the ultrasonic unit. Instruments in plastic or resin cassettes require slightly longer

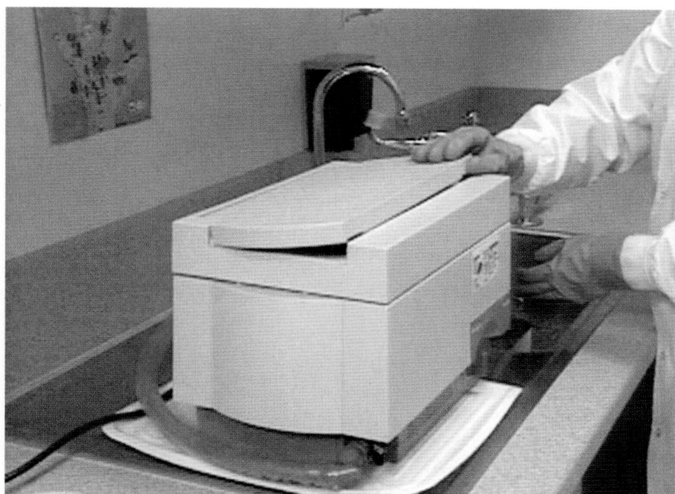

FIGURE 8-5 Keeping the ultrasonic cleaner covered while in use is important to reduce spatter and contaminated aerosols.

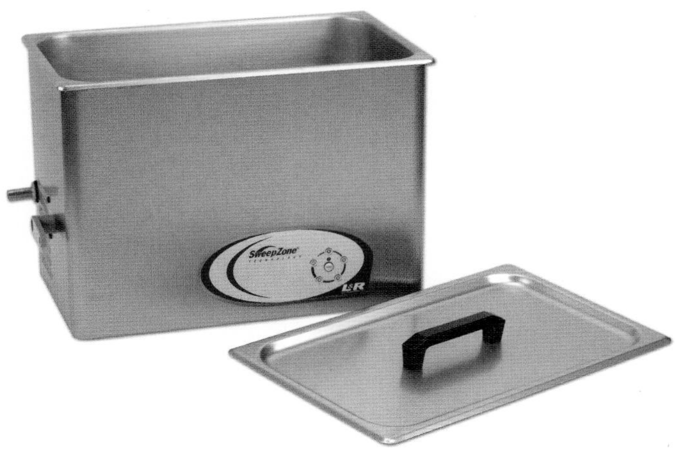

FIGURE 8-6 Ultrasonic cleaner used for precleaning contaminated items. (Courtesy L & R Manufacturing Company, Kearney, New Jersey.)

cleaning times because the cassette material absorbs some of the ultrasonic energy.

You should use ultrasonic solutions that are specially formulated for use only in the ultrasonic cleaner. Some ultrasonic cleaning products have enzyme activity (Figure 8-6). Other ultrasonic cleaning products have antimicrobial activity, which reduces the buildup of microbes in solutions with repeated use. Antimicrobial activity does not disinfect the instruments; it merely prevents microorganisms from increasing in number.

Do not use other chemicals such as plain disinfectants in the ultrasonic cleaner. Some disinfectants can *affix* the blood and debris onto the instruments, making subsequent cleaning more difficult. Specific ultrasonic solutions are available that remove difficult materials, such as cements, tartar, stains, plaster, and alginate (Figure 8-7). Refer to the ultrasonic unit manufacturer's instructions regarding the specific solution to be used.

Similar to the holding solution, the ultrasonic cleaning unit should be labeled with both a chemical label and a biohazard

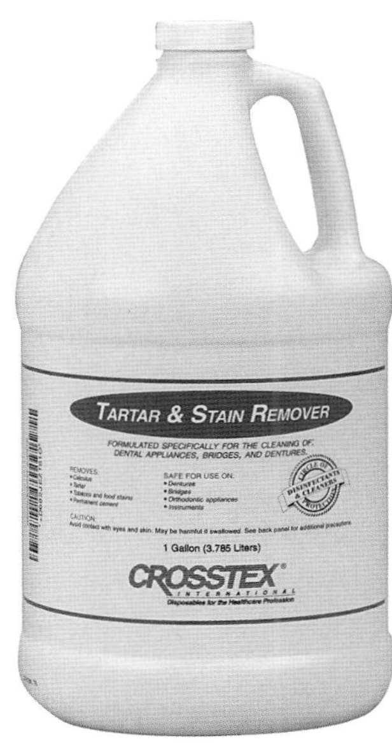

FIGURE 8-7 Special tartar and stain remover ultrasonic solution. (Courtesy Crosstex International, Inc., Hauppauge, New York.)

label because it contains a chemical along with contaminated instruments.

Care of the Ultrasonic Cleaner

The ultrasonic cleaner solution is highly contaminated and must be discarded at least once a day or sooner if it becomes visibly cloudy. When the solution is changed, the inside of the pan and lid should be rinsed with water, disinfected, rinsed again, and dried. All personal protective equipment (PPE) should be worn for changing of solutions in the ultrasonic cleaner.

Testing the Ultrasonic Cleaner

If you notice that the instruments are not being completely cleaned after processing in the ultrasonic cleaner, then the unit may not be properly functioning.

To determine whether the ultrasonic cleaner is properly working, hold a 5 × 5-inch sheet of lightweight aluminum foil vertically (like a curtain) half-submerged in the fresh, unused solution. Run the unit for 20 seconds, and then hold the foil up toward the light. The surfaces that were submerged in the solution should be evenly marked with a tiny pebbling effect over the entire surface. An area on the foil that is greater than ½-inch without pebbling indicates that a problem with the unit exists and that it needs servicing by the manufacturer.

Automated Washers and Disinfectors

Automated instrument washers and disinfectors look and work similar to a household dishwasher. However, the U.S. Food and Drug Administration (FDA) must approve them for use with dental instruments (Figure 8-8).

Automated washing and disinfecting units use a combination of very hot water recirculation and detergents to remove organic material. Then the instruments are automatically dried. These units are classified as thermal disinfectors because they

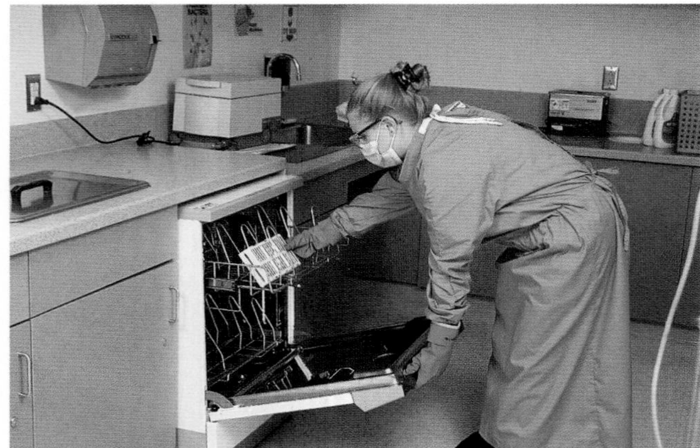

FIGURE 8-8 Miele Dental Thermal Disinfector provides safe and thorough instrument cleaning, disinfecting, and drying. Instruments must be packaged and sterilized after the cycle.

have a disinfecting cycle that subjects the instruments to a level of heat that kills most vegetative microorganisms.

Instruments processed in the automatic washers and disinfectors must be wrapped and sterilized before using on a patient.

Drying, Lubrication, and Corrosion Control

Instruments and burs made of carbon steel will rust during steam sterilization. Rust inhibitors, such as sodium nitrate or commercial products, are available as a spray or dip solution and will help reduce rust and corrosion.

Thoroughly drying the instrument using dry heat or unsaturated chemical vapor sterilization (see "Chemical Vapor Sterilization" section in this chapter) is an alternative to using rust inhibitors and does not cause rusting.

Hinged instruments may need to be lubricated to maintain proper opening. Take care to remove all excess lubricant before heat sterilization.

Packaging Instruments

Before sterilization, the instruments should be wrapped or packaged to protect them from becoming contaminated after sterilization. When instruments are sterilized without being packaged, they are immediately exposed to the environment as soon as the sterilizer door is opened. They can be contaminated by aerosols in the air, dust, improper handling, or contact with nonsterile surfaces.

An additional advantage of packaging instruments is that they can be grouped into special setups, such as crown and bridge, amalgam, prophy, or composite.

Packaging Materials

Sterilization packaging materials and cassettes are medical devices and therefore must be FDA approved. Using only products and materials that are labeled as *sterilization packaging* is critical. Never substitute products such as plastic wraps, paper, or zipper-lock freezer bags that are not registered for this purpose. These products may melt or prevent the sterilizing agent from reaching the instruments inside.

TABLE 8-2
Packaging Materials and Types of Sterilization

Packaging Material	Tips
Steam Sterilization	
Paper wrap	Do not use closed containers.
Nylon tubing	Do not use thick cloth.
Paper or plastic peel pouches	Some plastics melt.
Thin cloth	
Wrapped perforated cassettes	
Dry heat sterilizers	
Paper wrap	Some paper may scorch.
Appropriate type of nylon *plastic* tube	Some plastics melt.
Closed containers (use biologic indicator)	Use only materials approved for dry heat.
Unsaturated Chemical Vapor	
Paper wrap	Do not use closed containers.
Paper or plastic peel pouches	Do not use cloth (absorbs too much chemical vapor).
Wrapped perforated cassettes	Some plastics melt. Use only materials approved for chemical vapor.

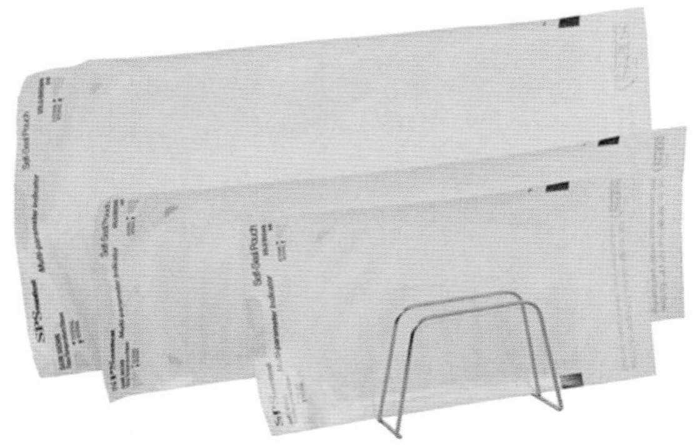

FIGURE 8-9 Self-seal packages provide an excellent wrap for sterilized materials. (Courtesy SPSmedical Supply Corporation, Rush, New York.)

Specific types of packaging material are available for each method of sterilization. You should use only the type of packaging material designed for the particular method of sterilization that you are using (Table 8-2).

A wide variety of sterilization packaging materials are available. Self-sealing or heat-sealed *poly bags* or tubes provide an excellent wrap (Figure 8-9). In addition, paper wraps and cloth wraps are available. If the package is not the self-sealing type, then you should use only sterilization indicator tape to seal the package.

TABLE 8-3
Advantages and Disadvantages of Sterilization Methods

Method of Sterilization	Advantages	Disadvantages
Steam autoclave	Sterilizes in a short time. Provides good penetration of steam. Is commonly used in dental offices. Can sterilize water-based liquids.	Damages some rubber and plastic items. Requires the use of distilled water. May rust non–stainless steel instruments and burs. Cannot use closed containers. Instruments may be wet after cycle.
Unsaturated chemical vapor	Sterilizes in a short time. Prevents corrosion. Instruments quickly dry after cycle.	Instruments must be dry. May damage plastic and rubber items. Requires special solution. Requires good ventilation. Cannot sterilize liquids. Cannot use closed containers. Cloth wrap may absorb chemicals.
Dry heat oven type (static air)	Prevents corrosion. Can use closed containers. Items are dry after cycle.	Requires long sterilization time. Requires predry instruments. Damages plastic and rubber. Cannot sterilize liquids.
Rapid heat transfer (forced air)	Is very fast. Prevents No corrosion. Items are dry after cycle.	Damages some plastics and rubber. Requires predry instruments. Cannot sterilize liquids.

Never use safety pins, staples, paper clips, or other sharp objects that could penetrate the packaging material.

The instruments are now ready for the sterilization process.

Reusing Wraps

Standard sterilization wraps are not to be reused; they are neither designed for reuse nor FDA registered for reuse. Reusing single-use sterilization wraps or bags can result in a loss of chemical indicator ability, insecure sealing of the package, and an inability of the package material to maintain sterility of the contents after processing.

Methods of Sterilization

Sterilization destroys all microbial forms, including bacterial spores. Sterile is an absolute term; there is no *partially* sterile or *almost* sterile.

All reusable items—critical and semicritical instruments—that come in contact with the patient's blood, saliva, or mucous membranes must be heat sterilized. The three most common forms of heat sterilization in the dental office are (1) steam sterilization, (2) unsaturated chemical vapor sterilization, and (3) dry heat sterilization (Table 8-3).

Although most reusable items can withstand heat processing, a few plastic items, such as rubber dam frames, shade guides, and x-ray film-holding devices, will be damaged by heat. For such items, a liquid sterilant must be used. A liquid sterilant is not recommended for use on any item that can withstand heat sterilization or is disposable.

Autoclaving

An **autoclave** is used to sterilize dental instruments and other items by means of steam under pressure. The autoclave is used for sterilization of a variety of dental instruments and accessories, including heat-resistant plastics, dental handpieces, instruments, cotton rolls, and gauze (Figure 8-10). Packaging material for autoclave sterilization must be porous enough to permit the steam to penetrate the packaging to the instruments inside. The packaging material may be fabric but most often is sealed film or paper pouches, nylon tubing, sterilizing wrap, or paper-wrapped cassettes.

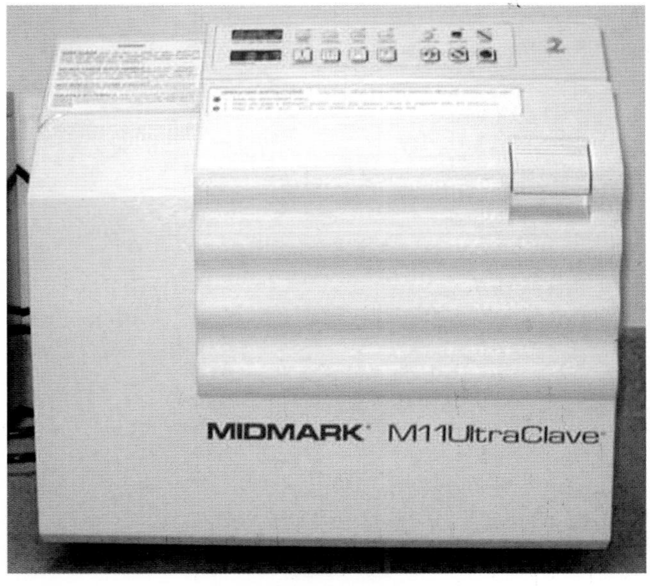

FIGURE 8-10 Steam autoclave.

Solid closed metal trays, capped glass vials, and aluminum foil cannot be used in an autoclave because they prevent the steam from reaching the inside of the pack.

A disadvantage of steam sterilization is that the moisture may cause corrosion on some high-carbon steel instruments. Distilled water should be used in autoclaves instead of tap water, which often contains minerals and impurities. Distilled water can minimize corrosion and pitting.

Operation Cycles

Dental office steam sterilizers usually operate through four cycles: (1) heat-up cycle, (2) sterilizing cycle, (3) depressurization cycle, and (4) drying cycle.

After water is added, the chamber is loaded, the door is closed, the unit is turned on, and the heat-up cycle begins to generate steam. The steam pushes out the air in the chamber, and when the set temperature is reached, the sterilizing cycle begins. The temperature is maintained for the set time, usually ranging from 3 to 30 minutes (Table 8-4).

All steam sterilizers operate in a similar manner, but different models and brands have different features. Various sizes of chambers and mechanisms of air removal, steam generation, drying, temperature displays, and recording devices are available (Figure 8-11).

Procedure 8-2 illustrates the use of an autoclave.

Flash Sterilization

Rapid or flash sterilization of dental instruments is accomplished by rapid heat transfer, steam, and unsaturated chemical vapor (Figure 8-12).

TABLE 8-4
Typical Steam Temperatures in Sterilizing Cycle

Temperature	Time
250° F (121° C)	30 minutes
250° F (121° C)	15 minutes
273° F (134° C)	10 minutes
273° F (134° C)	3 minutes

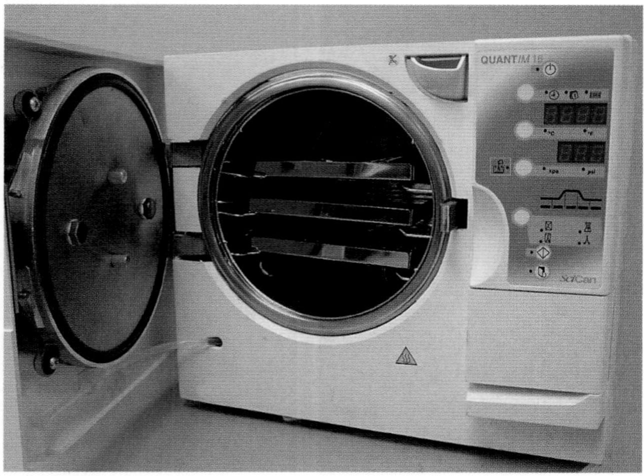

FIGURE 8-11 Postvacuum-type autoclave. (Courtesy SciCan Inc., Canonsburg, Pennsylvania.)

Flash sterilization may only be used on instruments that are placed in the chamber unwrapped. This presents a compromise because the sterility of the instruments is immediately defeated when the instruments are removed from the sterilizer.

Flash sterilization also should be used only for instruments that are to be promptly used after removal from the sterilizer. Using a method of sterilization in which the instruments can be packaged before use and remain packaged until the time of use is always the best policy.

Chemical Vapor Sterilization

Chemical vapor sterilization is very similar to autoclaving, except a combination of chemicals—alcohol, formaldehyde, ketone, acetone, and water—is used instead of water to create a vapor for sterilizing (Figure 8-13 and Procedure 8-3). OSHA requires a safety data sheet (SDS) on the chemical vapor solution because of the chemicals' toxicity.

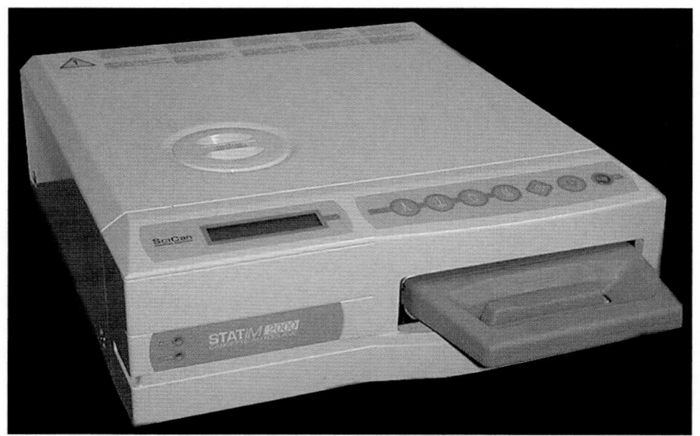

FIGURE 8-12 STATIM sterilizer. (Courtesy SciScan Inc., Canonsburg, Pennsylvania.)

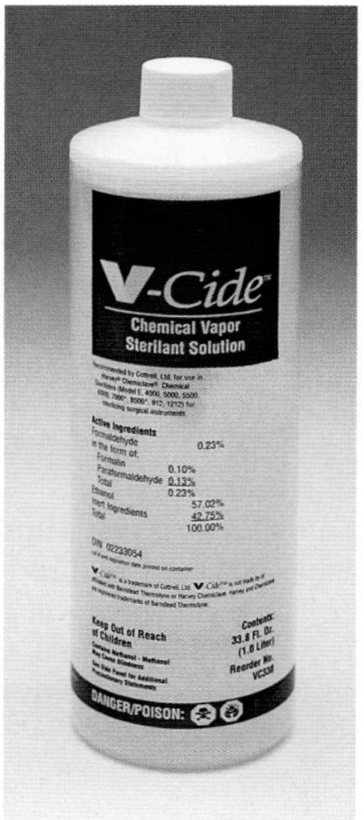

FIGURE 8-13 Sterilant solution used for a chemical vapor sterilizer. (Courtesy Certol, Commerce City, Colorado.)

Advantages

The major advantage of the chemical vapor sterilizer is that it does not rust, dull, or corrode dry metal instruments. The low water content of the vapor prevents destruction of items such as endodontic files, orthodontic pliers, wires, bands, and burs. A wide range of items can be routinely sterilized without damage.

Other advantages include the short cycle time and the availability of a dry instrument after the cycle.

Disadvantages

The primary disadvantage of the chemical vapor sterilizer is that adequate ventilation is essential because residual chemical vapors containing formaldehyde and methyl alcohol can be released when the chamber door is opened at the end of the cycle. These vapors can temporarily leave an unpleasant odor in the area and may be irritating to the eyes.

Packaging

Standard packaging for chemical vapor sterilization includes film pouches or paper bags, nylon see-through tubing, sterilization wrap, and wrapped cassettes. Packages should not be too thick or tightly wrapped to ensure adequate contact with the chemical vapors.

As in autoclaving, closed containers (such as solid metal trays and capped glass vials) and aluminum foil cannot be used in a chemical vapor sterilizer because they prevent the sterilizing agent from reaching the instruments inside.

Pressure, Temperature, and Time

The three major factors in chemical vapor sterilization are pressure, which should measure 20 pounds per square inch (psi); temperature, which should measure 270° F (131° C); and time, which should measure 20 to 40 minutes.

Dry Heat Sterilization

Dry heat sterilization operates by heating up air and transferring that heat from the air to the instruments. This form of sterilization requires higher temperatures than steam or chemical vapor sterilization. Dry heat sterilizers operate at approximately 320° F to 375° F (160° C to 190° C) and vary in the time of operation, depending on the manufacturer's instructions.

See Procedure 8-4: Sterilizing Instruments With Dry Heat.

The advantage of dry heat is that the instruments will not rust if they are thoroughly dry before they are placed in the sterilizer. Two types of dry heat sterilizers are static air and forced air.

Static Air Sterilizers

A **static air sterilizer** is similar to an oven; the heating coils are on the bottom of the chamber, and the hot air rises inside through natural convection. Heat is transferred from the static (nonmoving) air to the instruments in approximately 1 to 2 hours. The disadvantages of static dry heat are that the sterilization process is time-consuming and may not be effective if the operatory makes errors in calculating the correct processing time. The wrapping material must be heat resistant. Aluminum foil, metal, and glass containers may be used. Paper and cloth packs should be avoided because they may burn or discolor from the intense heat.

Forced Air Sterilizers

A **forced air sterilizer**, also called a rapid heat transfer sterilizer, circulates hot air throughout the chamber at a high velocity. This action permits rapid transfer of heat energy from the air to the instruments, reducing the time needed for sterilization. After the sterilizing temperature has been reached, exposure time in forced air sterilizers ranges from 6 minutes for unpackaged items to 12 minutes for packaged items.

Chemical Liquid Sterilization

Not all items can withstand heat sterilization. Some types of plastics, such as some rubber dam frames, shade guides, and x-ray film-holding devices, are damaged by heat sterilization. Thus a liquid sterilant, such as 2% to 3.4% glutaraldehyde, may be used for sterilization of these items (Procedure 8-5). Sterilization in glutaraldehyde requires a 10-hour contact time; anything less than 10 hours is disinfection, not sterilization (Figure 8-14). Biologic monitoring is not possible when using chemical liquid sterilants.

Be sure that you have an SDS for each of these products. All employees should be properly trained on how to handle such devices.

Sterilization Monitoring

To ensure that the sterilization process is actually effective in achieving complete sterilization of all dental instruments, a comprehensive monitoring program should be used.

Currently, three forms of sterilization monitoring are used: physical, chemical, and biologic. All three processes are unique, have different functions, and must be consistently used to ensure sterility.

Physical Monitoring

Physical monitoring refers to the use of a simple checklist process that verifies certain factors for every sterilization

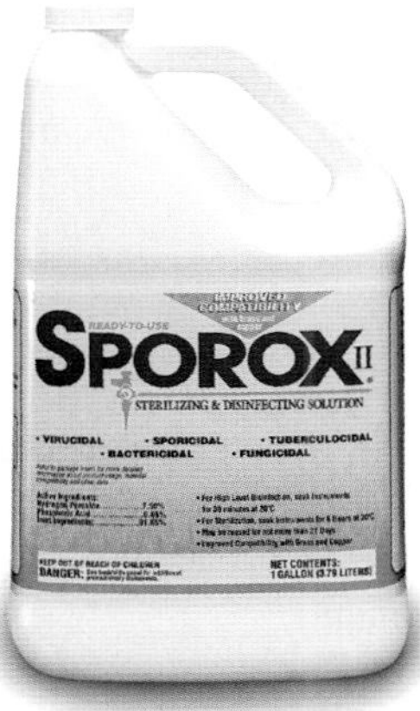

FIGURE 8-14 SPOROX® II is a high-level disinfectant and sterilant used for instruments that cannot tolerate heat sterilization. (Courtesy Sultan Chemists, Inc. Englewood, New Jersey.)

cycle. The cycle factors that should be monitored are the following:

- Level of solution
- Temperature
- Pressure
- Time

Although correct readings do not guarantee sterilization, an incorrect reading is the first signal of a problem.

Remember that the temperature recorded is for the chamber, not the inside of the pack. Therefore problems with overloading or improper packaging would not be detected from the reading on the gauges.

Chemical Monitoring

Chemical monitoring (external and internal) involves the use of a heat-sensitive chemical that changes color when exposed to certain conditions. The two types of chemical indicators are process indicators and process integrators.

Process Indicators

Process indicators (external) are placed outside the instrument packages before sterilization. Examples are autoclave tape and color change markings on packages or bags (Figure 8-15).

Process indicators simply identify instrument packs that have been exposed to a certain temperature; they do not measure the duration or the pressure. Process indicators are useful in distinguishing packages that were processed from those that were not. They can be used to prevent accidental use of unprocessed instruments.

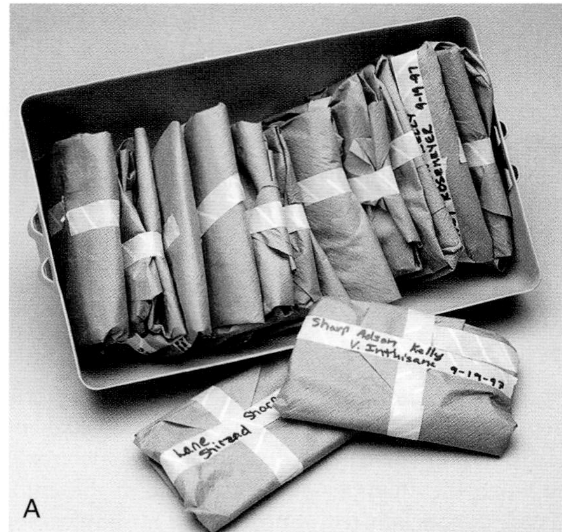

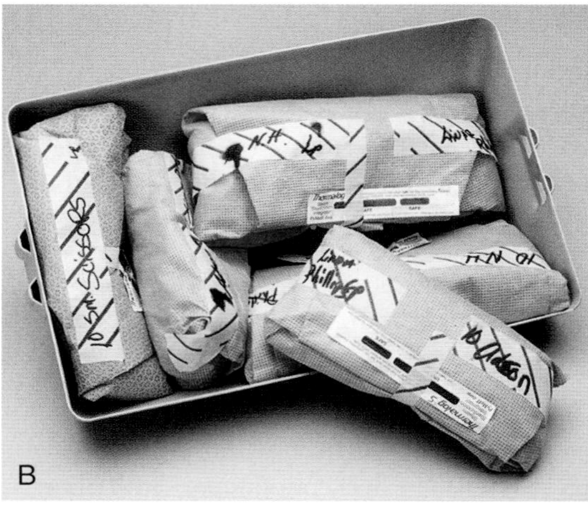

FIGURE 8-15 **A,** Unprocessed instruments. **B,** Wrapped instruments after processing. Note the color change in the tape. (From Proctor DB, Adams AP: *Kinn's the medical assistant: an applied learning approach,* ed 12, St. Louis, 2014, Saunders.)

Process Integrators

Process integrators (internal) are placed inside instrument packages. They respond to a combination of pressure, temperature, and time. Process integrators are also known as *multiparameter indicators.* All sterilization factors are integrated.

Examples of process integrators include strips, tabs, or tubes of colored liquid. The advantage of placing integrators inside each package is the assurance that the sterilizing agent penetrated the packaging (Figure 8-16).

Limitations

Process indicators and integrators provide immediate, visual control of sterilizing conditions. They do not indicate sterility and are not a replacement for biologic monitoring.

Biologic Monitoring

Biologic monitoring, or spore testing, is the only approved way to confirm whether sterilization has occurred and if all bacteria and endospores have been killed. The Centers for Disease Control and Prevention (CDC), the American Dental Association (ADA), and the Organization for Safety, Asepsis and Procedures (OSAP) recommend at least weekly biologic monitoring of sterilization equipment.

Several states also require routine biologic monitoring at weekly, monthly, or cycle-specific intervals, such as spore testing every 40 hours of use or every 30 days, whichever comes first. (Check the requirements in your state.)

See Procedure 8-6: Performing Biologic Monitoring.

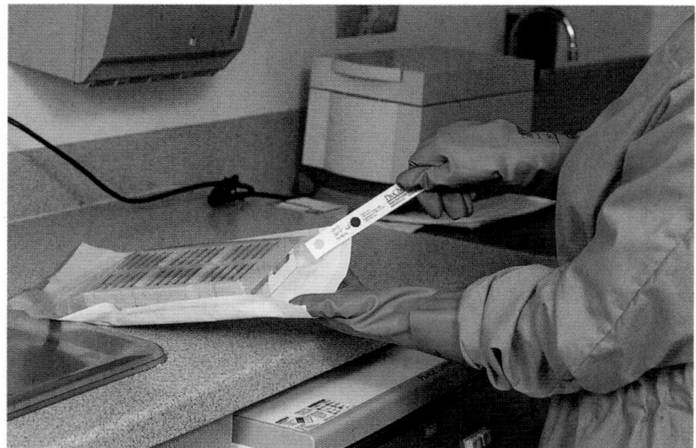

FIGURE 8-16 The dental assistant inserts the integrator strip into the sterilization pouch with the instruments.

Biologic indicators (BIs), also known as spore tests, are vials or strips of paper that contain harmless bacterial spores (spores are highly resistant to heat).

Three BIs are used in testing. Two BIs are placed inside instrument packs, and the sterilizer is operated under normal conditions. The third strip is set aside as a control.

After the load has been sterilized, all BIs are cultured. If the spores survive the sterilization cycle (a positive culture), then a sterilization failure has occurred. If the spores are killed (a negative culture), then the sterilization cycle was successful.

Culturing of the spore test is usually handled through the use of a mail-in monitoring service (Figure 8-17). If in-office culturing is performed, then the manufacturer's instructions must be carefully followed to avoid errors (Figure 8-18).

Maintaining accurate records of the results of each test is very important.

Sterilization Failures

Several factors can cause the sterilization process to fail, including improper instrument cleaning or packaging and sterilizer malfunction (Table 8-5).

The monitoring service will generally report a sterilization failure (a positive result) to the dental office immediately

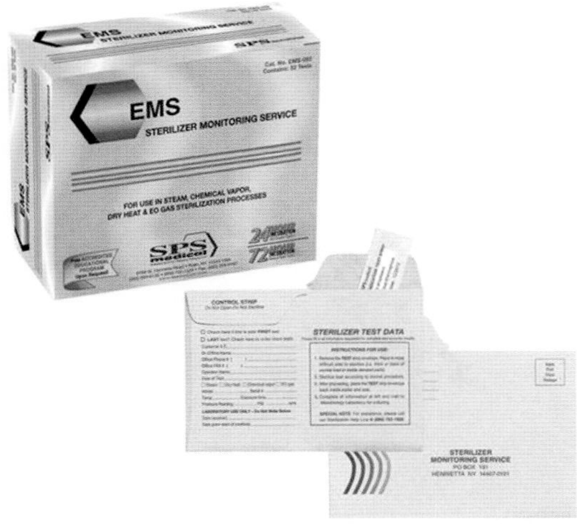

FIGURE 8-17 Using a mail-in service is a convenient method of biologic monitoring. (Courtesy SPSmedical Supply Corporation, Rush, New York.)

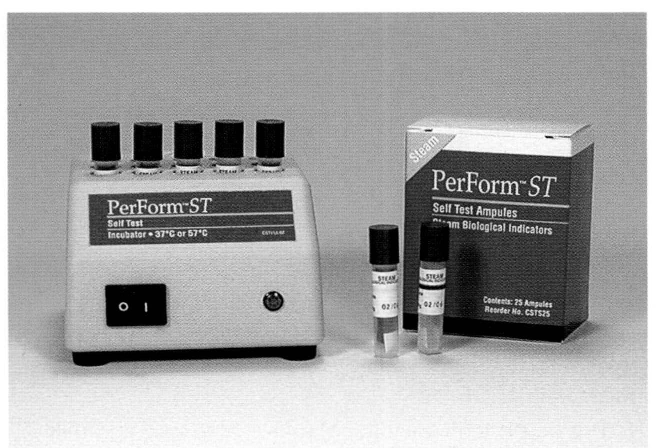

FIGURE 8-18 In-office biologic monitoring system. (Courtesy Certol, Commerce City, Colorado.)

TABLE 8-5
Results of Sterilization Errors

Errors	Examples	Results
Inadequate instrument cleaning	Dried blood and/or cement remain on the instruments.	Organisms may be insulated from the sterilizing agent.
Improper packaging	Wrap is excessive (too thick).	Prevents sterilizing agent from reaching the instruments.
	Packaging material is not compatible with the type of sterilizer.	Wrap may melt, or sterilizing agent may not penetrate the wrap.
	Container in the chemical vapor sterilizer or autoclave is closed.	Sterilizing agent cannot reach the inside surfaces.
Improper loading	Sterilizer is overloaded.	Increases the time to reach the proper temperature and can slow the penetration to the center of the load.
	No separation is allowed between the packages (too close together).	May prevent sterilizing agent from reaching all items and surfaces.
Improper timing	Operator makes a timing error.	Time to sterilize is insufficient.
	Timing is started before reaching the proper temperature (in nonautomatic units)	Time to sterilize is insufficient.
	Dry heat sterilizer door is opened during the cycle without starting over the time.	Time to sterilize is insufficient.
Improper temperature	Operator makes an error in operating the sterilizer.	Temperature is insufficient to sterilize.
	Sterilizer malfunctions.	Temperature is insufficient to sterilize.

by telephone. (A positive report indicates that sterilization did not occur.) If the culture is negative (a negative result), then the monitoring service will mail a report to the dental office to document that the cultures were read at 24, 48, and 72 hours. (A negative report indicates that sterilization did occur.)

Ethical Implications

Federal, state, and local agencies have issued regulatory actions to protect patients and members of the dental team from the transmission of disease in the dental office. Proper instrument processing is an integral component in preventing microorganisms from a previous patient from being transferred to the next patient.

As a member of the dental team, performing the procedures described in this chapter in a thorough and careful manner is your ethical and legal responsibility.

Procedure 8-1

Operating the Ultrasonic Cleaner

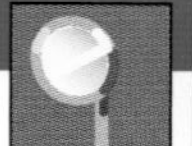
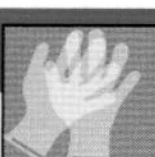
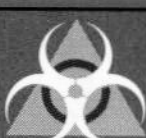
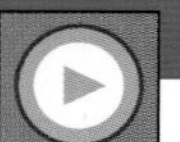

Goal

To prepare and use the ultrasonic cleaner effectively

Equipment and Supplies

- Ultrasonic cleaning unit
- Instruments
- Ultrasonic solution
- Clean towel

Procedural Steps

1. Put on protective clothing, mask, eyewear, and utility gloves.

Purpose: You will be handling sharp, contaminated instruments and using a chemical ultrasonic solution that could splash in your eyes.

2. Remove the lid from the container.

Purpose: The lid should remain on the ultrasonic device when not in use to prevent evaporation of the solution and to minimize airborne contamination.

3. Be certain the container has been filled with solution to the level recommended by the manufacturer.

Purpose: The instruments being cleaned must be completely submerged in the solution.

4. Place loose instruments in the basket or, if using cassettes, place the cassette in the basket.
5. Replace the lid, and turn the cycle to "On." The time of the cycle may vary, depending on the efficiency of the ultrasonic unit. The time ranges from 5 to 15 minutes.

Purpose: Instruments in resin or plastic cassettes require longer cleaning times because resin and plastic absorb some of the ultrasonic energy.

6. After the cleaning cycle, remove the basket and thoroughly rinse the instruments in a sink under tap water with minimal splashing. Hold the basket at an angle to allow water to run off into the sink to minimize splashing.

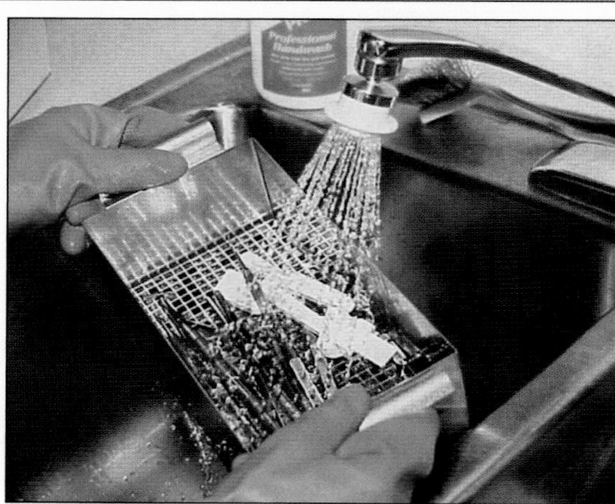

7. Gently turn the basket onto a towel, and remove the instruments or cassettes. Replace the lid on the ultrasonic cleaner.

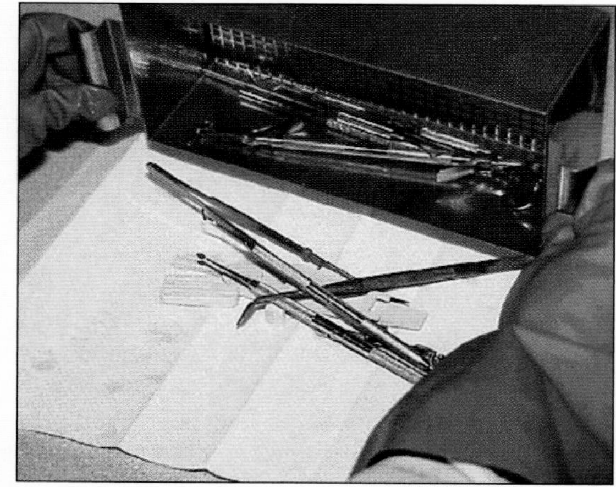

Procedure 8-2

Autoclaving Instruments

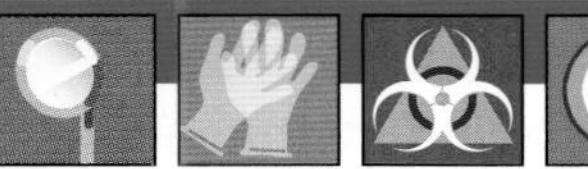

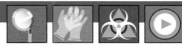

Goal

To prepare and autoclave instruments

Equipment and Supplies

- Appropriate PPE
- Autoclaving wrapping materials
- Process integrator
- Corrosion inhibitor solution (1% sodium nitrate)
- Tape to seal packages
- Pen or pencil to label packages
- Oven mitt

Procedural Steps

Wrap the Instruments

1. Instruments must be clean, but not necessarily dry, before wrapping for autoclaving.

Note: The exceptions are glass slabs and dishes, rubber items, and stones. These objects must be dry before being autoclaved.

2. Nonstainless instruments and burs may be dipped in a corrosion inhibitor solution (1% sodium nitrate) before being wrapped.

Note: An alternative for these instruments is sterilization by dry heat.

3. Insert the process integrator into the package.
4. Package, seal, and label the instruments.

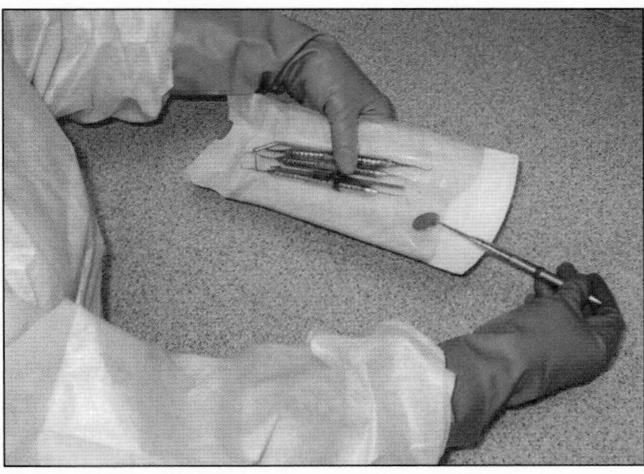

Load the Autoclave

1. Place bagged and sealed items in the autoclave.
2. Separate articles and packs from each other by a reasonable space. Tilt glass or metal canisters at an angle.

Purpose: A reasonable space between articles and packs permits the free flow of steam in and around all instrument packs.

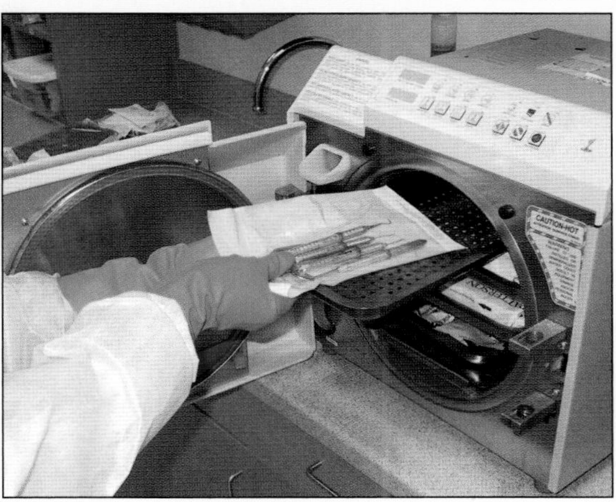

3. Place larger packs, which might block the flow of steam, at the bottom of the chamber.

Purpose: Large loads prevent the autoclave from reaching the correct temperature and pressure and make it difficult for the steam to flow properly.

4. Never overload the autoclave.

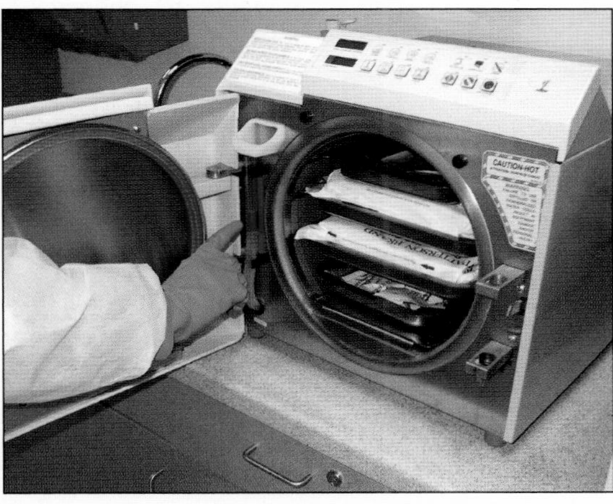

Purpose: Trapped air in the autoclave will inhibit the top-to-bottom flow of steam.

Operate the Autoclave

1. Read and follow the manufacturer's instructions. Most autoclaves require distilled water.

Purpose: Tap water often contains minerals that can damage the autoclave by forming deposits on the chamber's inner surfaces and can corrode metals.

2. Ensure that an adequate supply of water is available. If not, add distilled water.
3. Set autoclave controls for the appropriate time, temperature, and pressure.

Note: Pressure and temperature must be reached before timing begins. Duration of this warm-up time depends on the autoclave and the size of the load.

Continued

Procedure 8-2

Autoclaving Instruments—cont'd

4. At the end of the sterilization cycle, vent the steam into the room. Allow the contents of the autoclave to dry and cool.

Note: Most models automatically vent and cool. If the machine is not so equipped, then slightly open the door of the autoclave after the pressure has dropped within the chamber. Open the door with extreme caution because the contents and remaining steam are scalding. The contents should be allowed to dry and cool before they are removed.

Reassemble and Store the Trays

1. Wash your hands, and put on clean examination gloves for handling sterile packs and reassembling trays.
2. Remove sealed packs from the sterilizer, and place them in the clean area.

Important Note: Work only in the clean area of the sterilization center.

3. Place the sealed packs on the tray, and add the supplies necessary to perform the procedure.

Optional: In some practices, the necessary gloves and masks are added to the tray at this time. In other practices, these items are stored in the treatment room.

4. Store the prepared tray in the clean area until needed in the treatment room.

PPE, Personal protective equipment.

Procedure 8-3

Sterilizing Instruments With Chemical Vapor

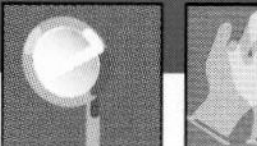
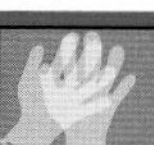

Goal

To prepare and sterilize instruments by chemical vapor sterilization

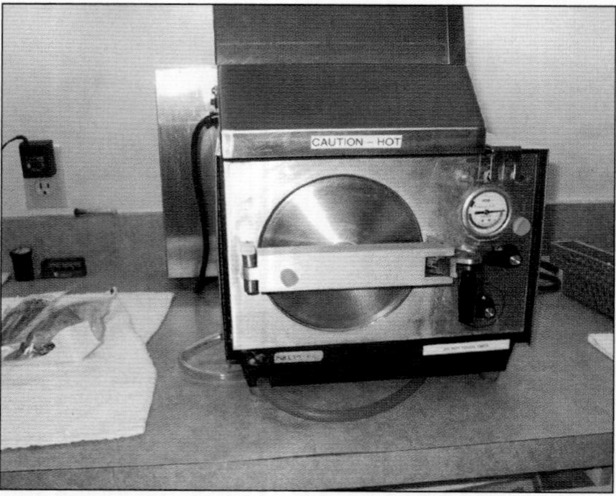

Equipment and Supplies

- Appropriate PPE
- Chemical vapor wrapping materials
- Precleaned and dried instruments
- Process integrator
- Tape to seal packages
- Pen or pencil to label packages

Procedural Steps

Wrap the Instruments

1. Ensure that the instruments are clean and dry before wrapping them for chemical vapor sterilization.

Purpose: If instruments are not absolutely dry, then they will rust.

2. Insert the appropriate process integrator into the test load instrument package.
3. Take care not to create packs that are too large to be sterilized throughout.

Purpose: Chemical vapor sterilization is not recommended for large loads or tightly wrapped instruments.

Load and Operate the Chemical Vapor Sterilizer

1. Read and follow the manufacturer's instructions.

Important Note: Always follow the precautions in the SDS.

2. Load the sterilizer according to the manufacturer's instructions.

Note: This step is similar to loading an autoclave.

3. Set the controls for the appropriate time, temperature, and pressure.

Note: Pressure and temperature must be reached before timing begins.

4. Follow the manufacturer's instructions for venting and cooling.
5. When the instruments are cool and dry, reassemble and store the preset tray.

PPE, Personal protective equipment; *SDS,* safety data sheet.

Procedure 8-4

Sterilizing Instruments With Dry Heat

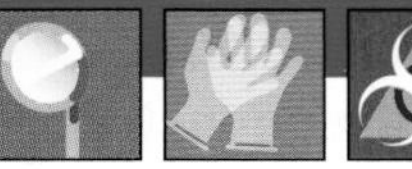
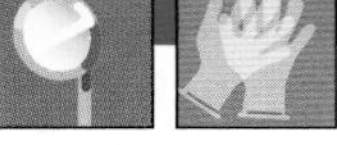
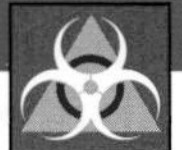

Goal

To prepare and sterilize instruments by dry heat sterilization

Equipment and Supplies

- Wrapping materials
- Precleaned instruments
- Process integrator for dry heat
- Tape to seal packages
- Pen or pencil to label packages

Procedural Steps

Wrap Instruments

1. Clean and dry instruments before wrapping.

Purpose: Wet instruments can rust during dry heat sterilization.

2. Prepare hinged instruments, such as surgical forceps, hemostats, and scissors, with their hinges opened.

Purpose: To allow heat to reach all areas during sterilization.

Load and Operate the Dry Heat Sterilizer

1. Read and follow the manufacturer's instructions.
2. Insert the process integrator into the test load package.
3. Load the dry heat chamber to permit adequate circulation of air around the packages.

Purpose: Sterilization does not occur unless heat reaches all areas of the instruments.

4. Set the time and temperature according to the manufacturer's instructions. Allow time for the entire load to reach the desired temperature.

Purpose: Timing does not start until the desired temperature has been reached throughout the entire load.

5. Do not place additional instruments in the load once the sterilization cycle has begun.

Purpose: Cooler instruments will significantly lower the temperature of the oven.

6. At the end of the sterilization cycle, allow the packs to cool and then handle them very carefully.

Purpose: Packs are very hot and could cause injury.

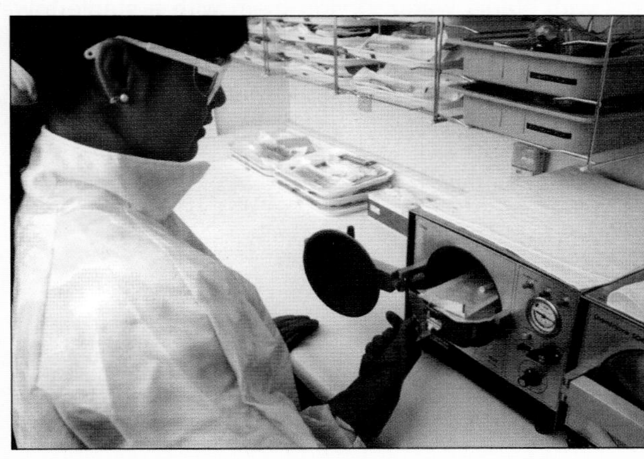

7. When the packs are cool, reassemble and store the preset tray.

Procedure 8-5

Sterilizing Instruments With Chemical Liquid

Goal

To prepare and sterilize instruments using a chemical sterilant

Equipment and Supplies

- Appropriate PPE
- Precleaned and dried items that cannot be heat sterilized
- Liquid chemical sterilant
- Sterile instrument tongs
- Sterile rinse water

Procedural Steps

Prepare the Solution

1. Use utility gloves, mask, eyewear, and protective clothing when preparing, using, and discarding the solution.

Purpose: Liquid sterilants are highly toxic and can lead to respiratory problems if not properly handled.

2. Follow the manufacturer's instructions for preparing and activating, using, and disposing of the solution.

Purpose: In many areas, glutaraldehyde is considered a hazardous material, requiring special disposal methods; it may not be dumped down the sink.

3. Prepare the solution for use as a sterilant. Label the containers with the name of the chemical, the date of preparation (to indicate the use life), and any other information that relates to the hazards of this product. Use life is the period of time during which a germicidal solution is effective after having been prepared for use.

Purpose: Some brands remain active for 30 days; others may have a longer or shorter use life.

4. Cover the container, and keep it closed unless you are putting instruments in or taking them out.

Purpose: Glutaraldehyde produces toxic fumes.

Continued

Procedure 8-5

Sterilizing Instruments With Chemical Liquid—cont'd

Use the Solution

1. Preclean, rinse, and dry the items to be processed.
2. Place the items in a perforated tray or pan. Place the pan in the solution, and cover the container. An alternative method is to use tongs and avoid splashing.
3. Be certain that all items are fully submerged in the solution for the entire contact time.

Purpose: The solution must be in contact with the items for the recommended contact time.

4. Thoroughly rinse processed items with water and dry. Place the items in a clean package.

Note: Sterility is best maintained by rinsing the processed items with sterile water, drying them with a sterile towel, and placing them in a sterile container.

Maintain the Solution

1. Periodically test the glutaraldehyde concentration of the solution with a chemical test kit (available from the manufacturer).
2. Replace the solution as indicated on the instructions or when the level of the solution is low or the solution is visibly dirty.
3. When you replace the used solution, discard all of the used solution, clean the container with a detergent, rinse with water, dry, and fill the container with a fresh solution.

Modified from Miller CH, Palenik CJ: *Infection control and management of hazardous materials for the dental team,* ed 4, St. Louis, 2010, Mosby.

PPE, Personal protective equipment.

Procedure 8-6

Performing Biologic Monitoring

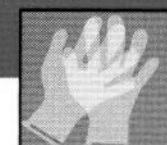
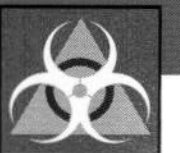

Goal

To assess sterilization using BIs (spore tests)

Equipment and Supplies

- Appropriate PPE
- Instruments
- Pencil
- Dual-species BI
- Sterilization log
- Mail-in envelope

Procedural Steps

1. While wearing all PPE, place the BI strip in the bundle of instruments and seal the package.

Purpose: Although the instruments have been precleaned, they are still contaminated.

2. Place the pack with the BI in the center of the sterilizer load.

Purpose: The center of the load is most difficult for the sterilizing agent to penetrate.

3. Place the remainder of the packaged instruments into the sterilizer, and process the load through a normal sterilization cycle.

Purpose: The monitoring evaluates what is considered the *normal* cycle.

4. Remove utility gloves, mask, and eyewear. Wash and dry hands.

Purpose: Removing all PPE and washing and drying hands prevent contamination of the sterilization log.

5. In the sterilization log, record the date of the test, type of sterilizer, cycle, temperature, time, and name of the person operating the sterilizer.

Purpose: Maintaining records is part of the exposure control program, and specific information is necessary in the event of a sterilization failure.

6. After the load has been sterilized, remove the processed BI strip.

Purpose: The BI strip has been exposed to the same sterilizing conditions as the instruments.

7. Mail the processed spore test strips and the control BI strip to the monitoring service.

Purpose: Obtaining and maintaining the results as part of the exposure control program is important.

BI, Biologic indicator; *PPE,* personal protective equipment.

Chapter Exercises

Multiple Choice

Circle the letter of the correct answer.

1. How many steps are involved in instrument processing?
   - **a.** 4
   - **b.** 5
   - **c.** 7
   - **d.** 10
2. The only certain method to determine sterilization is with the use of __________.
   - **a.** process indicators
   - **b.** process integrators
   - **c.** biologic monitoring
   - **d.** none of the above
3. Instruments that are not cleaned soon after use should be placed in a(n) __________.
   - **a.** ultrasonic cleaner
   - **b.** thermal disinfector
   - **c.** holding solution
   - **d.** rapid heat transfer unit
4. The ultrasonic cleaner solution should be changed at least __________.
   - **a.** after each patient
   - **b.** three times daily
   - **c.** once daily
   - **d.** once monthly
5. The ultrasonic cleaner should remain covered when __________.
   - **a.** not in use
   - **b.** in use
   - **c.** both of the above
6. The LEAST desirable method of precleaning instruments is __________.
   - **a.** hand scrubbing
   - **b.** ultrasonic cleaning
   - **c.** thermal disinfector
   - **d.** holding solutions
7. Which of the following can cause a sterilization failure when a dry heat sterilizer is used?
   - **a.** Improper cycle time
   - **b.** Overloading the chamber
   - **c.** Opening the door during the cycle
   - **d.** All of the above
8. The fastest method of sterilization is the __________ method.
   - **a.** autoclave
   - **b.** chemical vapor
   - **c.** dry heat static air
   - **d.** dry heat forced air
9. The method of sterilization that produces the greatest risk of rust and corrosion on the instruments is the __________ method.
   - **a.** autoclave
   - **b.** chemical vapor
   - **c.** dry heat static
   - **d.** dry heat forced
10. The method of sterilization that produces unpleasant fumes is the __________ method.
    - **a.** autoclave
    - **b.** chemical vapor
    - **c.** dry heat static
    - **d.** dry heat forced

Apply Your Knowledge

1. Mrs. Hansen is a new patient who has been referred to your office by a friend, who is also a patient in your office. Mrs. Hansen expressed concern about the sterilization procedures used in her previous dental office. What can you do to reassure Mrs. Hansen that your office takes instrument processing and sterilization very seriously?
2. On some days, you are so busy assisting with patient care at chairside that you are not always able to clean instruments soon after their use. You have noticed that dried blood and cement is not always removed during the ultrasonic cleaning process. What steps can you take to overcome this problem?
3. A new employee does not always wear her protective eyewear when operating the chemical vapor sterilizer. How could you help this new employee understand the importance of wearing all required PPE?

PART FOUR Dental Treatment

CHAPTER 9

Clinical Dentistry

http://evolve.elsevier.com/Robinson/essentials/

LEARNING OBJECTIVES

1. Pronounce, define, and spell the key terms.
2. Complete the following related to the clinical area of the dental office:
   - Describe the design and purpose of the clinical area of the dental office.
   - Identify the standard dental equipment located in the clinical area of the dental office.
3. Demonstrate the appropriate way of admitting and seating a patient.
4. Describe the proper positioning of the dental team.
5. Explain the clock concept of operating zones.
6. Demonstrate the transfer of instruments for the dentist and the clinical assistant.
7. Describe the dental assistant's role in expanded functions for restorative procedures.

KEY TERMS

carpal tunnel syndrome
cumulative trauma disorders
dental operatory
ergonomics
expanded function
grasp
operating zones
subsupine
supine

A smooth and efficient interaction between the dentist and the clinical dental assistant can determine the success of a dental practice. These two professions work closely together to accomplish four goals:

1. Increase patient comfort.
2. Provide quality dental care.
3. Reduce the time needed for dental treatment.
4. Minimize the stress and fatigue of the clinical team.

Clinical Area

The design of the clinical area depends on the physical size of the practice, the number of dentists associated with the practice, the number of dental assistants and dental hygienists on staff, and the number of patients seen daily.

The **dental treatment area,** also referred to as the dental operatory, is the center of the practice (Figure 9-1). Patients receive their treatment in this designated area. Most practices have two or more treatment areas for each dentist and then one additional treatment area for each dental hygienist.

Dental Treatment Area Equipment

The standard dental equipment in a general dental office is provided in Table 9-1. Specific descriptions and features are provided to help you learn and be familiar with their use for each patient.

Care of Dental Equipment

Dental equipment is expensive, complex, and delicate. It must always be carefully maintained in accordance with the manufacturer's instructions. The clinical staff assumes the responsibility for the daily care of equipment throughout the dental office.

Standard Procedure Routine

No matter what type of dental procedure in which you are assisting in, a standard procedure routine must be followed when admitting a patient, seating a patient, and positioning the dental team.

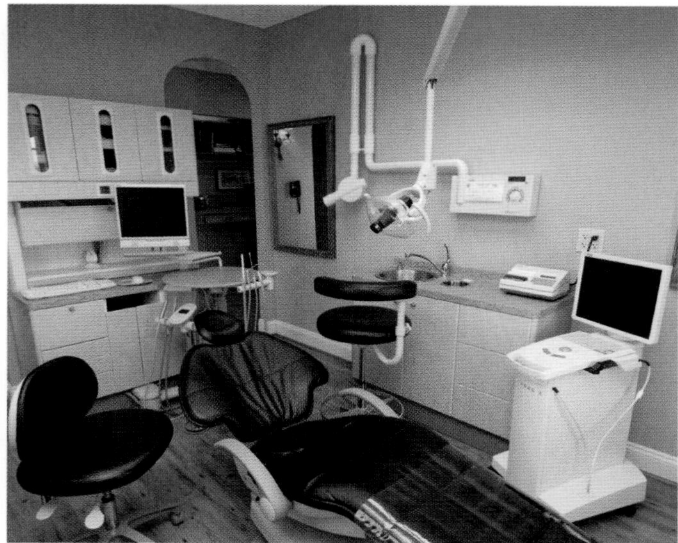

FIGURE 9-1 Dental treatment area. (Courtesy Patterson Dental, St. Paul, Minnesota.)

Admitting the Patient

Attention to detail when admitting a patient into the clinical area is very important in creating a positive experience for the patient. Always greet the patient by his or her last name, make sure to establish eye contact, smile, and introduce yourself if this is the patient's first appointment.

Once you enter the treatment area, place the patient's personal items in a safe and visible place, and initiate conversation to help the patient feel more comfortable and relaxed.

Positioning the Patient

The area of the mouth being treated and the type of procedure will determine the position of the patient chair. A patient can be placed in three different positions.

In the **upright position**, the back of the chair is placed at a 90-degree angle (Figure 9-2). This position is used for patient entry and dismissal. It may also be used when radiographs are exposed and when impressions are taken.

In the supine position, the chair back is lowered until the patient is almost lying down (Figure 9-3). Because of the contour of the chair, the patient will not appear flat. The patient's head and knees should be approximately at the same plane. The majority of dental procedures take place in this position.

The patient's head will be lower than the feet in the subsupine position and is recommended during an emergency situation, especially if a patient becomes unconscious.

See Procedure 9-1: Admitting and Seating the Patient.

Positioning the Dental Team

The manner in which the dentist and the clinical assistant position themselves around the patient allows for smooth and efficient team interaction (Figure 9-4). This concept was designed for the chairside assistant to work in close proximity with the dentist.

The rationale of this type of positioning of the dental team is to limit activities that can cause excessive reaching, bending,

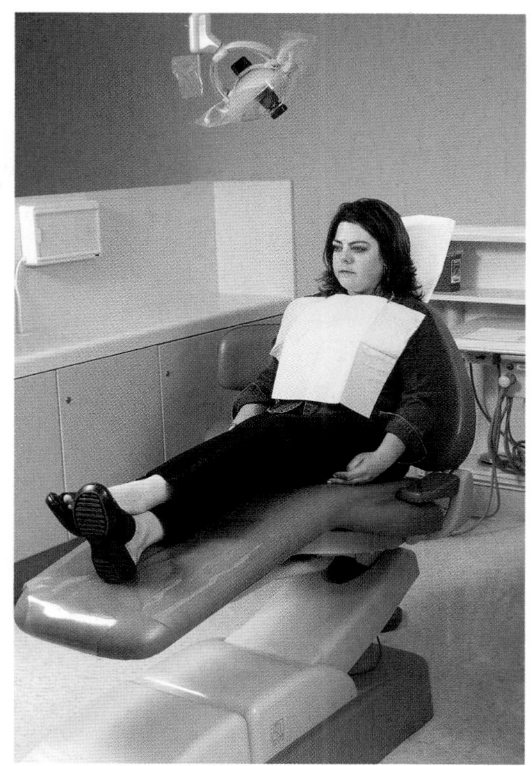

FIGURE 9-2 Patient positioned in an upright position.

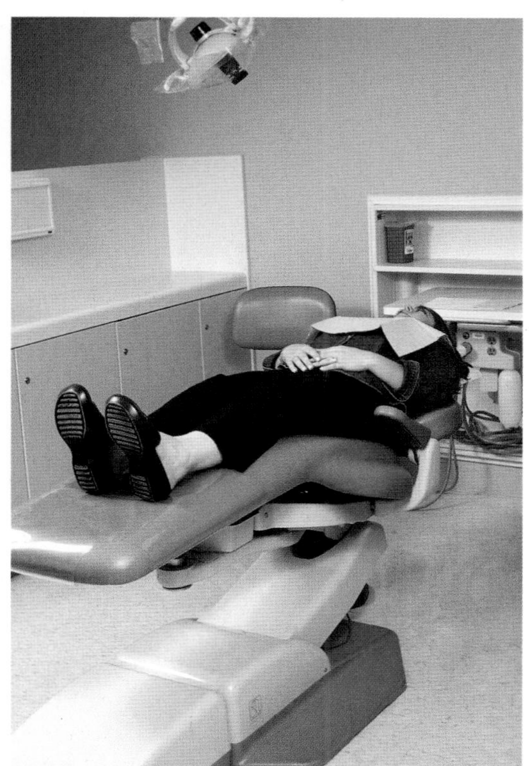

FIGURE 9-3 Patient positioned in a supine position.

TABLE 9-1
Dental Treatment Area Equipment

Type	Description	Features
Dental chair (Courtesy A-dec, Newberg, Oregon.)	Is designed to support the body with the patient's comfort in mind and to position the patient correctly for patient care.	• Adjustable headrest • Support for the arms • Controls to raise and lower the chair • Swivel chair • Adjustment controls to operate the chair
Operator's stool (Courtesy A-dec, Newberg, Oregon.)	Is designed to be ergonomically sound to support the body for a long period.	• Five casters for movement and balance • Adjustable seat • Broad base • Adjustable back
Assistant's stool (Courtesy A-dec, Newberg, Oregon.)	Is designed to be ergonomically sound and to provide stability, mobility, and comfort.	• Broad base with platform base • Wide-base seat • Abdominal bar • Foot bar for support
Operating light (Courtesy A-dec, Newberg, Oregon.)	Illuminates the oral cavity.	• Iridescent light • Track mounted
Air-water syringe	Is used in all procedures to rinse or dry a limited area or the complete mouth. Air is also used to keep the mouth mirror dry and clean.	• Provides a stream of water • Provides a stream of air • Provides a combined spray of air and water

TABLE 9-1
Dental Treatment Area Equipment—cont'd

Type	Description	Features
Oral evacuation system 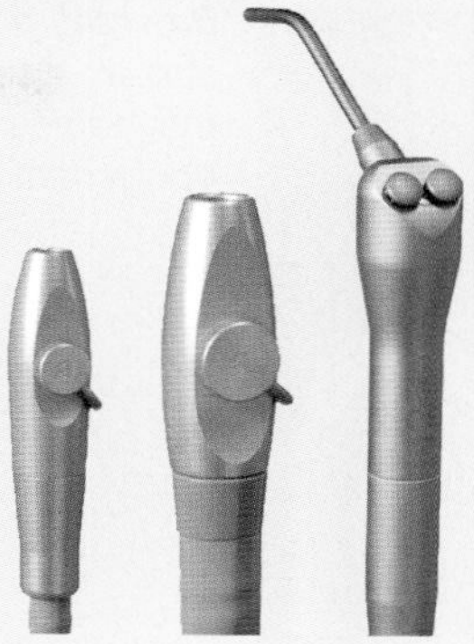 (Courtesy A-dec, Newberg, Oregon.)	Removes excess water, saliva, blood, and debris from the patient's mouth.	• Saliva ejector • High-volume evacuator (HVE) (air and water syringe)
Curing light 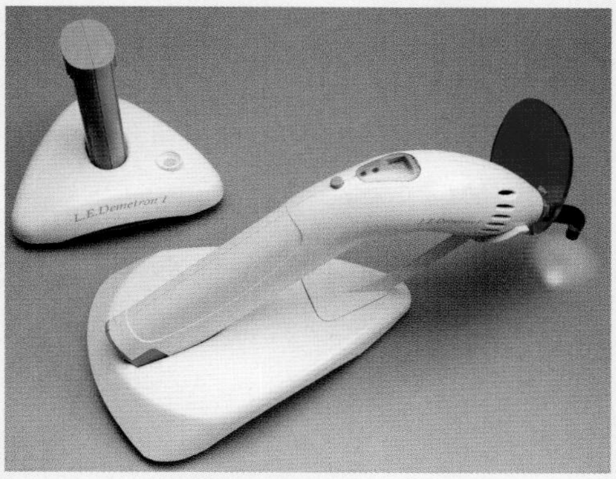 (From Boyd LRB: *Dental instruments: a pocket guide,* ed 4, St. Louis, 2012, Saunders.)	Electronically activated blue light polymerizes resins and composites.	• Lighted wand • Timer controlled
Amalgamator 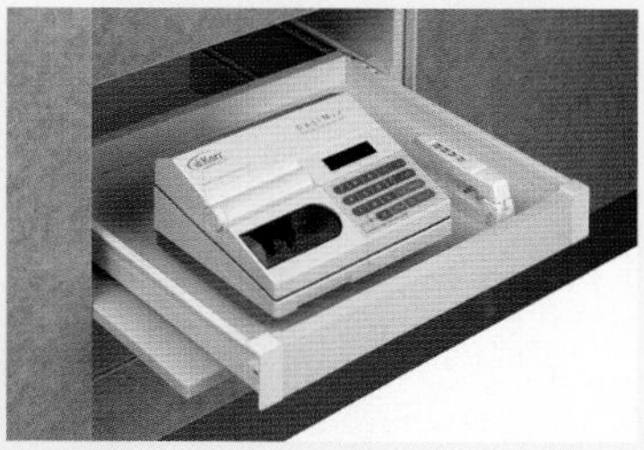 (Courtesy A-dec, Newberg, Oregon.)	Electronically triturates encapsulated dental materials.	• Covered for hazardous substance management • Timer
Rheostat 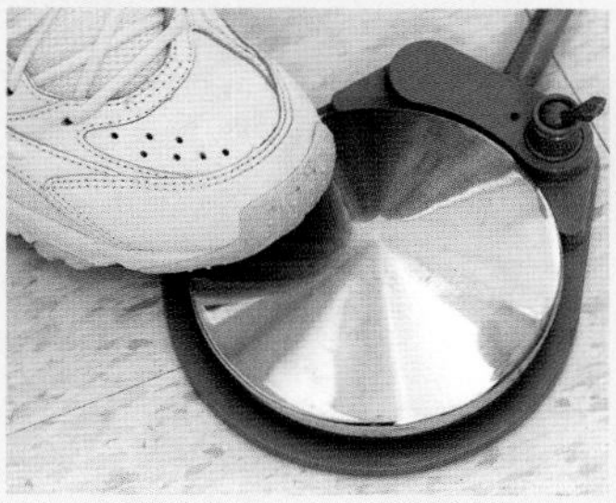	Is used to operate the slow- and high-speed handpieces.	• Foot controlled • Attached to the dental unit • Speed control by foot pressure

Continued

TABLE 9-1
Dental Treatment Area Equipment—cont'd

Type	Description	Features
Dental unit (Courtesy A-dec, Newberg, Oregon.)	Provides electrical and air-operated mechanics to the equipment.	• High- and low-speed handpieces • Air-water syringe • Saliva ejector • HVE

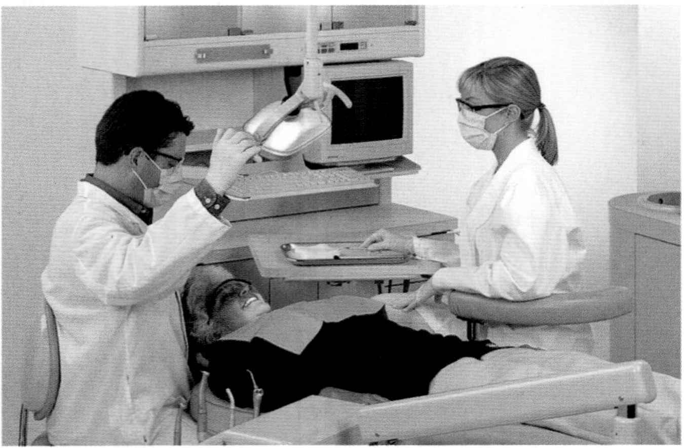

FIGURE 9-4 The dental team correctly positions themselves for a procedure. (Courtesy A-dec, Newberg, Oregon.)

and twisting. **Ergonomics** is the science that seeks to adapt working conditions to suit the worker. If this model is not followed, then specific areas of the body can be afflicted with injury when working in a dental environment.

Job-Related Injuries Associated With Dentistry

- **Carpal tunnel syndrome** (CTS)—problems associated with repetitive and forceful motion of the wrist
- **Cumulative trauma disorder** (CTD)—repetitive motion and overflexion and overextension of the wrist
- Shoulder and neck pain—strain or flexion of the shoulder for longer than 1 hour per day
- Neck and back pain—extension or elevation of the arm for an extended period
- Low back pain—twisting of the body over an extended period

Criteria for Proper Positioning of the Seated Operator (Figure 9-5)

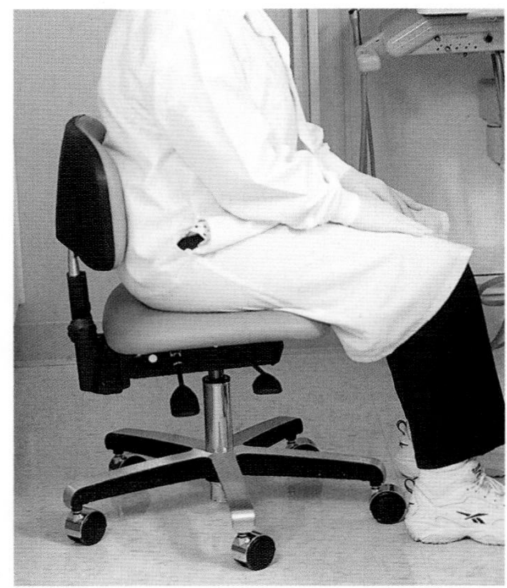

FIGURE 9-5 Proper positioning for a seated operator.

- The operator is seated in an unstrained position with back straight, feet flat on the floor, and thighs angled so that the knees are slightly lower than hip level.
- The operator should position elbows close to the sides, and the shoulders should be relaxed.
- The oral cavity should be positioned at the operator's elbow height.
- The operator's head should be positioned facing forward with eyes focused downward.

Criteria for Proper Positioning of the Clinical Assistant (Figure 9-6)

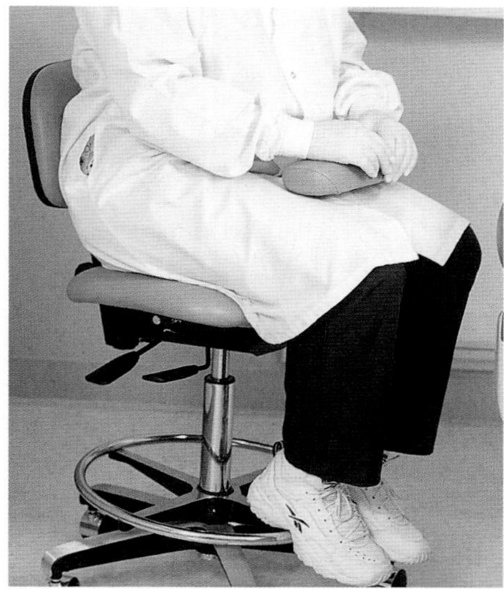

FIGURE 9-6 Proper positioning for a seated dental assistant.

- The clinical assistant is seated with a straight back and eye level approximately 4 to 5 inches higher than the operator.

Purpose: This added height allows for better visibility and easier access.

- The clinical assistant is seated with the abdominal bar adjusted to provide back or abdominal support.
- The feet should be placed on the platform near the base of the stool.
- The body is positioned facing toward the patient's head, with the hips and thighs level to the floor and parallel to the patient's shoulders.

Team Dentistry

Treatment areas can vary considerably in their design from office to office, but the type and location of equipment and the basic concepts required for practicing efficient and comfortable four-handed dentistry should be applied.

The use of **operating zones**, based on a *clock concept*, is the best way to identify the working positions of the dental team. The locations of the zones vary, depending on whether the operator ("operator" and "dentist" are used interchangeably) is right- or left-handed (Table 9-2).

Visualize a clock placed over the dental chair with the patient's face in the center of the circle and the top of the patient's head at the 12 o'clock position. The face of the clock is divided into four zones. Figure 9-7 illustrates the zones for a right-handed and a left-handed operator.

Instrument Transfer

The smooth, efficient transfer of instruments and dental materials is a team effort that requires coordination, communication, and practice between the dentist and the clinical assistant. The technique discussed is based on working with a right-handed dentist.

Basic Principles of Instrument Transfer

Instrument transfer, also referred to as *instrument exchange*, takes place in the transfer zone. The following principles are used to produce the most efficient instrument transfer:

- The clinical assistant understands the sequence of the procedure and is able to anticipate when a new instrument is required.
- A minimum of motion (involving only fingers, wrist, and elbow) should be used when transferring an instrument.
- Instruments are transferred in the **position of use**, which means that the working end of the instrument is directed toward the tooth being treated.
- The instrument is transferred so that the dentist can properly and firmly grasp the handle.
- The dentist must have a firm hold on the instrument.

Clinical Assistant's Transfer Technique

For transferring instruments throughout a procedure, a specific **single-handed technique** is designed to be used for its efficiency. This technique applies to hand instruments, dental handpieces, and the air-water syringe. Use the following basic principles to retrieve, transfer, and return instruments:

- The assistant will retrieve an instrument from the tray setup using the thumb, index finger, and middle finger of the left hand (Figure 9-8).
- The assistant retrieves the used instrument at the end of the handle or at the opposite end of the working end, using the last two fingers of the left hand (Figure 9-9).
- The assistant transfers the new instrument in the transfer zone and firmly positions it into the operator's grasp, making sure the working end of the instrument is directed toward the tooth surface or arch on which the operator is working (Figure 9-10).

Operator's Grasp in Receiving an Instrument

The manner in which the dentist holds an instrument is termed the **grasp**. The grasp is determined by the type of instrument, how it is used, and which arch is being treated. An understanding of these instrument grasps is essential for smooth instrument transfer and exchange of instruments (Figure 9-11).

Variations of Instrument Exchange

Because of their design or their use, certain instruments will be transferred differently.

See Procedure 9-2: Transferring Instruments Using the Single-Handed Technique and Procedure 9-3: Transferring Instruments Using the Two-Handed Technique.

Mirror and Explorer

When beginning a procedure, the dentist will signal that the procedure is about to begin by placing one hand on each side of the patient's mouth ready to receive the mirror and explorer. The clinical assistant will simultaneously deliver the mirror and the explorer, using a two-handed exchange. The dentist uses the

TABLE 9-2 Operating Zones

Zones	Location	Description
Static zone	RH 12:00-2:00 LH 10:00-12:00	Is directly behind the patient. A dental unit or a mobile cabinet is positioned in this area.
Operator's zone	RH 7:00-12:00 LH 12:00-5:00	Is to the side of the patient. The dentist is seated and moves in this area.
Assistant's zone	RH 2:00-4:00 LH 8:00-10:00	Is positioned on the opposite side of the patient from the operator. A mobile cabinet can be positioned to hold instruments and dental materials.
Transfer zone	RH 4:00-7:00 LH 5:00-8:00	Is directly over the patient's chest. The instruments and dental materials are exchanged in this area. Special caution must be taken not to transfer anything over the patient's face.

LH, Left-handed; *RH,* right-handed.

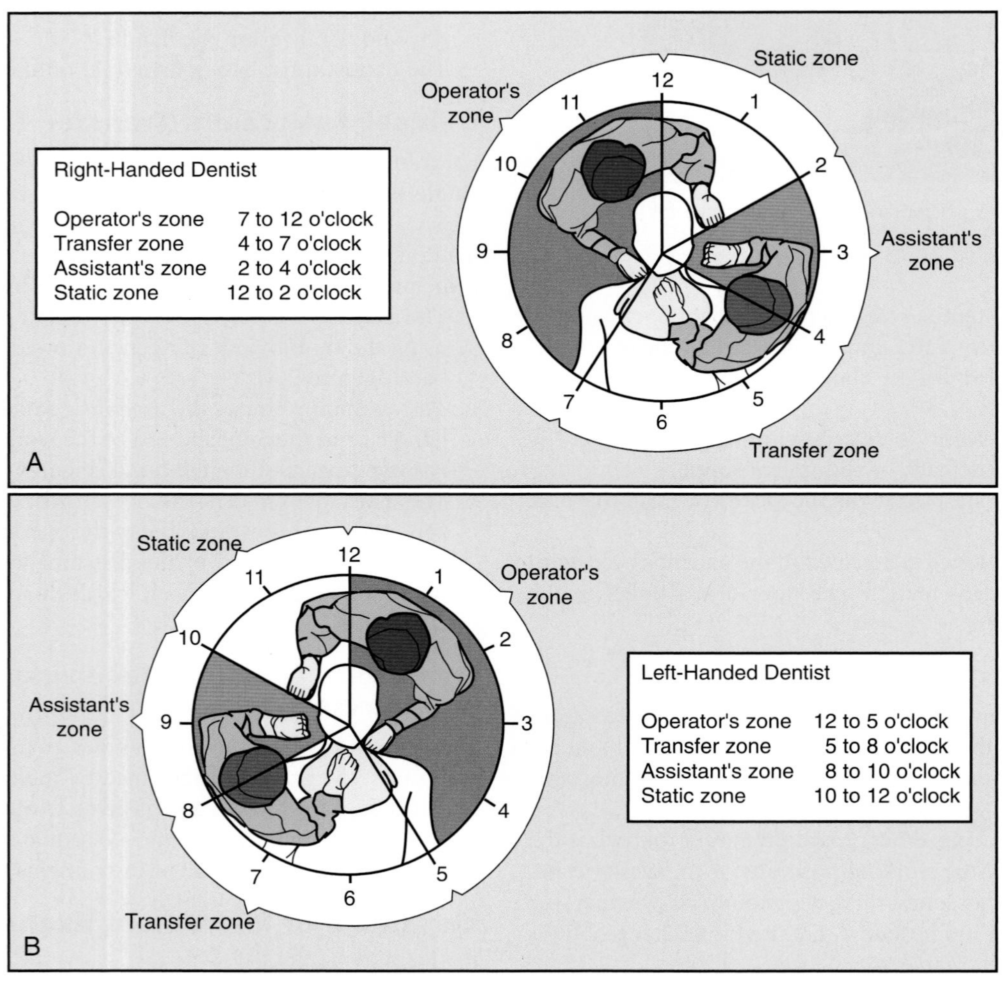

FIGURE 9-7 The clock concept for operating zones. **A,** Left zones for a right-handed dentist. **B,** Right zones for a left-handed dentist.

mouth mirror and the explorer to inspect the area to be treated (Figure 9-12).

Hinged Instruments

Instruments with hinges, such as forceps, scissors, and pliers, are designed to have both open and closed use. For pickup and transfer, these instruments are held at the hinge of the instrument and are transferred by directing the handle of the instrument into the dentist's palm or by positioning the handle of the scissors over the dentist's fingers (Figure 9-13).

Cotton Pliers

When cotton pliers are used to transfer small items to and from the oral cavity, a modification must be made to the

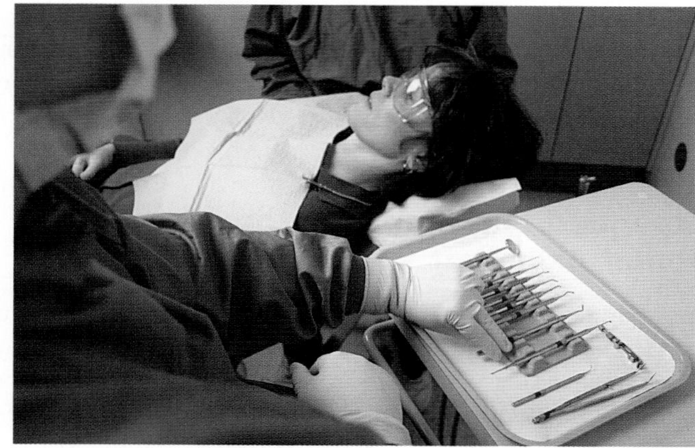

FIGURE 9-8 Retrieving an instrument from the tray setup.

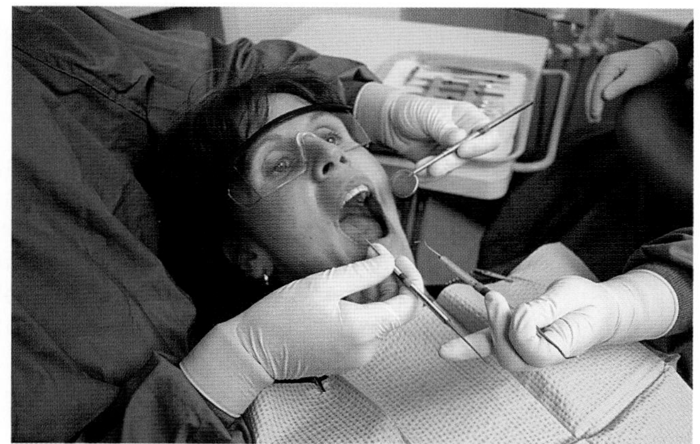

FIGURE 9-9 The used instrument is retrieved from the operator.

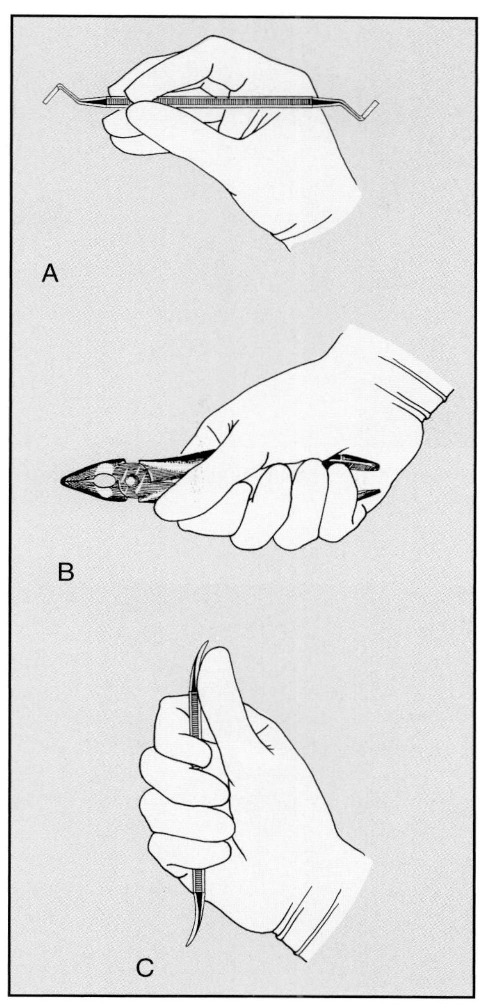

FIGURE 9-11 Basic instrument grasps used by the operator. **A,** Pen grasp. **B,** Palm grasp. **C,** Palm-thumb grasp.

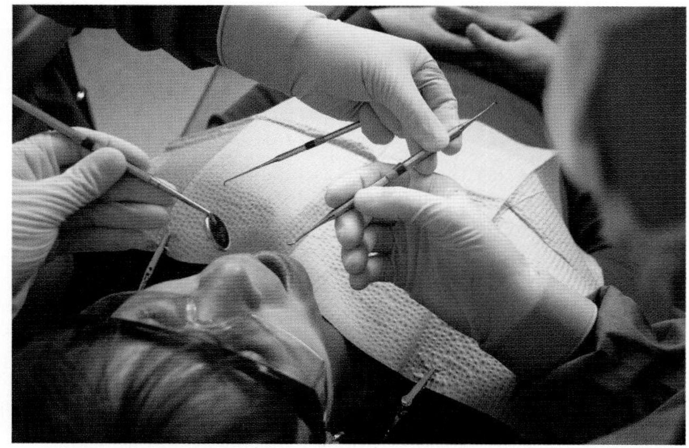

FIGURE 9-10 The new instrument is positioned in the operator's grasp.

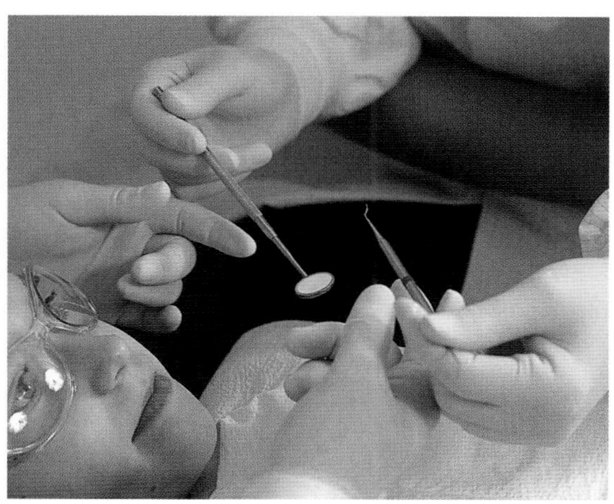

FIGURE 9-12 Transferring the mirror and explorer.

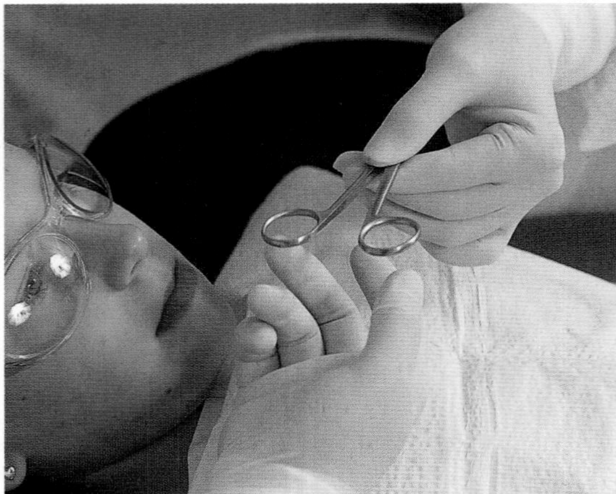

FIGURE 9-13 Transferring a hinged instrument.

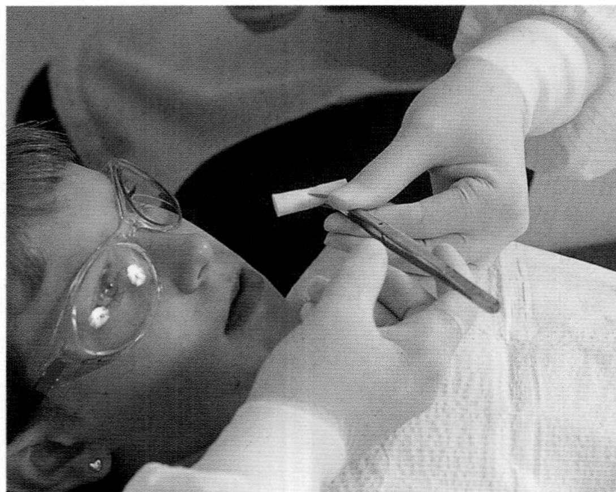

FIGURE 9-14 Transferring cotton pliers.

single-handed technique. The pliers are delivered to the dentist while pinching together the beaks to prevent dropping the item being held (Figure 9-14).

Transfer of Dental Materials

Dental materials are generally delivered to the dentist in the transfer zone near the patient's chin.

Cements and liners are delivered on the mixing slab or pad along with the applicator instrument. Hold the mixing pad in the right hand and a 2 × 2 gauze sponge in the left hand. The dentist can access the material, and the tip of the instrument can be wiped with the gauze as necessary.

Materials in syringes, such as etchants, composite resin materials, impression materials, and cements, are easily delivered directly to the dentist. The syringe is passed so that the dentist can grasp the syringe in the position of use with the tip turned upward for maxillary use and downward for mandibular use.

Amalgam is delivered to the dentist for placement into the prepared tooth. In some states, it is legal for the assistant to place the amalgam into the prepared tooth.

Delegating this task may be a matter of the dentist's preference or simply one of convenience. The team member who can conveniently see and reach the preparation should place the material directly into the cavity, thus eliminating unnecessary instrument exchanges.

Expanded Functions for the Dental Assistant

An expanded function is one in which the dentist delegates a specific intraoral task that is part of a clinical procedure to a credentialed expanded function dental assistant (EFDA) or a registered dental assistant (RDA). For a function to be delegated, it must be legal in that state to do so.

Most states require dental assistants to receive formal education before they are permitted to practice a delegated function. Training for expanded functions can take place in:

- Dental assisting programs
- Programs approved by the state dental board
- Continuing education courses approved by the state dental board

Types of Expanded Functions

Expanded functions that can be delegated to a dental assistant can take place in either a general dental office or specialty practices. As you take on the role of the operator for these functions, you must also take the responsibility of knowing more about the procedure and process. Listed is an overview of additional skills required to practice as the operator for an expanded function.

Fundamentals When Working as the Operator in Performing an Expanded Function

Dental Anatomy Review the patient's occlusion, landmarks of the oral cavity, tooth surfaces, anatomic features of the teeth, and line and point angles of tooth surfaces.

Operator Positioning Position yourself with the least amount of stress and strain on the body. This recommended position includes upright head position, straight back, elbows close to the body, and feet flat on the floor.

Mirror Skills Learn how to use the mouth mirror for indirect vision, retraction, and light reflection.

Use of a Fulcrum Establish a finger rest when using an instrument intraorally. This stabilization will prevent the possibility of slipping.

Learn Cavity Preparations Know specific cavity terms and classifications. This knowledge will help in the placement of matrix bands and wedges and in the application of dental materials.

Instrumentation Learn to adapt the working end of the instrument to each tooth surface, and then proceed by correctly moving the instrument to accomplish its task.

Application of Materials Each material is unique in how it is prepared and applied. Understand the application process for each type of restorative material.

Evaluate the Function Work with the dentist to have the same expectations and goals in the evaluation process of delegated expanded functions.

Procedure 9-1

Admitting and Seating the Patient

Procedural Steps

1. Pleasantly greet the patient in the reception area by name. Introduce yourself, and request that the patient follow you to the treatment area.
2. Place the patient's personal items, such as a jacket or handbag, in a safe place away from the procedure.
3. Initiate a conversation with the patient.

Purpose: Chatting about things other than the treatment may help the patient feel more comfortable and relaxed.

4. Ask whether the patient has any questions that you can answer about the treatment for the day. If you do not know the answer, then say so and offer to discuss the question with the dentist.

Purpose: Patients frequently ask the assistant questions about treatment that they are reluctant to ask the dentist. Willingness to answer these questions helps reassure the patient.

5. Ask the patient to sit on the side of the dental chair and then swing his or her legs onto the base of the chair.

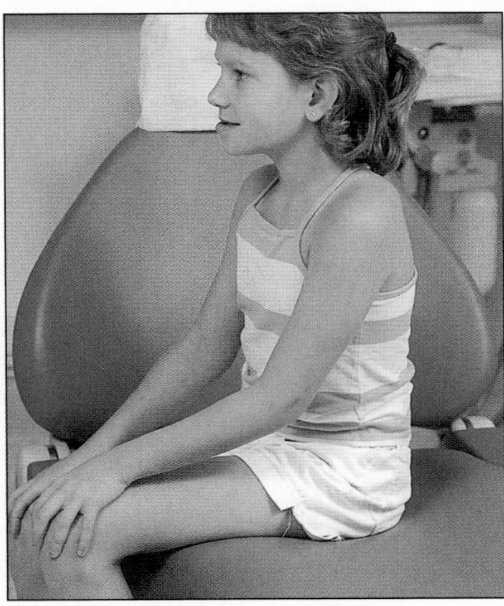

6. Lower or slide the chair arm into position.

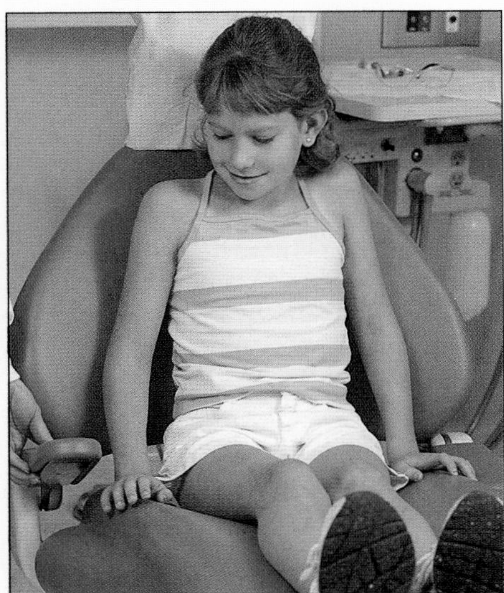

7. Place the disposable patient napkin over the patient's chest, and clasp the corners using a napkin chain.

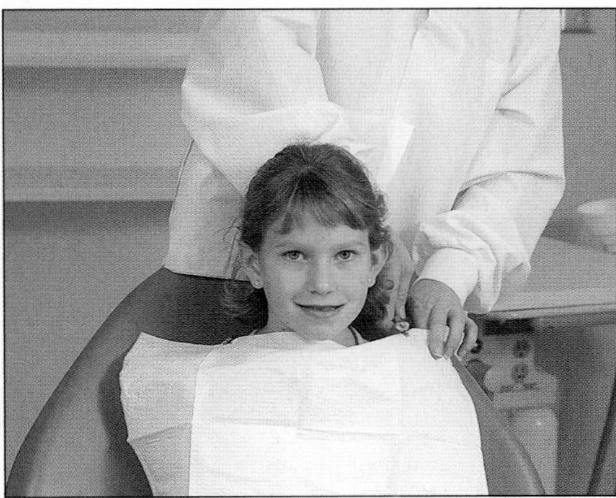

8. Inform the patient before adjusting the chair. Make the adjustments slowly until the patient and the chair are in the proper position for the planned procedure.

Note: Remember that the most common position for dental procedures is the supine position.

9. Position the operating light over the patient's chest, and turn it on.

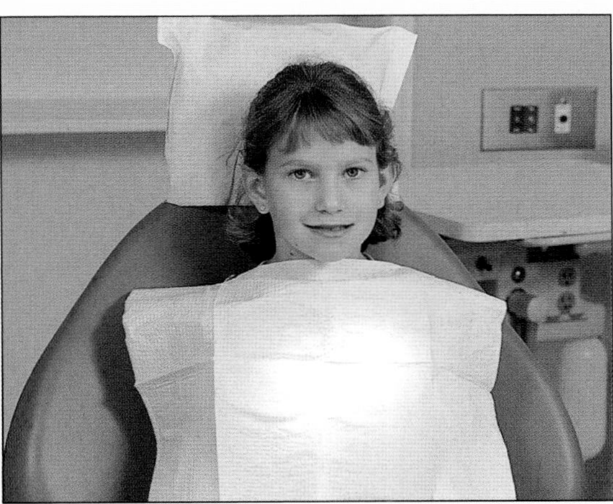

10. Once again, review the room to ensure that all treatment room preparations are organized and set out.
11. Wash your hands, and put on your personal protective equipment.
12. You are now ready to position yourself and to begin the procedure.

Procedure 9-2

Transferring Instruments Using the Single-Handed Technique

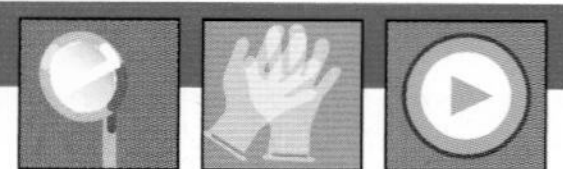

Procedural Steps

1. Retrieve the instrument from the tray setup using the thumb, index finger, and middle finger of your left hand.

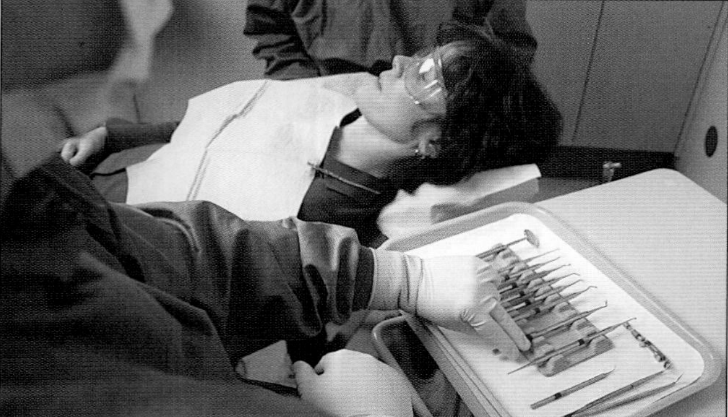

2. Grasp the instrument at the end of the handle or opposite the working end.

Note: Most instruments have two ends (double-ended instruments).

3. Transfer the instrument from the tray into the transfer zone, ensuring that the instrument is parallel to the instrument in the dentist's hand.
4. Using the last two fingers of your left hand, retrieve the used instrument from the dentist, tucking in the instrument toward the palm.

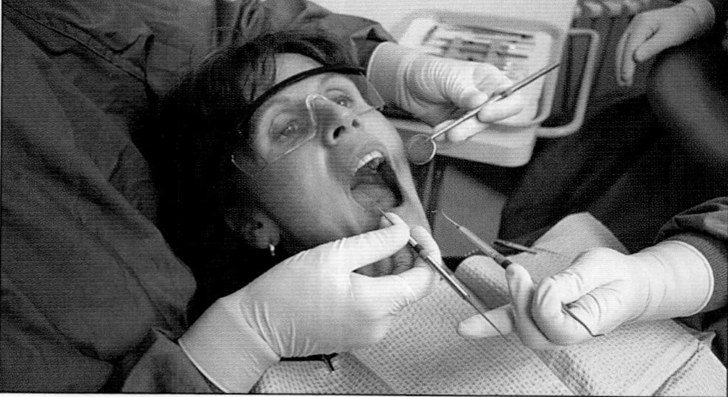

5. Firmly position the new instrument into the operator's fingers.

Note: When placing the instrument, make sure the working end is correctly positioned for the proper area of the mouth.

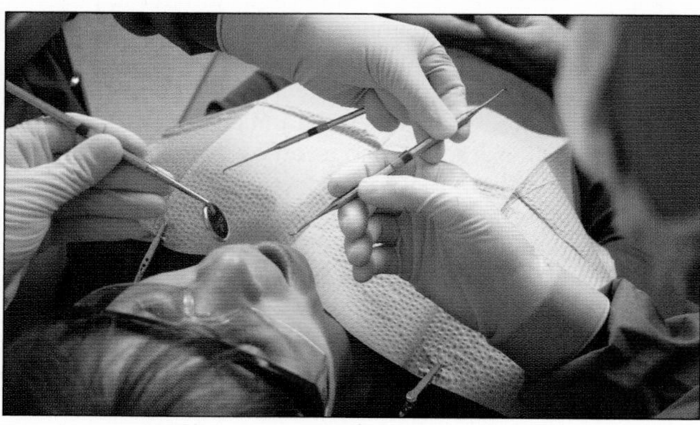

6. Place the used instrument back on the tray setup in its correct position of use.

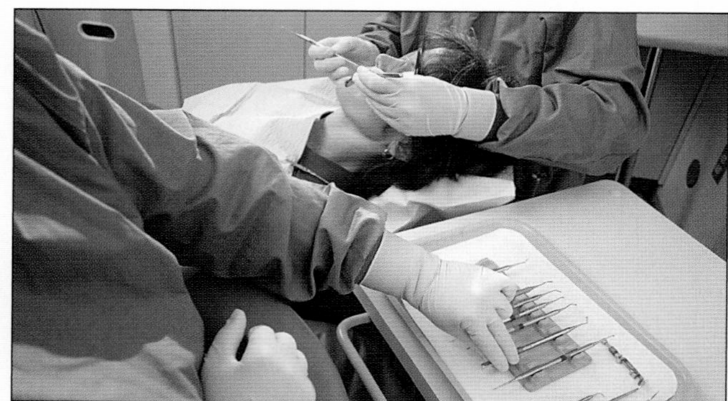

Procedure 9-3

Transferring Instruments Using the Two-Handed Technique

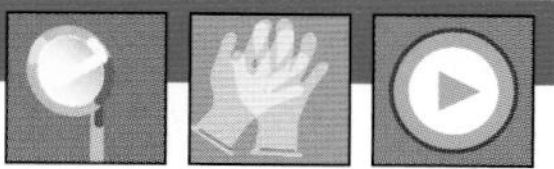

Procedural Steps

1. Using your right hand, grasp the instrument on the tray setup closer to the working end with your thumb and first two fingers.
2. With your left hand, retrieve the used instrument from the dentist, using the reverse palm grasp to hold the instrument before placing it back on the tray.
3. Deliver the new instrument to the dentist so that it is oriented with the working end in the appropriate position.
4. Return the used instrument to its proper position on the tray.

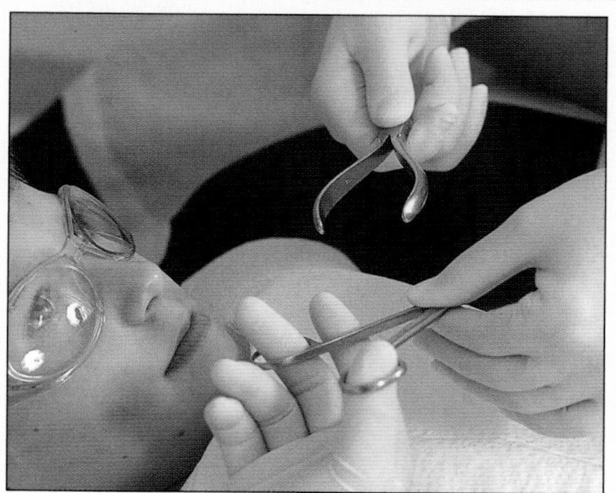

Chapter Exercises

Multiple Choice

Circle the letter next to the correct answer.

1. In the __________ position, the patient's head and knees are approximately on the same plane.
   - **a.** supine
   - **b.** subsupine
   - **c.** upright
2. The operator's stool __________ have a ring near the base to support the feet.
   - **a.** does
   - **b.** does not
3. In preparing to seat a patient, the __________.
   - **a.** arm on the patient chair is raised or moved out of the way
   - **b.** chair is in the supine position
   - **c.** headrest is removed
   - **d.** patient napkin is placed before the patient is seated
4. The dental unit houses the __________.
   - **a.** high-speed handpiece
   - **b.** low-speed handpiece
   - **c.** air-water syringe
   - **d.** a, b, and c
5. The work surface of the assistant's mobile unit is positioned in the __________ zone.
   - **a.** static
   - **b.** operator's
   - **c.** assistant's
   - **d.** transfer
6. The operator's zone for a right-handed dentist is from __________ o'clock.
   - **a.** 2 to 4
   - **b.** 4 to 7
   - **c.** 7 to 12
   - **d.** 12 to 2
7. When treating a tooth in the maxillary arch, the transfer of the next instrument should have the instrument's working end turned __________.
   - **a.** downward
   - **b.** upward
8. The assistant uses the __________ of the left hand when retrieving a used instrument from the dentist.
   - **a.** last two fingers
   - **b.** first three fingers
   - **c.** thumb and index fingers
9. Surgical forceps are best transferred using a __________ transfer.
   - **a.** single-handed
   - **b.** two-handed
10. During instrument exchange, the handles of the two instruments should be parallel to prevent __________.
    - **a.** injuring the patient
    - **b.** injuring the dental team
    - **c.** tangling
    - **d.** a, b, and c

Apply Your Knowledge

1. Your dentist has agreed to *finally* update the clinical equipment in the treatment areas. You are asked to meet with the sales representatives from three companies and make a decision concerning the type of patient chair, operator's stool, and assistant's stool. What are some of the features that should be considered when choosing this equipment?
2. Dr. Allen is on vacation for the week, and a temporary dentist is filling in. She is left-handed. What changes must be made in (1) the operating zones and (2) the methods of instrument transfer?
3. During a team meeting, Dr. Allen expresses some concerns about the clinical procedures taking longer than they should. Everyone agrees that the clinical team could "fine tune" some of their team dentistry skills. What areas could be reviewed and possibly modified?

CHAPTER 10

Moisture Control

http://evolve.elsevier.com/Robinson/essentials/

LEARNING OBJECTIVES

1. Pronounce, define, and spell the key terms.
2. Name the two basic types of rinsing procedures used in dentistry and demonstrate how to perform a mouth rinse.
3. List, describe, and demonstrate the two types of oral evacuation methods used in dentistry.
4. Complete the following related to common isolation techniques used in dentistry:
   - List the advantages and disadvantages of using cotton rolls.
   - Demonstrate the placement and removal of cotton rolls.
   - Discuss the use of dry angles in dentistry.
5. Complete the following related to the dental dam:
   - List the indications for use of a dental dam.
   - Describe the equipment used for preparation, placement, and removal of the dental dam.
   - Demonstrate the proper procedure to prepare, place, and remove the dental dam.

KEY TERMS

dental dam
evacuator
isolation
malaligned
septum

One of the key responsibilities of the clinical assistant is to maintain moisture control throughout a procedure. The tooth, surrounding tissue, and oral cavity can become a catch all for water, saliva, blood, and tooth fragments.

The type of procedure and access to the area will determine the best **isolation** method to use. This chapter describes several techniques and applications that will help you determine what works best for the situation.

Mouth Rinsing

The two basic types of rinsing procedures used in dentistry are limited-area rinsing and complete mouth rinsing.

Limited-area rinsing is frequently performed throughout a procedure because debris can accumulate during the preparation of a tooth. A limited-area rinse must be quickly and efficiently accomplished without causing any delay in the procedure and is routinely used when the dentist pauses for a closer inspection.

The **complete mouth rinse** is performed at the completion of a dental procedure and is always used to leave the patient with a comfortable and fresh feeling.

See Procedure 10-1: Performing a Mouth Rinse.

Oral Evacuation Methods

Throughout a dental procedure, the water from either the air-water syringe or from the high-speed handpiece is expressed to cool the tooth and remove debris. A specific type of oral evacuation method will be selected to remove the liquids and debris from the mouth.

Saliva Ejector

The saliva ejector is used to remove small amounts of saliva or water from the patient's mouth. This small strawlike tube has the flexibility to conform to many areas in the mouth (Figure 10-1). Placement of the saliva ejector is simple and comfortable for the patient. To maintain its position in the mouth, bend it in the shape of a candy cane and place it under the tongue on the opposite side on which you are working.

High-Volume Oral Evacuation

The **high-volume evacuator** (HVE) is a strong source of moisture control that is regularly applied during a dental procedure when the handpiece is being used.

The HVE system, also referred to as the oral **evacuator**, works on a vacuum principle similar to that of a household vacuum cleaner.

The HVE is used to:

- Maintain the mouth free from saliva, blood, water, and debris.
- Retract the tongue or cheek away from the procedure site.
- Reduce the bacterial aerosol caused by the high-speed handpiece.

HVE Tips

The most commonly used HVE tips are made of a durable plastic and are disposed of after a single use. HVE tips are also made of stainless steel, which must be sterilized before reuse (Figure 10-2).

HVE tips are available straight or with a slight angle in the middle. All types have two beveled working ends (**beveled** meaning slanted). The bevel is slanted downward for use in the **anterior** portion of the mouth. For use in the posterior portion of the mouth, the bevel is slanted upward.

When the HVE tip is placed into the handle of the suction unit, the tip is pushed into place through a plastic protective barrier, which will cover the HVE handle. If the incorrect end of the tip has been placed in the suction, do not turn it around; the HVE tip is now contaminated and must be replaced with a new tip.

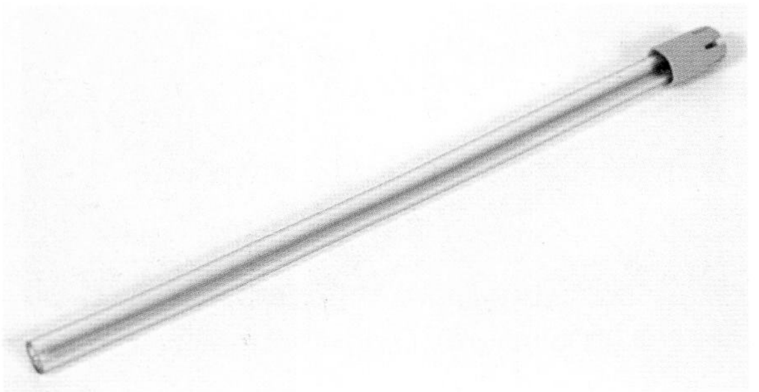

FIGURE 10-1 Saliva ejector.

Holding the Oral Evacuator

The oral evacuator can be held in one of two ways: the thumb-to-nose grasp or the pen grasp (Figure 10-3). Either method provides control of the tip, which is necessary for efficient use and patient comfort and safety. It is common to alternate between positions, depending on the area being treated or the resistance of the tissue to retract.

When assisting a right-handed dentist, hold the evacuator in the right hand. When assisting a left-handed dentist, hold the evacuator in the left hand. The other hand is then free to use the air-water syringe or to transfer instruments to the dentist as needed.

To be most efficient in HVE placement, position the HVE tip in the mouth first, and then allow the dentist to position the handpiece and the mouth mirror (Figure 10-4).

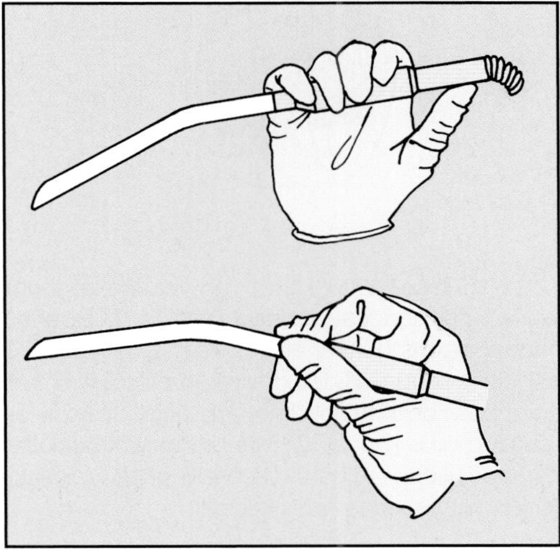

FIGURE 10-3 Methods of holding the oral evacuator tip. *Top,* Thumb-to-nose grasp. *Bottom,* Pen grasp.

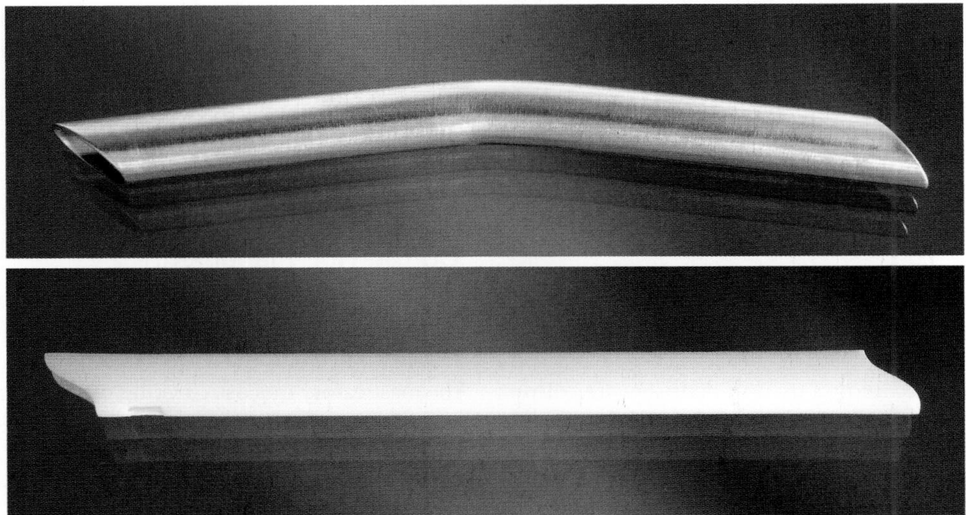

FIGURE 10-2 High-volume evacuator (HVE) tips. (From Boyd LRB: *Dental instruments: a pocket guide,* ed 5, St. Louis, 2015, Saunders.)

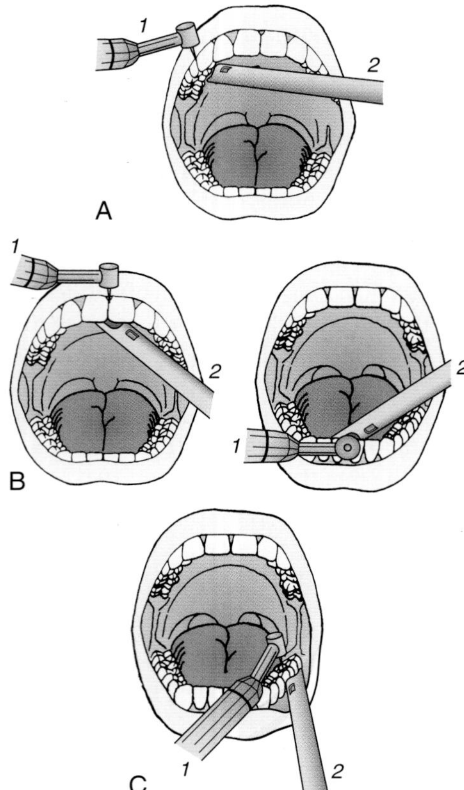

FIGURE 10-4 Placement of the high-volume evacuator (HVE) tip. **A,** Maxillary right buccal/occlusal surface. *1,* Operator's position with handpiece is buccal or occlusal; *2,* Assistant's position with suction tip is lingual. **B,** Maxillary/Mandibular central incisors; *1,* Operator's position with handpiece is facial; *2,* Assistant's position with suction tip is lingual. **C,** Mandibular left occlusal surface. *1,* Operator's position with handpiece is lingual/occlusal; *2,* Assistant's position with suction tip is buccal.

BOX 10-1 Advantages and Disadvantages of Cotton Rolls

Advantages

- Is easy to apply.
- Is comfortable for the patient.
- No additional equipment is needed for placement.

Disadvantages

- Does not prevent contamination of the area by saliva and moisture.
- Does not protect the patient from aspiration.
- If improperly removed, then dry cotton rolls may adhere to the oral mucosa, which can injure the tissue.
- Must be frequently replaced.
- Cotton rolls have limited retraction.

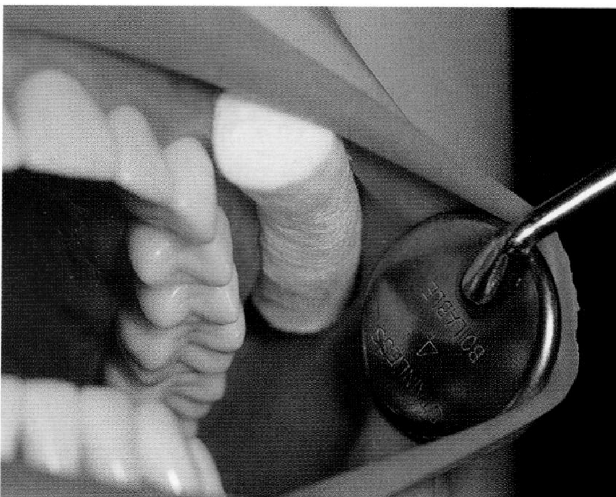

FIGURE 10-5 Cotton roll placement for the posterior maxillary arch.

See Procedure 10-2: Positioning the High-Volume Evacuator During a Procedure

Oral Evacuation Caution

Improper or careless placement of the HVE can cause soft tissue to be accidentally *sucked* into the tip, resulting in the possibility of damaging localized tissue. Keeping the tip at an angle with the soft tissue helps prevent this from occuring. If the soft tissue is accidentally sucked into the tip, then rotate the angle of the tip to break the suction or quickly turn off the vacuum control to release the tissue.

Isolation Techniques

The common isolation techniques used in dentistry are cotton rolls, dental dam, and dry angles. **Isolation**, as used here, means to keep the area isolated and dry.

Cotton Rolls

One method of ensuring a dry environment is with the use of **cotton rolls.**When placing a permanent restorative material, cementing a crown, or in the application of sealants, a clean and dry environment is necessary. Cotton rolls are available in a variety of sizes and are flexible to be formed to fit in an available space. Some cotton rolls have a light coating on the surface to make them slightly stiff. A softer type of cotton roll is not coated but is wrapped with a cotton thread.

There are advantages and disadvantages to using cotton rolls (Box 10-1).

Cotton Roll Placement

To isolate a specific area of the maxillary arch, a cotton roll is placed on the cheek side of the teeth in the **mucobuccal fold.** This fold securely holds the cotton roll in place and is the area where the masticatory mucosa covering the alveolar ridge turns upward and becomes the lining mucosa of the cheek (Figure 10-5).

Because of movement of the tongue and the tendency of saliva to pool in the floor of the mouth, cotton roll isolation is more difficult to achieve in the **mandibular arch.** Cotton rolls are placed in both the mucobuccal fold and the lingual side of the arch parallel to each other (Figure 10-6).

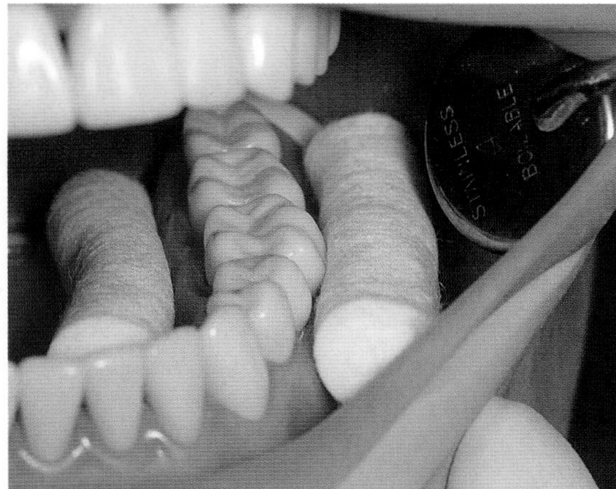

FIGURE 10-6 Cotton roll placement for the posterior mandibular arch.

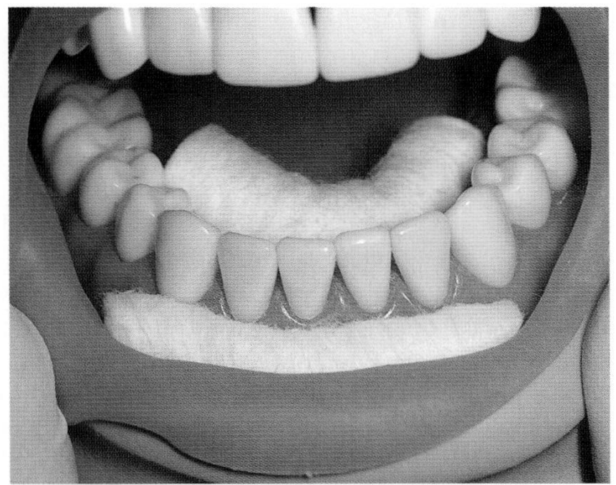

FIGURE 10-7 Cotton roll placement for the anterior section of the mandibular arch.

When the anterior portion of the mandible is isolated, cotton rolls are positioned in the lingual area, instructing the patient to raise his or her tongue for secure placement. The other cotton roll is placed between the lip and teeth (Figure 10-7).

Depending on the location, cotton rolls are placed and removed with cotton pliers or with gloved fingers. If the cotton roll becomes saturated before the procedure is completed, then it should be replaced as necessary.

See Procedure 10-3: Placing and Removing Cotton Rolls.

Related Aids

Dry Angles

A dry angle is a triangle-shaped absorbent pad to help isolate posterior areas in both the maxillary and mandibular arches. The pad is placed on the buccal mucosa over the Stensen duct (Figure 10-8). (This duct from the parotid gland is located opposite the maxillary second molar.)

These pads collect the flow of saliva and protect the tissue in this area. Follow the manufacturer's directions for placement and, if necessary, replace the pads if they become saturated before the procedure is completed. To remove, use water from the air-water syringe to wet the pad thoroughly before separating it from the soft tissue in the mucosa.

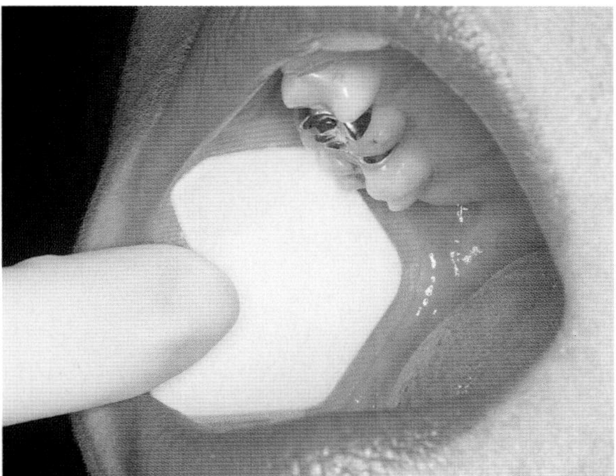

FIGURE 10-8 Application of a dry angle.

Dental Dam

The **dental dam** is a thin latex barrier used to isolate either a single tooth or several teeth during a dental procedure (Figure 10-9). These teeth are referred to as being isolated.

Indications for Using a Dental Dam

- Is an infection control protective barrier.
- Safeguards the patient's mouth against contact with debris, acid-etch materials, and other materials during treatment.
- Protects the patient from accidentally inhaling or swallowing debris, such as small fragments of a tooth or scraps of restorative material.
- Protects the tooth from contamination of saliva or debris if pulpal exposure accidentally occurs.
- Protects the oral cavity from exposure to infectious material when an infected tooth is opened during endodontic treatment.
- Provides moisture control that is essential for the placement of restorative materials.
- Improves access during treatment by retracting the lips, tongue, and gingiva.
- Provides better visibility because of the contrast of color of the dam and the tooth.
- Enhances dental team efficiency, discourages patient conversation, and may reduce the time required for some treatments.

Before placing the dental dam, review the patient's medical history for any indications of latex sensitivity or allergy. If this is an indication, then the dentist must be consulted before the application is continued.

The dental dam is applied after the local anesthetic has been administered and while the dentist is waiting for the anesthesia to take effect.

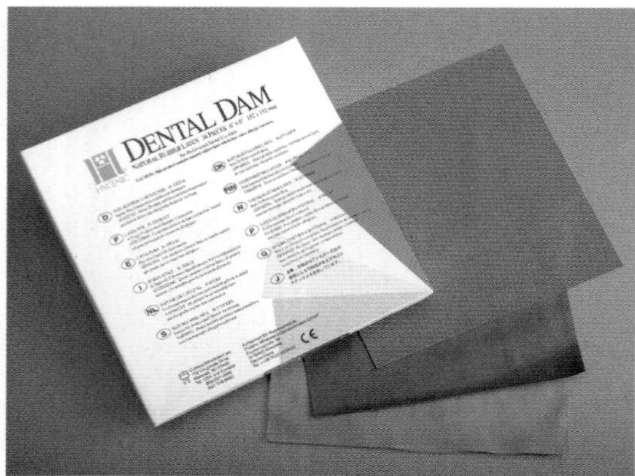

FIGURE 10-9 Dental dam. (From Boyd LRB: *Dental instruments: a pocket guide,* ed 5, St. Louis, 2015, Saunders.)

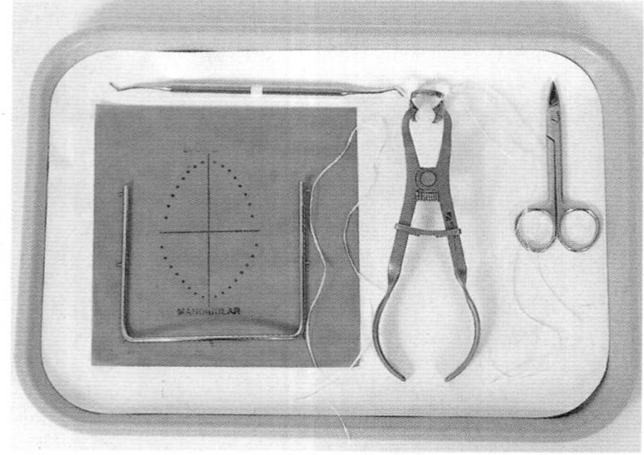

FIGURE 10-10 Dental dam tray setup for application.

The teeth to be isolated should be clean and free of plaque or debris. When indicated, tooth brushing or selective coronal polishing is performed before placing the dental dam (see Chapter 18). If not removed, the plaque or debris can become dislodged and may irritate the gingival tissue.

Dental Dam Equipment

The dental dam tray setup for application is in Figure 10-10. The equipment used for preparation, placement, and removal of the dental dam is described in Table 10-1.

Preparation of the Dental Dam Application

Each application of the dam is preplanned to accommodate the dentist's preferences, the tooth or teeth involved, and the procedure to be performed.

Several important factors are to be included when planning for punching the dental dam.

- The arch, its shape, and any irregularities, such as missing teeth or a fixed prosthesis
- Number of teeth to be isolated
- Identification of the anchor tooth and location of the key-punch hole
- Size and spacing of the other holes to be punched (the **anchor tooth** holds the dental dam clamp, and the **key-punch hole** covers the anchor tooth)

Maxillary Arch Applications

In preparing for the maxillary application, the dam material is stamped or marked. This mark automatically designates the margin of the dam for these holes. If the patient has a mustache or a thick upper lip, then allowing extra space for the anterior teeth area may be necessary.

Mandibular Arch Applications

In preparing for the mandibular application, the dam is stamped or marked. Because of the small size of the mandibular anterior teeth, the holes are punched closer together than those for posterior teeth.

Curve of the Arch

Making adjustments to accommodate an extremely narrow or wide arch is necessary. Failure to make such adjustments will increase the difficulty when inverting the edges of the punched holes of the dam into the gingival sulcus.

Bunching and stretching on the lingual aspect of the dental dam will occur if the curve of the arch is punched too narrow or too wide. Folds and stretching of the dam on the facial aspect occur if the arch is punched too curved or too narrow.

Malaligned Teeth

If a single tooth or teeth are **malaligned** within the dental arch, then special consideration is taken before the dental dam is punched. (Malaligned and **malposed** mean that the individual tooth is not in its normal position within the dental arch.)

If a tooth is lingually positioned, then the hole-punch size remains the same, but the hole is placed approximately 1 mm lingually from the normal arch alignment. If the tooth is facially positioned, then the hole-punch size remains the same, but the hole is placed approximately 1 mm facially from the normal arch alignment.

Teeth to be Isolated

Single-tooth isolation is commonly used for endodontic treatment. Some dentists choose to isolate only the tooth to be treated for selective restorative procedures, such as for Class I or Class V restorations. A different preference is to have two teeth isolated so that the posterior tooth acts as an anchor tooth to hold the clamp. When treating the posterior area, isolation of several teeth provides more stability and better visibility for the operator.

For **multiple-tooth isolation**, where optimal stability is needed, isolating the quadrant is desirable. Having multiple teeth isolated counteracts the pull on the dam that is created by the curvature of the teeth in the arch.

When anterior maxillary teeth are to be treated, maximum stability is achieved by isolating the six anterior teeth (canine to canine).

Key-Punch Hole

The **anchor tooth** holds the dental dam clamp. The **key-punch hole** is punched in the dental dam to cover the anchor tooth. A larger no. 5–size hole is necessary for the key punch because it must also accommodate the clamp.

TABLE 10-1
Dental Dam Equipment

Type of Equipment	Description of Equipment
Dam material 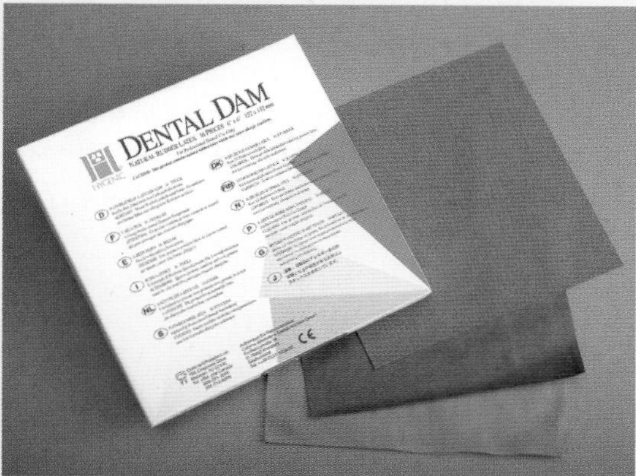 (From Boyd LRB: *Dental instruments: a pocket guide,* ed 5, St. Louis, 2015, Saunders.)	Comes in latex or latex-free material. Available sizes are 6 × 6 and 5 × 5. Comes in a wide range of colors and in three gauges of thickness (thin, medium, and heavy).
Dental dam frame 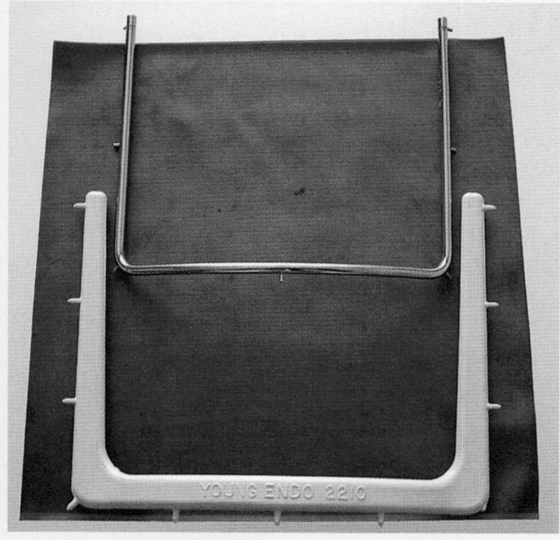 (From Boyd LRB: *Dental instruments: a pocket guide,* ed 5, St. Louis, 2015, Saunders.)	This U-shaped frame is made of plastic or metal that stretches the dam material away from the face and the worked area.
Dental dam napkin 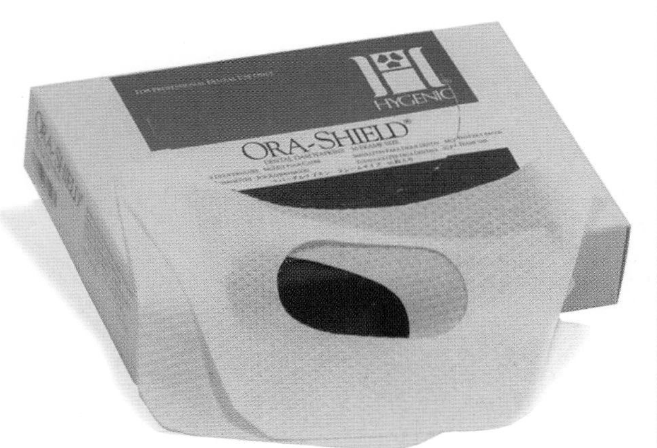 Heymann HO, Swift EJ Jr., Ritter AV: *Sturdevant's art and science of operative dentistry,* ed 6, St. Louis, 2013, Mosby.	This cotton absorbent sheet is placed between the dental dam and the patient.

Continued

TABLE 10-1
Dental Dam Equipment—cont'd

Type of Equipment	Description of Equipment
Lubricant	This water-soluble material can be placed on the underside of the dam around the punched area for easy placement between tight contacts.
Dental dam punch 5 Largest hole (clamped) 4 Large hole (molars) 3 Medium hole (premolars) 2 Small hole (maxillary anteriors) 1 Smallest hole (mandibular anteriors) (From Bird DL, Robinson DS: *Modern dental assisting,* ed 11, St Louis, 2015, Saunders.)	This hole-punch device is used to create holes in the dam that expose the teeth to be isolated. Different sizes are used for specific teeth.
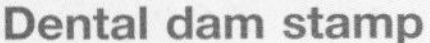 Dental dam stamp 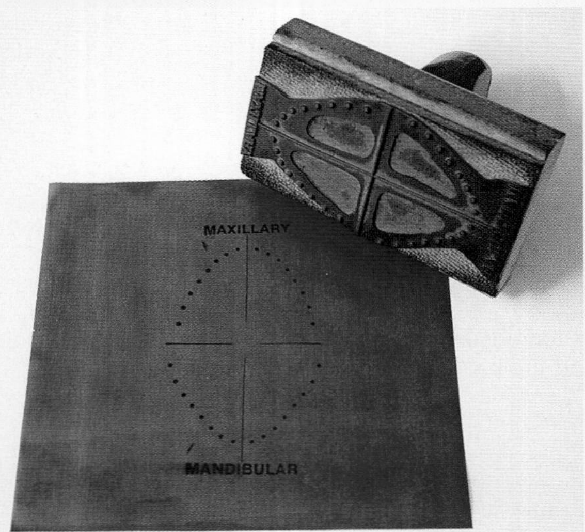 (From Boyd LRB: *Dental instruments: a pocket guide,* ed 5, St. Louis, 2015, Saunders.)	Stamp designed in the shape of a dental arch and imprints teeth on the dental dam to be punched.

TABLE 10-1
Dental Dam Equipment—cont'd

Type of Equipment	Description of Equipment
Dental dam forceps 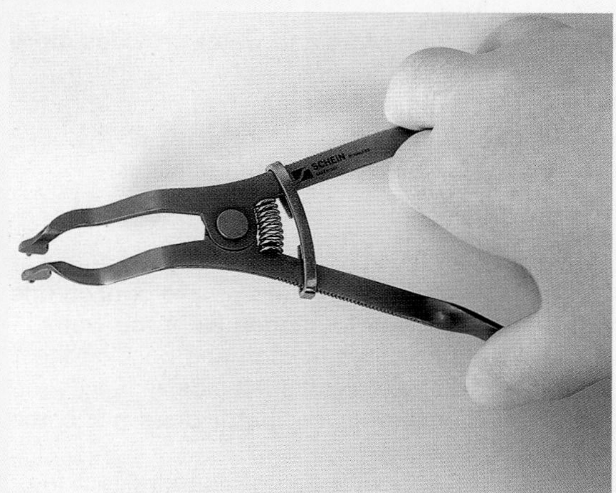 	This type of forceps is used to place and remove the dental dam clamp.
Dental dam clamps 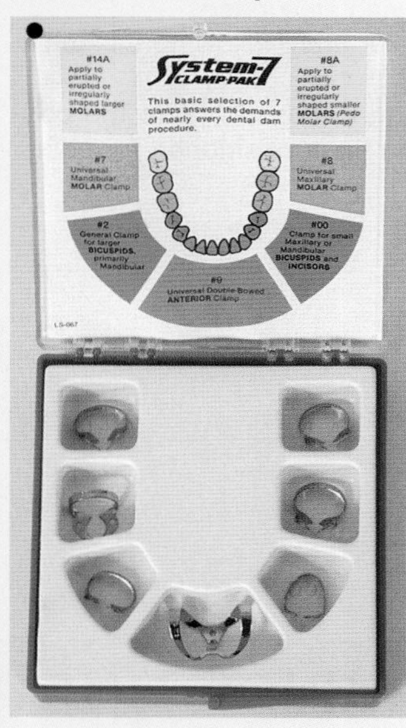 	This crown-shaped piece of metal anchors the dental dam material on a tooth. Many designs of clamps fit the contour of each tooth in the mouth. For safety purposes, always ligate the bow portion of a clamp with floss before placing in the mouth, which will prevent the clamp from being accidentally swallowed.

Hole Size and Spacing

The size of each hole selected on the dental dam punch must be appropriate for the tooth to be isolated. A correctly sized hole allows the dam to slip easily over the tooth and snugly fit in the cervical area, which is important to prevent leakage around the dam.

In general, the holes are spaced from 3.0 to 3.5 mm between the edges, not the centers, of the holes, which allowed adequate spacing between the holes to create a **septum** that slips between the teeth without tearing or injuring the gingiva.

The septum is the portion of the dental dam between the holes of the punched dam. During application, this portion of the dam is passed between the contacts. (*Septum* is singular, *septa* is plural.)

See Procedure 10-4: Preparation, Placement, and Removal of the Dental Dam (Expanded Function).

Ethical Implications

In the application of the dental dam, you may be asked to place it by yourself. If this is the case, then verify that applying a dental dam is a legal function in your state for dental assistants and that you have had special training in the application process.

Procedure 10-1

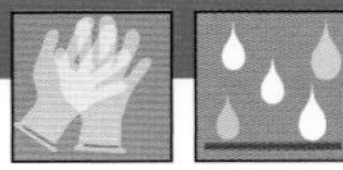

Performing a Mouth Rinse

Equipment and Supplies

- HVE tip
- Saliva ejector
- Air-water syringe

Procedural Steps

1. Decide which oral evacuation system will be best for the rinsing procedure.
2. Grasp the air-water syringe in your left hand and the HVE or saliva ejector in your right hand.

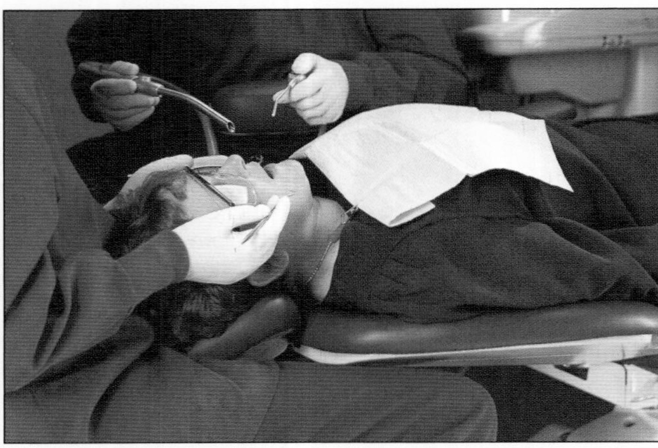

Limited-Mouth Rinse

1. Turn on the suction, and position the tip toward the site for a limited-area rinse.
2. Spray the combination of air and water onto the site to be rinsed.

Purpose: The combination of air and water provides more force to clean the area thoroughly.

3. Suction all fluid and debris from the area, being sure to remove all fluids.
4. Dry the area by pressing the air button only.

Full-Mouth Rinse

1. Have the patient turn toward you.

Purpose: Turning the head allows the water to pool on one side, making it easier for you to suction all of the water.

2. Turn on the HVE or the saliva ejector, and position the tip in the vestibule of the patient's left side.

Note: Carefully position the tip so that it does not come into contact with soft tissue.

3. With the HVE or saliva ejector tip positioned, direct the air-water syringe from the patient's maxillary right across to the left side, spraying all surfaces.
4. Continue along the mandibular arch, following the same sequence from right to left.

Purpose: This pattern of rinsing forces debris to the posterior mouth, where the suction tip is positioned for easier removal of fluids and debris.

HVE, High-volume evacuator.

Procedure 10-2

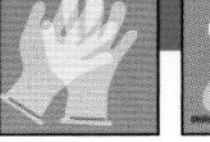

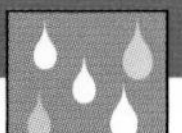

Positioning the High-Volume Evacuator During a Procedure

Equipment and Supplies

- Sterile HVE tip
- Plastic barrier cover for the HVE handle and hose
- Cotton rolls

Procedural Steps

1. Place the HVE tip in the holder by pushing the end of the tip into the holder through the plastic barrier.

Purpose: Leaves the opposite end exposed and ready for use.

2. If necessary, use the HVE tip or a mouth mirror to retract the cheek or tongue gently.

Posterior Placement

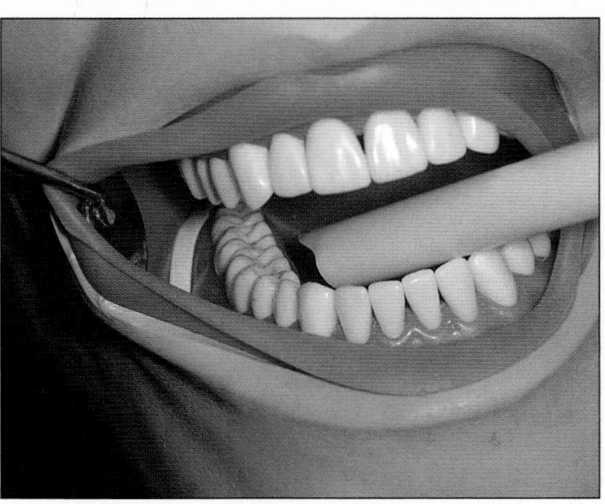

Procedure 10-2

Positioning the High-Volume Evacuator During a Procedure—cont'd

1. For a mandibular site, place a cotton roll under the suction tip.

Purpose: Provides patient comfort, aids in stabilizing tip placement, and prevents injury to the tissue.

2. Place the bevel of the HVE tip as close as possible to the tooth being prepared.

Purpose: Suction will draw the water into the tip immediately after it leaves the tooth being prepared.

3. Position the bevel of the HVE tip parallel to the buccal or lingual surface of the tooth being prepared.
4. Place the upper edge of the HVE tip so that it extends slightly beyond the occlusal surface.

Purpose: Suction will catch the water spray from the handpiece as it leaves the tooth being prepared.

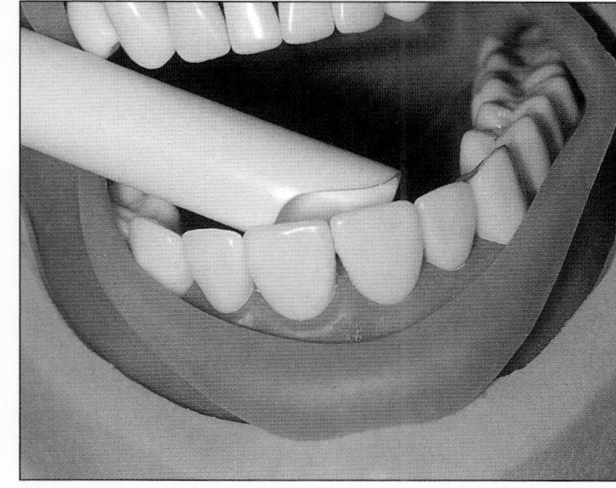

Anterior Placement

1. When the dentist is preparing the tooth from the lingual aspect, position the HVE tip so that it is parallel to the facial surface and slightly beyond the incisal edge.
2. When the dentist is preparing the tooth from the facial aspect, position the HVE tip parallel to the lingual surface and slightly beyond the incisal edge.

HVE, High-volume evacuator.

Procedure 10-3

Placing and Removing Cotton Rolls

Equipment and Supplies

- Basic setup
- Cotton rolls
- Air-water syringe

Maxillary Placement

1. Have the patient turn toward you with his or her chin raised.

Purpose: Provides better visualization and ease in the placement of the cotton roll.

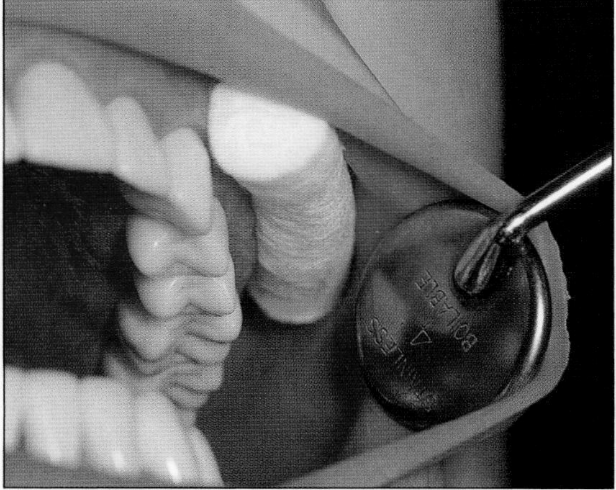

2. Using cotton pliers, pick up a cotton roll so that it is evenly positioned within the beaks of the cotton pliers.
3. Transfer the cotton roll to the mouth, and securely position it in the mucobuccal fold closest to the working field.

Note: Once you place the cotton roll with the pliers, you may want to use your gloved finger or the handle end of the cotton pliers to push the cotton roll into the mucobuccal fold.

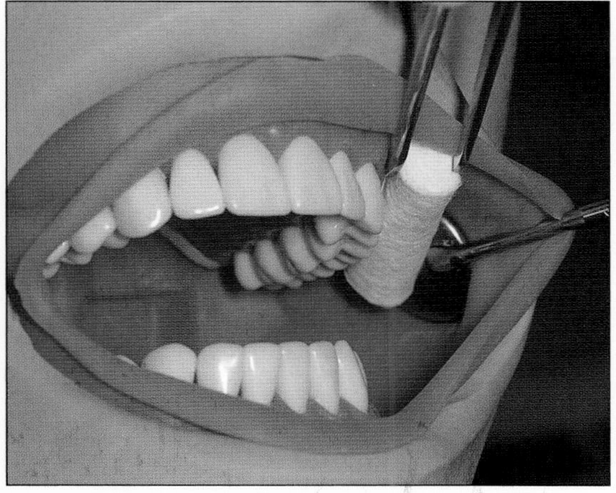

4. Maxillary placement can be used for any location on the maxillary arch.

Mandibular Placement

1. Have the patient turn toward you with his or her chin lowered.

Continued

Procedure 10-3

Placing and Removing Cotton Rolls—cont'd

Purpose: Provides better visualization and ease in the placement of the cotton roll.

2. Using the cotton pliers, pick up a cotton roll so that it is evenly positioned within the beaks of the cotton pliers.

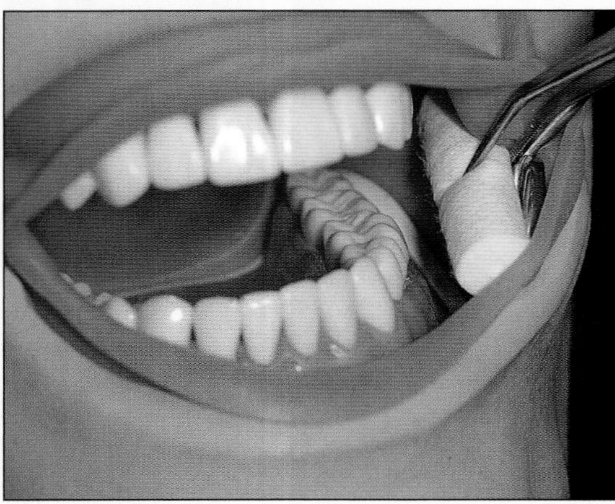

3. Transfer the cotton roll to the mouth, and securely position it in the mucobuccal fold closest to the working field.
4. Carry the second cotton roll to the mouth, and position it in the floor of the mouth between the working field and the tongue.

Note: Have the patient lift the tongue during placement and then relax the tongue to help secure the cotton roll in position.

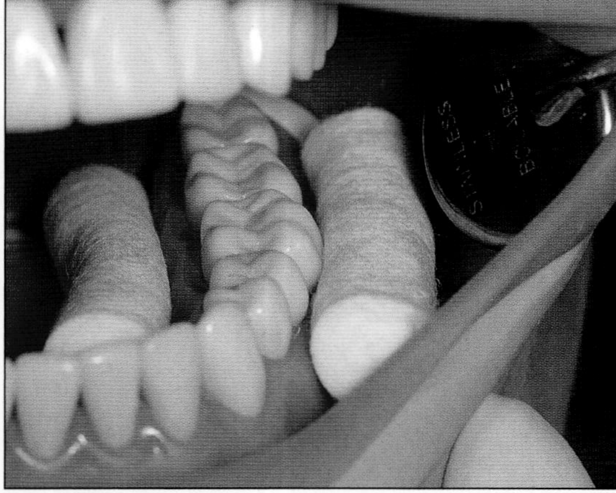

5. If you are placing cotton rolls for the mandibular anterior region, bend the cotton roll before placing for a contoured fit.

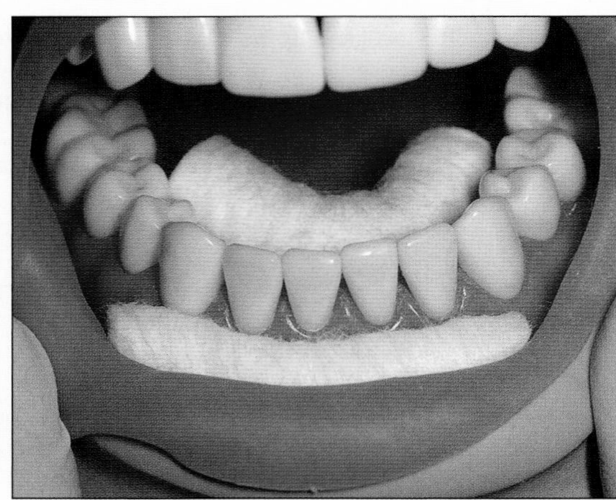

6. If using a saliva ejector for the procedure, then place it after the cotton roll is in position in the lingual vestibule.

Cotton Roll Removal

1. At the completion of a procedure, remove the cotton roll before the full-mouth rinse. If the cotton roll is dry, then moisten it with water from the air-water syringe.

Purpose: Dry cotton rolls will adhere to the lining of the oral mucosa, and tissue may become irritated when a dry cotton roll is pulled away from the area.

2. Using cotton pliers, retrieve the contaminated cotton roll from the site.
3. If appropriate for the procedure, then perform a limited rinse.

Procedure 10-4

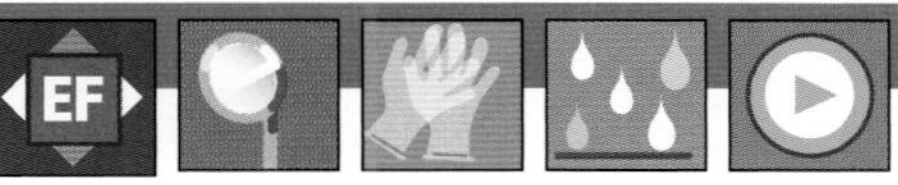

Preparation, Placement, and Removal of the Dental Dam (Expanded Function)

Equipment and Supplies

- Basic setup
- Precut 6 × 6 inch dental dam
- Dental dam stamp and inkpad or template and pen
- Dental dam punch
- Dental dam clamp or clamps with ligature attached
- Dental dam clamp forceps
- Young frame
- Dental dam napkin
- Dental tape or waxed floss
- Cotton rolls
- Lubricant for patient's lips
- Lubricant for dam
- Black spoon
- Crown and bridge scissors

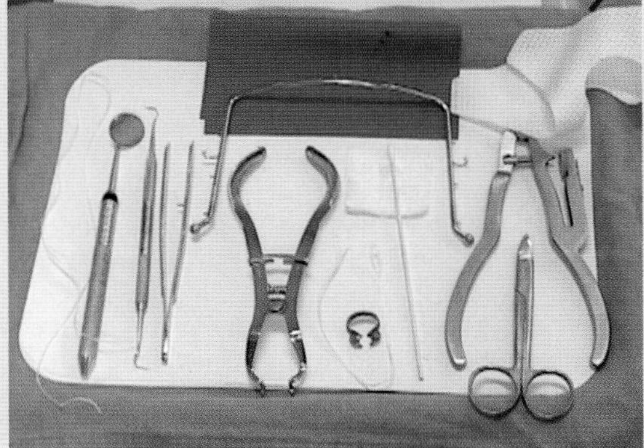

Patient Preparation

1. Check the patient's record for any contraindications to latex or past use, and identify the area to be isolated. Inform the patient of the need to place a dental dam, and explain the steps involved.
2. Assist the dentist in the administration of a local anesthetic. Ask the operator which teeth are to be isolated. Examine the area for any malposed teeth to be accommodated.
3. Apply lubricating ointment to the patient's lip with a cotton roll or a cotton-tip applicator.

Note: The patient's comfort is a concern throughout the placement and removal of the dental dam.

4. Use the mouth mirror and explorer to examine the site where the dam is to be placed. This area should be free of plaque and debris.

Purpose: If the dam is placed in an area with plaque and debris, then the dam could push the plaque and debris into the sulcus and irritate the gingival tissue.

Note: If debris or plaque is present, selective tooth brushing or coronal polishing is performed on these teeth before applying the dental dam.

5. Floss all contacts involved in the placement of the dental dam.

Purpose: Any tight contacts may tear the dam.

Punching the Dental Dam

1. Use a template or stamp to mark the teeth to be isolated on the dam.
2. Correctly punch the marked dam according to the teeth to be isolated. Be sure to use the correct size of punch hole for the specific tooth.
3. If teeth have tight contacts, then lightly lubricate the holes on the tooth surface (undersurface) of the dam.

Purpose: Lubrication eases placement of the dam over the contact area of the teeth.

Placing the Clamp and Frame

1. Select the correct size of clamp.

Note: The W7 clamp has been selected for this procedure.

2. Secure the clamp by tying a ligature of dental tape on the bow of the clamp.
3. Place the beaks of the rubber dam forceps into the holes of the clamp. Grasp the handles of the rubber dam forceps, and squeeze to open the clamp. Turn upward, and allow the locking bar to slide down to keep the forceps open for placement.
4. Place yourself in the operator's position, and adjust the patient for easy access.
5. Retrieve the rubber dam forceps. Position the lingual jaws of the clamp first, then the facial jaws. During placement, keep an index finger on the clamp to prevent the clamp from coming off before it has been stabilized on the tooth. Check the clamp for fit.

Purpose: Lingual jaw placement serves as a fulcrum for placement of the facial jaws.

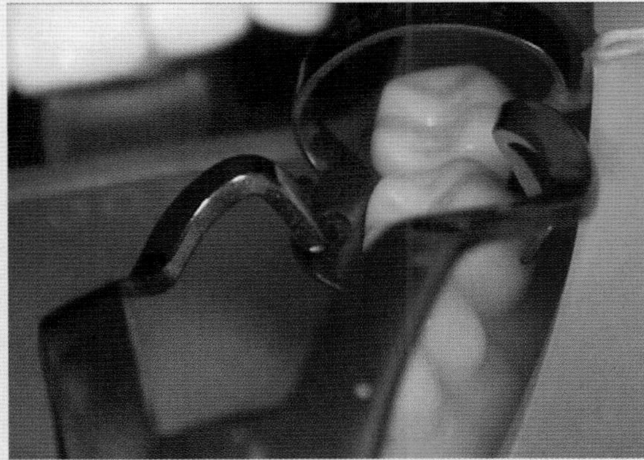

6. Transfer the dental dam to the site; stretch the punched hole for the anchor tooth over the clamp.

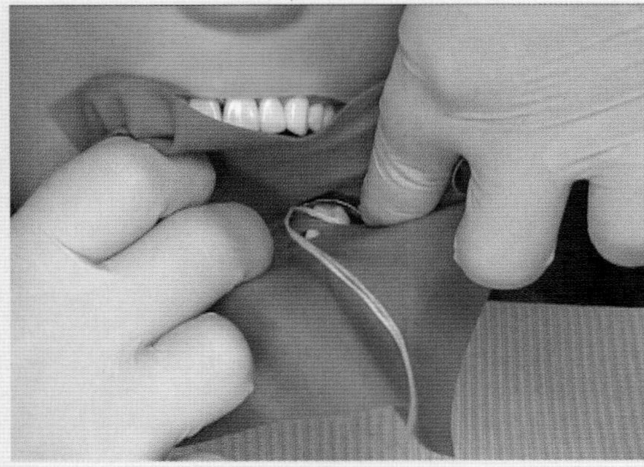

Continued

Procedure 10-4

Preparation, Placement, and Removal of the Dental Dam (Expanded Function)—cont'd

7. Using cotton pliers, retrieve the ligature and pull it through so that it is exposed and easy to grasp, if necessary.
8. Position the Young frame over the dam and slightly pull the dam, allowing it to hook onto the projections of the frame.

Purpose: This position ensures a smooth and stable fit.

9. Fit the last hole of the dam over the last tooth to be exposed at the opposite end of the anchor tooth.

Purpose: This position stabilizes the dam and aids in locating the remaining punch holes for the teeth to be isolated.

10. Using the index fingers of both hands, stretch the dam on the lingual and facial surfaces of the teeth so that the dam slides through each contact area.
11. With a piece of dental tape or waxed floss, floss through the contacts, pushing the dam below the proximal contacts of each tooth to be isolated.

Note: Slide the floss through the contact rather than pulling it back through the contact. This process will keep the dam in place.

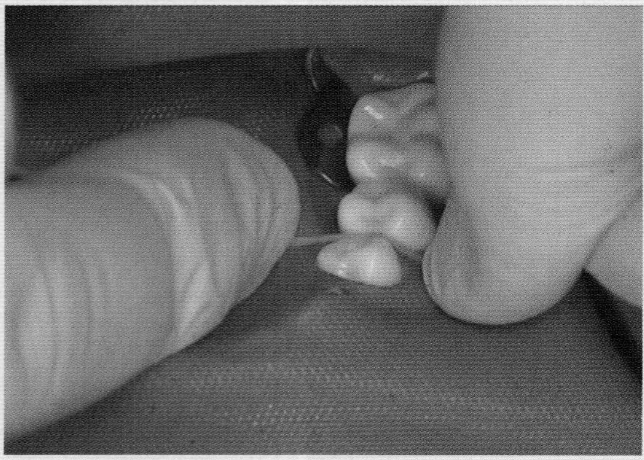

12. If the contacts are extremely tight, then use floss or a wedge placed into the interproximal area to separate the teeth slightly.
13. A ligature is placed to stabilize the dam at the opposite end of the anchor tooth.

Inverting the Dam

1. Invert, or reverse, the dam by gently stretching it near the cervix of the tooth.

Purpose: Inverting the dam creates a seal to prevent the leakage of saliva.

2. Apply air from the air-water syringe to the tooth being inverted to help in turning the dam material under.

Purpose: When the tooth surface is dry, the margin of the stretched dam usually inverts into the gingival sulcus as the dam is released.

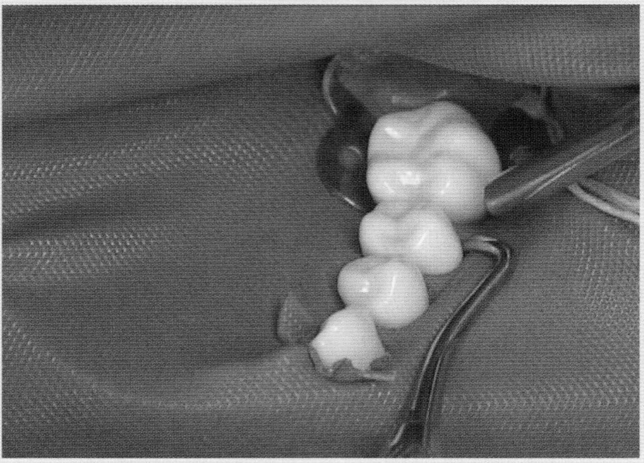

3. A black spoon or burnisher can be used to invert the edges of the dam.
4. When all punched holes are properly inverted, the dental dam application is complete.
5. If necessary for patient comfort, a saliva ejector may be placed under the dam and positioned on the floor of the patient's mouth on the side opposite the area being treated.
6. If the patient is uncomfortable and has trouble breathing only through the nose, then cut a small hole in the palatal area of the dam by pinching a piece of the dam with cotton pliers and cutting a small hole near the palatal area.

Removing the Dam

1. If a ligature was used to stabilize the dam, then remove it first. If a saliva ejector was used, then remove it.
2. Slide your finger under the dam parallel to the arch, and pull outward so that you are stretching the holes away from the isolated teeth. Working from posterior to anterior, use the crown and bridge scissors to cut from hole to hole, creating one long cut.

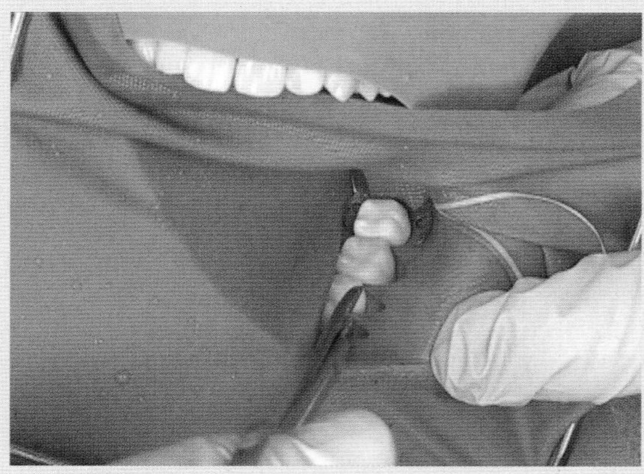

3. When all septa are cut, the dam is lingually pulled to free the dam from the interproximal space.

Procedure 10-4

Preparation, Placement, and Removal of the Dental Dam (Expanded Function)—cont'd

4. Using the dental dam forceps, position the beaks into the holes of the clamp, and open the clamp by squeezing the handle. Gently slide the clamp from the tooth.
5. Remove both the dam and the Young frame at one time.
6. Use a tissue or the dam napkin to wipe the patient's mouth, lips, and chin free of moisture.
7. Inspect the dam to ensure that the entire pattern of the torn septa of the dental dam has been removed.
8. If a fragment of the dental dam is missing, use dental floss to check the corresponding interproximal area of the oral cavity.

Purpose: Fragments of the dental dam left under the free gingiva can cause gingival irritation.

Chapter Exercises

Multiple Choice

Circle the letter next to the correct answer.

1. The dentist is placing a restoration on the facial surface of tooth #10; the HVE tip should be placed on the __________.
- **a.** facial surface
- **b.** lingual surface
- **c.** opposite side of where the dentist is working
- **d.** b and c

2. Hole size no. __________ is used for the anchor tooth, which holds the rubber dam clamp.
- **a.** 1
- **b.** 3
- **c.** 4
- **d.** 5

3. While placing the dental dam, you notice the contacts to be extremely tight. A(n) __________ may be used to help push the material interproximally.
- **a.** explorer
- **b.** tape or floss
- **c.** wooden wedge
- **d.** separating disc

4. The HVE handle should be held in a __________ grasp.
- **a.** palm
- **b.** pen
- **c.** thumb-to-nose
- **d.** b or c

5. The purpose of inverting the dental dam is to __________.
- **a.** prevent saliva leakage
- **b.** prevent the clamp from coming off
- **c.** stabilize the dam
- **d.** a, b, and c

6. If a patient's cheek or tongue is accidentally sucked into the HVE tip, then you should __________.
- **a.** inform the dentist
- **b.** quickly turn off the vacuum control
- **c.** rotate the angle of the tip to break the suction
- **d.** b or c

7. During oral evacuation for tooth #19, the bevel of the HVE tip should be positioned __________ the occlusal surface of the tooth being prepared.
- **a.** even with
- **b.** slightly below
- **c.** slightly above

8. Cotton roll isolation would not be the best selection for __________ procedures.
- **a.** restorative
- **b.** cementation
- **c.** sealant
- **d.** a and b

9. A limited rinse is one that __________.
- **a.** is completed at the beginning of the procedure
- **b.** is completed at the end of the procedure
- **c.** rinses the whole mouth
- **d.** rinses a specific area in the mouth

10. When using a saliva ejector, position the tip __________ on which you are working.
- **a.** in the buccal mucosa area
- **b.** under the tongue on the same side
- **c.** under the tongue on the opposite side
- **d.** in the palatal area

Apply Your Knowledge

1. You are assisting in an amalgam procedure and notice that the cotton rolls that were placed are saturated with saliva and debris. After removing the cotton rolls, you notice that the patient's mucosa is red and irritated. What caused this, and what should you say to the patient?

2. Dr. Stewart is restoring tooth #25 for a composite resin on the facial surface. Where is the best position for you to place the HVE tip during the tooth preparation?

3. How would you prepare the dental dam for placement for tooth #25?

PARTFIVE Patient Care

CHAPTER 11

The Dental Patient

http://evolve.elsevier.com/Robinson/essentials/

LEARNING OBJECTIVES

1. Pronounce, define, and spell the key terms.
2. Describe the role the dental assistant plays in providing quality patient care.
3. Complete the following related to the patient record:
   - Describe the forms of a patient record.
   - Demonstrate how to register a new patient.
   - Discuss the importance of having a medical history for a patient and how that influences the dental treatment plan.
   - Demonstrate how to obtain a medical-dental health history.
   - Describe how the Health Insurance Portability and Accountability Act (HIPAA) influences dental care.
4. Complete the following related to vital signs:
   - Define vital signs.
   - Describe the four vital signs commonly taken in the dental office.
   - Describe and demonstrate the procedures for taking a patient's temperature, pulse, respiration, and blood pressure.

KEY TERMS

blood pressure
brachial
carotid
demographics
diastolic
Health Insurance Portability and Accountability Act (HIPAA)
medically compromised
patient record
respiration
sphygmomanometer
stethoscope
systolic
temperature
thermometer
vital signs

Patients are the key reason a dental practice exists; therefore your primary responsibility to patients is to be an essential member of the dental team that provides quality patient care. This includes making patients feel welcome and comfortable in the practice, as well as maintaining the patient's safety and well-being during treatment.

The Dental Assistant's Responsibilities to the Patient

- Your alertness to variations in a patient's health is important. Recognition and implementation of less than 100% could have a lasting negative effect for the patient.
- Recognize that everyone has basic needs for approval and respect. Be willing to help a patient meet these needs in an acceptable manner.
- Make every effort to understand a patient. Realize that patients may be motivated by unknown factors and that those needs can be exaggerated in times of stress.
- Accept the patient as he or she is, and make the effort to be pleasant and respectful even when the patient may be irritable, anxious, uncooperative, or demanding.

Patient Record

Before treatment can begin, the dentist will request personal and clinical information from the patient. The patient record is an important legal document that maintains this information about a patient. Each patient has a separate record. Personal and clinical information is obtained by asking the new patient to complete the printed forms at the first visit.

Circumstances can exist during which a patient may be unable to complete the forms, such as a language barrier, not being able to read, or being visually impaired. When this type of circumstance is apparent, assist the patient by helping him or her complete the forms and by answering any questions necessary to help the patient provide the required data.

Patient Registration

The **patient registration form** is completed and primarily used for the business office in the management of the account. Information in the form must be complete and accurate and includes the following (Figure 11-1):

- Demographics: A patient must provide his or her full name, address, telephone number, employment information, and spousal information.
- **Responsible party:** Patients are not always responsible for payment of their own dental expenses. This section gathers information concerning the individual who accepts this responsibility. Information required here includes the responsible party's full name, address, home and work telephone numbers, and employment information. Be sure the responsible party signs the release of information and the assignment of benefits.
- **Insurance information:** This section gathers data required in completing dental insurance claims for the patient. The subscriber should provide specific insurance information, such as the group or policy number. Usually, the responsible party is also the insurance plan subscriber. Making a photocopy of the patient's insurance card is customary.

See Procedure 11-1: Registering a New Patient.

Clinical Information

The patient record also includes several forms that provide the dental team specific information about the patient's medical and dental history, dental treatment completed, and dental treatment planned as dictated by the dentist.

The patient's radiographs, laboratory prescriptions, and any correspondence will also be stored in the patient record. The patient must provide consent by signing a release-of-information form before a consultation between the dentist and the physician can take place.

Medical History

Questions regarding the patient's medical history, present physical condition, chronic conditions, allergies, and medications are asked. Each new patient must complete a medical history form before treatment can begin (Figure 11-2).

The patient's signature on the form indicates that he or she has provided the information and takes responsibility for its accuracy.

A complete and up-to-date medical history is important because it:

- Alerts the dentist to medical conditions and medications that may affect the type of treatment provided.
- Aids the dentist in identifying any special treatment needs.
- Alerts the dentist to any allergies that could pose a potential medical emergency.

Returning patients are asked to **update** their medical history at each visit. The patient should sign the form to indicate that the information is accurate and up to date (Figure 11-3).

The dentist may also wish to consult the patient's physician regarding health problems, particularly if the patient is medically compromised. (*Medically compromised* is defined as a patient with an illness or physical condition that may influence the way dental treatment is provided.)

Medication History

A medication history, which is an essential part of the medical history, is a record of all the medications a patient is currently taking. These include prescription medications, over-the-counter drugs, vitamins, and any other drugs. The medication history is particularly important in older patients, many of whom have chronic conditions and are taking several prescribed and over-the-counter medications.

The dentist needs to be aware of these medications because either the medicine or the condition for which it was prescribed may modify the selection of anesthetic, premedication, and procedures when providing dental treatment.

Allergies If the patient has any known allergies, then making the dental team aware of these is extremely important. An allergic reaction could increase with severity each time the individual comes into contact with the substance. For this reason, asking about both known and suspected allergies is important.

Of particular concern in the dental setting are allergies to latex, antibiotics, pain medications, and local anesthetic solutions.

Substances Used in a Dental Practice that Could Cause an Allergic Reaction

Latex—Latex gloves and the dental dam are routinely used in patient care.

Antibiotics—Antibiotic medications may be prescribed for patients who are at high risk for bacterial endocarditis, which is a severe bacterial infection of the cardiac valves and supporting structures caused by bloodborne pathogens gaining entry to the bloodstream.

Pain medication—Pain medication may be prescribed to manage postoperative pain.

Topical and local anesthetic solutions—It will be necessary for the dentist to select an alternative anesthetic solution that does not cause an allergic reaction.

Medical Alert If the patient has a predisposing medical condition that could affect decisions regarding dental treatment, then this information must be indicated on the inside cover of the patient record. Examples of this could include;

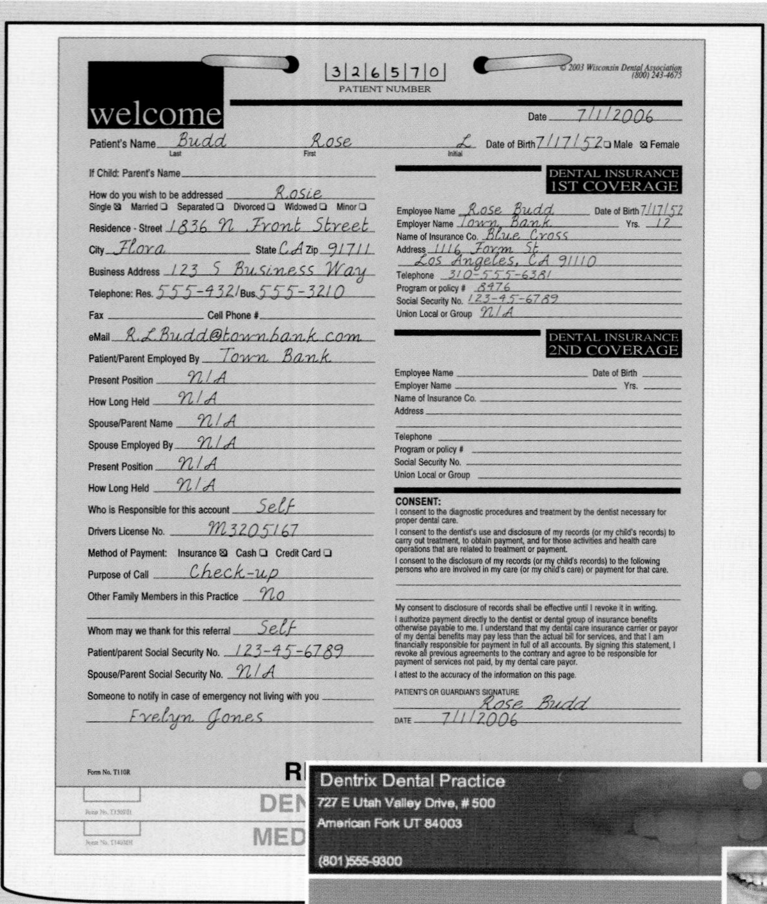

3 2 6 5 7 0
PATIENT NUMBER

© 2003 Wisconsin Dental Association (800) 243-4675

welcome

Date 7/1/2006

Patient's Name Budd (Last) Rose (First) L (Initial) Date of Birth 7/17/52 ☐ Male ☒ Female

If Child: Parent's Name

How do you wish to be addressed Rosie

Single ☒ Married ☐ Separated ☐ Divorced ☐ Widowed ☐ Minor ☐

Residence - Street 1836 N. Front Street

City Flora State CA Zip 91711

Business Address 123 S Business Way

Telephone: Res. 555-4321 Bus. 555-3210

Fax Cell Phone #

eMail R.L.Budd@townbank.com

Patient/Parent Employed By Town Bank

Present Position N/A

How Long Held N/A

Spouse/Parent Name N/A

Spouse Employed By N/A

Present Position N/A

How Long Held N/A

Who is Responsible for this account Self

Drivers License No. M3205167

Method of Payment: Insurance ☒ Cash ☐ Credit Card ☐

Purpose of Call Check-up

Other Family Members in this Practice No

Whom may we thank for this referral Self

Patient/parent Social Security No. 123-45-6789

Spouse/Parent Social Security No. N/A

Someone to notify in case of emergency not living with you

Evelyn Jones

DENTAL INSURANCE 1ST COVERAGE

Employee Name Rose Budd Date of Birth 7/17/52

Employer Name Town Bank Yrs. 12

Name of Insurance Co. Blue Cross

Address 1116 Form St. Los Angeles, CA 91110

Telephone 310-555-6381

Program or policy # 8476

Social Security No. 123-45-6789

Union Local or Group N/A

DENTAL INSURANCE 2ND COVERAGE

Employee Name Date of Birth

Employer Name Yrs.

Name of Insurance Co.

Address

Telephone

Program or policy #

Social Security No.

Union Local or Group

CONSENT:

I consent to the diagnostic procedures and treatment by the dentist necessary for proper dental care.

I consent to the dentist's use and disclosure of my records (or my child's records) to carry out treatment, to obtain payment, and for those activities and health care operations that are related to treatment or payment.

I consent to the disclosure of my records (or my child's records) to the following persons who are involved in my care (or my child's care) or payment for that care.

My consent to disclosure of records shall be effective until I revoke it in writing.

I authorize payment directly to the dentist or dental group of insurance benefits otherwise payable to me. I understand that my dental care insurance carrier or payor of my dental benefits may pay less than the actual bill for services, and that I am financially responsible for payment in full of all accounts. By signing this statement, I revoke all previous agreements to the contrary and agree to be responsible for payment of services not paid, by my dental care payor.

I attest to the accuracy of the information on this page.

PATIENT'S OR GUARDIAN'S SIGNATURE Rose Budd

DATE 7/1/2006

Form No. T110R

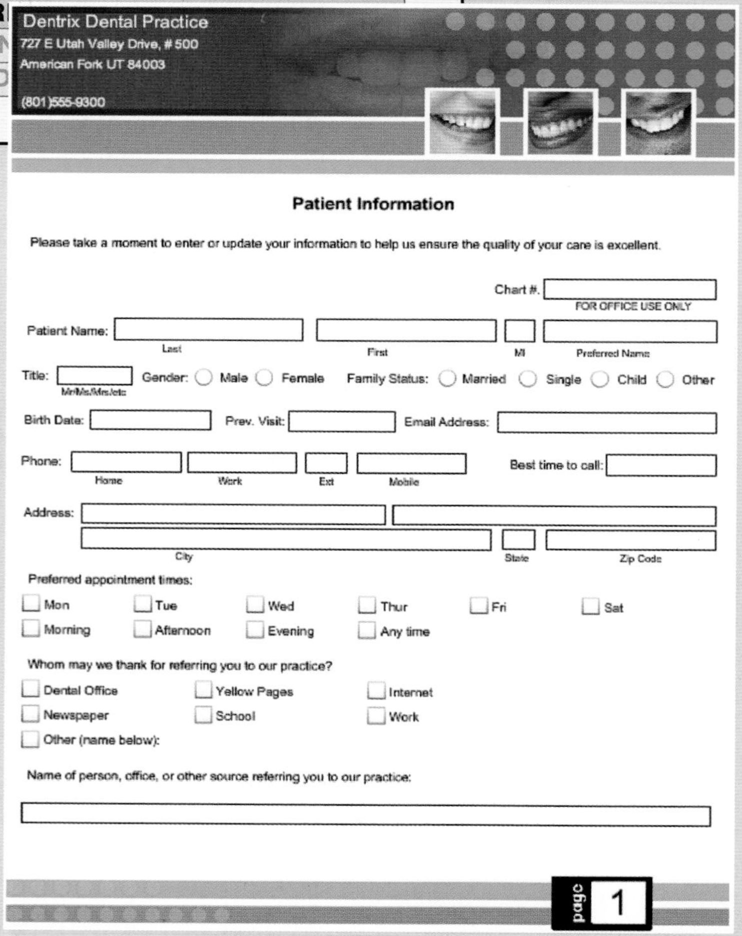

Registration Form

Registration forms provide demographic and financial information about the patient and the person or persons responsible for payment of dental fees. The form is divided into sections that help organize the information.

Paper: If this form is completed by the patient, ensure that all the information is legible and complete before it is stored in the file folder.

Electronic: The information and sections of the form are the same as the paper form, and information can feed into other areas of the patient's record.

Dentrix Dental Practice
727 E Utah Valley Drive, # 500
American Fork UT 84003
(801)555-9300

Patient Information

Please take a moment to enter or update your information to help us ensure the quality of your care is excellent.

Chart #: FOR OFFICE USE ONLY

Patient Name: Last First MI Preferred Name

Title: Mr/Ms/Mrs/etc Gender: ◯ Male ◯ Female Family Status: ◯ Married ◯ Single ◯ Child ◯ Other

Birth Date: Prev. Visit: Email Address:

Phone: Home Work Ext Mobile Best time to call:

Address: City State Zip Code

Preferred appointment times:

☐ Mon ☐ Tue ☐ Wed ☐ Thur ☐ Fri ☐ Sat

☐ Morning ☐ Afternoon ☐ Evening ☐ Any time

Whom may we thank for referring you to our practice?

☐ Dental Office ☐ Yellow Pages ☐ Internet

☐ Newspaper ☐ School ☐ Work

☐ Other (name below):

Name of person, office, or other source referring you to our practice:

page 1

FIGURE 11-1 Sample patient registration form. (From Gaylor LJ: *The administrative dental assistant,* ed 3, St. Louis, 2012, Saunders; form courtesy The Dental Record, Wisconsin Dental Association, Milwaukee, Wisconsin; Dentrix screenshot courtesy Henry Schein Practice Solutions, American Fork, Utah.)

3 2 6 5 7 0
PATIENT NUMBER

©04 Wisconsin Dental Association (800) 243-4675

welcome

Patient's Name Budd (Last) Rose (First) L (Initial) 7/17/52 (Date of Birth)

CIRCLE THE APPROPRIATE ANSWER, IF YOU DON'T KNOW THE CORRECT ANSWER PLEASE WRITE "DON'T KNOW" ON THE LINE AFTER THE QUESTION

1. Physician's Name Robert Alexander
   Address 1346 Medical Way Suite B
   Tel: ( )
2. Are you under a physician's care? .... YES NO
   Since when 3/95 Why
3. When was your last complete physical exam? 2003
4. Are you taking any medication or substances? .... YES NO
   (If yes, please list medications in comments section or on the back of this form.)
5. Do you routinely take health related substances? (Vitamins, herbal supplements, natural products) .... YES NO
6. Are you allergic to any medications or substances? (please list) .... YES NO
7. Do you have any other allergies or hives? .... YES NO
8. Do you have any problems with penicillin, antibiotics, anesthetics or other medications? .... YES NO
9. Are you sensitive to any metals or latex? .... YES NO
10. Are you pregnant or suspect you may be? .... YES NO
11. Do you use any birth control medications? .... YES NO
12. Have you ever been treated for or been told you might have heart disease? .... YES NO
13. Do you have a pacemaker, an artificial heart valve implant, or been diagnosed with mitral valve prolapse? .... YES NO
14. Have you ever had rheumatic fever? .... YES NO
15. Are you aware of any heart murmurs? .... YES NO
16. Do you have high or low blood pressure? (please circle) .... YES NO
17. Have you ever had a serious illness or major surgery? .... YES NO
    If so, explain
18. Have you ever had radiation treatment, chemo treatment for tumor, growth or other condition? .... YES NO
19. Do you have inflammatory diseases, such as arthritis or rheumatism? .... YES NO
20. Do you have any artificial joints/prosthesis? .... YES NO
21. Do you have any blood disorders, such as anemia, leukemia, etc? .... YES NO
22. Have you ever bled excessively after being cut or injured? .... YES NO
23. Do you have any stomach problems? .... YES NO
24. Do you have any kidney problems? .... YES NO
25. Do you have any liver problems? .... YES NO
26. Are you diabetic? .... YES NO
27. Do you have fainting or dizzy spells? .... YES NO
28. Do you have asthma? .... YES NO
29. Do you have epilepsy or seizure disorders? .... YES NO
30. Do you or have you had venereal disease? .... YES NO
31. Have you tested HIV positive? .... YES NO
32. Do you have AIDS? .... YES NO
33. Have you had or do you test positive for hepatitis? .... YES NO
34. Do you or have you had T.B.? .... YES NO
35. Do you smoke, chew, use snuff or any other forms of tobacco? .... YES NO
36. Do you regularly consume more than one or two alcoholic beverages a day? .... YES NO
37. Do you habitually use controlled substances? .... YES NO
38. Have you had psychiatric treatment? .... YES NO
39. Have you taken any prescription drugs fenfluramine, fenfluramine combined with phentermine (fen-phen), dexfenfluramine (redux), or other weight loss products? .... YES NO
40. Do you have any disease condition, or problem not listed? If so, explain
    None
41. Is there anything else we should know about your health that we have not covered in this form?
    None
42. Would you like to speak to the Doctor privately about any problem? .... YES NO

I CERTIFY THAT THE ABOVE INFORMATION IS COMPLETE AND ACCURATE

PATIENT'S / GUARDIAN'S SIGNATURE Rose Budd DATE 7/1/2006

DENTIST'S SIGNATURE Mary A. Edwards DATE 7/1/2006

ANEST.

MED. ALERT Penicillin Codeine

COMMENTS

estrogen
penicillin/codeine

infant
high 192/67

MED

Form No. T140MH

Medical History Form

A comprehensive medical history is necessary to ensure that the patient's medical needs are being met along with the dental needs. The medical history can alert the dentist to possible interactions between dental treatment and medical treatment, at which point the dentist may initiate contact with the patient's physician to ensure that any dental treatment is taking the patient's overall well-being into account.

Paper: The medical history form may use stickers, colored pens, stamps, or preprinted boxes to note any allergies or other conditions that may require special treatment. These should be done in a visual and highly consistent manner. To protect the patient's confidentiality, alerts should never be placed on the outside of the file folder where other patients may see them.

Electronic: The same sort of alerts can be placed within the patient file (see Individual Patient File screen) using colors and icons for quick and easy identification and accessible from a variety of different patient screens.

Dentrix Dental Practice
727 E Utah Valley Drive, # 500
American Fork UT 84003

(801)555-9300

Medical & Dental History Form

Patient Name: Last First MI Preferred Name

Please take a moment to let us know about your medical and dental history so we may serve you more effectively and in a way that watches out for your overall health and well-being.

Would you consider yourself to be in fairly good health?

○ Yes ○ No

Within the past year, have there been any changes in your general health?

○ Yes ○ No

What is the date (or approximate date) of your last medical exam?

Your Primary Care Physician's name, address, & phone number:

Please mark any of the following to indicate Yes in response to the question:

- ☐ Have you ever had complications following dental treatment?
- ☐ Are you currently under the care of a physician due to a specific condition?
- ☐ Have you been hospitalized within the last 5 years due to a surgery or illness?
- ☐ Are you currently taking any prescription or non-prescription medications?
- ☐ Do you use tobacco (smoking or chewing)?
- ☐ Do you require the use of corrective lenses (contacts or glasses)?
- ☐ Do you have any other conditions, diseases, etc., not listed above that we should be aware of?

If any of the previous questions are marked, please explain:

page 1

A

FIGURE 11-2 Medical-Dental Health History form. **A,** Medical health history *(front of form)*.

Continued

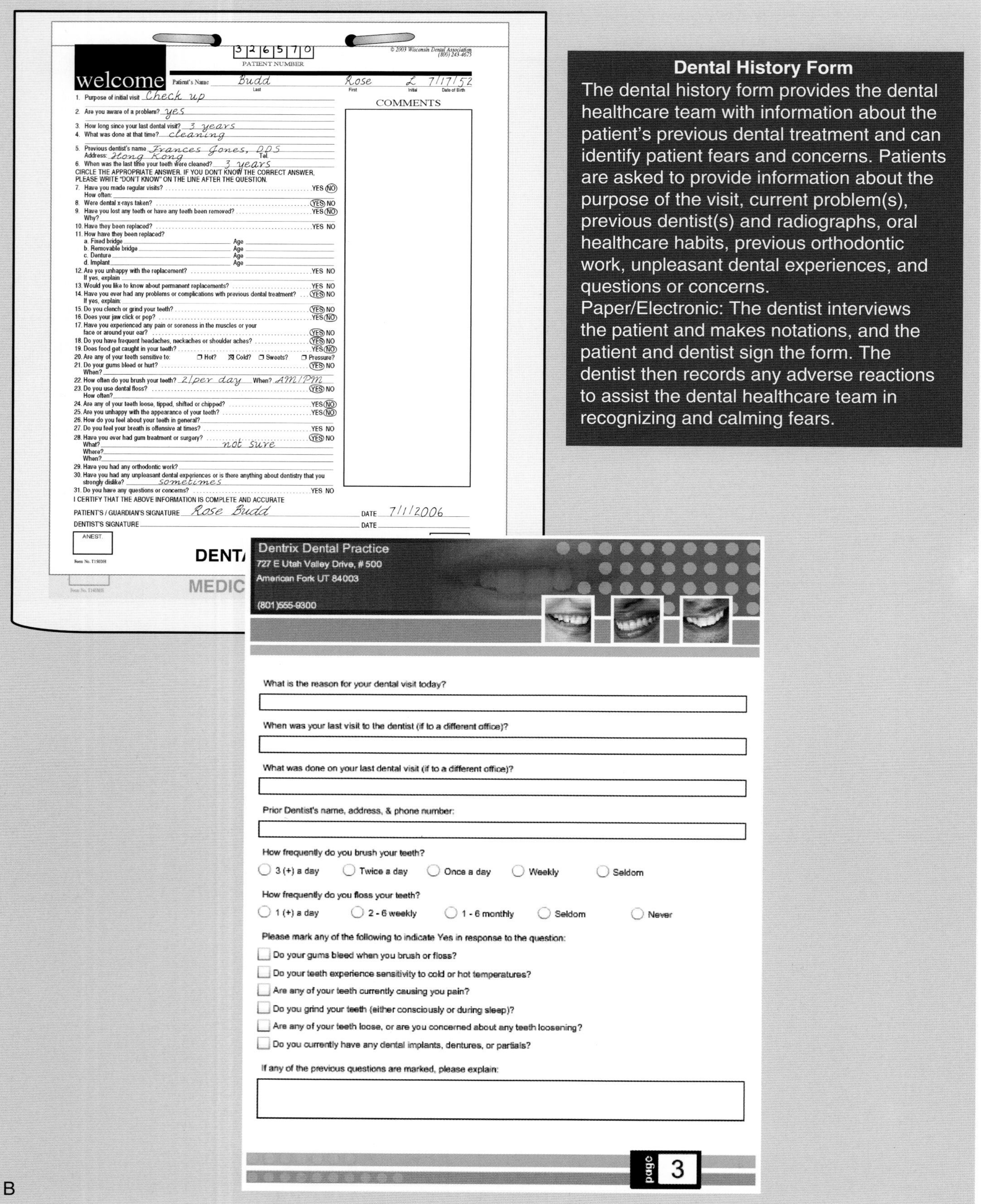

PATIENT NUMBER 3 2 6 5 7 0

© 2003 Wisconsin Dental Association (800) 243-4675

welcome

Patient's Name Budd (Last) Rose (First) L (Initial) 7/17/52 (Date of Birth)

1. Purpose of initial visit Check up
2. Are you aware of a problem? yes
3. How long since your last dental visit? 3 years
4. What was done at that time? cleaning
5. Previous dentist's name Frances Jones, DDS
   Address: Hong Kong Tel.
6. When was the last time your teeth were cleaned? 3 years

CIRCLE THE APPROPRIATE ANSWER. IF YOU DON'T KNOW THE CORRECT ANSWER, PLEASE WRITE "DON'T KNOW" ON THE LINE AFTER THE QUESTION.

7. Have you made regular visits? YES (NO)
   How often:
8. Were dental x-rays taken? (YES) NO
9. Have you lost any teeth or have any teeth been removed? YES (NO)
   Why?
10. Have they been replaced? YES NO
11. How have they been replaced?
    a. Fixed bridge Age
    b. Removable bridge Age
    c. Denture Age
    d. Implant Age
12. Are you unhappy with the replacement? YES NO
    If yes, explain
13. Would you like to know about permanent replacements? YES NO
14. Have you ever had any problems or complications with previous dental treatment? (YES) NO
    If yes, explain:
15. Do you clench or grind your teeth? (YES) NO
16. Does your jaw click or pop? YES (NO)
17. Have you experienced any pain or soreness in the muscles or your face or around your ear? (YES) NO
18. Do you have frequent headaches, neckaches or shoulder aches? (YES) NO
19. Does food get caught in your teeth? YES (NO)
20. Are any of your teeth sensitive to: ☐ Hot? ☒ Cold? ☐ Sweets? ☐ Pressure?
21. Do your gums bleed or hurt? (YES) NO
    When?
22. How often do you brush your teeth? 2/per day When? AM/PM
23. Do you use dental floss? (YES) NO
    How often?
24. Are any of your teeth loose, tipped, shifted or chipped? YES (NO)
25. Are you unhappy with the appearance of your teeth? YES (NO)
26. How do you feel about your teeth in general?
27. Do you feel your breath is offensive at times? YES NO
28. Have you ever had gum treatment or surgery? (YES) NO
    What? not sure
    Where?
    When?
29. Have you had any orthodontic work?
30. Have you had any unpleasant dental experiences or is there anything about dentistry that you strongly dislike? sometimes
31. Do you have any questions or concerns? YES NO

I CERTIFY THAT THE ABOVE INFORMATION IS COMPLETE AND ACCURATE

PATIENT'S / GUARDIAN'S SIGNATURE Rose Budd DATE 7/1/2006

DENTIST'S SIGNATURE DATE

COMMENTS

ANEST.

Form No. T150DH

DENT

MEDIC

Dental History Form

The dental history form provides the dental healthcare team with information about the patient's previous dental treatment and can identify patient fears and concerns. Patients are asked to provide information about the purpose of the visit, current problem(s), previous dentist(s) and radiographs, oral healthcare habits, previous orthodontic work, unpleasant dental experiences, and questions or concerns.

Paper/Electronic: The dentist interviews the patient and makes notations, and the patient and dentist sign the form. The dentist then records any adverse reactions to assist the dental healthcare team in recognizing and calming fears.

Dentrix Dental Practice
727 E Utah Valley Drive, # 500
American Fork UT 84003
(801)555-9300

What is the reason for your dental visit today?

When was your last visit to the dentist (if to a different office)?

What was done on your last dental visit (if to a different office)?

Prior Dentist's name, address, & phone number:

How frequently do you brush your teeth?
○ 3 (+) a day ○ Twice a day ○ Once a day ○ Weekly ○ Seldom

How frequently do you floss your teeth?
○ 1 (+) a day ○ 2 - 6 weekly ○ 1 - 6 monthly ○ Seldom ○ Never

Please mark any of the following to indicate Yes in response to the question:
☐ Do your gums bleed when you brush or floss?
☐ Do your teeth experience sensitivity to cold or hot temperatures?
☐ Are any of your teeth currently causing you pain?
☐ Do you grind your teeth (either consciously or during sleep)?
☐ Are any of your teeth loose, or are you concerned about any teeth loosening?
☐ Do you currently have any dental implants, dentures, or partials?

If any of the previous questions are marked, please explain:

page 3

B

FIGURE 11-2, cont'd **B,** Dental health history *(back of form)*. (From Gaylor LJ: *The administrative dental assistant,* ed 3, St. Louis, 2012, Saunders; form courtesy The Dental Record, Wisconsin Dental Association, Milwaukee, Wisconsin; Dentrix screenshot courtesy Henry Schein Practice Solutions, American Fork, Utah.)

PATIENT'S NAME ______________________ DATE OF BIRTH ______________

DATE	I HAVE REVIEWED THE ATTACHED HEALTH HISTORY. MY HEALTH AND MEDICATIONS HAVE CHANGED AS FOLLOWS (IF NO CHANGE, WRITE "NO CHANGE")	DENTIST'S SIGNATURE	PATIENT'S OR GUARDIAN'S SIGNATURE

FIGURE 11-3 Medical-dental health history update form.

ACKNOWLEDGEMENT OF RECEIPT OF NOTICE

As required by the Privacy Regulations, I hereby acknowledge that I have received a current copy of this practice's "NOTICE OF PRIVACY PRACTICES", revision date ______________.

As required by the Privacy Regulations, ______________________ from
Name of Staff Member
this practice has explained the "NOTICE OF PRIVACY PRACTICES" to my satisfaction.

As required by the Privacy Regulations, I am aware that this practice has included a provision that it reserves the right to change the terms of its notice and to make the new notice provisions effective for all protected health information that it maintains.

Requests:

☐ I wish to file a "Request for Restriction" of my Protected Health Information.

☐ I wish to file a "Request for Alternative Communications" of my Protected Health Information.

☐ I wish to object to the following in the "Notice of Privacy Practices":

____

____

I understand that this office may change their Notice of Privacy Practices and is not required to honor the terms of the original/previous version(s).

______________________ Signature ______________ Date

______________________ Print Name

(OFFICE USE ONLY)

Signed form received by: ______________________ Date: ______________

Good faith effort to obtain receipt: (Describe) ______________________

____

____

ITEM 066-6289/18243 © JULY2003

FIGURE 11-4 Example of a Notice of Privacy Practices form, acknowledging the receipt and understanding of the privacy practices established for a dental practice. (Courtesy Patterson Office Supplies, Champaign, Illinois.)

allergy to latex or high blood pressure. A brightly colored "ALERT" sticker is placed for the attention of the dental team. An alert sticker should never be placed on the outside of a patient record; doing so would violate dentist–patient confidentiality and the privacy of the patient.

Dental History

The patient's dental history offers important clues in reference to previous dental care. Questions can include how recently the patient received dental treatment, the frequency of dental visits, and the patient's attitude concerning the importance of the appearance of his or her own teeth and dental care.

See Procedure 11-2: Obtaining a Medical-Dental Health History.

Privacy Policy of the Health Insurance Portability and Accountability Act

The **Health Insurance Portability and Accountability Act (HIPAA)** requires that all dental practices have a written privacy policy. This policy must inform the patient that the office will not use or disclose protected health information (PHI) for any purpose other than treatment, diagnosis, and billing. The privacy policy must be available for patients to review, and all patients (new and existing) must sign an acknowledgment of receiving these privacy practices established for the office. The signed acknowledgment must be kept in the patient's record for a minimum of 6 years (Figure 11-4).

HIPAA states that additional authorization and consent from the patient would be required if the disclosure of documents were to be used for health care operations, research, or public need.

Being in a private or semiprivate area is necessary when reviewing a health history or any specific content of a patient record. Additional information about HIPAA can be found at: http://www.hhs.gov/ocr/privacy/hipaa/understanding/index.html.

Clinical Examination

The clinical examination form is the most comprehensive document in the patient record. This form provides all clinical data from the past, present, and future to the dental team. Each time a patient comes in for an appointment, this form is updated (Figure 11-5).

Treatment Plan

The treatment plan for a patient addresses the dental problems that were identified during the examination and the diagnosis portion of the patient visit (Figure 11-6).

Progress Notes

At the conclusion of each visit, details of what was discussed, diagnosed, or clinically completed are to be entered in the progress notes of the patient chart (Figure 11-7).

Vital Signs

Vital signs are indicators of a patient's overall health, and they include the **temperature**, pulse, respiration rate, and blood pressure.

Vital signs of each new patient should be taken to obtain a baseline reading and then should be completed at each subsequent visit. Monitoring the patient's vital signs during an emergency is essential, and all staff members should be competent in these skills. As a dental assistant, you must:

- Always be accurate in your recordings. Never estimate! If you are unsure of your findings, then either repeat the procedure or ask someone else to check them.
- Never rely on your memory; immediately record your findings.

Temperature

The temperature of the human body is the measurement of body heat. Normal body temperature varies by person, age, activity, and time of day. The average normal body temperature is generally accepted as 98.6° F (37° C). Some studies have shown that the normal body temperature can have a wide range, from 97° F (36.1° C) to 99° F (37.2° C).

Temperature is taken with a **thermometer** (*thermo,* meaning heat, and *meter,* meaning measure). A patient's oral temperature is commonly taken using a digital thermometer, which displays the body temperature (Figure 11-8).

See Procedure 11-3: Taking an Oral Temperature Reading With a Digital Thermometer.

Before taking an oral temperature, ask the patient if he or she has had anything hot or cold to drink, has been exercising, or has been smoking within the last 10 minutes. If the response is "yes," then wait before taking the temperature.

Pulse

A pulse is the beat of the heart. Expansion and compression happen every time the heart beats. By placing your index and middle fingers on a specific pulse location, it is possible to count the number of times the heart is beating per minute (Figure 11-9). The normal pulse rate in resting adults is between 60 and 100 beats per minute (bpm). The pulse rate is more rapid for a child (70 to 110 bpm). Table 11-1 shows different pulse locations.

See Procedure 11-4: Taking a Patient's Pulse.

Respiration

Respiration is the process of inhaling and exhaling, or breathing, and is the way the body takes in oxygen and releases carbon dioxide as a waste product. The normal respiration rate for a relaxed adult is 10 to 20 breaths per minute. For children and teenagers, the rate ranges from 18 to 30 breaths per minute. To measure a patient's respiration rate, you will also need to observe a rhythm and the depth of breath.

See Procedure 11-5: Measuring a Patient's Respiration.

Blood Pressure

The term **blood pressure** refers to the amount of work the heart has to exert to pump blood throughout the body. Blood pressure is the most complex vital sign to obtain. Once you understand the steps and have practiced the procedure, it will become less difficult. Blood pressure readings for adults are classified according to normal values and stages of hypertension (Figure 11-10).

The two readings for blood pressure are the **systolic** and the **diastolic**. The systolic pressure involves the left chamber of the heart, which pumps oxygenated blood into the vessels. The diastolic pressure reflects the heart at rest, when it is taking in blood to be oxygenated.

These readings are recorded as the **systolic pressure** (higher number) over the **diastolic pressure** (lower number). For example, 129/78 mm Hg indicates systolic pressure of 129 mm Hg and diastolic pressure of 78 mm Hg.

An **automated electronic blood pressure device** is used in many practices to simplify and speed the process (Figure 11-11). It is important that you carefully follow the steps and practice using this type of device until you are able to obtain an accurate reading while maintaining patient comfort.

See Procedure 11-6: Taking a Patient's Blood Pressure.

An accurate reading is obtained with the use of a **stethoscope** and a **sphygmomanometer**. The stethoscope is used to amplify the sounds of the blood pumped within the artery (Figure 11-12). These sounds heard are referred to as Korotkoff sounds, which are a series of sounds produced by the blood rushing back into the artery (Table 11-2). The sphygmomanometer is used to measure blood pressure (Figure 11-13).

The sphygmomanometer consists of a gauge attached to an inflatable rubber bladder enclosed in a cloth cuff. A closure, usually nylon tape (Velcro), is used to hold the cuff in place. A rubber bulb with a valve is used to inflate and deflate the bladder, which creates pressure to briefly control the blood flow in the artery. An **aneroid manometer** has a dial directly attached to the cuff.

Text continued on p. 154

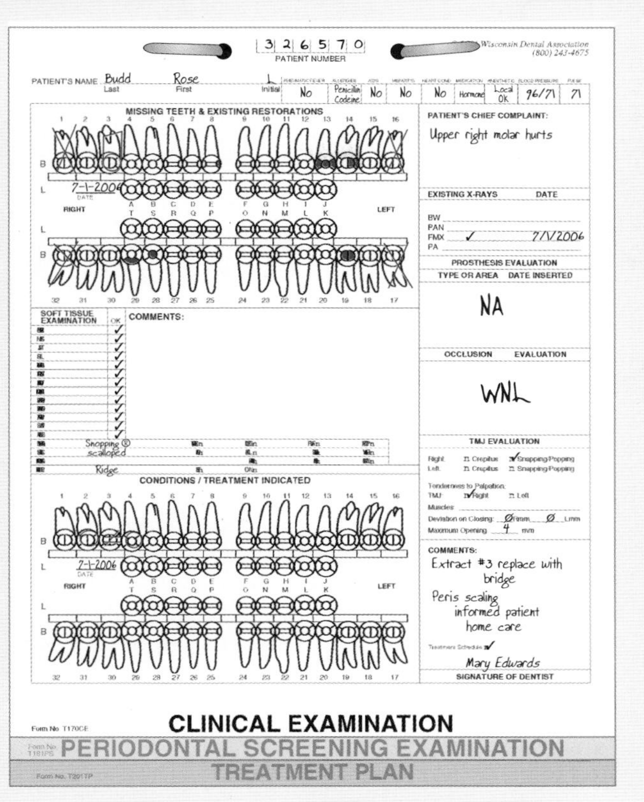

3 2 6 5 7 0
PATIENT NUMBER
Wisconsin Dental Association
(800) 243-4675

PATIENT'S NAME Budd (Last) Rose (First) L (Initial)

MISSING TEETH & EXISTING RESTORATIONS

7-1-2006 DATE

RIGHT LEFT

PATIENT'S CHIEF COMPLAINT:
Upper right molar hurts

EXISTING X-RAYS DATE
BW
PAN
FMX ✓ 7/1/2006
PA

PROSTHESIS EVALUATION
TYPE OR AREA DATE INSERTED
NA

OCCLUSION EVALUATION
WNL

TMJ EVALUATION

SOFT TISSUE EXAMINATION OK
COMMENTS:

Snapping
scalloped
Ridge

CONDITIONS / TREATMENT INDICATED

7-1-2006 DATE

RIGHT LEFT

COMMENTS:
Extract #3 replace with bridge
Peris scaling
informed patient
home care

Mary Edwards
SIGNATURE OF DENTIST

CLINICAL EXAMINATION
PERIODONTAL SCREENING EXAMINATION
TREATMENT PLAN

D C B Budd, Rose L.

Examination Form

The examination form illustrates the patient's dental condition at the time of his or her first visit to the dental practice. It is part of the permanent record and should not be altered. The form documents previous dental treatment, existing conditions, and missing teeth. In addition to oral hygiene information, the examination form lists periodontal findings and the result of soft tissue examination, plus temporomandibular joint (TMJ) and occlusal evaluation, the patient's chief complaint, and a record of dental images and their evaluation. The information is gathered and recorded with the assistance of a dental assistant and a dental hygienist and helps the dentist develop a treatment plan.

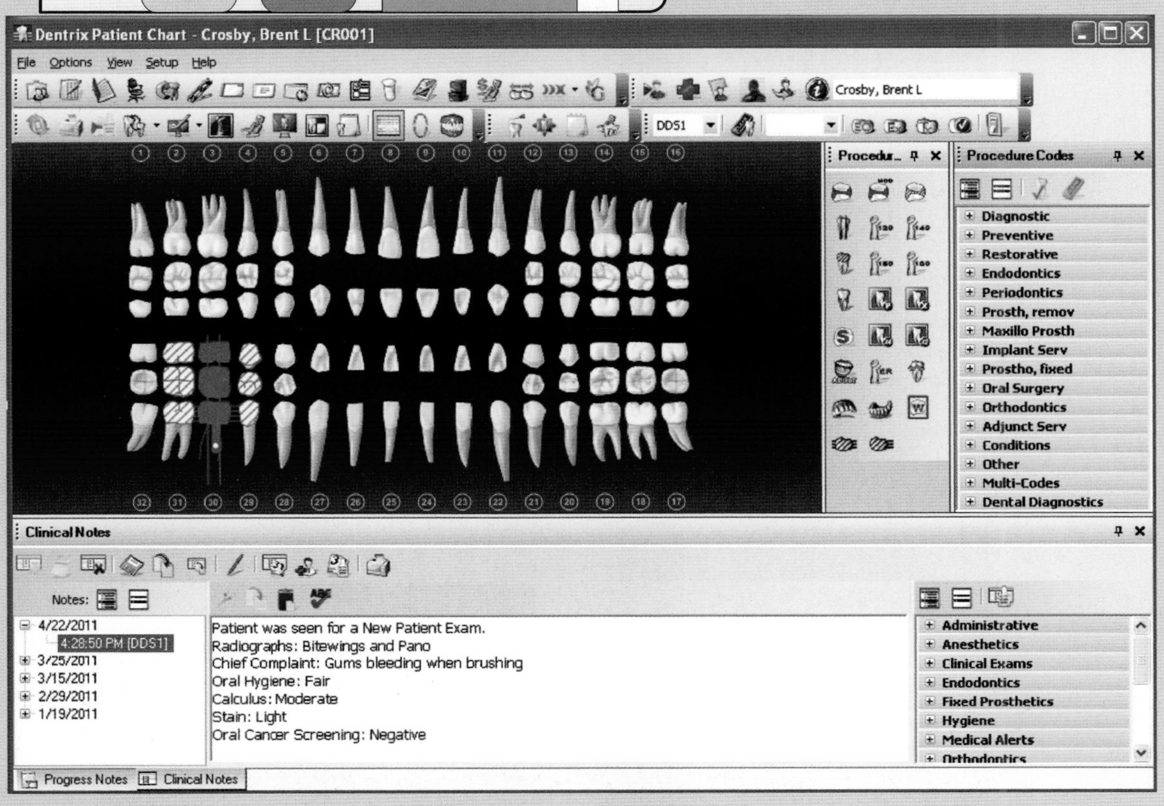

A

FIGURE 11-5 Example of a clinical examination form. (From Gaylor LJ: *The administrative dental assistant,* ed 3, St. Louis, 2012, Saunders; form courtesy The Dental Record, Wisconsin Dental Association, Milwaukee, Wisconsin; Dentrix screenshot courtesy Henry Schein Practice Solutions, American Fork, Utah.)

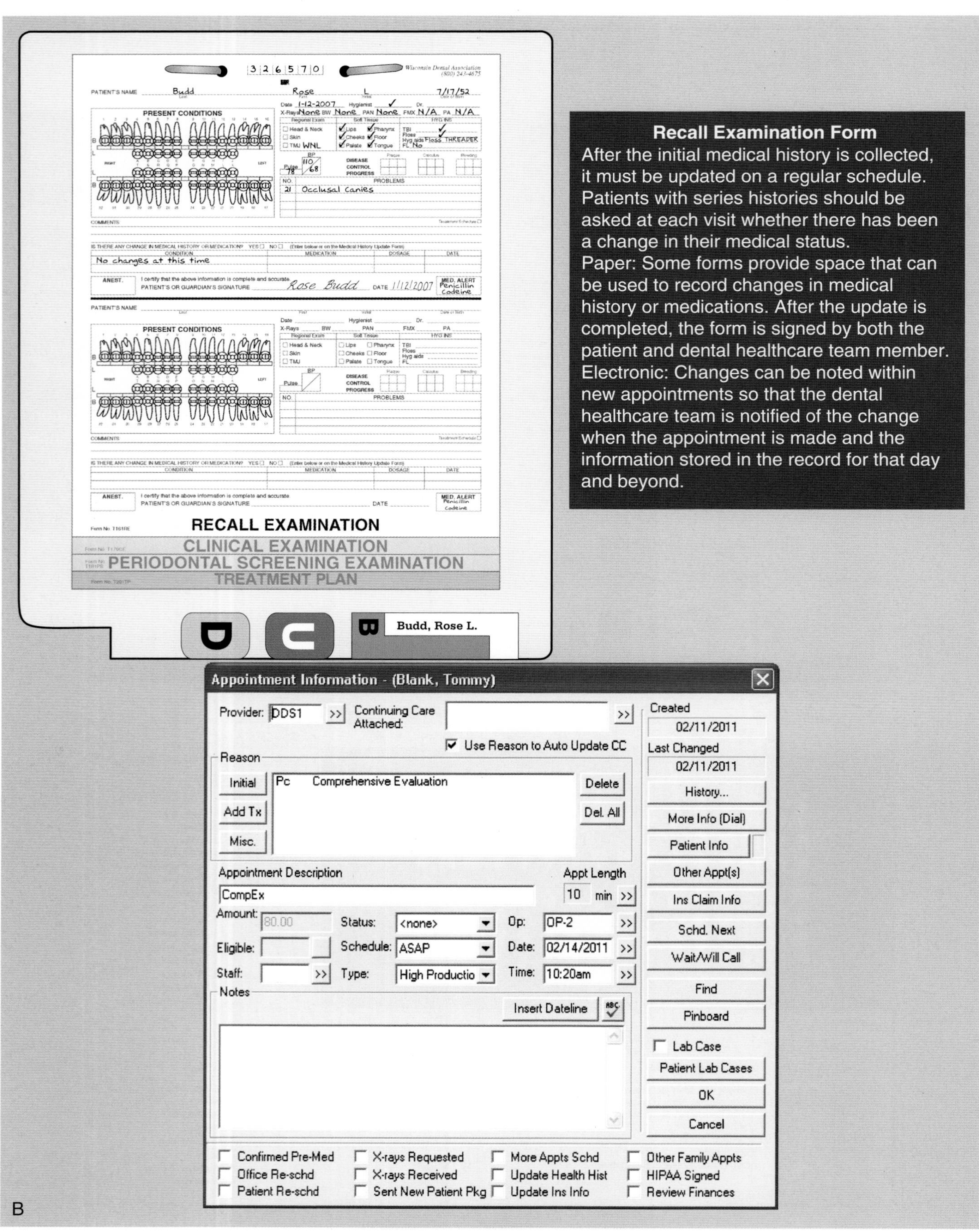

FIGURE 11-5, cont'd

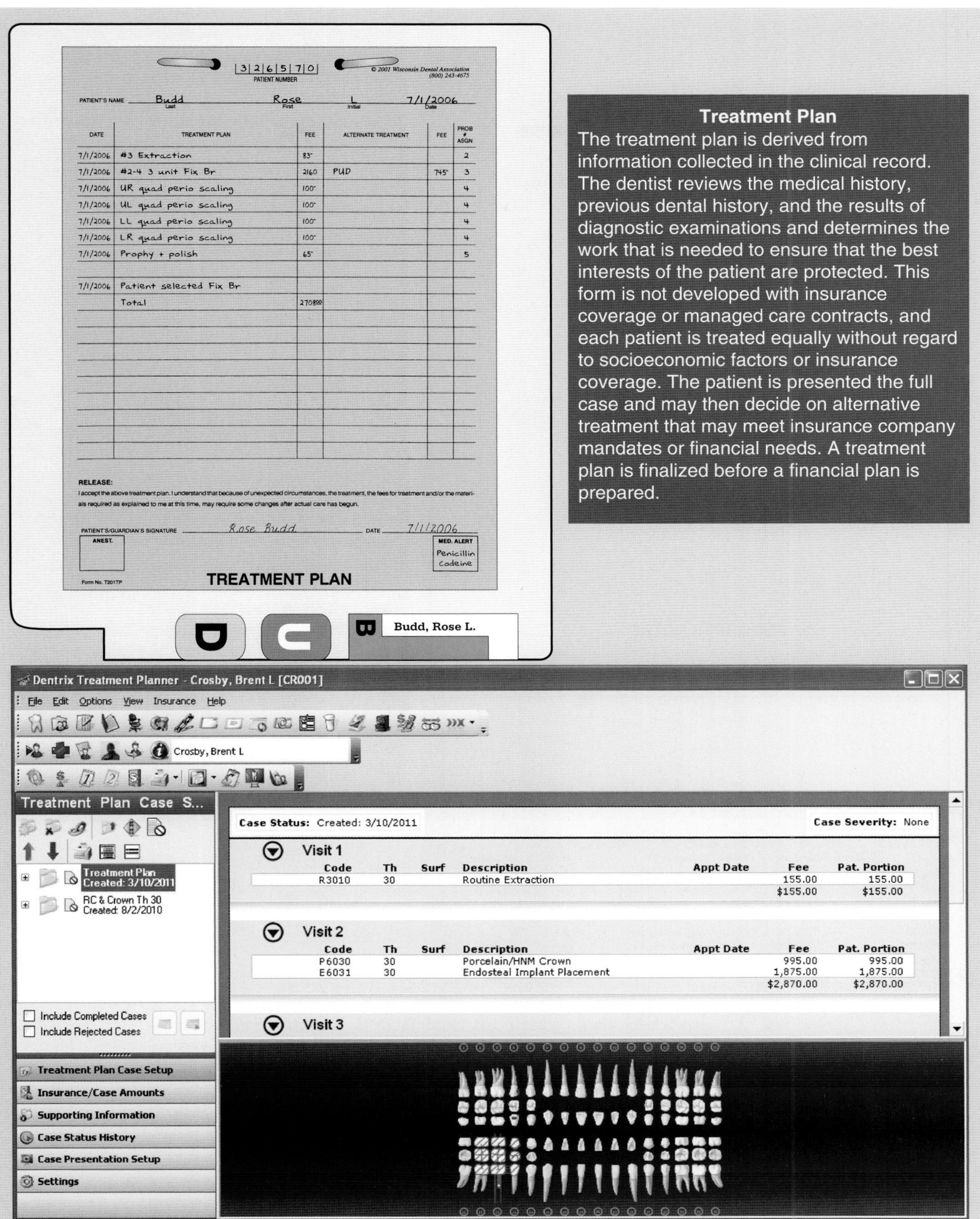

3 2 6 5 7 0
PATIENT NUMBER

© 2001 Wisconsin Dental Association
(800) 243-4675

PATIENT'S NAME Budd (Last) Rose (First) L (Initial) 7/1/2006 (Date)

DATE	TREATMENT PLAN	FEE	ALTERNATE TREATMENT	FEE	PROB # ASGN
7/1/2006	#3 Extraction	83-			2
7/1/2006	#2-4 3 unit Fix Br	2160	PUD	745-	3
7/1/2006	UR quad perio scaling	100-			4
7/1/2006	UL quad perio scaling	100-			4
7/1/2006	LL quad perio scaling	100-			4
7/1/2006	LR quad perio scaling	100-			4
7/1/2006	Prophy + polish	65-			5
7/1/2006	Patient selected Fix Br				
	Total	2708.00			

RELEASE:
I accept the above treatment plan. I understand that because of unexpected circumstances, the treatment, the fees for treatment and/or the materials required as explained to me at this time, may require some changes after actual care has begun.

PATIENT'S/GUARDIAN'S SIGNATURE Rose Budd DATE 7/1/2006

ANEST.

MED. ALERT Penicillin Codeine

Form No. T201TP

TREATMENT PLAN

Budd, Rose L.

Treatment Plan

The treatment plan is derived from information collected in the clinical record. The dentist reviews the medical history, previous dental history, and the results of diagnostic examinations and determines the work that is needed to ensure that the best interests of the patient are protected. This form is not developed with insurance coverage or managed care contracts, and each patient is treated equally without regard to socioeconomic factors or insurance coverage. The patient is presented the full case and may then decide on alternative treatment that may meet insurance company mandates or financial needs. A treatment plan is finalized before a financial plan is prepared.

FIGURE 11-6 Example of a treatment plan form. (From Gaylor LJ: *The administrative dental assistant,* ed 3, St. Louis, 2012, Saunders; form courtesy The Dental Record, Wisconsin Dental Association, Milwaukee, Wisconsin; Dentrix screenshot courtesy Henry Schein Practice Solutions, American Fork, Utah.)

Progress Notes Form

Progress notes are used to record the course of treatment for the patient.

Paper: Each form has space for the date, tooth number, and treatment. Space should also be provided for the initials and identification number (typically license number) of the treating dentist, assistant, or dental hygienist. (These requirements vary from state to state.) Entries on the progress notes include telephone conversations, missed appointments, prescriptions, and contact with insurance carriers or other health care providers. Directives, prognosis, and any difficulties during treatment are also noted. All entries must be supplied in ink, preferably black, and any corrections or deletions should be marked with a single line. Progress notes will also serve as a legal document, and the information must be accurate, complete, and legible.

Electronic: The electronic notes serve the same function as the form, but some of the information indicated within the paper form may be located elsewhere within the patient's electronic file and not necessarily duplicated within this section of the file, such as the provider's initials/signature and identification number, which are stored within that provider's own file.

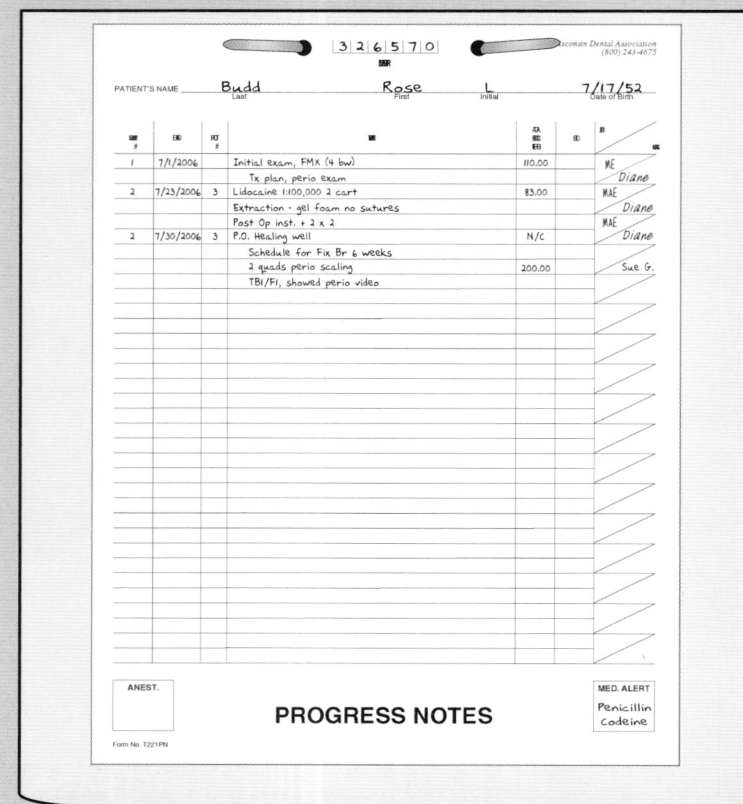

3 2 6 5 7 0

sconsin Dental Association
(800) 243-4675

PATIENT'S NAME Budd (Last) Rose (First) L (Initial) 7/17/52 (Date of Birth)

1	7/1/2006		Initial exam, FMX (4 bw)	110.00		ME
			Tx plan, perio exam			Diane
2	7/23/2006	3	Lidocaine 1:100,000 2 cart	83.00		MAE
			Extraction - gel foam no sutures			Diane
			Post Op inst. + 2 x 2			MAE
2	7/30/2006	3	P.O. Healing well	N/C		Diane
			Schedule for Fix Br 6 weeks			
			2 quads perio scaling	200.00		Sue G.
			TBI/FI, showed perio video			

ANEST.

PROGRESS NOTES

MED. ALERT
Penicillin
Codeine

Form No. T221PN

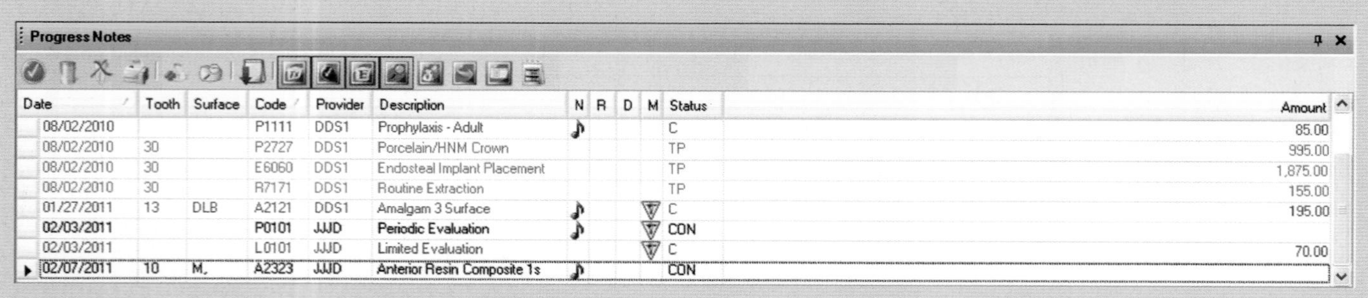

Progress Notes

Date	Tooth	Surface	Code	Provider	Description	N	R	D	M	Status	Amount
08/02/2010			P1111	DDS1	Prophylaxis - Adult					C	85.00
08/02/2010	30		P2727	DDS1	Porcelain/HNM Crown					TP	995.00
08/02/2010	30		E6060	DDS1	Endosteal Implant Placement					TP	1,875.00
08/02/2010	30		R7171	DDS1	Routine Extraction					TP	155.00
01/27/2011	13	DLB	A2121	DDS1	Amalgam 3 Surface					C	195.00
02/03/2011			P0101	JJJD	Periodic Evaluation					CON	
02/03/2011			L0101	JJJD	Limited Evaluation					C	70.00
02/07/2011	10	M,	A2323	JJJD	Anterior Resin Composite 1s					CON	

FIGURE 11-7 Example of the progress notes form. (From Gaylor LJ: *The administrative dental assistant,* ed 3, St. Louis, 2012, Saunders; form courtesy The Dental Record, Wisconsin Dental Association, Milwaukee, Wisconsin; Dentrix screenshot courtesy Henry Schein Practice Solutions, American Fork, Utah.)

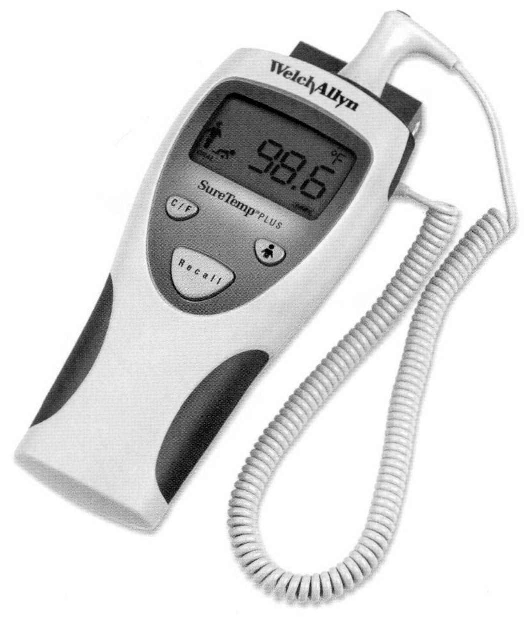

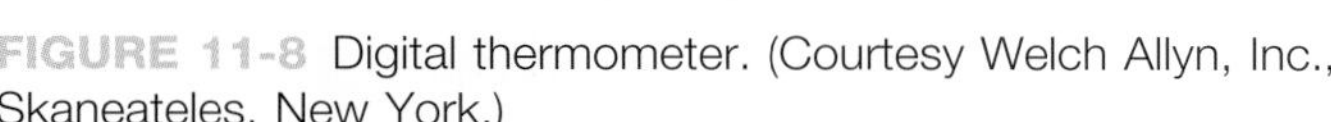
FIGURE 11-8 Digital thermometer. (Courtesy Welch Allyn, Inc., Skaneateles, New York.)

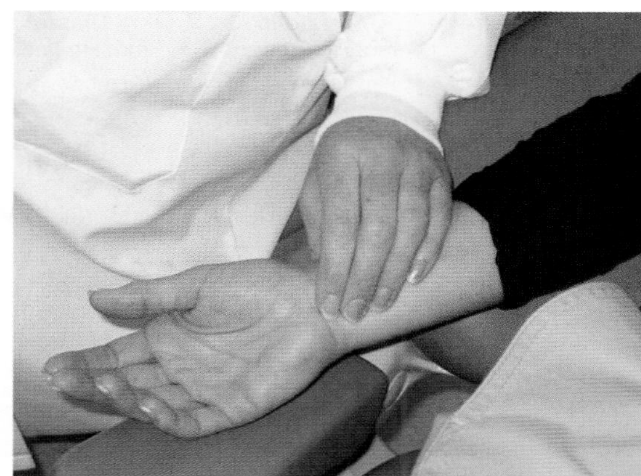
FIGURE 11-9 Taking a patient's pulse.

TABLE 11-1
Pulse Locations

Artery	Description and Location
Radial 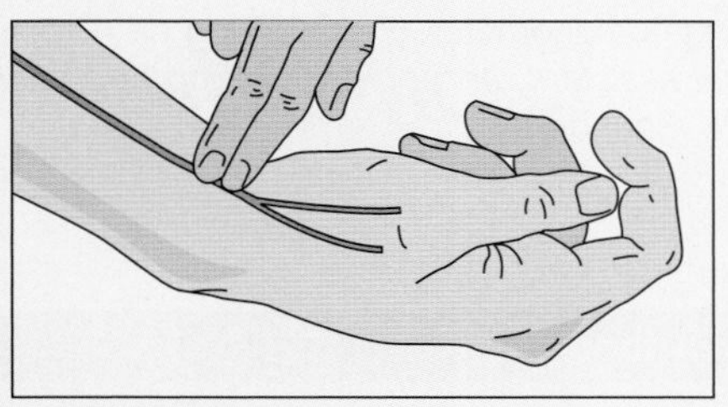	The radial artery is the most common site when taking a pulse. Place your index and middle fingers on the inner wrist on the thumb side.
Carotid 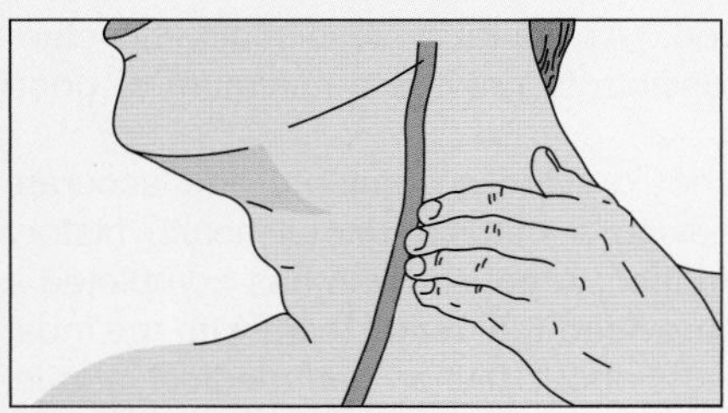	The carotid artery is the site used when performing cardiopulmonary resuscitation. The artery is located on either side of the trachea. Place your first three fingers under the chin and move to the side of the trachea in the groove of the neck.
Brachial 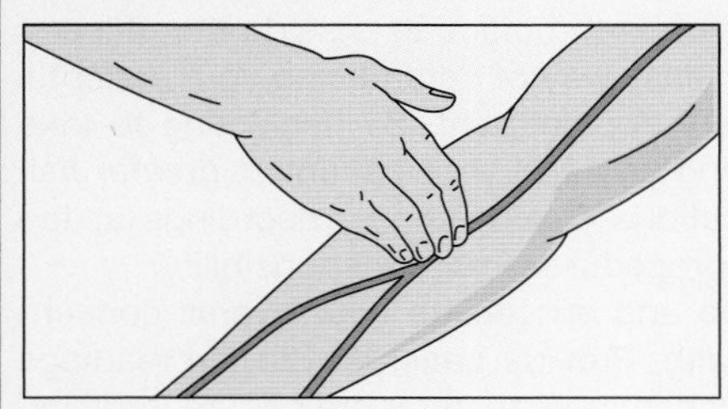	The brachial artery is the site used when establishing a blood pressure reading. Place your index and middle fingers on the inner part of the elbow at the antecubital space (where the arm bends).

Blood Pressure Category	Systolic mm Hg (upper #)		Diastolic mm Hg (lower #)
Normal	less than 120	and	less than 80
Prehypertension	120–139	or	80–89
High Blood Pressure (Hypertension) Stage 1	140–159	or	90–99
High Blood Pressure (Hypertension) Stage 2	160 or higher	or	100 or higher
Hypertensive Crisis (Emergency care needed)	**Higher than 180**	**or**	**Higher than 110**

* Your doctor should evaluate unusually low blood pressure readings.

This chart reflects blood pressure categories defined by the American Heart Association.

FIGURE 11-10 New blood pressure screening recommendations for adults. (Reprinted with Permission. www.heart.org. ©2014 American Heart Association, Inc.)

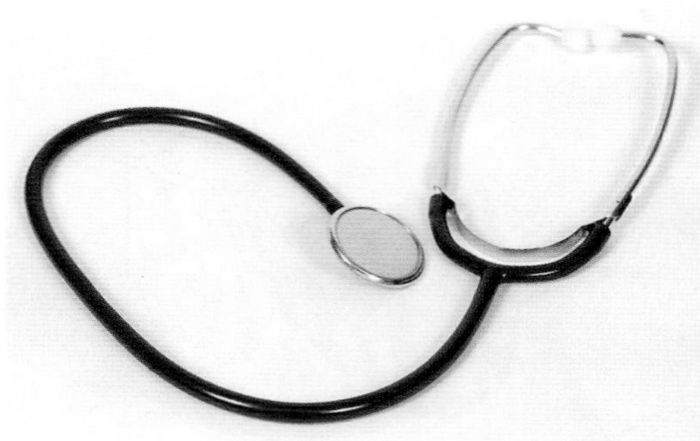

FIGURE 11-12 Stethoscope.

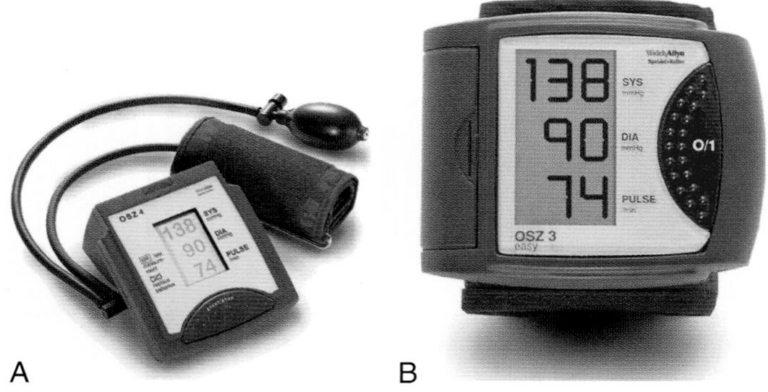

FIGURE 11-11 Automated electronic blood pressure devices. (Courtesy Welch Allyn, Inc., Skaneateles, New York.)

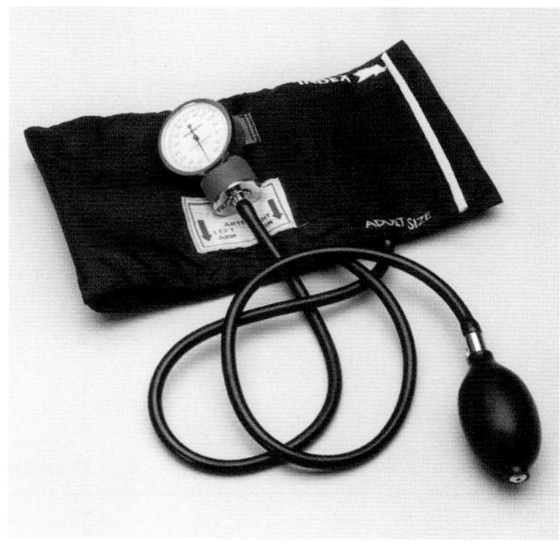

FIGURE 11-13 Sphygmomanometer. (From Young AP, Proctor DB: *Kinn's the medical assistant: an applied learning approach,* ed 11, St. Louis, 2011, Saunders.)

TABLE 11-2

Five Phases of Korotkoff Sounds in Blood Pressure Measurement

Phase	Description
I	Blood is beginning to flow back into the artery and can be heard as a sharp tapping sound. This is the systolic blood pressure reading.
II	The cuff deflates, and more blood flows. A swishing sound may be heard. This sound is softened and becomes prolonged into a murmur.
III	A large amount of blood is flowing into the artery. A distinct, sharp tapping sound returns and rhythmically continues.
IV	Blood is easily flowing, and the sound changes to a soft tapping. The sound becomes distinctly muffled and fainter.
V	At this point, the artery is fully open, and the sound disappears. This is the diastolic blood pressure reading.

Ethical Implications

Accurate information is crucial for the patient to receive proper care. One of the ethical standards that we are to uphold is "doing good." As dental professionals, this standard holds us responsible to provide a minimum of good care to our patients.

Your dentist cannot provide a complete and accurate diagnosis without having a medical-dental health history and a clinical examination. A patient who has completed a medical history has provided the dental team with the most up-to-date information about his or her medical status. Remember, a patient record is the patient's private information between you and the patient. This information is not to be used for discussion in the office or outside the office.

Vital signs are an easy way of determining your patient's health status at every appointment. By neglecting to take these, you are putting you and your patient at greater risk of medical complications. Taking these recordings at the beginning of every procedure is your responsibility.

Patients welcome and appreciate your overall concern about their total health. Provide patients with the readings of their vital signs. Patients like to compare past recordings.

Procedure 11-1

Registering a New Patient

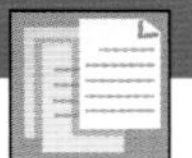

Equipment and Supplies

- Registration form
- Black pen
- Clipboard

Procedural Steps

1. Explain the need for the form to be completed. Give the registration form, along with a clipboard and a black pen, to the patient to be completed.
2. Review the completed form for the necessary information:
   a. Full name, birth date, and name of spouse or parent
   b. Home address and telephone number
   c. Occupation, name of employer, and business address and telephone number
   d. Name and address of person responsible for payment
   e. Method of payment (cash, check, or credit, assignment of benefits)
   f. Health insurance information (photocopy of both sides of the patient's insurance identification card)
   g. Name of the primary insurance carrier
   h. Group policy number

Purpose: This information is necessary for processing financial arrangements and insurance claims.

3. Verify that the patient has signed and dated the form.

Procedure 11-2

Obtaining a Medical-Dental Health History

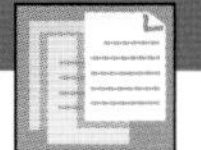

Equipment and Supplies

- Medical-Dental Health History form
- Black pen
- Clipboard

Procedural Steps

1. Explain the need for the information and the importance of fully completing the form.
2. Provide the patient with a black pen and the form on a clipboard.
3. Offer assistance to the patient in completing the form.

Purpose: The patient may not understand the terminology or may have a language barrier.

4. Ask the patient to return the form and clipboard to you after answering all the questions.
5. Thank the patient for completing the form, and request that the patient take a seat in the reception area.
6. Review the form for errors and/or any questions that may arise before handing it to the dental assistant.
7. Use the information from the patient's Medical-Dental Health History form to complete other documents. Remember that the information provided to you by the patient is confidential and must be maintained as such.

Procedure 11-3

Taking an Oral Temperature Reading With a Digital Thermometer

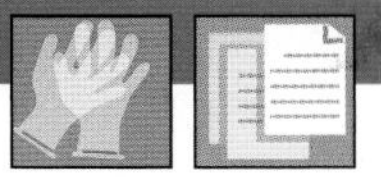

Equipment and Supplies

- Digital thermometer
- Probe cover
- Patient record for documenting temperature

Procedural Steps

1. Wash hands and don gloves.
2. Place a new sheath over the probe of the digital thermometer.
3. Turn on the thermometer. When the display indicates that it is ready, gently place the tip under the patient's tongue.
4. Tell the patient to close his or her lips over the thermometer and to refrain from talking or removing it from the mouth.

Purpose: Talking or removing the thermometer can alter the temperature reading.

5. Leave the thermometer in place until the display indicates a final reading; remove the thermometer from the patient's mouth.
6. Record the reading in the patient's record.
7. Turn off the thermometer, remove the sheath, and disinfect the thermometer as recommended by the manufacturer.

Date	Temp 99° F	Signature

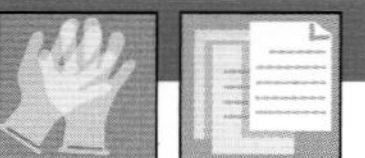

Procedure 11-4
Taking a Patient's Pulse

Equipment and Supplies

- Watch with a second hand
- Patient record to document findings

Procedural Steps

1. Seat the patient in an upright position.
2. Extend the patient's arm, resting it on his or her leg or on the armrest of the chair. Have the arm at or below the heart level.
3. Place the tips of your index and middle fingers on the patient's radial artery.

Note: Indicate in the patient's record whether you are using the right or left arm.

4. Feel for the patient's pulse before beginning to count.

Purpose: This makes it easier to maintain one position during counting (see Figure 11-9).

5. Count the pulse for 30 seconds; then multiply by 2 to compute the rate for a 1-minute reading.
6. Record the rate, along with any distinct changes in rhythm.

Date	Pulse rate—77 bpm (strong)	Signature

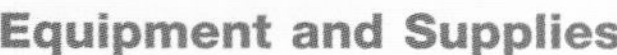

Procedure 11-5
Measuring a Patient's Respiration

Equipment and Supplies

- Watch with a second hand
- Patient record to document findings

Procedural Steps

1. In keeping your position with taking the pulse, glance up at the patient's chest to count the respiration.

Purpose: If the patient is aware that you are observing his or her breathing, they may exaggerate the depth or rate.

2. Count the rise and fall of the patient's chest for 30 seconds; then multiply by 2 to compute the rate for a 1 minute reading.
3. Enter the rate, rhythm, and depth of breathing in the patient record.

Date	Respiration—14 breaths/min (slightly sighing, moderate depth)	Signature

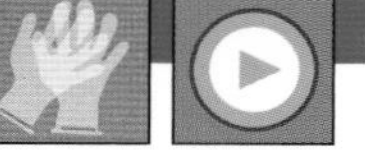

Procedure 11-6
Taking a Patient's Blood Pressure

Equipment and Supplies

- Stethoscope
- Sphygmomanometer
- Patient record to document the findings

Procedural Steps

1. Seat the patient with his or her arm extended at heart level and supported on the chair arm or on a table.

Purpose: The patient's arm should be at the same level as the heart.

2. If possible, roll up the patient's sleeve.

Purpose: Tight clothing can interfere with an accurate measurement and reading.

3. If you are taking the patient's blood pressure for the first time and you do not have a previous blood pressure reading to use for reference, then you will need to establish a basis to determine how high to inflate the cuff. To do this, first palpate the brachial artery to feel for the patient's pulse.

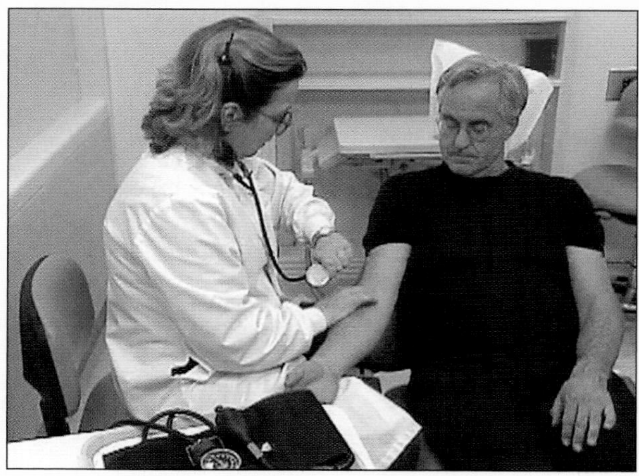

Procedure 11-6

Taking a Patient's Blood Pressure—cont'd

4. Take the patient's brachial pulse for 30 seconds, and then double the number for a 1-minute reading. Add 40 mm Hg to the reading to obtain your inflation level. For example, if the reading was 85, you would add 40, arriving at an inflation level of 125 mm Hg.
5. Expel any air from the cuff by opening the valve and gently pressing on the cuff.
6. Place the blood pressure cuff around the patient's arm approximately 1 inch above the antecubital space, making sure to center the arrow over the brachial artery.

Purpose: **Pressure must be directly applied over the artery for a correct reading.**

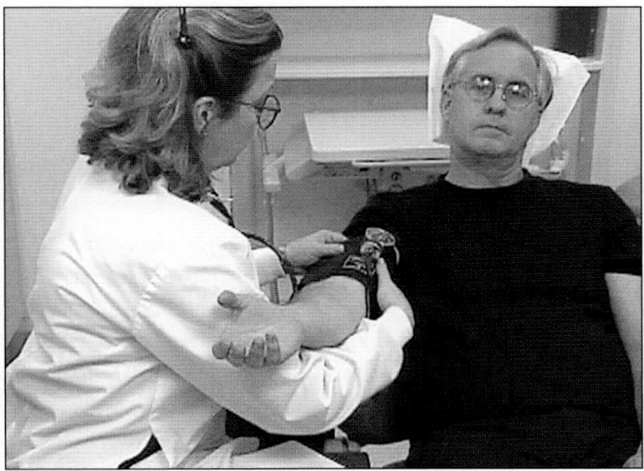

7. Tighten the cuff, using the Velcro closure to hold it in place.

Note: **Make sure that the cuff is tight enough that you can squeeze only a finger between the cuff and the arm.**

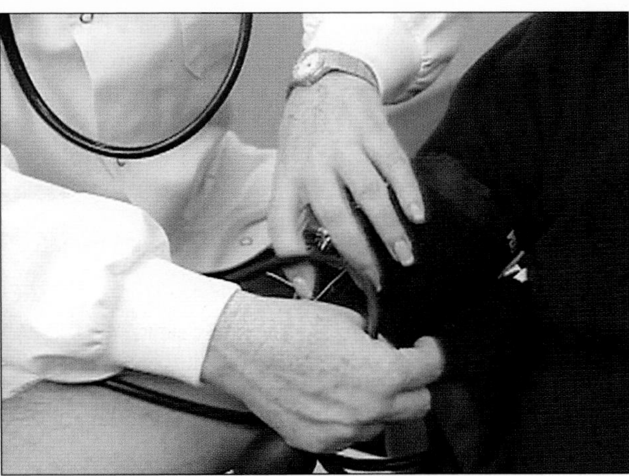

8. Place the earpieces of the stethoscope into your ears so that they are facing toward the front.
   Purpose: **This position of the earpieces is more comfortable and blocks out distracting noises while you are taking a blood pressure.**
9. Place the stethoscope disc over the site of the brachial artery, using slight pressure with the fingers.

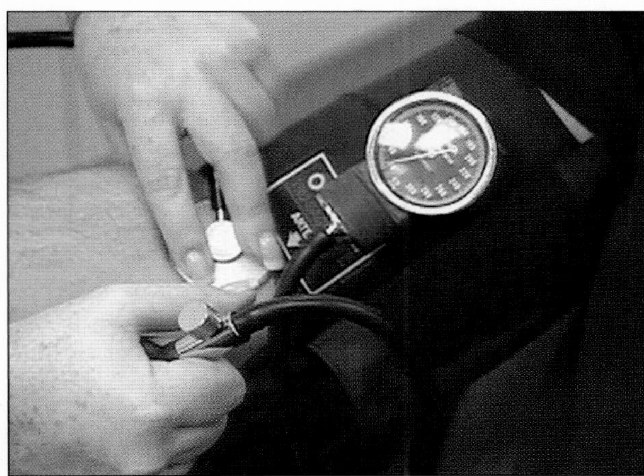

10. Grasp the rubber bulb with the other hand, locking the valve. Inflate the cuff to the noted reading.
    Note: **You need to inflate the bulb quickly.**
11. Slowly release the valve and listen through the stethoscope.
12. Note the first distinct thumping sound as the cuff deflates. This is the systolic pressure reading.

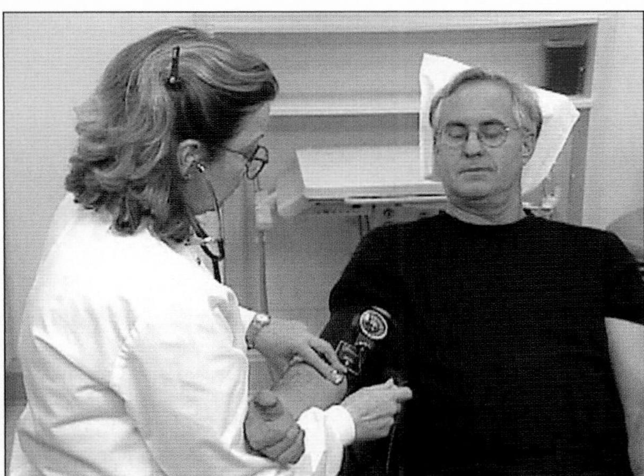

13. Slowly continue to release air from the cuff until you hear the last sound. This is the diastolic pressure reading.
14. Record the reading, indicating which arm was used.
15. Disinfect the stethoscope earpieces and diaphragm as recommended by the manufacturer. Return the setup to its proper place.

Date	Blood pressure 117/68 mm Hg R	Signature

Chapter Exercises

Multiple Choice

Circle the letter next to the correct answer.

1. When recording the blood pressure in the patient record, the first number you record is the __________ pressure.
   - a. diastolic
   - b. systolic
2. A normal respiration rate for a relaxed adult is __________ breaths per minute.
   - a. 10 to 20
   - b. 15 to 25
   - c. 20 to 26
   - d. 25 to 30
3. Financial information gathered on the registration form is primarily for __________.
   - a. collecting fees
   - b. filing insurance claims
   - c. making financial arrangements
   - d. a, b, and c
4. A medication history is a record of __________ that the patient is currently taking.
   - a. prescribed medications
   - b. the type of anesthetic the dentist uses
   - c. over-the-counter drugs
   - d. a and c
5. A patient's medical health history form should be completed or updated __________.
   - a. at each visit
   - b. at the recall visit
   - c. before initial treatment begins
   - d. b and c
6. The person who has agreed to pay the fees associated with the patient's dental care is known as the __________.
   - a. parent or guardian
   - b. patient
   - c. responsible party
   - d. spouse
7. The pulse is measured by placing the index and middle fingers on the __________ artery.
   - a. brachial
   - b. carotid
   - c. radial
   - d. all of the above
8. When blood pressure is obtained, the patient's arm (at the elbow) should be __________.
   - a. at the same level as his or her heart
   - b. higher than his or her heart
   - c. lower than his or her heart
   - d. a or c
9. The patient record includes the __________.
   - a. clinical examination form
   - b. medical-dental health history form
   - c. progress notes
   - d. a, b, and c
10. The patient's signature on the medical health history questionnaire indicates that he or she __________.
    - a. gives permission for the use of this information
    - b. is responsible for payment of the account
    - c. personally completed the form
    - d. takes responsibility for the accuracy of the information

Apply Your Knowledge

1. A new patient has completed her medical-dental health history form and has handed it to the administrative assistant. When you review this material, you notice that several questions are unanswered. How should you handle this matter?
2. A patient is coming in tomorrow to have his remaining teeth extracted for the purpose of a full denture. Discuss what "paperwork" you will need to complete with the patient before beginning the procedure.
3. You have recorded a patient's vital signs in her record and notice that her blood pressure today is 148/70 mm Hg. At the patient's last visit, it was 122/60. Is there anything to be concerned about? If so, what steps should be taken?

CHAPTER 12

The Dental Examination

http://evolve.elsevier.com/Robinson/essentials/

LEARNING OBJECTIVES

1. Pronounce, define, and spell the key terms.
2. List and describe the components of a dental examination, including the variety of examination techniques used in dentistry.
3. Describe what is included in and demonstrate the procedure for a soft tissue examination.
4. List and describe the two types of tooth diagrams.
5. Describe Black classification of cavities.
6. Identify charting symbols as related to dental needs and treatment.
7. Identify charting abbreviations used in dentistry and demonstrate the proper procedure for the charting of teeth.
8. Describe the importance of a treatment plan, as well as the various types.
9. Discuss how to record dental treatment and demonstrate the procedure to record the completed dental treatment.

KEY TERMS

cavity classifications
diagnosis
treatment plan

A thorough dental examination is necessary for the dentist to make a **diagnosis** (identification of disease) and to recommend to proceed with a **treatment plan** for the patient. A dental examination consists of many components of the oral cavity, which includes soft tissue, periodontal tissue and teeth, the facial structures and neck. Your role in this data-gathering process is very important. The assistant will prepare the setup, assist in the collection of information, and record the information in the patient's record as dictated by the operator.

Components of the Dental Examination

The dental examination begins after the patient has completed the medical and dental history form, and vital signs have been obtained and recorded by the dental assistant. Your role in assembling what is necessary for the dentist to diagnose a patient's dental status consists of gathering all completed forms that are necessary and then charting or recording the dentist's findings during the examination. The complete dental team (dentist, dental hygienist, and dental assistant) is responsible for gathering specific components of this information:

- Soft tissue examination
- Examination of the teeth
- Examination of the periodontal tissue
- Radiographs
- Impressions to create a diagnostic cast or model
- Photographs

Examination Techniques

The dentist will use a variety of techniques to accomplish a thorough examination. A review of examination techniques is provided in Table 12-1.

Recording the Dental Examination

Dental recording, also referred to as *charting,* can be described as "shorthand" for the dentist. The dentist will dictate his or her findings, and the assistant will record these findings on the patient's clinical examination form or in the patient's electronic chart. Symbols, abbreviations, and color-coding are all used to indicate various conditions. To chart the information dictated by the dentist accurately and quickly, it is imperative that you learn the dentist's preferred system.

Elements That Make Up a Charting System

- Tooth diagrams, numbering systems, and color coding
- Cavity classifications
- Charting symbols
- Abbreviations of tooth surfaces
- Abbreviations of treatments

TABLE 12-1
Examination Techniques

Technique	Description
Visual evaluation 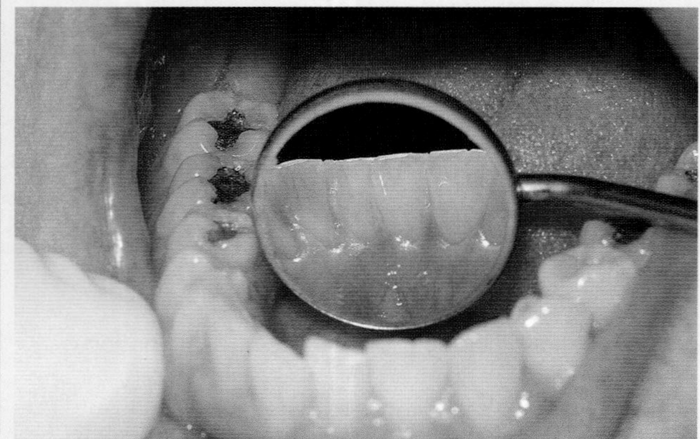	With the use of a mouth mirror, the dentist examines areas of the mouth and face that cannot be directly seen.
Palpation 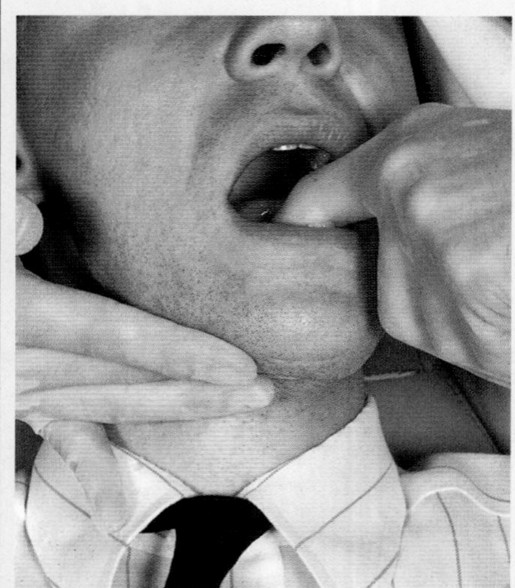	The examiner's hands are used to examine texture, size, and consistency of hard and soft tissue around the mouth and facial areas.
Instrumentation 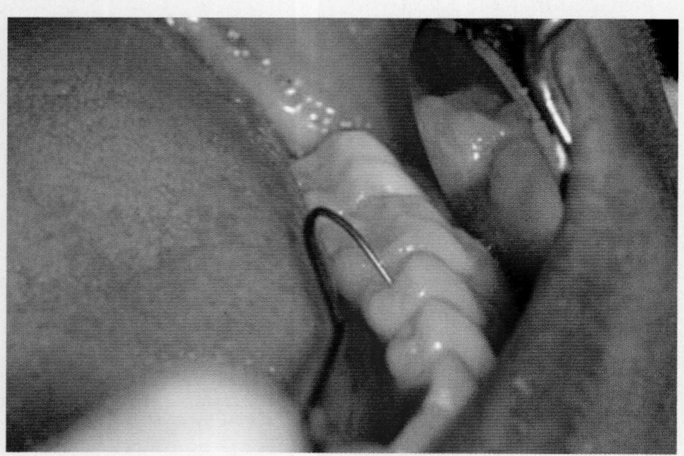	The examiner uses an instrument to examine hard tissue, such as teeth.

TABLE 12-1
Examination Techniques—cont'd

Technique	Description
Radiography 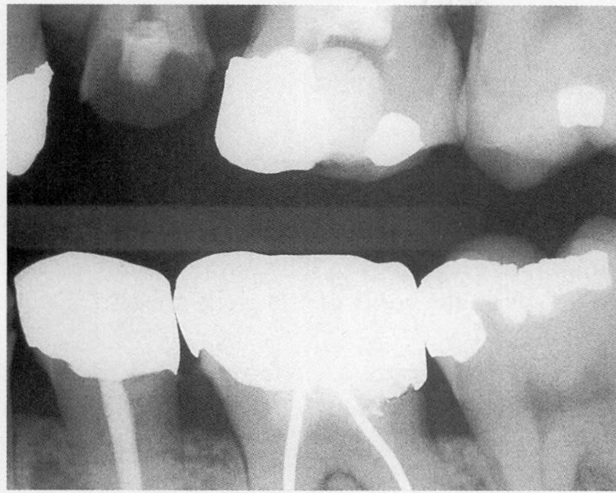	Radiographs provide a visual evaluation of areas that cannot be directly seen.
Intraoral imaging 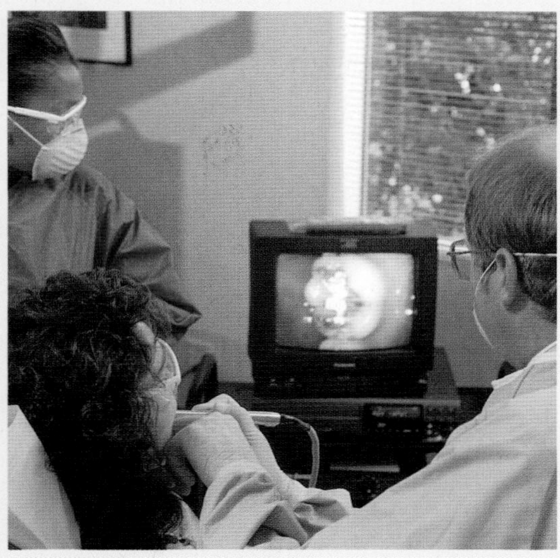	A miniature video camera projects an image on a screen. The magnification allows the dentist to better evaluate a specific tooth or area of the mouth, which makes it easier for the patient to understand what the dentist is discussing.
Photography 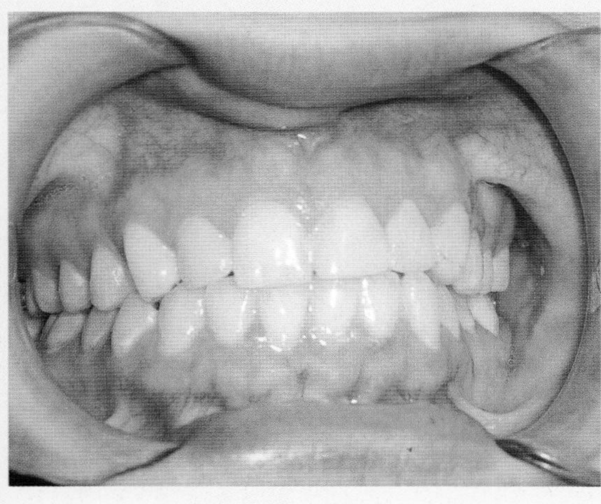	Photographs are an excellent tool for identification, treatment planning, case presentations, and patient education.

Oral Examination

A thorough oral examination includes more than simply checking the teeth. It includes a careful examination of the neck, face, and lips and all soft tissue within the mouth.

Soft Tissue Examination

The soft tissue examination involves a complete examination of the cheeks, mucosa, lips, palate, tonsil area, tongue, and floor of the mouth. This examination requires the use of visual examination and palpation. The purpose of this part of the examination is to detect any abnormalities in the head and neck area of a patient. See Procedure 12-1: Soft Tissue Examination (Expanded Function).

Examination of the Periodontal Tissue

It is recommended that a periodontal examination be a part of every adult patient's dental examination. It is common practice for the dental hygienist to perform the periodontal examination for a patient at a patient's scheduled recall appointment. After completing this appointment, the dental hygienist and dentist will confer to determine whether the patient should require a more thorough periodontal appointment. (For further discussion on the periodontal examination, see Chapter 24.)

Examination of the Teeth

A clinical examination of the teeth includes a thorough examination of each tooth. With the use of hand instruments, the dentist examines the surface of each tooth. The dentist dictates the findings to the dental assistant, who records them on the clinical examination form of the patient's record. Regardless of whether findings are manually recorded or entered in the patient's electronic record, it is essential that all entries are correctly entered and confirmed by the dentist.

Tooth Diagrams, Numbering Systems, and Color Coding

Tooth diagrams for recording dental conditions are available with a variety of diagram styles; with, the most commonly used diagrams being the anatomic and geographic designs.

In the **anatomic diagram**, the illustration resembles actual teeth. In some styles, the roots of the teeth are also included (Figure 12-1).

In the **geometric diagram**, a circle represents each tooth. The circle is divided to represent each tooth surface (Figure 12-2).

Tooth Numbering

To ensure greater accuracy, the teeth on the diagram are numbered in the appropriate sequence. The dentist selects the numbering system. (Numbering systems are discussed in Chapter 4.)

Tooth Arrangement

On the charting diagram, the teeth are arranged as if one is looking into the patient's mouth. Thus the right quadrants are

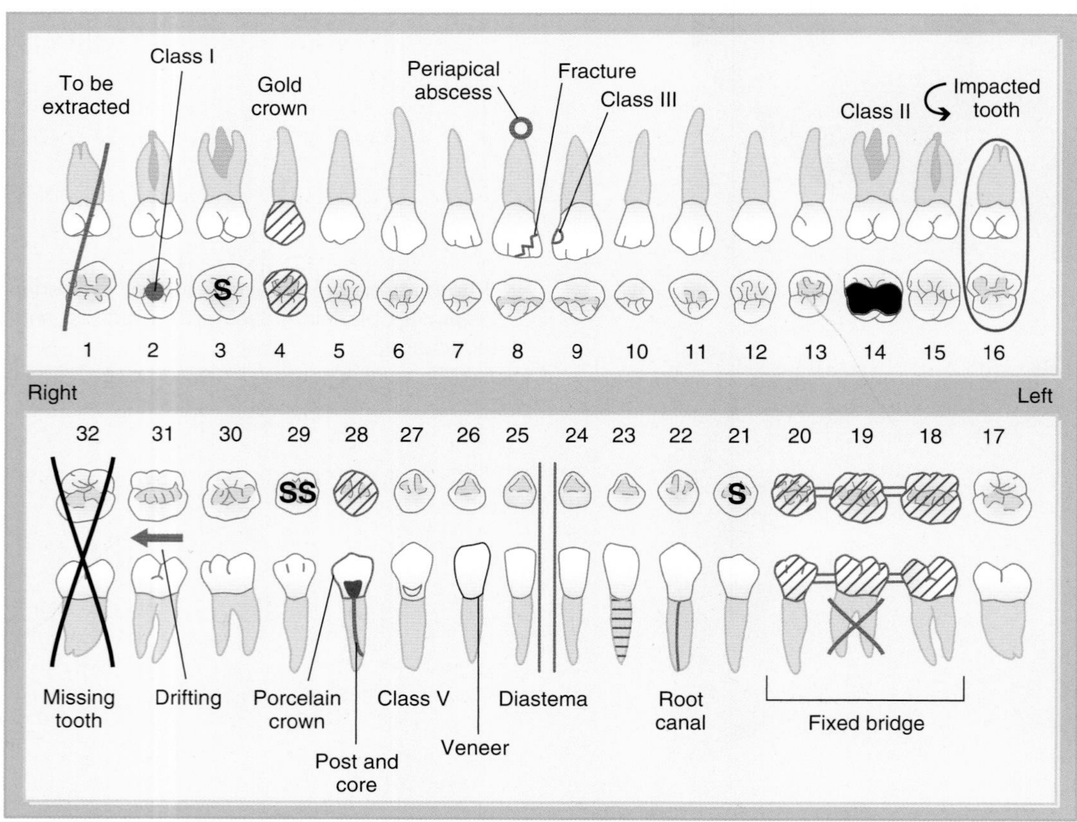

FIGURE 12-1 Anatomic diagram. *S,* Sealant; *SS,* stainless steel crown.

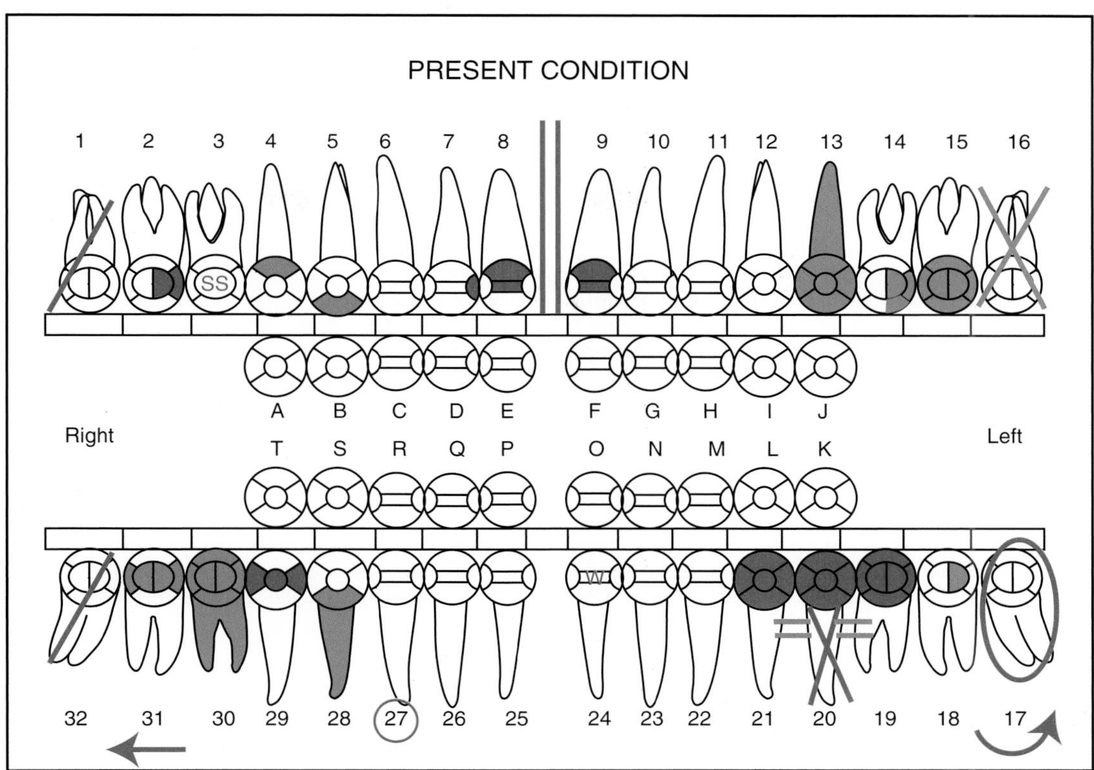

FIGURE 12-2 Geometric diagram. (From Gaylor LJ: The *administrative dental assistant*, ed 3, St. Louis, 2012, Saunders.)

on the left side of the page and the left quadrants are on the right side of the page.

Color Coding

Different colors are used to chart on the diagram to provide visual information about each entry. **Blue** or **black** represents dental treatment that has been completed. **Red** indicates dental needs detected and to be completed at future dental appointments.

Cavity Classifications

To better understand the types of restorations placed in teeth throughout the mouth, a standard cavity classification system was designed to describe the types and locations of decay requiring a restoration. G.V. Black (father of modern dentistry) developed the most commonly used system in the 1900s. Black's original classification included Classes I through V. Class VI was added later. Cavity classifications are described in Figure 12-3.

Charting Symbols

A wide variety of symbols and abbreviations are used in dentistry. Unlike the Universal Tooth Designation System and the Black cavity classifications, which are standardized, there are many ways of using symbols and color in charting. Each dentist has his or her individual preferences, and learning the dentist's preferred system is important.

The symbols shown in Table 12-2 commonly represent these conditions and materials either when charting by hand or when using a dental software program.

Charting Abbreviations

Treatment Abbreviations

When in doubt about the meaning or the use of an abbreviation, it is better to spell out the term or record what has taken place without using abbreviations. Abbreviations can be used to indicate the single surface or a combination of tooth surfaces.

Single surface abbreviations These and the other charting abbreviations involve the names of the tooth surfaces, such as **O** for occlusal (see Chapter 4 for names of all surfaces).

Combination of surfaces When two tooth surfaces are involved, such as distal and occlusal, the combined surfaces are referred to as **DO** for distal-occlusal. If three surfaces are combined, the same rule applies (e.g., **MOD** for mesial-occlusal-distal).

When referring to these combined surfaces, the letters are separately pronounced, for example, a **D-O cavity** or an **M-O-D restoration.**

See Procedure 12-2: Charting of Teeth.

Treatment Plan

Once the information has been gathered, recorded, and reviewed, the dentist will conclude with a diagnosis of the patient's dental conditions.

A written treatment plan is presented and described to the patient by the dentist, according to the patient's needs, priorities, and financial resources. If the patient agrees and accepts the plan, then the patient is required to provide a signature and date, verifying his or her understanding of the process.

Classification	Location and Description
Class I	Decay is diagnosed in the pits and fissures of the occlusal surfaces of molars and premolars, buccal or lingual pits of molars, and lingual pits of maxillary incisors. Because most of this type of decay is confined to a small area, the dentist will choose to restore these surfaces with composite (tooth-colored) resins. 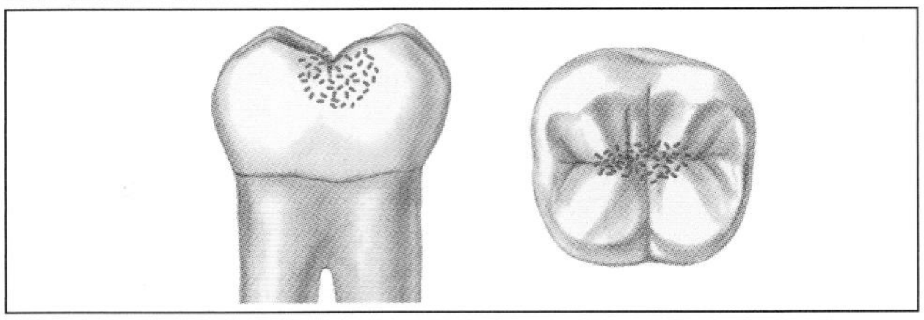
Class II	Decay is diagnosed in the proximal (mesial or distal) surfaces of premolars and molars. Because this surface area is harder to detect visually, a radiograph is used to detect the decay. The design of the restoration will most commonly include the occlusal surface and may possibly involve more than two surfaces. The type of dental material used to restore this classificationis either silver amalgam (chosen for its strength) or newer composite (tooth-colored) resins designed for posterior teeth (chosen for esthetic appeal). If the tooth has extensive decay, the dentist may choose to crown the tooth with a gold or porcelain inlay, onlay, or crown. 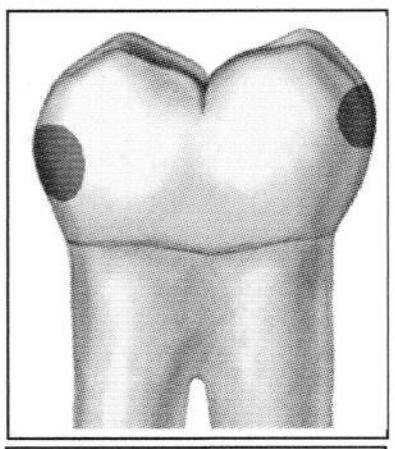
Class III	Decay is diagnosed in the proximal (mesial or distal) surfaces of incisors and canines. This decay is similar to that of Class II, except it involves anterior teeth. It is easier for the dentist to access these surfaces with less tooth structure affected. The type of dental material used to restore this classification is composite (tooth-colored) resins (for esthetic appearance). 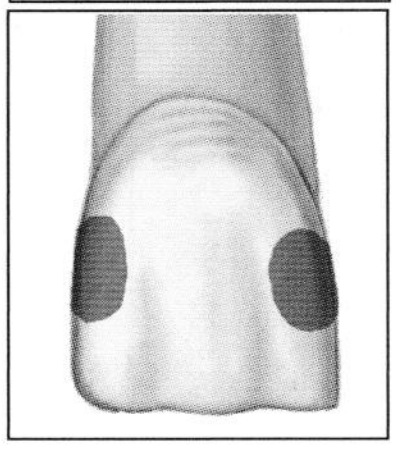
Class IV	Decay is diagnosed in the proximal (mesial or distal) surfaces of incisors and canines. The difference between Class IV and Class III decay is that Class IV involves the incisal edge or angle of the tooth. The type of dental material used to restore this classification is composite (tooth-colored) resins (for esthetic appearance). If the tooth has extensive decay, the dentist may choose to crown the tooth with a porcelain crown. 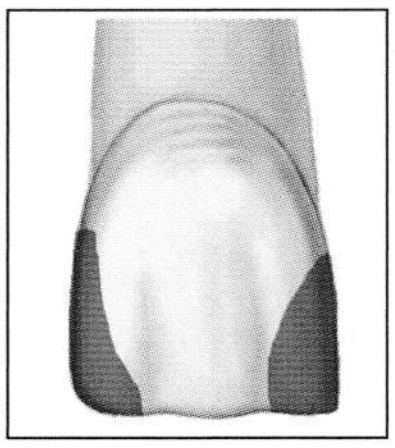
Class V	Decay is diagnosed in the gingival third of facial or lingual surfaces of any tooth.This is also referred to as a *smooth surface decay.* The type of dental material used to restore this classification depends on which teeth are affected. If the de-cay occurs in posterior teeth, the dentist may choose silver amalgam; if anterior teeth are involved, composite (tooth-colored) resin will most likely be used. 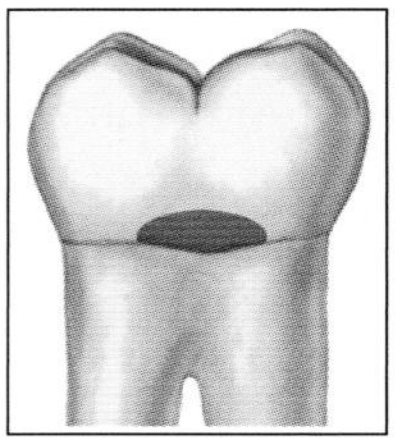 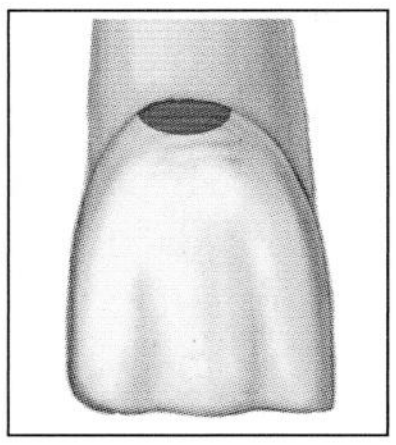
Class VI	Decay is diagnosed on the incisal edge of anterior teeth and the cusp tips of posterior teeth. Class VI decay is caused by abrasion (wear) and defects. The dental material is chosen based on which teeth are involved. 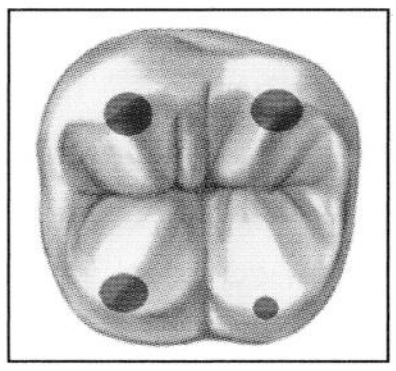

FIGURE 12-3 Black classification of cavities.

Types of Treatment Plans

Optional treatment plans can be presented to the patient for consideration. These plans can represent the following levels of care:

- **Level I—Emergency Care:** Relieves immediate discomfort, and provides relief to the patient.
- **Level II—Standard Care:** Relieves immediate discomfort and restores the teeth to normal function, which can include permanent restorations, root canal therapy, periodontal therapy, or fixed and removable prosthetics.
- **Level III—Optimum Care:** Relieves immediate discomfort, and restores the teeth and surrounding tissue to maximum function and esthetic acceptability. This treatment level can include cosmetic dentistry, orthodontics, periodontics, implants, and reconstructive surgery.

Text continued on p. 170

TABLE 12-2
Commonly Used Charting Symbols

Conditions	Explanation	Charting Symbol	Procedure
Missing Tooth	Tooth or teeth that are not present or congenitally missing	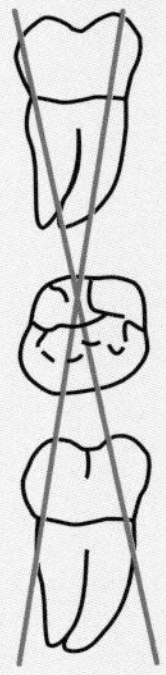	Draw a black/blue "X" through the tooth. It does not matter whether the tooth was extracted or is congenitally missing. If a quadrant, or arch, is edentulous, make one "X" over all teeth missing.
Impacted or Unerupted Tooth	Tooth or teeth that have not erupted and are not exposed in the mouth	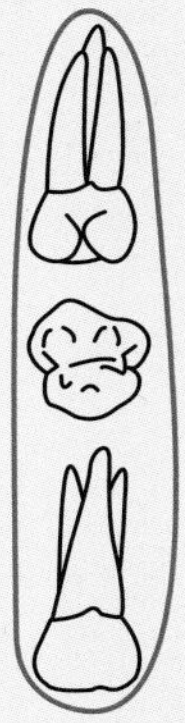	Draw a red circle around the whole tooth, including the root.
Tooth to Be Extracted	Tooth that has been diagnosed to be removed.	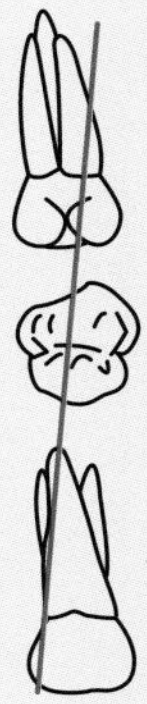	Draw a red diagonal line through the tooth. An alternative method is to draw two red parallel lines through the tooth.
Caries/Restore Class I	Decay affecting the pits and fissure of the occlusal surface	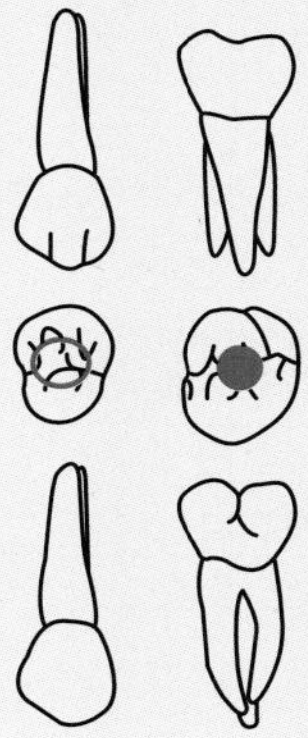	Outline the area involved if using composite and, if using amalgam, color in the area to complete in red and black/blue for the area already restored.

Continued

TABLE 12-2
Commonly Used Charting Symbols—cont'd

Conditions	Explanation	Charting Symbol	Procedure
Caries/Restore Class II	Decay affecting the occlusal and interproximal surfaces of posterior teeth	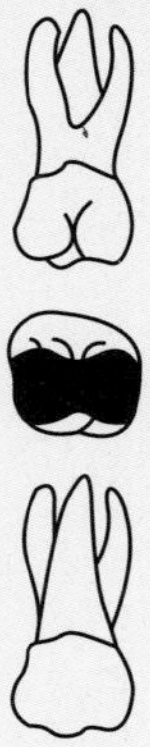	Outline the area involved if using composite and, if using amalgam, color in the area in red to complete and black/blue for the area already restored.
Caries/Restore Class III	Decay affecting the occlusal and interproximal surfaces of anterior teeth	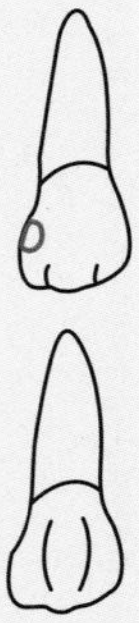	Outline the area to indicate composite in red to complete and black/blue for the area already restored.
Caries/Restore Class IV	Decay affecting the interproximal and incisal surface of an anterior tooth	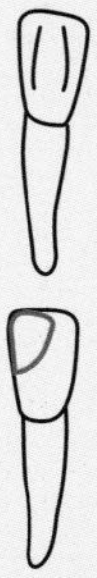	Outline the area to indicate composite in red to complete and black/blue for the area already restored.
Caries/Restore Class V	Decay affecting the gingival third of a tooth	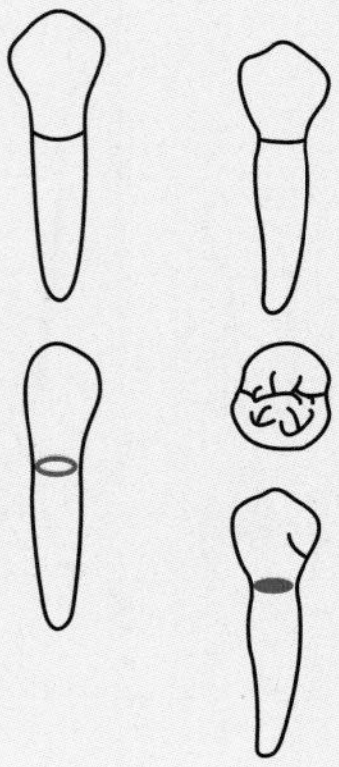	Outline the area involved if using composite and, if using amalgam, color in the area in red to complete and black/blue for the area already restored.

TABLE 12-2
Commonly Used Charting Symbols—cont'd

Conditions	Explanation	Charting Symbol	Procedure
Recurrent Decay	Decay is diagnosed from radiograph or from the margin of an existing restoration	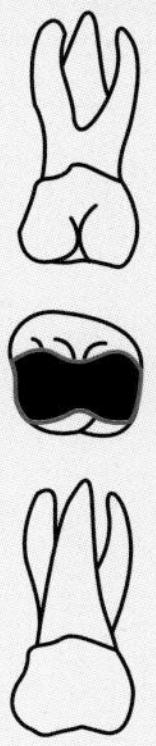	Outline the existing restoration in red to indicate decay in the area.
Sealant	Resin material placed in the pits and fissures of occlusal surface as a preventive means	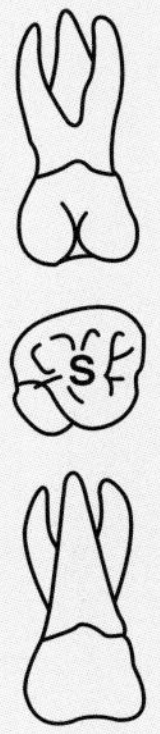	Place an "S" on the occlusal surface in red to complete and black/blue for already restored.
Periapical Abscess	Infection is within the pulp of a tooth.	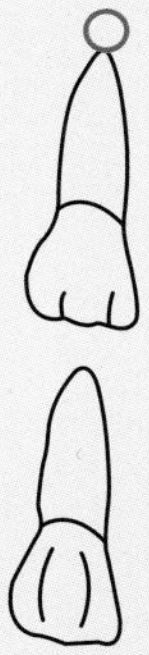	Draw a red circle at the apex of the root to indicate infection.
Root Canal	Disease has affected the pulp of the tooth and requires pulp therapy.	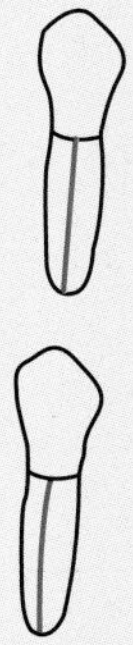	Draw a line through the center of each root involved in red to be completed and black/blue for already restored.
Veneer	Thin shell-like covering made from porcelain or composite to cover the facial aspect of a tooth surface	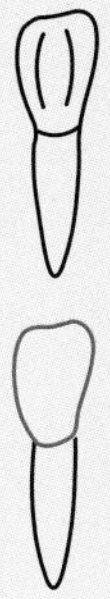	Outline the facial portion only in red to be completed and black/ blue for already restored.

Continued

TABLE 12-2
Commonly Used Charting Symbols—cont'd

Conditions	Explanation	Charting Symbol	Procedure
Inlay	Cast restoration made from either porcelain or gold for a conservative Class II restoration	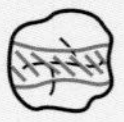	Outline the shape of the restoration in red or black/blue if using porcelain and place diagonal lines if using gold.
Onlay	Cast restoration made from either porcelain or gold for more coverage of the occlusal surface	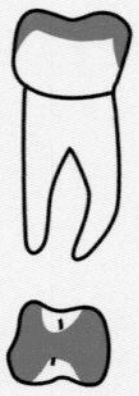	Outline the shape of the restoration in red or black/blue if using porcelain and place diagonal lines if using gold.
Porcelain Fused to Metal (PFM) Crown	Full crown of a single tooth using two types of materials, porcelain for esthetics and metal for strength	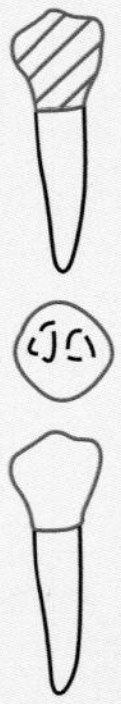	Outline the coronal portion of the tooth and add diagonal lines to indicate gold on the facial surface, in red to be completed and black/blue for already restored.
Gold Crown	Full crown of a single tooth using gold	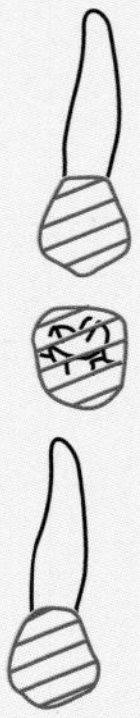	Outline the crown of the tooth and place diagonal lines in red to be completed and black/blue for already restored.
Stainless Steel Crown	Full metal crown used for primary molars	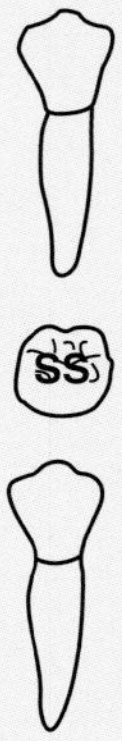 SS	Outline the crown of the tooth and place "SS" on the occlusal surface in red to be completed and black/blue for already restored.

TABLE 12-2
Commonly Used Charting Symbols—cont'd

Conditions	Explanation	Charting Symbol	Procedure
Post and Pore	Used for additional strength in an endodontically treated tooth	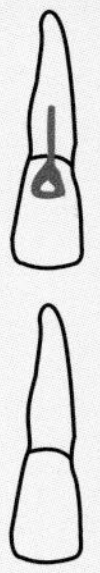	Draw a line through the root requiring the post; then continue the line into the gingival one third of the crown, making a triangle shape in red to be completed and black/blue for already restored.
Fixed Bridge	Cast unit to restore an area where one or more teeth are missing	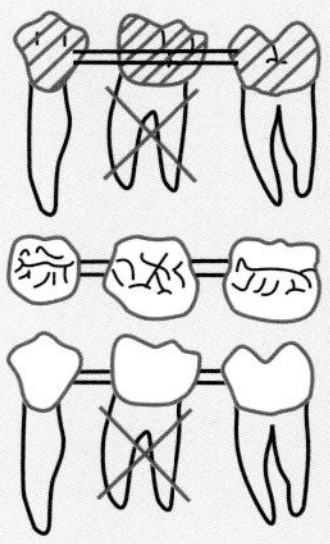	Draw an "X" through the root(s) of the missing tooth or teeth involved. Then draw a line to connect all teeth that make up the bridge. The type of material used to make the bridge will determine whether you outline the crowns for porcelain, use diagonal lines for gold, or use a combination of the two in red to be completed and black/blue for already restored.
Implant	Complete replacement of a tooth and root	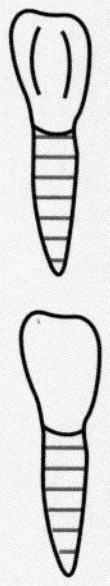	Draw horizontal lines through the root or roots of a tooth in red to be completed and black/blue for already placed.
Rotated Tooth	Tooth that has rotated from its normal position	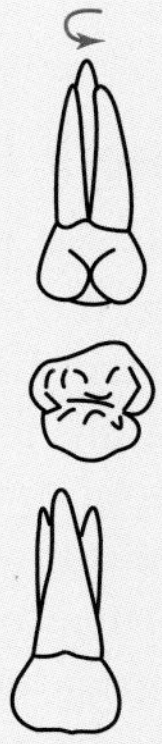	Indicate the direction the tooth has turned by placing a red arrow above the tooth
Drifting	Tooth or teeth that have shifted from their normal position	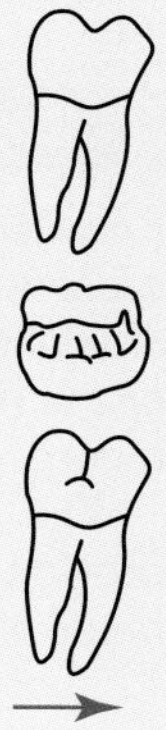	Place a red arrow that points to the direction in which a tooth is drifting.

Continued

TABLE 12-2
Commonly Used Charting Symbols—cont'd

Conditions	Explanation	Charting Symbol	Procedure
Diastema	Additional space existing between two teeth with no contact		Draw two red vertical lines between the teeth.
Fractured Tooth or Root	Surface of a tooth that has fractured due to trauma or extensive caries		If a tooth or a root is fractured, draw a red zigzag line where the fracture occurred.
Denture	Removal prosthetic to replace a full arch	CLD PUD PUD	Draw a complete line below the roots of the teeth connecting the teeth in red if denture is to be fabricated, or in blue/black if already fabricated.

From Bird DL, Robinson DS: *Modern dental assisting,* ed 11, St. Louis, 2015, Saunders.

Recording Dental Treatment

At the completion of every procedure, a specific sequence regarding treatment is followed when recording what was provided for the patient at the visit. This information is located in the patient's clinical record under "Treatment Provided." The chart entry should be clear and concise and should be entered in black ink.

Treatment Information to be Included in a Patient's Record

- Medical history update, including vital signs
- The tooth treated and the surfaces involved
- Anesthetic used
- Types of moisture control
- Types of dental materials used
- How well the patient tolerated the procedure
- Type of treatment to schedule patient's next appointment. Date and signature of dentist

See Procedure 12-3: Recording the Completed Dental Treatment.

About Fees

In most practices, a *super bill* is provided to the patient at the completion of a visit. This form is part of the bookkeeping system but is not part of the patient record. The information on this form is used to itemize what was completed during the appointment, providing the procedure(s), tooth number(s), and surfaces, as well as the fee charged for each procedure. This form also has an area to schedule the patient for his or her next appointment and the length of time required. The super bill can also be used to generate an insurance claim, if necessary.

Ethical Implications

Knowledge and skill in recording a patient's past and present dental conditions are very important. Charting is a critical skill for all dental assistants. If the dentist's dictation or the recording is not correctly documented in the patient record, then legally it is *not completed*.

The dentist must always review the patient record and provide his or her signature for verification on any entry made in a patient record.

Procedure 12-1

Soft Tissue Examination (Expanded Function)

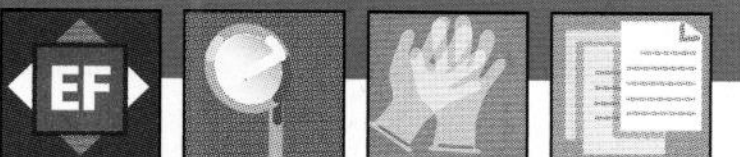

This procedure is legal for certified dental assistants to complete in many states.

Equipment and Supplies

- Gauze sponges (2 × 2 and 4 × 4)
- Tongue depressor (optional)
- Mouth mirror
- Patient record to document findings

Procedural Steps

Patient Preparation

1. When escorting the patient to the treatment area, observe the patient's general appearance, speech, and behavior.

Purpose: Unusual behavior or appearance must be immediately noted or called to the dentist's attention.

2. Seat the patient in the dental chair in an upright position. Drape the patient with a patient napkin.
3. Explain the procedure to the patient.

Purpose: The patient who knows what to expect will be more comfortable and more willing to participate in the examination.

Extraoral Features

1. Examine the face, neck, and ears for asymmetry and/or abnormal swelling.

Purpose: The two sides of the face should be symmetric.

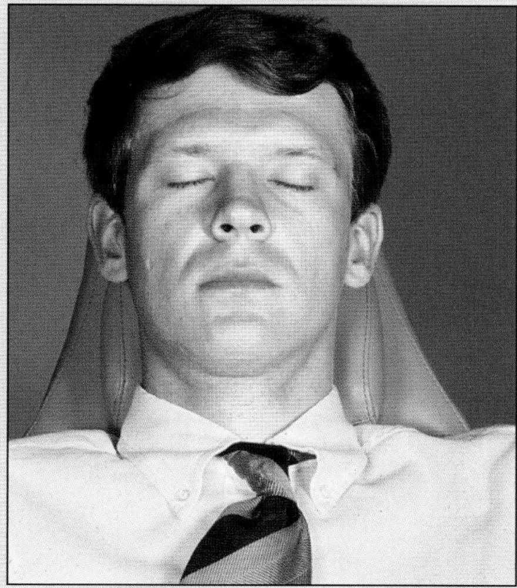

2. Look for abnormal tissue changes, skin abrasions, and discoloration.

Purpose: Unusual bruising, scratches, or cuts may require further evaluation of the area.

3. Evaluate the texture, color, and continuity of the vermilion border, the commissures of the lips, the philtrum, and the smile line.

Purpose: Lumps, dryness, and cracking of the tissue are deviations from normal and may indicate the need for further evaluation of the area.

4. Document all findings in the patient record.

Cervical Lymph Nodes

1. Position yourself behind the patient so that you can easily place your fingers just below the patient's ears.
2. To examine the right side of the neck, use your left hand to steady the patient's head. Using your fingers and thumb of your right hand, gently follow the chain of lymph nodes downward, starting in front of the right ear and continuing to the clavicle (collarbone).

Purpose: You are looking for swelling, abnormal formation, and tenderness of the area.

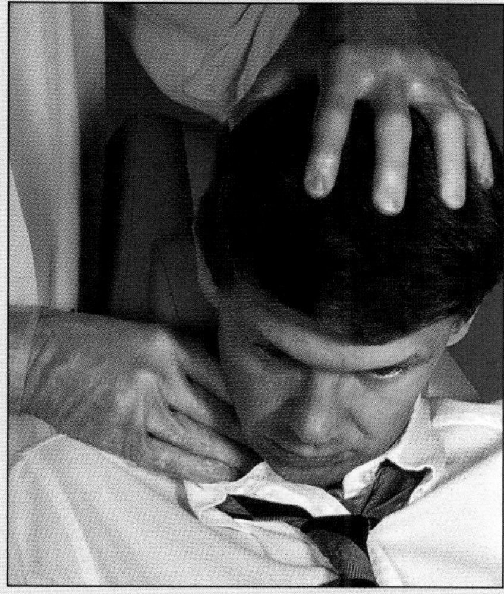

3. To examine the left side of the neck, use your right hand to steady the patient's head. Using your fingers and thumb of your left hand, gently follow the chain of lymph nodes downward, starting in front of the left ear and continuing to the clavicle (collarbone).
4. Document all findings in the patient record.

Continued

Procedure 12-1

Soft Tissue Examination (Expanded Function)—cont'd

Temporomandibular Joint

1. To evaluate the temporomandibular joint (TMJ) movements in centric, lateral, protrusive, and retrusive movements, ask the patient to open and close the mouth normally and then to move the jaw from side to side.
2. To further evaluate the movement of the TMJ, gently place your fingers just in front of the external opening of the ear. Ask the patient to open and close the mouth normally.

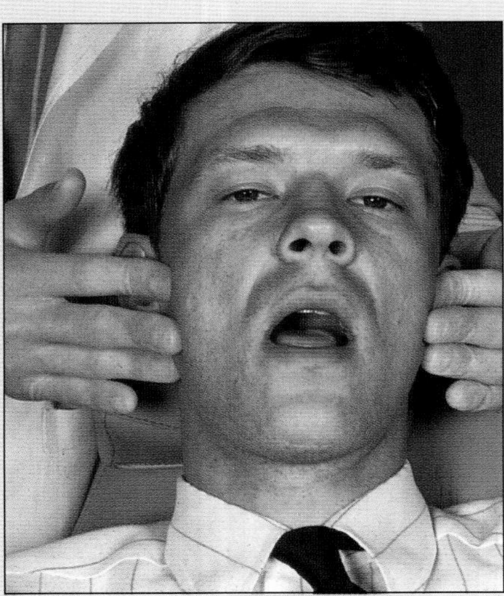

3. To determine whether there is noise in the TMJ during movement, listen as the patient opens and closes the mouth. A stethoscope placed on the joint may be used.
4. Note in the patient record any abnormalities or patient comments on pain, tenderness, or other problems related to opening and closing of the mouth.

Indications of Oral Habits

1. Look for indications of oral habits, such as thumb sucking, tongue-thrust swallow, mouth breathing, and tobacco use.

Purpose: These habits can affect the patient's oral health.

2. Look for signs of other oral habits, such as bruxism, grinding, and clenching. Indications include abnormal wear on the teeth and problems in the TMJ.

Interior of the Lips

1. Ask the patient to open his or her mouth slightly.
2. Examine the mucosa and labial frenum of the upper lip by gentle retraction of the lip with your thumbs and index fingers.
3. Examine the mucosa and labial frenum of the lower lip by gentle retraction of the lip with your thumbs and index fingers.
4. Gently palpate the tissue to detect lumps or similar abnormalities.

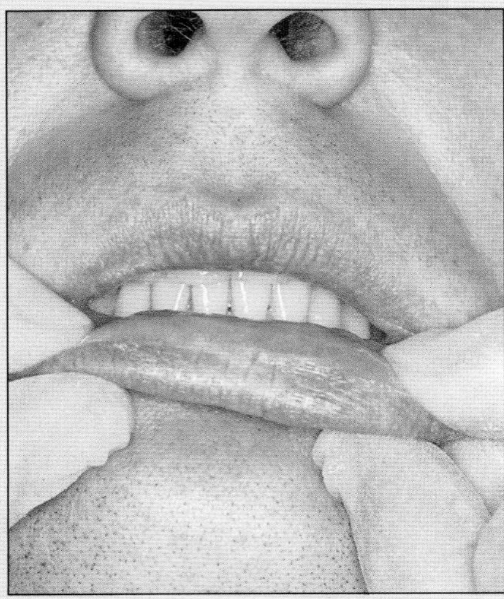

Oral Mucosa and Tongue

1. Gently palpate the tissue of the buccal mucosa by placing the thumb of one hand inside the patient's mouth and the index and third fingers of your other hand on the exterior of the cheek.

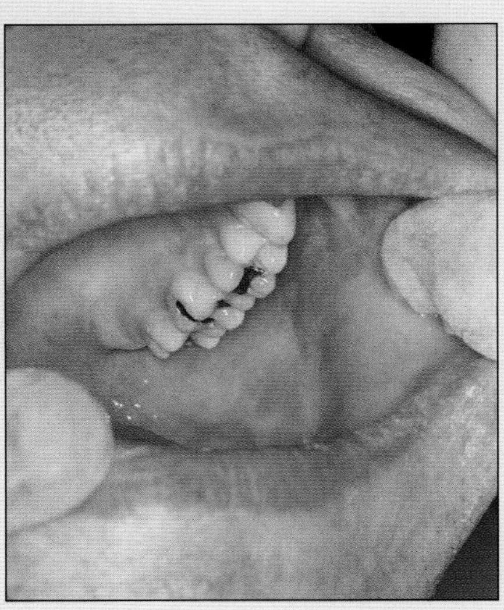

Procedure 12-1

Soft Tissue Examination (Expanded Function)—cont'd

2. Examine the tissue covering the hard palate.

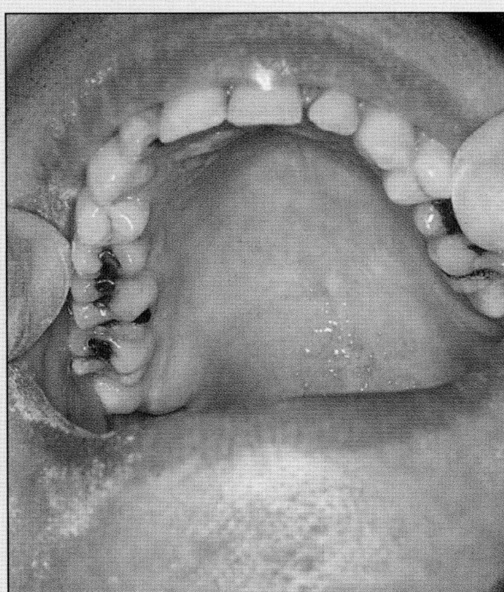

3. Visually examine the buccal mucosa and the opening of the Stensen duct. A warm mouth mirror may be used to view the flow of saliva from the duct.

Purpose: The mouth mirror is warmed to prevent fogging.

4. Ask the patient to extend his or her tongue and then to relax it. Using sterile gauze, gently grasp the tip of the tongue and pull it forward.
5. Observe the dorsum (top) of the tongue for color, papillae, presence or lack of a coating, and abnormalities.
6. Gently move the tongue from side to side to examine the lateral (side) and ventral (underneath) surfaces.

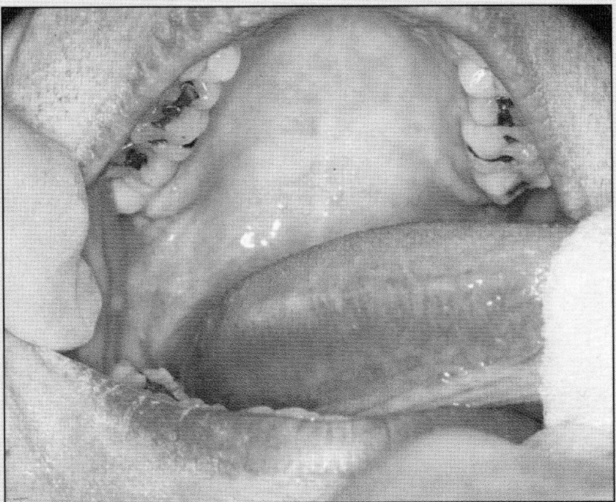

7. Use a warm mouth mirror to observe the posterior area.

Caution: **To avoid triggering the gag reflex, this mirror is very carefully placed and is moved very little.**

8. Examine the uvula, base of the tongue, and posterior area of the mouth by placing a mouth mirror or tongue depressor firmly at the base of the tongue.

Caution: Firm but gentle placement reduces the possibility of triggering the gag reflex.

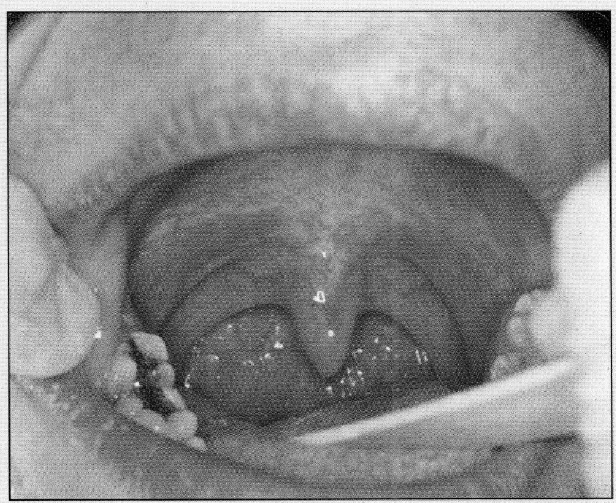

9. With the mouth mirror firmly depressing the base of the tongue, ask the patient to say "ahh."

Purpose: The oropharynx expands, allowing a better view of the upper portion of the throat.

Floor of the Mouth

1. With the patient's teeth closed, palpate the soft tissue of the face above and below the mandible.

Purpose: Tori and other abnormalities can be detected.

2. Gently palpate the interior of the floor of the mouth by placing the index finger of one hand on the floor of the mouth and placing the fingers of the other hand on the outer surface under the chin.

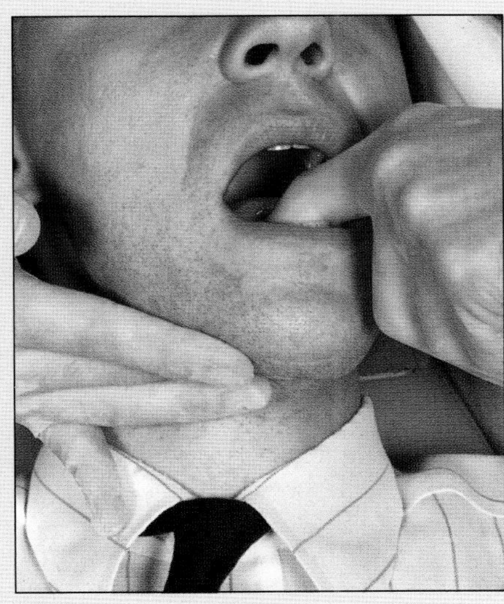

Continued

Procedure 12-1

Soft Tissue Examination (Expanded Function)—cont'd

3. Instruct the patient to touch the tongue to the hard palate.

Purpose: The floor of the mouth, lingual frenum, and salivary ducts can be visually examined.

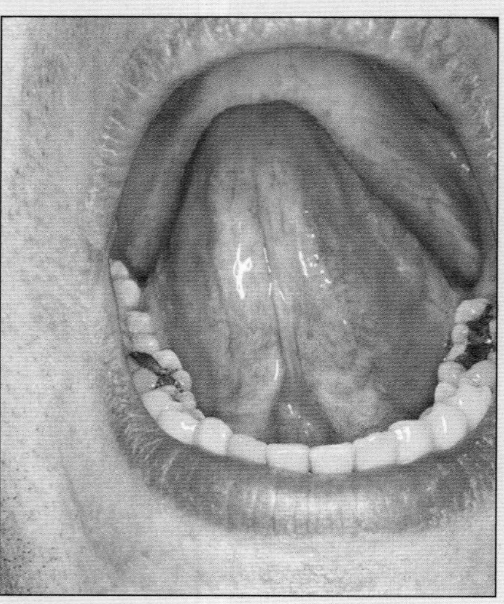

4. Observe the quantity and consistency of the flow of saliva. Depending on the patient's general health, diet, and medications, the saliva may vary in consistency from watery to thick and ropy.
5. Accurately document all information in the patient record.

Date	Extraoral examination: no changes, schedule for a 6-month examination.	Signature

Procedure 12-2

Charting of Teeth

Equipment and Supplies

- Mouth mirror
- Explorer
- Cotton pliers
- Periodontal probe
- Gauze sponges (2 × 2)
- Dental floss
- Articulating paper
- Articulating paper holder
- Air-water syringe
- Pencil or pen (red and black)
- Clinical examination form

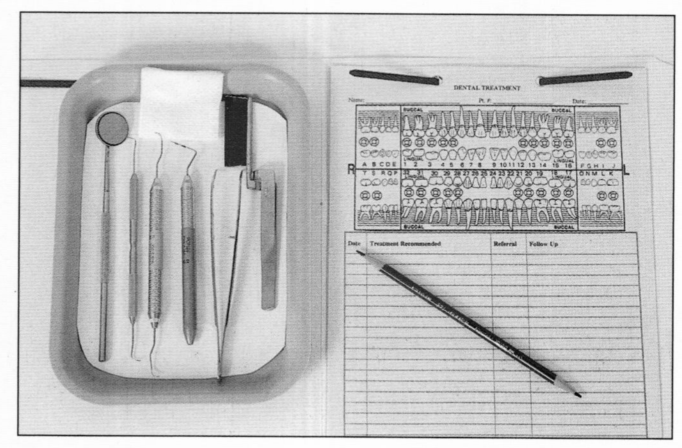

Procedural Steps

Patient Preparation

1. The patient is seated and draped with a patient napkin.
2. The patient is placed in a supine position.

Purpose: The dentist has better intraoral vision and instrumentation with the patient in a supine position.

Examination of the Teeth and Occlusion

1. Ensure that colored pencils or pens, the clinical examination form, and a flat surface are readily available.

Purpose: The more organized you are, the fewer errors and stops will be made.

2. Throughout the procedure, use the air syringe to clear the mouth mirror, and adjust the operating light as necessary.

Purpose: Better visualization is provided for the dentist as the teeth are examined.

3. Transfer the mirror and the explorer to the dentist. The dentist will begin with tooth #1 and will continue to #32. The dentist will examine every surface of each tooth.
4. Record the specific notations as the dentist calls them out.
5. The dentist will examine the patient's occlusion (bite). Place the articulating paper within the holder and transfer the instrument with the paper correctly positioned for that side of the mouth.

Procedure 12-2

Charting of Teeth—cont'd

Note: The holder is positioned closest to the cheek with the paper between the teeth.

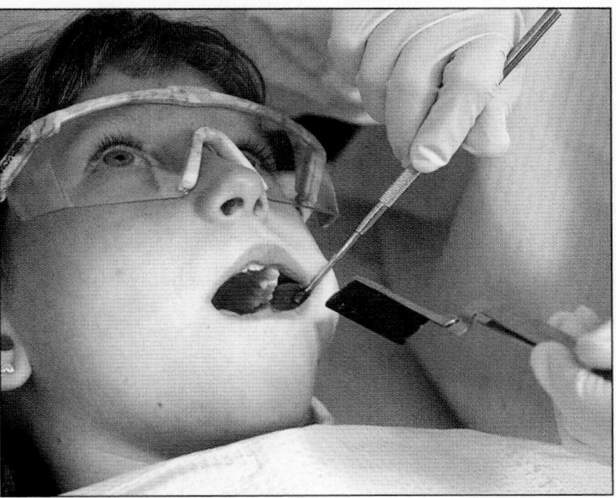

6. Any marks made by the paper will remain on the patient's occlusal and incisal surfaces.

Purpose: The dentist will look for any abnormal markings to indicate improper occlusion.

7. At the completion of the procedure, rinse and dry the patient's mouth.
8. Accurately document all information in the patient record and sign.

Date	Intraoral examination. Patient has MO decay on tooth #4. Reschedule patient for a 2-unit appointment.	Signature

Procedure 12-3

Recording the Completed Dental Treatment

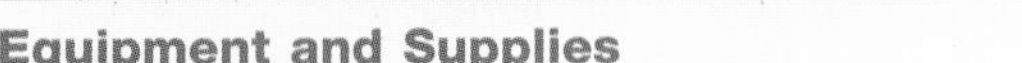

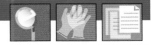

Equipment and Supplies

- Black ink pen
- Patient's record

Procedural Steps

1. In the Date column, record the date the treatment was provided, using numbers in a month/date/year format, such as 9/7/16.
2. In the Progress Notes column, record all areas of the dental procedure, such as the tooth, the surfaces of the tooth restored, the type and amount of anesthetic agent, the dental materials used, and the patient's tolerance of the appointment.
3. If appropriate, then describe the procedure that was performed with appropriate details, such as whether the tooth was prepared for a crown.

Purpose: The treatment is documented, which serves as a reference for future appointments.

4. After entering the complete treatment, sign the entry.

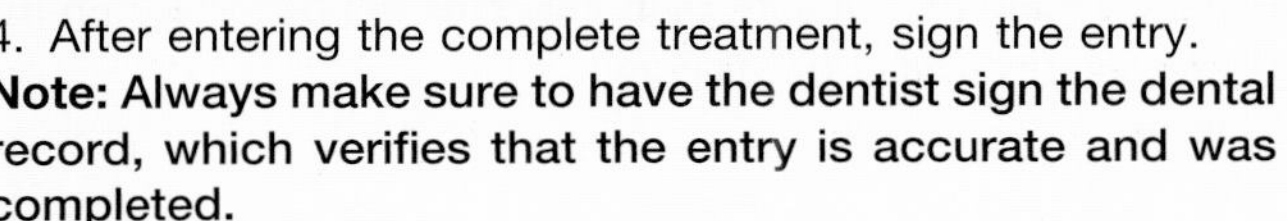

Note: Always make sure to have the dentist sign the dental record, which verifies that the entry is accurate and was completed.

5. Return the completed dental record to the business office.

Purpose: The patient returns to the business office area to make payment for services and to schedule any additional appointments.

DATE	PROGRESS NOTES
9/7/16	New patient examination, reviewed health history. Vital signs: BP 117/76, temp 98.4°F, resp 21, pulse 76. Intraoral and extraoral examination, 4 bite-wing radiographs, preliminary impression. Schedule patient for cleaning and composite resin on #12. E. Campbell, DDS/L. Stewart, CDA

Chapter Exercises

Multiple Choice

Circle the letter next to the correct answer.

1. Charting a condition that requires treatment, should be color-coded in __________.
   - **a.** green
   - **b.** red
   - **c.** black
   - **d.** pencil
2. An intraoral imaging system is used to __________.
   - **a.** visualize soft tissue in areas that are hard to reach
   - **b.** magnify conditions in the mouth
   - **c.** replace radiographs
   - **d.** make a commercial for a dental product
3. The abbreviation PFM represents __________.
   - **a.** patient faints momentarily
   - **b.** porcelain filling on mesial
   - **c.** porcelain fused to metal
   - **d.** protrusive forward movement
4. During the soft tissue examination, the dentist may use __________ to pull the tongue forward gently.
   - **a.** cotton pliers
   - **b.** Howe pliers
   - **c.** sterile gauze
   - **d.** suture material
5. If using the Universal Numbering System when looking at a charting diagram, the patient's right quadrant will be located on the __________ side of the diagram.
   - **a.** left
   - **b.** right
6. During routine charting of a patient, the dentist indicates that the patient should receive a gold crown for tooth #4. This should appear as a crown outlined with __________.
   - **a.** blue and blue diagonal lines
   - **b.** red and red diagonal lines
   - **c.** blue and colored in solid blue
   - **d.** red and colored in solid red
7. On which tooth would a class III cavity classification charting be commonly seen?
   - **a.** #3
   - **b.** #12
   - **c.** #24
   - **d.** #29
8. A small red circle at the tip of the root apex indicates __________.
   - **a.** an abscess
   - **b.** an impacted tooth
   - **c.** completed endodontic treatment
   - **d.** root caries
9. According to the Black classification, Class __________ cavities are also known as smooth surface cavities.
   - **a.** I
   - **b.** II
   - **c.** V
   - **d.** VI
10. Treatment entries in the patient's chart must be recorded __________.
    - **a.** by a computer entry
    - **b.** in ink to make it permanent
    - **c.** in pencil in case it needs to be corrected
    - **d.** a or b

Apply Your Knowledge

1. When charting the findings for a patient, Dr. Campbell prefers to call out cavity classifications. If Dr. Campbell indicated a Class II on the "distal of tooth #4," a Class III on the "mesial of tooth #6," a Class IV on the "distal of tooth #7," and a Class I on the "lingual of tooth #8," how would these be charted?
2. Dr. Campbell is dictating her findings on a patient during a recall appointment and indicates that tooth #12 has recurrent decay. When you look at the chart, you notice that tooth #12 has an MO amalgam. How would recurrent decay appear?
3. If a dental examination is more than simply "checking someone's teeth," then what else would it include?

CHAPTER 13

Medical Emergencies in the Dental Office

http://evolve.elsevier.com/Robinson/essentials/

LEARNING OBJECTIVES

1. Pronounce, define, and spell the key terms.
2. Discuss the standard of care for handling medical emergencies, including demonstration of cardiopulmonary resuscitation and the Heimlich maneuver.
3. Describe the assigned roles of dental office staff members during a medical emergency.
4. List the emergency telephone numbers considered essential during a medical emergency.
5. Discuss the need for updating emergency supplies, checking on expiration dates on emergency drugs, and taking responsibility for the maintenance of the oxygen equipment.
6. Differentiate between a sign and a symptom of a medical emergency.
7. Discuss the protocol for emergency responses and demonstrate how to respond to specific types of emergencies that could occur in the dental office, such as:
   - An unconscious patient.
   - A patient with breathing difficulty.
   - A patient experiencing a seizure.
   - A patient experiencing a diabetic emergency.
   - A patient experiencing chest pain.
   - A patient experiencing a cerebrovascular accident (stroke).
   - A patient experiencing an allergic reaction.

KEY TERMS

acute myocardial infarction
allergen
anaphylaxis
angina pectoris
antigen
asthma
cerebrovascular accident (CVA)
diabetes
emergency
epilepsy
hyperglycemia
hyperventilation
hypoglycemia
postural hypotension
signs
symptoms
syncope

An **emergency** is a condition or circumstance that requires immediate action to be taken for a person who has become suddenly ill or injured. When a medical emergency occurs, there is no time to refer to a medical resource for answers. You must be prepared to respond immediately.

The population seen in the typical dental practice is diverse in age, with a wide range of medical conditions. For this reason, it is important for all personnel within the dental office to gain knowledge, confidence, and competency in:

- Understanding legal responsibilities when assisting in an emergency
- Assessing the patient during dental treatment to detect any change that might prevent a medical emergency
- Being prepared for a medical emergency
- Continuing to assess the patient's condition throughout a medical emergency
- Having knowledge of the specific drugs recommended for a medical emergency
- Having specific equipment ready for use in an emergency and knowing how to use it

Preventing Emergencies

The easiest way for the dental office staff to help in preventing a potential medical emergency is requesting that each patient complete an updated medical history. By having the patient provide changes in his or her health status and prescription medications, the dental team can feel confident in a patient's health status. Once an update is completed, the patient will provide his or her signature to verify the information legally.

Knowledge of any chronic disorders, allergies, heart problems, and current medications allows the dentist to plan an individual dental treatment based on a patient's specific needs.

Legal Responsibilities

Handling a medical emergency must be taken seriously by not allowing the legal implications to intimidate or prevent you from doing your job.

In a professional situation, the law requires a health care worker to act or behave in a definable way known as the **standard of care.** A comparison of individuals with similar training and experience and how they would respond under similar circumstances, with similar equipment, and in the same setting determines the standard of care.

The standard of care for handling medical emergencies requires that the dental assistant become certified in:

- Cardiopulmonary resuscitation (CPR) (see Procedure 13-1)
- Heimlich maneuver (see Procedure 13-2)
- Obtaining and recording vital signs (see Chapter 11)

Emergency Preparedness

Every member of the dental team must be prepared for an emergency. A standardized procedure for the management of emergencies must be established and observed.

Assigned Roles

In the management of an emergency, the combined efforts of trained staff members are most efficient when each person takes on a specific role. The dentist is responsible for defining these roles. Most commonly, staff members will take on roles related to where they are commonly located in the office. Although primary roles are assigned, staff members must be versatile and trained and prepared to fill other roles, if necessary.

Staff Roles During an Emergency

- Front desk staff member (business assistant) will call for help and remain on the telephone at all times to obtain appropriate medical assistance and to provide directions to the office.
- The dentist, clinical assistant, or dental hygienist will remain with the patient for assessment or to assist with basic life support.
- Additional clinical staff members (dental assistant or dental hygienist) will retrieve the oxygen and emergency drug kit.
- Additional dental team members will respond to the needs of other patients in the office.

Routine Drills

Training must be kept current at all times. A mock emergency should be created monthly in the dental office, enabling staff members to practice their roles, take part in cross-training, and be able to refine the emergency plan.

Emergency Telephone Numbers

A list of emergency telephone numbers should be posted next to each telephone throughout the office. Maintaining a current list of these telephone numbers is an important part of emergency preparedness. The list should include numbers for the local police, fire, and emergency medical service (EMS).

In areas of the United States and Canada, all three agencies can be reached by dialing 9-1-1. However, emergency services vary widely, depending on the geographic area and the population served. An important part of emergency preparedness is to know:

- How quickly can the local EMS get to your office?
- What life support capabilities will they have? (Not all EMS services carry the same equipment or provide the same level of service.)
- What, if any, limitations and restrictions do they have? (Local restrictions may control the services the EMS is permitted to provide in a prehospital situation.)

Listing telephone numbers of the nearest hospital, physicians, and oral surgeons is also important. These professionals might be able to offer the life support necessary when you are waiting for the EMS or another type of emergency response.

Emergency Supplies

In a dental office, a portable standardized emergency kit is maintained with emergency drugs and supplies (Figure 13-1). The clinical staff is assigned the responsibility for maintaining and replacing outdated supplies on a routine schedule.

An emergency drug kit must be readily accessible for the dentist. The types of drugs that are normally in an emergency

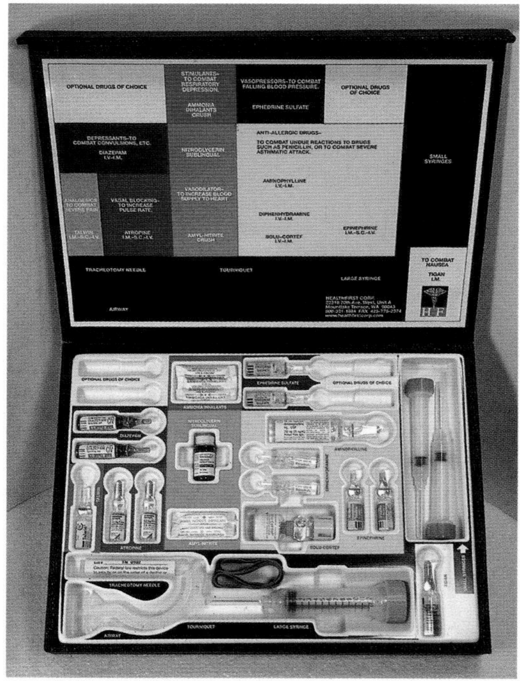

FIGURE 13-1 Standardized color-coded basic emergency kit.

TABLE 13-1
Drugs Used in Medical Emergencies

Drug	Common Examples	Use	Route
Oxygen	N/A	Respiratory distress	Inhaled
Respiratory stimulant	Spirits of ammonia	Fainting	Inhaled
Epinephrine 1:1000	Epi-Pen	Allergic reaction	IM, IV, SC
Diphenhydramine	Benadryl	Allergic reaction	IV, deep IM
Chlorpheniramine	Chlor-Trimeton	Allergic reaction	IM, IV
Nitroglycerin	Nitrostat	Angina	Sublingually
Albuterol	Ventolin	Bronchospasm with asthma	Inhaled
Diazepam	Valium	Seizures	IM, IV
Glucose	Orange juice, sugar, icing	Hypoglycemia	Orally
Morphine	Astramorph	Pain and anxiety	IM, IV, SC
Methoxamine	Vasoxyl	Blood pressure	IM, IV
Hydrocortisone insufficiency; severe allergic reaction	Solu-Cortef	Adrenocortical	IM, IV
Atropine	Atropair	Bradycardia	IM, IV, SC

IM, Intramuscularly; *IV,* intravenously; *N/A,* not applicable; *SC,* subcutaneously.

kit are provided in Table 13-1, along with their use and route of administration.

Oxygen is the most frequently used *drug* in a medical emergency. The ideal agent for resuscitation of a patient who is unconscious but still breathing is 100% oxygen.

Oxygen tanks (always color-coded green) must be checked weekly for any leaks. A portable unit of oxygen may be stored where it can be quickly moved into a treatment room, if necessary. *Note:* If the dental office is equipped with a nitrous oxide and oxygen unit, then oxygen from this unit can be used for emergency situations.

To maintain readiness in an emergency situation, it is necessary to:

- Routinely check supplies for their condition to determine whether they are properly working (rubber tubing, oxygen masks, intravenous [IV] needles and syringes, ventilation masks, and blood pressure equipment).
- Examine each drug in the emergency kit for its expiration date. (Drugs past the expiration date should be immediately replaced.)
- Perform weekly checks of the oxygen tank(s).

Patient Assessment

The dental staff must be aware that a medical emergency can occur at any time. For this reason, ongoing observation of the patient in the reception area, when moving to and from the dental treatment area, during a dental procedure, or when the patient is dismissed cannot be overemphasized.

Signs and Symptoms

When an emergency does occur, recording the **signs** and **symptoms** in the patient's record is important. A sign is what you observe in a patient, such as a rapid pulse rate or a change in skin color. Because you actually observe them, signs are considered more reliable than symptoms.

A symptom is the patient's report to you of what he or she is feeling or experiencing. The patient, for example, may say, "I feel dizzy," or "I am having difficulty breathing," or "My arm hurts."

Vital Signs

By being alert and using your eyes, ears, and hands, you can obtain a significant amount of information about your patient. Monitoring vital signs (pulse, respiration, blood pressure, and temperature) is important. Observing the patient's skin color gives an indication of blood circulation, and noticing the patient's face and eyes helps in assessing the patient's level of consciousness.

An accurate assessment of vital signs, also known as *diagnostic signs*, is essential for proper patient management during an emergency. During an emergency, vital signs should be reassessed every 10 to 15 minutes to determine whether the patient's condition is remaining constant, improving, or deteriorating. (How to obtain vital signs is discussed in Chapter 11.)

Emergency Responses

Diagnosis of a specific condition is not your job. As a dental assistant, your responsibility is to recognize the symptoms and signs of a significant medical complaint, communicate this information to the dentist, and then assist with appropriate support and transportation procedures. Specific responses could include:

"The patient's breathing is rapid and shallow [or slow and deep]."
"The patient is perspiring."
"The patient is pale."

"The patient's skin is clammy."

"The patient is confused."

When you assess a medical emergency situation, a primary factor in determining the mode of treatment is the consciousness of the patient. Medical emergencies described in this chapter and commonly encountered in the dental office are summarized in Procedures 13-3 through 13-9.

Syncope

Syncope, commonly known as fainting, is one of the most frequent medical emergencies in the dental office. Syncope is the imbalance in the blood distribution of the brain and larger vessels within the body. This reduced blood flow to the brain causes the patient to lose consciousness. Both **psychologic** factors and **physical** factors can contribute to syncope.

Psychologic and Physical Factors Contributing to Syncope

Psychologic

Stress
Apprehension
Fear
Sight of blood or instruments

Physical

Maintaining one position in the dental chair for a long period
Being in a confined environment
Skipping meals or being hungry
Experiencing fatigue or exhaustion

This situation is usually harmless to the patient as long as someone is there to protect them when they become unconscious. Syncope is one emergency that can be prevented by closely observing the patient.

A patient may complain of symptoms, and you may notice signs for several minutes before the patient actually loses consciousness.

Postural Hypotension

Postural hypotension, also known as *orthostatic hypotension*, is unconsciousness that can occur when the patient too quickly assumes an upright position. The lack of sufficient blood flow to the brain causes postural hypotension, and it may occur in a patient immediately after a sudden change in position, after receiving nitrous oxide and/or oxygen or IV sedation, or if the patient is pregnant.

The duration of unconsciousness is brief—usually only seconds to minutes. If unconsciousness persists longer, then there may be other causes, and appropriate action must be immediately taken.

See Procedure 13-3: Responding to the Unconscious Patient.

Hyperventilation

Hyperventilation is rapid or deep breathing. A person inhales oxygen and exhales carbon dioxide, but when hyperventilating, the excessive breathing creates low levels of carbon dioxide in the blood. The patient will usually remain conscious.

This medical emergency commonly occurs when a patient is extremely anxious or apprehensive before or during dental treatment. To prevent or reduce hyperventilation, the dental team should be alert at all times and be prepared to help the patient deal with severe apprehension in a positive manner.

Asthmatic Attack

Asthma is a chronic pulmonary (breathing) disease involving the airways of the lungs. This disorder can affect all ages. Asthma is characterized by a sudden onset of recurring periods of wheezing, chest tightness, shortness of breath, and coughing attacks. An allergic reaction, severe emotional stress, or respiratory infection can trigger an asthmatic attack.

Patients with asthma are aware of the sudden onset and should carry an inhaler that contains medication (a bronchodilator) used to relieve the first symptoms of an attack. Identifying asthma in the patient's medical history is very important; the patient should bring the inhaler with him or her to each dental appointment.

See Procedure 13-4: Responding to the Patient with Breathing Difficulty.

Epilepsy

Epilepsy is a neurologic disorder characterized by clusters of nerve cells or neurons in the brain that abnormally signal and cause recurrent episodes of seizures. In most patients, epileptic seizures are controlled with medication; however, under stressful conditions, a seizure may still occur.

There are many different types of seizures. Generally, seizures are categorized on the basis of what part of the brain is involved in a seizure. People might experience one type or more than one type of seizure. There are four primary categories of seizures:

- **Generalized seizures**, also referred to as *grand mal seizures*, affect the entire brain.

Types of Generalized Seizures

- **Absence seizures** may cause the person to appear to be staring into space with or without slight twitching of the muscles.
- **Tonic seizures** cause stiffening of the muscles of the body, generally those in the back, legs, and arms.
- **Clonic seizures** cause repeated jerking movements of muscles on both sides of the body.
- **Myoclonic seizures** cause jerks or twitches of the upper body, arms, or legs.
- **Atonic seizures** cause a loss of normal muscle tone, which often leads the affected person to fall down or to drop the head involuntarily.
- **Tonic-clonic seizures** cause a combination of symptoms, including stiffening of the body and repeated jerks of the arms and/or legs, as well as a loss of consciousness.

- **Partial seizures**, also referred to as *petit mal seizures*, affect a part of the brain. A person experiencing a partial seizure will often stay awake and be aware throughout the seizure. Although the person may know what is happening, he or she may be unable to speak and/or move until the seizure is over.
- **Nonepileptic seizures** are not related to epilepsy at all. Rather, they are caused by other things such as diabetes, a high fever, or something else entirely.
- **Status epilepticus** is a continuing seizure and one of the few reasons emergency personnel should be contacted.

See Procedure 13-5: Responding to the Patient Experiencing a Seizure.

Diabetes

Diabetes is a disorder of a person's metabolism; that is, the way the body uses digested food for energy. With the help of a hormone called insulin, cells throughout the body absorb glucose and use it for energy. Diabetes develops when the body does not make sufficient insulin or is unable to use insulin effectively; consequently, the blood glucose level, a type of sugar in the blood, becomes too high.

The disease is classified into two categories:

Type 1 diabetes, previously known as *juvenile diabetes*, is usually diagnosed in children and young adults. The body does not make insulin, and the patient is insulin dependent.

Type 2 diabetes, previously known as *adult-onset diabetes*, is commonly diagnosed in adults. Because of an increase in obesity in children, type 2 diabetes is increasing in children and young adults. The patient is treated with lifestyle changes, oral medications (pills), and possibly insulin.

When the balance shifts, with too much or too little food ingested, insulin levels change, resulting in hyperglycemia (too much blood sugar) or hypoglycemia (too little blood sugar).

Hyperglycemia is a condition in which the glucose (sugar) level in the blood abnormally increases. (Hyperglycemia means blood sugar that is abnormally high.) If left untreated, hyperglycemia may progress to diabetic ketoacidosis and a life-threatening diabetic coma.

Hypoglycemia, also known as *insulin shock*, is an abnormal decrease in the glucose level in the blood. (Hypoglycemia means blood sugar that is abnormally low.) Hypoglycemia can rapidly manifest itself. The most common causes of hypoglycemia are missing a meal, taking an overdose of insulin without adequate food intake, and excessively exercising without an appropriate adjustment of insulin and food intake.

See Procedure 13-6: Responding to the Patient Experiencing a Diabetic Emergency.

Angina Pectoris

Angina pectoris, commonly referred to as *angina*, is a symptom of an underlying heart problem in which severe chest pain occurs because the heart muscle is deprived of adequate oxygen. Although painful, angina pectoris does not usually lead to the death of the patient or to permanent heart damage. It does, however, indicate that the person has some degree of coronary artery disease.

Because the signs and symptoms of angina and a myocardial infarction are similar, distinguishing between angina and myocardial infarction is important.

Criteria for Distinguishing Angina from Myocardial Infarction

- Pain from angina will usually last from 3 to 8 minutes.
- Pain from angina is relieved or promptly eased with the administration of nitroglycerin.
- A patient with angina should include this information on his or her medical history.
- Although the patient has a history of angina, when an attack strikes, remembering that pain from angina could be myocardial infarction is important.

Acute Myocardial Infarction

During an acute myocardial infarction, commonly known as a *heart attack*, the muscles of the heart are affected as a result of insufficient oxygen. If this damage is severe, then the patient can die; however, prompt medical treatment can help limit damage to the heart.

Although other conditions exhibit similar symptoms, time is important, and the response of the dental team must be swift and prudent. Unexplained chest pain should be treated as a potential acute myocardial infarction.

See Procedure 13-7: Responding to the Patient with Chest Pain.

Cerebrovascular Accident

A cerebrovascular accident (CVA), commonly known as a *stroke*, is an interruption of blood flow to the brain. If the interruption lasts long enough, then it can cause damage to the brain, resulting in the loss of brain function. There are three types of strokes: (1) *ischemic stroke*, caused by an obstruction in a blood vessel that supplies blood to the brain; (2) *hemorrhagic stroke*, caused by a weakened blood vessel that bleeds into the brain; and (3) *transient ischemic attack (TIA)*, caused by a temporary clot, often referred to as a "mini stroke." Prompt treatment is crucial. Early action can minimize brain damage and potential complications.

See Procedure 13-8: Responding to the Patient Experiencing a Cerebrovascular Accident (Stroke).

Allergic Reactions

An **allergy**, also known as *hypersensitivity*, is an altered state of reactivity in body tissue in response to specific antigens. An antigen is a foreign substance from the environment such as a chemical, bacteria, virus, or pollen that causes an immune response through the production of antibodies. An antigen that can trigger the allergic state is known as an allergen.

Although the patient's health history is the major factor in determining the risk of an allergic reaction, every new drug or dental material introduced to a patient can possibly produce a reaction. Of particular concern is the increasing incidence of allergic reactions to latex, which is used in examination gloves and dental dams.

The two most important factors to consider when managing an allergic reaction are the speed with which symptoms appear and the severity of the reaction.

A **localized allergic response**, also known as a *cellular response*, is usually slow to develop. Mild symptoms can include itching, erythema (redness of the skin), and large hives.

The symptoms of **anaphylaxis**, also known as a *systemic reaction*, are very serious and quickly develop. These symptoms include swelling, blockage of air passages, and a drop in blood pressure. Without appropriate care, the patient may die within a few minutes.

See Procedure 13-9: Responding to the Patient Experiencing an Allergic Reaction.

Documentation of an Emergency

When a medical emergency arises in the dental office, the dentist will record all the events that occurred from the beginning of treatment throughout the crisis in the patient record. After such an emergency, the dentist will enter extensive notes in the patient's record explaining exactly what happened, the treatment provided, and the patient's condition at the time he or she left the office.

If an emergency is not fully resolved while the patient is in the office, then the dentist may telephone the patient, family, or patient's physician the next day to inquire about the patient's health.

Besides the patient record, the dentist is required to maintain records of office preparedness protocols and practices. These records are essential and could be used as valuable evidence if any legal problems arise.

Ethical Implications

As a health care professional, you are obligated to follow through and assist in a medical emergency. The *Good Samaritan* law tells us that we must ethically do all that we can do within our limitations.

Because there are so many new drugs and procedures to follow with medical conditions, it is advantageous to update your medical emergency knowledge and skills by attending continuing education courses yearly.

Remember to be alert to every patient who walks in the office. An emergency may take place when you least expect it.

Procedure 13-1

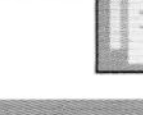

Performing Cardiopulmonary Resuscitation (CPR) (One Person)

Equipment and Supplies

Mannequin approved by the American Heart Association (AHA) and equipped with a printout for demonstration of proper technique (for instruction purposes and mock emergency drills).

Procedural Steps for Adult, Child, Infant CPR

Determine Unresponsiveness

Approach the victim and check for signs of circulation, such as normal breathing, coughing, or movement in response to stimulation. Pinch or tap the victim and ask, "Are you OK?"

Initiate Assistance

1. If there is no response, **call for assistance** and ask someone to call 911; obtain an AED/defibrillator if available.
2. If you are alone and your patient is an adult, phone 911 first and then begin compressions.
3. If the patient is a child, give 2 minutes of compression first, then call 911.

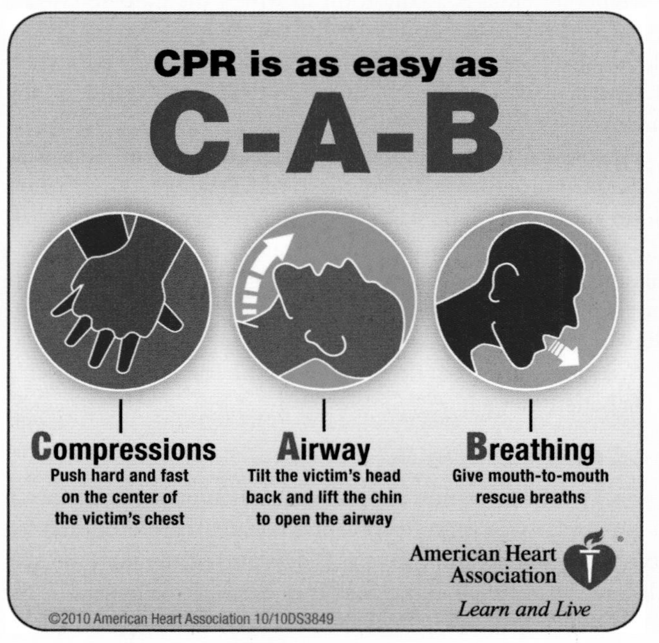

(Copyright American Heart Association.)

Procedure 13-1

Performing Cardiopulmonary Resuscitation (CPR) (One Person)—cont'd

Initiate Compressions

4. Kneel at the victim's side opposite the chest. Move your fingers up the ribs to the point where the sternum and the ribs join. Your middle finger should fit into the area, and your index finger should be next to it across the sternum.
5. Place the heel of your hand on the chest midline over the sternum, just above your index finger. Place your other hand on top of your first hand, and lift your fingers upward off the chest.

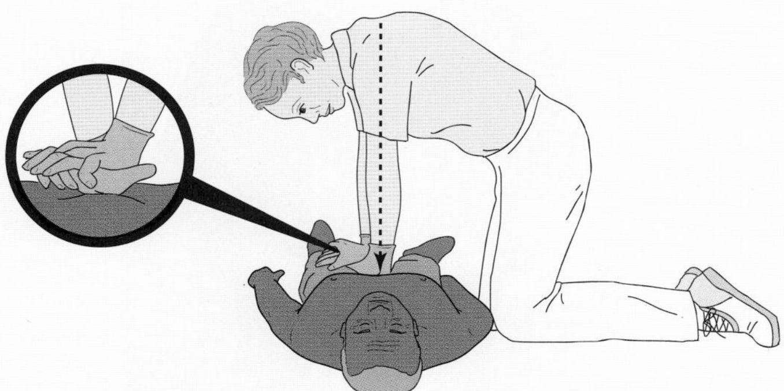

(From Sorrentino SA, Remmert LN: *Mosby's essentials for nursing assistants,* ed 5, St. Louis, 2014, Mosby.)

6. Bring your shoulders directly over the victim's sternum as you compress downward, and keep your arms straight.
7. Provide 30 chest compressions at a rate of 100/minute with adequate depth. Specific techniques to remember during compressions are as follows:
   - Push hard and fast.
   - Allow complete chest recoil after each compression.
   - Minimize interruptions in compressions.
   - Avoid excessive ventilation.
   - If multiple rescuers are available, they should rotate the task of compressions every 2 minutes.
8. For adults and children over 8, compress the chest a depth of at least 2 inches (5 cm).
9. For infants compress the chest a depth of about 1½ inches (4 cm).

Airway and Ventilation

10. Opening the airway (followed by rescue breaths to improve oxygenation and ventilation) should be completed only if there are two rescuers and one of the rescuers is trained in CPR.
11. Once chest compressions have been started, a trained rescuer should deliver rescue breaths by mouth-to-mouth or bag-mask to provide oxygenation and ventilation, as follows:
    - Deliver each rescue breath over 1 second.
    - Give a sufficient tidal volume to produce visible chest rise.
    - Use a compression to ventilation ratio of 30 chest compressions to 2 ventilations.
    - Repeat ongoing cycles of CPR until EMS arrives, the person starts breathing, someone comes with an AED, or another trained rescuer takes over.
12. Document emergency response in the patient record.

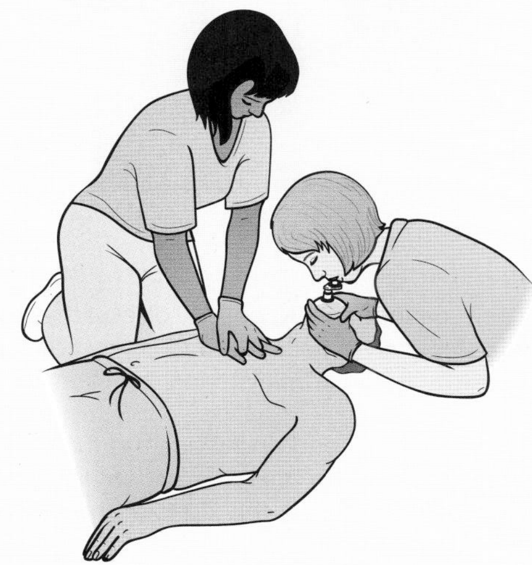

(From Sorrentino SA, Remmert LN: *Mosby's essentials for nursing assistants,* ed 5, St. Louis, 2014, Mosby.)

Procedure 13-2

Responding to a Patient with an Obstructed Airway

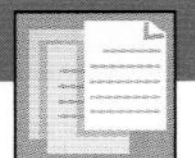

Signs and Symptoms

- Patient grasping at the throat (the universal sign of choking)
- Ineffective cough
- High-pitched breathing sound
- Respiratory difficulty
- Change in skin color

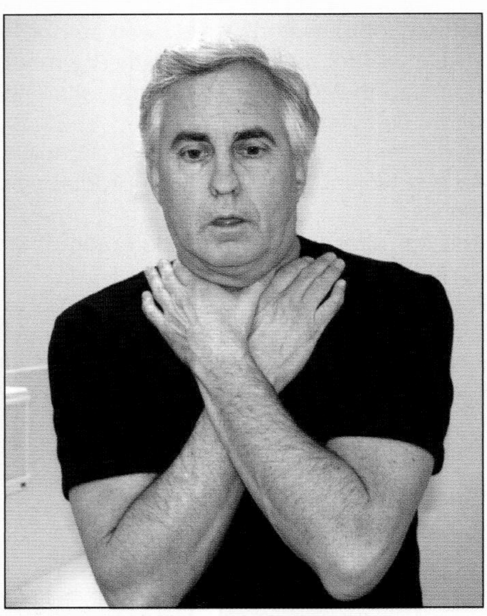

Procedural Steps

Care of the Patient

1. If the patient cannot speak, cough, or breathe, then the airway is completely blocked. Immediately call for assistance, and begin administering the Heimlich maneuver.
2. Make a fist with one hand and place the thumb side of your hand against the patient's abdomen, just above the navel and below the xiphoid process of the sternum.
3. Grasp your fist with the other hand and forcefully thrust both hands into the abdomen, using an inward and upward motion.
4. Repeat these thrusts until the object is expelled.

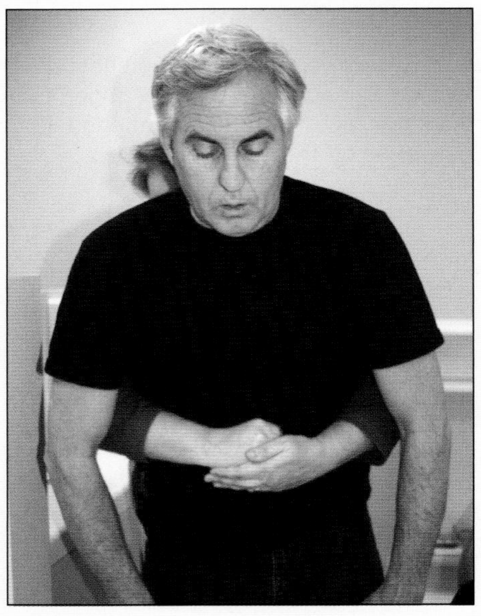

Responding to the Conscious Seated Patient

1. Do not try to move the patient out of the dental chair before administering the Heimlich maneuver.

Purpose: Patient movement may cause the lodged item to be swallowed.

2. Place the heel of one hand at the patient's abdomen above the navel and well below the xiphoid process.
3. Place your other hand directly over your first hand. Administer a firm, quick, upward thrust into the patient's diaphragm.
4. Repeat this maneuver 6 to 10 times as needed until the object is dislodged or until advanced emergency assistance arrives.

Procedure 13-3

Responding to the Unconscious Patient

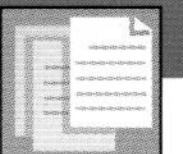

Syncope (Fainting)

Signs and Symptoms

- Feeling of warmth or flushing (flushed)
- Nausea
- Rapid heart rate
- Perspiration
- Pallor (pale skin color)
- Lower blood pressure

Response Steps

1. Place the patient in a subsupine position with the head lower than the feet.

Purpose: This position causes blood to flow away from the stomach and back toward the brain and is frequently sufficient to revive the patient.

2. Call for emergency assistance (9-1-1).
3. Loosen any binding clothes on the patient.

Procedure 13-3

Responding to the Unconscious Patient—cont'd

4. Have an ammonia inhalant ready to administer by waving it under the patient's nose several times.
5. Have oxygen ready to administer.
6. Monitor and record the patient's vital signs.

Postural Hypotension

Signs and Symptoms

- Low blood pressure
- Altered state of consciousness to possible loss of consciousness

Response Steps

1. Place the patient in a subsupine position with the head lower than the feet.

Purpose: This position causes blood to flow away from the stomach and back toward the brain and is frequently sufficient to revive the patient.

2. Establish an airway.
3. Slowly move the patient into an upright position.
4. If the patient does not immediately respond, then call for emergency assistance (9-1-1).
5. Monitor and record vital signs.

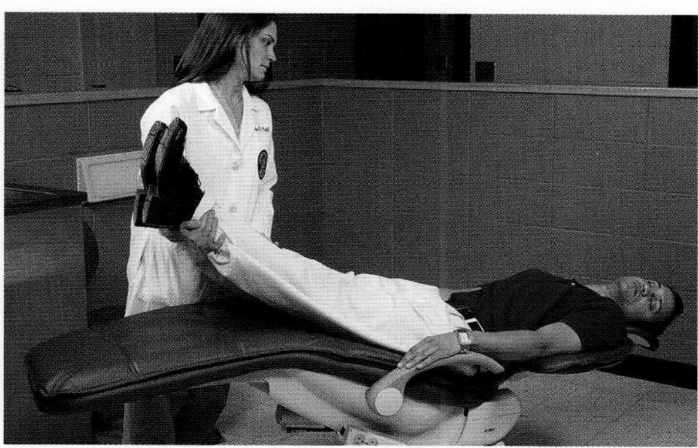

(From Hupp JR, Ellis E III, Tucker M: *Contemporary oral and maxillofacial surgery,* ed 6, St. Louis, 2014, Mosby.)

Procedure 13-4

Responding to the Patient with Breathing Difficulty

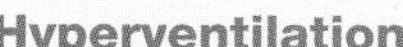

Hyperventilation

Signs and Symptoms

- Rapid, shallow breathing
- Lightheadedness
- Tightness in the chest
- Rapid heartbeat
- Lump in the throat
- Panic-stricken appearance

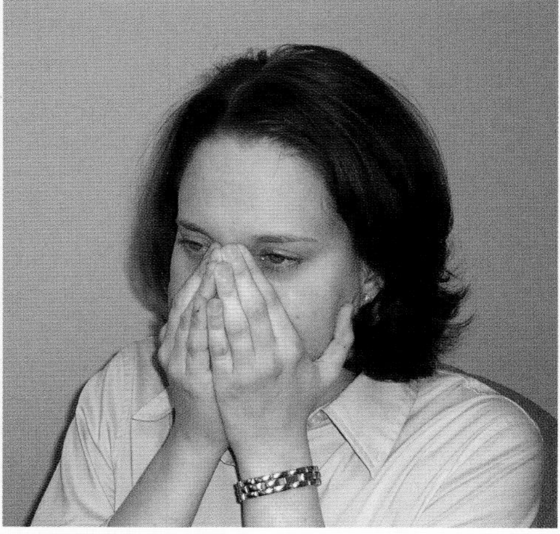

Response Steps

1. Place the patient in a comfortable position.
2. Use a quiet tone of voice to calm and reassure the patient.
3. Have the patient breathe into his or her cupped hands.

Note: Some sources recommend breathing into a paper bag, but a patient's cupped hands have been found to be quicker and more effective.

Asthma Attack

Signs and Symptoms

- Coughing
- Wheezing
- Increased anxiety
- Pallor
- Cyanosis (bluish skin around the nails)
- Increased pulse rate

Response Steps

1. Call for assistance.
2. Position the patient as comfortably as possible (upright is usually best).
3. Have the patient self-medicate with his or her inhaler.
4. Administer oxygen as needed.
5. Assess and record vital signs.

From Bird DL, Robinson DS: *Modern dental assisting,* ed 11, St. Louis, 2015, Saunders.

Procedure 13-5

Responding to the Patient Experiencing a Seizure

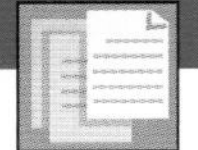

Generalized Seizure

Signs and Symptoms

- Unconsciousness
- Increased body temperature
- Rapid heart rate
- Increased blood pressure

Response Steps

1. Call for emergency assistance (9-1-1).
2. If a seizure occurs while the patient is in the dental chair, then quickly remove all materials from the mouth and place the patient in a supine position.

Purpose: The patient could inflict self-harm if something is in his or her mouth. Do not place anything in the patient's mouth during a seizure.

3. Protect the patient from self-injury during movements of the convulsion.
4. Prepare to use an anticonvulsant medication (diazepam) from the drug kit.
5. Initiate basic life support (CPR), if needed.
6. Monitor and record vital signs.

Partial Seizure

Signs and Symptoms

- Intermittent blinking
- Mouth movements
- Blank stare
- Unresponsive to surroundings; seems to be in his or her "own world"

Response Steps

1. Call for emergency assistance (9-1-1).
2. Prevent injury to the patient.
3. Monitor and record vital signs.
4. Refer the patient for medical consultation.

CPR, Cardiopulmonary resuscitation.

Procedure 13-6

Responding to the Patient Experiencing a Diabetic Emergency

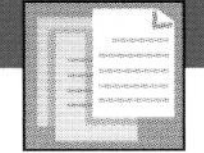

Hyperglycemia

Signs and Symptoms

- Excessive urination
- Excessive thirst, dry mouth, and dry skin
- Acetone breath (fruity smell)
- Blurred vision and headache
- Rapid pulse
- Lower blood pressure
- Loss of consciousness

Response Steps

1. Call for emergency assistance (9-1-1).
2. If the patient is conscious, then ask when he or she last ate, whether the patient has taken his or her medication and/or insulin, and whether he or she has brought medication or insulin to their dental appointment.

Purpose: If the patient has already eaten but has not taken insulin, then the patient may immediately need insulin.

3. Retrieve the patient's insulin, if it is available. If able, then the patient should self-administer the insulin.
4. Provide basic life support (CPR) if the patient becomes unconscious.
5. Monitor and record vital signs.

Hypoglycemia

Signs and Symptoms

- Mood changes
- Hunger
- Perspiration
- Increased anxiety
- Possible unconsciousness

Response Steps

1. Call for emergency assistance (9-1-1).
2. If the patient is conscious, then ask when he or she last ate, whether the patient has taken his or her medication and/or insulin, and whether he or she has brought medication or insulin to the dental appointment.
3. If the patient is conscious, then provide a glucose tablet, concentrated juice, or cake icing.

Purpose: These substances will be rapidly absorbed into the bloodstream.

4. Provide basic life support (CPR) if the patient becomes unconscious.
5. Monitor and record vital signs.

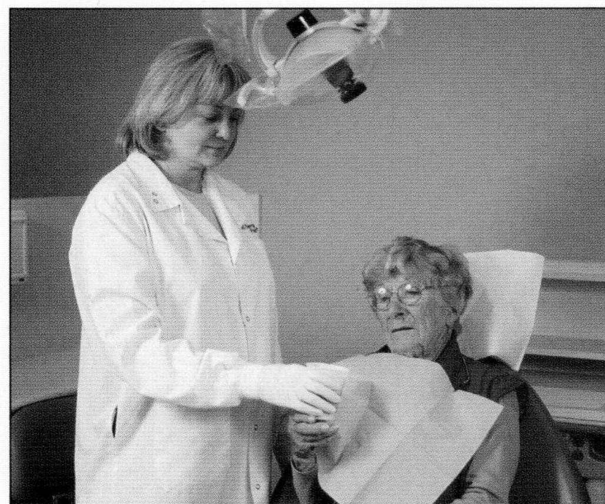

CPR, Cardiopulmonary resuscitation.

Procedure 13-7

Responding to the Patient with Chest Pain

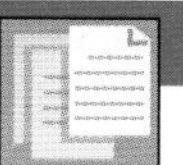

Angina

Signs and Symptoms

- Tightness or squeezing sensation in the chest
- Sharp pain radiating to the left shoulder
- Sharp pain radiating to the left side of the face, jaws, and teeth

Response Steps

1. Call for emergency assistance (9-1-1).
2. Position the patient upright.
3. If possible, have the patient self-medicate with personal nitroglycerin supply (tablets, spray, or topical cream). If this is not possible, then obtain nitroglycerin from the office emergency kit.
4. Administer oxygen.
5. Monitor and record vital signs.

Acute Myocardial Infarction (Heart Attack)

Signs and Symptoms

- Chest pain ranging from mild to severe
- Pain in the left arm, jaw, and teeth
- Shortness of breath and sweating
- Nausea and vomiting
- Pressure, aching, or burning feeling of indigestion
- Generalized feeling of weakness

Response Steps

1. Call for emergency assistance (9-1-1).
2. Initiate basic life support (CPR) if the patient becomes unconscious.
3. Medicate with nitroglycerin from the office emergency kit.
4. Administer oxygen.
5. Monitor and record vital signs.

CPR, Cardiopulmonary resuscitation.

Procedure 13-8

Responding to the Patient Experiencing a Cerebrovascular Accident (Stroke)

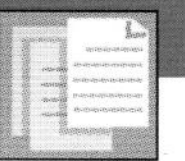

Signs and Symptoms

- Paralysis
- Speech problems
- Vision problems
- Possible seizure
- Difficulty swallowing
- Headache
- Unconsciousness

Response Steps

1. Call for emergency assistance (9-1-1).
2. Initiate basic life support (CPR) if the patient becomes unconscious.
3. Monitor and record vital signs.

THINK YOU ARE HAVING A STROKE?
CALL 9-1-1 IMMEDIATELY!

F.A.S.T. is an easy way to remember the sudden signs of stroke. When you can spot the signs, you'll know that **you need to call 9-1-1 for help right away.** *F.A.S.T. is:*

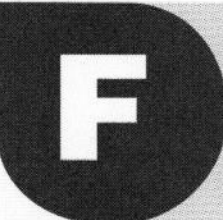

Face Drooping
Does one side of the face droop or is numb? Ask the person to smile. Is the person's smile uneven?

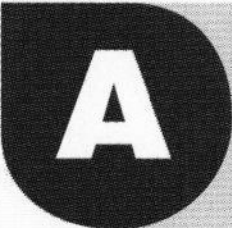

Arm Weakness
Is one arm weak or numb? Ask the person to raise both arms. Does one arm drift downward?

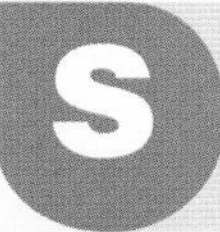

Speech Difficulty
Is speech slurred? Is the person unable to speak or hard to understand? Ask the person to repeat a simple sentence, like "The sky is blue." Is the sentence repeated correctly?

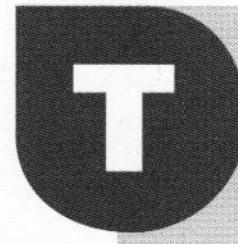

Time to call 9-1-1
If someone shows any of these symptoms, even if the symptoms go away, call 9-1-1 and get the person to the hospital immediately. Check the time so you'll know when the first symptoms appeared.

CPR, Cardiopulmonary resuscitation.

Procedure 13-9

Responding to the Patient Experiencing an Allergic Reaction

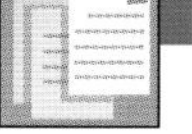

Localized Rash

Signs and Symptoms

- Itching
- Erythema (skin redness)
- Hives

Response Steps

1. Call for emergency assistance (9-1-1).
2. Prepare an antihistamine for administration.
3. Be prepared to administer basic life support (CPR), if necessary.

Continued

Procedure 13-9

Responding to the Patient Experiencing an Allergic Reaction—cont'd

4. Refer the patient for medical consultation.

Purpose: If the patient has an allergic reaction once, he or she may become increasingly hypersensitive and have a life-threatening response the next time.

Anaphylaxis

Signs and Symptoms

- Feeling physically ill
- Nausea and vomiting
- Shortness of breath
- Heart arrhythmia (irregular heartbeats)
- Sudden drop in blood pressure
- Loss of consciousness

Response Steps

1. Call for emergency assistance (9-1-1).
2. Place the patient in a supine position.
3. Start basic life support (CPR) if the patient becomes unconscious.
4. Prepare to assist in the administration of epinephrine.
5. Administer oxygen.
6. Monitor and record vital signs.

CPR, Cardiopulmonary resuscitation.

Chapter Exercises

Multiple Choice

Circle the letter next to the correct answer.

1. An acute allergic reaction that can be life threatening is known as __________.

a. acidosis
b. anaphylaxis
c. angina
d. asthmatic attack

2. A sign of syncope is __________.

a. tightness in the chest
b. increased blood pressure
c. rapid heart rate
d. wheezing

3. The severe pain of __________ can be relieved by the administration of nitroglycerin.

a. a cerebrovascular accident
b. an acute myocardial infarction
c. an asthmatic attack
d. angina pectoris

4. The abbreviation EMS stands for __________.

a. early medical station
b. emergency medical service
c. essential medical standards
d. everything medically standard

5. A patient may __________ if he or she is extremely anxious about dental treatment.

a. hyperventilate
b. hypoventilate
c. become hyperglycemic
d. become hypoglycemic

6. The standard of care for handling medical emergencies requires that all dental personnel be certified in __________.

a. basic first aid
b. cardiopulmonary resuscitation (CPR)
c. Heimlich maneuver
d. b and c

7. An allergic reaction is caused by an __________.

a. allergen
b. analgesic
c. antihistamine
d. none of the above

8. Cake frosting or orange juice can be administered in an emergency response to an increase in the level of blood sugar in the patient with __________.

a. asthma
b. hyperglycemia
c. hypoglycemia
d. postural hypotension

9. An ammonia inhalant is used to treat a patient who is experiencing __________.

a. a CVA
b. a mild allergic reaction
c. an angina attack
d. syncope

10. During an asthma attack, breathing can be eased by administering a(n) __________.

a. bronchodilator
b. insulin
c. antihistamine
d. a or c

Apply Your Knowledge

1. You are newly employed in a dental office, and while assisting the dentist in a restorative procedure, the dental hygienist calls out that she immediately needs assistance. What would be your role in this medical emergency?

2. You are currently certified in CPR but have been told that the American Red Cross has made changes to next year's protocol. How would you go about getting recertified and learning about the new changes you should follow?

3. You are assisting the dentist in a surgical procedure. It has been a very long procedure, and you are not used to standing. Your breathing becomes rapid, you can feel your pulse racing, and you are starting to perspire. What do you think is happening, and what should you do?

4. Your patient, Alice Jones, ran from her car into the office, knowing that she was 15 minutes late for her 11:30 appointment. You seat her and assist the dentist in administering the anesthetic. You notice that she is restless, perspiring, and complaining of hunger. What is going on, and how should you respond?

CHAPTER 14

Pain and Anxiety Control

http://evolve.elsevier.com/Robinson/essentials/

LEARNING OBJECTIVES

1. Pronounce, define, and spell the key terms.
2. Discuss the importance of pain and anxiety control in dentistry.
3. Describe the composition and application of topical anesthetics, as well as demonstrate how to apply a topical anesthetic.
4. Complete the following related to local anesthesia techniques:
   - Describe the composition and application of local anesthetics.
   - Demonstrate how to assemble the local anesthetic syringe.
   - Assist in the administration of local anesthesia.
   - Discuss how to prevent needle stick injuries with local anesthetics.
5. Complete the following related to pain and anxiety control methods used in dentistry:
   - Describe relaxation techniques.
   - List the indications for use of nitrous oxide analgesia in dentistry.
   - Discuss the contraindications and safety precautions related to nitrous oxide.
   - Assist in the administration and monitoring of nitrous oxide–oxygen sedation.
   - Discuss other types of anxiety control used in dentistry.

KEY TERMS

analgesia	duration	sedation
anesthetics	induction	syringe
antianxiety	nitrous oxide–oxygen	vasoconstrictor

The dental profession has access to a wide range of pain and anxiety control procedures to provide oral health care to millions of individuals who would otherwise remain untreated because of their fear of pain. Pain and anxiety control is defined as the exposure of chemical, physiological, and psychological approaches to prevent and treat preoperative, operative, and postoperative pain and anxiety.

For most dental procedures, pain control is accomplished with the application of a topical and local anesthetic agent.

Some patients arrive for their appointment and are apprehensive about receiving dental treatment. This type of patient may require additional means to help control their anxiety. The administration of **nitrous oxide–oxygen** and/or **antianxiety** drugs may be prescribed to provide comfort to the patient when receiving dental care.

A new direction for confronting anxiety with a patient is introducing relaxation techniques. Relaxation techniques can help reduce levels of stress hormones, as well as pain and anxiety. By asking the patient to imagine having a pleasant experience or being in a soothing place while following a deep breathing technique can help reduce the fear.

Use of **intravenous sedation** or **general anesthesia** is recommended for a patient with the need for invasive or extensive dental treatment or for one who is medically or physically compromised.

The dental assistant must be familiar with the procedures, types of equipment, and the range of **anesthetics** used in all areas of dentistry.

Topical Anesthesia

Topical anesthesia is a procedure during which a highly concentrated anesthetic agent is topically applied to the area where a local anesthetic injection is to take place. This provides a temporary numbing effect on the nerve endings on the surface of the oral mucosa. Topical anesthetic agents are available in the form of ointments, liquids, sprays, and patches (Figure 14-1).

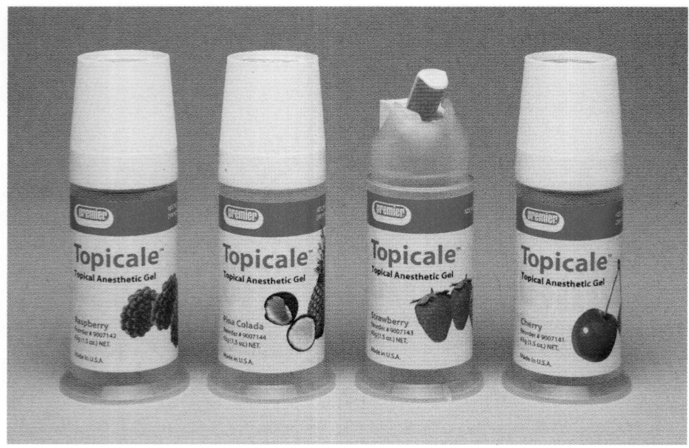

FIGURE 14-1 Topical anesthetics. (Courtesy Premier Dental Products Company, Plymouth Meeting, Pennsylvania.)

Topical Anesthetic Ointment

Topical anesthetic ointment can lessen or even eliminate that initial "pinch" from an injection. For maximum effectiveness, the topical anesthetic is applied to the dried mucosal surface at the site of the injection with a cotton-tip applicator for 2 to 5 minutes.

See Procedure 14-1: Applying a Topical Anesthetic Ointment.

Local Anesthesia

Local anesthesia is a procedure that was first introduced in the 1800s. A local anesthetic agent is the most frequently used form of pain control in dentistry and is the drug of choice to reduce or relieve associated pain that may take place during and immediately after a dental procedure. This type of anesthesia provides a safe, effective, and dependable method for a suitable duration in virtually all forms of dental treatment.

Local Anesthetic Agents

The chemical makeup of local anesthetic agents blocks the ability of the nerve membrane to generate an impulse. Because of this block, the impulse does not transmit the feeling of pain to the brain. To receive local anesthesia, the agent is injected near the nerve that specifically affects the tooth receiving dental treatment.

Local anesthetic agents are broadly classified under two chemical groups: amides and esters. The amides were first introduced to clinical practice in the 1940s and provide the standards by which all other local anesthetic agents are measured. Amide local anesthetics available for dental anesthesia include lidocaine, mepivacaine, articaine, and prilocaine.

Induction and Duration of an Anesthetic

Induction is the time frame from when the injection is given to the complete effective numbing sensation. **Duration** is the time frame from when the injection is given until the numbing sensation is gone. Duration varies among anesthetic agents, between pulp and soft tissues, and between maxillary infiltration and mandibular blocks. Duration will also vary from patient to patient. In general, local anesthetic agents follow this time frame:

- Short-acting duration local anesthetic agents can last approximately 30 minutes
- Intermediate-acting duration local anesthetic agents will last approximately 60 minutes (most local anesthetic agents are in this group and are used for general dental procedures)
- Long-acting duration local anesthetic agents, will last approximately 90 minutes

Vasoconstrictors

A **vasoconstrictor** is an added drug that has been added to the local anesthetic agent to slow down the intake of the anesthetic agent and increase the duration of action. The action of a vasoconstrictor can:

- Prolong the effect of the anesthetic agent by decreasing blood flow in the immediate area of the injection
- Decrease bleeding in the area, which is beneficial during surgical procedures

The most common vasoconstrictors used are epinephrine, levonordefrin, and Neo-Cobefrin. The ratio of vasoconstrictor to anesthetic solution is supplied as 1:50,000, 1:100,000, or 1:200,000. A concentration of 1:100,000 indicates that one part of the vasoconstrictor is diluted in 100,000 parts of anesthetic solution. The lower the second number, the larger the amount of epinephrine in the solution.

Health Conditions Affecting the Selection of a Local Anesthetic Agent

- Hypertension
- Cardiovascular disease
- Hyperthyroidism
- Liver disease
- Kidney disease
- Pregnancy

Health Status of the Patient

Local anesthetic agents and vasoconstrictors are considered safe drugs when properly administered. Certain health conditions may affect the dentist's choice in the type of anesthetic solution and whether or not that solution contains a vasoconstrictor. Health conditions are noted in the patient's medical history, and the dentist must be alerted to the health conditions when selecting a local anesthetic agent.

Local Anesthesia Techniques

The location and the nerves of the tooth or teeth to be anesthetized determine the type of injection method to be used. The two principal methods used in dentistry are infiltration anesthesia and block anesthesia.

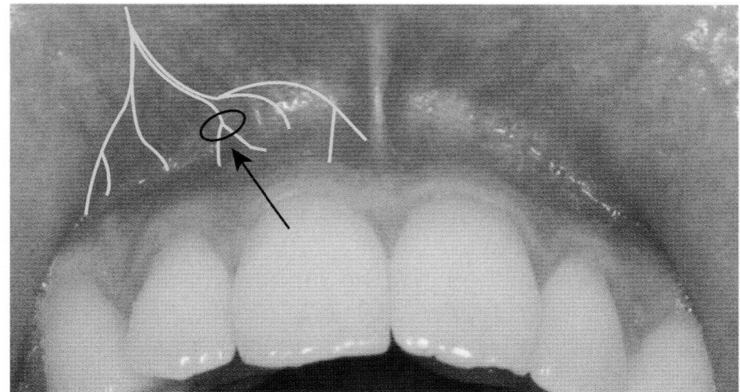

FIGURE 14-2 Infiltration injection. (From Malamed SF: *Handbook of local anesthesia*, ed 6, St. Louis, 2013, Mosby.)

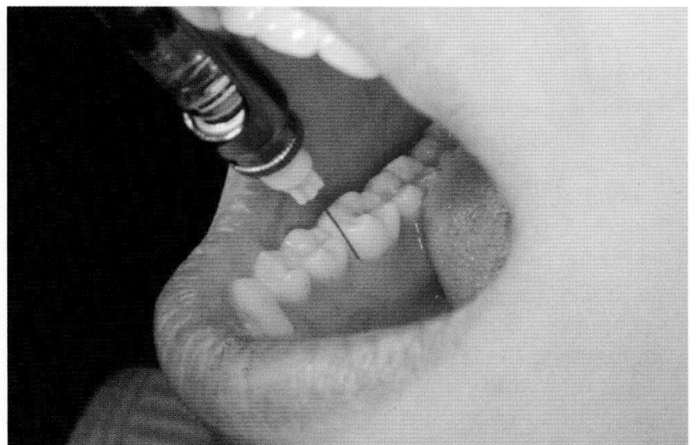

FIGURE 14-3 Periodontal ligament injection into the gingival tissue. (From Malamed SF: *Handbook of local anesthesia*, ed 6, St. Louis, 2013, Mosby.)

Infiltration Anesthesia

Infiltration anesthesia involves injecting the anesthetic solution into the tissue near the apices of the tooth to be treated (Figure 14-2). Infiltrating a maxillary tooth is possible because the alveolar cancellous bone is porous and allows the solution to diffuse through the bone and reach the nerve at the apices of the tooth.

Periodontal Ligament Injection

An alternative infiltration technique involves directly injecting the anesthetic solution under pressure into the periodontal ligament and surrounding gingival tissue (Figure 14-3). This type of injection can be completed with the use of a conventional syringe or a specialized periodontal ligament injection syringe.

Block Anesthesia

Block anesthesia involves injecting the anesthetic solution around a larger nerve, which means numbing a larger area (Figure 14-4). Because the mandibular bone is dense and the nerve system is designed differently from that of the maxillary bone, the anesthetic solution is injected into a **nerve trunk**.

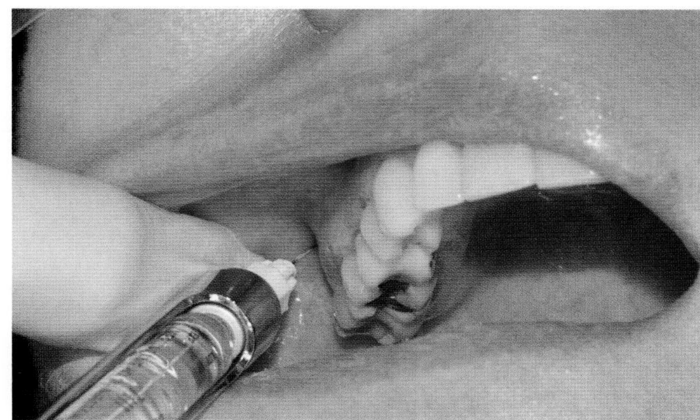

FIGURE 14-4 Block injection. (From Logothesis DD: *Local anesthesia for the dental hygienist,* St. Louis, 2012, Mosby.)

Mandibular nerve block is obtained by injecting the anesthetic agent into the inferior alveolar nerve, which numbs one half of the lower jaw including the teeth, tongue, and lip.

Buccal nerve block provides anesthesia to the buccal soft tissues closest to the mandibular molars.

Incisive nerve block is given at the site of the mental foramen, numbing the anterior teeth.

Preparing the Anesthetic Syringe

When gathering the appropriate setup (Table 14-1) to assemble the anesthetic syringe, the dental assistant will need to inquire information from the treatment plan about the procedure before assembly: (1) the type of anesthetic and (2) the needle length and needle gauge.

See Procedure 14-2: Assembling the Local Anesthetic Syringe.

Duration of Injectable Amide Local Anesthetics

ANESTHETIC	PULPAL	SOFT TISSUE
Lidocaine hydrochloride with epinephrine 1:50,000	60 minutes	180–300 minutes
Mepivacaine hydrochloride with epinephrine 1:20,000	60 minutes	180–300 minutes
Articaine hydrochloride with epinephrine 1:200,000	45–60 minutes	120–300 minutes
Prilocaine hydrochloride with epinephrine 1:200,000	60–90 minutes	180–480 minutes

Data from Malamed SF: *Handbook of local anesthesia*, ed 6, St. Louis, 2013, Mosby.

Transferring the Anesthetic Syringe

The transfer of an anesthetic syringe should take place in the transfer zone just below the patient's chin. If the patient is apprehensive or if the dentist is anesthetizing a child, then behind the patient's head may be a more suitable zone for transferring the syringe.

Always be alert to infection control and protocol. The transfer of a sterile syringe is appropriate, but once the syringe has been used, it becomes contaminated, and the dentist will need to recap and retrieve the syringe for additional injections.

TABLE 14-1
Local Anesthetic Setup

Part	Description
Anesthetic syringe 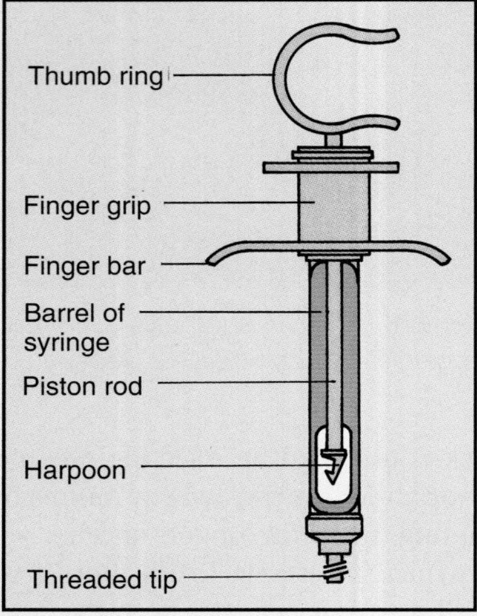 	The thumb ring, finger grip, and finger bar make it possible for the dentist to hold the syringe firmly when giving the injection. The harpoon is pushed into the rubber stopper of the anesthetic cartridge; by pulling back, the piston rod retracts the rubber stopper. This action makes aspiration possible. An aspirating syringe is used to administer the local anesthetic agent to enable the dentist to aspirate (aspirate means to draw back) after insertion of the needle. The piston rod pushes down on the rubber stopper of the anesthetic cartridge and pushes the anesthetic solution out through the needle. The barrel of the syringe holds the anesthetic cartridge in the syringe. The cartridge is loaded into the syringe through the large open area on the side of the barrel. The other side has a large window, enabling the dentist to watch for blood in the cartridge as he or she aspirates. The hub is the threaded tip where the needle is screwed onto the syringe.
Disposable needle 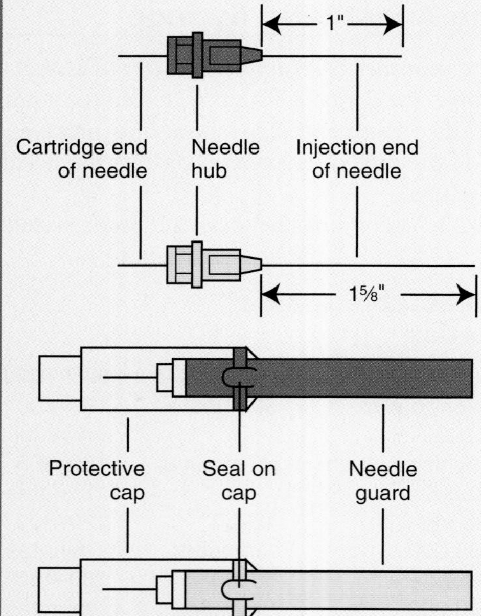 (Modified from Boyd LRB: *Dental instruments: a pocket guide,* ed 5, St. Louis, 2015, Saunders.)	The sterile needle comes as a sealed unit and is never used if the seal has been previously broken. The lumen is the hollow center of the needle through which the anesthetic solution flows. The cartridge end is the shorter end of the needle and has a clear or white plastic protective cap. This end of the needle fits onto the threaded tip of the syringe and punctures the rubber diaphragm of the anesthetic cartridge. The needle hub is attached to the threaded tip of the syringe. Needles with a self-threading plastic hub are pushed and screwed onto the syringe. Needles with a prethreaded metal hub are threaded into place. Needle length: The injection end of the needle comes in two lengths—1 inch or 1⅝ inch. Most commonly, the 1-inch "short" needle is used for maxillary injections and infiltration injections. The "long" 1⅝-inch needle is used for mandibular block injections. Needle gauge: Needle gauge refers to the thickness of the needle. Gauges are numbered; the larger the gauge number, the thinner the needle. Because a longer needle needs more strength, it is commonly used in a lower gauge number. The most commonly used gauge numbers are 25, 27, and 30.

TABLE 14-1
Local Anesthetic Setup—cont'd

Part	Description
Anesthetic cartridge Aluminum cap; Glass cartridge; Color-coded band; Rubber diaphram; Silicone rubber stopper (From Logothesis DD: *Local anesthesia for the dental hygienist,* St. Louis, 2012, Mosby.)	Local anesthetic solutions are supplied in glass cartridges with a rubber stopper at one end and an aluminum cap at the other. Cartridges are supplied in blister packs already sterilized and sealed.
Color coding (see below)	A color-coding system designed by the American Dental Association (ADA) has created standardization for all injectable local anesthetic products.

Color coding

Local Anesthetic Solution	Color of Cartridge Band
Articaine HCl 4% with epinephrine 1:100,000	Gold
Bupivacaine 0.5% with epinephrine 1:200,000	Blue
Lidocaine HCl 2%	Light blue
Lidocaine HCl 2% with epinephrine 1:50,000	Green
Lidocaine HCl 2% with epinephrine 1:100,000	Red
Mepivacaine HCl 3%	Tan
Mepivacaine HCl 2% with levonordefrin 1:20,000	Brown
Prilocaine HCl 4%	Black
Prilocaine HCl 4% with epinephrine 1:200,000	Yellow

Anesthetic syringe and color coding illustrations from Malamed SF: *Handbook of local anesthesia,* ed 6, St. Louis, 2013, Mosby.

Patients should never be left alone after the anesthesia has been given. Continually observe the patient to ensure that the he or she is not in distress or developing an allergic reaction.

See Procedure 14-3: Assisting in the Administration of Local Anesthesia.

Local Anesthetic Cautions

Needlestick injuries are serious, and care must be taken to prevent such accidents when handling a contaminated syringe. An important precautionary directive from the Centers for Disease Control and Prevention (CDC) states that contaminated needles used in dental procedures should be recapped by a recapping device or by a single-handed scoop technique (Figure 14-5).

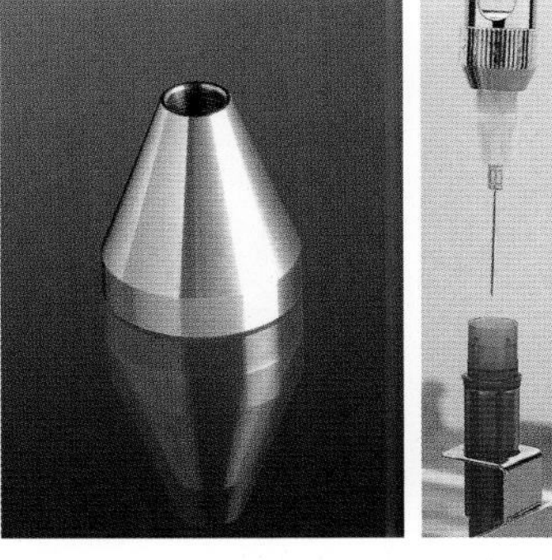

FIGURE 14-5 Needle recapping devices. (Left photo from Boyd LRB: *Dental instruments: a pocket guide,* ed 5, St Louis, 2015, Saunders. Right photo courtesy Hu-Friedy Mfg. Co., LLC, Chicago, IL.)

A **recapping device** allows the dentist to slide the needle into the guard without touching it.

With a **single-handed scoop technique**, the needle guard is placed on the tray, and the end of the needle is slid into its cover. Once the end of the needle is covered, the other hand may safely be used to complete bringing the cap into position.

Pain and Anxiety Control Methods

Many people have some form of pain or anxiety when it comes to receiving dental care. Several methods described in this section are used to reduce the pain and anxiety during preoperative, operative, and postoperative care.

Relaxation Techniques

Fear can be minimized during a dental procedure when the staff is empathetic (understanding) toward patients. Several techniques can be used to help alleviate the fear before and during dental treatment.

- Devices such as headsets with music or a video can distract and calm the patient before the injection and throughout the procedure.
- Having the patient slowly and deeply breathe supplies the body with oxygen and other chemicals that relax the central nervous system and help reduce discomfort.

Nitrous Oxide Analgesia

Nitrous oxide **analgesia** is one of the most common forms of in-office pain control. The gas is inhaled through the nose and primarily acts as a sedative to help eliminate fear and to relax the patient. The terms *inhalation sedation*, *nitrous oxide–oxygen analgesia*, and *psychosedation* are all interchangeably used to describe nitrous oxide. In this discussion, the term *nitrous oxide analgesia* will be used.

The combination of nitrous oxide and oxygen gases produces nitrous oxide analgesia (Figure 14-6). The patient inhales a combination of nitrous oxide gas and oxygen through a nosepiece, feeling the effect almost immediately. The mix produces a pleasant, relaxing experience for the patient with easy onset, minimal side effects, and rapid recovery (Table 14-2).

When used alone, nitrous oxide analgesia dulls the perception of pain, such as during injection of a local anesthetic agent

TABLE 14-2
Nitrous Oxide Analgesia Equipment

Equipment	Description
Cylinders	Nitrous oxide and oxygen are dispensed in steel cylinders, which are color-coded green for oxygen and blue for nitrous oxide. Cylinders should be stored in an upright position, away from a heat source, and secured to the wall (or a portable unit) to prevent them from falling on the valve stem, which could cause the cylinder to explode.
Gas machines	Nitrous oxide gas machines are available as a portable or a central system. Components of gas machines include the following: • Yokes, which hold the cylinder in the machine • Control valves, which are used to control the flow of each gas • Flow meter, which indicates the rate of flow of the gas The greater the flow of gas, the higher the ball rises. Separate color-coded flow meters are used for nitrous oxide and for oxygen. • Pressure gauge, which indicates the pressure of cylinder contents • Masks, which are the nasal inhalers through which the patient breathes the gases Masks are supplied in sizes for adults and children. They are also available in a disposable variety, which is discarded after a single use, and in rubber, which can be sterilized or disinfected for reuse. • Gas hose, which carries the gases from the reservoir bag to the mask or nosepiece • Reservoir bag, which is where the two gases are combined and from which the patient draws for breathing

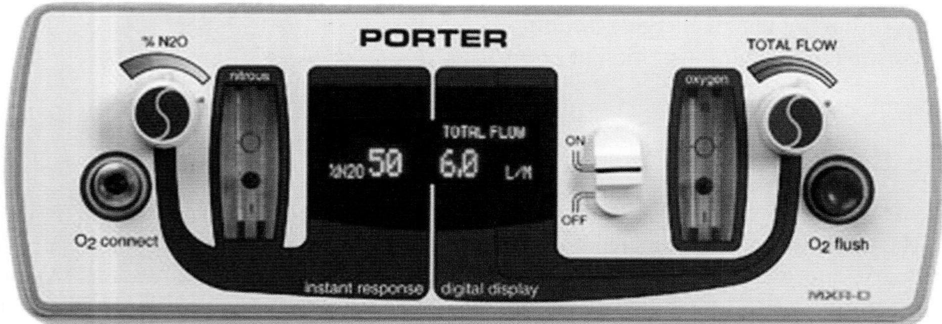

FIGURE 14-6 Nitrous oxide gas–oxygen (N_2O)system unit. (From Boyd LRB: *Dental instruments: a pocket guide,* ed 5, St. Louis, 2015, Saunders.)

or simple procedure. However, it must be used in conjunction with an effective local anesthetic solution to achieve total pain control for most dental procedures.

After the completion of treatment, the flow of nitrous oxide is discontinued, and complete oxygen is delivered through the nosepiece for approximately 5 minutes. Some patients may require more time on 100% oxygen to oxygenate (clear) or completely recover from the effects of the nitrous oxide analgesia. Indications and contraindications for the use of nitrous oxide should be considered before use.

Indications for Using Nitrous Oxide Analgesia

- Administration is relatively simple and is easily managed by the dentist.
- Special training is required for the dentist and the dental assistant; the services of an anesthetist or other special personnel are not necessary.
- Nitrous oxide–oxygen sedation has an excellent safety record with minimal side effects.
- The patient is awake and able to communicate at all times.
- Recovery is rapid and complete within a matter of minutes.
- Nitrous oxide–oxygen sedation may be used with patients of all ages.

Contraindications for Using Nitrous Oxide Analgesia

- Pregnancy: Although no evidence indicates that enough nitrous oxide crosses the placenta to damage the fetus, nitrous oxide analgesia is administered to a pregnant patient only with the permission of her obstetrician.
- Nasal obstruction: Cold or allergy symptoms can prevent the patient from obtaining the benefit of the drug.
- Emphysema or multiple sclerosis: These diseases cause breathing difficulties. Increased oxygen during the administration of nitrous oxide analgesia may lower the stimulus to breathe as often as necessary.
- Emotional instability: This reaction can be intensified because of the altered perception of reality produced by the nitrous oxide analgesia.

Safety Precautions with Nitrous Oxide

Nitrous oxide is used only during patient treatment. It is never unnecessarily administered or used for recreational purposes.

For staff and patient safety, the maximum allowable amount of nitrous oxide in the dental environment is 50 parts per million (ppm). Without proper precautions, hazardous concentrations of nitrous oxide in the dental environment can reach 900 ppm.

Masks are designed to have a **scavenger system** attached for the protection of the dental team. A scavenger system should always be used to reduce the amount of nitrous oxide exhaled into the air by the patient and thus breathed by members of the dental team (Figure 14-7). The use of a scavenger system is recommended to reduce the amount of nitrous oxide released into the treatment area.

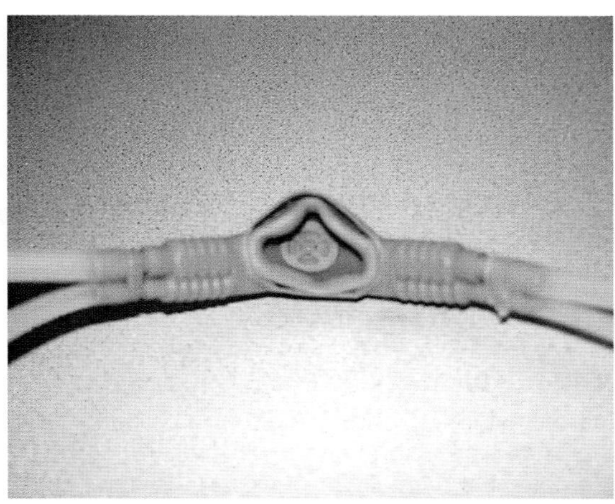

FIGURE 14-7 Scavenger system attached to the mask and evacuation unit to redirect unused nitrous oxide gas.

Patient Assessment and Monitoring

In specific states, credentialed dental assistants are allowed to assess and monitor nitrous oxide–oxygen analgesia under the direct supervision of the dentist. Before the administration of nitrous oxide analgesia begins, the patient must be informed about what to expect. This includes:

- Explaining the process of administering the gases
- Describing how to use the mask and explaining the importance of nasal breathing
- Describing the sensations of warmth and tingling that the patient may experience
- Reassuring the patient that he or she will remain conscious, aware, and in control of his or her actions

The baseline is the ratio of nitrous oxide to oxygen that is most effective for each patient. At the baseline, the patient is conscious and cooperative but pleasantly relaxed. The dentist determines the volumes of nitrous oxide and oxygen and the time necessary for the patient to reach baseline. The least amount of nitrous oxide should always be used. For most patients, 30% nitrous oxide or less is effective. Small children typically require less. Once the baseline has been determined, this information is recorded on the patient's record at each appointment.

See Procedure 14-4: Assisting in the Administration and Monitoring of Nitrous Oxide–Oxygen Sedation (Expanded Function).

Antianxiety Agents

Antianxiety drugs are prescribed for the relief of anxiety. In larger doses, these drugs can produce sleep, sedation, and anesthesia. Antianxiety agents can be orally or intravenously administered or by inhalation (gases). Before administering any form of an antianxiety drug, the dentist is required to have specialized training in the choice of agents and the method of delivery.

Antianxiety agents commonly prescribed include secobarbital (Seconal), chlordiazepoxide (Librium), and diazepam

(Valium), which can suppress mild to moderate anxiety. Chloral hydrate (Noctec) is a sedative that is often used for sedating children.

When these drugs are prescribed, the patient will be asked to take the drug orally 30 to 60 minutes before the appointment. Patients must be informed that these drugs induce drowsiness and that they should not drive themselves to and from the appointment.

Indications for the Use of Antianxiety Drugs

- The patient is apprehensive about a procedure.
- The procedure is long and/or difficult.
- The patient is mentally or physically compromised.
- The patient is a very young child in need of extensive treatment.

Analgesic Agents

Analgesic agents are drugs that dull the perception of pain without producing unconsciousness. They may be prescribed to relieve a toothache or to relieve postoperative pain. Patients may be less anxious if they are assured of adequate pain control.

Mild analgesic drugs, such as aspirin, ibuprofen, or acetaminophen, are used for the relief of low-intensity pain. These analgesic agents provide adequate pain relief for many types of dental pain, including a toothache or the discomfort that may follow the extraction of a tooth.

Strong analgesic drugs can include a narcotic drug and are only to be prescribed for patients with severe pain, such as that which follows extensive surgical procedures. Examples of narcotic drugs include codeine, oxycodone (Percodan), meperidine (Demerol), morphine, and hydromorphone (Dilaudid). Narcotic drugs are capable of producing physical and psychologic dependence, and their extended use should be avoided.

Prescriptions

A prescription is a written order authorizing the pharmacist to supply a certain drug to a patient. The prescription, itself, is made up of the components shown in Figure 14-8. When the dentist prescribes medication, a record of the prescription is recorded in the patient's record.

Under no circumstance may a dental assistant prescribe medication. Medicine is dispensed only with explicit instructions and under the direct supervision of the dentist.

Brand names or **trade names** of a drug are controlled by the business firm as a registered trademark; for example, Tylenol is a brand name of acetaminophen. Brand names are always capitalized.

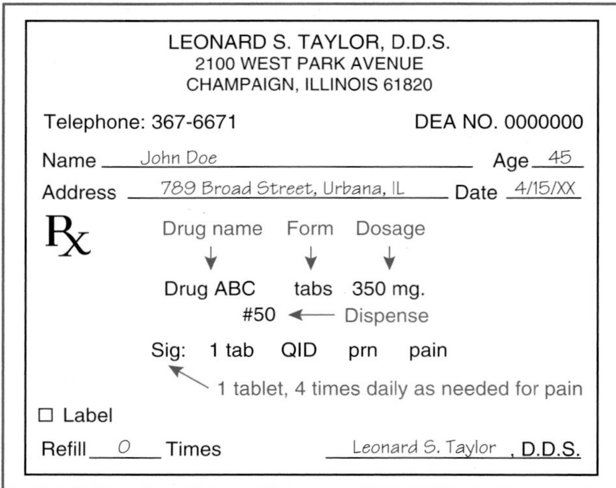

LEONARD S. TAYLOR, D.D.S.
2100 WEST PARK AVENUE
CHAMPAIGN, ILLINOIS 61820

Telephone: 367-6671 DEA NO. 0000000

Name John Doe Age 45

Address 789 Broad Street, Urbana, IL Date 4/15/XX

℞ Drug name Form Dosage

Drug ABC tabs 350 mg.

#50 ← Dispense

Sig: 1 tab QID prn pain

1 tablet, 4 times daily as needed for pain

☐ Label

Refill 0 Times Leonard S. Taylor, D.D.S.

FIGURE 14-8 Sample prescription blank. (Courtesy Patterson Office Supplies, Champaign, Illinois.)

Generic names are those drug names that any business firm may use. All common and unprotected names fall into this second group. Generic names are not capitalized.

For example, Valium is the brand name of a drug used to treat anxiety. The generic name for Valium is diazepam.

Documentation of Anesthesia and Pain Control

Keeping accurate records is an essential aspect of pain and anxiety analgesia. The following information is always documented in the progress notes section of the patient record:

- Preoperative and postoperative vital signs
- Tidal volume if inhalation sedation is provided
- Time anesthesia began and ended
- Peak concentration administered
- Postoperative time (in minutes) for patient recovery
- Adverse events or patient complaints

Ethical Implications

Prescribed drugs come in many forms and are supplied in many applications. The drugs used in dentistry provide a great range in helping patients feel at ease from anxiety or relief from pain. Drugs can also pose great potential for harming patients. Caution must always be taken when preparing and assisting in the administration of drugs.

A patient of the practice may have a substance abuse problem and may come to your office "under the influence" or may even try to solicit prescriptions from the dentist. Pay special attention to managing the prescription pads, controlled substances, and nitrous oxide in your office.

Procedure 14-1

Applying a Topical Anesthetic Ointment

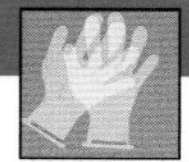

Equipment and Supplies

- 2 × 2-inch gauze squares
- Topical anesthetic ointment
- Sterile cotton-tip applicator

Procedural Steps

Preparation

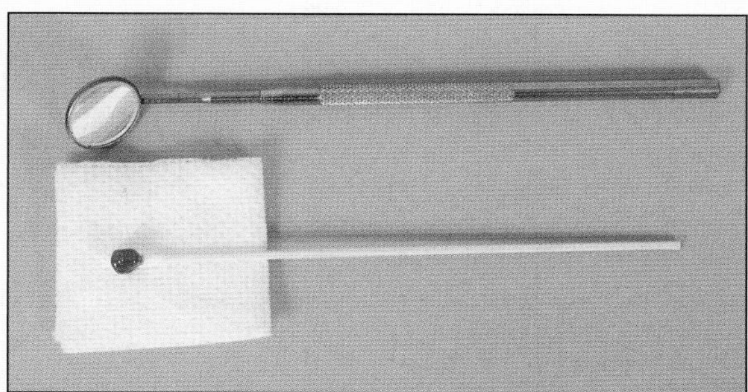

1. Place a small amount of topical ointment on the end of the cotton-tip applicator. Replace the cover of the ointment.

Note: Never insert the same applicator into the ointment after it has been used and contaminated.

2. Explain the procedure to the patient.

Purpose: Patients are more comfortable and less anxious when they are well informed and know what to expect.

3. Determine the injection site, and gently dry the site with a 2 × 2 gauze square.

Purpose: Drying the site allows the ointment to penetrate the surface area better and not become diluted by saliva, which would decrease its effectiveness.

Placement

1. Place the ointment directly on the injection site.

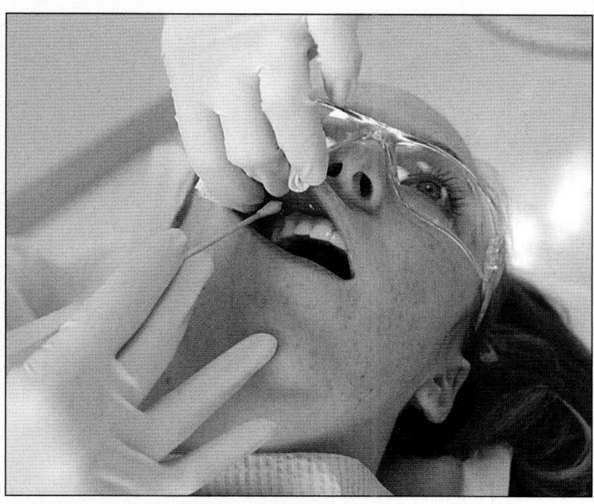

2. Allow the applicator to remain on the site for 3 to 5 minutes.
3. Remove the applicator just before the dentist gives the injection.

Purpose: The site should not be wet with saliva, which would decrease the effect of the ointment.

Procedure 14-2

Assembling the Local Anesthetic Syringe

Equipment and Supplies

- Sterile syringe
- Sealed disposable needle or needles
- Sterile local anesthetic cartridges

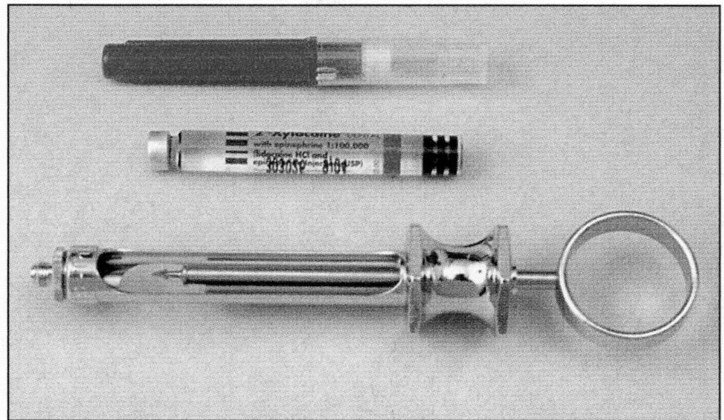

Procedural Steps

Selecting the Anesthetic Set-up

1. The location of the injection will determine the needle length. The dentist determines the type of anesthetic solution.

Purpose: The choices of anesthetic solution and needle length depend on the patient's medical and dental history and the procedure.

2. Organize supplies, and position the items at chairside out of the patient's view.
3. Wash hands before preparing the syringe.

Loading the Anesthetic Cartridge

1. Hold the syringe in one hand, and use the thumb ring to pull back the plunger.

Continued

Procedure 14-2

Assembling the Local Anesthetic Syringe—cont'd

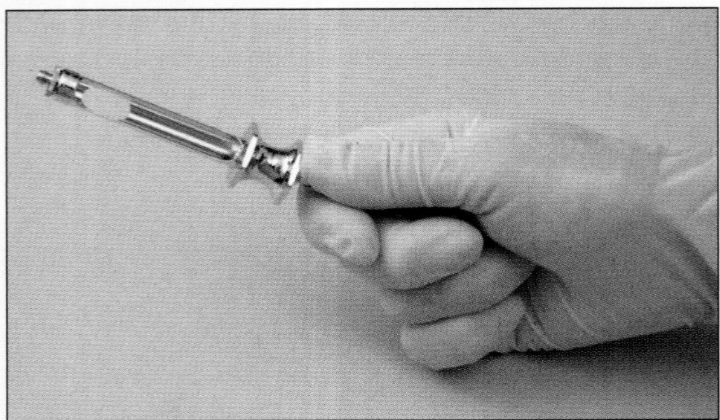

2. With the other hand, load the anesthetic cartridge into the syringe. The stopper end goes in first, toward the plunger.

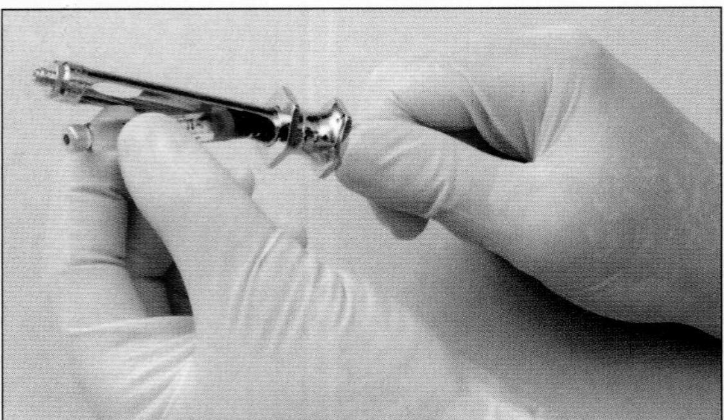

3. Release the thumb ring, and allow the harpoon to engage into the stopper.
4. Use gentle finger pressure to engage the piston forward until the harpoon is engaged into the stopper.

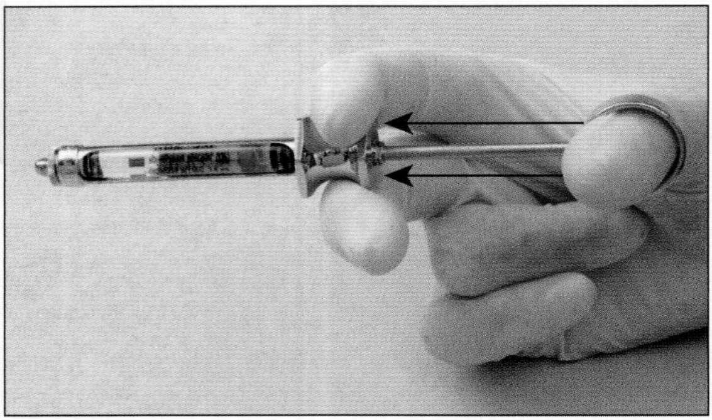

Note: DO NOT hit the piston with the palm of your hand in an effort to engage the harpoon. This could lead to fracturing of the glass cartridge.

5. To ensure that the harpoon is securely in place, gently pull back on the plunger.

Purpose: The harpoon must be securely engaged so that the dentist can aspirate during the injection.

Placing the Needle on the Syringe

1. Break the seal on the needle, and remove the protective cap from the needle. The protective guard (clear plastic) is removed at this time. The needle guard is not yet removed.
2. Screw the needle into position on the syringe. Take care to position the needle so that it is straight and firmly attached.

Purpose: If the needle is not correctly positioned, then the anesthetic solution may leak or may not flow properly.

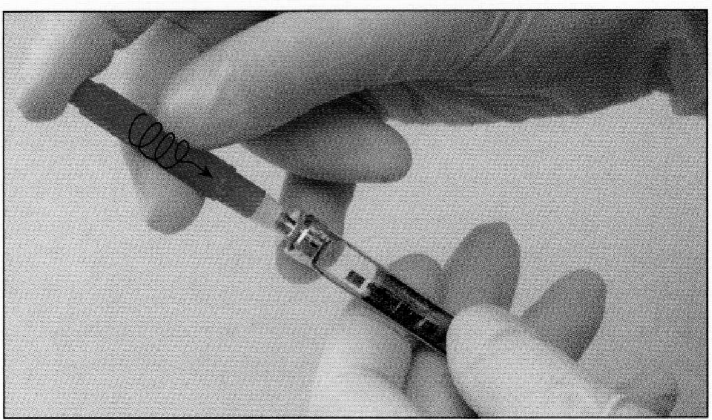

3. Place the prepared syringe on the tray ready for use and out of the patient's sight.

Note: Previous teaching suggested that the needle be attached to the syringe before placing the anesthetic cartridge. Stanley Malamed recommends the above sequence of steps because it virtually eliminates the possibility of a broken cartridge or leakage of anesthetic solution during the procedure.

Photos from Malamed SF: *Handbook of local anesthesia,* ed 6, St. Louis, 2013, Mosby.

Procedure 14-3

Assisting in the Administration of Local Anesthesia

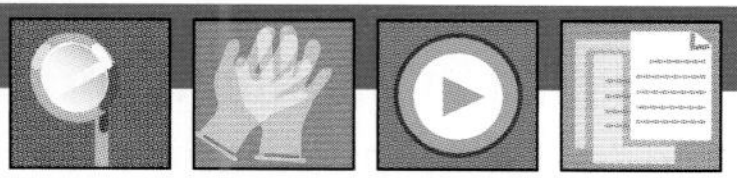

Equipment and Supplies

- Topical anesthetic ointment
- Sterile cotton-tip applicators
- Sterile gauze sponges
- Sterile assembled local anesthetic syringe

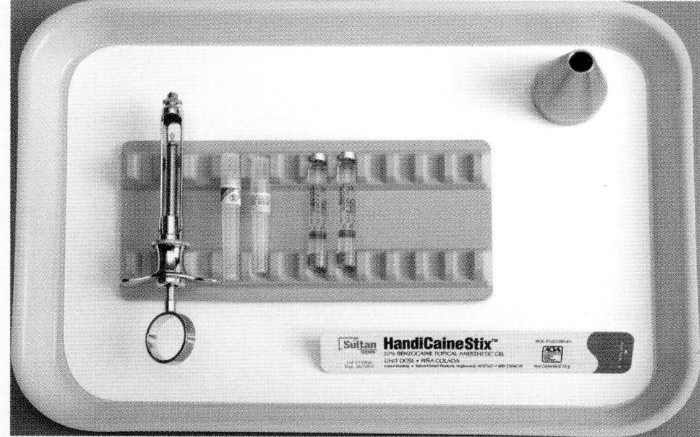

(From Boyd LRB: *Dental instruments: a pocket guide,* ed 5, St. Louis, 2015, Saunders.)

Procedural Steps

1. Apply a topical anesthetic solution to the appropriate area of injection (see Procedure 14-1).
2. Loosen the needle guard.
3. Transfer the syringe to the operator by placing the thumb ring over the dentist's thumb.

Note: This exchange takes place just below the patient's chin and out of the patient's line of vision.

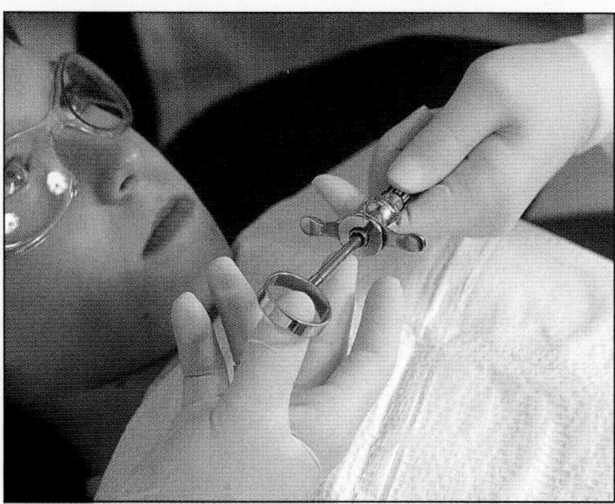

4. While the dentist is giving the injection, monitor the patient for any adverse reactions, and project a calming and relaxed manner.
5. The dentist will return the contaminated syringe to the tray and will replace the needle guard by using a one-handed scoop technique or a recapping device.

Purpose: This step prevents the possibility of a needle stick injury.

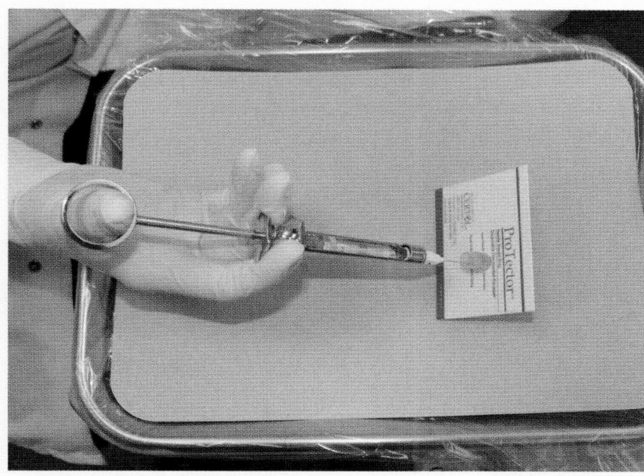

(From Logothesis DD: *Local anesthesia for the dental hygienist,* St. Louis, 2012, Mosby.)

6. After the injection is completed, have the patient turn toward you. Rinse the patient's mouth using the air-water syringe and the high-volume evacuator or saliva ejector.
7. Continue monitoring the patient throughout the procedure for any adverse effects.
8. At the completion of the procedure, instruct the patient about the numbness and not to bite his or her lip or cheek.
9. Before leaving the dental treatment area, remove the used needle with the needle guard still in place, and dispose of it in the sharps container.
10. Remove the anesthetic cartridge, and dispose of it with the medical waste. Place the syringe on the tray to be returned to the sterilization center.
11. Record the type and amount of anesthesia used for the procedure.

Procedure 14-4

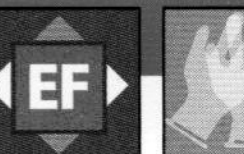
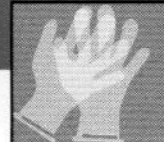
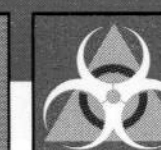
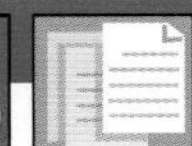

Assisting in the Administration and Monitoring of Nitrous Oxide–Oxygen Sedation (Expanded Function)

Equipment and Supplies

- Nitrous oxide–oxygen sedation system
- Scavenger-type masks (adult and child sizes)
- Equipment for measuring vital signs

Procedural Steps

1. Check the tanks for an adequate supply of gases. Select and place the appropriate size of mask on the tubing.
2. Seat the patient, update the medical history, and take and record vital signs.
3. Review the use of nitrous oxide with the patient.

Purpose: Informing the patient before administration helps eliminate fear of the unknown.

4. Place the patient in a supine position.
5. Have the patient position the mask over his or her nose and adjust the fit.

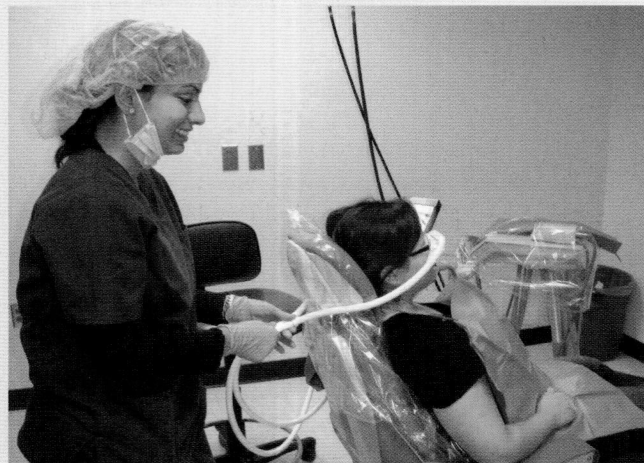

6. Tighten the tubing once it is comfortable for the patient.

Purpose: Tightening the tubing eliminates the need for the patient to hold the mask in place and to prevent leakage from around the mask.

7. If the mask pinches or causes discomfort, then place a gauze square under the edge.

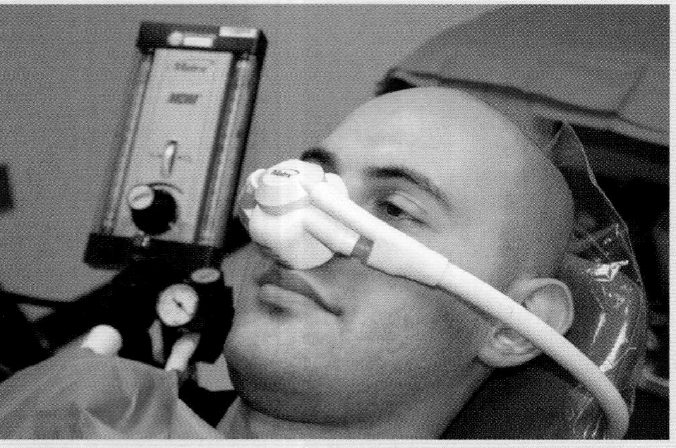

Administration

1. At the dentist's instructions, begin adjusting the flow meter for oxygen flow only. The patient is given 100% oxygen for at least 1 minute.

Nitrous oxide–oxygen

2. At the dentist's direction, adjust the flow of nitrous oxide in increments of 0.5 to 1 liters per minute, and reduce the oxygen flow by a corresponding amount.

Note: Most machines automatically perform this function.

3. At 1-minute intervals, the previous step is repeated until the dentist determines that the patient has reached the baseline reading.

Purpose: This slow process minimizes the risk of administering too much nitrous oxide.

4. Note the patient's baseline level.
5. Closely monitor the patient throughout the procedure.

Oxygenation

1. Toward the end of the procedure, nitrous oxide is depleted and 100% oxygen is administered, as directed by the dentist.

Purpose: Oxygenation of patients for a minimum of 5 minutes helps prevent diffusion hypoxia, which creates a feeling of lightheadedness.

2. After the oxygenation is complete, remove the mask. Slowly position the patient upright.

Purpose: Bringing the patient upright too quickly may cause postural hypotension (fainting).

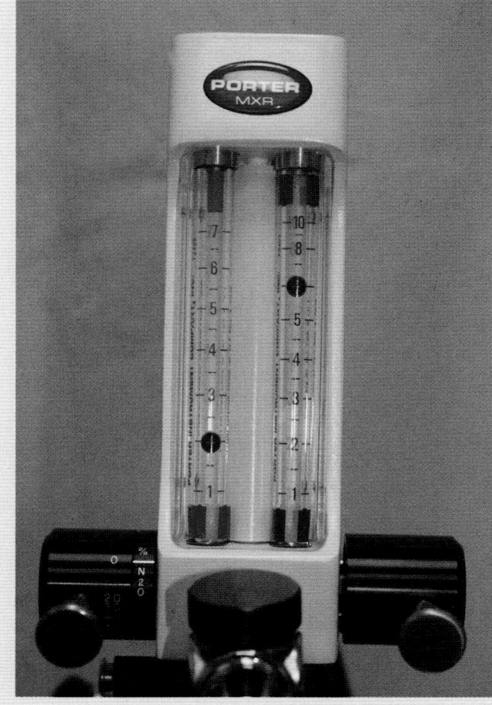

3. Record the patient's baseline levels of nitrous oxide and oxygen and his or her response during analgesia.

Purpose: This documentation provides a legal record of care and serves as a reference for future care and the administration of nitrous oxide–oxygen sedation (analgesia).

Photos from Malamed SF: *Sedation: a guide to patient management,* ed 5, St Louis, 2009, Mosby.

Chapter Exercises

Multiple Choice

Circle the letter next to the correct answer.

1. __________ is a health disorder to which the dentist should be alerted when selecting an anesthetic with a vasoconstrictor.
   a. Arthritis
   b. Paralysis
   c. Liver disease
   d. Migraine headaches
2. Oxygen and nitrous oxide gases are supplied in steel cylinders. The color-coding for the nitrous oxide tanks is __________.
   a. yellow
   b. blue
   c. green
   d. red
3. Anesthetic cartridges should be __________.
   a. maintained in the refrigerator until their use
   b. sterilized before use
   c. maintained in their packaging
   d. disinfected before use
4. A vasoconstrictor is a drug that has been added to local anesthetic agents to cause the blood vessels to __________.
   a. expand
   b. constrict
   c. bleed
   d. dissolve
5. __________ anesthesia is achieved by the dentist injecting the anesthetic solution into the nerve trunk.
   a. Block
   b. Infiltration
   c. Topical
   d. Analgesia
6. A __________-inch needle is selected when administering infiltration of a local anesthetic.
   a. 1
   b. 1⅝
   c. 2
   d. 2⅝
7. Topical anesthetics should remain on the oral mucosa for __________.
   a. 30 seconds
   b. 1 minute
   c. 2 to 5 minutes
   d. 7 to 10 minutes
8. __________ is the most commonly used form of topical anesthetic for a local anesthesia procedure.
   a. Patch
   b. Liquid
   c. Ointment
   d. Spray
9. After a procedure, the contaminated needle is discarded in the?
   a. Sharps container
   b. Sterilization center
   c. Treatment room
   d. Garbage
10. Before applying topical anesthetic ointment, __________.
    a. gently dry the tissue
    b. thoroughly rinse the area
    c. blow air on the site from the air-water syringe
    d. tightly pull the mucosa

Apply Your Knowledge

1. You are assisting in a restorative procedure for teeth #2, #3, and #5. As you prepare the local anesthetic setup, what should be retrieved for the setup? Remember the type of injection and how many teeth will be involved.
2. The dentist has just completed administering the injection, and he transfers a contaminated uncapped syringe back to you over the patient's chest. Will you receive the syringe? If not, what will you do?
3. A patient is receiving nitrous oxide–oxygen sedation analgesia during a procedure. The patient has no indication in the record about any adverse effects, but your patient seems anxious and fidgety. What is your sense of the situation, and how do you handle this situation?

PART SIX Dental Imaging

CHAPTER 15

Radiation Safety and Production of X-Rays

http://evolve.elsevier.com/Robinson/essentials/

LEARNING OBJECTIVES

1. Pronounce, define, and spell the key terms.
2. Explain the uses of dental radiology and discuss the benefits of x-rays.
3. Define *x-rays,* discuss the anatomic structure of matter, and describe ionization.
4. Describe the properties of x-ray beams.
5. Differentiate among the types of radiation.
6. Complete the following related to radiation measurement and radiation exposure:
   - Describe how to measure radiation using both the standard and the metric system.
   - Discuss radiation exposure.
   - Define *absorbed dose* and determine dose equivalents.
7. Complete the following related to radiation hazards and protection:
   - Define *maximum permissible dose*.
   - Explain the ALARA principle.
8. Discuss the biologic effects of radiation, including the differences between somatic and genetic effects of x-rays.
9. Discuss the methods used to protect patients from radiation.
10. Discuss the methods used to protect the operator from radiation.
11. Identify the various components of the dental x-ray machine.
12. Define *radiopaque* and *radiolucent*.
13. List and describe the four factors that affect the quality of a radiograph.

KEY TERMS

absorbed dose
acute radiation exposure
ALARA principle
anode
background radiation
cathode
cervical collar
chronic radiation exposure
collimation
collimator
contrast
control panel
cumulative effects
density
digital imaging
dose equivalence
filter
filtration
focusing cup
F-speed film
genetic changes
ionization
latent period
leakage radiation
maximum permissible dose (MPD)
object-film distance (OFD)
photon
position indicator device (PID)
primary radiation
radiation monitoring
radiolucent
radiopaque
scatter radiation
secondary radiation
somatic changes
source-film distance
tubehead

BOX 15-1 Benefits of Dental Radiographs

- Detect dental decay in the early stages.
- Identify bone loss in the early stages.
- Locate abnormalities in surrounding hard and soft tissues.
- Evaluate growth and development.
- Document the condition of a patient at a specific time.
- Obtain information during a dental procedure, such as a broken root tip during an oral surgical procedure.

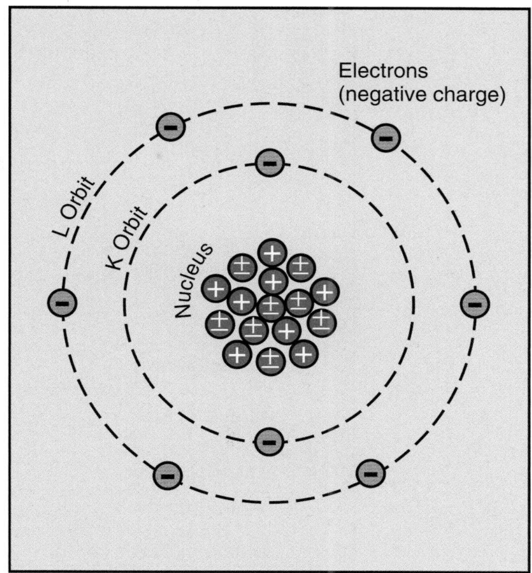

FIGURE 15-1 Diagrammatic representation of an oxygen atom.

Dental images are essential in the practice of dentistry and may be produced on conventional x-ray film or by digital technology. Regardless of the technique used, a quality image is necessary to identify and diagnose conditions that otherwise may go undetected.

Dental images, commonly known as x-ray images, are part of the patient's permanent dental record. Radiation, which is used to produce all dental images, has the ability to cause damage to all types of living tissue. Any exposure to radiation, no matter how small, has the potential to cause harm to the operator and to the patient.

The benefits of using x-ray images in dentistry certainly outweigh the risks when proper safety procedures are followed (Box 15-1). This chapter discusses radiation hazards, the production of x-ray images, and the methods used to protect the patient and operator from the harmful effects of exposure to radiation.

Radiation Physics

An understanding of the basic principles of radiation physics and how x-ray images are produced will help the dental assistant to practice safely and to produce high-quality images.

Definition

X-ray beams can be defined as weightless bundles of energy (photons) without an electrical charge that travel in waves at the speed of light.

Atomic Structure

The basic anatomic structure of matter is important because it directly relates to the ways in which x-ray beams are produced, emitted (given off) from the machine, and absorbed by the body tissue of both patient and the operator.

All matter is made of atoms. Atoms are extremely minute and consist of (1) an inner core, or nucleus, that possesses a positive electrical charge; and (2) a number of negatively charged particles called *electrons* that orbit around the nucleus. The nucleus of an atom consists of positively charged subatomic particles called *protons* and subatomic particles called *neutrons* that have no charge.

The arrangement within the atom is similar to that of the solar system. The atom has a nucleus as its center, similar to the sun, and the electrons revolve around it like planets (Figure 15-1). The electrons remain stable in their orbit unless disturbed or removed.

In the neutral or stable atom, the number of orbiting electrons (−) equals the number of protons (+) in the nucleus; hence the atom is electrically neutral.

Atoms, in turn, join to form molecules. A molecule is the smallest particle of a substance that retains the property of the original substance.

Ionization

Ionization is the harmful effect of x-ray beams in humans that results in a disruption of cellular structure and causes permanent damage to living cells and tissue. When x-ray beams strike a patient's tissue, ionization results.

During ionization, electrons are removed from electrically stable atoms by collisions with photons. (A **photon** is a minute bundle of pure energy that has no weight or mass.) The atoms that lose electrons become positive ions. Negative electrons become negative ions. As such, they are unstable structures capable of interacting with (and damaging) other atoms, tissue, or chemicals.

Properties of X-Ray Beams

X-ray beams are a form of energy that can penetrate matter and have unique properties (Table 15-1). Similar to visible light and radar, radio, and television waves, x-ray beams belong to a group called *electromagnetic radiation* (Figure 15-2). Electromagnetic radiation is made of photons that travel through space at the speed of light in a straight line with a wavelike motion.

The shorter the wavelength of radiation, the greater its energy. Because of the high energy of short wavelengths, they are able to penetrate matter more easily than longer wavelengths. The unique properties of x-ray beams make them especially valuable in dentistry.

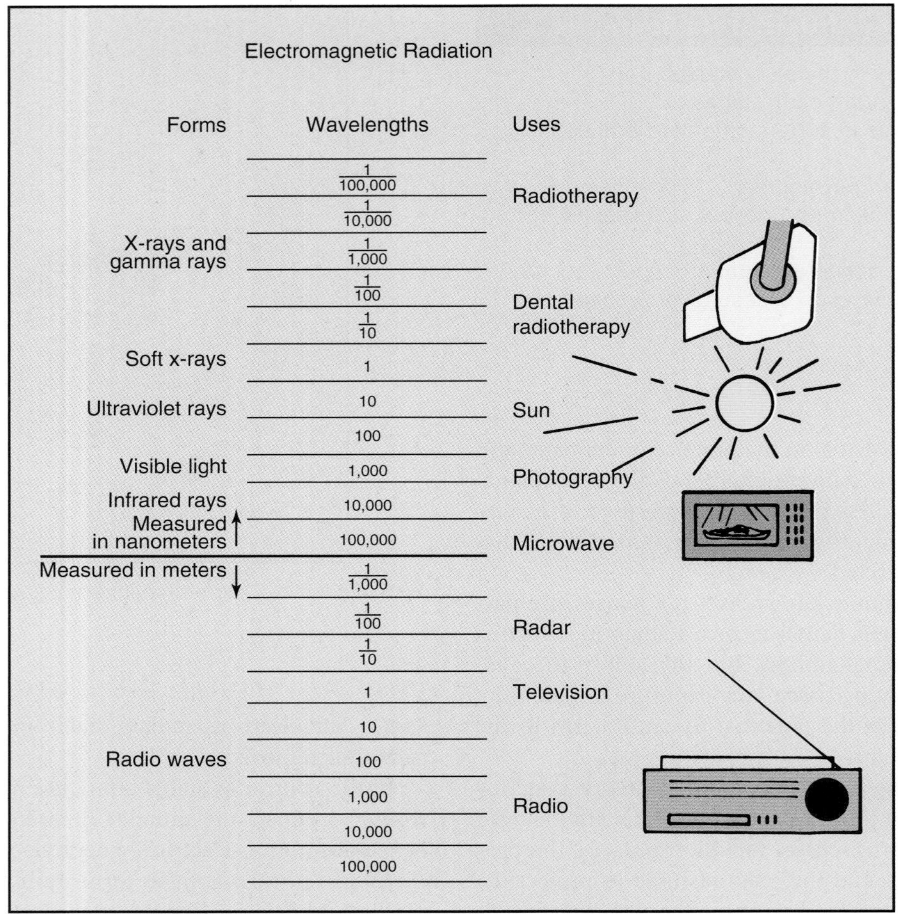

FIGURE 15-2 Electromagnetic spectrum, showing the various wavelengths of radiation typically used.

TABLE 15-1
Properties of an X-Ray Beam

Property	Comment
Appearance	Is invisible.
Mass	Has no mass or weight.
Charge	Has no charge.
Speed	Travels at the speed of light.
Path of travel	Travels in a straight line but can be deflected or scattered.
Focusing ability	Cannot be focused.
Penetrating ability	Penetrates solids, liquids, and gases.
Absorption	Can be absorbed by matter.
Ionization ability	Causes ionization.
Fluorescence	Can cause certain substances to fluoresce (glow).
Effect on film	Produces an image on photographic film.
Effect on living tissue	Causes biologic changes in living cells.

Types of Radiation

Primary radiation, also known as the central ray or primary beam, is the stream of radiation as it is emitted from the x-ray unit. The primary beam travels in a straight line and contains powerful short wavelengths. It is the short wavelengths in the dental ray that produce diagnostically useful radiographs (Figure 15-3, **A**).

Secondary radiation in dentistry is given off after the primary beam comes into contact with the soft tissue of the head, the bones of the skull, and the teeth. Secondary radiation is less penetrating than primary radiation because the rays become weaker after they contact the tissue; however, the patient still may absorb these rays (Figure 15-3, **B**).

Scatter radiation is a form of secondary radiation that occurs when an x-ray beam is deflected from its path during impact with the patient. (*Deflected* means turned aside.) Scatter radiation travels in all directions and is impossible to confine. Without adequate protective barriers, the operator and others nearby may be affected by exposure to scatter radiation (Figure 15-3, **C**).

Leakage radiation is radiation that escapes in all directions from a faulty x-ray tubehead. Equipment should be frequently checked and immediately repaired when necessary.

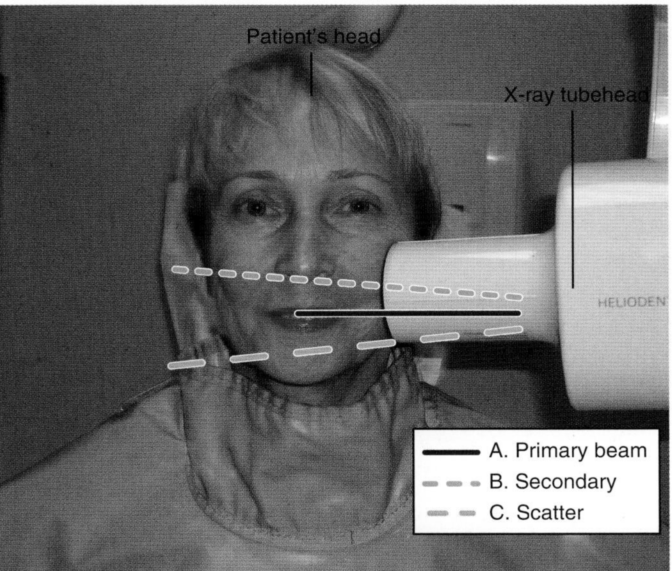

FIGURE 15-3 Types of radiation interaction with the patient. **A**, Primary. **B**, Secondary. **C**, Scatter.

TABLE 15-2
Equivalent Traditional and SI Units of Radiation Measurement

Measurement	Traditional System	SI System
Radiation exposure	1 roentgen (R)	1 coulomb per kilogram (C/kg)
Absorbed dose	100 radiation absorbed doses (rad)	1 gray (Gy)
Dose equivalence	100 roentgen equivalents [in] man (rem)	1 sievert (Sv)

SI, Système Internationale d'Unités.

Radiation Measurement

Just as distance can be measured in miles or kilometers and time can be measured in hours or minutes, radiation is also measured. Two sets of systems are currently used to define the way radiation is measured. The older system is referred to as the **traditional**, or **standard** system. The newer system is the metric equivalent known as the **Système Internationale d'Unités (SI)**.

Traditional units of radiation measurement include:

- Roentgen (R)
- Radiation absorbed dose (rad)
- Roentgen equivalent [in] man (rem)

SI units include:

- Coulomb/kilogram (C/kg)
- Gray (Gy)
- Sievert (Sv)

Both systems are presented here, and the units are compared in Table 15-2.

Radiation Exposure

The term *radiation exposure* refers to the amount of radiation to which a person is exposed and is measured in SI units as coulombs per kilogram (C/kg). The traditional term is the roentgen (R). One C/kg equals 1 (R).

Absorbed Dose

The amount of radiation energy actually absorbed by tissue is the absorbed dose. The SI unit of **absorbed dose** is called a gray (Gy). The traditional system used the term radiation-absorbed dose (rad) as the unit of measurement. The conversions for rad and Gy are as follows:

$$1\,\text{Gy} = 100\,\text{rad}$$

$$1\,\text{rad} = 0.01\,\text{Gy}$$

Dose Equivalence

The **dose equivalence** measurement is used to compare the biologic effects of different types of radiation.

The SI unit of dose equivalence is the sievert (Sv). The traditional unit is a roentgen equivalent [in] man (rem): 1 Sv = 100 rem. Technically, some differences exist between the units of radiation measurement; however, in dental radiology, the units are virtually interchangeable. Conversions for the rem and Sv are as follows:

$$1\,\text{rem} = 0.01\,\text{Sv}$$

$$1\,\text{Sv} = 100\,\text{rem}$$

Radiation Hazards and Protection

We are exposed to radiation every day of our lives. **Background radiation** comes from natural sources, such as radioactive materials in the ground and cosmic radiation from space. Exposure from medical or dental sources is an additional risk. Because of their concern, patients frequently ask, "I've heard x-rays are bad for me. Do you really have to take them?" The dental assistant must anticipate this patient reaction and be able to explain to the patient the risks and diagnostic benefits of dental radiation, the safety precautions used during radiographic exposure, and the benefits of detecting disease that might not otherwise be detected, all of which far outweigh the risks from receiving small doses of radiation.

Note: Two important concepts are basic to radiation protection. The first is the concept of maximum permissible dose, and the second is the ALARA principle.

Maximum Permissible Dose

The **maximum permissible dose (MPD)** is the exposure limit for those who are occupationally exposed to radiation when observing all safety practices. This amount of radiation to the whole body produces very little chance of injury.

The MPD for whole-body exposure for an occupationally exposed person (e.g., dental radiographer) is 0.05 Sv (5 rem).

Occupationally exposed women who are pregnant are allowed an MPD of only 0.005 Sv (0.5 rem) per year. This is the same dose limit that applies to the general population.

Dental personnel should strive for an occupational dose of zero by adhering to strict radiation protection practices.

ALARA Principle

The ALARA principle or concept states that all exposure to radiation must be kept **A**s **L**ow **A**s **R**easonably **A**chievable. Every possible method of reducing exposure to radiation should be used. The radiation protection measures detailed in this chapter can be used to minimize exposure to both the patient and the operator.

Biologic Effects of Radiation

X-ray beams in sufficient doses may produce harmful effects in humans. Exposure to radiation can bring about changes in body chemicals, cells, tissues, and organs. The effects of the radiation may not become evident for many years after the time when the x-ray beams were absorbed. This time lag is called the latent period.

Some tissue in the body is more sensitive to the effects of radiation than others. Table 15-3 compares the relative sensitivity of specific cells and tissues. Note that tissues of the head and face that are exposed to dental x-ray beams are fairly high on the list.

TABLE 15-3
Relative Radiation Sensitivity of Cells and Tissue

Sensitivity to Radiation	Cell Type or Tissue
High	Small lymphocyte Bone marrow Reproductive cells Intestinal mucosa
Fairly high	Skin Lens of the eye Oral mucosa
Medium	Connective tissue Small blood vessels Growing bone and cartilage
Fairly low	Mature bone and cartilage Salivary gland Thyroid gland Kidney Liver
Low	Muscle Nerve

Modified from Miles DA, Van Dis ML, Williamson GF, Jensen CW: *Radiographic imaging for the dental team,* ed 4, St. Louis, 2009, Saunders.

Cumulative Effects

Exposure to radiation has a cumulative effect (builds up) over a lifetime. This damage can be compared with the wrinkles and injury damage that can occur to the skin from repeated exposure to the rays of the sun over the years.

Acute and Chronic Radiation Exposure

Acute radiation exposure occurs when a large dose of radiation is absorbed in a short time, such as in a nuclear accident.

Chronic radiation exposure occurs when small amounts of radiation are repeatedly absorbed over a long period. It may be years after the original exposure that the effects of chronic x-ray exposure are observed.

Genetic and Somatic Effects

X-ray exposure affects both genetic and somatic cells. Genetic cells are the reproductive cells (sperm and ova). Damage to genetic cells is passed on to succeeding generations. These genetic changes are referred to as **genetic mutations.**

All other cells in the body belong to the group of somatic tissue. (*Somatic* means referring to the body.) X-ray exposure can damage somatic tissue, but the damage caused by somatic changes is not passed on to future generations (Figure 15-4).

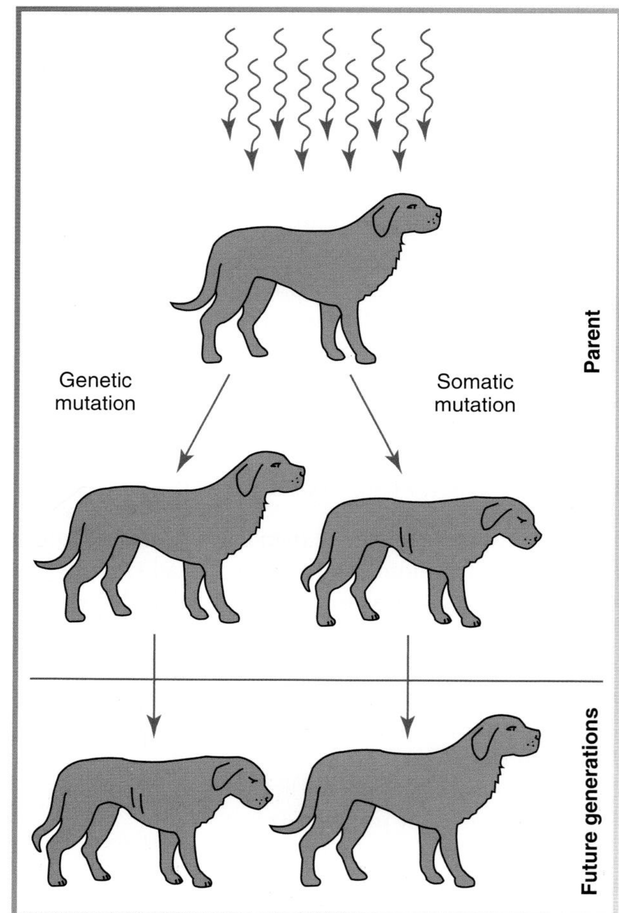

FIGURE 15-4 Comparison of somatic and genetic effects of radiation. (From Iannucci JM, Jansen Howerton L: *Dental radiography: principles and techniques,* ed 4, St. Louis, 2012, Saunders.)

Patient Protection

Minimizing Genetic Effects

Although the radiation dose to reproductive cells from dental radiography is very small, every patient must wear a lead apron and a thyroid collar during every radiographic procedure. Because of any possible risk of radiation during pregnancy, women of childbearing years are asked to let dental personnel know if they are pregnant. The exact amount of x-radiation that may produce damage to a developing human embryo or fetus is unknown. Nevertheless, postponing nonemergency radiographs until after pregnancy is advisable. In case of a dental emergency, a minimal number of films can be taken. As with all patients, the lead apron must cover the pregnant patient's entire abdomen.

Prescribing Radiographs

Every patient has different dental needs; therefore every patient should be individually evaluated for dental radiographs. The dentist is responsible for prescribing, or ordering, dental radiographs. Radiographs should never be taken at predetermined intervals. For example, the dentist who prescribes four bitewing radiographs every 6 months for every patient is not considering the individual needs of each patient.

To limit the amount of radiation a patient receives, the dentist must use professional judgment about the number, type, and frequency of dental radiographs (Box 15-2).

Fast-Speed Film

When using the conventional film-based technique, fast-speed film is the single most effective method of reducing a patient's exposure to x-ray beams. The faster the film speed, the less radiation is necessary for each exposure.

The film speed is determined by the amount of x-radiation needed to produce a high-quality radiograph. Film speed is rated in a range from A to F. Currently, F-speed film, or InSight, (Figure 15-5) is the fastest intraoral film available. Before the introduction of F-speed film, E-speed, or Ektaspeed, was the fastest film available. F-speed film provided an additional 20% reduction in exposure over E-speed films (and 60% reduction in exposure from earlier D-speed film, or Ultra-Speed). The film speed is determined by the size of the crystals in the emulsion that coats the film. Larger crystals (F speed) are more sensitive to radiation and need less radiation.

Film sizes and types of radiographs are discussed in Chapter 16.

BOX 15-2 Patient Protection

To ensure patient protection, the dentist should:

- Prescribe only the necessary radiographs.
- Use proper equipment (filters, collimators, and position indicator devices [PIDs]).
- Use the fastest-speed dental film.
- Use film-holding instruments.
- Use good film exposure techniques.
- Use lead aprons and thyroid collars for all patients.

Digital Imaging

Digital imaging requires **significantly less x-radiation** than conventional film-based radiography because the sensor used to capture the image is more sensitive to x-ray beams than is conventional film (Figure 15-6). Exposure times for digital images are 70% to 80% less than those required with conventional film. It is no longer a matter of *if* but rather *when* most dental practices will be using digital imaging. Digital radiography is discussed in greater detail in Chapter 16.

Proper Equipment

Another factor limiting the amount of radiation the patient receives is the use of proper equipment. The dental x-ray tubehead must be equipped with the appropriate aluminum filter, lead collimator, and position indicator device. The other components of the dental x-ray unit and tubehead are discussed in detail in Chapter 16.

Filtration

The purpose of the aluminum filter is to filter out longer-wavelength, low-energy x-rays from the x-ray beam (Figure 15-7). Low-energy, longer-wavelength x-rays are harmful to the patient and are not useful in producing a diagnostic image.

Filtration of the x-ray beam results in higher energy and a more penetrating, useful beam.

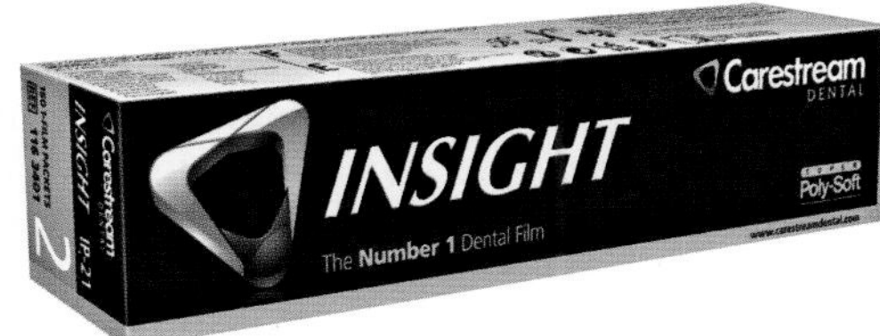

FIGURE 15-5 InSight intraoral dental film. (Courtesy Carestream Health, Inc., Rochester, New York.)

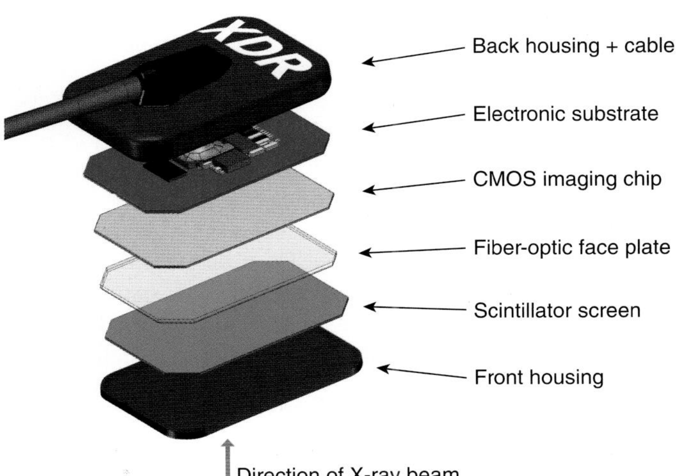

FIGURE 15-6 Exploded view of a solid-state image receptor. *CMOS*, Complementary metal-oxide semiconductor. (Courtesy of XDR Radiology, Los Angeles, California.)

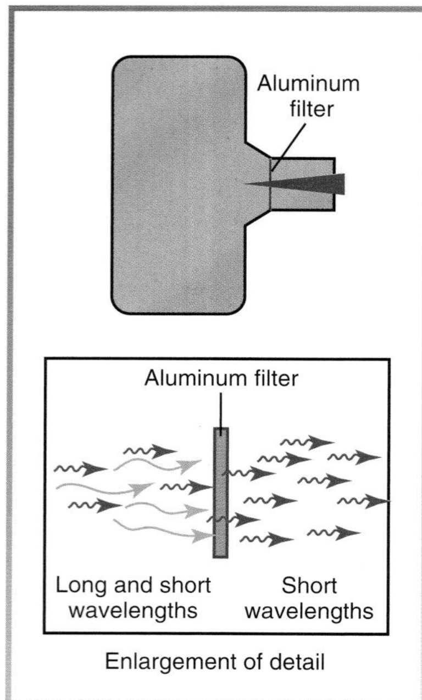

FIGURE 15-7 Aluminum discs are placed in the path of the x-ray beam to filter out low-energy long wavelengths, which are harmful to the patient. (From Iannucci JM, Jansen Howerton L: *Dental radiography: principles and techniques,* ed 4, St. Louis, 2012, Saunders.)

Collimation

Collimation is used to restrict the size and shape of the x-ray beam and to reduce patient exposure. The **collimator** is a lead plate with a hole in the center. It is placed directly over the opening in the machine housing where the x-ray beam exits the tubehead. The collimator may have a round or a rectangular opening. The rectangular collimator restricts the size of the x-ray beam to slightly larger than No. 2 intraoral film. (Film size is discussed in Chapter 16.) The round collimator produces a beam that is 2¾ inches in diameter—considerably larger than No. 2 intraoral film. When the shape and size of the beam are changed to a rectangle, the amount of tissue exposed can be reduced by more than one half (Figure 15-8).

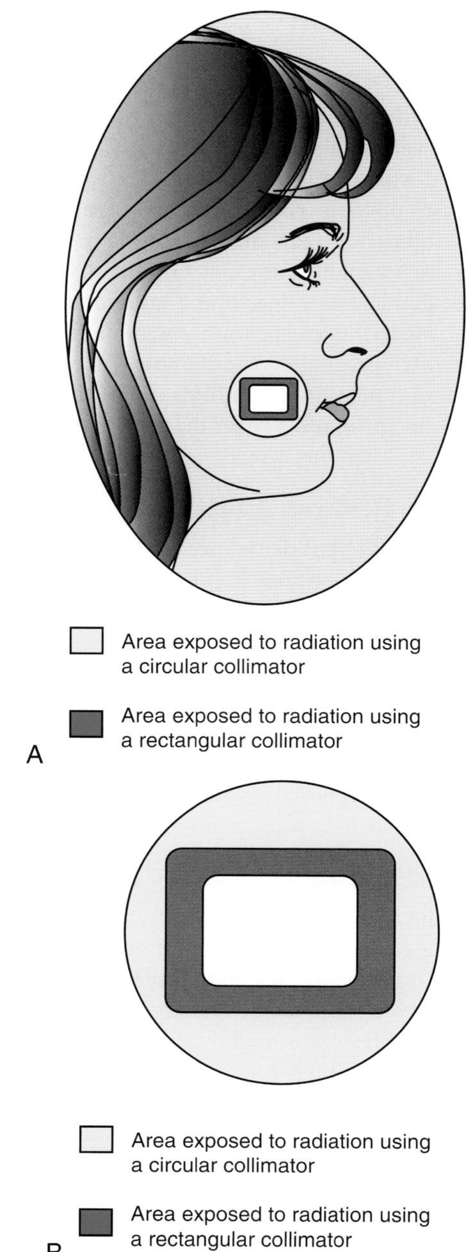

FIGURE 15-8 **A** and **B,** Rectangular collimation.

Position Indicator Device

The **position indicator device (PID)** is used to aim the x-ray beam at the film in the patient's mouth, thereby minimizing the amount of radiation to the patient's face. PIDs used in dentistry are usually 8, 12, or 16 inches long. The radiographic technique being used determines the length selected (see Chapter 16). To minimize patient exposure, the long PID is preferred because less divergence (spread) of the x-ray beam occurs (Figure 15-9).

Proper Film Exposure Technique

Unnecessary radiation exposure to patients is caused by the need for retakes. Every time a film must be retaken because of error in operator exposure technique or a processing error, the patient is exposed to double the amount of radiation. (Exposure techniques are discussed in Chapter 16.)

Film-Holding Instruments

Patients are sometimes asked to use their finger to hold the film in their mouth. This technique is not acceptable because the patient's hands and fingers are exposed to radiation.

A variety of film-holding instruments can be used to keep the patient's hand and fingers from being exposed to the x-ray beams (Figure 15-10). Film holders also hold the film in a stable position and aid the operator in properly positioning the film in the PID. (The technique for using film holders is discussed in Chapter 16.)

Lead Aprons and Thyroid Collars

The thyroid gland is susceptible to radiation during dental x-ray procedures. The function of lead aprons and thyroid collars is

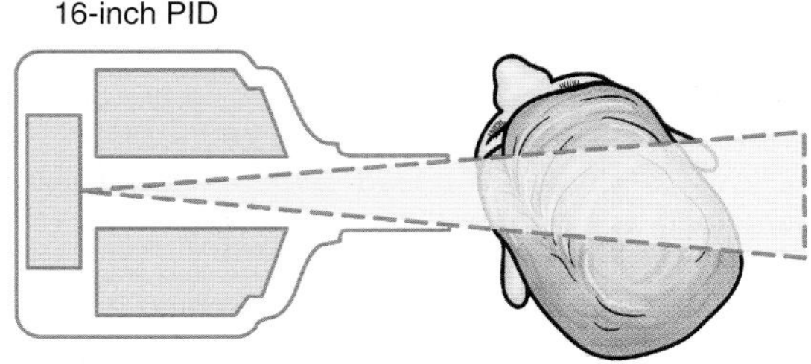

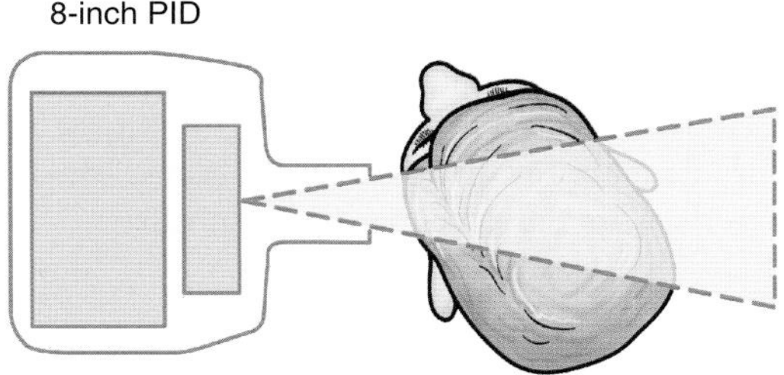

FIGURE 15-9 Compared with a short (8-inch) position indicator device (PID), a longer (16-inch) device is preferred because it produces less divergence of the x-ray beam. (Modified from Frommer H, Stabulas-Savage J: *Radiology for the Dental Professional,* ed 9, St Louis, 2011, Mosby.)

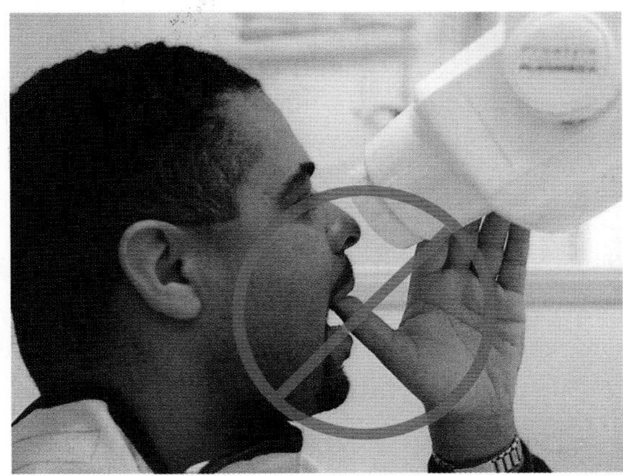

FIGURE 15-10 The patient's fingers are unnecessarily exposed to radiation when film holders are not used.

to reduce radiation exposure to the gonads and thyroid gland. A lead apron and thyroid collar must be used on all patients for all exposures (Figure 15-11). This rule applies to all patients, regardless of the patient's age or sex or the number of films to be taken. The lead apron should cover the patient from the thyroid and extend over the lap area.

The thyroid collar, also known as a **cervical collar**, covers the thyroid gland during the exposure and reduces radiation exposure to the gland. Most thyroid collars are part of the lead apron; however, they are also available as separate items.

The lead apron and the thyroid collar should be hung up or laid over a rounded bar rather than folded when not in use. (Folding eventually cracks the lead and allows radiation leakage.)

Most states now have laws that require the use of lead aprons during dental radiographic exposures.

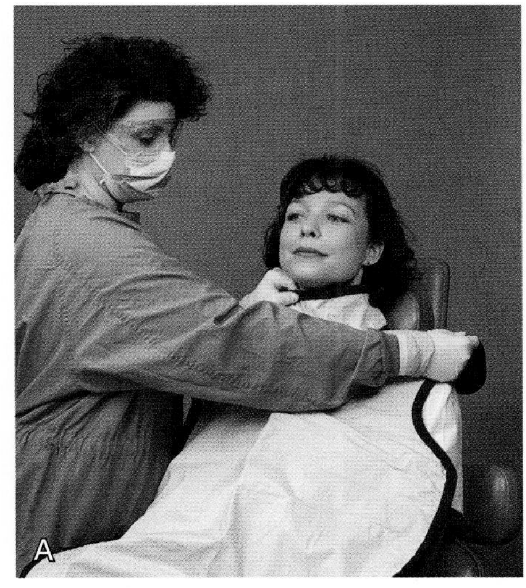

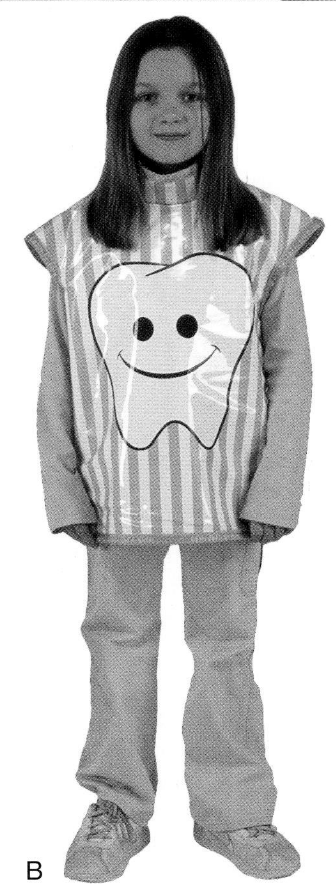

FIGURE 15-11 **A,** The lead apron and the thyroid collar must be large enough to cover the seated patient from the neck to above the knees. **B,** Children are more sensitive to radiation than adults; therefore the use of leaded aprons with thyroid collars is especially important for this population. (**B**, Courtesy Dentsply Rinn Corporation, http://rinncorp.com/.)

If the Patient is Unable to Hold the Film

If the patient is a child who is unable to cooperate, the child is seated on the parent's lap in the dental chair. Both the parent and the child are covered with the lead apron, and the parent holds the film in place (Figure 15-12). If the patient is an adult

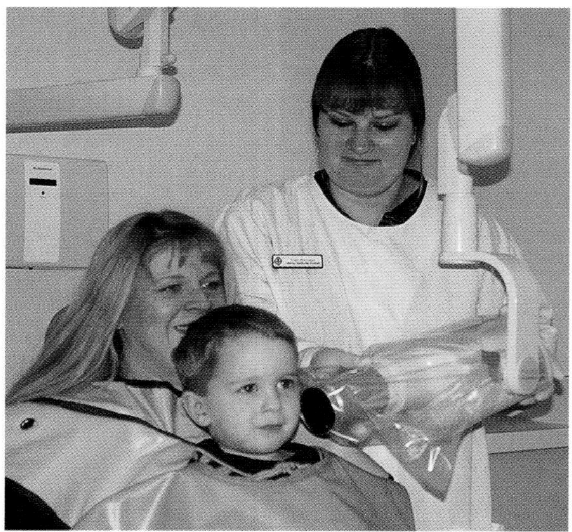

FIGURE 15-12 Child sitting on a parent's lap while a dental x-ray image is taken.

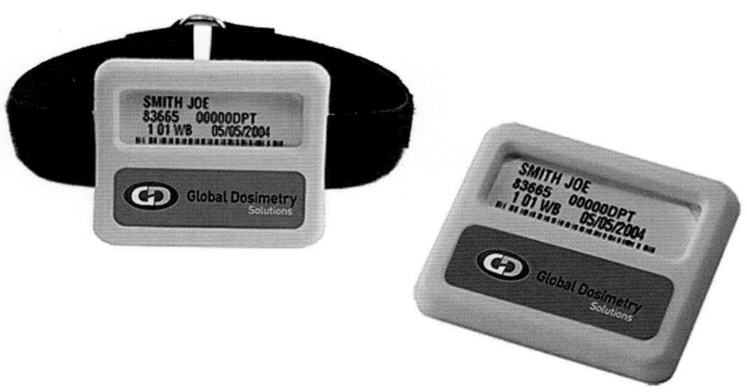

FIGURE 15-13 A film badge is used to monitor the amount of radiation that reaches the dental radiographer. (Courtesy of Global Dosimetry Solutions, Irvine, California.)

with disabilities, ask the caregiver to hold the film in place, and give the caretaker a lead apron to wear. Having the parent or caregiver hold the film is acceptable because this is a single exposure for that individual. If the dental assistant were to hold the film in this manner, he or she would have repeated exposures and would suffer the cumulative effects of radiation.

Protection of the Operator

Radiation Monitoring

Radiation monitors can be worn by the operator or placed on x-ray equipment or on walls. Radiation monitoring protects the operator by identifying occupational exposure to radiation.

Personnel Monitoring

A film badge (pocket dosimeter) is used to measure the amount of occupational exposure. The badge contains a film packet, similar to dental film, embossed with the wearer's name and identification number (Figure 15-13).

BOX 15-3 Rules of Radiation Protection

1. Never stand in the direct line of the primary beam.
2. Always stand behind a lead barrier or a proper thickness of drywall. If a lead barrier is not available, then stand at a right angle to the beam.
3. Never stand closer than 6 feet from the x-ray unit during an exposure, unless you are behind a barrier.

Employees are provided their own individual badge to be worn at all times while at work. Film badges should not be worn outside of the office, especially in bright sunlight. Film badges must be removed when the person being monitored is having medical or dental x-ray images taken because the badge is intended to measure only occupational exposure.

Equipment Monitoring

Dental x-ray machines should be monitored for leakage radiation. (Leakage radiation is any radiation, with the exception of the primary beam, that is emitted from the dental tubehead.) Dental x-ray equipment can be monitored through the use of a film device that can be obtained from the manufacturer or from the state health department.

Rules of Operator Protection

An assistant who fails to follow the rules of radiation protection may suffer the results of chronic radiation exposure. By following the rules of radiation protection, dental personnel can keep their radiation exposure to zero (Box 15-3).

Dental X-Ray Machine

Components of the Dental X-Ray Machine

Dental x-ray machines may vary slightly in size and appearance, but all have three primary components: the tubehead, an extension arm, and the control panel (Figure 15-14).

Tubehead

The primary function of the tubehead is to house the dental x-ray tube. The tubehead is made of metal and has a protective lead lining to prevent any radiation from escaping. (Lead is very effective at blocking radiation.)

Components of the dental x-ray tube The dental x-ray tube is made of glass and is approximately 6 inches long and 1½ inches in diameter (Figure 15-15). The air has been removed from the tube to create a vacuum. This vacuum environment allows electrons to flow with minimal resistance between the electrodes (cathode and anode).

Cathode. The cathode (−) is a tungsten filament. Tungsten is a metal capable of withstanding the intense heat given off during the generation of x-ray beams. Electrons are generated in the x-ray tube at the cathode. The hotter the filament becomes, the more electrons are produced.

Focusing cup. The focusing cup, also a part of the cathode, keeps the electrons suspended in a cloud at the cathode. When the exposure button is pressed, the circuit within the tubehead is completed, and the electrons very rapidly cross from the

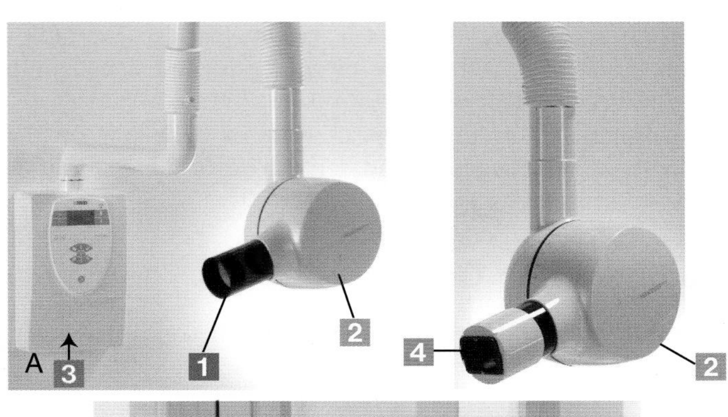

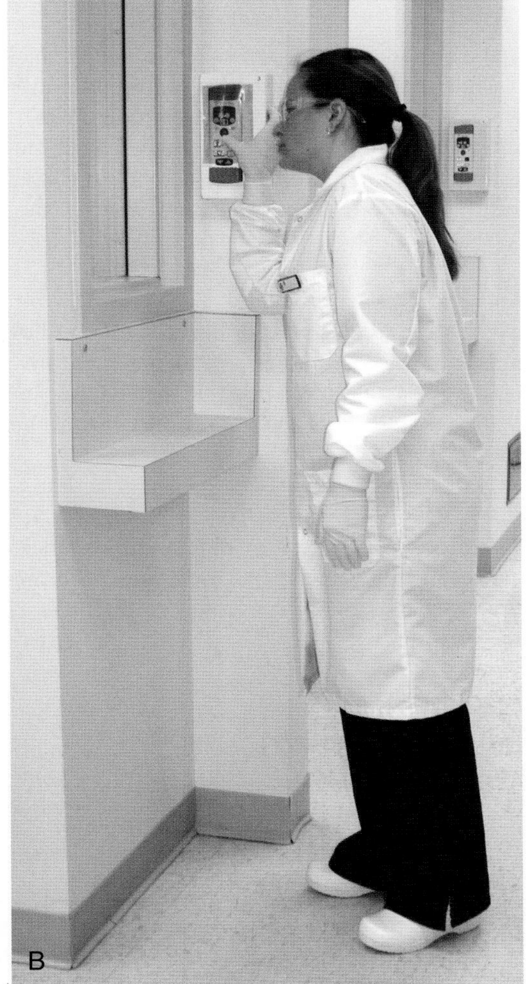

FIGURE 15-14 **A,** Dental x-ray unit. (1) Position indicator device (PID) (round); (2) tube head; (3) imaging with digital panel; (4) rectangular PID. **B,** The operator stands at the control panel located outside the x-ray room. (**A,** Courtesy Dentsply Sirona, Charlotte, NC.)

cathode (−) to strike the anode (+). This process occurs because positive and negative attract each other.

Anode. The **anode** (+) acts as the target for the electrons. It consists of a **tungsten target** (a small block of tungsten) that is embedded in the larger copper stem. The copper around the target conducts the heat away from the target, thus reducing wear and tear on the target.

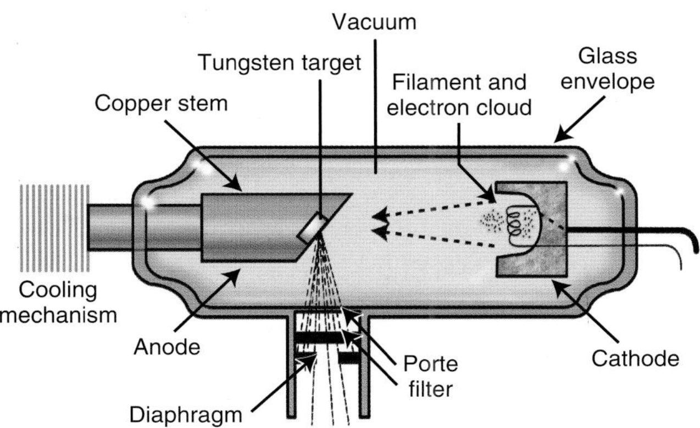

FIGURE 15-15 Schematic drawing of a dental x-ray tube. (Modified from Frommer H, Stabulas-Savage J: *Radiology for the Dental Professional,* ed 9, St. Louis, 2011, Mosby.)

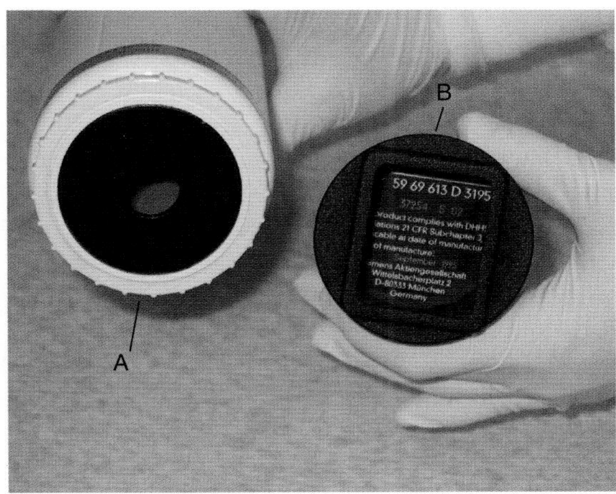

FIGURE 15-16 **A,** Collimator. **B,** Filter.

The oil in the x-ray tube absorbs approximately 99% of the energy generated by this process, and this energy is given off as heat. The remaining 1% exits the tubehead as x-ray beams through the window (opening) as a divergent beam toward the patient. The center portion of this x-ray beam is known as the *central ray,* or *primary beam.*

Collimator. The collimator, similar to the filter, is a metal disc, usually lead; it has a small opening in the center to control the size and shape of the x-ray beam as it leaves the tubehead (Figure 15-16).

Filter. The filter is an aluminum disc located at the port of the tubehead where the PID is connected. The filter removes low-energy, long-wavelength x-ray beams, which may be absorbed by the patient but are not necessary for producing the radiograph.

Position indicator device. The PID, which is lined with lead, is placed against the patient's face during film exposure to aim the x-ray beam at the film in the patient's mouth. The PID may be rectangular or cylindrical.

Extension Arm

The extension arm, which is hollow, encloses the wire between the tubehead and the control panel. It also plays an important role in positioning the tubehead.

The tubehead is attached to the extension arm by means of a yoke that can be horizontally turned 360 degrees. (**Horizontally** means to move in a side-to-side motion; **vertically** means to move in an up-and-down direction.) This design permits maximum flexibility in positioning the tubehead.

If the tubehead drifts, then the arm should be immediately repaired. The patient or the operator must never hold the tubehead in place during exposure.

Control Panel

The **control panel** of an x-ray unit contains the master switch and two indicator lights, an exposure timer, an mA selector, and the kV selector. A single, centrally located control panel may be used to operate several tubeheads located in separate treatment rooms.

Master switch and indicator lights The master switch turns the machine on and off. An orange indicator light shows when the master switch is on. The x-ray machine may be safely left on all day; it does not produce radiation unless the electronic timer is being pushed.

The red emission indicator light comes on only when the electronic timer is being pushed and radiation is being emitted.

Exposure timer The timer is electronically controlled to provide precise exposure time, and x-ray beams are generated only while the exposure timer is pressed.

Exposure time is measured in fractions of a second called *impulses* (1 impulse = $\frac{1}{60}$ second).

Milliamperage selector The mA selector controls the number of electrons produced. Increasing the mA increases the quantity of electrons available for the production of x-ray beams.

Kilovoltage selector The kV selector is used to control the penetrating power, or the quality, of the x-ray.

Image Characteristics

Images that appear on radiographs are referred to as being radiolucent or radiopaque (Figure 15-17).

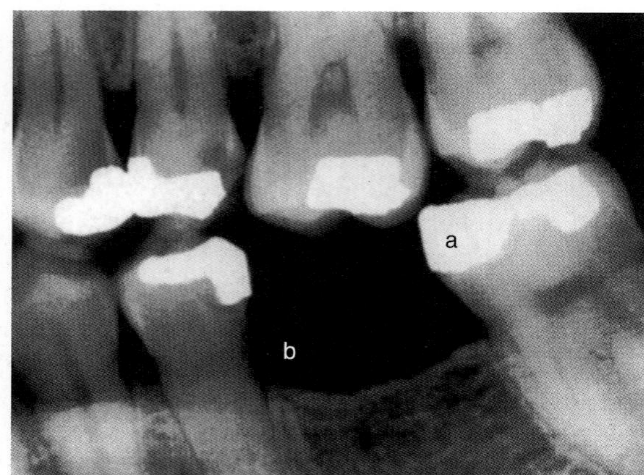

FIGURE 15-17 Bite-wing radiograph shows radiopaque (white *a*) area of amalgam restoration and radiolucent (black *b*) areas of air and cheek tissue.

Radiolucent structures appear dark or black on the radiograph. Air spaces, soft tissues of the body, and dental pulp appear as radiolucent images.

Radiopaque structures appear white or light gray on the radiograph. Metal, enamel, and dense areas of bone appear as radiolucent images.

Radiographic Quality

Four factors affect the quality of a radiograph: contrast, density, image detail, and image distortion (Table 15-4).

Contrast

The image on a radiograph appears in a range of shades from black to white, with multiple shades of gray in between. The difference between the shades of gray are called **contrast**. The ideal contrast of a film clearly shows the white of radiopaque metal restorations, the radiolucent black of air, and the many shades of gray between. Contrast is controlled by the kilovolt peak (kVp) setting.

Density

Density is the overall blackness or darkness of a radiograph. A radiograph with the correct density enables the dentist to view black areas (air space), white areas (enamel, dentin, and bone), and gray areas (soft tissue). The mA setting controls the density (Box 15-4).

Image Distortion

Image distortion is influenced by object-film distance, source-film distance, and movement. (As used here, *distortion* means not accurately showing position, length, or width.)

TABLE 15-4
Visual Characteristics and Influencing Factors

Visual Characteristics	Influencing Factors	Effect of Influencing Factors
Density	mA	↑ mA = ↑ density ↓ mA = ↓ density
	kVp	↑ kVp = ↑ density ↓ kVp = ↓ density
	Time	↑ time = ↑ density ↓ time = ↓ density
	Subject thickness	↑ thickness = ↓ density ↓ thickness = ↑ density
Contrast	kVp	↑ kVp = long-scale contrast; low contrast ↓ kVp = short-scale contrast; high contrast

mA, Milliamperage; *kVp,* kilovoltage peak.

BOX 15-4 Factors Affecting the Density of a Radiograph

1. Amount of radiation reaching the film
2. Distance from the x-ray tube to the patient
3. Processing times and temperatures (see Chapter 16)
4. Patient thickness (the term *patient thickness* refers to the patient's body size)

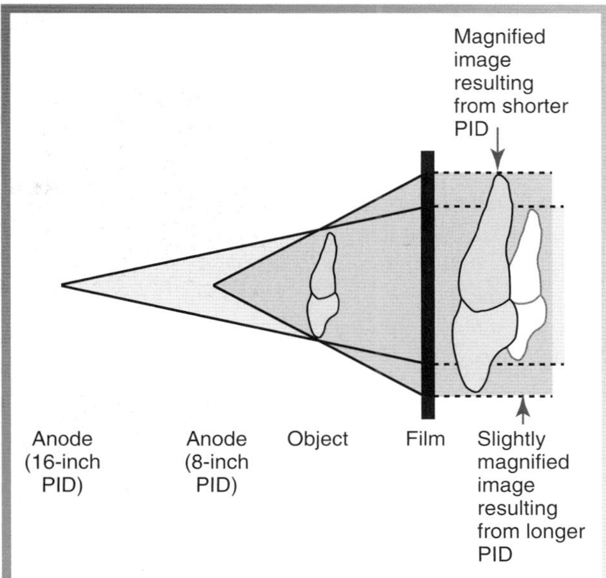

FIGURE 15-18 A long position indicator device PID (16 inches) and a long target-film distance result in less magnification. (From Iannucci JM, Jansen Howerton L: *Dental radiography: principles and techniques,* ed 4, St. Louis, 2012, Saunders.)

Object-Film Distance

The term **object-film distance (OFD)** describes the distance between the teeth (object) being radiographed and the radiographic film.

In dental radiography, placing the film close to the teeth reduces distortion or the lack of sharpness that results when the film is placed at a greater distance from the teeth.

Source-Film Distance

Source-film distance (also known as the target-film distance) is the distance between the source of the x-ray beams (focal spot on the tungsten target) and the film. The length of the PID determines the source-film distance. A longer PID reduces distortion as a result of magnification (Figure 15-18).

The x-ray film should always be placed as close to the tooth as possible. The closer the placement of the film to the tooth, the less image enlargement will be seen on the film.

Movement

Movement of the patient, film, or tubehead can result in an image that is blurred (not sharp) or an image that lacks detail. Therefore it is very important that the patient remains still and does not move the film during exposure (Box 15-5).

BOX 15-5 Documentation

Exposure of dental radiographs must always be documented in the patient's dental record, which should include the following information:

- Informed consent
- Number and type of radiographs exposed
- Rationale for exposing such radiographs
- Diagnostic information obtained from the radiograph

Ethical Implications

Following all radiation safety procedures and being aware of the legal implications involved in taking dental radiographs are the ethical and legal responsibilities of the dental assistant. Federal and state regulations control the use of dental x-ray equipment. For example, the Consumer-Patient Radiation Health and Safety Act is a federal law that establishes guidelines for the proper maintenance of x-ray equipment and requires persons taking dental radiographs to be properly trained and certified. Some state regulations require dental offices, clinics, and dental schools to be inspected every 1 to 3 years to check the safety of the x-ray equipment.

As a dental assistant, being informed about the specific radiation safety requirements in your state is your responsibility.

Chapter Exercises

Multiple Choice

Circle the letter next to the correct answer.

1. The ALARA goal can be achieved by __________.
   - **a.** well-trained and competent operators
   - **b.** using fast-speed film
   - **c.** placing lead aprons on all patients
   - **d.** all of the above
2. The fastest film speed used in dentistry is __________.
   - **a.** C
   - **b.** D
   - **c.** E
   - **d.** F
3. Dental film badges are used to record __________.
   - **a.** the radiation received by the operator
   - **b.** the radiation received by the patient
   - **c.** the number of films taken
   - **d.** all of the above
4. Dental personnel should strive for __________ exposure to radiation.
   - **a.** zero
   - **b.** the maximum possible dose
   - **c.** 0.05 rem
   - **d.** 0.01 Sv
5. The process in which cells are altered by exposure to radiation is __________.
   - **a.** electromagnetic force
   - **b.** ionization
   - **c.** matter
   - **d.** photon
6. Which of the following has an influence on radiation safety?
   - **a.** Safe equipment
   - **b.** Skilled operator
   - **c.** Lead apron and thyroid collars
   - **d.** All of the above
7. Dental radiographs are used to __________.
   - **a.** detect dental decay in the early stages
   - **b.** detect bone loss in the early stages
   - **c.** evaluate growth and development
   - **d.** accomplish all of the above
8. Which of the following are characteristics of x-ray beams? They are __________.
   - **a.** invisible
   - **b.** weightless
   - **c.** travel in straight lines
   - **d.** all of the above
9. Which of the following affects the density of a radiograph?
   - **a.** Amount of radiation reaching the film
   - **b.** Distance from the x-ray tube to the patient
   - **c.** Size of the patient's body
   - **d.** All of the above
10. The results of radiation that are passed on to future generations are called __________ effects.
    - **a.** somatic
    - **b.** genetic
    - **c.** acute
    - **d.** cumulative
11. The term for images that appear dark or black on radiographs is __________.
    - **a.** radiopaque
    - **b.** radiolucent
12. Filters in dental x-ray units are made from __________.
    - **a.** lead
    - **b.** aluminum
    - **c.** steel
    - **d.** tungsten
13. The purpose of a collimator is to __________.
    - **a.** remove long wavelengths of radiation
    - **b.** remove short wavelengths of radiation
    - **c.** restrict the diameter of the beam
    - **d.** enlarge the diameter of the beam
14. The purpose of the filters in dental x-ray machines is to __________.
    - **a.** remove long wavelengths of radiation
    - **b.** remove short wavelengths of radiation
    - **c.** restrict the diameter of the beam
    - **d.** enlarge the diameter of the beam
15. The purpose of the PID is to __________.
    - **a.** aim the x-ray beam at the film
    - **b.** generate x-rays
    - **c.** minimize the amount of radiation
    - **d.** accomplish all of the above

Apply Your Knowledge

1. Mr. Lopez indicates a reluctance to have the recommended full-mouth series of dental radiographs taken. On careful questioning, you determine that his reluctance is because of his lack of understanding about the effects of radiation. How would you manage this situation?
2. Your dentist employer has given you the responsibility of selecting a new dental x-ray unit for your office. One of the choices you must make is the type of collimator in the new machine. What things would you consider? Why?
3. Mrs. Collins brings her 3-year-old son, Dennis, into your dental office to be seen on an emergency basis. He fell and cracked his front tooth, and the dentist asks you to take an x-ray image. Dennis is too small to sit in the chair himself and is unable to hold the film holder in his mouth. What are you going to do?
4. You have a friend who is not in the dental profession but is very concerned about your safety because you work around x-ray machines on a daily basis. What can you tell her?
5. As a child, you probably played "shadow casting" using sunlight or a flashlight. Try this experiment using a flashlight and a wall. Shine the light on the wall, and place one hand between the light beam and the wall. If you move your hand closer to the wall and away from the light source, the shadow is close to the actual size of your hand. If you move your hand away from the wall and nearer to the light source, the image of your hand is magnified (larger) but is distorted in shape. How does this experiment on shadow casting relate to dental radiography?

CHAPTER 16

Oral Radiography

http://evolve.elsevier.com/Robinson/essentials/

LEARNING OBJECTIVES

1. Pronounce, define, and spell the key terms.
2. Identify the three types of intraoral views.
3. Discuss the components of film-based radiography, including the film packet and x-ray film.
4. Describe the care of dental films, including storage and film care during exposure.
5. Describe and practice infection control techniques in film-based dental radiography and demonstrate how to practice infection control during film exposure.
6. Complete the following related to intraoral radiography techniques:
   - Compare and contrast the paralleling technique and the bisecting angle technique.
   - Assemble the XCP (Extension-Cone Paralleling) instruments.
   - Describe vertical and horizontal angulation.
7. Complete the following related to the full-mouth radiographic survey:
   - Produce full-mouth radiographic survey using paralleling technique.
   - Produce four-film radiographic survey using bite-wing technique.
8. Describe the basic principles of the occlusal technique and produce maxillary and mandibular radiographs using occlusal technique.
9. Identify errors in exposure and processing technique, and describe the steps for prevention.
10. Demonstrate the infection control techniques necessary during film processing, both in the darkroom and with use of a daylight loader.
11. List the steps in manual processing and in automatic processing of dental radiographs, as well as the steps in duplicating radiographs.
12. Mount a full series of periapical and bite-wing dental radiographs.
13. Describe the advantages and disadvantages of digital radiography and describe the two main technologies used in digital dental imaging.
14. Complete the following related to panoramic imaging:
    - Describe the purposes, uses, advantages, and disadvantages of panoramic imaging.
    - Describe the equipment used in panoramic imaging.
    - Demonstrate how to prepare equipment for panoramic radiography.
    - Demonstrate how to prepare a patient for panoramic radiography.
    - Demonstrate how to position a patient for panoramic radiography.
    - Discuss common errors and infection control in panoramic imaging.
    - Practice infection control with digital sensors and phosphor storage plates.
15. Discuss informed consent, documentation, and ownership of dental radiographs when it comes to dental radiography.

KEY TERMS

automatic processing techniques
bisecting angle technique
bite-wing image
cassette
charge-coupled device (CCD)
diagnostic quality image
digital image
digitizes
film duplicating
horizontal angulation
latent image
manual processing
occlusal technique
panoramic radiography
paralleling technique
periapical views
phosphor storage plates (PSPs)
point of entry
radiograph
scanning
sensor-holding device
vertical angulation

In the previous chapter, you learned that any exposure to radiation has the potential to damage your or the patient's living tissue. In this chapter, you will learn how to prevent unnecessary radiation exposure to the patient when you produce diagnostic quality films or images and prevent the need for retakes. As a dental assistant, being competent with all forms of dental radiography is important, including digital technology and film-based techniques, dental x-ray equipment, x-ray film and processing, and infection control as it relates to dental radiography. Developing the clinical skills to avoid technique errors and recognizing them when they do occur are also critical, as well as knowing how to prevent errors in the future.

Digital imaging has revolutionized dental radiology and is rapidly replacing traditional film-based techniques (Figure 16-1). When discussing digital radiography, the term **digital image** is used instead of radiograph, film, or x-ray. A **radiograph** is an image on conventional dental film.

Intraoral Views

Types of Intraoral Views

Whether you are using a digital or a film-based technique, there are three types of intraoral views: (1) periapical, (2) bite-wing, and (3) occlusal. Each type of intraoral view provides specific information (Table 16-1).

Film-Based Radiography

Placing a film in the patient's mouth and then exposing it to an x-ray beam captures the image on film to make dental radiographs. The **latent image** (invisible) on the film becomes visible

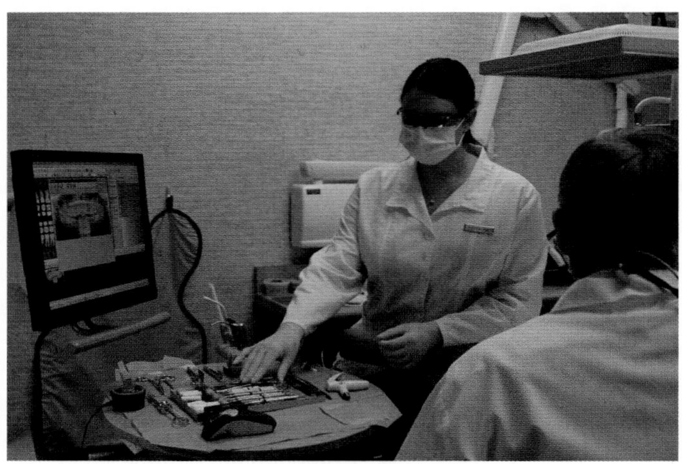

FIGURE 16-1 A rear-mounted computer monitor allows the dental team to refer to the images and the patient record. A flat screen computer monitor is mounted from the ceiling, so patients can watch videos of their choice during dental treatment. (Courtesy Dr. Jeffrey Elliot, Santa Rosa, California.)

TABLE 16-1
Types of Dental Images

Type	Primary Uses	Example
Periapical	Shows images of the entire length of the tooth, plus 3 to 4 mm beyond the apices. Is used to diagnose abscesses and other pathologic conditions around the root area of the teeth. Is also used to identify unerupted teeth.	
Bite-wing	Shows images of the crowns of the teeth on both arches on one film. A bite-wing survey (BWX) can consist of two or four films and is used to diagnose interproximal caries, recurrent caries, pulpal pathologic conditions, and conditions of the crestal bone.	
Occlusal	Is used to locate impactions, supernumerary teeth, pathologic conditions, and fractures of the maxilla or mandible. No. 4 film is used.	

Occlusal radiograph from Miles DA, Van Dis ML, Williamson GF, et al: *Radiographic imaging for the dental team,* ed 4, Philadelphia, 2009, Saunders.

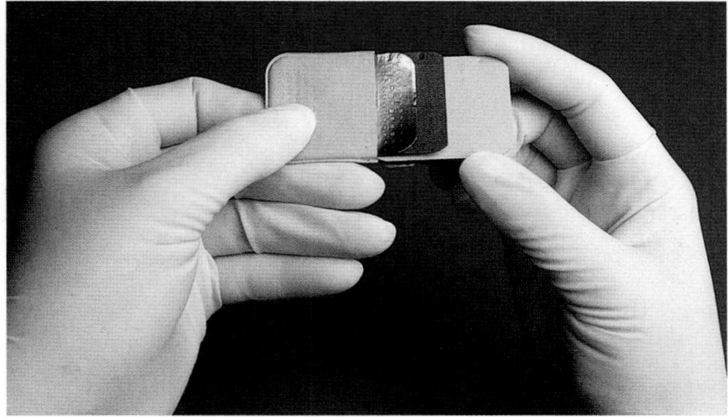

FIGURE 16-2 Contents of a dental film packet: lead foil, radiographic film, and black paper.

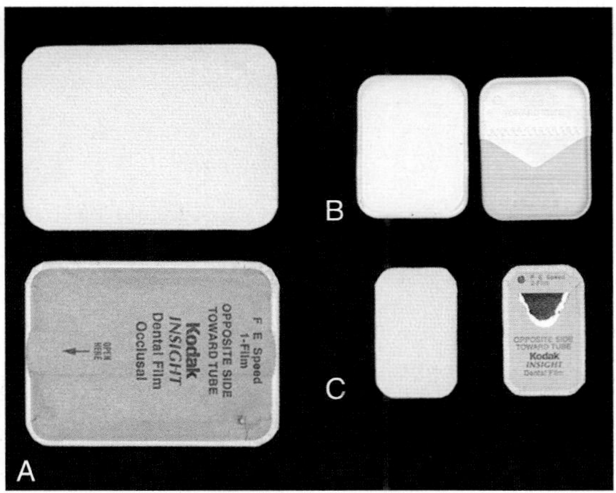

FIGURE 16-3 The white side of the film packet faces the tube. **A,** Size 4 occlusal film. **B,** Size 2 film. **C,** Size 1 film.

only after the film is processed in a darkroom (a light-tight room) or in an automatic film-processing machine. Once the film is processed and dried, it becomes a radiograph; it is placed into a film mount and is ready to be viewed and interpreted by the dentist.

Intraoral Dental X-Ray Film

Film Packets

A film packet consists of an outer wrap, a lead foil, black paper, and one or two films (Figure 16-2). The front of the packet is white. This side is always placed toward the position indicator device (PID). The back, which is colored and has the tab used for opening the packet before processing, is always placed away from the PID. A small circle on the back indicates where the embossed dot, or raised bump, is on the film. Later, this dot will help in mounting and determining the right side from the left.

Within the packet, the film is protected on either side by a sheet of black paper; a thin sheet of lead foil absorbs most of the x-ray beams that pass through the film, thus protecting the patient.

Double-Film Packets

Double-film packets contain two pieces of film between the black paper lining. This makes it possible to produce a duplicate set of the radiographs without exposing the patient to additional radiation or having to go through the **film duplicating** process.

Double-film packets are useful when the insurance company requests radiographs or when a patient is referred to a specialist.

Intraoral Dental X-Ray Film

Intraoral dental film consists of a semiflexible plastic film base coated on both sides with an emulsion containing x-ray–sensitive crystals of silver bromide, silver halide, and silver iodine embedded in gelatin. The size of the crystals determines the film speed. (Film speed is discussed in Chapter 15.) These are numbered from 0 to 4, with 0 being the smallest (Figure 16-3 and Table 16-2).

TABLE 16-2
Commonly Used Film Sizes

Size	Uses
0	Usually for children younger than 3 years of age
1	Anterior film for adult full-mouth surveys
2	Adult BWXs and adult posterior periapical radiographs
3	Less common, but used for adult BWX radiographs
4	Occlusal radiographs

BWX, Bite-wing survey.

Care of Dental Films

Film Storage

All dental films should be stored according to the manufacturer's instructions to protect it from light, heat, moisture, chemicals, and scatter radiation. The box of radiographic film is marked with an expiration date.

Film Care During Exposure

Films to be exposed are dispensed before the radiographic procedure begins. They are placed on a clean towel just outside the room where the films are to be exposed.

Never leave films, whether exposed or unexposed, in the room where additional films are being exposed. Doing so could result in the new films being exposed to scatter radiation, which results in film fog and reduces their diagnostic value.

Infection Control in Dental Radiography

Dental radiographic procedures present special infection control challenges (Box 16-1). The operator contacts the patient's saliva while placing and removing the film packets or sensors and touches many things while exposing and processing

BOX 16-1 Surfaces Likely to be Contaminated During X-Ray Procedures

- X-ray tubehead
- Position indicator device (PID)
- X-ray control panel
- Exposure button
- Computer keyboard
- Digital sensors and cables
- Phosphor storage plates (PSPs)
- Lead apron
- Dental chair controls
- Operatory counter surfaces
- Darkroom equipment
- Sleeves on automatic processors

film. Protective measures and barriers used while producing radiographs are illustrated in Figure 16-4. Dental film is now available with plastic barriers over the packet. The film is exposed as usual, and then the plastic barrier cover is removed before entering the darkroom for processing. The infection control protocol is more efficient and effective when the dental assistant plans for the procedure before the patient is seated (Box 16-2).

See Procedure 16-1: Practicing Infection Control During Film Exposure.

Intraoral Radiography Techniques

Regardless of whether you are using conventional film-based or digital systems, two basic techniques are used to obtain **periapical views**: (1) the **paralleling technique** and (2) the **bisecting**

BOX 16-2 CDC Guidelines for Dental Radiology

1. Wear gloves when exposing radiographs and handling contaminated film packets. Use other PPE (e.g., protective eyewear, mask, gown) as appropriate if spattering of blood or other body fluids is likely (IA, IC).
2. Use heat-tolerant or disposable intraoral devices whenever possible (e.g., film-holding and positioning devices). Clean and heat sterilize heat-tolerant devices between patients (IB).
3. Transport and handle exposed film in an aseptic manner to prevent contaminating the developing equipment (II).
4. The following apply for digital radiography sensors:
   a. Use FDA-cleared barriers. (IB)
   b. Clean and heat sterilize, or high-level disinfect, between patients; barrier protect semicritical items. If an item cannot tolerate these procedures, then, at a minimum, protect it between patients with an FDA-cleared barrier, and clean and disinfect with an EPA-registered hospital disinfectant with intermediate-level (i.e., tuberculocidal claim) activity. Consult the manufacturer for methods of disinfecting and sterilizing digital radiography sensors and for protecting associated computer hardware (IB).

CDC, Centers for Disease Control and Prevention; *EPA,* U.S. Environmental Protection Agency; *FDA,* U.S. Food and Drug Administration; *PPE,* personal protective equipment.

Modified from *Guidelines for infection control in dental health care settings—2003,* Atlanta, Georgia, 2003, Department of Health & Human Services, Centers for Disease Control and Prevention.

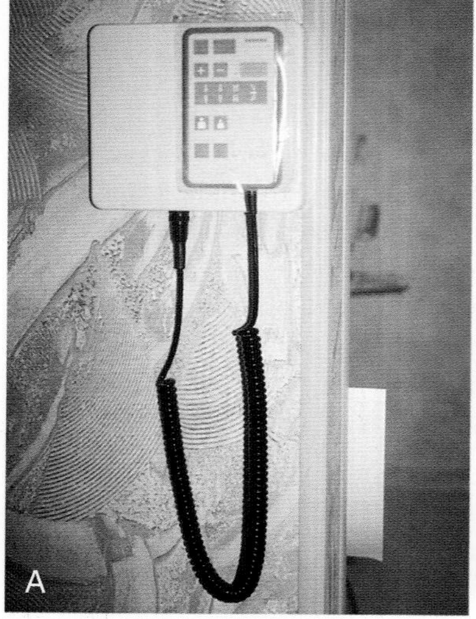

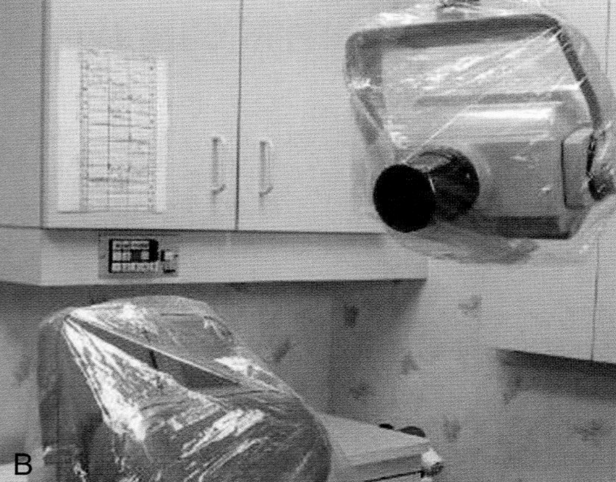

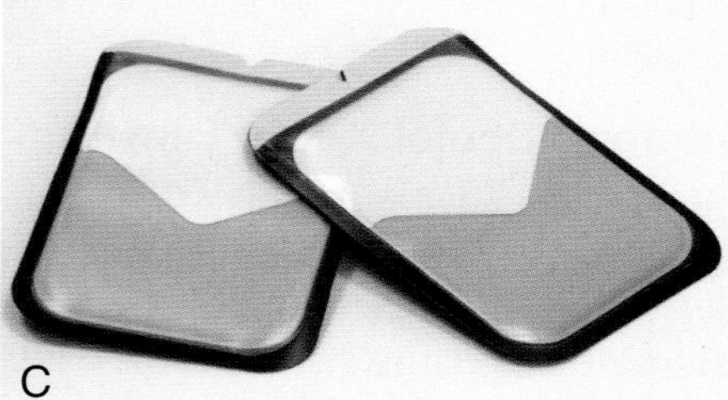

FIGURE 16-4 **A,** X-ray equipment with barriers in place. **B,** Radiography operatory with barriers in place. **C,** Protective barrier on x-ray film.

angle technique. The paralleling technique is preferred because it provides a more accurate image of the teeth and surrounding structures. The bisecting angle technique is discussed in this chapter as a supplemental method (Figure 16-5).

Paralleling Technique

Basic Principles

Two basic principles define the paralleling technique: (1) the film is placed parallel to the long axis of the teeth being radiographed, and (2) the x-ray beam is directed at right angles (perpendicular) to the film or sensor and the long axis of the tooth.

Film- or Sensor-Holding Instruments

To place and keep the film packet or sensor in its proper position in relation to the tooth, the paralleling technique requires the use of film- or sensor-holding instruments. A variety of film- or sensor-holding instruments are available (Figure 16-6).

A commonly used type of film- or sensor-holding device is the Rinn extension-cone paralleling (XCP) instrument (Figure 16-7). In addition to film or sensor positioning, these instruments include a localizing ring, also known as an *aiming ring,* which facilitates aligning the PID with the film or sensor in both horizontal and vertical planes. This alignment increases the accuracy and reduces the need for unnecessary retakes. The procedures that follow at the end of this chapter include the use of XCP film- and sensor-holding instruments; however, the basic principles of placement and paralleling are similar, regardless of the film- or sensor-holding instrument that is used.

See Procedure 16-2: Assembling Extension-Cone Paralleling (XCP) Instruments.

Using the Paralleling Technique

Important factors to be considered in exposing periapical views include the dental chair position, film or sensor position and placement, point of entry of the x-ray beam, vertical and horizontal angulation, and the use of a film- or sensor-holding instrument.

Dental chair position The dental chair is positioned so that the patient's head is straight. For most exposures, this means that the patient is seated in an upright position. This position is adjusted so that the occlusal plane of the jaw being radiographed is parallel to the floor when the film or sensor is in position.

Film or sensor placement and position The film or sensor is placed in a vertical position for anterior projections and in a horizontal position for posterior periapical projections. The film or sensor is held in position by the patient closing on a bite-block or other film- or sensor-holding device.

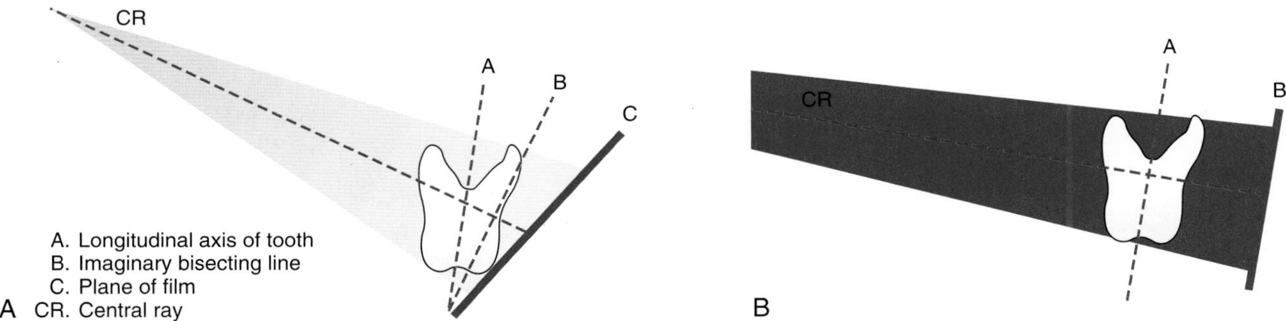

FIGURE 16-5 Intraoral x-ray techniques. **A,** Bisecting angle technique. **B,** Paralleling technique.

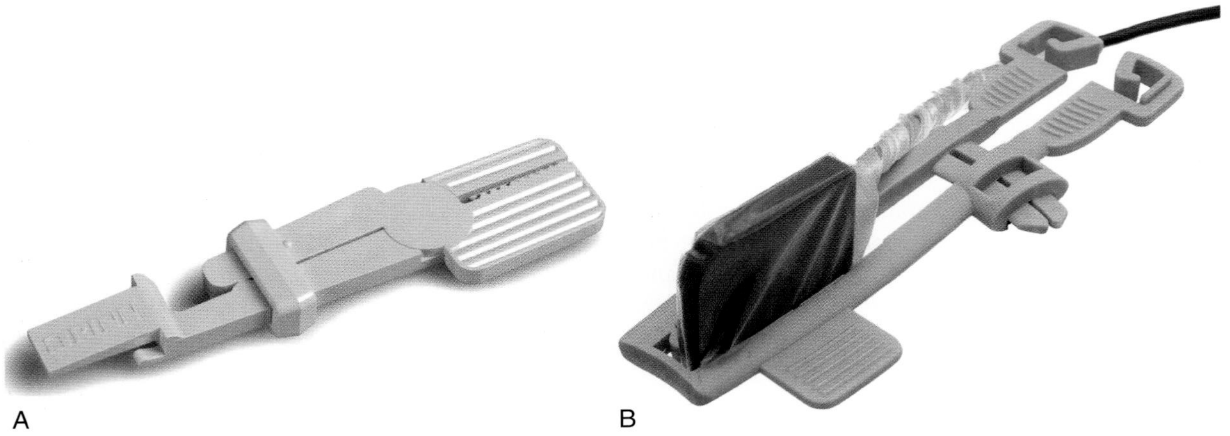

FIGURE 16-6 **A,** Snap-a-Ray Xtra Film and phosphor plate holder for the bisecting technique. **B,** The EeZee-Grip Digital Sensor Holder for the bisecting technique. (Courtesy Dentsply Rinn, Elgin, Illinois.)

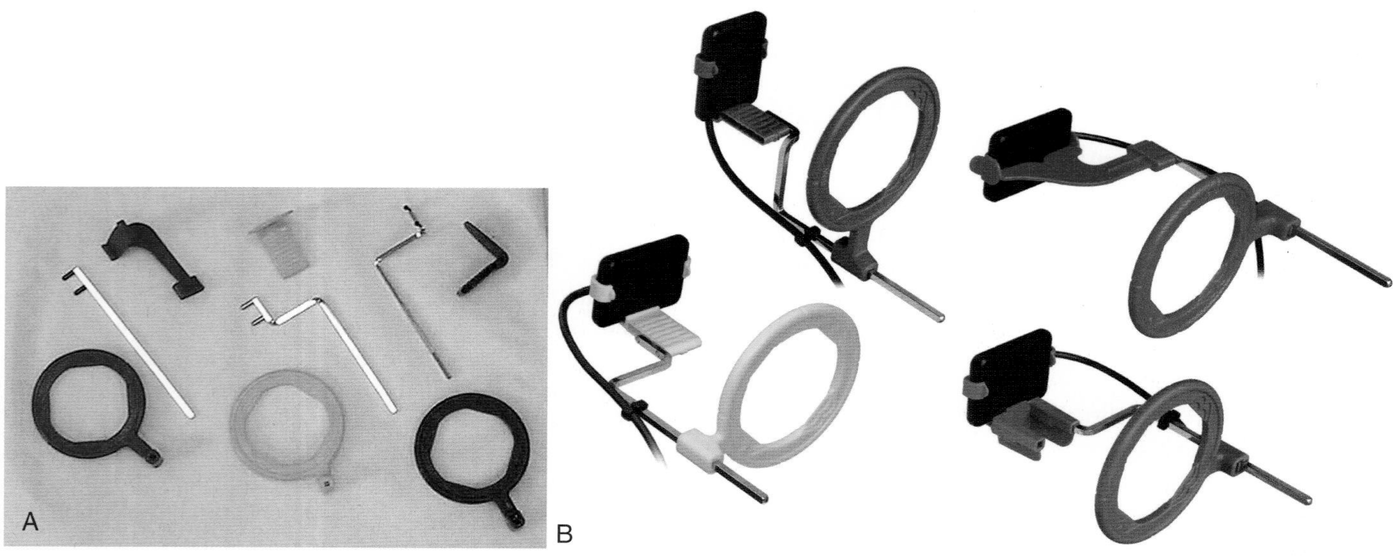

FIGURE 16-7 Rinn extension-cone paralleling (XCP) instruments are color-coded for easy assembly. **A,** The red instruments are for bite-wing placement, the yellow are for posterior placement, and the blue are for anterior placement. **B,** Rinn sensor suitable for Gendex, VisualiX, USB/GX Cygnus, and Visiodent.

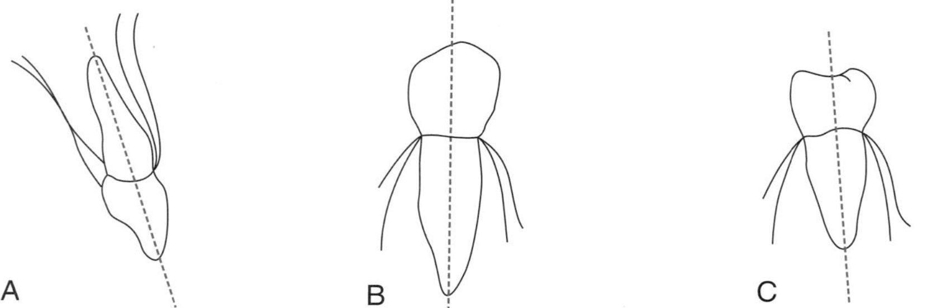

FIGURE 16-8 **A,** The apices of the maxillary teeth tilt inward toward the palate. **B,** The apices of the mandibular premolars are nearly vertical. **C,** The apices of the mandibular molars tilt slightly inward. (From Haring JI, Jansen Howerton L: *Dental radiography: principles and techniques,* ed 3, St. Louis, 2006, Saunders.)

When conventional film is used, the film is placed so that the raised dot is toward the occlusal surface and is facing the PID. This technique places the front of the film packet toward the PID, prevents the dots from becoming superimposed over the apex of a tooth, and later helps in mounting the processed film. The film position must be parallel to the entire tooth, not just parallel to the crown. This is an important concept to understand. Although the crowns of the teeth appear to tilt one way, the entire structure actually tilts another. For example, the apices of most of the maxillary teeth tilt inward toward the palate. The mandibular premolars are more nearly vertical, and the mandibular molars tilt slightly inward (Figure 16-8).

To achieve parallelism between the long axes of the teeth and the film or sensor, the film or sensor must be placed slightly away from the teeth toward the midline of the oral cavity. In addition, film or sensors that are placed too close to the teeth may not record enough tissue in the area of the root apices. The film or sensor must be positioned away from the teeth, with the patient biting near the anterior edge of the bite-block.

Point of entry The **point of entry** is the position on the patient's face at which the central x-ray beam is aimed. The goal is to cover the film or sensor completely with the beam of radiation.

Vertical angulation **Vertical angulation** is the movement of the tubehead in an up-and-down direction, similar to nodding your head "yes" (Figure 16-9). In the paralleling technique, the vertical angulation must be perpendicular to the film or sensor and to the long axes of the teeth, or the images will be elongated or foreshortened (Figures 16-10 and 16-11).

Horizontal angulation **Horizontal angulation** is the movement of the tubehead in a side-to-side direction, similar to shaking your head "no" (Figure 16-12). In the paralleling technique, the horizontal angulation of the x-ray beam must be directed through the contacts of the teeth and be as perpendicular (at a right angle with the film or sensor) to the horizontal plane of the film or sensor as possible. Failure to do this will cause overlapping of proximal contacts (Figure 16-13).

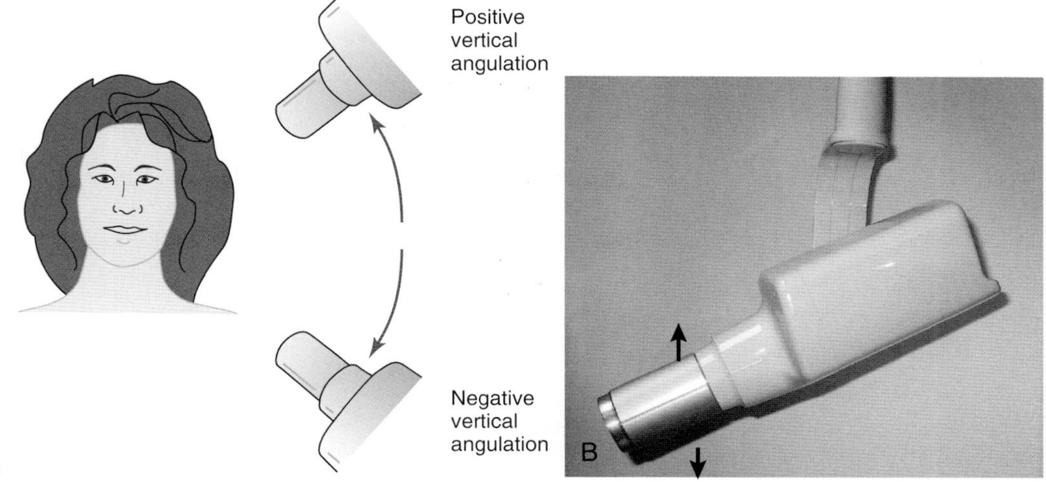

FIGURE 16-9 Vertical angulation of the position indicator device (PID) refers to PID placement in an up-and-down (head-to-toe) direction.

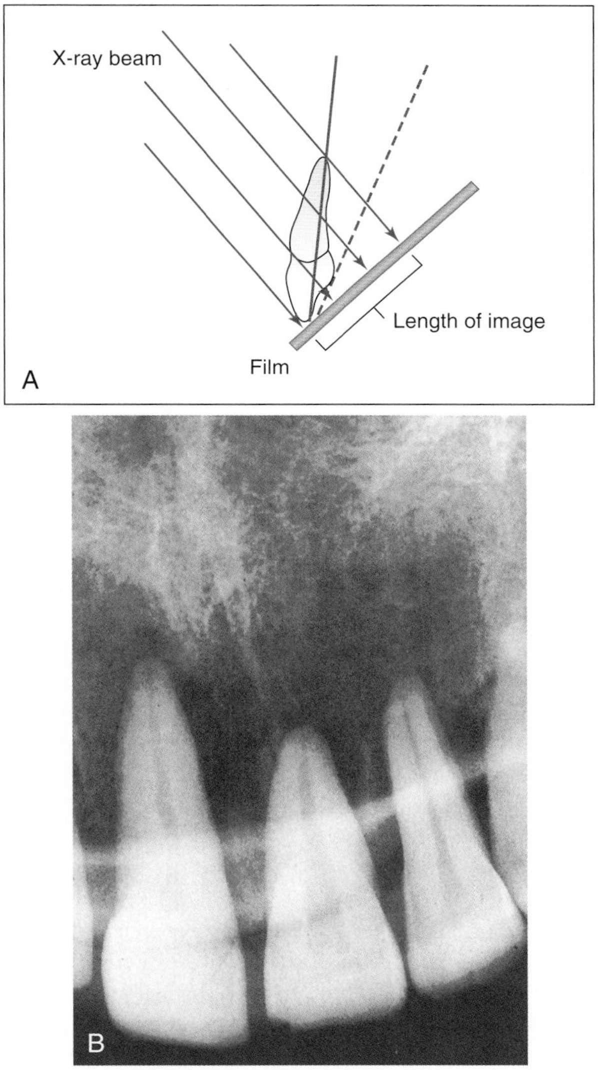

X-ray beam
Length of image
Film
A
B

FIGURE 16-10 **A,** If the vertical angulation is too steep, then the image on the film is shorter than the actual tooth. **B,** Foreshortened image. (From Haring JI, Lind LJ: *Radiographic interpretation for the dental hygienist,* Philadelphia, 1993, Saunders.)

X-ray beam
Length of image
Film
A
B

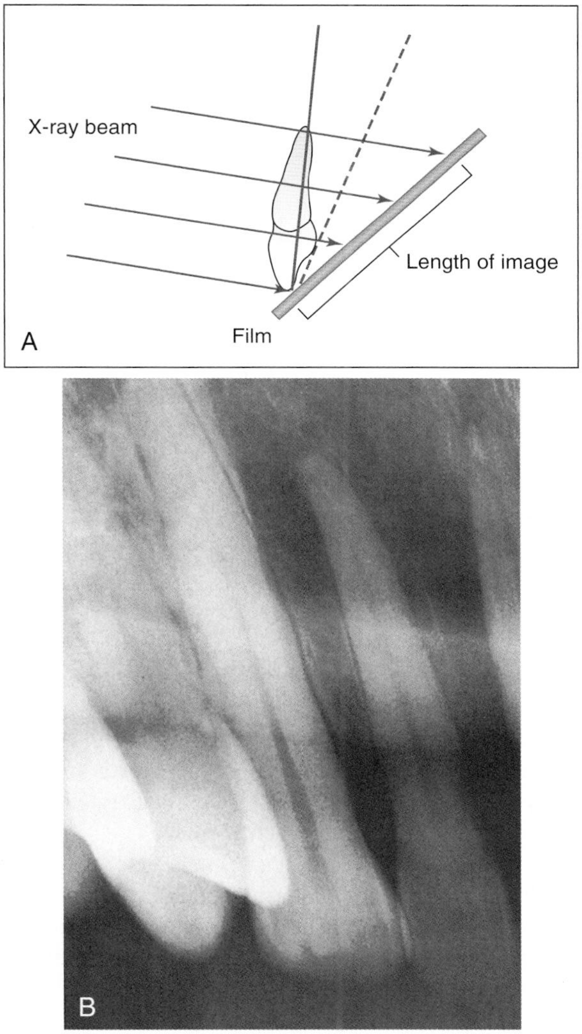

FIGURE 16-11 **A,** If the vertical angulation is too flat, then the image on the film is longer than the actual tooth. **B,** Elongated image. (From Haring JI, Lind LJ: *Radiographic interpretation for the dental hygienist,* Philadelphia, 1993, Saunders.)

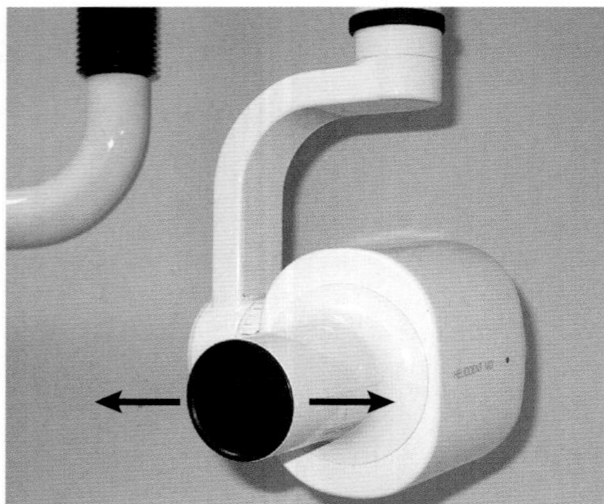

FIGURE 16-12 The arrows indicate movement in a horizontal direction.

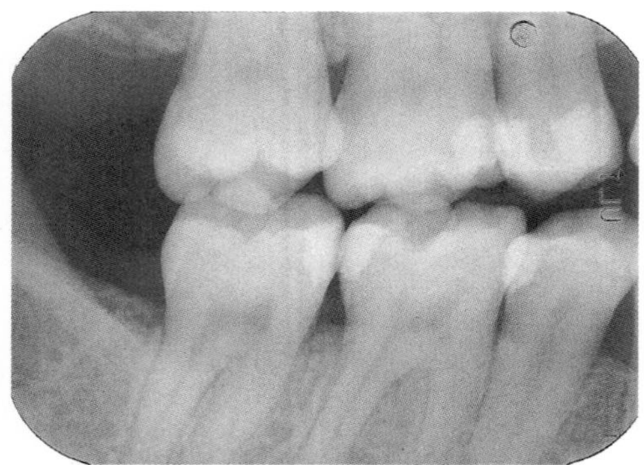

FIGURE 16-13 Overlapped contact areas.

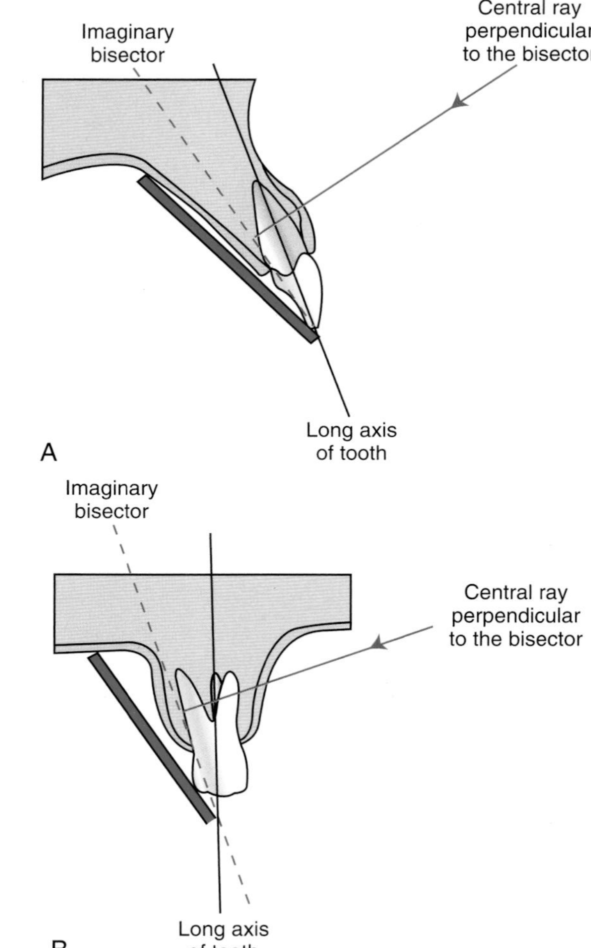

FIGURE 16-14 **A,** Anterior tooth with the central ray perpendicular to the *imaginary* bisector of the angle between the long axis of the tooth and the film plane. **B,** A posterior tooth using the bisecting angle concept. (From Miles D, Van Dis ML, Williamson GF, et al: *Radiographic imaging for the dental team,* ed 4, Philadelphia, 2009, Saunders.)

Bisecting Angle Technique

The bisecting angle technique can be used in some special circumstances, for example, in difficult or unusual anatomy, such as in patients with a very shallow palate or a very short lingual frenum or when palatal or mandibular tori (bone growths) are present. In addition, small children and some endodontic views may require the use of this technique. Using the proper technique, diagnostic images can be obtained with this method.

Basic Principles

The bisecting angle technique is based on the geometric principle of bisecting a triangle (bisecting means dividing into two equal parts; Figure 16-14).

The angle formed by the long axis of the teeth and the film or sensor is bisected, and the x-ray beam is directed at a right angle (perpendicular) to the bisecting line.

In this technique, the film or sensor is placed close to the crowns of the teeth to be radiographed and extends at an angle into the palate or floor of the mouth. Film or sensor holders for the bisecting angle technique, including some with alignment indicators, are commercially available.

Patient Positioning

The patient's midsagittal plane should be perpendicular to the floor, which means that the patient's head is upright for maxillary film and is slightly tipped back for the mandibular arch.

A No. 2 film or sensor is used in both the anterior (in a vertical position) and posterior (in a horizontal position) regions. Only three films are needed in the maxillary anterior region because all four maxillary incisors can be imaged on the No. 2 film or sensor.

Beam Alignment

The x-ray beam is directed to pass between the contacts of the teeth being radiographed in the horizontal dimension, just as it does in the paralleling technique. The vertical angle, however, must be directed at 90 degrees to the imaginary bisecting line. Too much vertical angulation will produce images that are too short (foreshortened), and too little vertical angulation will result in images that are too long (elongated). The beam must be centered to prevent cone cutting. A short or a long PID can be used (Table 16-3).

Full-Mouth Radiographic Survey

A full-mouth radiographic survey (FMX) consists of a specified number of periapical and bite-wing views. A complete full-mouth survey may have as few as 10 or as many as 18 periapical views, plus whatever bite-wing views are indicated. The number and size of the film or sensor to be used depend on the:

- Dentist's instructions
- Number of teeth present
- Size of the oral cavity
- Anatomic structures within the mouth
- Age of the patient
- Level of patient cooperation

The procedure described here includes positioning and steps for each exposure in one half of the maxillary arch and one half of the mandibular arch with the use of the paralleling technique and XCP film- or sensor-holding instruments (Box 16-3).

TABLE 16-3
Vertical Angulations for the Bisecting Angle Technique

Teeth Being Imaged	Vertical Angulations (in degrees)
Maxillary incisors	−40 to −50
Maxillary cuspids	−45 to −55
Maxillary premolars	−30 to −40
Maxillary molars	−20 to −30
Mandibular incisors	−15 to −25
Mandibular cuspids	−20 to −30
Mandibular premolars	−10 to −15
Mandibular molars	−5 to 0

If the patient positioning is correct, then these vertical angulations will produce reasonable film images for most patients.

When the opposite side of each arch is radiographed, the same procedures are followed. The completed radiographic survey is shown in Figure 16-15.

See Procedure 16-3: Producing a Full-Mouth Radiographic Survey Using the Paralleling Technique.

Producing Bite-Wing Views

Bite-wing views are always parallel films, regardless of the technique used for the periapical radiographs.

See Procedure 16-4: Producing a Four-Film Radiographic Survey Using the Bite-Wing Technique.

The film or sensor is positioned (by a bite tab or a holding device) parallel to the crowns of both the upper and the lower teeth, and the central ray (CR) is directed perpendicular to the film or sensor.

The premolar **bite-wing image** should include the distal halves of the crowns of the cuspids, both premolars, and often the first molars on both the maxillary and the mandibular arches. The molar film should be centered over the second molars.

Correct horizontal angulation is crucial to the diagnostic value of a bite-wing view. Even a slight amount of overlapping of the proximal (contact) surfaces on the image may lead to a misdiagnosis.

BOX 16-3 Guidelines for Film Placement

- The white side of the film always faces the teeth.
- Anterior films are always vertically placed.
- Posterior films are always horizontally placed.
- The identification dot on the film is always placed in the slot of the film holder (dot in the slot).
- The film holder is always positioned away from the teeth and toward the middle of the mouth.
- The film is always centered over the areas to be examined.
- The film is always placed parallel to the long axis of the teeth.

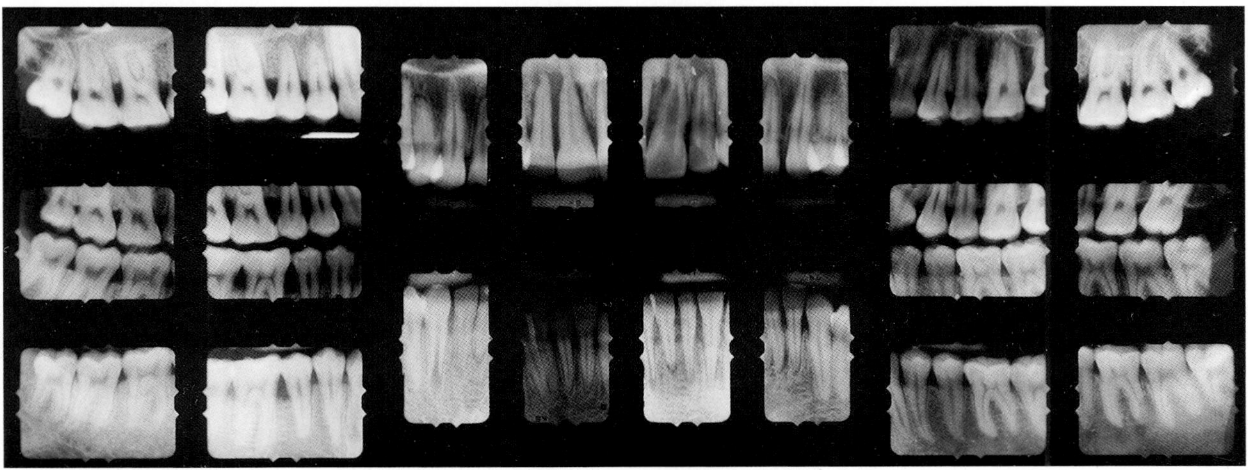

FIGURE 16-15 Mounted full-mouth series with eight anterior films using the paralleling technique.

BOX 16-4 Uses for Occlusal Radiographs

- To locate retained roots of extracted teeth
- To locate supernumerary (extra) unerupted or impacted teeth
- To locate salivary stones in ducts of the submandibular gland
- To locate fractures of the maxilla and mandible
- To examine the area of a cleft palate
- To measure changes in the size and shape of the maxilla or mandible

Occlusal Technique

The **occlusal technique** is used to examine large areas of the upper or lower jaw (Box 16-4). The occlusal technique is so named because the patient bites or *occludes* the entire film. This technique requires the use of conventional dental film. In adults, No. 4 intraoral film is used, but No. 2 film is used in children. The occlusal technique is used when large areas of the maxilla or mandible must be radiographed.

See Procedure 16-5: Producing Maxillary and Mandibular Radiographs Using the Occlusal Technique.

Basic Principles

The basic principles of the occlusal technique are as follows:

1. Film is positioned with the white side facing the arch being exposed.
2. Film is placed in the mouth between the occlusal surfaces of the maxillary and mandibular teeth.
3. Film is stabilized when the patient gently bites on the surface of the film.
4. Vertical angulation between 35 and 65 degrees is used.

Exposure and Technique Errors

A **diagnostic quality image** is one that has been properly placed, exposed, and processed. Only diagnostic quality images are of benefit to the dentist, and retakes require the patient to be subjected to additional radiation. It is important for the dental assistant to recognize errors, identify their causes, and know how to correct the problem (Figure 16-16).

Processing Radiographs

Processing dental film consists of a series of steps that change the latent (invisible) image into a visible image on the radiograph. Most practices now use an automatic processor on their films. However, in some dental offices, knowing how to process the film manually is necessary. This section discusses both methods.

Infection Control During Film Processing

After completing the exposures, remove your gloves and wash your hands. Carefully carry the paper cup or plastic bag containing the contaminated films to the processing area. Be careful not to touch the contaminated films with your bare hands. Regardless of whether you use a manual or an automatic processor with a daylight loader, you must remember that the used film packets are considered contaminated and should be appropriately handled.

See Procedure 16-6: Practicing Infection Control in the Darkroom and Procedure 16-7: Practicing Infection Control With the Use of the Daylight Loader.

TABLE 16-4
Maintenance of Processing Solutions

Type of Processing Chemicals	Schedule of Maintenance
Manual chemicals	Solutions should be changed every 3 to 4 weeks.
Automatic chemicals	Solutions should be changed every 2 to 6 weeks.
Replenisher chemicals	Developer and fixer solutions should be replenished daily in both manual and automatic processing. Follow the manufacturer's instructions for the amount to remove and replace.

Processing Solutions

Processing solutions are considered to be hazardous chemicals and are subject to special chemical labeling and disposal requirements. Always wear your personal protective equipment when handling these chemicals, and check disposal requirements specific to your state (see Chapter 6).

Care and Maintenance of Processing Solutions

You must always follow the manufacturer's instructions for storing, mixing, and using the processing solution (developer, fixer, and replenisher). These solutions deteriorate with exposure to air, continued use, and chemical contamination. Overused and old solutions cause radiographs to be too light and nondiagnostic (Table 16-4).

Developer Solution

The first step in processing begins with the developer solution. The developer solution softens the emulsion. After developing, partially processed films are rinsed in water to remove any remaining chemical.

Note: There must be no exposure to light at this point in the processing or the film will turn black.

Fixer Solution

The fixer solution removes the unexposed silver halide crystals and creates white-to-clear areas on the radiograph.

After the films have been fixed, they are thoroughly washed in water to remove any remaining chemicals.

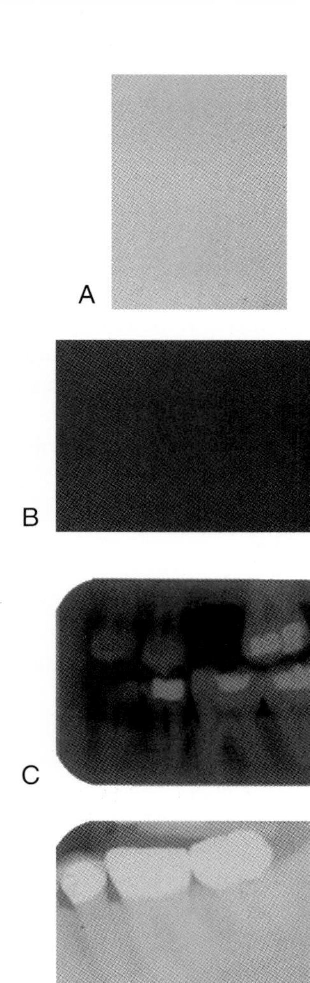

A

Cause: Unexposed
Correction: Be sure machine is on. Listen for exposure sound.

B

Cause: Exposed to white light
Correction: Do not unwrap film in light. Check darkroom for light leaks.

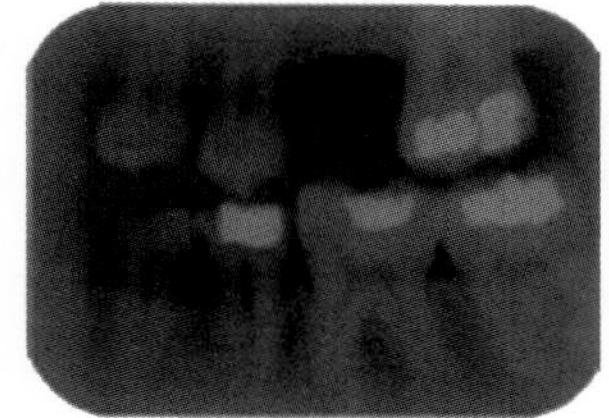

C

Cause: Overexposed
Correction: Check exposure settings, and decrease as necessary.

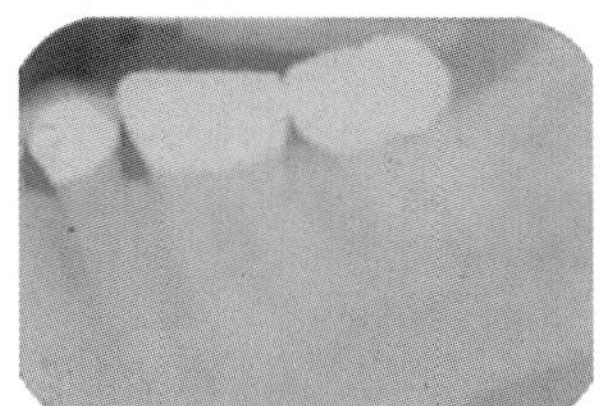

D

Cause: Underexposed
Correction: Check exposure settings, and increase as necessary.

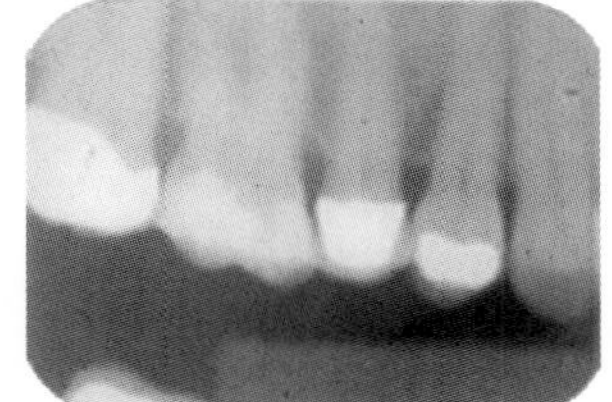

E

Cause: Incorrect image receptor placement
Correction: No more than $^1/_8$ inch of film extends beyond incisal/occlusal surfaces.

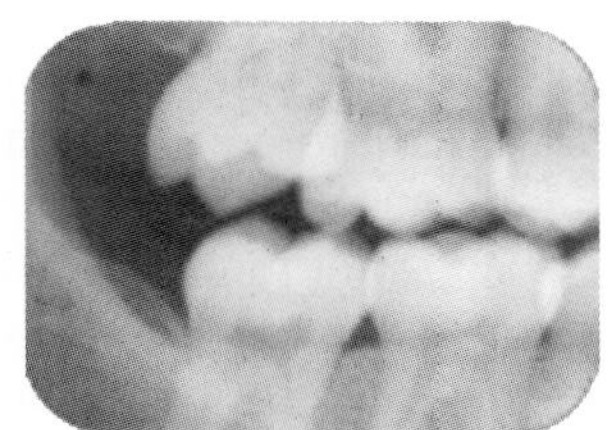

F

Cause: Incorrect horizontal angulation
Correction: Direct central ray through interproximal spaces.

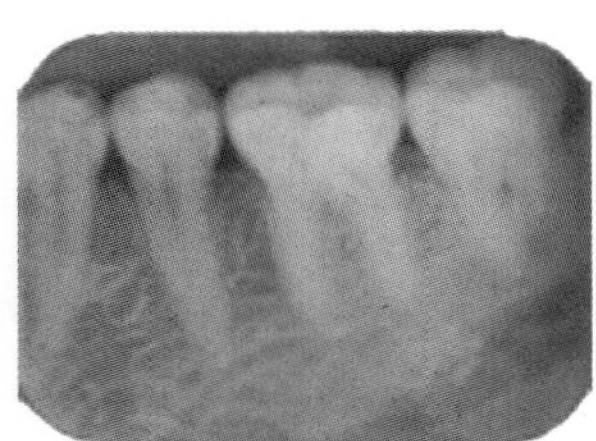

G

Cause: Vertical angulation too steep
Correction: Use XCP instruments to avoid excessive angulation.

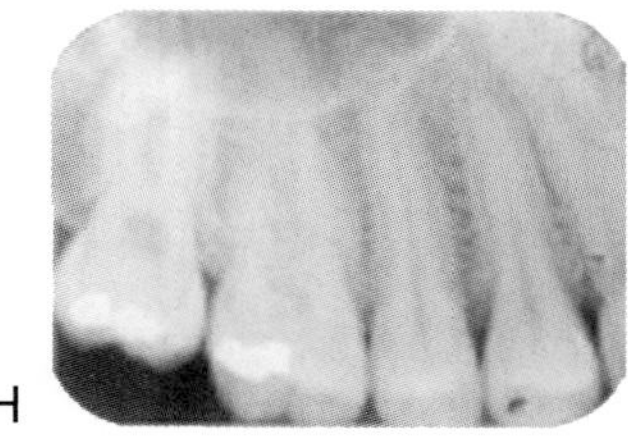

H

Cause: Vertical angulation too flat
Correction: Use XCP instruments to avoid insufficient angulation.

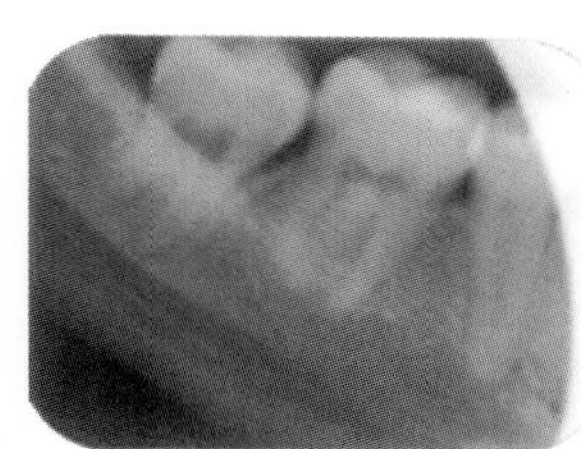

I

Cause: PID not properly aligned
Correction: Always check film for bending before exposure.

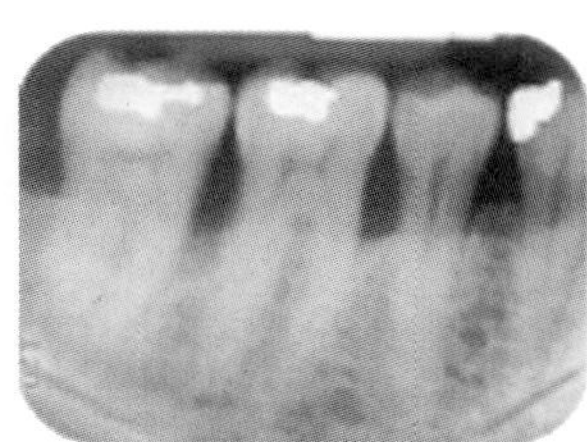

J

Cause: Film excessively bent
Correction: Always check film for bending before exposure.

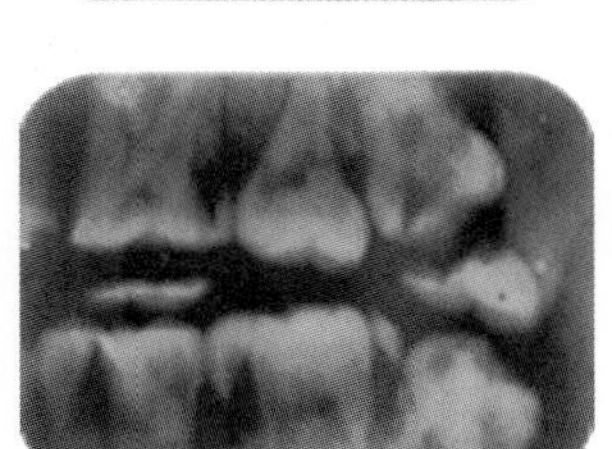

K

Cause: Film exposed twice
Correction: Always separate exposed and nonexposed films.

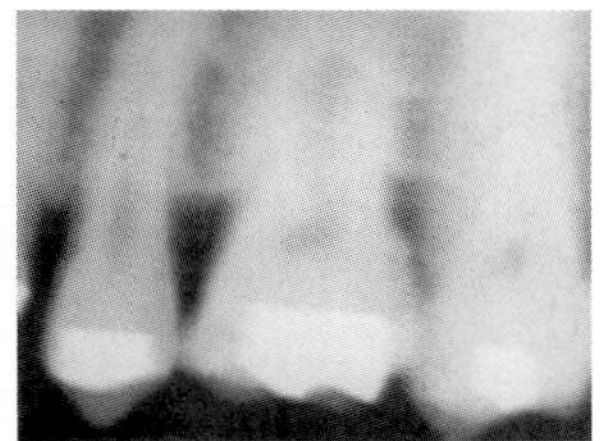

L

Cause: Patient movement
Correction: Stabilize patient's head before exposure. Instruct patient not to move.

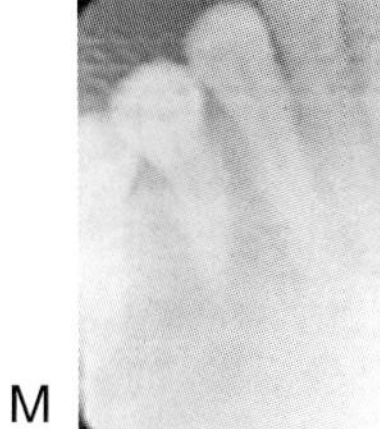

M

Cause: Film placed in mouth backwards
Correction: Check film placement; white side always faces PID.

FIGURE 16-16 Radiographic exposure errors. **A,** Clear. **B,** Black. **C,** Dark. **D,** Light. **E,** No apices. **F,** Overlapped contacts. **G,** Foreshortened image. **H,** Elongated image. **I,** Cone cut. **J,** Distorted image with dark lines on corners. **K,** Double image. **L,** Blurred image. **M,** Light image with herringbone pattern. *XCP,* Extension-cone paralleling; *PID,* position indicator device. (Radiographs from Iannucci J, Jansen Howerton L: *Dental radiography: principles and techniques,* ed 4, St. Louis, 2012, Saunders.)

Replenisher Solution

Replenishers are solutions of developer and fixer that are added to compensate for the loss of volume and the strength of the solutions that results from use.

Manual Processing

Manual processing depends on a combination of:

1. Solution temperature
2. Time in the solution

   Note: Both are critical for the successful processing of film.

See Procedure 16-8: Manual Processing of Dental Radiographs.

Darkroom

Manual film processing requires that the darkroom (Figure 16-17) be light-tight and have adequate working space and good ventilation and be clean and dry at all times. It should be equipped with the following:

- Items required for infection control (e.g., gloves, disinfectant spray, paper towels)
- Disposal container for contaminated film packets or barriers
- Recycle container for lead foil pieces (*Caution:* Lead should not be thrown in the trash.)
- Separate processing tanks for the developer solution, the rinse water, and the fixer solution
- Hot and cold running water supply, with mixing valves to adjust the temperature
- Safelight and a source of white (normal) light. (A safelight is a device that provides enough illumination in the darkroom to work without the danger of fogging the film. Red light bulbs are not safelights.)
- Timer accurate to minutes and seconds
- Accurate thermometer that floats in the tanks to indicate the temperature of solutions
- Stirring rod or paddle to mix the chemicals and to equalize the temperature of solutions
- Safe storage space for chemicals
- Film hangers
- Film-drying rack and film dryer

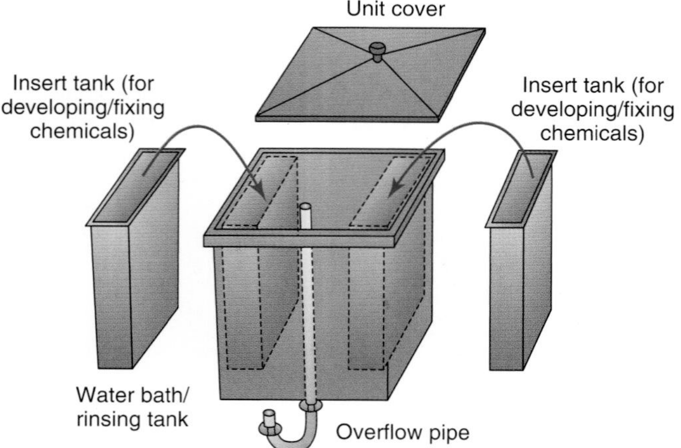

FIGURE 16-17 Processing tanks showing developing and fixing tank inserts in a bath of running water.

Processing Tanks

In most darkrooms, the developer solution is in the tank on the left, the water bath (rinse) is the center tank, and the fixer solution is in the tank on the right. Always check the location of each chemical before processing.

Keep the tank covered except when placing and removing films to prevent evaporation of the solutions.

Automatic Film Processing

Automatic film processing is a simple method used to process dental x-ray films (Box 16-5 and Figure 16-18).

See Procedure 16-9: Automatic Processing of Dental Radiographs Using the Daylight Loader.

An automatic film processor consists of a series of rollers that transport the films through the steps and solutions necessary for complete processing (Figure 16-19).

The temperature of the developer in automatic processors ranges from 85° F to 105° F (29.4° C to 40.5° C), which significantly reduces the developing and overall processing time. Automatic film processing requires only 4 to 6 minutes to develop, fix, wash, and dry a film, whereas manual processing and drying techniques require approximately 1 hour.

Units with a daylight loading capability do not require a darkroom because they have light-tight baffles into which the hands are placed while the film is opened and inserted into the rollers. In a daylight loading unit, the exposed film is unwrapped and processed within the machine.

An automatic processor without daylight loading capability requires the use of a darkroom while unwrapping and placing films into the processor.

Care of the Automatic Processor

The automatic processor must be routinely cleaned and disinfected according to the manufacturer's directions. In addition, automatic processors must have routine preventive maintenance.

The two most common causes of automatic processor breakdown are (1) failure to keep the rollers clean and (2) inadequate replenishing of chemicals. The manufacturer's recommendations for daily and monthly cleaning of the automatic processor must be carefully followed.

BOX 16-5 Advantages of Automatic Film Processing

- Less processing time is required.
- Time and temperature are automatically controlled.
- Less equipment is required.
- Less space is needed.

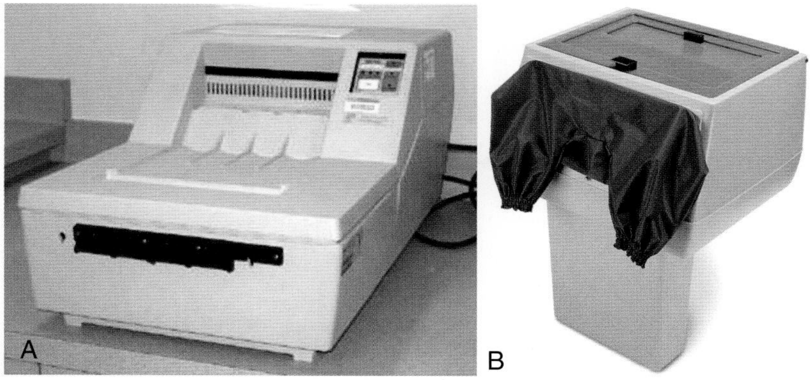

FIGURE 16-18 Automatic film processors. **A,** Without the daylight loader. **B,** With the daylight loader. (**B,** Courtesy Air Techniques, Inc., Melville, New York.)

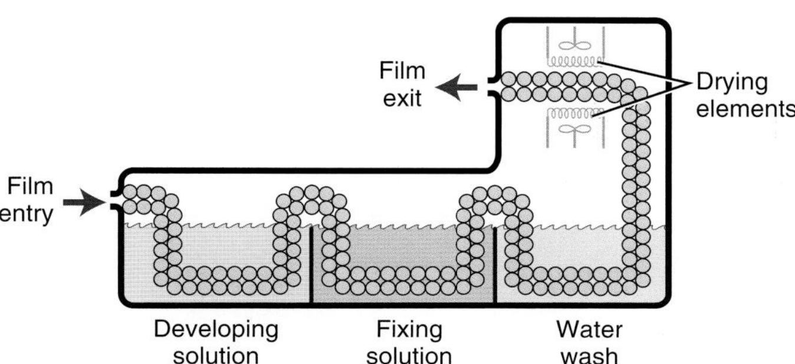

FIGURE 16-19 Workings of an automatic film processor. The operator opens the film packet in the darkroom and inserts the film into the opening. The film is carried on rollers through the processing solutions. The finished film is returned in 4 to 5 minutes. A series of rollers transports the film through developing, fixing, and washing stations. (From White SC, Pharoah MJ: *Oral radiology: principles and interpretation,* ed 7, St. Louis, 2014, Mosby.)

Processing Errors

Proper processing of exposed film is as important as the exposure technique used in producing diagnostic quality radiographs. Dental assistants should readily recognize errors and understand how to avoid them (Figure 16-20).

Duplicating Radiographs

Duplicate radiographs are identical copies of an intraoral or an extraoral radiograph; they may be necessary when:

- Referring a patient to a specialist
- Filing insurance claims
- A patient changes dentists

Equipment and Film Requirements

To duplicate radiographs, you will need a special duplicating type of film and a duplicating machine (Figure 16-21).

Duplicating film is only used for duplication and is never exposed to x-ray beams. Duplicating film is available in periapical sizes and in 5 × 12-inch and 8 × 10-inch sheets.

The duplicating machine uses white light to expose the film. Because the film is light sensitive, the duplication process is performed in the darkroom with the safelight.

Note: The longer the duplicating film is exposed to light, the lighter the duplicate films will become. This is the opposite of x-ray films, which will become darker when exposed to light.

Steps in Duplicating Radiographs

1. Turn on the safelight, and turn off the white light.
2. Place the radiographs on the duplicator machine glass.
3. Place the duplicating film on top of the radiographs with the emulsion side (darker side) against the radiographs.
4. Turn on the light in the duplicating machine for the manufacturer's recommended time.

Purpose: The light passes through the radiographs and strikes the duplicating film.

5. Remove the duplicating film from the machine, and process it normally, using manual or **automatic processing techniques.**

Mounting Radiographs

Processed radiographs are arranged in anatomic order in holders, called *mounts,* to make it easy for the dentist to study and review the film (see Procedure 16-10: Mounting Dental Radiographs). The mount is always labeled with the patient's name and the date that the radiographs were exposed. The dentist's name and address should also be on the mount.

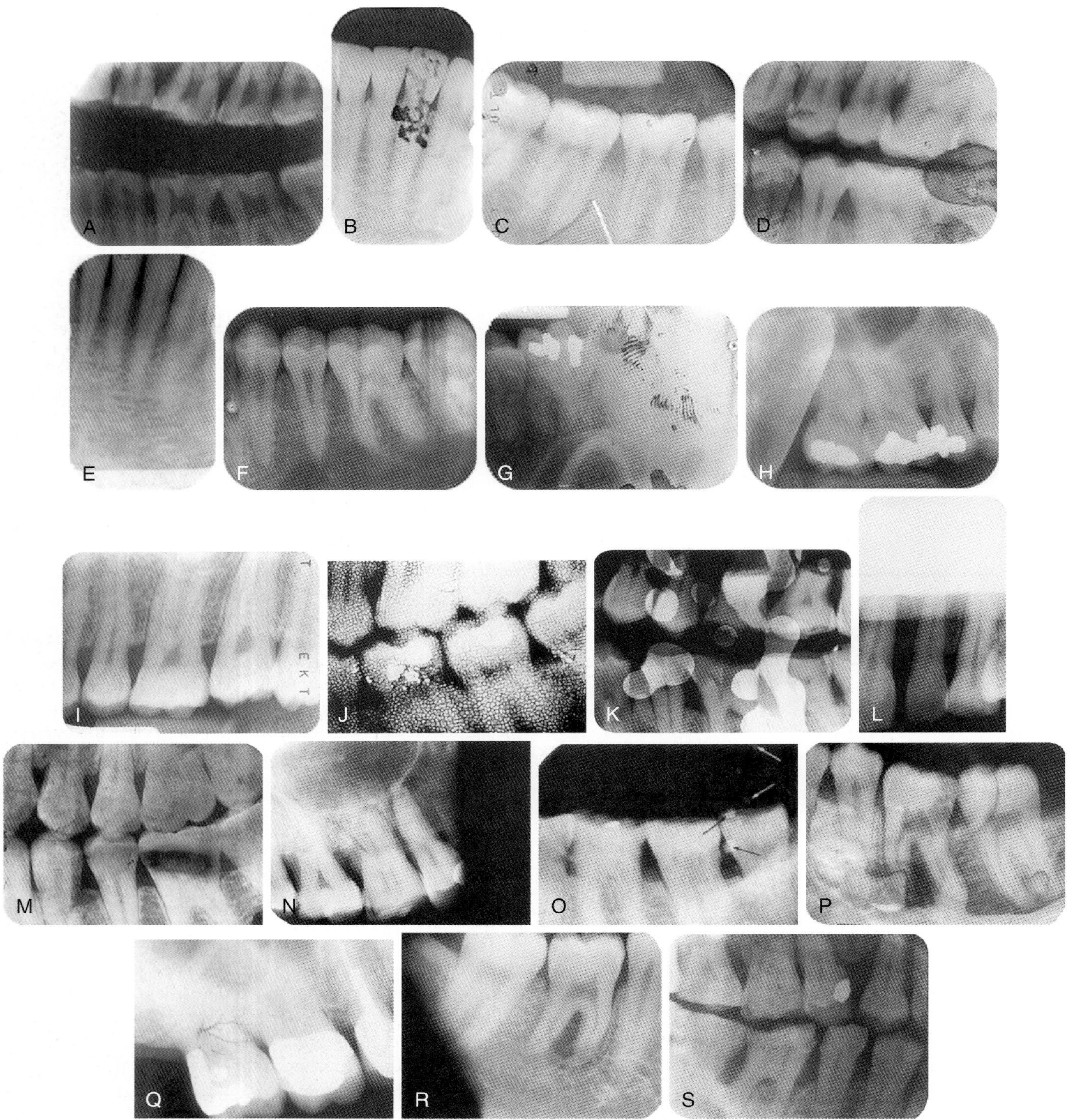

FIGURE 16-20 Radiograph processing errors. **A,** Overdeveloped. **B,** Developer splash. **C,** Scratched film. **D,** Water spots. **E,** Solution too low. **F,** Roller marks. **G,** Fingerprints. **H,** Overlapped films. **I,** Underdeveloped. **J,** Reticulation. **K,** Fixer spots. **L,** Developer cutoff. **M,** Number of errors. **N,** Fixer cutoff. **O,** Air bubbles. **P,** Black fingerprint. **Q,** Static electricity. **R,** Exposure to light. **S,** Fogged film. (From Iannucci J, Jansen Howerton L: *Dental radiography: principles and techniques,* ed 4, St. Louis, 2012, Saunders.)

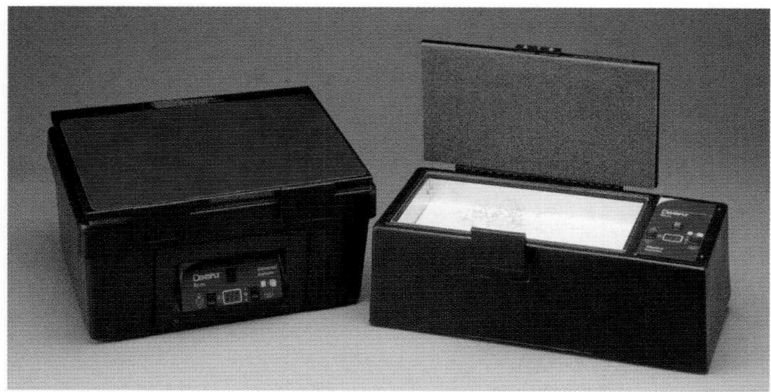

FIGURE 16-21 Film duplicator. (Courtesy DENTSPLY Rinn, Elgin, Illinois.)

Selecting the Mount

Mounts are available in many sizes with different numbers and sizes of windows (openings) to accommodate the number and sizes of exposures in the patient's radiographic survey. The mounts most commonly used for radiographic surveys are available in black, gray, and clear plastic.

Methods of Mounting Films

Two methods can be used when mounting radiographs. Both methods rely on the identification of the raised (embossed) dot found on the film:

1. In method 1, the films are placed in the mount with the raised dots facing up (convex). The American Dental Association (ADA) recommends this method of mounting radiographs. Radiographs are viewed as if the viewer is looking directly at the patient; the patient's left side is on the viewer's right, and the patient's right side is on the viewer's left.
2. In method 2, the radiographs are placed in the mount with the raised dots facing down (concave). Radiographs are viewed as if the viewer is inside the patient's mouth and is looking out; the patient's left side is on the viewer's left, and the patient's right side is on the viewer's right.

Note: Knowing how the dentist prefers to have radiographs mounted is very important. Mistakes in mounting radiographs can result in errors in the dental treatment.

Tips for Mounting Radiographs

Images of normal anatomy can help you correctly place the films in the mount (Figure 16-22). Using dental restorations and missing teeth as aids is also helpful in mounting films. To mount the films with the raised dot facing up, remember that it should look like a pimple, not a dimple.

Digital Radiography

Digital radiography is a type of x-ray imaging that uses digital x-ray sensors to replace traditional photographic x-ray film. It produces enhanced computer images of the teeth and other oral structures and conditions. Digital dental images can be taken inside (intraoral) or outside (extraoral) of the mouth.

Digital imaging has revolutionized radiology in dentistry. There are many reasons for the steady increase in the use of digital technologies:

- Digital imaging eliminates chemical processing. Therefore processing errors are eliminated, and no hazardous wastes such as processing chemicals and lead foil are used.
- Images can be electronically transferred to other health care providers without any distortion of the original image.
- Digital imaging requires significantly less x-radiation than conventional radiography because the image receptors are more sensitive to x-ray beams than conventional film. Exposure times for digital imaging are 50% to 80% less than those required for radiography using conventional film.
- Most digital imaging systems use a standard dental x-ray machine. However, the exposure timer must be calibrated to allow exposures in a time frame of a second. A standard x-ray unit that is adapted for digital radiography can still be used for conventional radiography.
- Digital imaging allows enhancements, measurements, and corrections to be made that are not possible with film (Table 16-5 and Box 16-6).

Types of Digital Imaging Systems

There are two primary technologies in digital dental imaging: (1) *solid-state technology* and (2) *phosphor storage plate technology.*

Solid-State Technology

With the solid-state system, a *sensor,* or a **charge-coupled device (CCD)**, is the image receptor. It contains an x-ray–sensitive silicon chip with an electronic circuit embedded in the silicon (Figure 16-23). The image is recorded on the sensor (instead of film) and is then sent to a computer that **digitizes** (converts to numbers) the electronic impulses, allowing the computer to produce a diagnostic image on a monitor almost instantaneously.

Intraoral sensors used in digital radiography may be wired or wireless. *Wired* means that the imaging sensor is held by a fiberoptic cable to a computer that records the generated signal. *Wireless* means that the sensor is not linked by a cable. The concept of wireless is similar to a remote control for a television (Figure 16-24).

Phosphor Storage Plate Technology

This technique uses reusable **phosphor storage plates (PSPs)** as the image receptor. They are thin flexible plates the size and shape of conventional x-ray film that has been coated with phosphor crystals. During exposure, the PSPs absorb and store the electrons from x-ray beams and release this energy as light (phosphorescence), creating a latent image on the plate. The plate must be scanned before the image can be viewed on the computer.

The scanner *reads* the information on the plate by using a bright light beam to release the electrons from the plate and convert it into a digital image on the computer.

Exposure

Before using them on a patient, the plates are inserted into specially designed barrier envelopes that are impervious to oral fluids and light (Figure 16-25). The barrier envelopes are then sealed closed, and the imaging plates are ready to be positioned

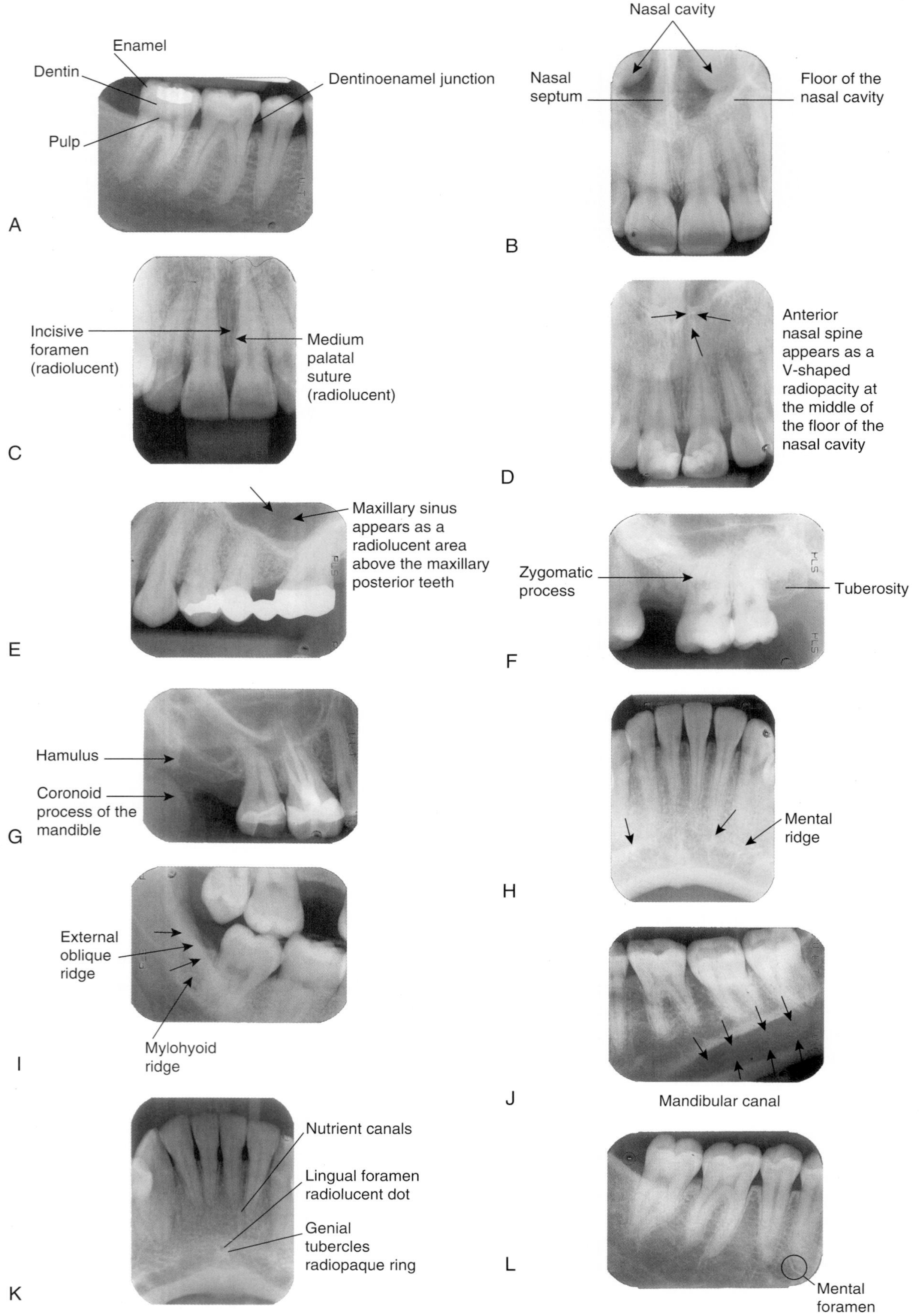

FIGURE 16-22 Radiographic landmarks of normal anatomy. **A,** Structures of the tooth. **B** through **D,** Maxillary structures. Radiographic landmarks of normal anatomy. **E** through **G,** Maxillary structures. **H** through **L,** Mandibular structures.

TABLE 16-5
Advantages and Disadvantages of Digital Radiography

Advantages	
Gray-scale resolution	Gray-scale resolution is excellent, which is important because an accurate diagnosis is often based on contrast. The dentist may manipulate the contrast on the computer.
Reduced radiation exposure to the patient	Digital radiographic systems require 50% to 80% less radiation exposure than conventional x-ray units.
Faster viewing of images	Images are almost immediately ready for viewing.
Lower equipment and film costs	Costs for x-ray film and processing solutions are eliminated. No environmental concerns related to disposal of processing chemicals are present.
Patient education	Patients can see and understand conditions within the teeth. Can increase the patient's willingness to accept treatment plans.
Disadvantages	
Initial setup costs	Digital radiography systems require an initial investment estimated at $10,000, depending on the type of computer and other auxiliary features.
Quality of images	Not everyone agrees, but the images appear to be satisfactory to diagnose dental disease.
Sensor size	Some patients find the sensors bulky and complain about the thickness. Some patients tend to gag more frequently than when traditional film is used.
Infection control	The sensor must be protected with disposable control barriers because the digital sensor cannot be heat sterilized.

BOX 16-6 Infection Control Steps in Digital Imaging

Treatment Area

1. Place barriers or disinfect the x-ray machine, dental chair, work area, computer, mouse, and lead apron.
2. Before seating the patient, gather positioning devices, cotton rolls, paper towels, and disposable cup.

Preparation of the Patient and Operator

1. Before gloving, seat the patient and adjust the chair and headrest. Ask the patient to remove objects from the face and mouth. Place the lead apron.
2. Wash your hands, put on gloves, and assemble positioning devices.

Exposure of Images

1. After each exposure, dry the image receptor.
2. Never place a positioner on uncovered surfaces.

After Exposure of Images

1. Before removing your gloves, dispose of all contaminated items (such as cotton rolls).
2. Place the positioner device in an area for contaminated instruments.
3. Remove your gloves, wash your hands, and remove the lead apron.

in the patient's mouth using the same placement and positioning techniques used with conventional film.

After exposure, the imaging plates are carefully removed from the contaminated barrier envelope using the same precautions as when handling contaminated x-ray films.

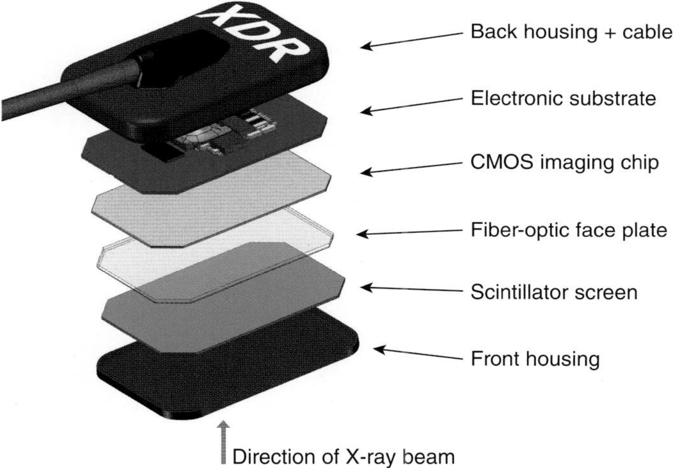

FIGURE 16-23 Enlarged view of a digital sensor. (Courtesy of XDR Radiology, Los Angeles, California.)

Scanning the Phosphor Storage Plate

Exposed PSP receptors must be scanned to release stored energy, digitize the image, and display it on a computer monitor. After exposure, scanning should take place as soon as possible because the electrons creating the image are released over time and the latent image will fade. Plates with exposed images that were exposed at the proper settings may be stored for 12 to 24 hours and will retain acceptable quality.

Erasing the Phosphor Storage Plate

After the digital image has been transferred into the computer, the plates must be erased to remove the previous image and be

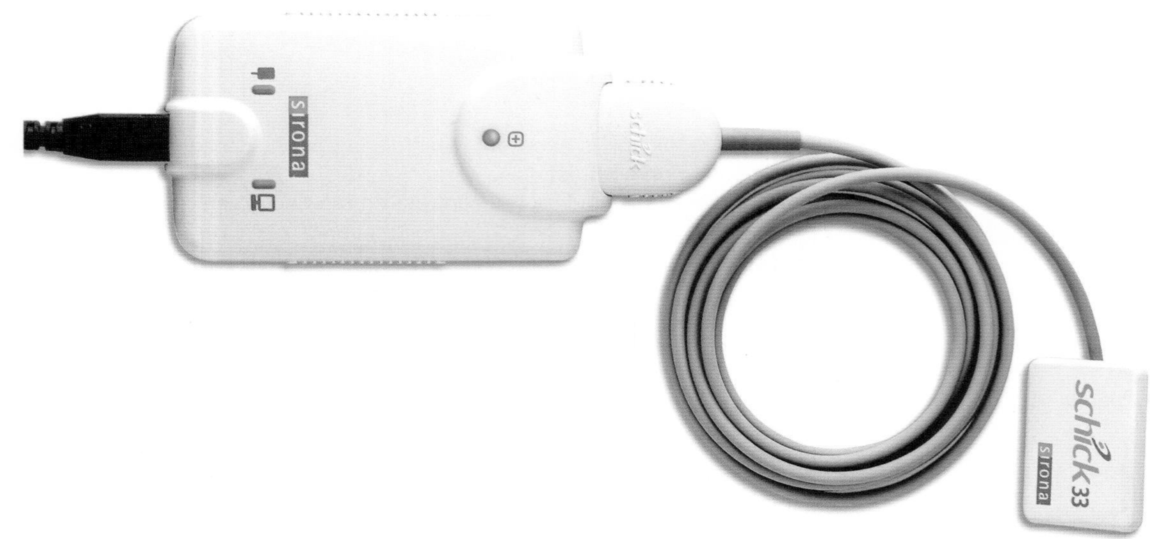

FIGURE 16-24 Cable sensor. (Courtesy Dentsply Sirona, Charlotte, NC.)

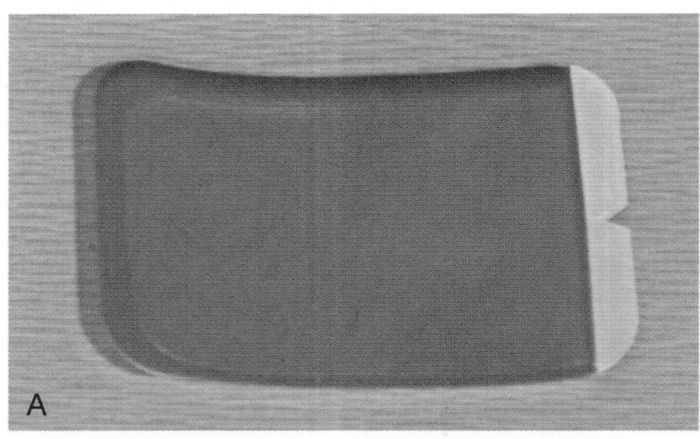

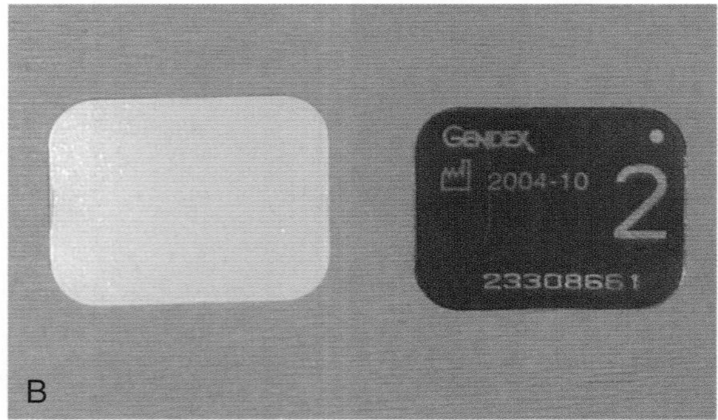

FIGURE 16-25 **A,** Barrier envelope for the phosphor storage plate. **B,** Front and back sides of a phosphor storage plate. (From Bird DL, Robinson DS: *Modern dental assisting,* ed 11, St. Louis, 2015, Saunders.)

ready for the next use. A semidark environment is recommended when handling the plates. The more intense the background light and the longer the plates are exposed to background light, the greater the loss of electrons, degrading the image. *Note:* Red safelights found in most darkrooms are not safe for PSPs, which are most sensitive to the red light spectrum.

Erasing the images is done by flooding the plates with bright light, such as on a dental view box with the phosphor side of the plate facing the light for 1 or 2 minutes. More intense light sources can be used for shorter periods. Some manufacturers integrate automatic plate-erasing lights in their system. Inadequate plate erasure results in double images and results in a nondiagnostic image. PSPs are expensive and must be handled with care to ensure that they do not become scratched or exposed to dust.

Computer

The computer stores the incoming electronic signal and converts it from the sensor or PSP to shades of gray that are viewed on the computer monitor. Digital imaging technology allows the dentist to manipulate the image to enlarge it and change the contrast and density of the image without additional radiation exposure to the patient.

The image is recorded on the computer in 0.5 to 120 seconds—significantly less time than is required for conventional film processing. This speed of image recording is extremely useful during certain types of dental procedures, such as surgical implants or root canal therapy. This speed of recording is also excellent for patient education and case presentation. Images may be permanently stored in the computer, printed on a hard copy for the patient record, electronically transmitted to insurance companies or referring dentists, and used for legal purposes.

Procedures

Positioning of the sensor or PSP for periapical and bite-wing projections is the same as the technique used in conventional film placement. Step-by-step procedures for the use of digital radiography systems vary by manufacturer. Referring to the manufacturer's instruction booklet for information concerning the operation of the system, equipment preparation, patient preparation, and exposure factors is critical.

Sensor Preparation

The technique for the placement of the intraoral sensor in the mouth of the patient is similar to the technique used in

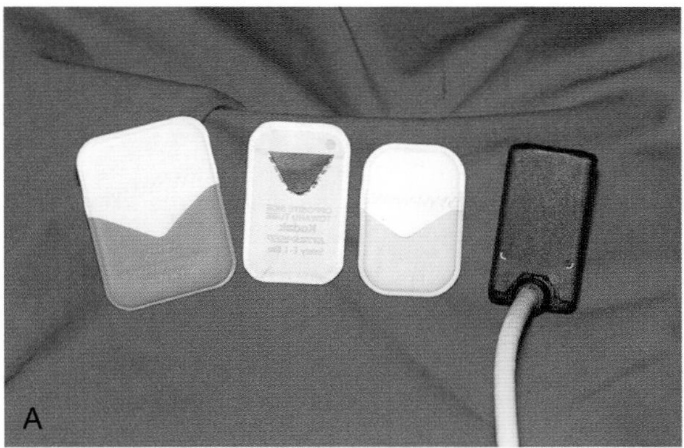

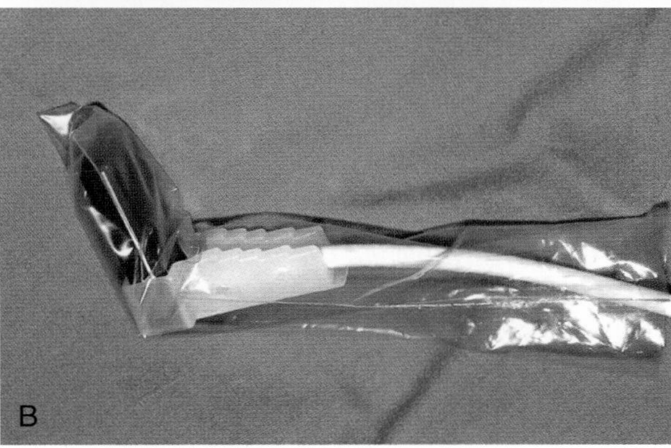

FIGURE 16-26 **A,** Size of the electronic sensor is compared with size Nos. 0, 1, and 2 traditional intraoral film. **B,** Electronic sensor is protected with a plastic barrier and is ready for positioning into the patient's mouth in the same manner as used with conventional film and holder. (Courtesy Dr. Michael Danford, Santa Rosa, California.)

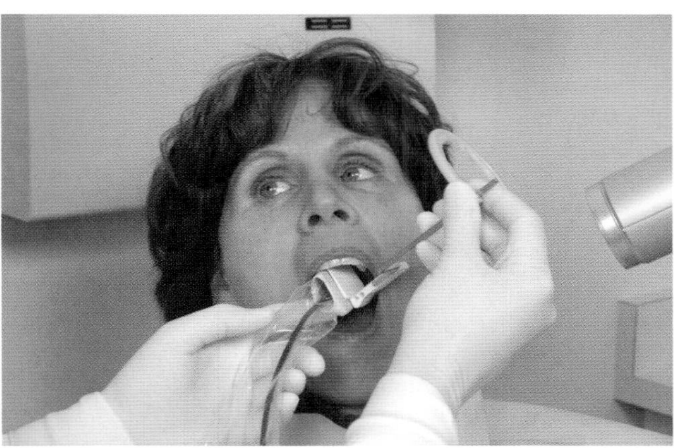

FIGURE 16-27 Sensor is being placed in the patient's mouth.

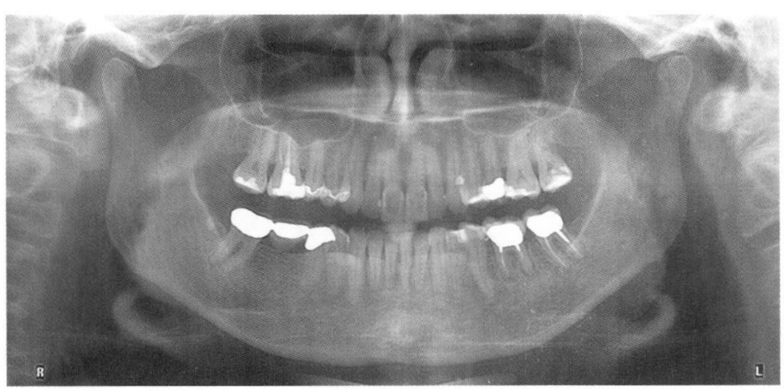

FIGURE 16-28 Panoramic radiograph. (From White SC, Pharoah MJ: *Oral radiology: principles and interpretation,* ed 7, St. Louis, 2014, Mosby.)

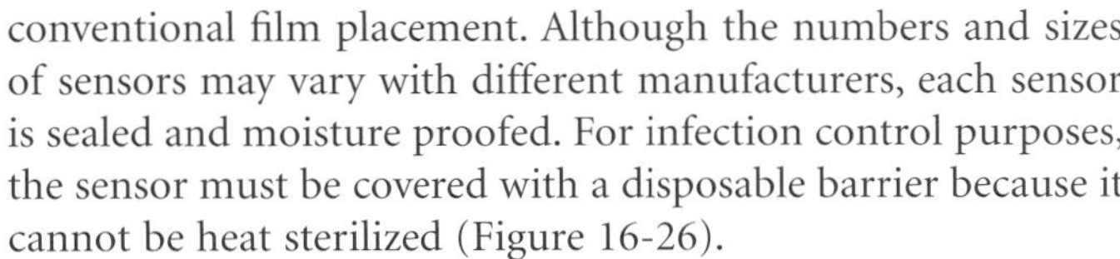

conventional film placement. Although the numbers and sizes of sensors may vary with different manufacturers, each sensor is sealed and moisture proofed. For infection control purposes, the sensor must be covered with a disposable barrier because it cannot be heat sterilized (Figure 16-26).

Sensor Placement

The sensor is held in the mouth by special film-holding devices. The paralleling technique is the preferred exposure method because of the dimensional accuracy of the images. Paralleling technique film holders must be used to stabilize the sensor in the mouth. As with conventional intraoral film, the sensor is centered over the area of interest (Figure 16-27).

Common Errors

As with film-based techniques, errors can happen when the operator fails to place the image receptor or align the x-ray beam properly. Correct vertical and horizontal angulation is essential. Digital imaging does not prevent operator errors resulting in foreshortening, elongation, closed contacts, and cone cuts. The quality of digital images is still based on the skill of the operator.

Radiation Safety and Protection

Although the amount of radiation to the patient from digital imaging is less than from film-based techniques, it is still ionizing radiation, and the operator must still follow the **ALARA** (**A**s **L**ow **A**s **R**easonably **A**chievable) principle. As always, the patient should be protected with a thyroid collar (for intraoral imaging only) and lead apron, and the operator should be behind an adequate barrier or at a 6-foot distance and between a 90- and a 135-degree angle to the beam.

Extraoral Radiography

Panoramic Radiographs

Panoramic radiographs allow the dentist to view the entire dentition and related structures on a single large film. The images on a panoramic film are not as well defined or clear as the images on intraoral films (Figure 16-28). Therefore bite-wing films are used to supplement a panoramic radiograph to detect dental caries or periapical lesions (Box 16-7).

Panoramic units may use panoramic film or be digital. In **panoramic radiography**, both the film and the tubehead rotate around the patient, producing a series of individual images. When these images are combined to present a single

BOX 16-7 Panoramic Radiographs in Dentistry

Are used to:
- Locate impacted teeth.
- Observe tooth eruption patterns.
- Detect lesions in the jaw.
- Detect features in the bone.
- Provide an overall view of the mandible and maxilla.

Are not used to:
- Substitute for intraoral films.
- Diagnose dental caries.
- Diagnose periodontal disease.
- Diagnose periapical lesions.

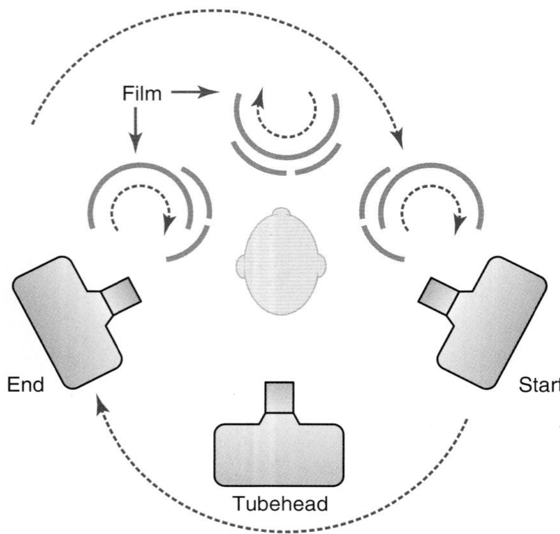

FIGURE 16-29 The film and tubehead move around the patient in opposite directions. (Courtesy of Dr. Robert M. Jaynes, Assistant Professor, Oral Radiology Group, The Ohio State University College of Dentistry.)

image, an overall view of the maxilla and mandible is created (Figure 16-29).

Advantages and Disadvantages

As with all radiographic techniques, panoramic radiography has both advantages and disadvantages (Table 16-6).

Equipment

Many styles of panoramic x-ray units are available. Although each manufacturer's panoramic unit is slightly different, all machines have similar components. The primary components of the panoramic unit include the panoramic x-ray tubehead, head positioner, and exposure controls (Figure 16-30).

Tubehead The panoramic x-ray tubehead is similar to an intraoral tubehead in that it has a filament to produce electrons and a target to produce radiographs. Unlike the intraoral tubehead, the vertical angulation of the panoramic tubehead is not adjustable.

TABLE 16-6
Advantages and Disadvantages of Panoramic Radiography

Advantages	
Field size	The entire maxilla and mandible can be visualized on one panoramic film.
Ease of use	Learning how to expose a panoramic radiograph is relatively quick and easy.
Patient acceptance	Most patients prefer the panoramic radiograph because they do not have to hold uncomfortable film in their mouths.
Less radiation exposure	The patient receives less radiation exposure as compared with the full-mouth radiographic survey (FMX).
Disadvantages	
Image sharpness	The images seen on a panoramic radiograph are not as sharp as those visualized on an intraoral film.
Focal trough limitations	Structures must be within the focal trough or they will appear out of focus.
Distortion	Even when the proper technique is used, some overlapping of the teeth and distortion of the images will always be noted.
Cost of equipment	Compared with the cost of an intraoral radiograph unit, a panoramic unit is more expensive.

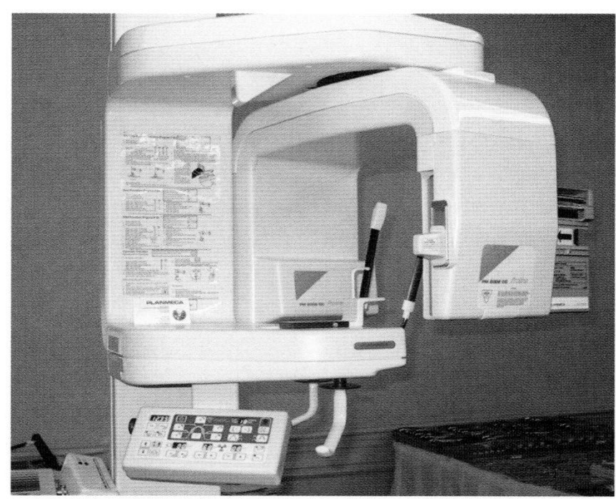

FIGURE 16-30 Primary components of a panoramic unit.

Head positioner Each panoramic unit has a head positioner that is used to align the patient's teeth as accurately as possible. Each head positioner consists of a chin rest, a notched bite-block, a forehead rest, and lateral head supports or guides (Figure 16-31). Each panoramic unit is unique, and the operator must follow the manufacturer's instructions to position the patient correctly.

Exposure controls Exposure controls allow the milliamperage and kilovoltage settings to be adjusted to accommodate

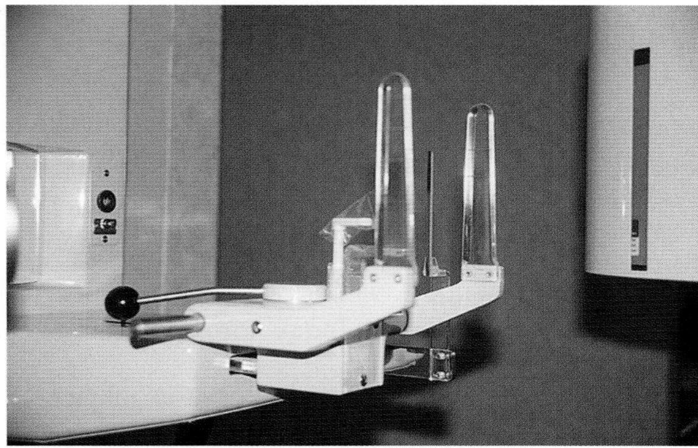

FIGURE 16-31 Head positioner, consisting of a notched bite-block, forehead rest, and lateral head supports, is used to position the patient's head.

patients of different sizes. Step-by-step procedures for exposure of a panoramic film include equipment preparation.

See Procedure 16-11: Preparing the Equipment for Panoramic Radiography, Procedure 16-12: Preparing the Patient for Panoramic Radiography, and Procedure 16-13: Positioning the Patient for Panoramic Radiography.

Common Errors

To produce a diagnostic panoramic radiograph and minimize patient exposure, you must avoid mistakes and follow the guidelines for exposing panoramic radiographs (Box 16-8).

Infection Control

See Procedure 16-14: Practicing Infection Control With Digital Sensors, and Procedure 16-15: Practicing Infection Control With Phosphor Storage Plates.

Informed Consent

Informed consent includes explaining to the patient the purpose of taking radiographs and helping the patient understand the risks and benefits of dental radiographs. An example would be informing the patient of the conditions and diseases that might go undetected without radiographs and what the consequences might be. If the patient is a minor or a legally incompetent adult, then the parent or guardian must give consent.

Documentation

Exposure of dental radiographs must always be documented in the patient dental record and should include the following information:

- Informed consent
- Number and type of radiographs exposed
- Rationale for exposing such radiographs
- Diagnostic information obtained from the radiographs

BOX 16-8 Guidelines for Exposing Panoramic Radiographs

1. Use a plastic barrier on the bite-block.
2. Use the manufacturer's recommendations for exposure factors.
3. Explain the procedure to the patient.
4. Place the proper type of lead apron.
5. Ask the patient to remove all radiolucent objects.
6. Ask the patient to sit or stand as straight as possible.
7. Ask the patient to place his or her anterior teeth in the groove on the bite-block.
8. Position the patient with the midsagittal plane perpendicular to the floor.
9. Position the patient with the Frankfort plane parallel to the floor.
10. Ask the patient to close the lips on the bite-block and to swallow and place the tongue against the roof of the mouth.
11. Ask the patient to remain still during the exposure.

Ownership of Dental Radiographs

Although the patient or the insurance company paid the fee for the radiographs, the dentist owns the dental radiographs. Radiographs are diagnostic aids and are considered a part of the patient's permanent record.

Patients have a right to reasonable access to their records, including a copy of the radiographs. If a patient moves or transfers to another dentist, then the patient can request in writing that his or her radiographs or digital images be forwarded to that dentist. Duplicate radiographs should be made and forwarded to the new dentist, and the original radiographs and digital images should be retained in the patient's record.

Ethical Implications

You must be aware of the laws in your state regarding the use of ionizing radiation in dentistry and must comply with all licensing or certification requirements.

Exposing patients to radiation has health and safety considerations and implications for the proper diagnosis of dental disease and treatment planning. In addition, legal action is a possibility if an improper diagnosis is made or if a lack of treatment results because of dental radiographs that are not properly exposed or processed.

Procedure 16-1

Practicing Infection Control During Film Exposure

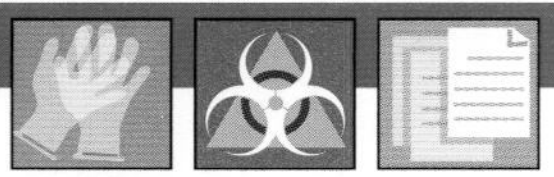

Goal

To perform all infection control practices during film exposure

Equipment and Supplies

- Barriers for the operatory
- Paper towels
- X-ray film or digital sensors (sizes as necessary)
- Packaged film- or sensor-holding device
- Sensor or phosphor storage plate (PSP) barriers (optional)
- Lead apron with thyroid collar
- Disposable container for exposed films (labeled with the patient's name)
- Surface cleaner or disinfectant

Procedural Steps

1. Wash and dry your hands.
2. Place surface barriers on equipment and work area.

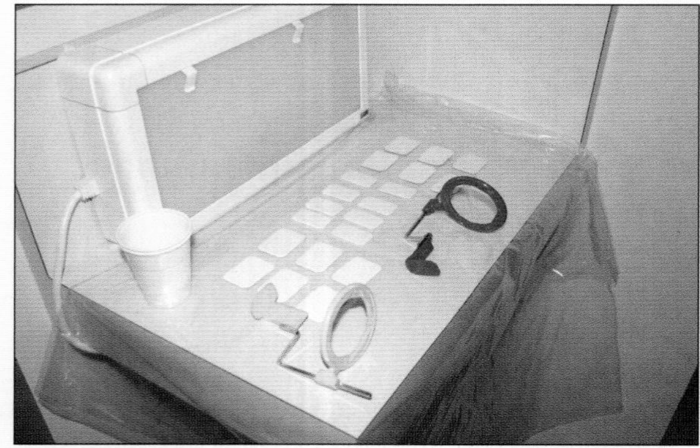

3. Set out the packaged film- or sensor-holding device, film, labeled container for exposed film, paper towel, and other miscellaneous items you might need.

Purpose: **Once gloved, you should not have to leave the operatory area for additional materials.**

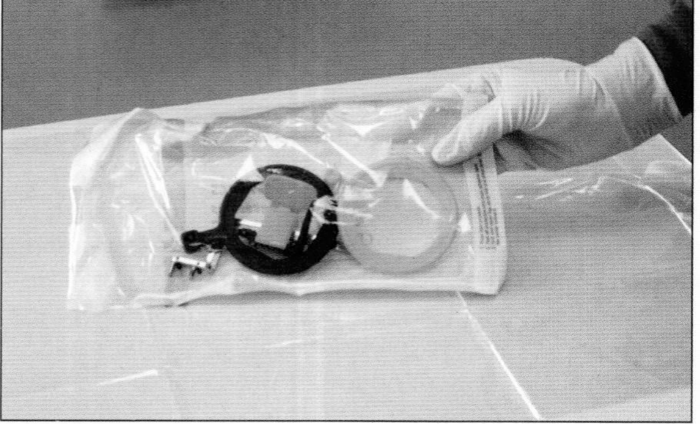

4. Seat the patient, and place the lead apron.
5. Wash and dry your hands, and don gloves.
6. After each exposure, wipe the excess saliva from the film or sensor using a paper towel.

Note: **If you are using a digital sensor, then be very careful not to damage or dislodge the barrier between exposures.**

7. Place each exposed film or PSP into the container, being careful not to touch the external surface.

Purpose: **Your contaminated gloves will contaminate the outer surface of the container.**

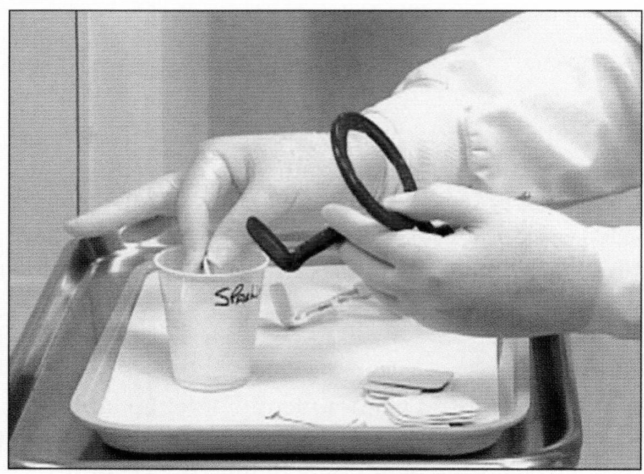

8. After the exposures are complete, remove the lead apron and dismiss the patient.

Note: **To remove the lead apron and still maintain aseptic technique, you can wear overgloves to remove the apron, or you can take off your gloves and remove the apron barehanded. If you remove the lead apron while gloved, then you must disinfect the lead apron.**

9. While still gloved, remove barriers, taking care not to touch the surfaces underneath.

Purpose: **You must wear gloves while removing barriers because they are contaminated. If you touch a surface underneath the barrier while you are removing it, then that surface will become contaminated and must be disinfected.**

10. Dispose of barriers and paper towels.
11. Place the film- or sensor-holding device on a tray to be returned to the instrument-processing area.
12. Wash and dry your hands.
13. Take the exposed films to the processing area.

Procedure 16-2

Assembling Extension-Cone Paralleling (XCP) Instruments

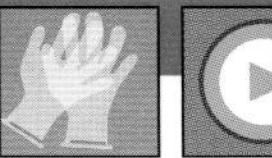

Goal

To assemble Rinn XCP instruments for all areas of the mouth in preparation for radiographic surveys

Equipment and Supplies

- Rinn XCP instruments (for film or digital sensors)

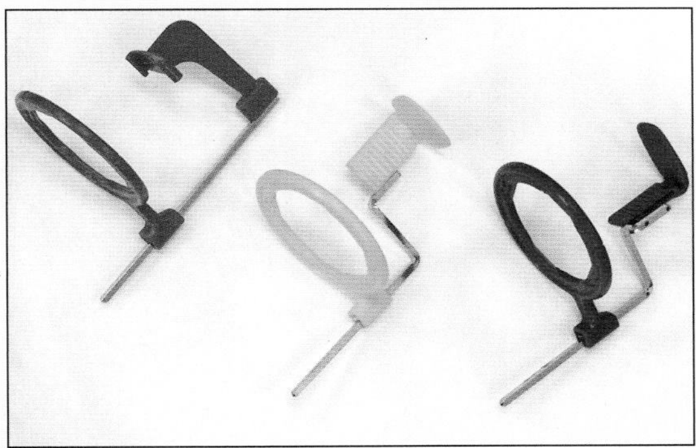

Procedural Steps

Anterior Assembly

1. Lay out the blue parts for the anterior XCP instrument.

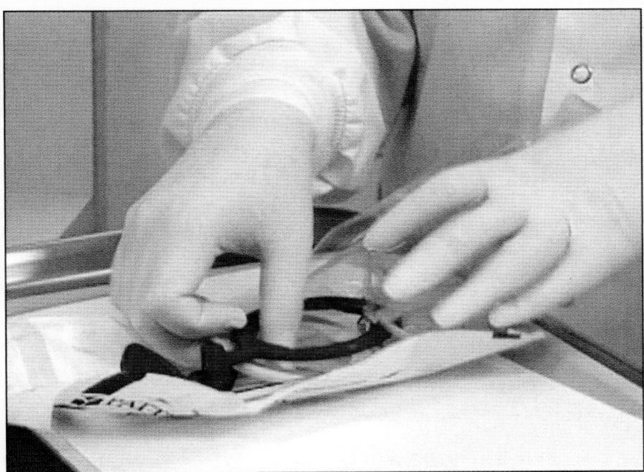

2. Assemble the anterior XCP instrument by inserting the two prongs of the blue anterior indicator arm into the openings in the blue anterior bite-block.

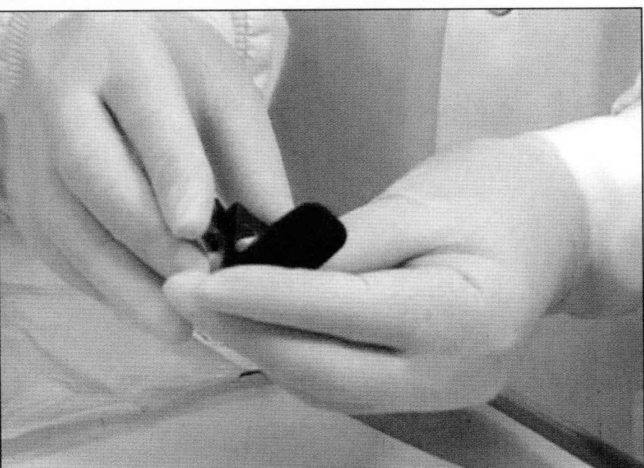

3. Insert the anterior indicator arm into the opening on the blue anterior aiming ring.

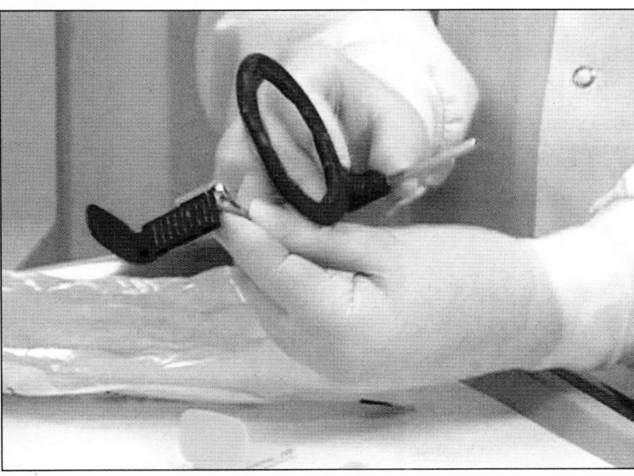

4. Flex the plastic backing of the blue bite-block to open the film slot for easy insertion of the anterior film packet.

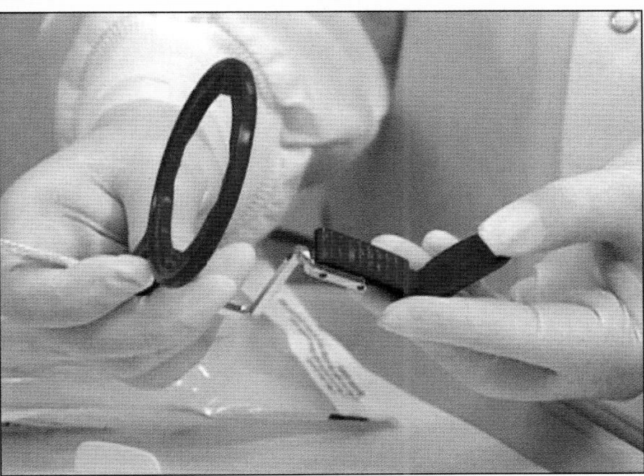

5. The blue anterior XCP instrument is correctly assembled when the film is seen centered in the middle of the aiming ring.

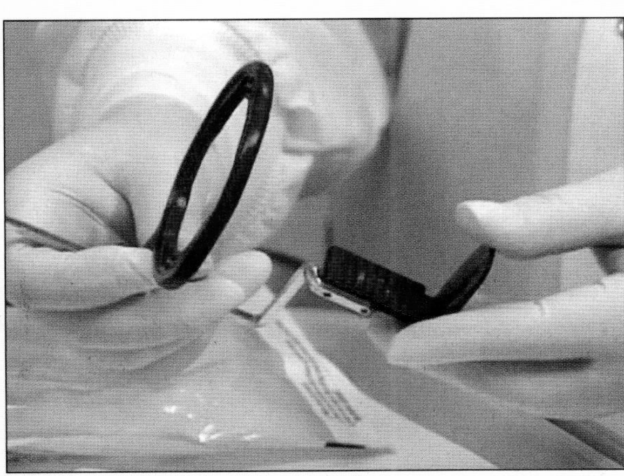

Continued

Procedure 16-2

Assembling Extension-Cone Paralleling (XCP) Instruments—cont'd

Posterior Assembly

1. Lay out the yellow parts for the posterior XCP instrument.
2. Assemble the yellow posterior XCP instrument by inserting the two prongs of the yellow posterior indicator arm into the openings in the yellow posterior bite-block.

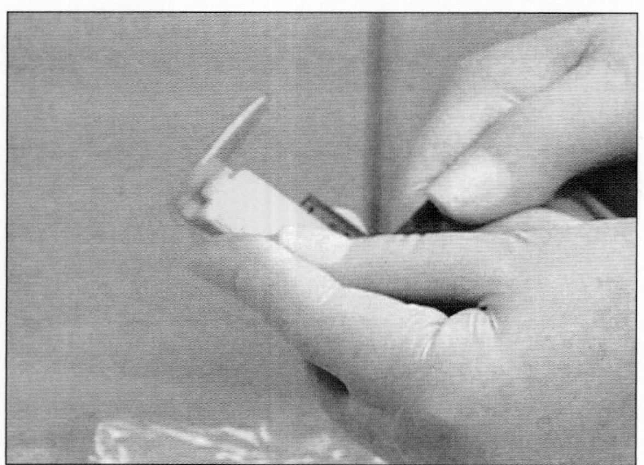

3. Insert the yellow posterior indicator arm into the opening on the yellow posterior aiming ring.

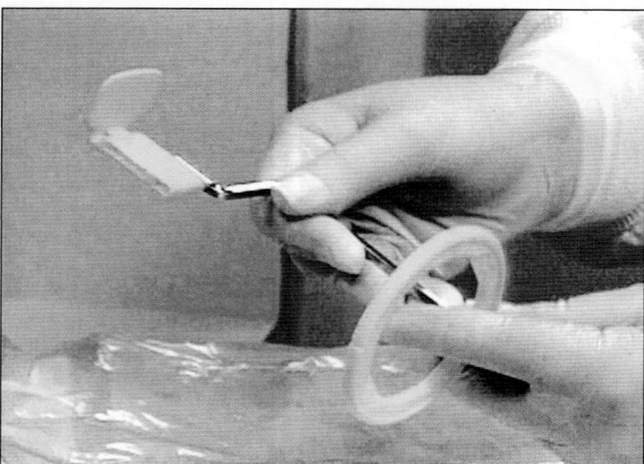

4. Flex the plastic backing of the yellow bite-block to open the film slot for easy insertion of the posterior film packet.

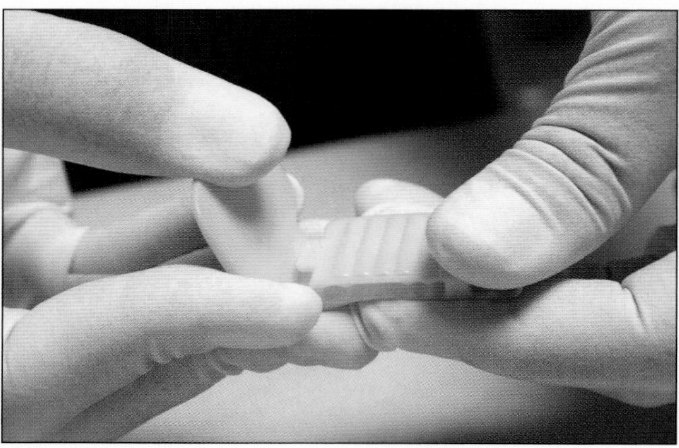

5. The posterior XCP instrument is correctly assembled when the film is seen centered in the middle of the aiming ring.

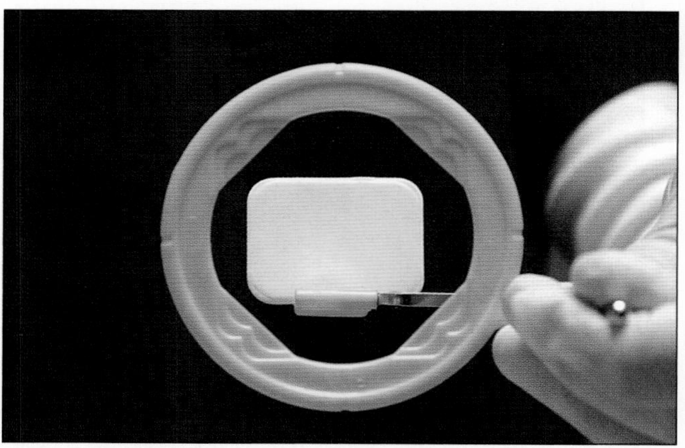

Procedure 16-3

Producing a Full-Mouth Radiographic Survey Using the Paralleling Technique

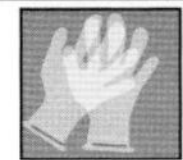
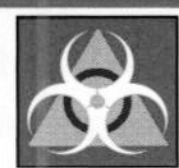
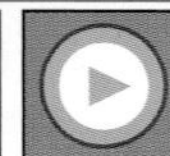
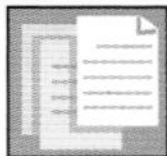

Goal

To follow the proper steps to produce a full-mouth radiographic survey (FMX) using the paralleling technique

Equipment and Supplies

- Appropriate number and size of x-ray films or sensors
- Appropriate infection control materials (paper cup, barriers, paper towel, and impervious surface cover)
- Lead apron and thyroid collar
- Sterile packaged extension-cone paralleling (XCP) instruments
- Cotton rolls
- Patient chart

Procedural Steps

Preparation Before Seating Patient

1. Prepare the operatory with all infection control barriers.

Purpose: Any object that is touched and was not covered with a barrier must be disinfected after the patient is dismissed.

2. Determine the number and type of views to be exposed through a review of the patient's chart, directions from the dentist, or both.
3. If you are using film or phosphor storage plates (PSPs), then label a paper cup with the patient's name and the date. Place it outside the room where the x-ray machine will be used.

Purpose: This is the transfer cup for storing and moving exposed films or PSPs.

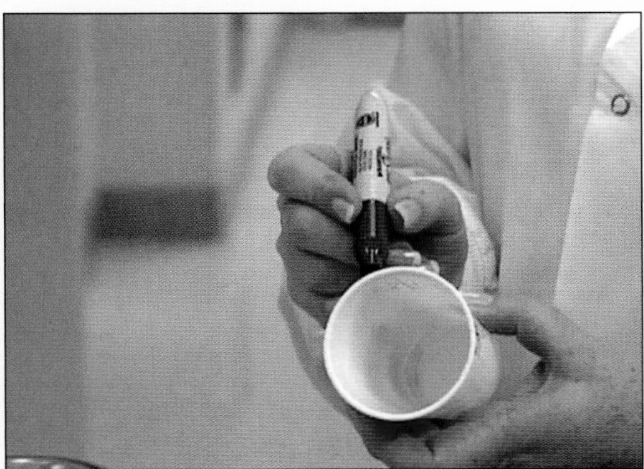

4. Turn on the x-ray machine, and check the basic settings (kilovoltage, milliamperage, and exposure time).
5. Wash and dry your hands.
6. Dispense the desired number of films, and store them outside the room where the x-ray machine is being used.

Purpose: This step prevents fogging caused by scatter radiation.

Positioning the Patient

1. Comfortably seat the patient in the dental chair with his or her back in an upright position and the head supported.
2. Ask the patient to remove eyeglasses and bulky earrings.

Purpose: These objects may cause radiopaque images to be superimposed on the radiographs.

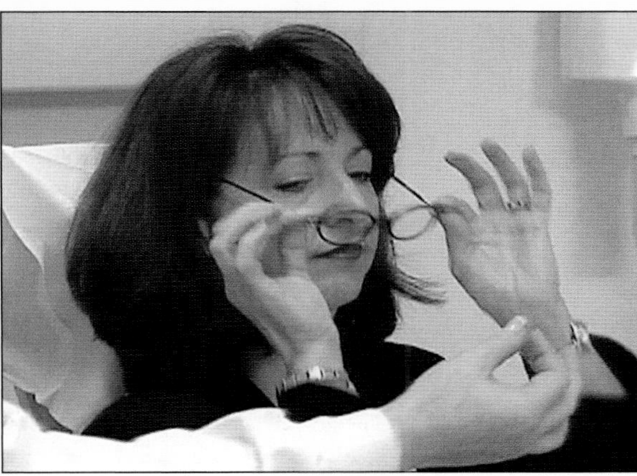

3. Ask the patient to remove prosthetic appliances or objects from the mouth.

Note: Always wear gloves when handling a prosthetic appliance.

4. Position the patient so that the occlusal plane of the jaw being x-rayed is parallel to the floor when the mouth is open.
5. Drape the patient with a lead apron and a thyroid collar.
6. Wash and dry your hands, and put on clean examination gloves.
7. Open the package and assemble the sterile film- or sensor-holding instruments.

Purpose: Allowing the patient to observe you washing your hands, putting on clean gloves, and opening the sterile package of instruments assures the patient that appropriate infection control measures are being taken.

Maxillary Canine Region

1. Vertically insert the No. 1 film packet or sensor into the anterior bite-block.

Note: Not all digital sensors are available in the No. 1 size.

2. Position the film packet or sensor with the canine and first premolar centered. Position the film as far posterior as possible.
3. With the film- or sensor-holding instrument and film in place, instruct the patient to close the mouth slowly but firmly.
4. Position the localizing ring and position indicator device (PID); then make the exposure.

Continued

Procedure 16-3

Producing a Full-Mouth Radiographic Survey Using the Paralleling Technique—cont'd

Note: The image of the lingual cusp of the first premolar is usually superimposed on the distal surface of the canine because of the curvature of the maxillary arch. This contact area must be opened on the view of the premolar region.

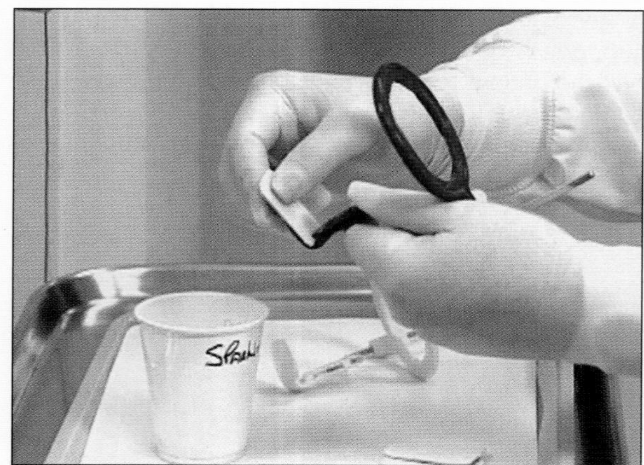

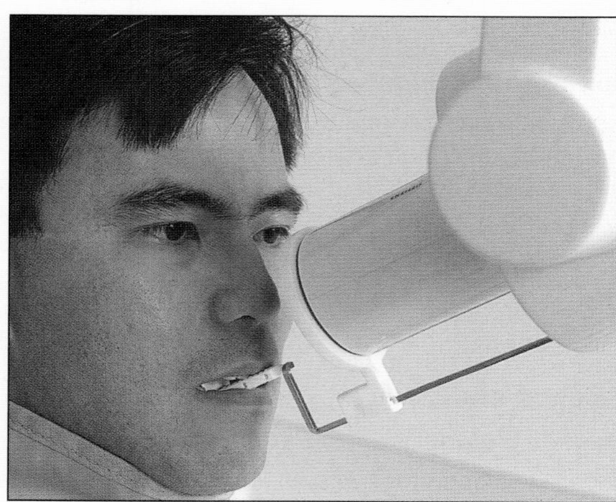

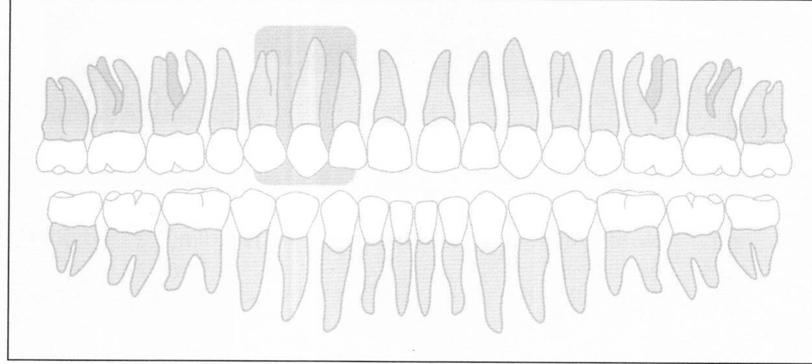

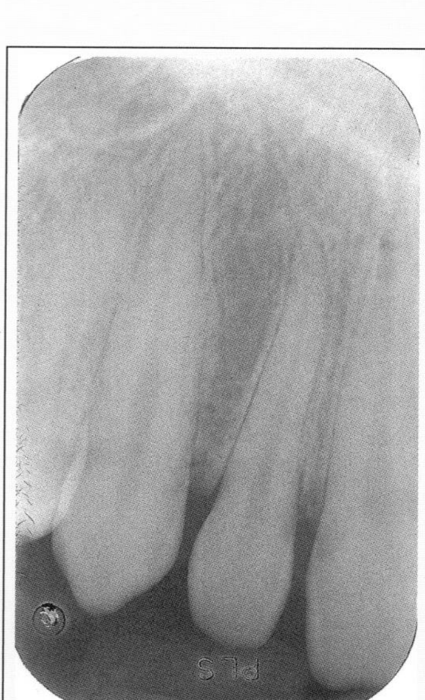

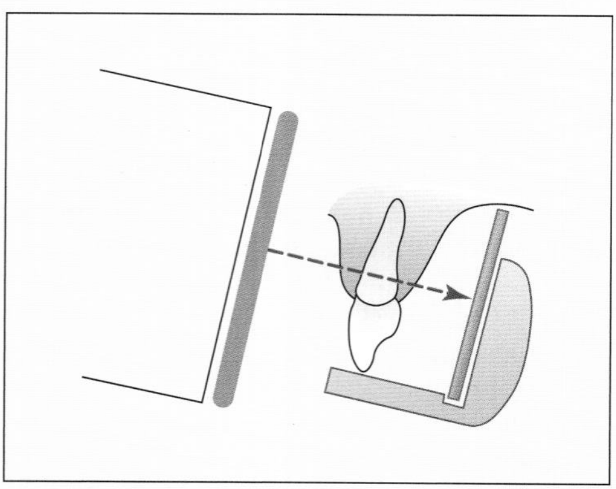

Procedure 16-3

Producing a Full-Mouth Radiographic Survey Using the Paralleling Technique—cont'd

Maxillary Central or Lateral Incisor Region

1. Vertically insert the No. 1 film packet or sensor into the anterior block.

Note: Not all digital sensors are available in the No. 1 size.

2. Center the film packet or sensor between the central and lateral incisors. Position the film or sensor as posterior in the mouth as possible.
3. With the instrument and film in place, instruct the patient to close the mouth slowly but firmly.
4. Position the localizing ring and PID; then make the exposure.

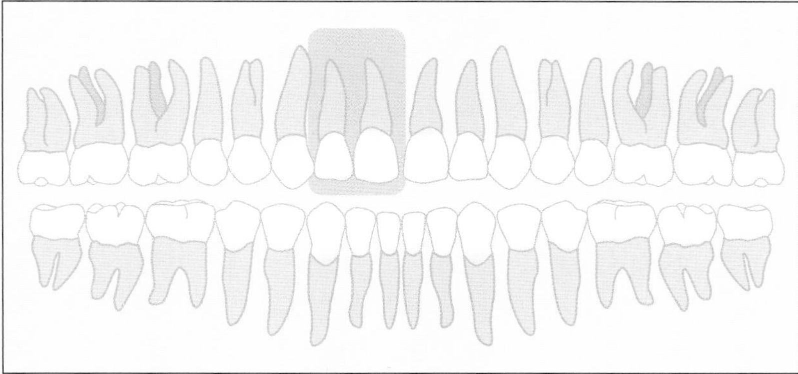

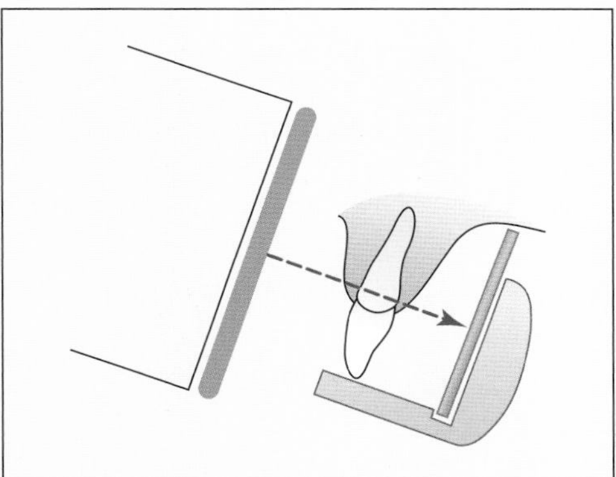

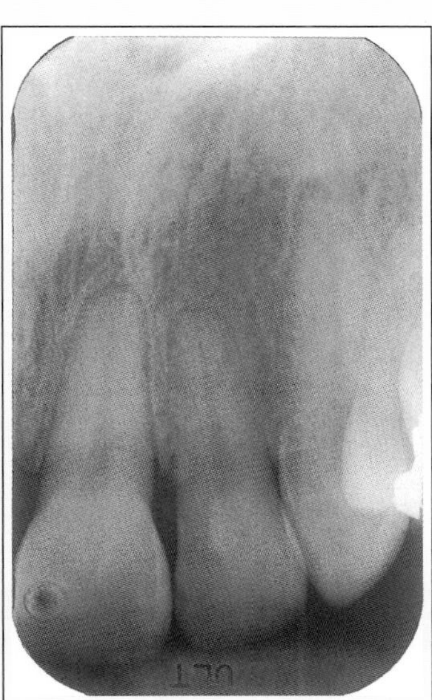

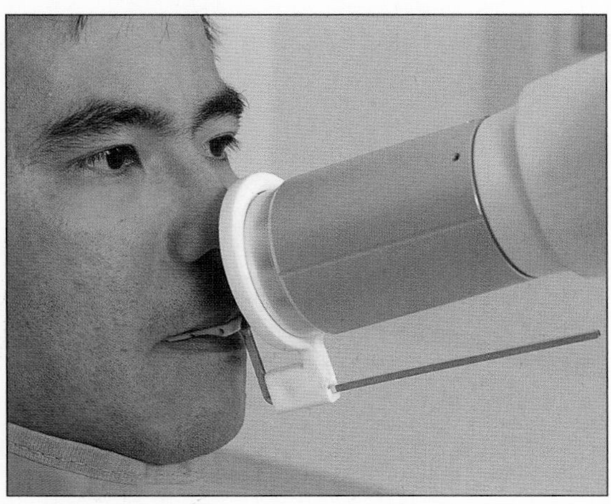

Continued

Procedure 16-3

Producing a Full-Mouth Radiographic Survey Using the Paralleling Technique—cont'd

Mandibular Canine Region

1. Vertically insert the No. 1 film packet or sensor into the anterior block.

Note: Not all digital sensors are available in the No. 1 size.

2. Center the film or sensor on the canine. Position the film or sensor as far in the lingual direction as the patient's anatomy will allow.

Note: **A cotton roll may be placed between the maxillary teeth and the bite-block to prevent rocking of the bite-block on the canine tip and to increase patient comfort.**

3. With the instrument and film in place, instruct the patient to close the mouth slowly but firmly.
4. Position the localizing ring and PID; then make the exposure.

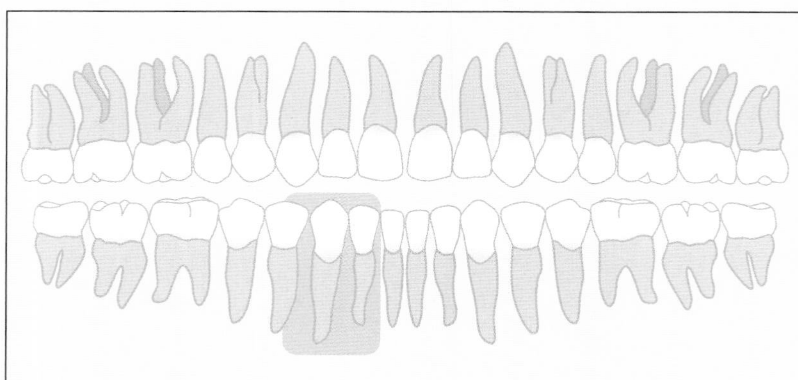

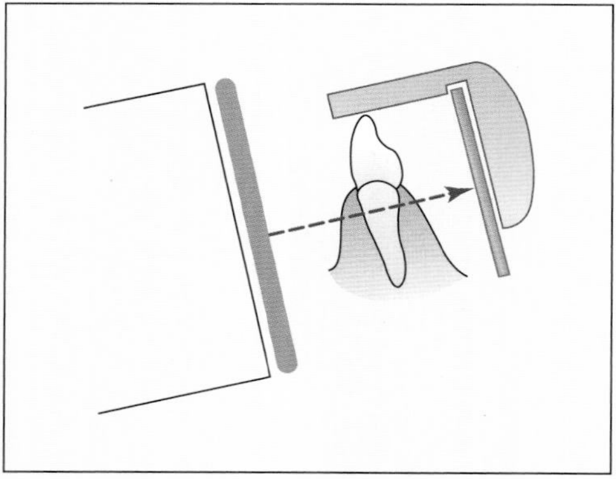

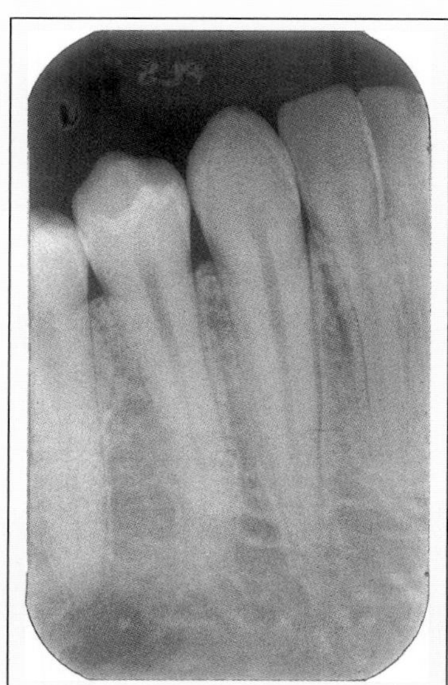

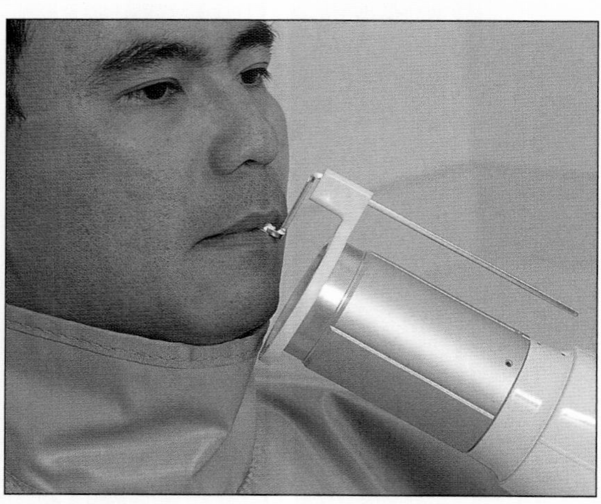

Procedure 16-3

Producing a Full-Mouth Radiographic Survey Using the Paralleling Technique—cont'd

Mandibular Incisor Region

1. Vertically insert the No. 1 film packet or sensor into the anterior bite-block.

Note: Not all digital sensors are available in the No. 1 size.

2. Center the film or sensor packet between the central incisors. Position the packet as far in the lingual direction as the patient's anatomy will allow.

Note: A cotton roll may be placed between the maxillary teeth and the bite-block to prevent rocking of the bite-block on the canine tip and to increase patient comfort.

3. With the instrument and film in place, instruct the patient to close the mouth slowly but firmly.
4. Slide the localizing ring down the indicator rod to the patient's skin surface.
5. Position the localizing ring and PID; then make the exposure.

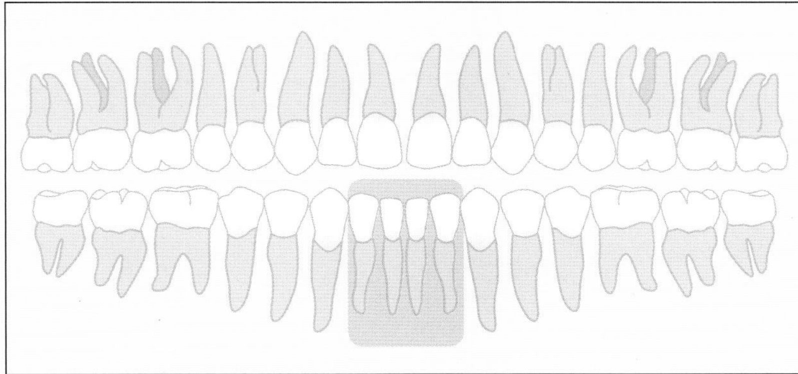

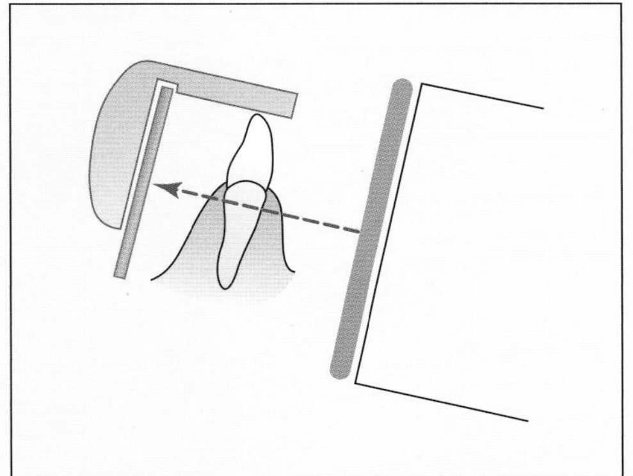

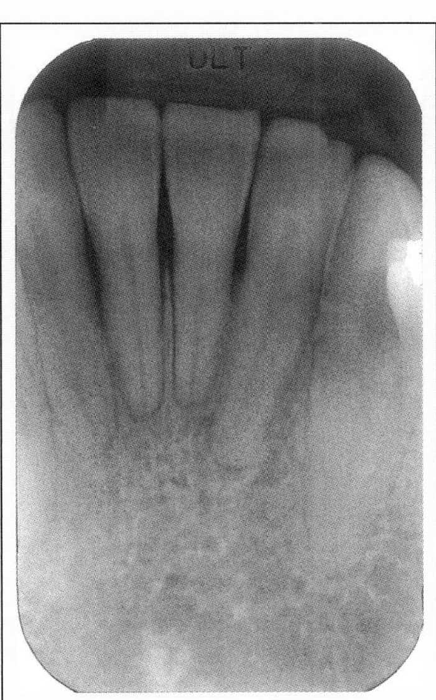

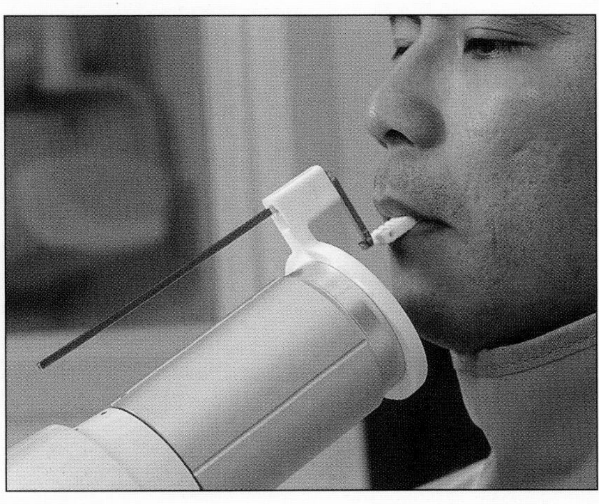

Continued

Procedure 16-3

Producing a Full-Mouth Radiographic Survey Using the Paralleling Technique—cont'd

Maxillary Premolar Region

1. Horizontally insert the film or sensor into the posterior bite-block, pushing the film or sensor all the way into the slot.
2. Center the film or sensor on the second premolar. Position the film in the midpalatal area.
3. With the instrument and film in place, instruct the patient to close the mouth slowly but firmly.
4. Position the localizing ring and PID; then make the exposure.

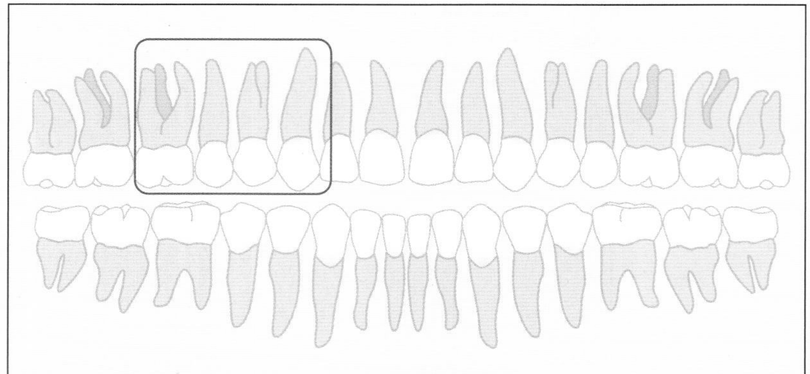

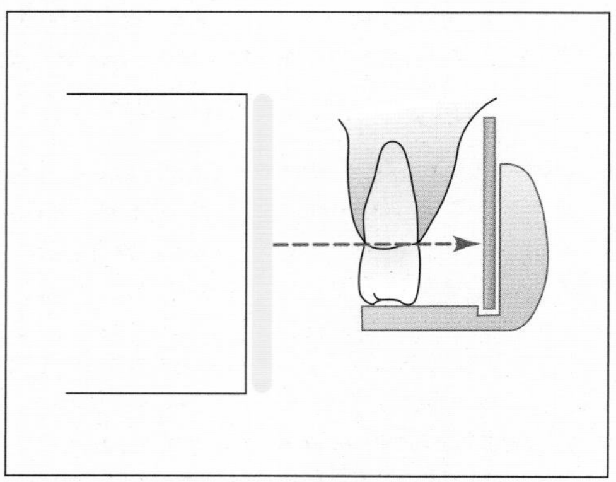

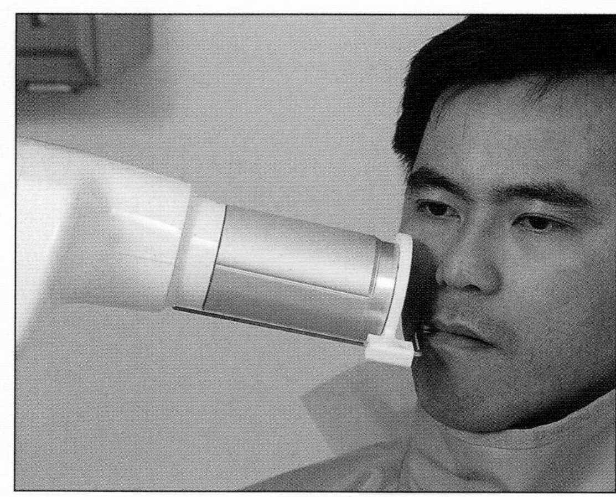

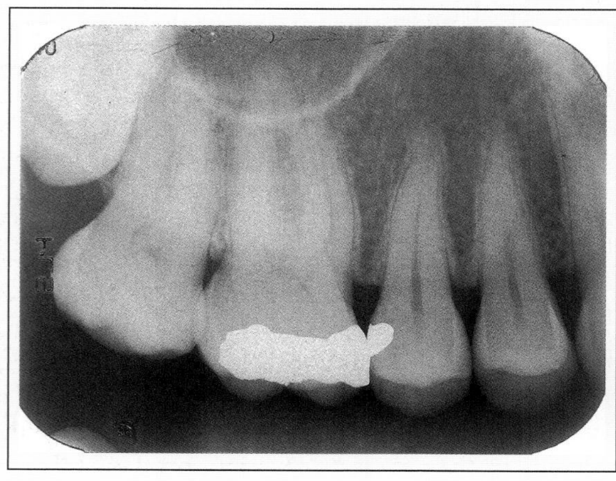

Procedure 16-3

Producing a Full-Mouth Radiographic Survey Using the Paralleling Technique—cont'd

Maxillary Molar Region

1. Horizontally insert the film or sensor into the posterior bite-block.
2. Center the film or sensor on the second molar. Position the film or sensor in the midpalatal area.
3. With the instrument and film in place, instruct the patient to close the mouth slowly but firmly.
4. Position the localizing ring and PID; then make the exposure.

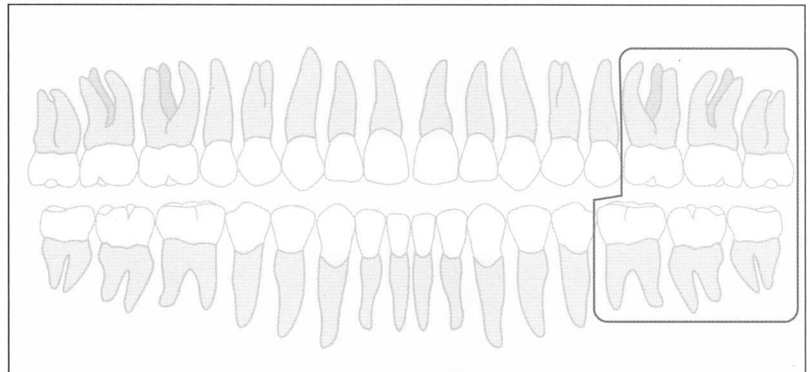

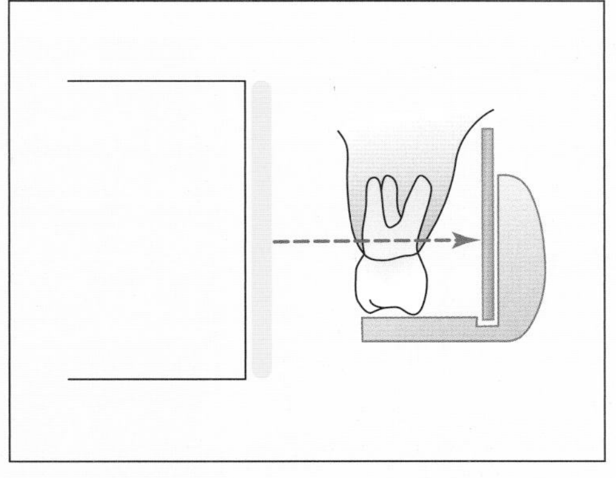

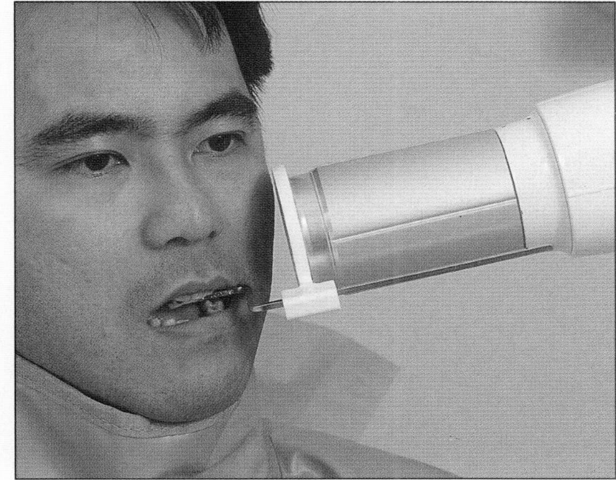

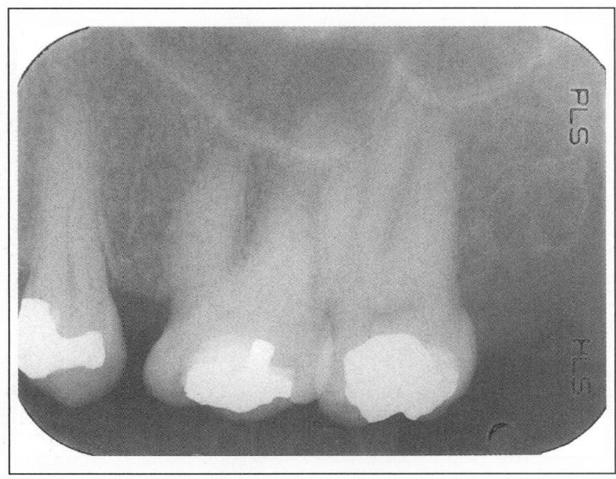

Continued

Procedure 16-3

Producing a Full-Mouth Radiographic Survey Using the Paralleling Technique—cont'd

Mandibular Premolar Region

1. Horizontally insert the No. 2 film or sensor into the posterior bite-block.
2. Center the film or sensor on the contact point between the second premolar and the first molar. Position the film or sensor as far lingual as the patient's anatomy will allow.
3. With the instrument and film in place, instruct the patient to close the mouth slowly but firmly.
4. Slide the localizing ring down the indicator rod to the patient's skin surface.
5. Position the localizing ring and PID; then make the exposure.

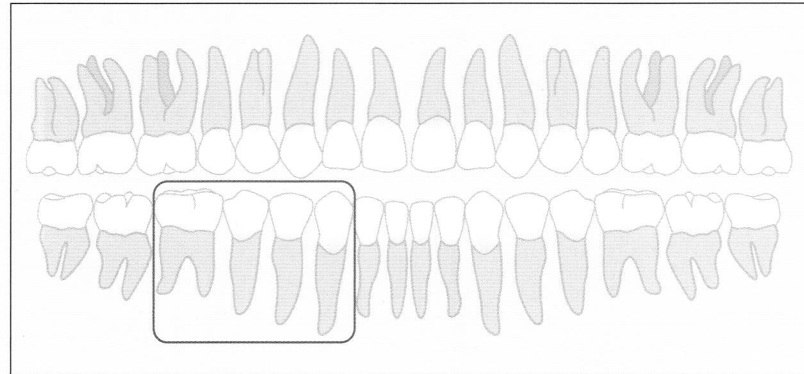

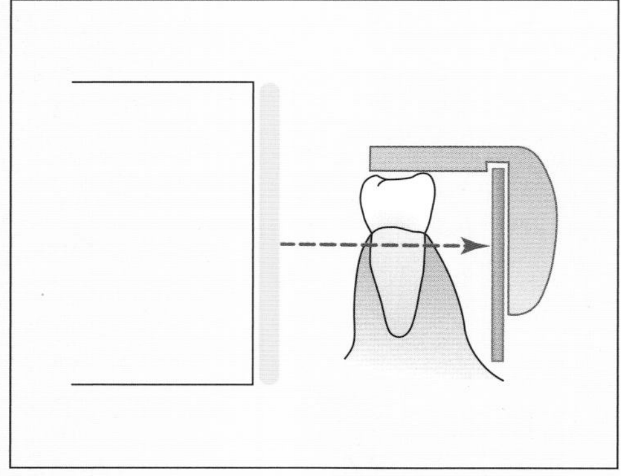

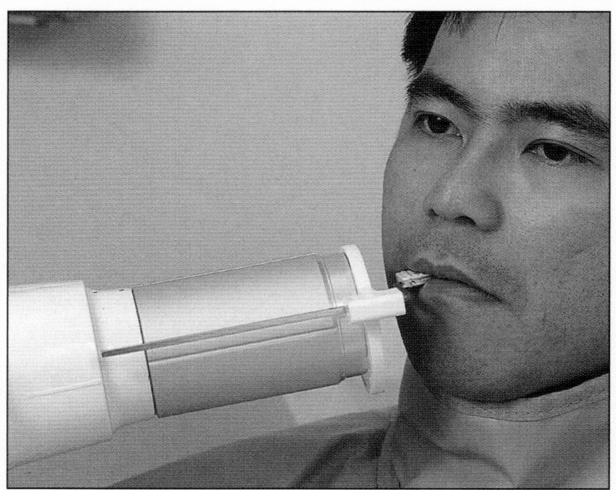

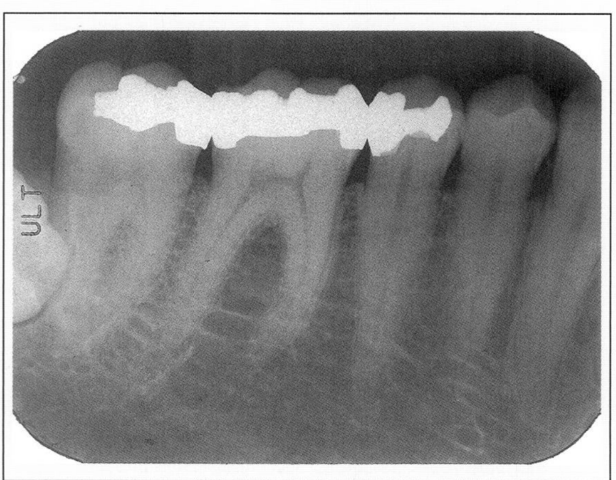

Procedure 16-3

Producing a Full-Mouth Radiographic Survey Using the Paralleling Technique—cont'd

Mandibular Molar Region

1. Horizontally insert the No. 2 film or sensor into the posterior bite-block.
2. Center the film or sensor on the second molar. Position the film or sensor as far lingual as the tongue will allow.

Note: This position will be closer to the teeth than the position for the premolar and anterior views.

3. With the instrument and film in place, instruct the patient to close the mouth slowly but firmly.
4. Slide the localizing ring down the indicator rod to the patient's skin surface.
5. Position the localizing ring and PID; then make the exposure.

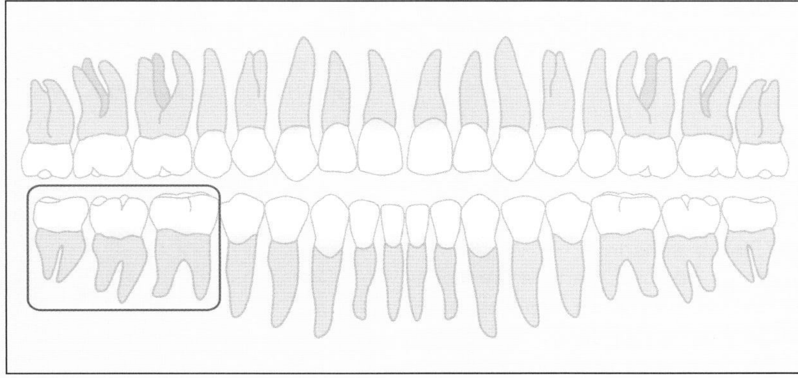

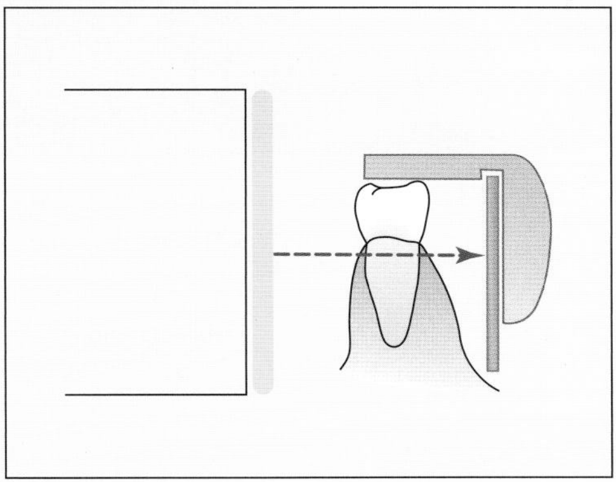

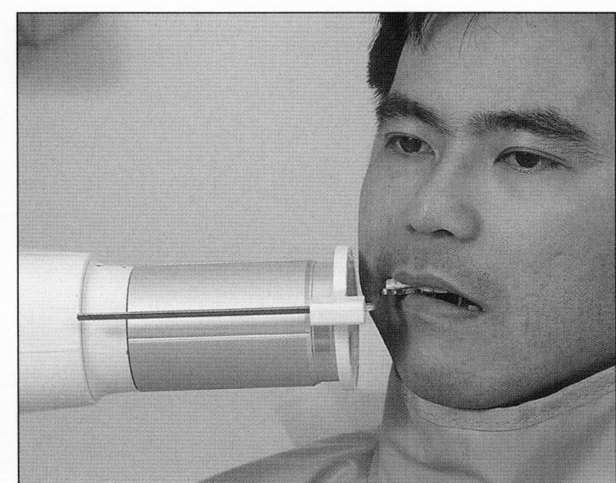

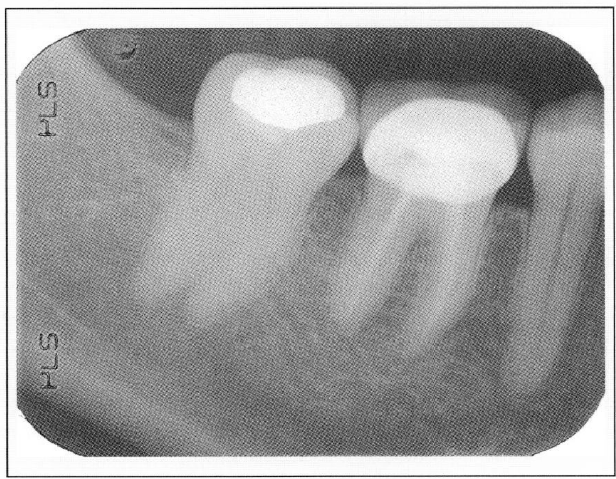

Procedure 16-4

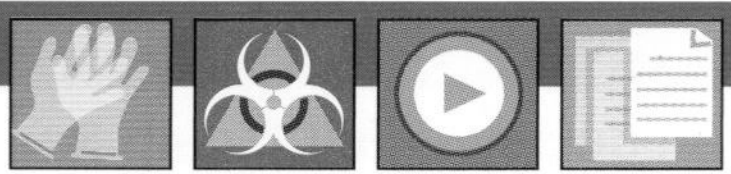

Producing a Four-Film Radiographic Survey Using the Bite-Wing Technique

Goal

To produce a four-view series of radiographs using the bite-wing technique

Equipment and Supplies

- Four No. 2 films, digital sensors, or phosphor storage plates (PSPs)
- Paper cup
- Lead apron and thyroid collar
- Bite-wing tab or film- or sensor-holding device

Procedural Steps

Premolar Bite-Wing Exposure

1. Set vertical angulation at –10 degrees.

Purpose: A positive angulation means that the position indicator device (PID) points downward, which places the beam so that it is nearly perpendicular to both the upper and the lower halves of the film or sensor.

2. Position the patient so that the occlusal plane is parallel to the floor. If necessary, ask the patient to lower or raise the chin.

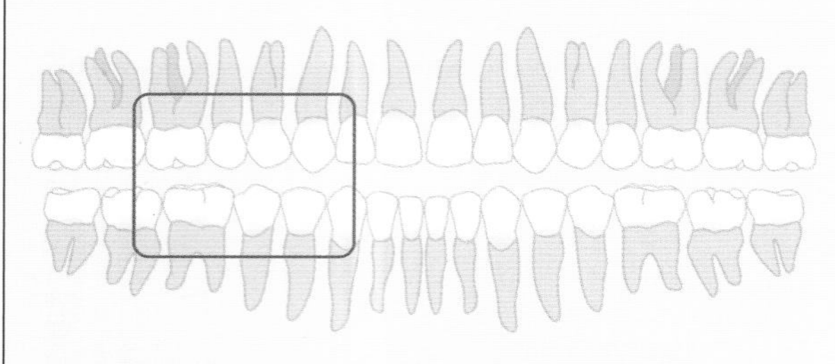

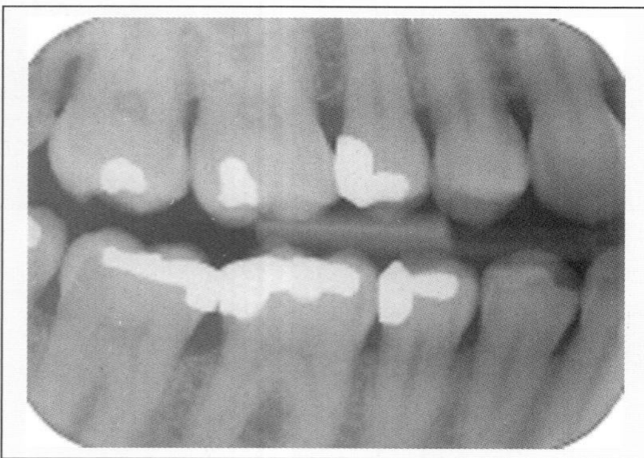

3. Position the film or sensor in the patient's mouth by placing the lower half between the tongue and the mandibular teeth. Position the film or sensor with the anterior border at the middle of the canine.
4. Hold the film or sensor in place by pressing the tab over the occlusal aspect of the mandibular teeth.

Purpose: This step prevents the film or sensor from slipping out of position.

5. Ask the patient to close the mouth slowly. Take care not to allow the patient to close on the fingertip of your glove.
6. Do not pull the film or sensor too tightly against the lower teeth as the patient closes the mouth.

Purpose: Doing so can cause the film or sensor to push against the lingual aspect of the maxillary alveolar ridge and force the film down into the floor of the mouth.

7. Stand in front of the patient to set the horizontal angulation. To better visualize the curvature of the arch, place your index finger along the premolar area. Align the open end of the PID parallel with your index finger and the curvature of the arch in the premolar area.

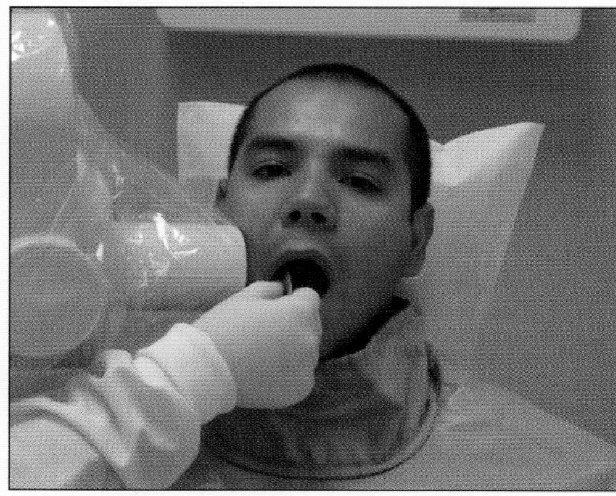

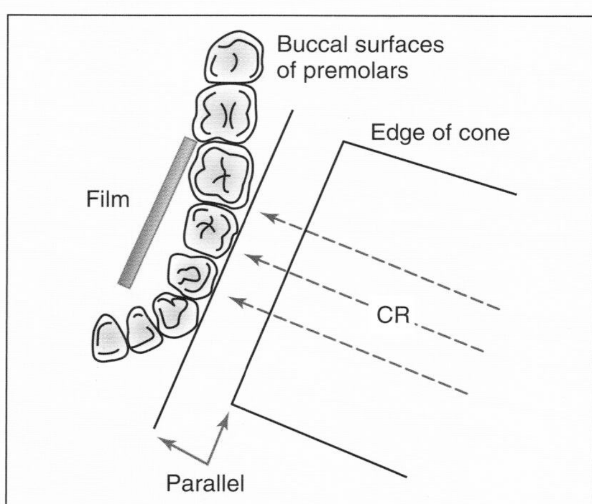

Molar Bite-Wing Exposure

1. Set vertical angulation at –10 degrees.

Purpose: A positive angulation means that the PID points downward. This angulation places the beam so that it is nearly perpendicular to both upper and lower halves of the film.

2. Position the patient so that the occlusal plane is parallel with the floor. If necessary, ask the patient to lower or raise the chin.

Procedure 16-4

Producing a Four-Film Radiographic Survey Using the Bite-Wing Technique

3. Position the film in the patient's mouth by placing the lower half between the tongue and the mandibular teeth. Center the film or sensor on the second molar; the front edge of the film or sensor should be aligned with the middle of the mandibular second premolar.
4. Hold the film or sensor in place by pressing the tab over the occlusal aspect of the mandibular teeth.

Purpose: This step prevents the film or sensor from slipping out of position.

5. Ask the patient to close the mouth slowly. Take care not to allow the patient to close on the fingertip of your glove.
6. Do not pull the film too tightly against the lower teeth as the patient closes the mouth.

Purpose: Doing so can cause the film or sensor to push against the lingual aspect of the maxillary alveolar ridge and force the film down into the floor of the mouth.

7. Stand in front of the patient to set the horizontal angulation. To better visualize the curvature of the arch, place your index finger along the premolar area. Align the open end of the PID parallel with your index finger and the curvature of the arch in the molar area.

Purpose: Different film placement and horizontal angulations are needed to open the proximal contact areas.

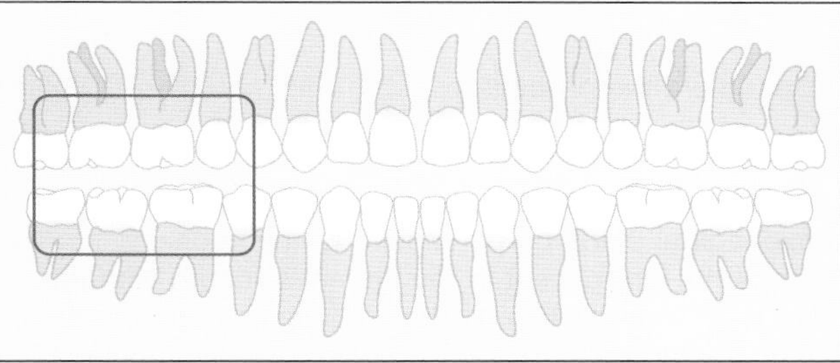

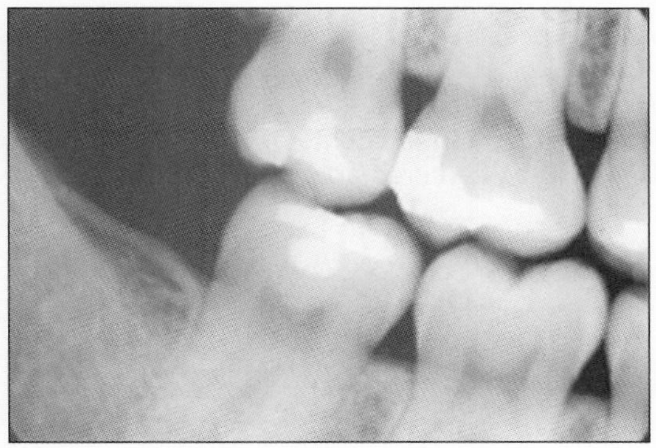

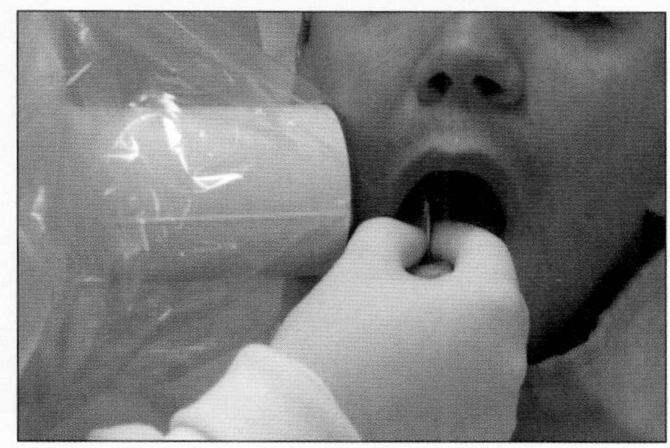

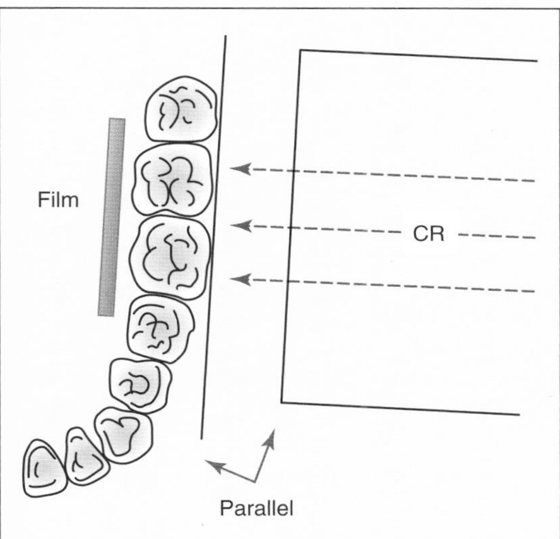

8. Make certain that the PID is positioned far enough forward to cover both the maxillary and the mandibular canines to prevent a cone cut.

Purpose: To check for a cone cut, stand directly behind the tubehead and look along the side of the PID. No portion of the film or sensor should be visible; the film or sensor should be covered by the PID.

9. Direct the central ray through the contact areas.
10. Make the exposure.

Procedure 16-5

Producing Maxillary and Mandibular Radiographs Using the Occlusal Technique

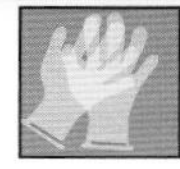
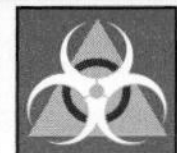
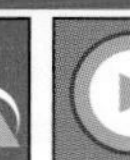
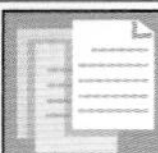

Goal

To follow the steps of the occlusal technique in producing diagnostic quality maxillary and mandibular radiographs

Equipment and Supplies

- Two No. 4 films
- Paper cup
- Lead apron and thyroid collar

Procedural Steps

Maxillary Occlusal Technique

1. Ask the patient to remove prosthetic appliances or objects from the mouth.
2. Place the lead apron and thyroid collar.
3. Position the patient's head so the film plane is parallel to the floor and the midsagittal plane is perpendicular to the floor.
4. Place the film packet in the patient's mouth with the white side of the film on the occlusal surfaces of the maxillary teeth. The long edge of the film is placed in a side-to-side direction.
5. Place the film as far posterior as possible.
6. Position the PID so that the central ray (CR) is directed at –65 degrees through the center of the film. The top edge of the PID is placed between the eyebrows on the bridge of the nose.

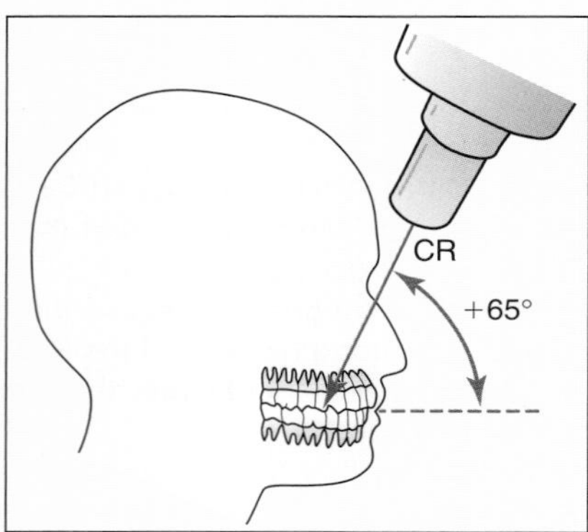

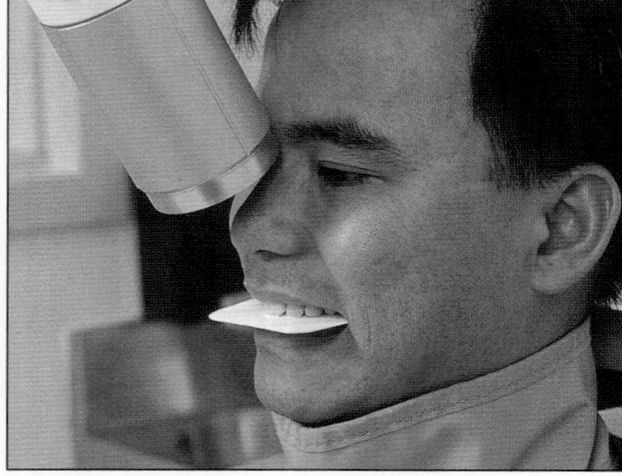

7. Press the activating button on the x-ray machine, and make the exposure.

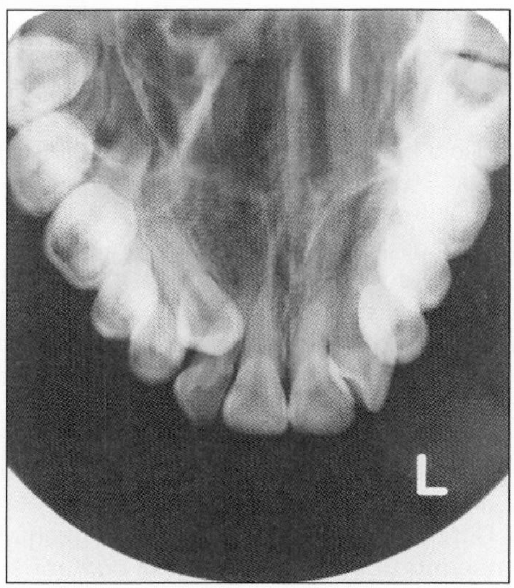

8. Document the procedure.

Mandibular Occlusal Technique

1. Recline the patient, and position the head with the midsagittal plane perpendicular to the floor.
2. Place the film packet in the patient's mouth with the white side of the film on the occlusal surfaces of the mandibular teeth. The long edge of the film is placed in a side-to-side direction.
3. Position the film as far posterior on the mandible as possible.
4. Position the PID so that the CR is directed at a 90-degree angle to the center of the film packet. The PID should be centered approximately 1 inch below the chin.

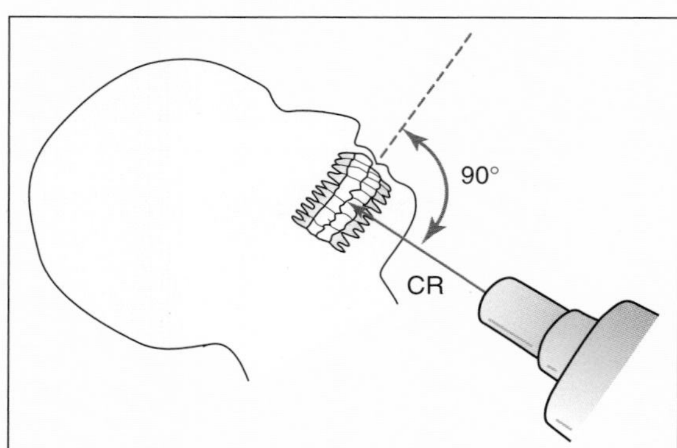

Procedure 16-5

Producing Maxillary and Mandibular Radiographs Using the Occlusal Technique—cont'd

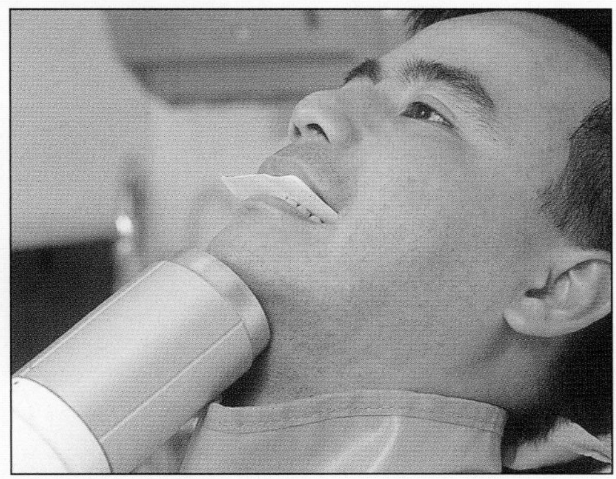

5. Press the exposure button, and make the exposure.

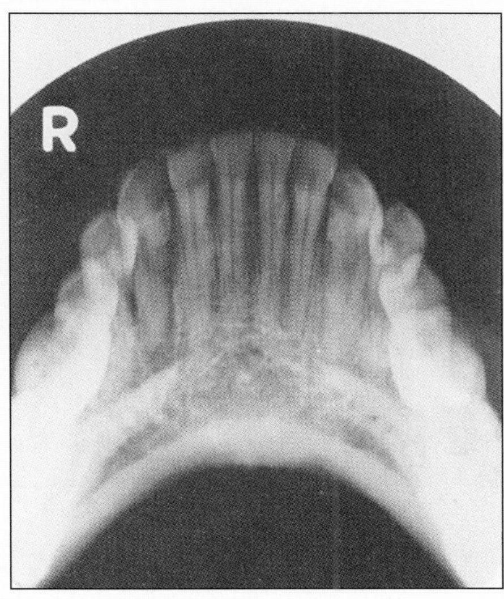

6. Document the procedure.

Procedure 16-6

Practicing Infection Control in the Darkroom

Goal

To practice infection control measures when in the darkroom

Equipment and Supplies

- Paper towels
- Clean gloves
- Clean paper cup
- Container for lead foil

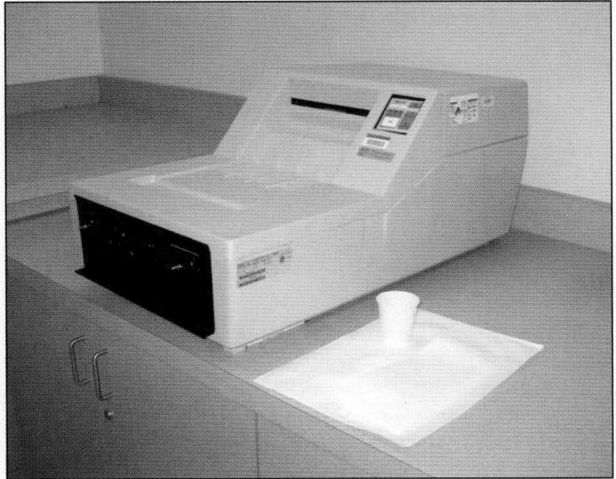

Procedural Steps

1. Place a paper towel and a clean cup on the counter near the processor.

Purpose: The paper towel provides a barrier for the work surface, and the cup is used to discard the opened film packets.

2. Wash your hands, and put on a new pair of gloves, preferably the type that does not contain powder.

Purpose: Powder remaining on the hands can cause artifacts on the exposed film.

3. Turn on the safety light, and then turn off the white light. Open the film packets and allow each exposed film to drop onto the paper towel. Be careful that the unwrapped films do not come into contact with the gloves.

Purpose: The film must remain free from contamination. A contaminated film may remain contaminated even after processing.

Continued

Procedure 16-6

Practicing Infection Control in the Darkroom—cont'd

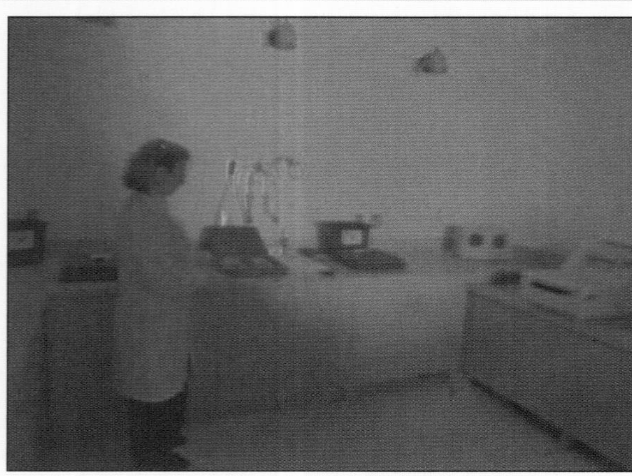

4. Remove the lead foil from the packet, and place it in the foil-recycling container.

Purpose: Lead foil is considered an environmental hazard and should not be discarded with the general waste.

5. Place the empty film packets into the clean cup.
6. Discard the cup. Remove your gloves by turning them inside out; then discard them.
7. Place the films into the processor or on developing racks with your bare hands.

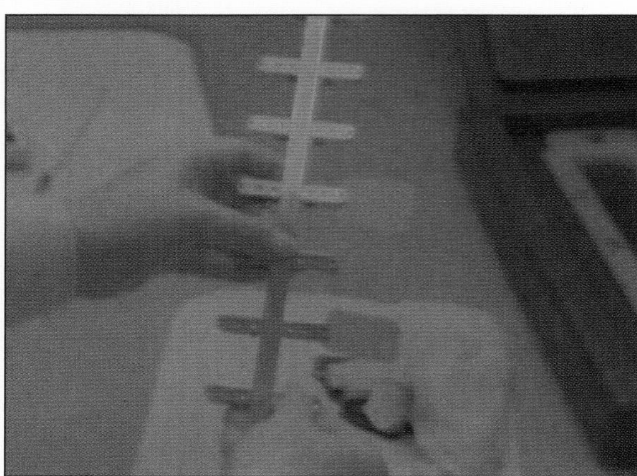

Note: If you used films with plastic barriers, then you would have already removed the protective barrier in the operatory with gloved hands. You would then open the packets with your bare hands and feed the films into the processor.

Procedure 16-7

Practicing Infection Control With the Use of the Daylight Loader

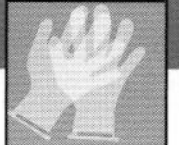
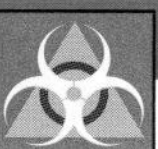

Goal

To practice infection control measures when using the daylight loader in processing dental radiographic films

Equipment and Supplies

- Paper towels
- Clean gloves
- Clean cup
- Container for lead foil

Procedural Steps

1. Wash and dry your hands, and then place a paper towel or a piece of plastic as a barrier to cover the bottom of the daylight loader.

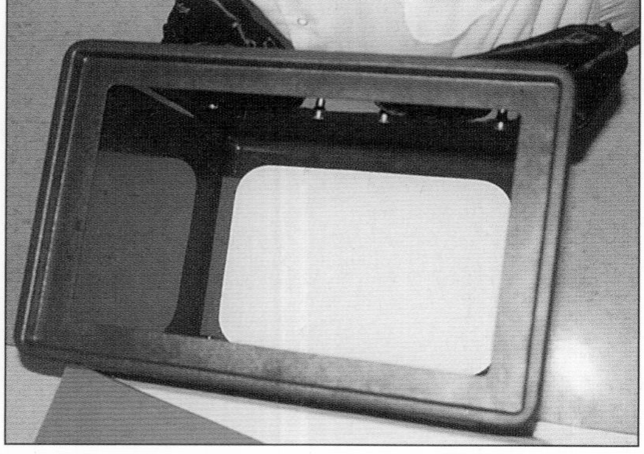

2. Place the following into the bottom of the daylight loader.
   a. Cup containing the contaminated film
   b. Clean pair of gloves
   c. Second empty paper cup

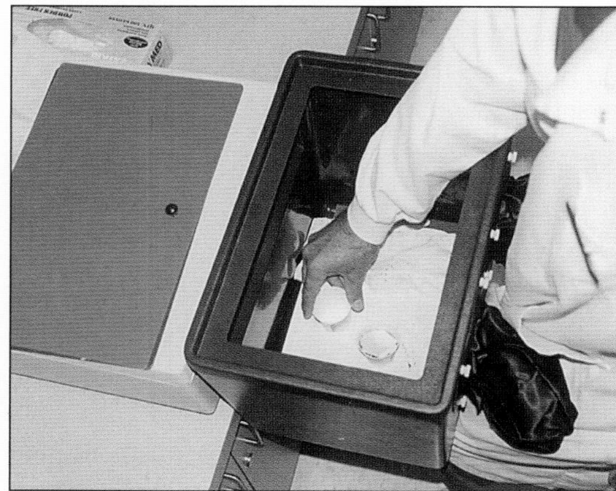

3. Close the top of the daylight loader.
4. Put your clean hands through the sleeves of the daylight loader; then put on the gloves.

Purpose: Clean hands prevent contamination of the sleeves. Contaminated gloves should never be placed through the sleeves of the daylight loader.

Procedure 16-7

Practicing Infection Control With the Use of the Daylight Loader—cont'd

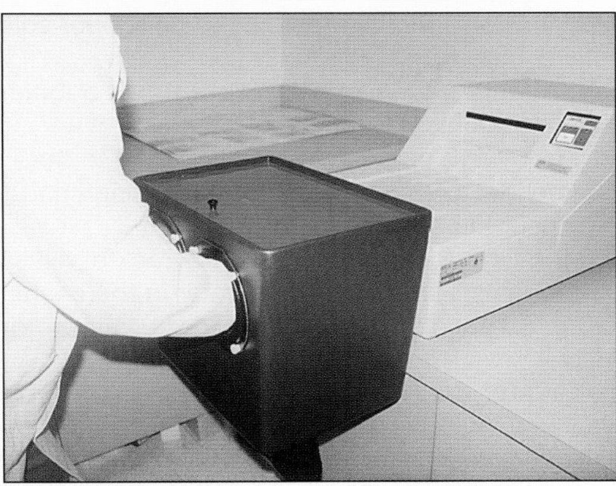

5. Open the packets, and allow the films to drop onto the clean barrier.

Purpose: The clean barrier keeps dust or powder from the film.

6. Place the contaminated packets into the second cup, and place the lead foil into the foil-recycling container.

Purpose: The cup confines the contaminated film packets and makes disposal easier.

7. After you open the last packet, remove your gloves by turning them inside out. Insert the films into the developing slots.

Purpose: The film remains uncontaminated and eliminates the question of whether organisms can survive in the solutions.

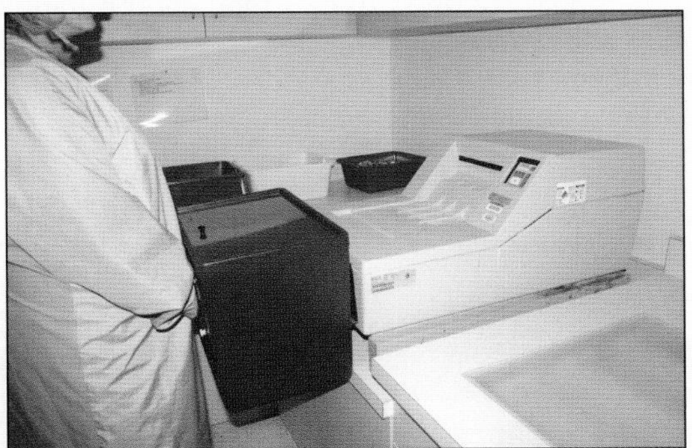

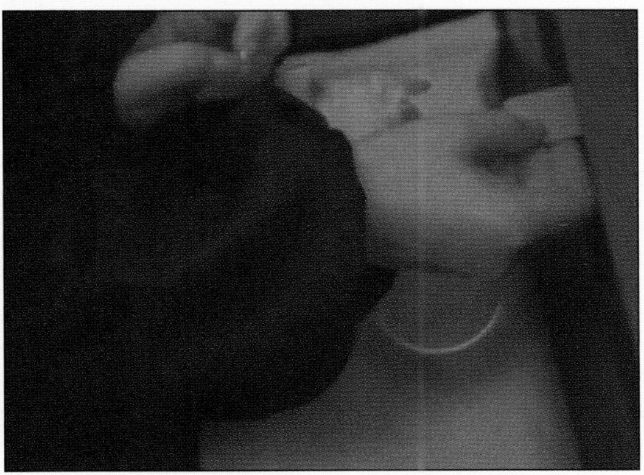

8. After you insert the last film, pull your ungloved hands through the sleeves.
9. Open the top of the loader, and then carefully pull the ends of the barrier over the paper cup and used gloves and discard.

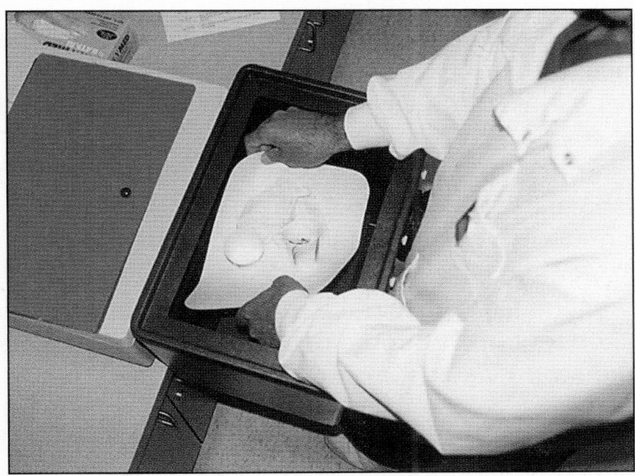

Note: Be careful not to touch the contaminated parts of the barrier with your bare hands.

Procedure 16-8

Manual Processing of Dental Radiographs

Goal

To process dental radiograph films using a manual tank

Equipment and Supplies

- Fully equipped darkroom
- Surface barriers or disinfecting solution for counters
- Exposed films
- Film rack
- Timer
- Pencil
- Film dryer (optional)

Procedural Steps

Preparation

1. Follow all the infection control steps discussed in this chapter.

Continued

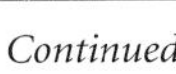

Procedure 16-8

Manual Processing of Dental Radiographs—cont'd

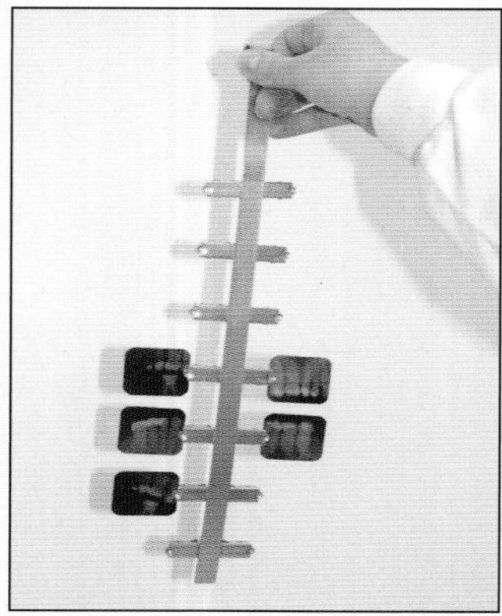

2. Stir solutions with the corresponding paddle.

Purpose: The chemicals are heavy and tend to settle to the bottom of the tank. Do not interchange mixing paddles, or cross-contamination will occur.

3. Check the temperature of the solutions, and refer to the processing chart to determine the times.

Purpose: The temperature of the solution determines the processing time.

4. Label the film rack with the patient's name and date of exposure.
5. Turn on the safelight, and then turn off the white light.
6. Wash your hands, and put on gloves.
7. Open the film packets, and allow the films to drop onto the clean paper towel. Take care not to touch the films.

Purpose: The films have not been contaminated. Films that have been touched become contaminated and may remain contaminated even after processing.

Processing

1. Attach each film to the film rack so that the films are parallel and not touching each other.
2. As you immerse the film rack in the developer solution, slightly agitate (jiggle) the rack.

Purpose: Agitating the film rack prevents air bubbles from forming on the film.

3. Start the timer. The timer is set according to the recommendations stated on the processing chart (e.g., 5 minutes if the solution is 68° F).
4. When the timer goes off, remove the rack of films and rinse the rack in the circulating water in the center tank for 20 to 30 seconds. Allow the excess water to drip off the films.

Purpose: Water dripping from the racks into the fixer will dilute it.

5. Insert the rack of films into the fixer tank, and set the timer for 10 minutes.

Purpose: For permanent fixation, the film is kept in the fixer for a minimum of 10 minutes. However, films may be removed from the fixing solution after 3 minutes for viewing; this is a wet reading. Films must be returned to the fixer to complete the process.

6. Return the rack of films to the center tank of circulating water for at least 20 minutes.

Purpose: Incomplete washing will cause the films to turn brown eventually.

7. Remove the rack of films from the water, and place it in the film dryer. If a film dryer is not available, then hanging the films to air-dry is recommended.

Purpose: Films may be air-dried at room temperature in a dust-free area or placed in a heated drying cabinet. Films must be completely dried before they can be handled for mounting and viewing.

8. When the films are completely dry, remove them from the rack and mount and label.

Procedure 16-9

Automatic Processing of Dental Radiographs Using the Daylight Loader

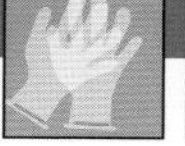
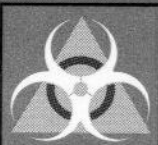
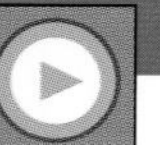

Equipment and Supplies

- Automatic x-ray processor with the daylight loader
- Exposed dental films
- Chemical disinfection spray
- Two disposable cups or containers for lead foil and film packets
- Paper towel

Procedural Steps

1. At the beginning of the day, turn on the machine and allow the chemicals to warm up according to the manufacturer's recommendations.

Purpose: The heating unit must warm the chemicals to the correct temperature to ensure that the films will be of diagnostic quality.

2. Follow the infection control steps discussed in the "Infection Control in Dental Radiography" section earlier in this chapter.

Purpose: Film packets are contaminated because they have been in the patient's mouth.

3. Wash and dry your hands.
4. Open the lid on the daylight loader, and place a paper towel over the bottom. Then place two disposable cups on the towel.

Purpose: The paper towel will act as a surface barrier on the bottom of the daylight loader. One disposable cup is for the lead foil in the film packet; the other is used to dispose of the paper towel, film packets, and gloves.

5. Put on gloves, and slide your gloved hands through the sleeves of the daylight loader.

Procedure 16-9

Automatic Processing of Dental Radiographs Using the Daylight Loader—cont'd

6. Remove the film from its packet, and check to ensure that the black paper has not stuck to the film. If the black paper is left on the film or if double film packets have not been separated, then the films will be ruined and the automatic processor could jam.
7. Feed the film into the machine.

Note: Open the film packets, and feed films in one at a time to prevent having films overlap during loading.

8. While the film is feeding into the machine, remove the lead foil from the packet and place it in one of the disposable cups. Then drop the empty packet onto the paper towel.
9. Keep the films straight as they are slowly fed into the machine. Allow at least 10 seconds between insertion of each film into the processor and the insertion of the next film. Place films in alternate film slots when possible.
10. After the last film is inserted into the machine, carefully remove your gloves and drop them into the center of the paper towel. While touching only the corners and underside of the paper towel, wrap the paper towel over the contaminated film packets and gloves. Place the wrapped paper towel into the second cup.

Purpose: Handling the paper towel only by the corners and underside will help eliminate cross-contamination during film-processing procedures.

11. Remove the cup containing the lead foil, and take it to the foil-recycling container.
12. Remove the processed radiographs from the film recovery slot on the outside of the automatic processor. Allow 4 to 6 minutes for the automated process to be completed.

Note: When processing extraoral films, carefully remove the film from the cassette. Handle all films only by the edges to prevent fingerprints and scratches on the films.

Procedure 16-10

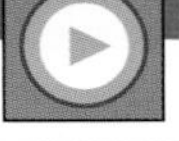

Mounting Dental Radiographs

Goal

To mount a full-mouth series of dental radiographs

Equipment and Supplies

- Appropriate size of film mount
- Pencil
- View box
- Paper towel
- Processing for full-mouth series of radiographs

Procedural Steps

1. Place a clean paper towel over the work surface in front of the view box.

Purpose: To keep the films clean.

2. Turn on the view box.
3. Label and date the film mount.

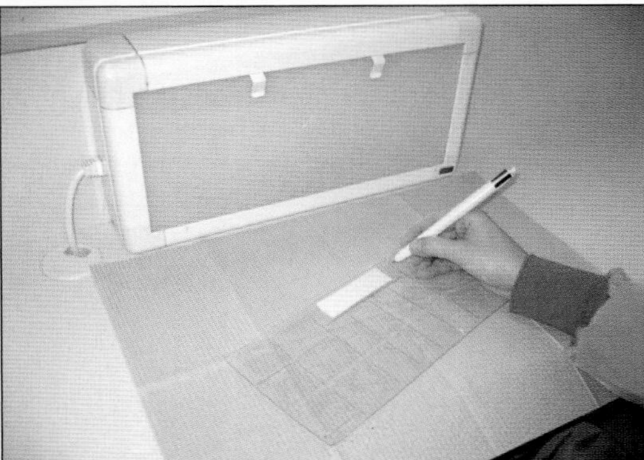

4. Wash and dry your hands.

Purpose: Washing and drying the hands prevents finger marks on the radiographs.

5. Identify the embossed dot on each radiograph; place the film on the work surface with the dot facing up.

Purpose: The American Dental Association (ADA) recommends mounting with the dot up.

6. Sort the radiographs into three groups: bite-wing, anterior periapical, and posterior periapical views.
7. Arrange the radiographs on the work surface in anatomic order. Use your knowledge of normal anatomic landmarks to distinguish maxillary from mandibular radiographs.
8. Arrange all maxillary radiographs with the roots pointing upward and all mandibular radiographs with the roots pointing downward.
9. Place each film in the corresponding window of the film mount. The following order is suggested for film mounting:
   a. Maxillary anterior periapical films
   b. Mandibular anterior periapical films
   c. Bite-wing films
   d. Maxillary posterior periapical films
   e. Mandibular posterior periapical films

Continued

Procedure 16-10

Mounting Dental Radiographs—cont'd

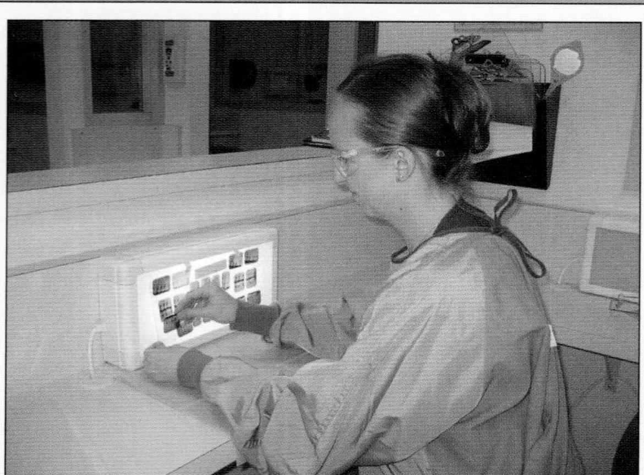

10. Check the mounted radiographs to ensure that (1) the dots are all properly oriented, (2) the films are properly arranged in anatomic order, and (3) the films are secure in the mount.

Procedure 16-11

Preparing the Equipment for Panoramic Radiography

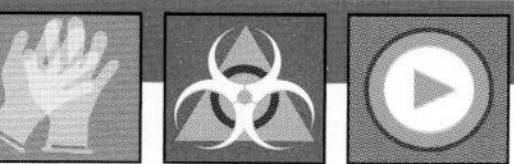

Goal

To prepare the equipment necessary for a panoramic radiograph

Equipment and Supplies

- Extraoral film
- Cassette
- Infection control barriers

Procedural Steps

1. Load the panoramic cassette in the darkroom under safelight conditions. Handle the film only by its edges to prevent fingerprints.

Purpose: The panoramic film is sensitive to light, and the remainder of the film in the box will be ruined if exposed to light.

2. Place all infection control barriers and containers.
3. Cover the bite-block with a disposable plastic barrier. If the bite-block is not covered, it must be sterilized before it is used on the next patient.

Purpose: The bite-block is considered a semicritical item and must be disposable or sterilized.

4. Cover or disinfect (or both) any part of the machine that comes in contact with the patient.

Purpose: Parts of the machine touching the patient but not intraorally used are considered noncritical items and must be disinfected with a high-level disinfectant.

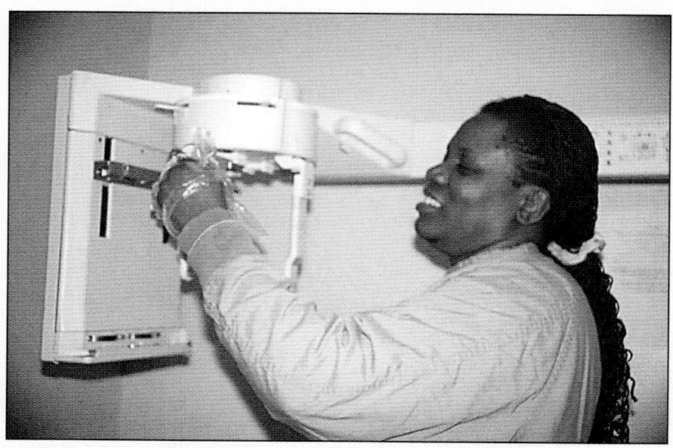

5. Set the exposure factors (kilovoltage, milliamperage) according to the manufacturer's recommendations.
6. Adjust the machine to accommodate the height of the patient, and properly align all movable parts.
7. Load the cassette into the carrier of the panoramic unit.

Procedure 16-12

Preparing the Patient for Panoramic Radiography

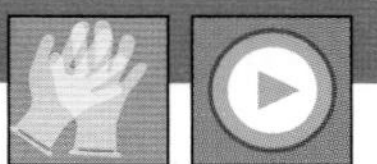

Goal

To prepare a patient for a panoramic x-ray image

Equipment and Supplies

- Double-sided lead apron (or style recommended by the manufacturer)
- Plastic container

Procedural Steps

1. Explain the procedure to the patient. Give the patient the opportunity to ask questions.

Purpose: The patient has the right to be informed and give consent to the procedure.

2. Ask the patient to remove all objects from the head and neck area, including eyeglasses, earrings, lip-piercing and tongue-piercing objects, necklaces, napkin chains, hearing aids, hairpins, and complete and partial dentures. Place the objects in a container.

Purpose: If not removed, these objects will appear on the radiograph and could superimpose diagnostic information.

3. Place a double-sided (for protecting the front and back of the patient) lead apron on the patient, or use the style of lead apron recommended by the manufacturer.

Note: A thyroid collar is not recommended for all panoramic units because it blocks part of the beam and obscures important anatomic structures. Refer to the manufacturer's instructions for the unit you use.

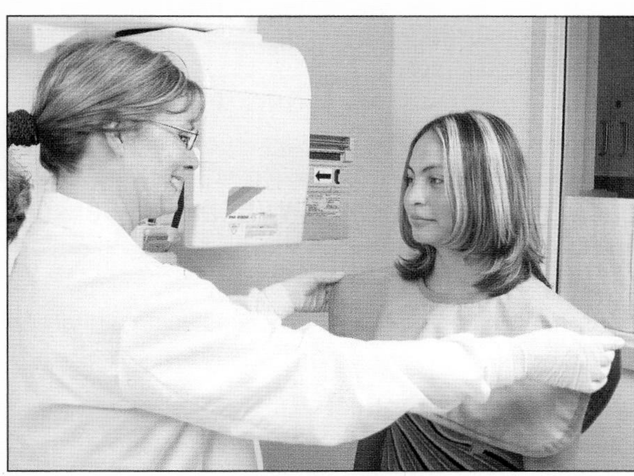

Procedure 16-13

Positioning the Patient for Panoramic Radiography

Goal

To position the patient for a panoramic radiograph

Procedural Steps

1. Instruct the patient to sit or stand "as tall as possible" with the back straight and erect.

Purpose: The spinal column is very dense; if the spine is not straight, then a white shadow will appear over the middle of the radiograph and obscure diagnostic information.

2. Instruct the patient to bite on the plastic bite-block and then slide the upper and lower teeth into the notch (groove) on the end of the bite-block.

Purpose: The groove aligns the teeth in the focal trough.

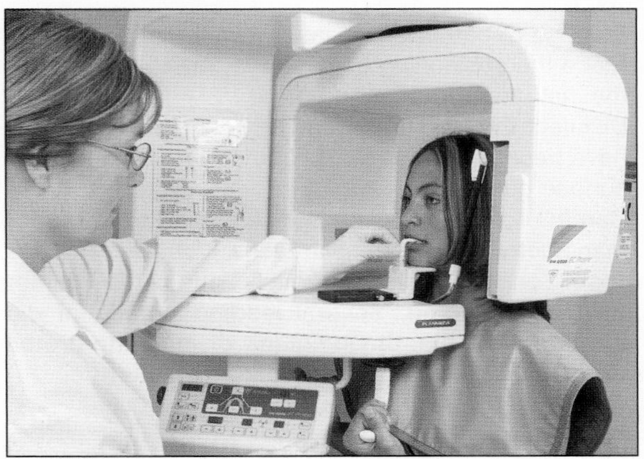

3. Position the midsagittal plane (the imaginary line that divides the patient's face into right and left sides) perpendicular to the floor.

Purpose: If the patient's head is tipped or tilted to one side, then a distorted image will result.

4. Position the Frankfort plane (the imaginary plane that passes through the top of the ear canal and the bottom of the eye socket) parallel with the floor.

Purpose: The occlusal plane will be positioned at the correct angle.

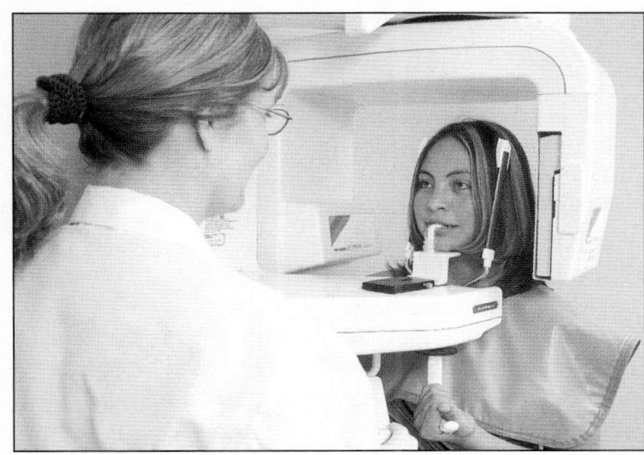

5. Instruct the patient to position the tongue on the roof of the mouth and then close the lips around the bite-block.

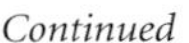
Continued

Procedure 16-13

Positioning the Patient for Panoramic Radiography—cont'd

Purpose: If the tongue is not placed on the roof of the mouth, a radiolucent shadow will be superimposed over the apices of the maxillary teeth.

6. After the patient has been positioned, instruct him or her to remain still while the machine rotates during exposure.

Purpose: Any movement of the patient will result in a blurred image on the radiograph.

7. Expose the film, and proceed with film processing.
8. Document the procedure.

DATE	PROCEDURE	OPERATOR
1/25/16	Exposed panoramic radiograph	DLB

Procedure 16-14

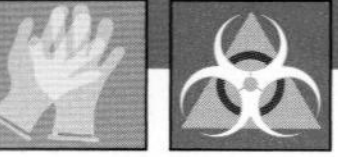
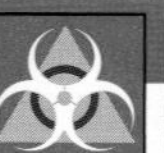
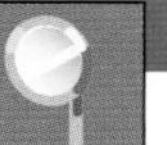

Practicing Infection Control With Digital Sensors

Goal

To perform all infection control practices using digital sensor exposure

Equipment and Supplies

- Barriers for the operatory, including the sensor, computer keyboard, and mouse
- Paper towels or gauze squares
- Digital sensor (sizes as necessary)
- Packaged positioning device
- Wraps or cushions for sensor (optional)
- Sensor and cable barriers
- Lead apron with thyroid collar
- Surface cleaner or disinfectant

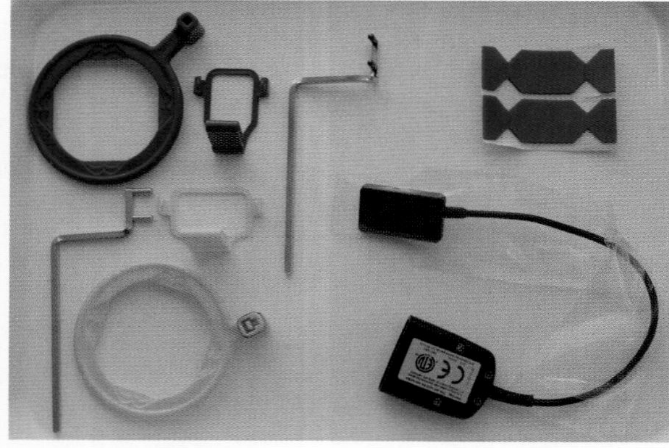

Procedural Steps

1. Wash and dry your hands.
2. Place surface barriers on equipment, computer keyboard and mouse, and work area.
3. Set out the packaged positioning device, barriers for the sensor and cable, a paper towel or gauze squares, and miscellaneous items you might choose.

Purpose: Once gloved, you should not have to leave the operatory area for additional materials.

4. Secure the barrier around the digital sensor.

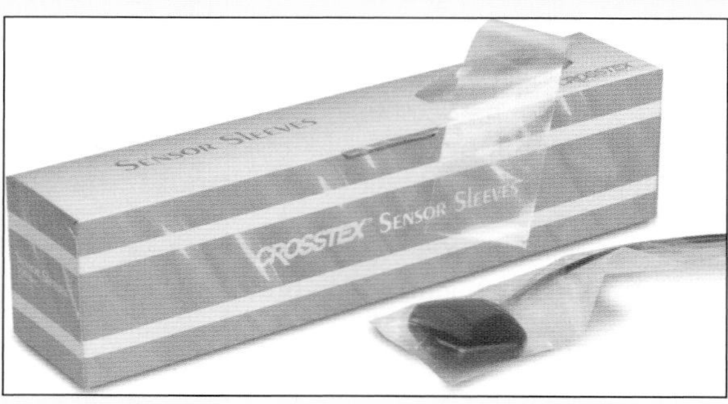

Purpose: Sensors are reused on patients and cannot be heat sterilized. Therefore protecting them with FDA-cleared barriers is essential.

5. Seat the patient, and place the lead apron.
6. Wash and dry your hands, and don gloves.
7. After all exposures are complete, remove the lead apron and dismiss the patient.

Note: To remove the lead apron and still maintain the aseptic technique, you can wear overgloves to remove the apron or you can take off your gloves and remove the apron bare handed.

8. Put on utility gloves, and remove barriers from the x-ray equipment, taking care not to touch the surfaces underneath.

Purpose: Chemical-resistant utility gloves are necessary when performing surface disinfection. If you touch a surface underneath the barrier while you are removing it, then that surface will be contaminated and must be disinfected.

9. Dispose of barriers and paper towels.
10. Place the positioning device on a tray to be returned to the instrument-processing area.
11. Disinfect the lead apron and any surfaces that may have become contaminated during the removal of surface barriers.
12. Carefully disinfect the sensor according to the manufacturer's recommendations.

Purpose: Sensors are very expensive and can be damaged if improperly handled. Several leading brands of digital sensors are available. Cleaning and disinfecting protocols may vary according to the individual manufacturer.

13. Wash and dry your hands.

Courtesy Crosstex, Hauppauge, New York.
FDA, U.S. Food and Drug Administration.
(From Bird DL, Robinson DS: *Modern dental assisting,* ed 11, St. Louis, 2015, Saunders.)

Procedure 16-15

Practicing Infection Control With Phosphor Storage Plates

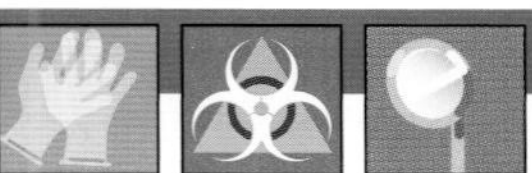

Goal

To perform all infection control practices when using phosphor storage plates (PSPs)

Equipment and Supplies

- Barriers for the operatory
- Barriers for the computer and mouse
- Paper towels or gauze
- Cotton rolls
- PSPs (sizes as necessary)
- Barrier PSP envelopes
- Packaged positioning device
- Lead apron with thyroid collar
- Black transfer box
- Paper cup
- Image scanner
- Surface cleaner or disinfectant

Procedural Steps

1. Turn on the computer.
2. Log on to link the patient's images to his or her chart.
3. Choose the image layout you wish to use.

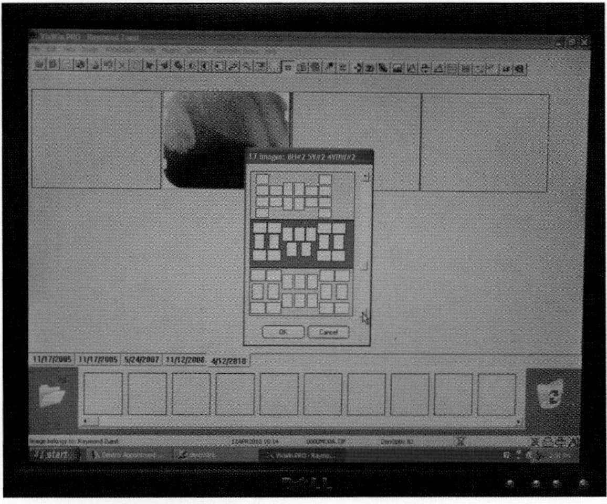

4. Wash and dry your hands.
5. Place surface barriers on equipment and work area.

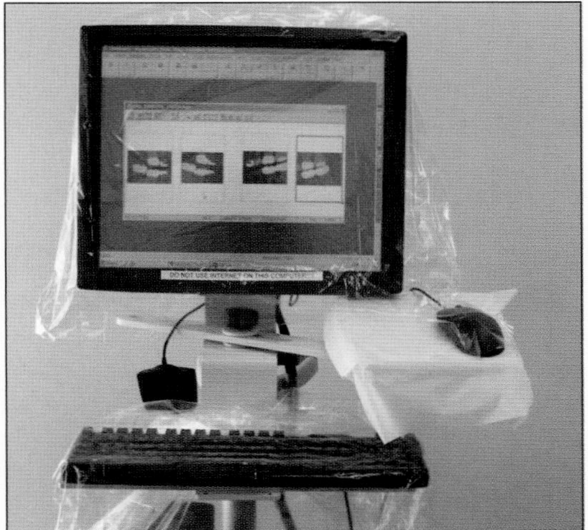

6. Slide the PSPs into barrier envelopes. Seal the barrier envelope by removing the protective strip and by gently pressing to seal the edge.

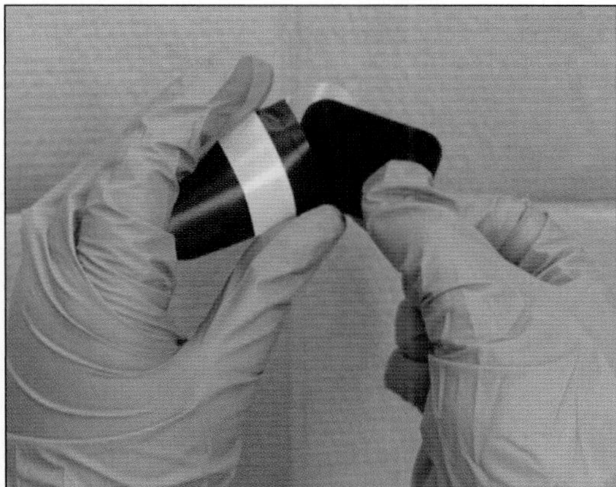

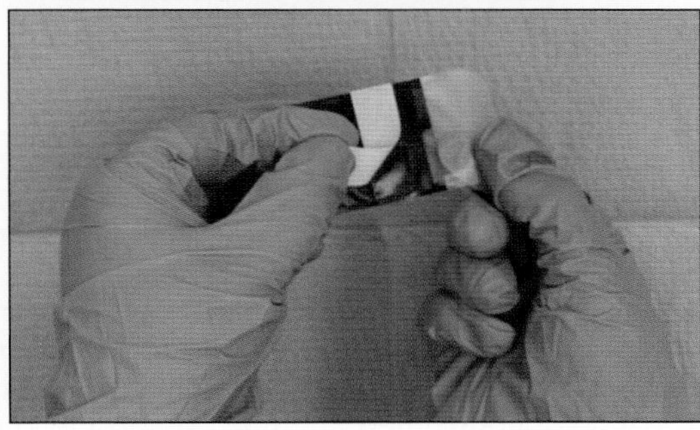

7. Set out the packaged positioning device, paper cup, transfer box, paper towel, and other miscellaneous items you might need.

Purpose: Once gloved, you should not have to leave the operatory area for additional materials.

Exposures

1. Seat the patient, and place the lead apron.
2. Wash and dry your hands, and don gloves.
3. Place the PSP into the film holder for each exposure.

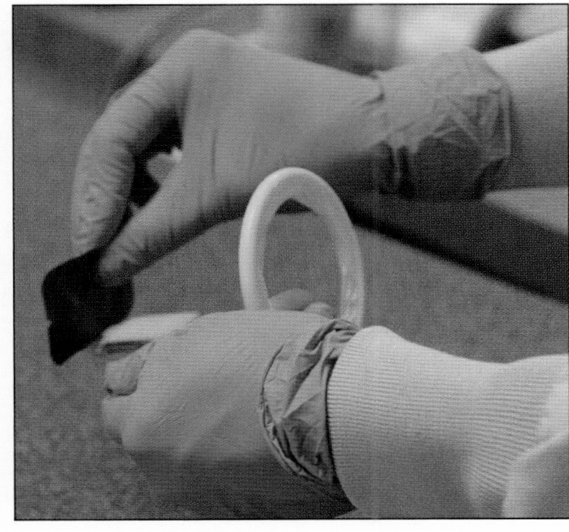

Continued

Procedure 16-15

Practicing Infection Control With Phosphor Storage Plates—cont'd

4. After each exposure, wipe excess saliva from the PSP envelope using a paper towel.
5. Place each exposed PSP into the paper cup labeled with the patient's name or directly into the black transfer box.

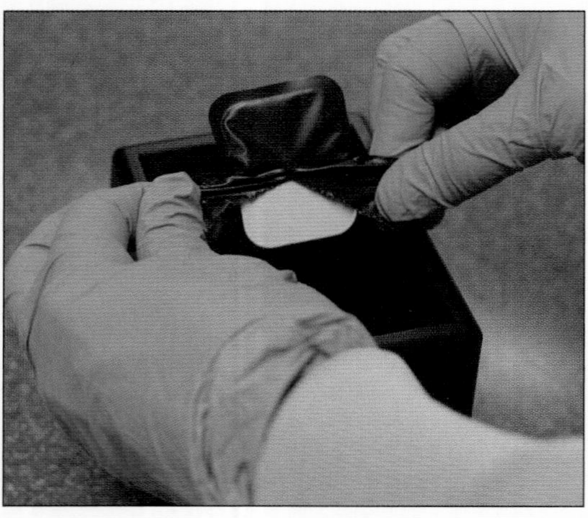

6. After the exposures are complete, remove the lead apron and dismiss the patient.
7. While still gloved, remove barriers, taking care not to touch the surfaces underneath.

Purpose: You must wear gloves while removing barriers, because they are contaminated. If you touch a surface underneath the barrier while you are removing it, then that surface will be contaminated and must be disinfected.

8. Dispose of barriers and paper towels.
9. Place the used positioning device on a tray to be returned to the instrument-processing area.

Preparing PSPs for Scanning

Note: If scanning is immediately performed after exposure, the black transfer box step is not necessary, and the PSPs can be immediately scanned. The black transfer box is necessary because PSPs should not be exposed very long to bright light or warmth because this exposure will release the energy before it is read by the scanner.

1. While gloved, remove each PSP from the paper cup, carefully open the sealed envelope, and allow the PSP to drop into the black transfer box. Use care not to touch the outside of the transfer box to avoid contamination.

Purpose: Gloves must be worn because the PSP envelopes are contaminated.

2. Dispose of the contaminated envelopes.
3. Remove your gloves, and wash and dry your hands.

Scanning the PSP

1. Scanning machines vary greatly, depending on the manufacturer; therefore reading the specific instructions for the specific machine being used is critical.

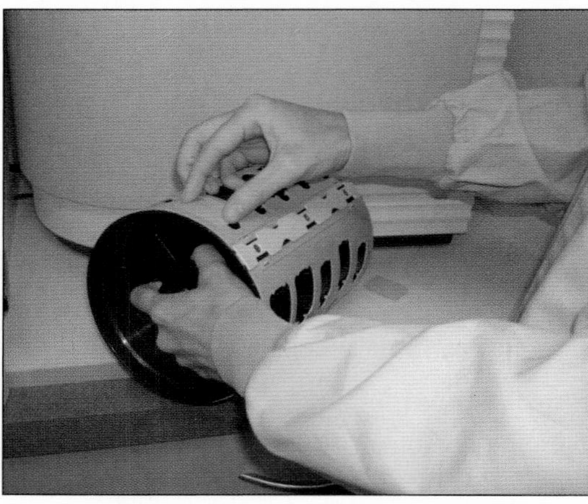

2. Insert the PSP into the scanner according to the manufacturer's instructions.

Purpose: The scanning machine will convert the fluorescent signal into a digital image that will appear on the monitor.

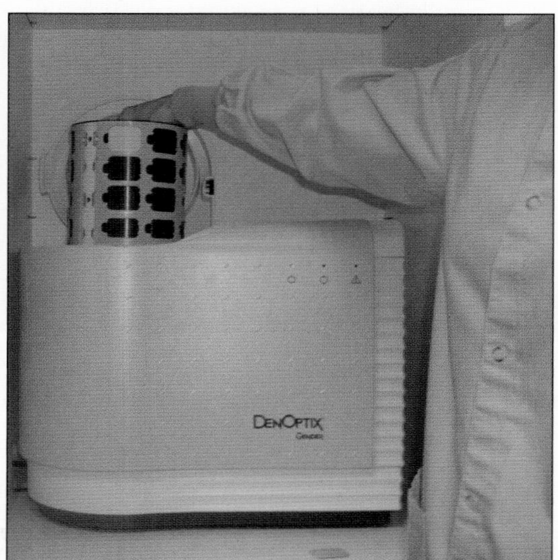

3. When the imaging is complete, log off the system.
4. Document the procedure in the patient's record.

Photos from Bird DL, Robinson DS: *Modern dental assisting,* ed 11, St. Louis, 2015, Saunders.

Chapter Exercises

Multiple Choice

Circle the letter next to the correct answer.

1. Images on radiographs that appear black are called __________.
  a. radiopaque
  b. radiolucent

2. The overall darkness of a radiographic image is called the __________.
  a. density
  b. contrast
  c. sharpness
  d. gray tones

3. The colored side of the film packet is always placed __________ the PID.
  a. away from
  b. toward

4. If the dentist suspects an abscess, then what type of radiograph would most likely be needed?
  a. bite-wing
  b. periapical
  c. occlusal

5. The image that exists on the film after exposure and before processing is called the __________ image.
  a. ghost
  b. latent
  c. hidden
  d. radiation

6. The type of radiograph that shows the crowns of the teeth on both arches at one time is called a __________ view.
  a. bite-wing
  b. occlusal
  c. periapical

7. The film size that is usually used for children younger than 3 years is __________.
  a. 0
  b. 1
  c. 2
  d. 3

8. The radiographic technique that requires the film to be placed at a right angle to the teeth is the __________ technique.
  a. paralleling
  b. bisection angle

9. Bite-blocks for holding the film in the patient's mouth should be __________.
  a. sterilized
  b. disposable
  c. either of the above

10. What processing error would cause the film to be too dark?
  a. Insufficient processing time
  b. Insufficient fixing time
  c. Developer temperature too warm
  d. Developer temperature too cold

11. What technique error would cause the image of the teeth on the radiograph to look too long?
  a. Foreshortening
  b. Closed contacts
  c. Elongation
  d. Incorrect vertical angulation

12. What technique error would cause closed contacts?
  a. Excessive vertical angulation
  b. Insufficient vertical angulation
  c. Incorrect horizontal angulation

13. Which type of radiograph shows the maxillary and mandibular teeth on one film?
  a. Periapical view
  b. Bite-wing view
  c. Panoramic view

14. Digital radiography requires __________ radiation than traditional machines.
  a. more
  b. less

15. An advantage of panoramic radiographs is the excellent detail of the images.
  a. True
  b. False

Apply Your Knowledge

1. After exposing and processing a maxillary premolar radiograph, you notice that the teeth appear unusually short on the film, and the dentist asks you to retake the image. What change will you make when you retake the image?

2. You are preparing to take an FMX on an adult patient. What materials would you set out, and where would you place surface barriers?

3. An 18-year-old patient is scheduled for a prophy and bite-wing films. How many films would you take?

4. Recently, you noticed that the radiographs have streaks on them when they come out of the automatic processor. What could be the problem?

5. Mrs. Li has been a patient in your office for almost 5 years and is now moving out of the area. Mrs. Li comes into the office and wants her radiographs to take with her. She said she paid for the radiographs and that they belong to her. How would you handle this situation?

PART SEVEN Preventive Dentistry

CHAPTER 17

Preventive Care

http://evolve.elsevier.com/Robinson/essentials/

LEARNING OBJECTIVES

1. Pronounce, define, and spell the key terms.
2. Describe the goal of preventive dentistry and name the components of a comprehensive dental program.
3. Describe the role of bacterial dental biofilm and dental calculus in dental caries and periodontal disease.
4. Educate a patient on tooth brushing and assist a patient with dental floss.
5. Describe home care techniques and the use of special interdental aids.
6. Complete the following related to fluoride:
   - Explain the uses of systemic and topical fluoride in preventive dentistry.
   - Apply topical fluoride gel or foam.
   - Apply fluoride varnish.
   - Explain the process of demineralization and remineralization of the teeth.
   - Identify the recommended concentration of fluoride in community water.
   - Identify types of self-applied fluoride.
7. Name the six key nutrients and describe their primary functions.
8. Discuss the role of cariogenic foods in causing dental caries.
9. Describe the MyPlate concept.
10. Discuss how to educate and motivate patients in the aspects of preventive dental care.

KEY TERMS

active learning
biofilm
calculus
demineralization
dental decay
disclosing agents
fluoride
fluoride varnish
fluorosis
interdental aids
MyPlate
oral biofilm
plaque
preventive dentistry
remineralization
sodium fluoride
stannous fluoride
systemic fluorides
topical fluorides
white spot

The goal of preventive dentistry is to achieve and maintain optimal oral health for a lifetime. Through a comprehensive oral health program and a partnership between the patient and dental professionals, optimal oral health can become a reality for everyone.

This chapter discusses the components of a comprehensive preventive dentistry program (Table 17-1).

Process of Dental Disease

To educate patients effectively, you must first understand how dental diseases occur and how preventive dentistry is effective in reducing these occurrences.

Bacterial Dental Biofilm

Bacterial dental **biofilm** (also known as **plaque** or **oral biofilm**) is a sticky, soft deposit of bacterial colonies that adhere to the teeth. Plaque biofilm naturally forms as soon as 1 hour after brushing. Biofilm forms on both supragingival and subgingival surfaces. The formation of biofilm involves three basic steps (Table 17-2). **Supragingival** biofilm is above the gingival margin, and **subgingival** biofilm is below the gingival margin. Plaque that remains on the teeth can harden and become *calculus* or *tartar*. The bacteria found in biofilm are the primary cause of **dental caries** and **periodontal disease.**

TABLE 17-1
Comprehensive Preventive Dentistry Program

Preventive Measure	Description
Nutrition	Dietary counseling extends beyond the narrow scope of limiting sugar consumption and may include a discussion of nutrition from the standpoint of oral health and general health.
Patient education	Education motivates patients, provides them with information, and assists them in developing the skills necessary to practice good oral hygiene.
Biofilm control	Daily removal of bacterial biofilm from the teeth and adjacent oral tissue is the goal.
Fluoride therapy	Therapy includes professionally applied fluorides, at-home fluoride therapy, and consumption of fluoridated community water.
Sealants	Sealants are most frequently applied to difficult-to-clean occlusal surfaces of the teeth. Decay-causing bacteria are then prevented from reaching into occlusal pits and fissures. (Chapter 18 discusses sealants.)

Dental Calculus

Dental **calculus** is mineralized bacterial biofilm that forms a hard mass on the surface of the natural teeth and on dentures and other dental prostheses. Calculus occurs at every age and on both permanent and primary teeth. Calculus plays an important role in periodontal disease. The rough surface of the subgingival calculus holds the disease-causing bacterial biofilm close to the gingival tissue, continuing the inflamed state of the tissue.

Understanding the interrelationship between the removal of biofilm, calculus, and good oral health is important for the patient.

Dental Caries

Dental caries, also known as **dental decay**, occurs when the bacteria in the biofilm convert sugar from the foods we eat into acid. After time, the acid attacks the tooth and causes **demineralization** (loss of calcium and phosphate) of the enamel. The earliest sign of demineralization appears as a **white spot** on the tooth (Figure 17-1, **A**). As the biofilm continues to attack the tooth, the areas of demineralization can turn into areas of caries (decay; Figure 17-1, **B**).

Periodontal Disease

Periodontal disease can range from **gingivitis** (inflammation of the gingivae) to extensive bone loss around the teeth (periodontitis). Dental biofilm is the primary cause of periodontal diseases (Figure 17-2). Periodontal diseases are discussed in Chapter 24.

TABLE 17-2
Stages in the Formation of Biofilm

Stage	Description
Pellicle formation	The pellicle is a thin layer of glycoproteins from the saliva that forms over tooth surfaces and restorations. It reforms on the teeth within minutes after brushing and/or polishing. It serves to keep the tooth surfaces moist and may even provide a barrier against acids in biofilm.
Bacteria attach to the pellicle	Bacteria colonize within the pellicle and begin to grow and multiply and produce acids. Organisms in the first few hours are gram-positive cocci and rods (see Chapter 5).
Bacteria multiply and mature	The longer the biofilm remains on the teeth, the greater the numbers and types of bacteria. Eventually *Streptococcus mutans* and *Streptococcus sanguinis* dominate the colonies. These bacteria are primarily responsible for dental caries and periodontal disease.

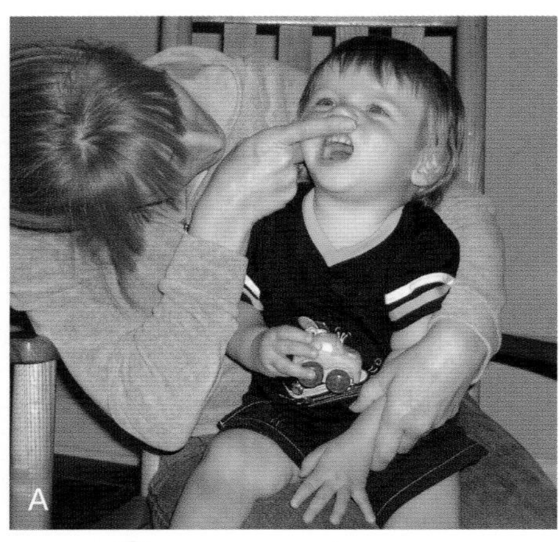

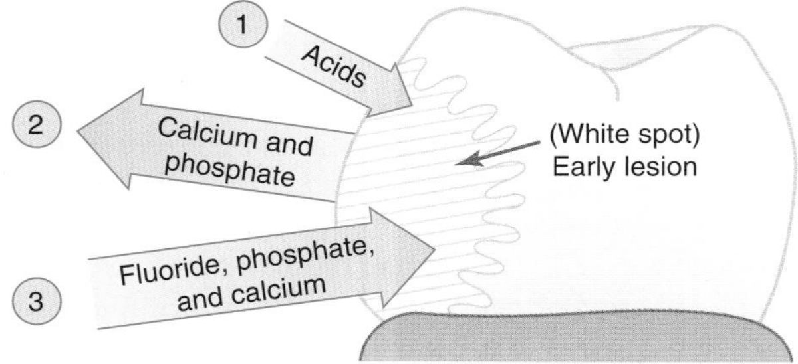

1. The tooth is attacked by acids in plaque and saliva.
2. Calcium and phosphate dissolve from the enamel in the process of demineralization.
3. Fluoride, phosphate, and calcium reenter the enamel in a process called remineralization.

B

FIGURE 17-1 **A,** The mother lifts the child's lip to look for early signs of decay. **B,** Process of caries development. (**A,** From Bird DL, Robinson DS: *Modern dental assisting,* ed 11, St. Louis, 2015, Saunders.)

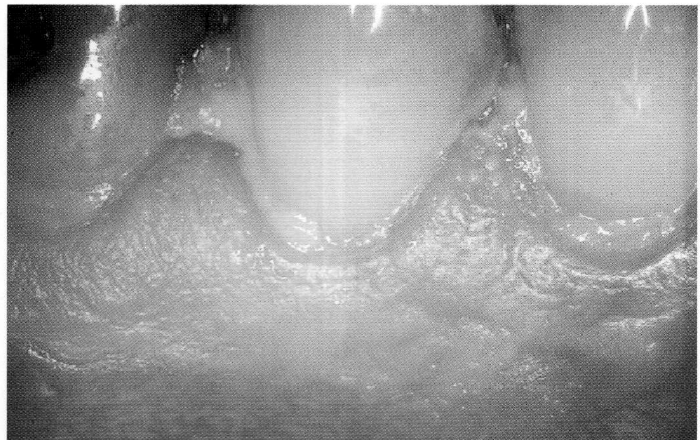

FIGURE 17-2 Buildup of bacterial biofilm on tooth surfaces affects the gingival tissues.

Tooth Brushing

Many different toothbrushes and brushing methods are in use today. The dental professional will assess the patient's needs and recommend the toothbrush and brushing method best suited to the individual patient.

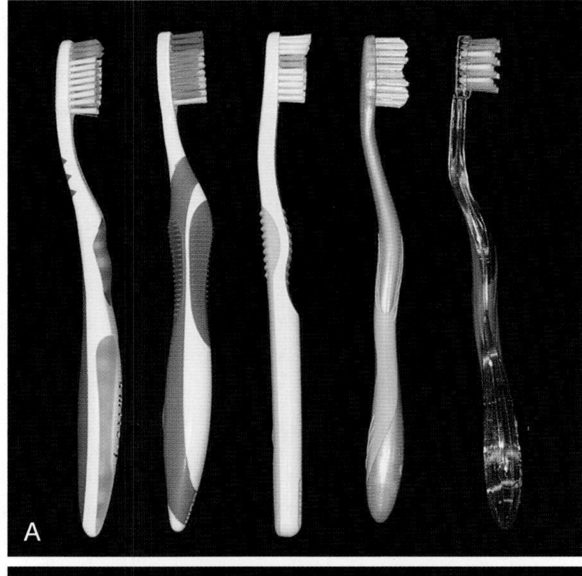

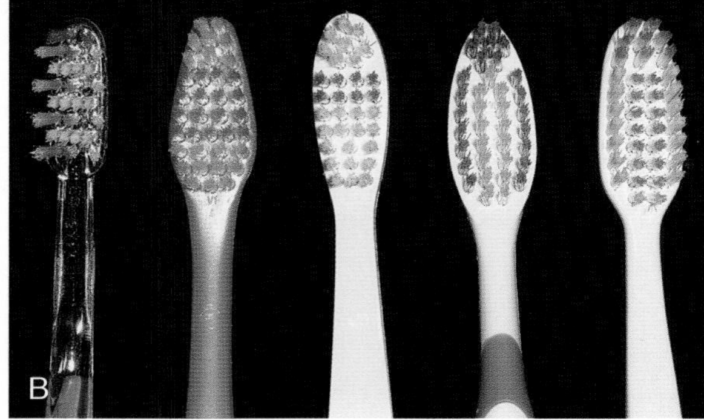

FIGURE 17-3 Examples of manual toothbrushes. (From Newman M, Takei T, Klokkevold P, et al, editors: *Carranza's clinical periodontology,* ed 12, St. Louis, 2015, Saunders.)

How Often to Brush

There is no single answer when patients ask, "How often should I brush?" The answer is based on complete biofilm removal rather than on the number of brushings.

To control bacterial biofilm and to prevent halitosis (mouth odor), at least two brushings and flossings are recommended each day. Bacteria thrive in warm, moist, dark environments; therefore the mouth should be cleaned before going to bed at night. The longer the bacteria remain undisturbed, the more damaging the biofilm becomes.

Toothbrush Selection

The size and style of the toothbrush are highly personal decisions. Many styles of head size, tuft shape, and handle angle and shape are available (Figure 17-3). Soft-bristled brushes are generally recommended for use and are less likely to cause damage to the soft tissue or any exposed cementum or dentin. Soft bristles also adapt to the contours of the tooth better. Toothbrushes should be replaced as soon as the bristles show signs of wear; generally, every 8 to 12 weeks.

A powered toothbrush may be substituted for a manual toothbrush if the biofilm is not removed with the manual brush. Suggest that the patient use a timer to ensure that adequate time

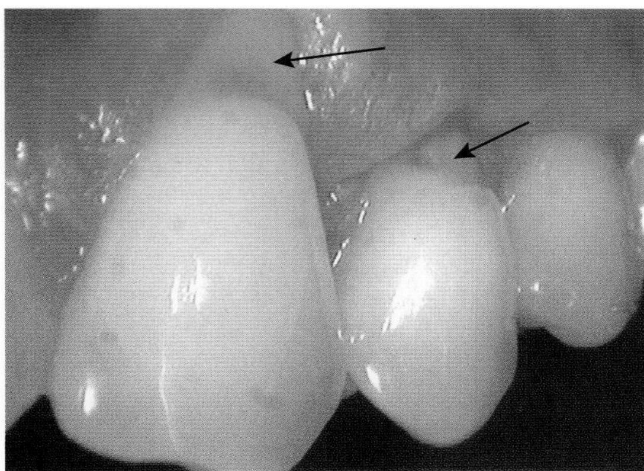

FIGURE 17-4 Improper brushing techniques can result in abrasion *(arrows)* of the tooth surface, causing gingival recession. (Courtesy Dr. Robert Meckstroth.)

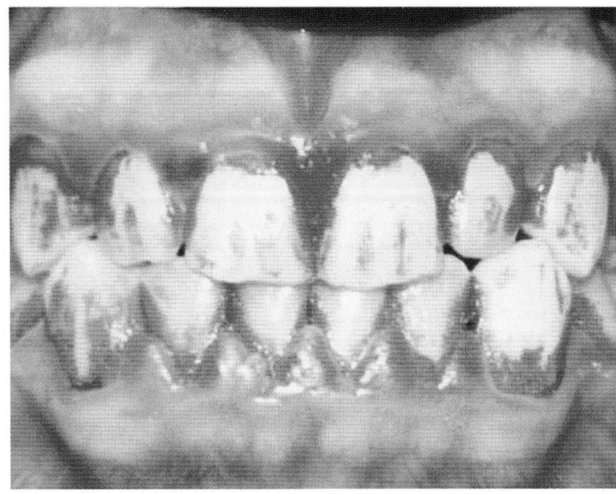

FIGURE 17-5 Dental biofilm made visible with a disclosing agent.

is spent brushing. Powered toothbrushes are also useful for physically handicapped individuals who are unable to clean their teeth with a manual brush. They may be useful for a patient with orthodontic bands and brackets and for some patients with periodontal problems.

Tooth Brushing Precaution

The patient should be cautioned about the damage that may be caused by vigorously scrubbing the teeth. Over time, hard scrubbing may cause abnormal abrasion (wear) of the tooth structure, gingival recession, and exposure of the root surface (Figure 17-4).

Disclosing Agents

Because biofilm is difficult to see, some people find it easier to learn tooth brushing and other biofilm removal techniques with the aid of a disclosing agent. **Disclosing agents** temporarily color the biofilm (usually red) to make it visible and therefore easier to remove (Figure 17-5).

Disclosing agents are artificially sweetened and may be candylike tablets or may be formulated in a solution that is wiped over the teeth using a cotton-tip applicator. All ingredients in the tablet or solution are nontoxic and harmless if swallowed. However, they stain clothing, so be careful with their use (Box 17-1).

BOX 17-1 Instructions for Use of Disclosing Tablets

- Be aware that the disclosing agent will temporarily color the tongue and gingivae along with the biofilm. In addition, the acquired pellicle will appear as a pale-stained surface sheen.
- Chew the tablet, and swish the resulting solution around in the mouth for at least 30 seconds.
- Spit the excess liquid into a bowl of running water.
- Rinse the mouth with plain, cool water. Red remaining on the teeth indicates biofilm, which must be removed.
- After the biofilm has been removed, any remaining stain on the tissue will soon be rinsed away by the saliva.

Bass Method of Sulcular Tooth Brushing

Several brushing techniques are commonly used. The Bass method (named after Dr. C. Bass, a pioneer in preventive dentistry) is the most commonly recommended technique (Table 17-3). This method is very effective in removing biofilm directly beneath the gingival margin. The gingival margin is most important in controlling gingival inflammation.

Note: Adding a rolling stroke after sulcular brushing modifies the Bass technique.

Brushing the Tongue

Bacteria on the tongue and tooth surfaces must also be removed by brushing. The easiest method is to place the toothbrush at the back of the tongue and sweep forward several times across the dorsum (top) of the tongue.

Care of the Toothbrush

When brushing is completed, the toothbrush should be thoroughly rinsed to remove excess water. The toothbrush should then be placed in a position with good air circulation to permit air-drying.

Flossing

Removing biofilm from between the teeth is a critical part of good oral health. Dental floss is the most effective tool for most people to use in removing biofilm from between the proximal surfaces of the teeth and in reducing interproximal bleeding.

Dental floss comes in several different types: waxed or unwaxed, thick or extra fine, or even in a tufted texture that changes shape when tightened. Research has shown no difference in the effectiveness of waxed or unwaxed floss for removing biofilm. It depends on how well the dental floss is used.

Dental floss is even available in various colors and flavors. However, colored and flavored dental flosses are no more effective in removing biofilm, although they may motivate patients

TABLE 17-3
Bass Method of Sulcular Brushing

Positioning the toothbrush	Place the toothbrush with the bristles directed straight into the gingival sulcus. The brush should be placed at a 45-degree angle to the long axis of the tooth.
Strokes	Press lightly so that the tips of the bristles go into the sulcus and embrasures. Vibrate the brush back and forth with very short strokes. Count at least 10 vibrations. Then reposition the brush over the next two or three teeth.
Cleaning the occlusal surfaces	Place the bristles on the occlusal surface, and move the brush in back-and-forth or small circular motions.
Cleaning the lingual surfaces	Hold the brush in a vertical position, and use gentle back-and-forth strokes.

Figure of positioning the toothbrush from Newman MG, et al: *Carranza's clinical periodontology,* ed 12, St. Louis, 2015, Saunders. Figures of cleaning occlusal and lingual surfaces from Carranza FA Jr: *Glickman's clinical periodontology,* ed 8, Philadelphia, 1996, WB Saunders.

to floss more routinely (Figure 17-6). The choice of dental floss is based on the patient's manual skills, needs, and preferences.

See Procedure 17-1: Assisting the Patient With Dental Floss (Expanded Function).

Home Care Techniques

Once the patient is motivated to want to learn and use **biofilm control** skills, he or she must learn how to perform them correctly. The dental professional will work with the patient to develop a program of oral hygiene that the patient will routinely follow at home. The goal of the program is to thoroughly remove biofilm at least once daily. After it has been thoroughly removed, it takes approximately 24 hours for biofilm to form again. Many home care techniques are used for biofilm removal;

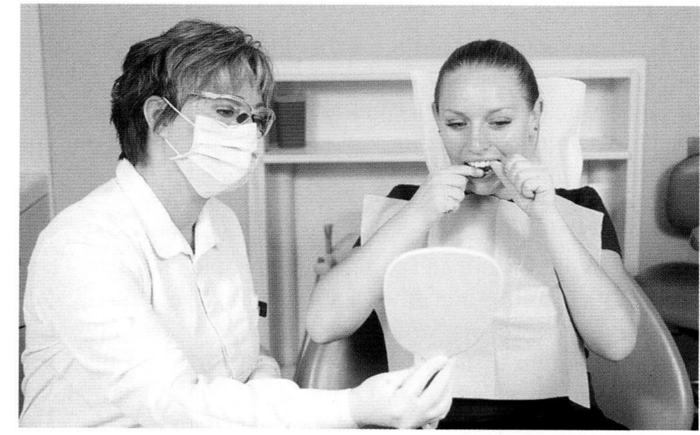

FIGURE 17-6 The dental assistant helps the patient with flossing.

TABLE 17-4
Interdental Aids

Interdental Aid	Description
Interproximal brushes	These small brushes are inserted between the teeth from the facial side and are moved with short back-and-forth strokes. This process is repeated from the lingual side.
Rubber and wooden-tip stimulators	Stimulators are used to remove interproximal biofilm and to provide gingival stimulation.
Floss holder	Is used to make flossing easier for individuals who have arthritis or poor manual dexterity or for those patients who believe their hands are too large.
Floss threader	Is used to remove biofilm and debris from under fixed bridges and orthodontic appliances.
Water irrigation device	Is used to clean debris from orthodontic brackets. A water irrigation device does not remove biofilm and should not be used in place of brushing and flossing.

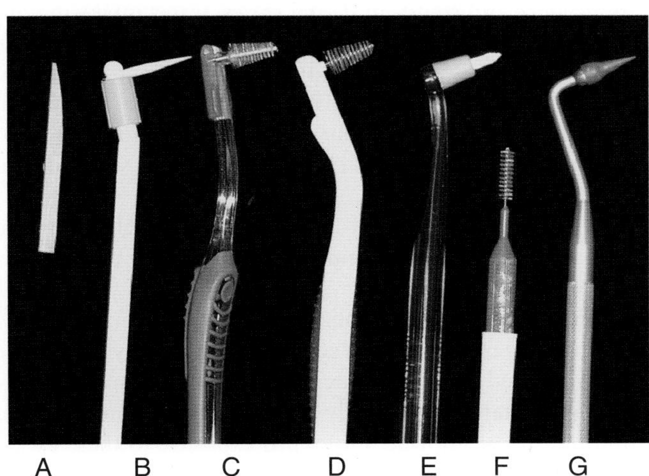

FIGURE 17-7 Types of interdental aids. Interproximal cleaning devices include (**A** and **B**) wooden tips, (**C** through **F**) interproximal brushes, and (**G**) rubber-tip stimulator. (From Newman M, Takei T, Klokkevold P, et al, editors: *Carranza's clinical periodontology,* ed 12, St. Louis, 2015, Saunders.)

the technique selected must be based on the needs and abilities of the individual patient.

Special **interdental aids** are recommended for cleaning between teeth with large or open interdental spaces. These devices may be used in addition to dental floss but are not a substitute (Table 17-4 and Figure 17-7).

Fluoride

Fluoride is a naturally occurring mineral that is found in many forms. It may be present in the water from wells; in the food we eat, which has absorbed fluoride from the soil; and as additives in many different products we use.

Fluorides are effective in strengthening the enamel's resistance to dental decay. However, to achieve the maximum benefits of fluoride, an ongoing supply of both systemic and topical fluoride must be available throughout life (Box 17-2).

BOX 17-2 Benefits of Fluoride

- Prevents demineralization.
- Helps early lesions to remineralize.
- Hardens tooth structure.
- Increases enamel resistance.

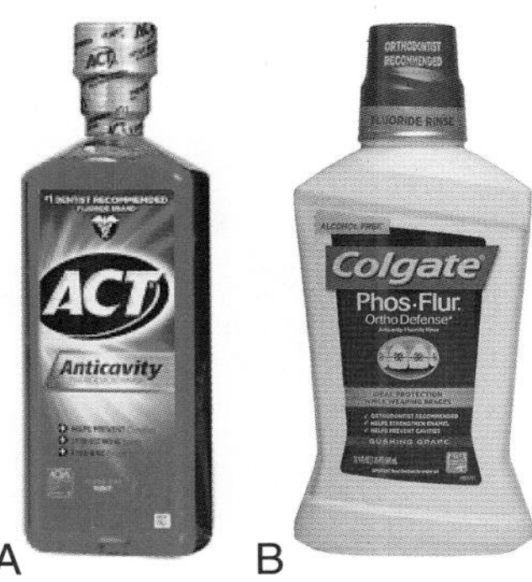

FIGURE 17-8 Samples of over-the-counter 0.04% sodium fluoride rinses with the American Dental Association Seal of Acceptance. (A, Courtesy of Chattem, Inc., Chattanooga, Tennessee. B, Courtesy Colgate Oral Pharmaceuticals, New York, New York.)

Systemic fluorides, also known as dietary fluorides, are those consumed in water, foods, beverages, or supplements.

Topical fluorides are directly applied to the teeth in the form of fluoridated toothpaste, fluoride mouth rinses, and topical applications (Figure 17-8).

See Procedure 17-2: Applying a Topical Fluoride Gel or Foam (Expanded Function).

Fluoride varnish is a concentrated topical fluoride within a resin or synthetic base that is painted on the teeth to prolong fluoride exposure (Figure 17-9). Fluoride varnish can be used instead of a fluoride gel; two to three professional applications a year are effective in preventing decay.

See Procedure 17-3: Applying Fluoride Varnish (Expanded Function).

Demineralization and Remineralization

Demineralization is the loss of minerals (calcium, phosphorus, and fluoride), causing a breakdown of the enamel. Demineralization leads to a *white spot,* which is actually the early lesion and, with further demineralization, will form caries (Figure 17-10).

When biofilm is present, the teeth are exposed to tooth acid formed by bacteria within the biofilm. These acid attacks cause demineralization. When fluoride is present in the outer layers of the enamel, the tooth is more resistant to demineralization.

Remineralization is the reverse process. Minerals are restored to the tooth surface that has been demineralized. When

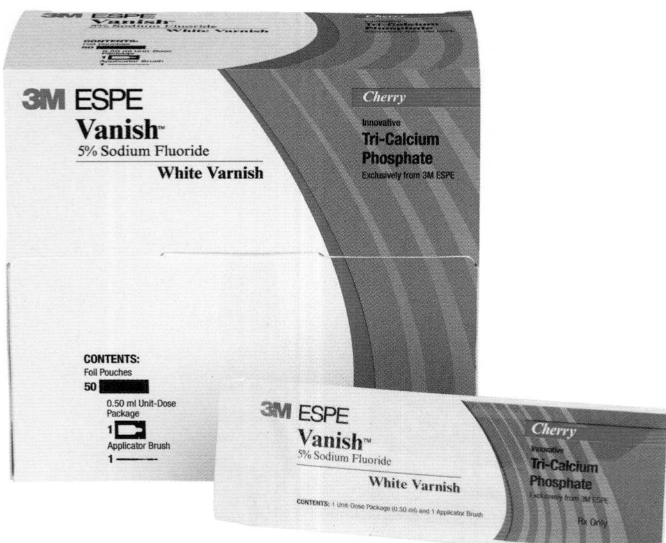

FIGURE 17-9 Fluoride varnish with tricalcium phosphate. (Photo courtesy of 3M, St. Paul, Minnesota.)

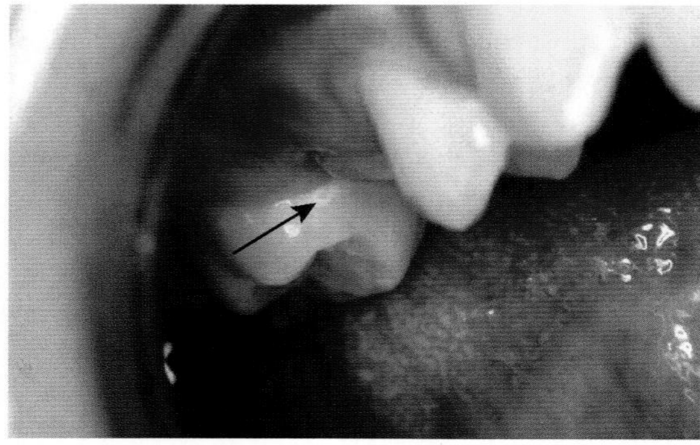

FIGURE 17-10 Early carious lesion or white spot of demineralization. (Courtesy Dr. John Featherstone, University of California, San Francisco, School of Dentistry.)

early remineralization occurs, the white *spot* hardens and may even be harder than the enamel around it. However, if the carious lesion has progressed too far, then remineralization cannot halt the process, and the tooth must be restored by a dentist. A toothache and possible loss of the tooth will result. Fluoride, itself, cannot remineralize tooth structure, but it acts as a catalyst to repair damaged enamel by using calcium, phosphorus, and fluoride from the saliva.

Safe Use of Fluoride

Fluorides added to the public water supply and present in dental products carry little or no risk when used as directed. Fluoride is beneficial in small amounts, but it can be harmful if instructions for use are not followed.

Long-term overexposure to fluoride, even at low concentrations, can result in dental **fluorosis** in children younger than 6 years of age who have developing teeth. (Fluorosis appears as white spots on the teeth. These spots do not weaken the teeth and are primarily a cosmetic problem.)

Children should always be supervised when brushing or using fluoride rinses and should not be allowed to swallow fluoride toothpaste or fluoride rinses.

It is important for any dental professional responsible for the application of fluoride to know how much fluoride he or she is giving to patients.

Sources of Systemic Fluoride

Fluoridated Water

For more than 40 years, fluoride has been safely added to the communal water supply. Most major cities in the United States are fluoridated, and efforts to fluoridate additional communities are ongoing.

In September 2010, the U.S. Department of Health and Human Services (DHHS) convened a panel of scientists from across the U.S. government to review new information related to fluoride intake and to develop new recommendations for community water fluoridation.

These scientists reviewed the best available information on prevalence and trends in dental caries, water intake in children in relation to outdoor air temperature, changes in the percentages of U.S. children and adults with dental fluorosis, and new assessments by the U.S. Environmental Protection Agency (EPA) that have examined cumulative sources of fluoride exposure and the risks of children developing severe dental fluorosis.

This new information led DHHS to propose changing the recommended level for community water systems to 0.7 milligrams per liter (mg/L).

Levels of fluoride in controlled water fluoridation are so low that the danger of ingesting an acutely toxic quantity of fluoride from fluoridated water is nonexistent. However, some communities have water that naturally contains more than twice the optimum level of fluoride. Prolonged exposure to these excessive amounts may cause dental fluorosis.

Other Dietary Sources

Foods and Beverages Because many processed foods and beverages are prepared with fluoridated water, they must be considered as sources of dietary fluoride. In children who regularly drink them, processed juices and juice-flavored drinks can be a major source of dietary fluoride.

Toothpaste and Mouth Rinses Toothpaste and mouth rinses containing fluoride should not be a source of systemic fluoride; with proper use, any excess toothpaste or rinse is spit out and never swallowed.

Prescribed Dietary Fluoride Supplements

Dietary fluoride supplements in the form of tablets, drops, or lozenges may be prescribed by the dentist for children ages 6 months to 16 years who live where no source of fluoridated water is available. Before prescribing, the dentist will take the following factors under consideration:

- Fluoride level of the child's drinking water
- Child's exposure to multiple water sources (e.g., a child whose home water source is not fluoridated but who attends a daycare center or a school in a fluoridated area)
- All potential sources of fluoride (e.g., many juices and prepared foods for young children)

The parents and patient must be willing to cooperate on an ongoing basis because supplementation is recommended until 16 years of age.

Topical Fluoride

Topical fluoride application is an essential part of a comprehensive dental preventive program. **Stannous fluoride** and **sodium fluoride** are very effective in reducing dental decay. Topical fluorides are available in forms that are self-applied by the patient and in professionally applied formulations.

Types of Self-Applied Fluoride

Fluoride-Containing Toothpastes

Toothpastes containing fluoride are the primary source of topical fluoride (Table 17-5). A major benefit of this fluoride is that the brushing action brings it into close contact with the surfaces of the teeth. Daily brushing with fluoride-containing toothpaste benefits patients of all age groups. Children younger than 6 or 7 years should be carefully supervised because ingestion of fluoride-containing toothpaste may cause dental fluorosis and nausea (Figure 17-11).

Fluoride Mouth Rinses

Fluoride mouth rinses are most effective when used after brushing and flossing. Over-the-counter, nonprescription rinses are designed to be used on a daily basis. Prescription rinses are often used for their antibiofilm properties. Rinses containing stannous fluoride are effective in reducing dental hypersensitivity (sensitivity of the tooth).

Mouth rinses containing fluoride may be recommended as an additional source of topical fluoride for high-risk patients (Box 17-3).

Brush-On Fluoride Gel

Brush-on gels are available with and without prescriptions. High-risk patients may use these at home by brushing them on the teeth or by applying them at home with a reusable custom tray.

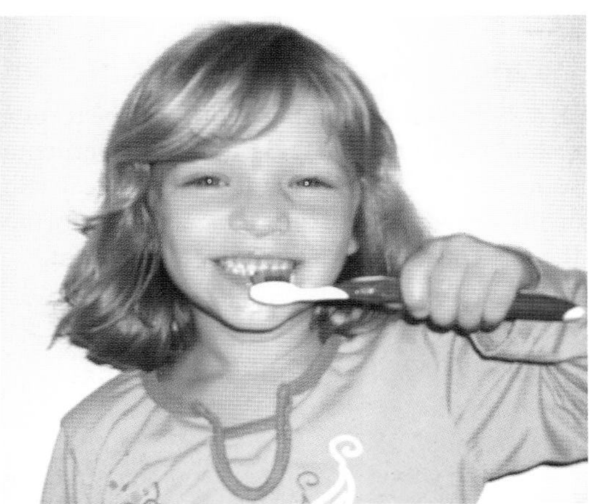

FIGURE 17-11 Children younger than 8 years of age should be carefully supervised while they are brushing to ensure that all areas of their teeth have been thoroughly cleaned and that they do not swallow fluoride-containing toothpaste. (From Bird DL, Robinson DS: *Modern dental assisting,* ed 11, St. Louis, 2015, Saunders.)

BOX 17-3 Patients at High Risk for Dental Decay

This group includes patients who:

- Have already experienced dental decay.
- Live in areas where the public water supply is not fluoridated.
- Are prone to root caries.
- Have illnesses or are taking medications that slow the flow of saliva.
- Are undergoing chemotherapy or radiation treatments that damage the tissue and affect the flow of saliva.

TABLE 17-5
Types of Self-Applied Fluorides

Type	Form	Comments
Sodium fluoride (NaF) 0.24%	Dentifrices (gel or paste)	Is approved by the American Dental Association (ADA).
Sodium monofluorophosphate (Na_2PO_3F) 0.76%	Dentifrices (gel or paste)	Is approved by the ADA.
Neutral NaF 0.025%	Mouth rinse	Is sold over the counter without a prescription.
Neutral NaF 0.20%	Mouth rinse	A prescription is required.
NaF 1.1%	Brush-on gel	Is not intended for use as a dentifrice; the teeth must be brushed first, then the gel is used.
Stannous fluoride (SnF_2) 0.4% in glycerin base	Brush-on gel	Is not intended for use as a dentifrice; the teeth must be brushed first, then the gel is used.

The patient is instructed to use the tray at bedtime. A small amount of the brush-on gel is placed in the tray, and the tray is placed over the teeth for the amount of time recommended by the manufacturer.

If water in the area is fluoridated, then the patient is instructed to rinse and spit to prevent consuming excess fluoride. If the water in the area is not fluoridated, then the patient is told not to rinse after the application.

Professional Topical Fluoride Applications

Professional topical fluoride applications may be recommended for some children soon after the eruption of permanent teeth and for some patients at high risk for dental decay (Box 17-3). Professionally applied topical fluoride may be performed by the dentist, the hygienist, or a qualified dental assistant.

Professionally Applied Topical Fluoride: 1-Minute versus 4-Minute Applications

Although the most update of fluoride occurs in the first minute, research shows that the full 4 minutes provides the best topical benefit. The American Dental Association (ADA) states that "*...there are considerable data on caries reduction for professionally applied topical fluoride gel treatments of 4 minutes or more. In contrast, there is laboratory, but no clinical equivalency data on the effectiveness of 1-minute fluoride gel applications.*"

Upon examining current information on this topic, dental professionals need to determine whether professional topical fluoride applications are appropriate for all their patients, based on the caries risk factors.

Nutrition

Good nutrition depends on an adequate supply of the nutrients that are properly used by the body. (Nutrients are substances that supply the elements necessary to meet the body's requirements for energy, growth, maintenance, and well-being.)

All nutrients are available through a well-balanced diet. Each nutrient has a specific role, and one nutrient cannot perform the functions of another nutrient. For optimal health, the foods we eat must meet our nutrient requirements and energy needs.

Supplements and vitamin pills cannot make up for foods that are not nutritionally adequate. When food intake exceeds the body's energy needs, the excess is stored as fat and the individual gains weight.

Key Nutrients

The six key nutrients are carbohydrates, proteins, fats, water, vitamins, and minerals (Tables 17-6 through 17-9).

Cariogenic Foods

Any food that contains sugars or other carbohydrates that can be metabolized by bacteria in biofilm is described as being cariogenic. (*Cariogenic* means producing or promoting dental decay.)

A major factor in determining the cariogenicity (ability to cause dental caries) of a carbohydrate is how long the food remains in the mouth. Refined carbohydrates such as candy and other sweets are cariogenic (caries producing) because their sugars are readily available.

Sugary liquids such as soft drinks quickly leave the mouth and are not as cariogenic as are sticky foods that stay in the mouth longer. Foods such as crackers, although not sweet, are cariogenic because they stick to the teeth and remain in the mouth long enough to be broken down into sugars that can be used by the bacteria in biofilm.

Complex carbohydrates such as fruits and vegetables are less cariogenic because they leave the mouth before they are converted into simple sugars.

Dietary Guidelines

The Dietary Guidelines Issued by the U.S. Department of Agriculture (USDA) are important in helping find ways to reduce the rates of death and disease related to obesity, diabetes, cardiovascular disease, cancer, and other chronic illnesses. On June 2, 2011, the USDA unveiled the government's new food icon, MyPlate (Figure 17-12).

MyPlate

The MyPlate icon replaced the familiar USDA's MyPyramid guide that had been used for the past 19 years. MyPlate is now being displayed on food packaging and is used in nutrition education in the United States. The MyPlate icon emphasizes the fruit, vegetable, grain, protein, and dairy food groups. Understanding these guidelines is important when planning your own dietary intake and in providing nutrition counseling to your patients (Box 17-4). The MyPlate icon is intentionally simple and designed to help consumers think about building a healthy plate at meal times and to help them seek more

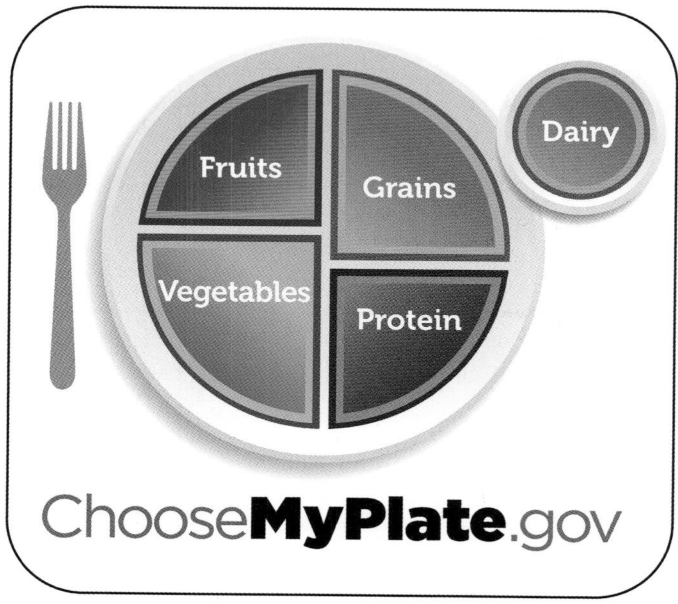

FIGURE 17-12 MyPlate. United States Department of Agriculture, Choose MyPlate. www.choosemyplate.gov

TABLE 17-6
Six Key Nutrients

Nutrient	Description
Carbohydrates	Carbohydrates are used by the body as the chief source of energy. Each gram of carbohydrate supplies 4 calories. Calories are the basic unit used to measure the body's energy needs and use.
Complex carbohydrates	Primarily found in grains, vegetables, and fruits, complex carbohydrates are important because they provide energy, vitamins, minerals, and fiber.
Refined carbohydrates	Are found in processed foods, such as sugar, syrup, jelly, bread, crackers, cookies, candy, cake, and soft drinks. In contrast to complex carbohydrates, most refined carbohydrates supply only empty calories, and many are high in fat. (Empty calories are calories that provide only energy and no other nutrients.)
Proteins	Proteins are the only nutrients that can build and repair body tissue; this is their primary function. When other sources are not available, proteins can be used to meet energy needs. Proteins come from animal sources (meat, cheese, milk, and eggs) and plant sources (beans and nuts). Each gram of protein supplies 4 calories.
Fats	Fats facilitate absorption of the fat-soluble vitamins A, D, E, and K. They also provide essential fatty acids; however, daily fat requirements are filled by fats contained in other foods such as meat (where they naturally occur) and in processed foods (where they are added during preparation). Fats, which come from both animal and plant sources, provide large amounts of energy in a small amount of food. Each gram of fat supplies 9 calories.
Water	Often called the forgotten nutrient, water is important because it helps build tissue and aids in regulating body temperature. An daily adequate supply is essential because we can live longer without food than we can without water.
Vitamins	Vitamins are organic substances that are necessary in very small amounts for proper growth and development and for optimal health. (Organic substances consist of matters of plant or animal origin.)
Fat-soluble vitamins	Are stored in body fat and are not destroyed by cooking. The functions, sources, and deficiency symptoms of fat-soluble vitamins are described in Table 17-7.
Water-soluble vitamins	Naturally present in food, water-soluble vitamins are easily destroyed during food preparation. These vitamins are not stored in the body and must be consumed each day. The functions, sources, and deficiency symptoms of water-soluble vitamins are described in Table 17-8.
Minerals	Minerals are the components of the bones and teeth that make them rigid and strong. They also play an important role in maintaining other bodily functions. The functions, sources, and deficiency symptoms of the major minerals are described in Table 17-9.

BOX 17-4 Dietary Guidelines for Americans

Eat a variety of foods. Food contains combinations of nutrients, and a varied diet, in the recommended proportions, will ensure an adequate supply of the key nutrients.

Maintain a healthy weight. Food intake should be balanced with exercise to maintain optimal health.

Choose a diet with plenty of grain products, vegetables, and fruits. These foods are important because they are a good energy source and provide a variety of nutrients and fiber.

Choose a diet low in fat, saturated fat, and cholesterol. Less than 30% of your daily caloric intake should come from fats. (Remember, fats have 9 calories per gram!)

Use sugars in moderation. Sugars primarily provide empty calories that can contribute to weight gain, and sugars are associated with dental disease. When calculating sugar intake, remembering that 4 grams equals a teaspoonful of sugar is helpful.

Use salt and sodium in moderation. In some people, salt is associated with hypertension (high blood pressure) and other health problems. Many processed foods have a high sodium content.

If you drink alcoholic beverages, do so in moderation. In addition to its intoxicating characteristics, alcohol contains 7 empty calories per gram.

information to plan their own dietary intake by visiting www.ChooseMyPlate.gov.

The MyPlate icon depicts a place setting with a plate and glass divided into five food groups. MyPlate is divided into sections of approximately 30 percent grains, 30 percent vegetables, 20 percent fruits and 20 percent protein, accompanied by a smaller circle representing dairy, such as a glass of low-fat or nonfat milk or a yogurt cup.

MyPlate makes recommendations, such as "Make half your plate fruits and vegetables," "Switch to 1% or skim milk,"

TABLE 17-7
Fat-Soluble Vitamins

Vitamin	Important Functions	Best Sources	Deficiency Symptoms
Vitamin A	Promotes growth. Promotes the health of the eyes. Maintains the structure and functioning of the cells of the skin and mucous membranes. Promotes the health of oral structures.	Fish liver oil Liver Green and yellow vegetables Fruit (yellow) Butter, milk, cream, cheese Egg yolk	Retarded growth Night blindness Increased susceptibility to infection Changes in skin and mucous membranes
Vitamin D	Helps absorb calcium from the digestive tract, and builds calcium and phosphorus into bones and teeth.	Vitamin D–irradiated milk Fish liver oil Sunshine on skin	Rickets Poor tooth development
Vitamin E	Promotes growth. Protects vitamin A and essential fatty acids from oxidation. Aids in the formation of red blood cells, muscles, and other tissue.	Wheat germ oil Vegetable oils Green vegetables Milk fat, butter Egg yolk	Undetermined Undetermined
Vitamin K	Promotes normal clotting of the blood. Helps maintain normal liver function.	Green leafy vegetables Liver Soybean and other vegetable oils Synthesized by intestinal bacteria	Hemorrhage

TABLE 17-8
Water-Soluble Vitamins

Vitamin	Important Functions	Best Sources	Deficiency Symptoms
Thiamine (B1)	Promotes growth. Promotes normal appetite and digestion. Maintains good muscle tone and healthy functioning of the heart and nerves.	Yeast Wheat germ Organ meats Meat Dried beans and peas Whole grain or enriched products	Beriberi Retarded growth Loss of appetite and weight Nerve disorders Lowered resistance to fat digestion Digestive disorders
Riboflavin (B2)	Helps release energy from carbohydrates, proteins, and fats. Promotes growth. Helps maintain healthy skin and oral tissues. Promotes.	Liver and other organ meats Meat, poultry, fish Milk Eggs Yeast Green vegetables Whole grain or enriched products	Lesions around mouth, particularly at corners Retarded growth
Niacin	Helps other cells use nutrients. Is necessary for the normal function of digestive tract and nervous system.	Meat, poultry, fish Milk, butter Whole grain or enriched products The body can convert tryptophan in protein into niacin.	Pellagra Glossitis Digestive disturbances Mental disorders
Folic acid (Folacin)	Is essential to health; is found in all body cells. Aids in the formation of hemoglobin and red blood cells.	Liver and organ meats Yeast Dark-green leafy vegetables Dried beans and peas	Digestive disorders Disorders of the hematopoietic system

TABLE 17-8
Water-Soluble Vitamins—cont'd

Vitamin	Important Functions	Best Sources	Deficiency Symptoms
Pantothenic acid	Aids in the metabolism of carbohydrates, proteins, and fats. Aids in the formation of hormones and nerve-regulating substances.	Yeast Liver and other organ meats Eggs Whole grain or enriched products	Fatigue, sleep disturbances Headache, malaise Nausea, abdominal distention
Vitamin B12	Aids in the formation of red blood cells and in blood regeneration. Is used in the treatment of pernicious anemia.	Liver and other organ meats Muscle meats, fish Milk, cheese Eggs	Not yet known
Biotin	Helps release energy from carbohydrates. Aids in the formation of fatty acids.	Liver and other organ meats Milk Egg yolk Yeast	Dermatitis, glossitis Loss of appetite, nausea Loss of sleep Muscular pains Hyperesthesia and paresis
Vitamin B6	Aids in the absorption and metabolism of proteins and fats. Assists in the formation of red blood cells.	Meat (especially liver), fish Yeast Milk Eggs	Similar to those found in biotin deficiencies
Vitamin C	Is essential in the formation and maintenance of the capillary walls, in strengthening the walls of blood vessels, and in preventing the tendency to bleed easily. Is essential in healing. Acts as a detoxifying agent. Is important to maintain healthy gums.	Citrus fruits, melons, berries, and other fruits Tomatoes and other raw vegetables	Scurvy Tendency to bruise easily

TABLE 17-9
Minerals Required for Health

Mineral	Important Functions	Best Sources	Deficiency Symptoms
Calcium	Promotes normal development and maintenance of bones and teeth. Promotes clotting of the blood. Promotes normal muscle activity.	Milk and milk products Sardines and other whole canned fish Leafy green vegetables	Retarded growth Poor tooth formation Slow clotting time of blood Increased susceptibility to fracture
Phosphorus	Aids in the formation of bones and teeth. Releases energy from carbohydrates, proteins, and fats. Maintains healthy nerve tissue and normal muscle activity.	Meat, poultry, fish Milk and milk products Dried beans and peas	Weakness, loss of appetite Retarded growth Porous bones Poor tooth formation
Magnesium	Builds bones. Releases energy from muscle glycogen. Aids in the conduction of nerve impulses to muscles.	Raw, leafy green vegetables Nuts and seeds Whole grains and soybeans	Muscular twitching and tremors Irregular heartbeat Insomnia Leg and foot cramps, shaky hands

Continued

TABLE 17-9
Minerals Required for Health—cont'd

Mineral	Important Functions	Best Sources	Deficiency Symptoms
Potassium	Promotes muscle contraction. Maintains fluid and electrolyte balance. Aids in the release of energy.	Oranges, bananas Meat Bran Peanut butter	Abnormal heart rhythm, muscular weakness Lethargy Kidney and lung failure
Chloride	Regulates balance of body fluids. Activates enzymes in saliva.	Table salt	Very rare Disturbed balance in body fluids
Sodium	Regulates balance of body fluids.	Table salt	Difficulty is primarily caused by excess. May cause excess fluid retention in the body. Can lead to high blood pressure.
Iron	Aids in the formation of hemoglobin.	Liver and other organ meats Red meat Egg yolks Leafy green vegetables Dried fruit	Anemia, characterized by weakness, dizziness, loss of weight, gastric disturbances, and pallor
Copper	Aids in the formation of red blood cells.	Liver and other organ meats Oysters Dried beans and peas Corn oil margarine	Anemia Faulty development of bone and nervous tissue
Zinc	Is a constituent of approximately 100 enzymes.	Meat, especially liver Eggs Seafood	Delayed wound healing Diminished taste sensation
Iodine	Is part of the thyroid hormones.	Seafood Iodized salt	Goiter (enlarged thyroid)
Fluoride	Aids in the formation of decay-resistant teeth. Maintains bone strength.	Fluoridated water	Excessive dental decay
Chromium	Aids in the metabolism of glucose.	Meat Cheese Yeast Whole grain breads and cereals	Possibly abnormal sugar metabolism
Selenium	Is an antioxidant and interacts with vitamin E.	Meat, poultry, seafood Milk Egg yolk	Not known in humans
Manganese	Promotes functioning of the central nervous system. Promotes normal bone structure.	Nuts and whole grains Vegetables and fruits Tea, instant coffee	Not known in humans
Molybdenum	Is part of the enzyme xanthine oxidase.	Liver and other organ meats Cereal grains	Not known in humans

"Make at least half your grains whole," and "Vary your protein food choices." The guidelines also recommend portion control while still enjoying food, as well as reducing sodium and sugar intakes.

The MyPlate icon is currently available in 20 languages: English, Arabic, Chinese (simplified and traditional), Filipino-Tagalog, French, German, Hindi, Indonesian, Italian, Japanese, Korean, Malay, Pashto, Portuguese, Russian, Spanish, Thai, Urdu, and Vietnamese.
www.choosemyplate.gov.

Preventive Dental Care

Patient Education

Patient education in oral health is the responsibility of all members of the dental health care team. Beginning with the initial examination, patient education is provided at every visit. An oral health education program is based on motivation and education.

Motivation

The dental health professional should work with the patient to increase his or her motivational level so that the patient wants

BOX 17-5 Active Patient Education

1. Establish open communication and a safe learning environment.
2. Listen to the patient's concerns regarding his or her oral health.
3. Jointly decide on an oral hygiene regimen.
4. Present the skills to be learned one at a time and as simply as possible. When possible, use visual aids, such as disclosing tablets, to clarify the point.
5. Give the patient an opportunity to practice new skills; for example, provide a toothbrush and guide the patient as he or she practices using a new brushing technique.
6. Provide reinforcement and encouragement until the patient has mastered these skills; for example, use a disclosing tablet to demonstrate that all of the biofilm has been removed.
7. Listen to the patient regarding his or her understanding of the information.
8. Encourage the patient to continue these new actions at home until the desired habit pattern has been formed.

to learn and is willing to do the things necessary to achieve and maintain oral health. The lower the patient's level of motivation, the less is his or her chance of success with an oral hygiene program.

The first step is to help the patient recognize that he or she has a problem that needs to be solved. Then it is necessary for the patient to be willing to accept a role in solving the problem. As an example, the patient may not know that improper tooth brushing can damage the teeth and gums. Once the patient recognizes the problem and is willing to change his or her behavior, he or she will be more motivated to learn how to use proper techniques.

Education

Oral health education is not a lecture. It is listening more than talking and involves more problem solving than instruction. It is creating in the patient an awareness of the need to return regularly for professional prophylaxis, examination, and treatment.

It is helping parents recognize the importance of preventive steps, such as the placement of sealants and the use of fluorides.

It is counseling to increase the patient's awareness of the role of nutrition in achieving optimal dental and general health.

In your role as a dental health educator, you must be enthusiastic about helping others achieve optimal oral health.

Acceptance

The patient can more easily learn when he or she feels safe, accepted, and respected. Encouragement is freely given, and correction is structured in a positive manner. Most importantly, the patient is never scolded, embarrassed, or teased because of his or her ignorance or errors.

Active Learning

The most productive form of learning occurs when the patient is actively participating in the process, using as many of his or her senses as possible. Teaching biofilm control is an ideal situation for **active learning** (Box 17-5).

Ethical Implications

Dental health professionals are concerned not only with treating oral diseases but also with preventing them. A comprehensive dental treatment plan must include a plan for disease prevention that consists of nutritional counseling, patient education, biofilm control, fluoride therapy, and dental sealants when indicated.

Procedure 17-1

Assisting the Patient With Dental Floss (Expanded Function)

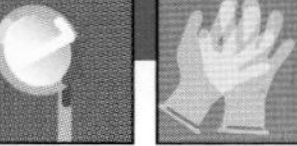

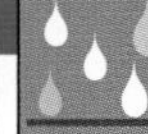
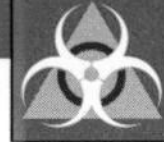
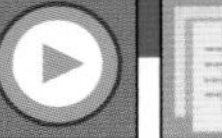
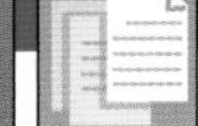

Prerequisites for Performing this Procedure

- Infection control protocol
- Patient communication skills
- Understanding of tooth morphologic form and structure
- Understanding of oral anatomy
- Manual dexterity

Equipment and Supplies

- Hand mirror for patient
- Dental floss

Procedural Steps

Preparing the Floss

1. Cut a piece of floss approximately 18 inches long. Wrap the excess floss around the middle fingers of both of your hands, leaving 2 to 3 inches of working space exposed.

Continued

Procedure 17-1

Assisting the Patient With Dental Floss (Expanded Function)—cont'd

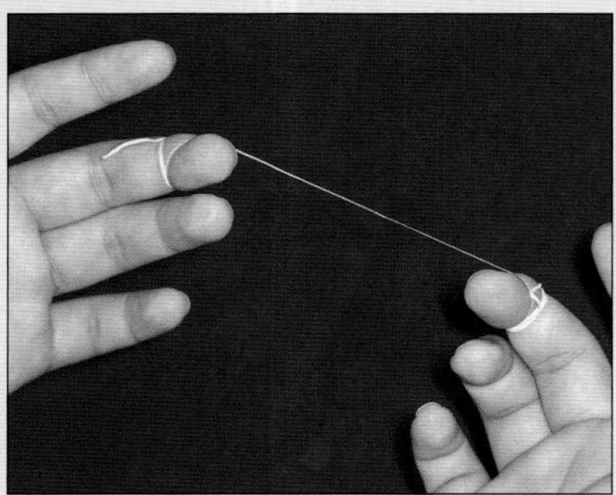

2. Tightly stretch the floss between your fingers, and use your thumb and index finger to guide the floss into place.
3. Tightly hold the floss between the thumb and forefinger of each hand. These fingers control the floss, and they should be no farther than 12 inches apart.

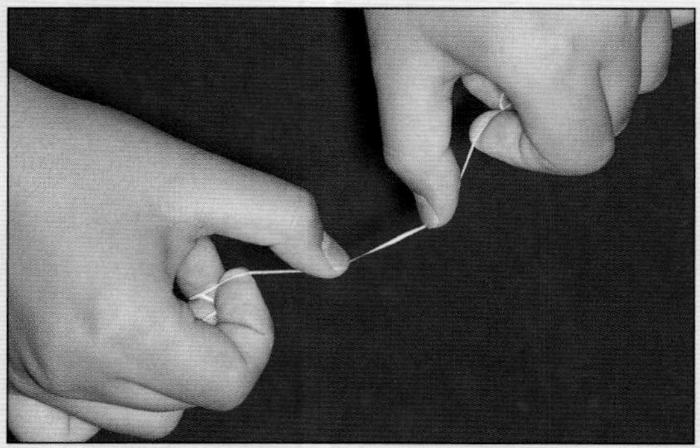

Flossing the Teeth

4. Gently pass the floss between the patient's teeth, using a sawing motion. Guide the floss to the gumline. Do not force or snap the floss past the contact area.

Purpose: The floss may cut or injure the tissue.

5. Curve the floss into a C shape against one tooth. Gently slide it into the space between the gingiva and the tooth. Use both hands to move the floss up and down on one side of the tooth.

Purpose: This step demonstrates how to remove biofilm from difficult-to-reach proximal areas.

6. Repeat these steps on each side of all the teeth in both arches, including the posterior surface of the last tooth in each quadrant.

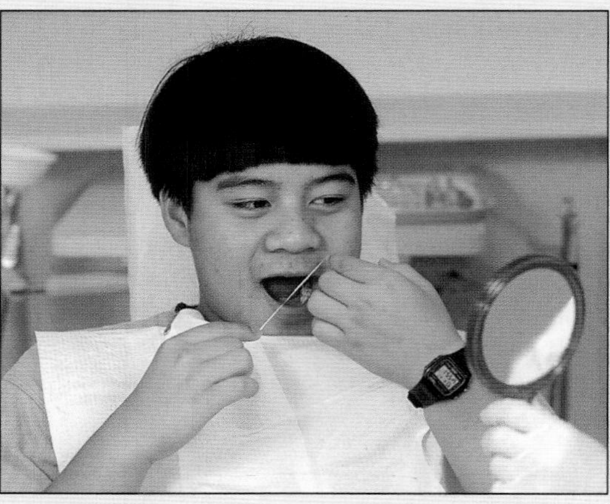

7. As the floss becomes frayed or soiled, move a fresh area into the working position.

Note: This procedure is described as it would be performed by the patient at home.

Documentation

DATE	PROCEDURE	OPERATOR
2/20/16	Provided flossing demonstration and instruction. Patient practiced technique and did well.	DLB/43

Photos from Bird DL, *Robinson DS: Modern dental assisting,* ed 11, St. Louis, 2015, Saunders.

Procedure 17-2

Applying a Topical Fluoride Gel or Foam (Expanded Function)

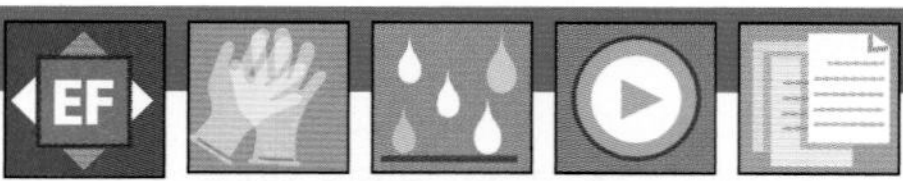

Prerequisites for Performing this Procedure

- Infection control protocol
- Patient communication skills
- Knowledge of oral anatomy
- Moisture control techniques

Equipment and Supplies

- Fluoride gel or foam
- Disposable trays of appropriate sizes
- Saliva ejector
- Cotton rolls
- Air-water syringe
- Timer

Procedure 17-2

Applying a Topical Fluoride Gel or Foam (Expanded Function)—cont'd

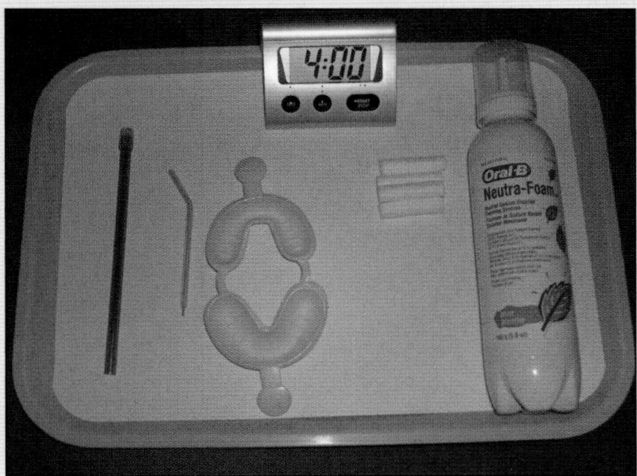

Procedural Steps

Selecting the Tray

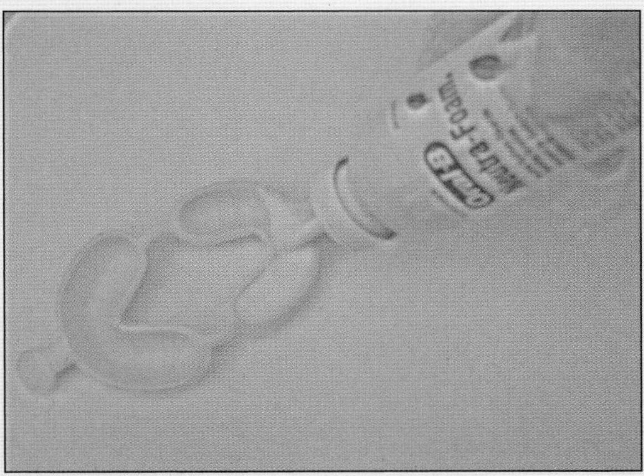

1. Select a disposable tray that is the appropriate size for the patient's mouth. The tray must be long and sufficiently deep to cover all erupted teeth completely without extending beyond the distal surface of the most posterior tooth.

Purpose: Trays are available in sizes to fit primary, mixed, and adult dentition. If the patient's mouth can accommodate it, then you may use a double-arch tray, which saves time by simultaneously treating both arches. Remember, trays are discarded after a single use, and if you try a tray in the mouth but do not use it, then that tray must also be discarded.

Preparing the Teeth

2. Check to see whether calculus is present; if it is not, then no preparation is required.

Purpose: Fluoride easily diffuses through the acquired pellicle and bacterial biofilm.

3. If calculus is present, then request that the dentist or dental hygienist remove it.

Purpose: Calculus prevents fluoride from reaching the enamel of the tooth.

Note: The presence of biofilm will not affect the uptake of fluoride.

Applying the Topical Fluoride

4. Seat the patient in an upright position, and explain the procedure.

Purpose: Having the patient upright prevents the gel from going into the throat.

5. Instruct the patient not to swallow the fluoride.
6. Select the appropriate tray, and load it with a minimal amount of fluoride, following the guidelines according to the patient's age.

Reminder: Containers that are handled with gloved hands during the appointment should be surface-disinfected during treatment room cleanup.

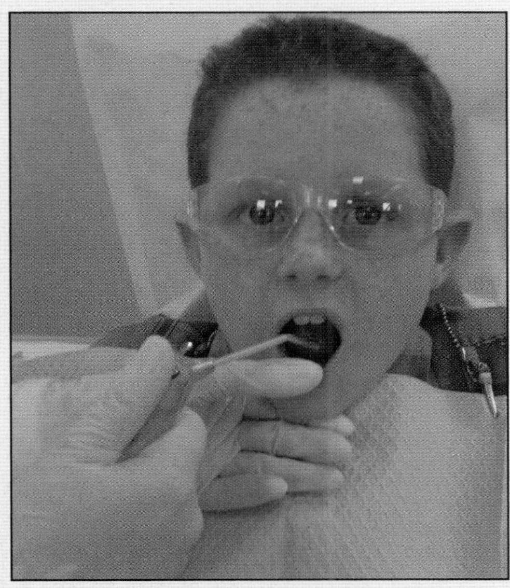

7. Dry the teeth using air from the air-water syringe.

Purpose: For fluoride to be maximally effective, the teeth must be dry when the fluoride is applied.

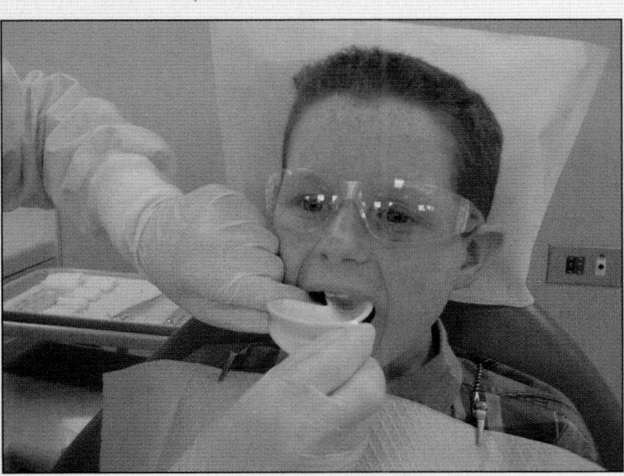

Continued

Procedure 17-2

Applying a Topical Fluoride Gel or Foam (Expanded Function)—cont'd

8. Insert the tray, and place cotton rolls between the arches. Ask the patient to bite up and down gently on the cotton rolls.

Purpose: This step allows the fluoride to be squeezed over all the tooth surfaces.

9. Promptly place the saliva ejector, and tilt the patient's head forward.

Purpose: This step prevents the patient from swallowing the fluoride.

10. Set the timer for the appropriate amount of time in accordance with the manufacturer's instructions. During this time, do not leave the patient unattended.

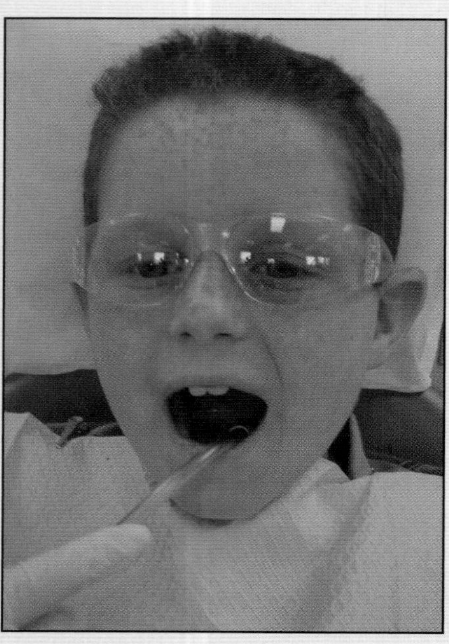

11. On completion, remove the tray, but do not allow the patient to rinse or swallow. Promptly use the saliva ejector or the high-volume oral evacuator tip to remove excess saliva and solution. Do not allow the patient to close the lips tightly around the saliva ejector.

Purpose: Removing excess saliva and fluoride solution will make the patient more comfortable and less likely to rinse with water.

12. Instruct the patient not to rinse, eat, drink, or brush the teeth for at least 30 minutes.

Purpose: These activities could disturb the action of the fluoride.

Documentation

DATE	PROCEDURE	OPERATOR
1/25/16	Applied APF fluoride gel. Instructed patient not to eat for 30 min.	DLB/43

Photos from Bird DL, Robinson DS: *Modern dental assisting,* ed 11, St. Louis, 2015, Saunders.

Procedure 17-3

Applying Fluoride Varnish (Expanded Function)

EF

Prerequisites for Performing this Procedure

- Infection control protocol
- Patient communication skills
- Knowledge of oral anatomy

Equipment and Supplies

- 5% sodium fluoride varnish (unit dose)
- Cotton-tip applicator or syringe applicator
- 2 × 2 gauze squares or cotton rolls
- Saliva ejector

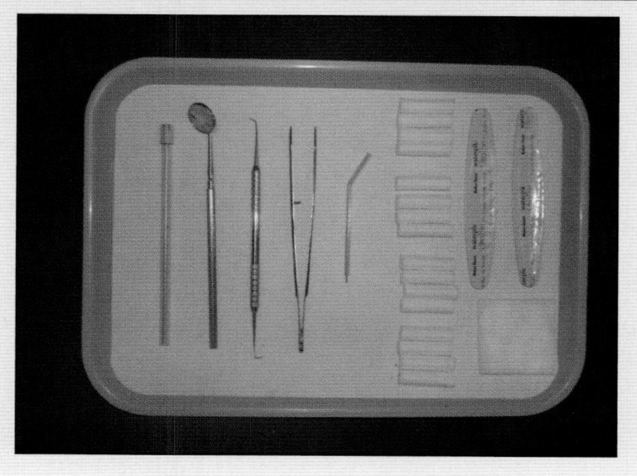

Procedure 17-3

Applying Fluoride Varnish (Expanded Function)—cont'd

Procedural Steps

1. Obtain informed consent from the patient or parent or legal guardian in the case of a minor patient.

Purpose: Informed consent is a legal requirement for the provision of any dental treatment.

2. Gather supplies and single-unit dose for application.

Purpose: Once you begin the procedure, you will not be able to stop in the middle to get something you forgot to set out.

3. Recline the patient to an ergonomically correct position.

Purpose: You will have better access to the oral cavity and will be in a comfortable position.

4. Wipe the teeth to be varnished with the gauze or cotton roll, and insert the saliva ejector.

Note: The varnish is not moisture sensitive and can be applied in the presence of saliva.

Purpose: The saliva ejector is for patient comfort only.

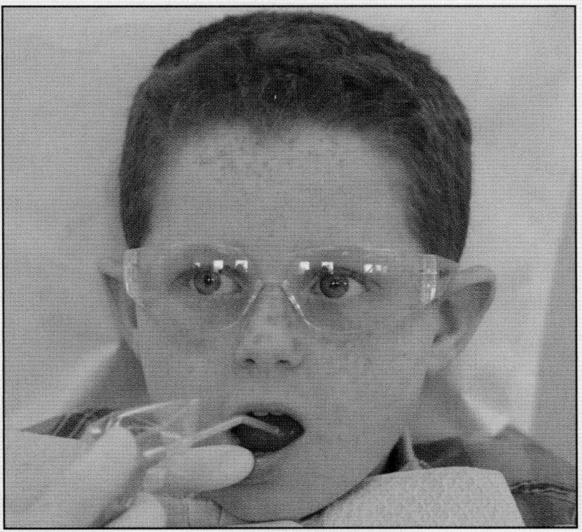

5. Using a cotton-tip applicator, brush, or syringe-style applicator, apply 0.3 to 0.5 ml of varnish (unit dose) to the clinical crowns of teeth; application time is 1 to 3 minutes.

Note: Refer to the manufacturer's instructions for specific application time.

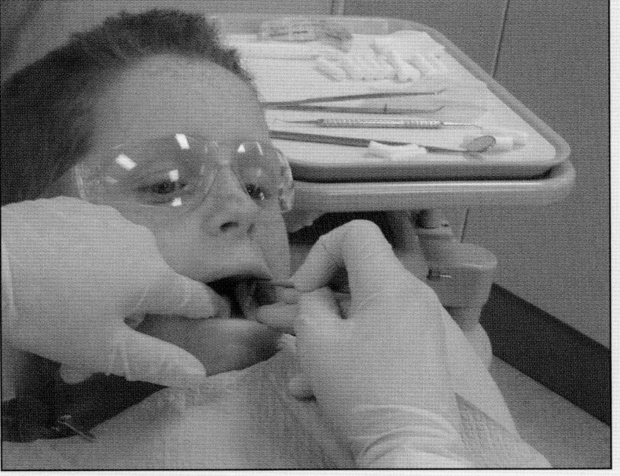

6. Dental floss may be used to draw the varnish interproximally.

Purpose: This step provides varnish protection for hard-to-reach surfaces.

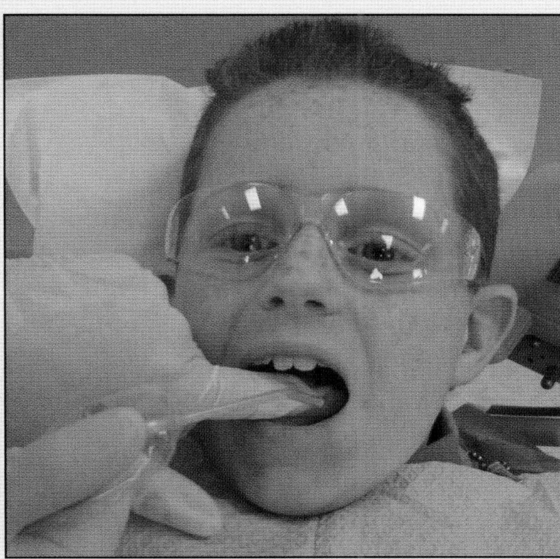

7. Allow your patient to rinse after the procedure has been completed.

Purpose: This step removes any residual taste.

8. Remind the patient to avoid eating hard foods, drinking hot or alcoholic beverages, brushing, and flossing for at least 4 to 6 hours, or preferably until the next day after the application. Drink through a straw for the first few hours after application.

Purpose: This step prolongs the contact of the varnish. Varnish can be removed the next day with tooth brushing and flossing.

Documentation

DATE	PROCEDURE	OPERATOR
1/25/16	Applied 0.3 ml of 5% sodium fluoride varnish (insert brand name) on facial and lingual surfaces of teeth #6 to #14, and #19 to #30.	DLB 43

From Bird DL, Robinson DS: *Modern dental assisting,* ed 11, St. Louis, 2015, Saunders.

Chapter Exercises

Multiple Choice

Circle the letter next to the correct answer.

1. What type of motion should be used when brushing the occlusal surfaces of the teeth?
a. Back-and-forth
b. CA circular
c. Sweeping stroke
d. a and b

2. The patient learns most effectively when he or she __________.
a. feels safe and accepted
b. is actively involved
c. recognizes that he or she has a problem to be solved
d. all of the above

3. The most effective way to remove biofilm from proximal tooth surfaces is by __________.
a. flossing
b. oral irrigation
c. rinsing
d. tooth brushing

4. When brushing the lingual surfaces of the anterior teeth, the head of the toothbrush is placed in a __________ position.
a. horizontal
b. vertical

5. A stiff-bristled brush should not be used on cementum or dentin because the surface is __________.
a. stained by the abrasive
b. soft and easily grooved
c. a and b

6. Once biofilm has been thoroughly removed, it takes approximately __________ hours to form again.
a. 6
b. 12
c. 24
d. 36

7. Fluoridated toothpaste is a source of __________ fluoride.
a. systemic
b. topical

8. In community water fluoridation, the recommended concentration of fluoride to water is __________ mg/L.
a. 3
b. 5
c. 1
d. 0.07

9. Prolonged exposure to excessive amounts of fluoride may cause __________.
a. dental decay
b. dental fluorosis
c. periodontal disease
d. all of the above

10. Only energy and no nutrients are provided by __________.
a. carbohydrates
b. empty calories
c. fat
d. protein

Apply Your Knowledge

1. Mrs. Barbara Lucas brings her three daughters—ages 9, 7, and 3 years—into your office for a routine prophy and examination. Eli, the youngest, is very excited when her older sister, Carmen, receives tooth brushing instruction. Eli wants to use the same fluoride toothpaste as her sister, and she wants to brush her teeth by herself. Is there anything you would want to discuss with Mrs. Lucas regarding Eli's brushing?

2. Because dental biofilm is invisible, it can be difficult for patients to realize it is there. What can you use to make your home care demonstrations more effective?

3. Mrs. Slovin has telephoned your office with a concern that her child has been invited to participate in a school-based fluoride rinse program in her son's second-grade class. What would you do in this situation?

4. You and two of the other dental assistants in your office have decided to improve your eating habits and lose a little weight; however, you want to make certain you get enough nutrients. Where could you find information about nutrition and personalized food plans?

CHAPTER 18

Coronal Polishing and Dental Sealants

http://evolve.elsevier.com/Robinson/essentials/

LEARNING OBJECTIVES

1. Pronounce, define, and spell the key terms.
2. Complete the following related to coronal polishing:
   - Explain the difference between a prophylaxis and a coronal polishing.
   - Explain the indications for and the contraindications to a coronal polish procedure.
3. Complete the following related to stains of the teeth:
   - Name and describe the types of extrinsic stains.
   - Describe the two categories of intrinsic stains.
   - Discuss air-powder polishing and rubber cap polishing.
4. Complete the following related to equipment for rubber-cup polishing:
   - Demonstrate the grasp and positioning for the prophy angle.
   - Demonstrate the fulcrum or finger rest used in each quadrant during a coronal polish procedure.
   - Discuss why bristle brushes must be used with special care.
   - Describe four types of abrasives used for polishing teeth.
5. Describe the process of rubber-cup coronal polishing, and demonstrate the proper seating positions for the operator and the assistant during a coronal polish procedure.
6. Explain the purposes for the placement and application of dental sealants.
7. Identify the two types of dental sealant polymerization.
8. Explain the precautions for the placement of dental sealants.

KEY TERMS

air-powder polishing
biofilm
calculus
clinical crown
dental sealants
endogenous
etching
exogenous
fulcrum
light-cured
oral prophylaxis
pits and fissures
rubber-cup polishing

Coronal Polishing

Coronal polishing (rubber-cup polish) is used to remove **biofilm** and stains from the coronal surfaces of the teeth. Biofilm is a dense nonmineralized complex mass of colonies in a gel-like matrix. Coronal polishing is performed with the use of a dental handpiece, a rubber cup, and an abrasive agent. There are specific indications for and contraindications to performing a coronal polish procedure (Table 18-1).

Coronal polishing is not a substitute for an oral prophylaxis. An **oral prophylaxis**, commonly known as a prophy or a cleaning, is the complete removal of calculus, debris, stains, and biofilm from the teeth. (**Calculus** is a hard mineralized deposit attached to the teeth.) In almost every state, the dentist and the registered dental hygienist are the only members of the dental team licensed to perform an oral prophylaxis.

In some states, coronal polishing is delegated to registered or to expanded function dental assistants who have had special training in this procedure. Coronal polishing is strictly limited to the clinical crowns of the teeth (Table 18-2 and Box 18-1). (The **clinical crown** is that portion of the tooth that is visible in the oral cavity.)

Stains of the Teeth

Stains are primarily esthetic problems and vary in type and difficulty of removal. Food, chemicals, and bacteria cause stains.

TABLE 18-1
Indications for and Contraindications to Coronal Polishing

Indications	Contraindications
Before placement of dental sealants	When no stain is present
Before placement of the dental dam	Patients who are at high risk of dental caries, such as nursing bottle caries, root caries, or areas of thin demineralized enamel (small amounts of enamel are removed during the polishing procedure)
Before application of topical fluoride	Patients who are at risk for transient bacteremia and the prophylactic administration of antibiotics as discussed in Chapter 11 (unless these medications have been given)
Before cementation of orthodontic bands	Sensitive teeth (abrasive agents can increase the areas of sensitivity)
Before application of acid etching solution on enamel (if indicated by the manufacturer's instructions) Before cementation of crowns and bridges	Newly erupted teeth (mineralization of the surfaces may be incomplete)

TABLE 18-2
Possible Damaging Effects of Coronal Polish

Tooth Surfaces	Gingival Tissue	Restorations
Newly erupted teeth are incompletely mineralized, and excessive polishing with an abrasive could remove a small amount of surface enamel. Avoid polishing exposed cementum in areas of recession because cementum is softer than enamel and is more easily removed. Avoid polishing areas of demineralization because of the possibility of loss of surface enamel.	The potential to damage the gingival tissue exists if the cup is run at a high speed and is applied too long. The potential to force particles of the polishing agent into the sulcus and to create a source of irritation exists with fast rotation.	Abrasive pastes can leave scratches or rough surfaces on gold, composite restorations, acrylic veneers, and porcelain-filled surfaces.

BOX 18-1 Benefits of Coronal Polishing

- Fluoride is better accepted into the enamel.
- Etching agent works better, and the sealants adhere better.
- Smooth tooth surfaces are easier for the patient to keep clean.
- Formation of new deposits is slowed.
- Patients appreciate the smooth feeling and the clean appearance.

Stains of the teeth occur in three basic ways:

1. Directly adhere to the surface of the tooth.
2. Embedded in calculus and plaque deposits.
3. Incorporated within the tooth structure.

Before coronal polishing is undertaken to remove stains, distinguishing between extrinsic and intrinsic stains is important (Figure 18-1).

Extrinsic stains are those that occur on the *external* surfaces of the teeth and *may* be removed by scaling and/or polishing (Table 18-3).

Intrinsic stains are those that occur *within* the enamel and *cannot* be removed by polishing (Table 18-4). Intrinsic stains may be **endogenous** (occurring during tooth development), or they may be **exogenous** (occurring after eruption).

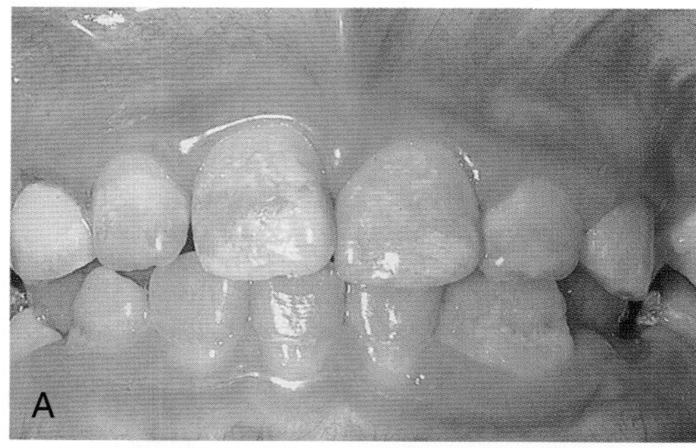

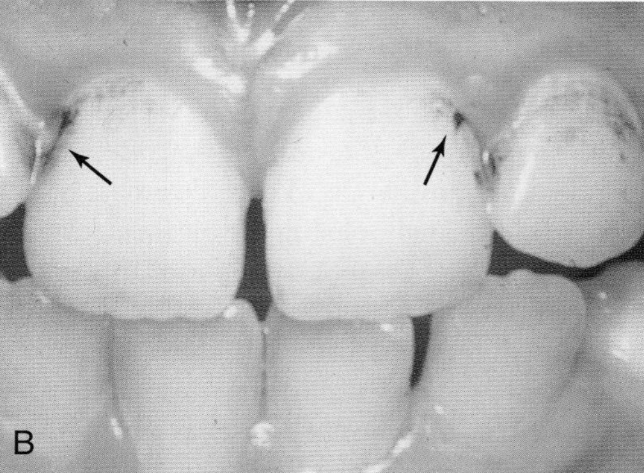

FIGURE 18-1 **A,** Intrinsic staining from dental fluorosis. **B,** Brown and yellow extrinsic stains *(arrows)*. (Courtesy Dr. Frank Hodges.)

TABLE 18-3
Extrinsic Stains

Type of Stain	Appearance	Cause
Black stain	Is a thin black line on the teeth near the gingival margin; is more common in girls. Is frequently found in clean mouths. Is difficult to remove.	Is caused by natural tendencies.
Tobacco stain	Is a very tenacious dark brown or black stain.	Is caused by the products of coal tar in the tobacco and from the penetration of tobacco juices into pits and fissures, enamel, and dentin of the teeth. The use of any tobacco-containing products causes tobacco stains on the teeth and restorations.
Brown or yellow stain	Is most commonly found on the buccal surfaces of the maxillary molars and the lingual surfaces of the lower anterior incisors.	Is caused by poor oral hygiene or the use of a toothpaste with inadequate cleansing action.
Green stain	Appears as a green or green-yellow stain, usually occurring on the facial surfaces of the maxillary anterior teeth. Is the most common stain in children.	Is caused by poor oral hygiene when bacteria or fungi are retained in the bacterial plaque.
Antiplaque agents	Is a reddish-brown stain that appears on the interproximal and cervical areas of the teeth. Can also appear on restorations, in plaque, and on the surface of the tongue.	Is caused by the use of prescription mouth rinses that contain chlorhexidine. (Chlorhexidine is a disinfectant with broad antibacterial action.)
Food and drink	Is a light brownish stain and is lessened with good oral hygiene.	Is caused by tea, coffee, colas, soy sauce, berries, and other foodstuffs.

TABLE 18-4
Intrinsic Stains

Type of Stain	Appearance	Cause
Pulpless teeth	Not all pulpless teeth discolor. A wide range of colors exists: light yellow, gray, reddish brown, dark brown, or black; sometimes an orange or greenish color is seen.	Blood and pulpal tissue break down as a result of bleeding in the pulp chamber or death of the pulp tissue. Pigments from the blood and tissue penetrate the dentin and show through the enamel.
Tetracycline antibiotics	Is a light green to dark yellow or a gray-brown discoloration that depends on the dose, the length of time the drug was used, and the type of tetracycline.	Can occur in the child when the mother is given tetracycline during the third trimester of pregnancy or when given to the child in infancy and early childhood.
Dental fluorosis	Also termed *mottled enamel*, dental fluorosis is the result of ingestion of excessive fluoride during the mineralization period of tooth development.	Varying degrees of discoloration range from a few white spots to extensive white areas or distinct brown stains. (Fluorosis is discussed and illustrated in Chapter 17.)
Imperfect tooth development	Teeth are yellowish-brown or gray-brown and appear translucent or opalescent and vary in color.	May result from genetic abnormality or environmental influences during development.
Silver amalgam	Appears as a gray or black discoloration around a restoration.	Metallic ions from the amalgam penetrate the dentin and enamel.
Other systemic causes	Appears as a yellowish or greenish discoloration in the teeth.	Causes include conditions of prolonged jaundice early in life and erythroblastosis fetalis (Rh incompatibility)

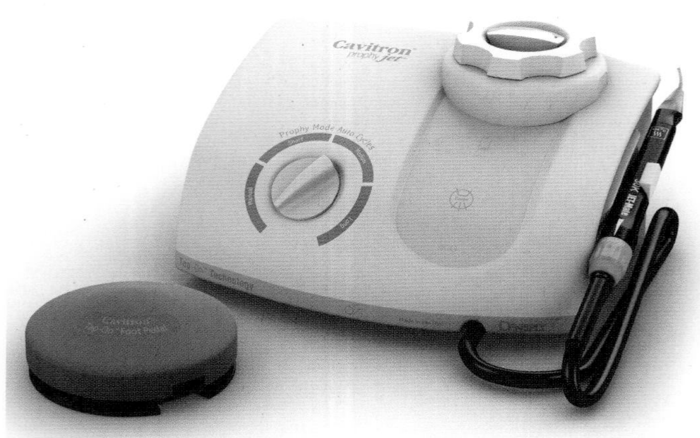

FIGURE 18-2 The air-powder polishing technique uses a specially designed handpiece with a nozzle that delivers a precise mixture of air, water and sodium bicarbonate. The powder and water, under pressure, rapidly and efficiently remove stains and biofilm without contacting tooth enamel. The flow rate of the powder is adjusted to control the rate of abrasion. (Courtesy Dentsply Sirona, York, PA.)

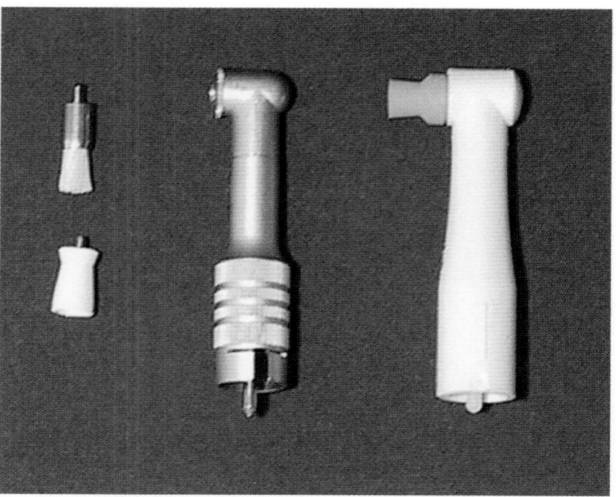

FIGURE 18-3 Various types of prophy angles.

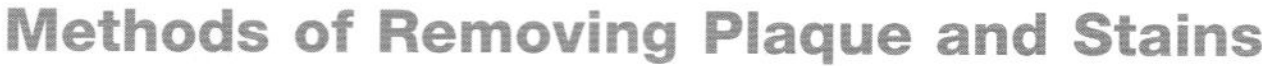

Methods of Removing Plaque and Stains

Every stain removal technique has the potential for damage by removing a small amount of enamel from the surfaces of the teeth being polished. In addition, injury to the gingivae is also a potential; therefore these techniques must always be carried out with the utmost caution.

Two methods of stain removal are the **air-powder polishing** and the **rubber-cup polishing** techniques.

Remember, you must check the regulations in your state to see whether the coronal polishing procedure can be delegated to a qualified dental assistant and, if so, which technique is permitted.

Air-Powder Polishing

The air-powder polishing technique uses a specially designed handpiece with a nozzle that delivers a high-pressure stream of warm water and sodium bicarbonate. The powder and water, under high pressure, rapidly and efficiently remove stains; the flow rate is adjusted to control the rate of abrasion (Figure 18-2).

Rubber-Cup Polishing

Rubber-cup polishing is the most common technique for removing stains and plaque and for polishing teeth. An abrasive polishing agent is placed in a rubber polishing cup that is slowly and carefully rotated by a prophy angle attached to the slow-speed handpiece. (This form of coronal polishing is described in this chapter.)

Equipment for Rubber-Cup Coronal Polishing

Polishing Cups

Soft, webbed polishing cups are used to clean and polish the smooth surfaces of the teeth (Figure 18-3). The polishing cup is attached to the reusable prophy angle by a snap-on or screw-on attachment.

Polishing cups are made from both natural and synthetic rubber. Natural rubber polishing cups are more resilient and do not stain the teeth. Synthetic rubber polishing cups are stiffer than natural polishing cups. If synthetic polishing cups are used, then white synthetic cups are preferable because black synthetic cups may stain the teeth. Synthetic polishing cups should be used for patients with an allergy to latex products.

Prophylaxis Angle and Handpiece

The prophylaxis angle, commonly called a *prophy angle*, attaches to the slow-speed handpiece (see Chapter 19). The reusable prophy angle must be properly cleaned and sterilized after each use. (Handpiece maintenance is discussed in Chapter 19.) When attaching the polishing cup or brush to the reusable type of prophy angle, be certain that the polishing cup or brush is securely fastened. If a polishing cup or brush falls off during the procedure, then the patient could swallow or inhale it.

A disposable angle is available that is discarded after a single use. This disposable angle is manufactured with a polishing cup or a brush already attached.

Handpiece Grasp

The handpiece and prophylaxis angle are held in a pen grasp with the handle resting in the V-shaped area of the hand between the thumb and index finger (Figure 18-4). A proper grasp is important because if the grasp is not secure and comfortable, then the weight and balance of the handpiece can cause hand and wrist fatigue (Box 18-2).

Fulcrum and Finger Rest

The terms **fulcrum** and finger rest are interchangeably used to describe the placement of the third, or ring, finger of the hand that is holding the instrument or handpiece.

The fulcrum provides stability for the operator and must be placed in such a way as to allow movement of the wrist and forearm.

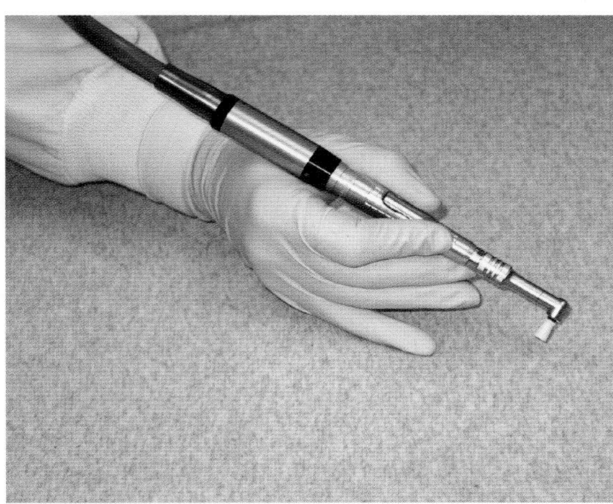

FIGURE 18-4 Close-up view of hand with handpiece and proper grasp.

BOX 18-2 Handpiece Operation

1. For polishing, a low-speed handpiece that operates to a maximum of 20,000 revolutions per minute (rpm) is recommended. Rationale: The low speed minimizes frictional heat and gingival trauma from the polishing cup.
2. The rheostat (foot pedal) controls the speed of the handpiece and is similar to the gas pedal in an automobile.
3. The toe of the foot is used to activate the rheostat. The sole of the foot remains flat on the floor.
4. To produce a slow, even speed, steady pressure is applied with the toe on the rheostat.

BOX 18-3 Bristle Brush Polishing Stroke

1. Soak stiff brushes in hot water to soften them.
2. Apply a mild abrasive polishing agent to the brush, and spread the polishing agent over the occlusal surfaces to be polished using a light wiping stroke.
3. Use the free hand and fingers to both retract and protect the cheek and tongue from the revolving brush.
4. Establish a firm finger rest, and bring the brush almost into contact with the tooth surface before activating the brush. Use the slowest speed, and then lightly apply the revolving brush to the occlusal surfaces. Use care to avoid contacting the gingivae.
5. Use a short-stroke brushing motion from the inclined planes to the cusps of the tooth.
6. Frequently move from tooth to tooth to avoid generating frictional heat.
7. Frequently replenish the supply of polishing agent to minimize frictional heat.

BOX 18-4 Factors Influencing the Rate of Abrasion

- Amount of abrasive agent that is used (the more agent that is used, the greater the degree of abrasion.)
- Amount of pressure that is applied to the polishing cup (the lighter the pressure, the less abrasion)
- Rotation speed of the polishing cup (the slower the rotation of the cup, the less abrasion)

The fulcrum is repositioned throughout the procedure as necessary and may be intraoral or extraoral, depending on a variety of circumstances such as:

- Presence or absence of teeth
- Area of the mouth being polished
- How wide the patient can open the mouth

Improper movement of the hand and fingers greatly increases operatory fatigue and, over time, can cause painful inflammation of the ligaments and nerves of the wrist.

Bristle Brushes

Bristle brushes are made from natural or synthetic materials and may be used to remove stains from deep **pits and fissures** of the enamel surfaces. Bristle brushes can cause severe gingival lacerations and must be used with special care (Box 18-3). Brushes are not recommended for use on exposed cementum or dentin because these surfaces are soft and easily abraded.

Abrasives

Dental abrasives (polishing materials) are used to remove stains and to polish natural teeth, prosthetic appliances, restorations, and castings.

Abrasives are available in various grits. (Grit refers to the degree of coarseness of an abrasive agent.) Abrasives are available in extra coarse, coarse, medium, fine, and extra fine. The coarser the agent, the more abrasive the surface.

Even a fine-grit abrasive agent removes small amounts of the enamel surface. Therefore the goal is to always use the abrasive agent that produces the least amount of abrasion to the tooth surface (Box 18-4).

Abrasives are available in commercial premixed pastes or in powders that are mixed with water or mouthwash to form slurry used in the polishing cup. Powder abrasives should be as wet as possible (but not runny) to minimize frictional heat. If the mixture is too wet, then splatter will occur and keeping the material in the cup will be difficult. The commercial type of premixed paste is packaged ready to use.

Table 18-5 contains some of the most commonly used dental abrasives.

Rubber-Cup Coronal Polishing

Rubber-Cup Polishing Stroke

1. Begin with the distal surface of the most posterior tooth in the quadrant, and work forward toward the anterior.
2. The stroke should be from the gingival third toward the incisal third of the tooth (Figure 18-5).
3. Fill the polishing cup with the polishing agent, and spread it over several teeth in the areas to be polished.

TABLE 18-5
Commonly Used Abrasives

Agent	Action
Silex	Is fairly abrasive and is used for cleaning more heavily stained tooth surfaces.
Super-fine silex	Is used to remove light stains on tooth enamel.
Fine pumice	Is a mild abrasive and is used for more persistent stains, such as tobacco stains.
Zirconium silicate	Is used for cleaning and polishing tooth surfaces. Zirconium silicate is highly effective and does not abrade tooth enamel.
Chalk	Is also known as whiting and is precipitated by calcium carbonate. Chalk is frequently incorporated into toothpaste and polishing pastes to whiten the teeth.
Commercial premixed preparations	Premixed preparations contain an abrasive, water, a humectant to keep the preparation moist, a binder to prevent separation of the ingredients, flavoring agents, and color. Some commercial preparations are available in small plastic containers or individual packets that contribute to the cleanliness and sterility of the procedure.
Fluoride prophylaxis paste	Replaces some of the fluoride that is lost from the surface layer during the polishing process. A fluoride prophylaxis paste is not a substitute for the topical application of fluoride. Its use is contraindicated before acid etching of the enamel when followed by bonding of sealants or other bonded materials.

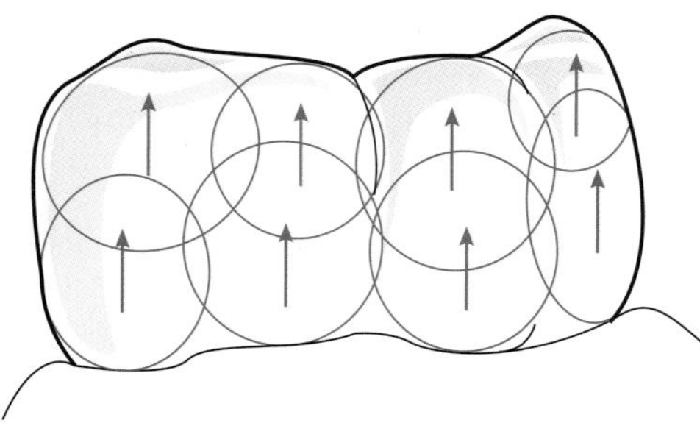

FIGURE 18-5 Use overlapping strokes to ensure complete coverage of the tooth.

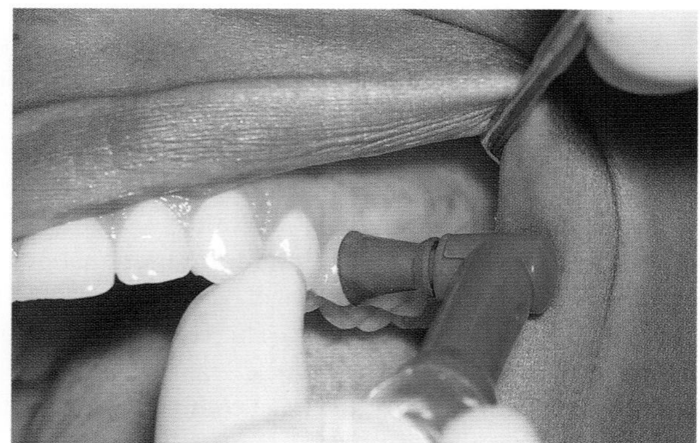

FIGURE 18-6 Stroke from the gingival third to the incisal third with just enough pressure to make the cup flare.

4. Establish a finger rest, and place the cup almost in contact with the tooth.
5. Use the slowest speed, and then lightly apply the revolving cup to the tooth surface for 1 to 2 seconds.
6. Use light but enough pressure to make the edges of the polishing cup slightly flare (Figure 18-6).
7. Move the cup to another area on the tooth, using a patting, wiping motion and an overlapping stroke to avoid creating frictional heat that could harm the tooth.
8. Frequently reapply the polishing agent, as needed.
9. Turn the handpiece to adapt the polishing cup to fit every area of the tooth to ensure that the cup covers all areas of the tooth.
10. If two polishing agents with different degrees of coarseness are being used, then always use a separate polishing cup for each abrasive. Use the coarsest abrasive agent first and finish with the finest (least abrasive). Always rinse between polishing agents. The finer abrasive agent will remove scratches left by the coarser abrasive agent.

Positioning the Patient and Operator

Proper positioning of both the operator and the patient is necessary so that the coronal polishing procedure may be performed with maximum comfort and efficiency for the patient and the operator.

Positioning the Patient

- The dental chair is adjusted so that the patient is approximately parallel to the floor with the back of the chair slightly raised.
- The movable headrest is adjusted for patient comfort and operator visibility.
- For access to the mandibular arch, position the patient's head with the chin down. (When the mouth is open, the lower jaw should be parallel to the floor.)
- For access to the maxillary arch, position the patient's head with the chin up.

Positioning the Operator

- The operator positions described in this chapter are in reference to the face of a clock. (This concept is discussed in Chapter 9.)

- The operator should be comfortably seated at the patient's side and must be able to move around the patient to gain access to all areas of the oral cavity.
- The seated operator's feet should be flat on the floor with the thighs parallel to the floor.
- The operator's arms should be at waist level and even with the patient's mouth.
- When performing a coronal polish procedure, the right-handed operator generally begins by being seated at the 8 o'clock to 9 o'clock position.
- When performing a coronal polish procedure, the left-handed operator generally begins by being seated at the 3 o'clock to 4 o'clock position.

Tip: For maximum support and safety, place the fulcrum as close as possible to the area you are polishing, preferably on the same dental arch.

Sequence of Polishing

If full-mouth coronal polishing is indicated, then it must be performed in a predetermined sequence to ensure that no area is missed. The best sequence is based on the operator's preference and the individual needs of the patient.

One very effective sequence is described here. The positions and fulcrums described are for a right-handed operator. The concepts of direct and indirect vision are discussed in Chapter 9.

To maintain patient comfort throughout the procedure, the patient's mouth is rinsed with water from the air-water syringe as necessary. The assistant removes excess water and debris by using the high-volume evacuator (HVE) tip.

Procedure 18-1 describes coronal polishing for all tooth surfaces and quadrants.

Flossing after Coronal Polishing

Dental floss and tape have two purposes after coronal polishing. The first is to polish the interproximal tooth surface. The second is to remove any abrasive agent or debris that may be lodged in the contact area.

To polish these areas, an abrasive is placed on the contact area between the teeth, and the floss or tape is worked through the contact area with a back-and-forth motion. Because both operator and patient preferences vary, many kinds of floss and tape are available. When properly used, floss and tape are effective. After the interproximal surfaces are polished, a fresh piece of dental floss or tape is used to remove any remaining abrasive particles between the teeth.

If necessary, a floss threader can be used to pass the floss under any fixed bridgework to gain access to the abutment teeth. Flossing is discussed further in Chapter 17.

Evaluation of Polishing

When you have completed polishing and flossing, evaluate the effectiveness of your technique by reapplying the disclosing agent. Then use a mouth mirror to determine whether the following criteria have been met:

- No disclosing agent remains on any of the tooth surfaces.
- Teeth are uniformly glossy and reflect light from the mirror.
- No evidence of trauma to the gingival margins or any other soft tissue in the mouth is noted.

Pit and Fissure Sealants

Dental sealants are highly effective in preventing dental caries in the pit and fissure areas of the teeth. Although fluorides have the ability to increase the resistance of enamel to decay, the pits and fissures do not benefit from the effects of fluoride as much as smooth enamel surfaces do. Studies have shown 100% caries protection when dental sealants are properly placed and retained on the tooth surface (Figure 18-7).

Dental sealants are made of a resin material and are applied to the pits and fissures of teeth to prevent dental caries. A dental sealant is successful only if it firmly adheres to the enamel surface and protects the pits and fissures from the oral environment. Pits and fissures are the fossae and grooves that failed to fuse during development (see Chapter 4).

The narrow width and uneven depth of pits and fissures make them ideal places for the accumulation of acid-producing bacteria (Figure 18-8). Saliva, which helps remove food particles from other areas of the mouth, cannot clean deep pits and fissures in molars. The pits and grooves on the teeth are so small that even a single toothbrush bristle is too large to enter and clean pits and fissures (Figure 18-9). The sealant acts as a physical barrier that prevents oral bacteria and dietary carbohydrates from creating the acidic conditions that cause demineralization

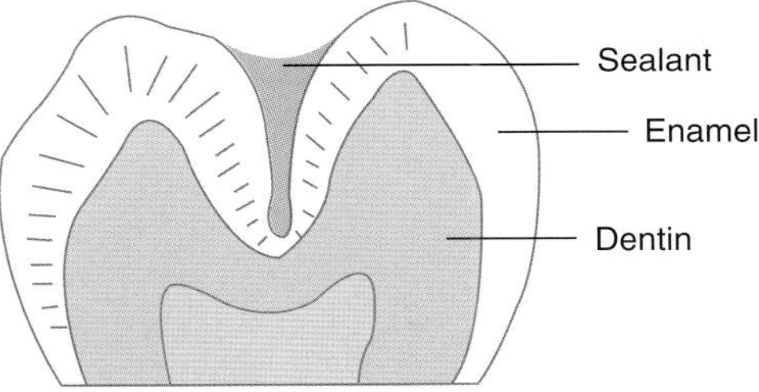

FIGURE 18-7 Sealants act as a physical barrier to oral bacteria and carbohydrates. (From *Preventing pit and fissure caries: a guide to sealant use*, Boston, 1986, Massachusetts Department of Public Health and Massachusetts Health Research Institute.)

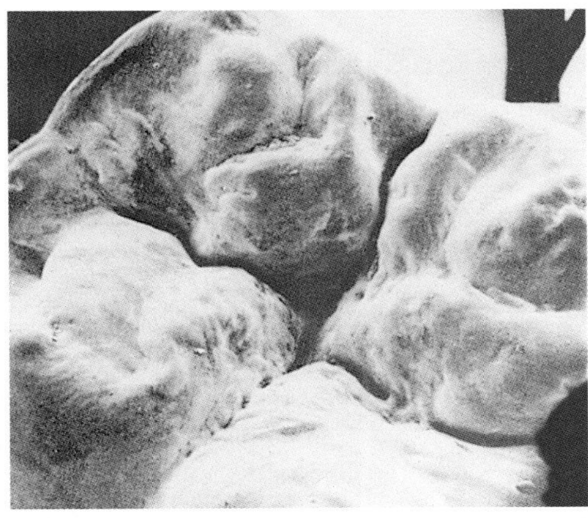

FIGURE 18-8 Scanning electron micrograph (SEM) of occlusal pits and fissures. (From Daniel SJ, Harfst SA, Wilder RS: *Mosby's dental hygiene: concepts, cases, and competencies*, ed 2, St. Louis, 2008, Mosby.)

and ultimately dental caries. Placement of a dental sealant is a noninvasive technique that preserves the tooth structure and also prevents dental decay (Figure 18-10). Table 18-6 contains indications for and contraindications to the placement of pit and fissure sealants.

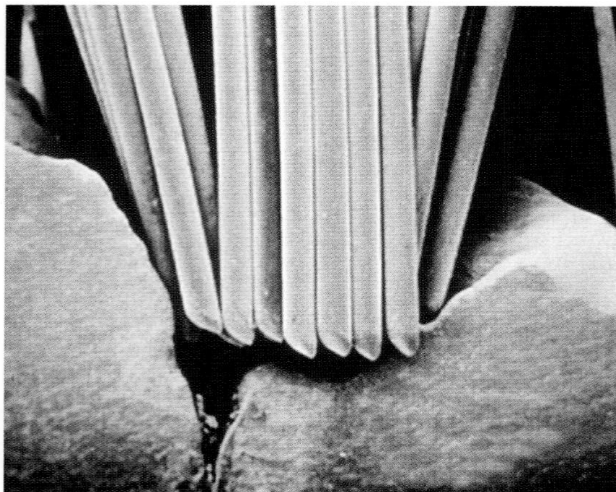

FIGURE 18-9 Micrograph showing toothbrush bristle in a groove.

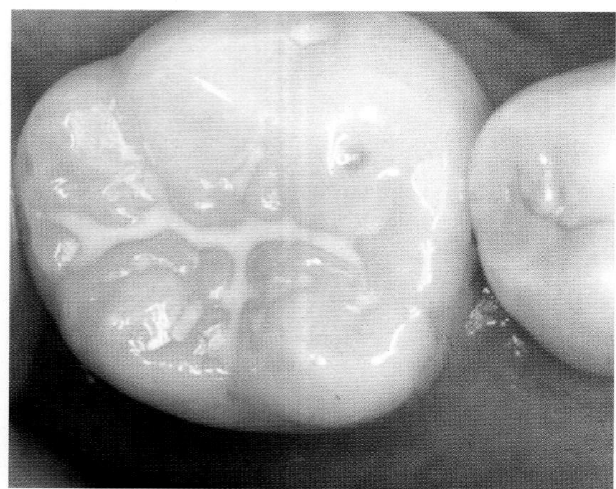

FIGURE 18-10 Molar with a properly placed sealant.

In many states, the application of dental sealants is a duty that may be delegated to the educationally qualified dental assistant (Table 18-7).

See Procedure 18-2: Application of Dental Sealants (Expanded Function).

Types of Sealant Materials

A wide variety of sealant materials is available. The dental assistant should have a thorough understanding of the types and characteristics of the various sealant products.

Method of Polymerization

One major difference among these materials is the method of polymerization (setting or curing). Some brands are self-cured, whereas others are light-cured. Both types are comparable in bond strength and rate of retention.

Self-cured materials are supplied as a two-part system (base and catalyst). When these pastes are mixed together, they quickly polymerize (harden), usually within 1 minute. The material must be in place before the initial setting occurs (Figure 18-11).

TABLE 18-6
Indications for and Contraindications to the Placement of Pit and Fissure Sealants

Indications	Contraindications
Deep pits and fissures are present.	Pits and fissures are not deep and are easily cleaned.
The tooth has recently erupted (within the past 4 years).	The occlusal surface is decayed, and a restoration must be placed to repair the tooth.
Sealant placement is used in conjunction with a preventive program, such as fluoride therapy.	The proximal surfaces are decayed. The occlusal surface will be included in the restoration of the decayed proximal surface. A restoration is already in place.

TABLE 18-7
Guidelines for Sealant Placement

Steps	Principle
Maintenance of a dry tooth surface	Saliva contamination will interfere with retention of the sealant by the tooth. A dry field may be maintained by using a rubber dam, cotton roll holders, cotton rolls, and dry angles.
Preparation of the tooth	The tooth must be cleaned with a prophy brush (bristle) and a mixture of pumice and water. The pumice must not contain oil or fluoride because both would interfere with the conditioning of the tooth. After cleaning, the surfaces must be thoroughly rinsed and dried.
Conditioning of the tooth	Conditioning the tooth is a very critical step because retention of the sealant relies on proper conditioning. The tooth is etched or conditioned with a solution of phosphoric acid. After conditioning, the tooth is rinsed and dried. Once the tooth is conditioned, it must not be contaminated with water or saliva. If contamination occurs, then repeating the entire etching process will be necessary.
Sealant placement	Using a dispenser or brush applicator, adequate amounts of sealant are placed to cover all fissures on the occlusal surface. A thin layer of sealant is carried into the buccal and lingual inclines of the occlusal surface to seal supplementary fissures. Follow the manufacturer's directions.

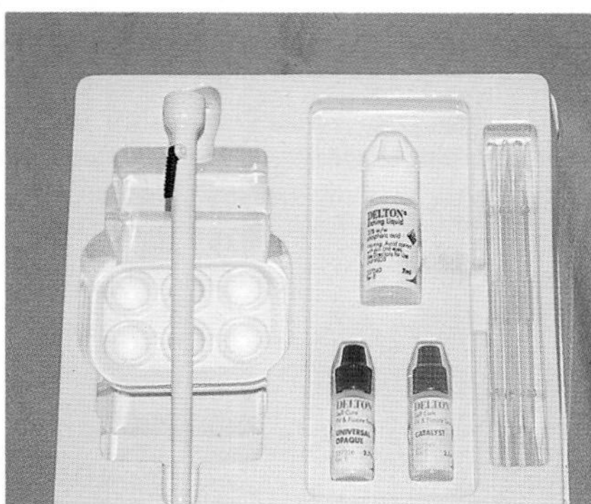

FIGURE 18-11 Universal liquid and catalyst shown with mixing wells and a mixing stick. (From Darby ML, Walsh MM: *Dental hygiene: theory and practice,* ed 4, St. Louis, 2015, Saunders.)

BOX 18-5 Questions Commonly Asked by Patients

Q. Do sealants hurt?
A. No. Sealants are easy and painless to apply.
Q. Does it take long to apply sealants?
A. It takes only a few minutes to seal each tooth.
Q. How long will sealants last?
A. Sealants hold up well under the force of normal chewing and usually last several years. During your regular dental visits, your dentist will check the condition of the sealants and reapply them if necessary.

BOX 18-6 Storage and Usage Tips for Sealant Materials

- Immediately replace caps on syringes and bottles after use.
- Do not expose materials to air or light.
- Do not store materials in proximity to eugenol-containing products.
- Most etchant and sealant materials are designed for use at room temperature. Check the manufacturer's recommendations.
- The shelf life of most sealant products at room temperature ranges from 18 to 36 months.
- Some brands of sealants must be stored in a refrigerator.

Light-cured sealants do not require mixing. They cure when exposed to ultraviolet light. Currently, a one-step delivery system is available in which the material is provided in a light-protected preloaded syringe and is ready for direct application to the tooth. After the material is applied to the tooth, the curing light activates the setting of the material.

Color

Sealants may be clear, tinted, or opaque (white). Tinted or opaque sealants are more popular because they are easier to see during application and during checks for sealant retention on subsequent office visits. Some brands have a tint that is visible during the application but then turns clear after polymerization.

Storage and Use

Because products and recommendations differ among manufacturers, it is very important that you read the instructions specific to the brand being used. Box 18-5 lists common questions patients have regarding sealants, and Box 18-6 lists some general tips on sealant materials.

Precautions for Dental Personnel and Patients

Etchant Precautions

Etching agents contain phosphoric acid. Patients and dental personnel should always wear protective eyewear when using etchants. Avoid contact with oral soft tissue, eyes, and skin. In case of accidental contact, immediately flush with large amounts of water. If eye contact is involved, immediately rinse with plenty of water and seek medical attention.

Sealant Precautions

Sealant material contains acrylate resins. Do not use sealants on patients with known acrylate allergies. To reduce the risk of an allergic response, minimize exposure to these materials. In particular, prevent exposure to uncured resin. Using protective gloves and a no-touch technique is recommended. If skin contact occurs, then wash the skin with soap and water. Acrylates may penetrate gloves. If the sealant contacts the gloves, then remove and discard the gloves, immediately wash the hands with soap and water, and put on new gloves. If accidental eye contact or prolonged contact with oral soft tissue should occur, then flush with large amounts of water. If irritation persists, contact a physician.

Protective glasses should be used by operators when ultraviolet or visible light-cured resins are used. Protective eyewear should also be provided for the patient during sealant procedures.

Ethical Implications

The delegation of additional functions to dental assistants varies widely. In some states, the application of dental sealants and coronal polish is considered to be an expanded function for dental assistants. In other states, however, dental assistants are allowed only to assist with the application of coronal polish and the placement of dental sealants. Some states allow dental assistants to apply coronal polish but not the placement of sealants. Checking the regulations in your state and practicing accordingly are your professional responsibilities. Whether or not you are legally allowed to actually place sealants, you can certainly educate your patients about the importance of sealants, explain the placement process, and answer their questions.

No states allow a dental assistant to perform a dental prophylaxis. This procedure must be performed by a dentist or a dental hygienist and should not be confused with coronal, or rubber-cup, polishing.

Procedure 18-1

Rubber-Cup Coronal Polishing (Expanded Function)

Equipment and Supplies

- Sterile or disposable prophy angle
- Snap-on or screw-on polishing cup accessory
- Snap-on or screw-on bristle brush
- Prophy paste or other abrasive in slurry
- High-volume evacuator (HVE) tip or saliva ejector
- Disclosing agent (tablets, gel, or solution)
- Cotton-tip applicator (if disclosing solution is used)
- Dental tape
- Dental floss
- Bridge threader
- Air-water syringe and sterile tip

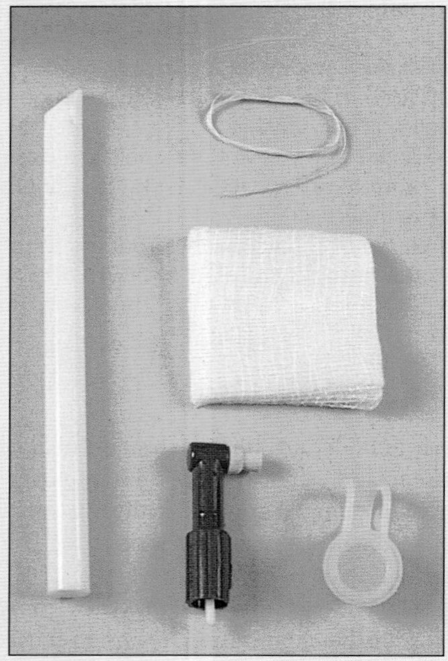

Procedural Steps

1. Check the patient's medical history for any contraindications to the coronal polish procedure.
2. Seat and drape the patient with a waterproof napkin. Ask the patient to remove any dental prosthetic appliance that he or she may be wearing. Provide the patient with protective eyewear.
3. Explain the procedure to the patient, and answer any questions.
4. Inspect the oral cavity for lesions, missing teeth, and tori.
5. Apply a disclosing agent to identify the areas of plaque.

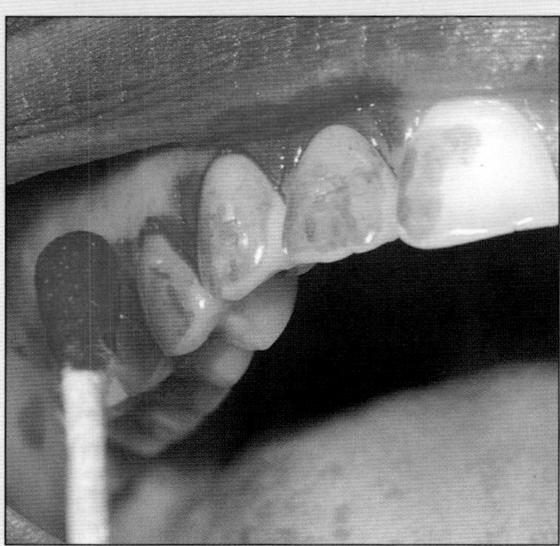

Maxillary Right Posterior Quadrant, Buccal Aspect

1. Sit in the 8 o'clock to 9 o'clock position, or move to the 11 o'clock to 12 o'clock position.
2. Ask the patient to tilt the head up and turn slightly away from you.
3. Hold the dental mirror in your left hand. Use it to retract the cheek or to gain indirect vision of more posterior teeth.

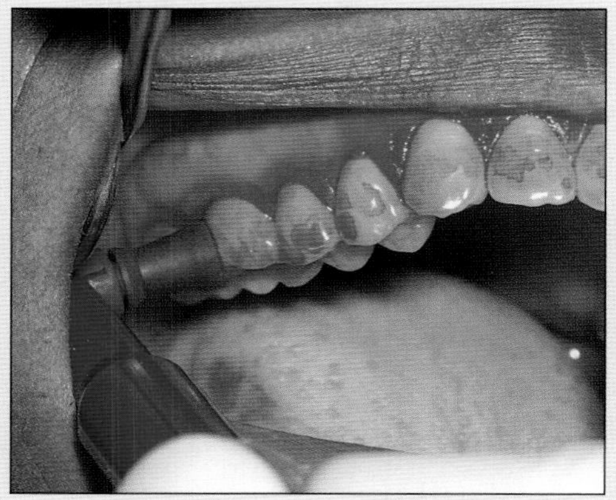

4. Establish a fulcrum on the maxillary right incisors.

Maxillary Right Posterior Quadrant, Lingual Aspect

1. Remain seated in the 8 o'clock to 9 o'clock position, or move to the 11 o'clock to 12 o'clock position.
2. Ask the patient to turn the head up and toward you.
3. Hold the dental mirror in your left hand. Use direct vision in this position; the mirror provides a view of the distal surfaces.
4. Establish a fulcrum on the lower incisors, and reach up to polish the lingual surfaces.

Procedure 18-1

Rubber-Cup Coronal Polishing (Expanded Function)—cont'd

Maxillary Anterior Teeth, Facial Aspect

1. Remain in the 8 o'clock to 9 o'clock position.
2. Position the patient's head so that it is slightly tipped up and facing straight ahead. Make necessary adjustments by slightly turning the patient's head toward or away from you.
3. Use direct vision in this area.
4. Establish a fulcrum on the incisal edge of the teeth, adjacent to the ones being polished.

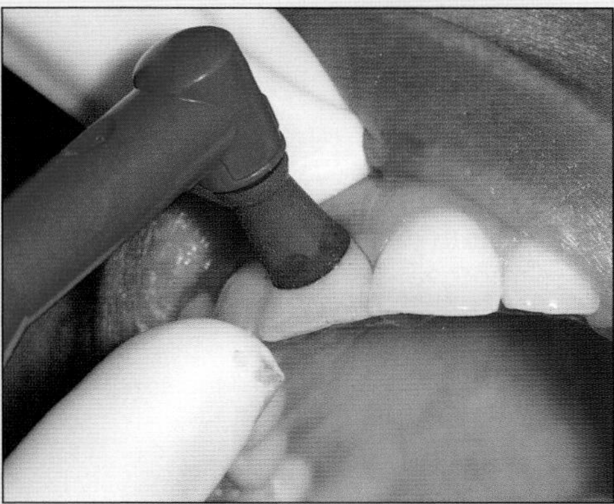

Maxillary Anterior Teeth, Lingual Aspect

1. Remain in the 8 o'clock to 9 o'clock position, or move to the 11 o'clock to 12 o'clock position.
2. Position the patient's head so that it is slightly tipped upward.
3. Use the mouth mirror to gain indirect vision and to reflect light on the area.

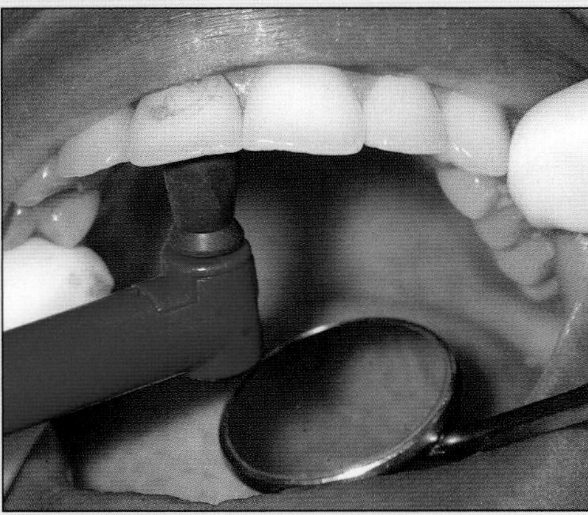

4. Establish a fulcrum on the incisal edge of the teeth, adjacent to the ones being polished.

Maxillary Left Posterior Quadrant, Buccal Aspect

1. Sit in the 9 o'clock position.
2. Position the patient's head so that it is tipped upward and slightly turned toward you to improve visibility.
3. Use the mirror to retract the cheek and to gain indirect vision.
4. Rest your fulcrum finger on the buccal occlusal surface of the teeth toward the front of the sextant.

Alternative: Rest your fulcrum finger on the lower premolars, and reach up to the maxillary posterior teeth.

Maxillary Left Posterior Quadrant, Lingual Aspect

1. Remain in the 8 o'clock to 9 o'clock position.
2. Ask the patient to turn the head away from you.
3. Use direct vision in this position. Hold the mirror in your left hand for a combination of retraction and reflecting light.
4. Establish a fulcrum on the buccal surfaces of the maxillary left posterior teeth or on the occlusal surfaces of the mandibular left teeth.

Maxillary Left Posterior Quadrant, Lingual Aspect

1. Remain in the 8 o'clock to 9 o'clock position.
2. Ask the patient to turn the head away from you.
3. Use direct vision in this position. Hold the mirror in your left hand for a combination of retraction and reflecting light.
4. Establish a fulcrum on the buccal surfaces of the maxillary left posterior teeth or on the occlusal surfaces of the mandibular left teeth.

Mandibular Left Posterior Quadrant, Buccal Aspect

1. Sit in the 8 o'clock to 9 o'clock position, or move to the 11 o'clock to 12 o'clock position.
2. Ask the patient to turn the head slightly toward you.
3. Use the mirror to retract the cheek and for indirect vision of the distal and buccal surfaces.
4. Establish a fulcrum on the incisal surfaces of the mandibular left anterior teeth, and reach back to the posterior teeth.

Mandibular Left Posterior Quadrant, Lingual Aspect

1. Remain in the 9 o'clock position.
2. Ask the patient to turn the head slightly away from you.
3. For direct vision, use the mirror to retract the tongue and to reflect more light to the working area.

Continued

Procedure 18-1

Rubber-Cup Coronal Polishing (Expanded Function)—cont'd

4. Establish a fulcrum on the mandibular anterior teeth, and reach back to the posterior teeth.

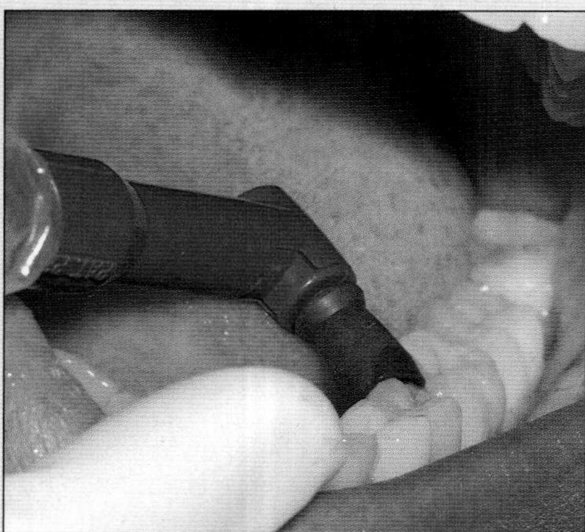

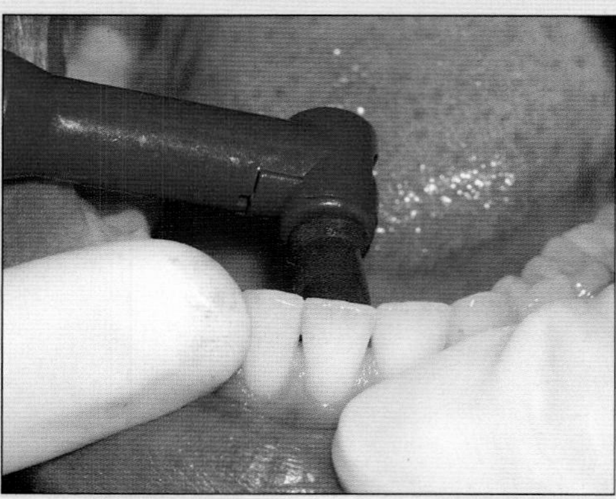

Mandibular Right Quadrant, Buccal Aspect

1. Sit in the 8 o'clock position.
2. Ask the patient to turn the head slightly away from you.
3. Use the mirror to retract tissue and to reflect light. The mirror may also be used to view the distal surfaces in this area.
4. Establish a fulcrum on the lower incisors.

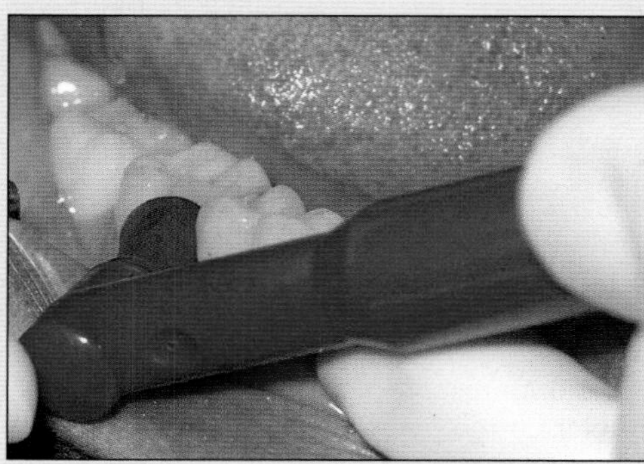

Mandibular Anterior Teeth, Facial Aspect

1. Sit in the 8 o'clock to 9 o'clock position, or move to the 11 o'clock to 12 o'clock position.
2. As necessary, instruct the patient to make adjustments in the head position by turning toward or away from you or by tilting the head up or down.
3. Use your left index finger to retract the lower lip. Both direct and indirect vision can be used in this area.
4. Establish a fulcrum on the incisal edges of the teeth adjacent to the ones being polished.

Mandibular Anterior Teeth, Lingual Aspect

1. Sit in the 8 o'clock to 9 o'clock position, or move to the 11 o'clock to 12 o'clock position.
2. As necessary, instruct the patient to make adjustments in the head position by turning toward or away from you or by tilting the head up or down.
3. Use the mirror to gain indirect vision, to retract the tongue, and to reflect light onto the teeth. Direct vision is often used in this area when the operator is seated in the 12 o'clock position, but indirect vision can also be helpful.
4. Establish a fulcrum on the mandibular cuspid incisal area.

Mandibular Right Quadrant, Lingual Aspect

1. Remain in the 8 o'clock position.
2. Ask the patient to turn the head slightly toward you.
3. Retract the tongue with the mirror.
4. Establish a fulcrum on the lower incisors.

Mandibular Right Quadrant, Lingual Aspect

1. Sit in the 8 o'clock to 9 o'clock position, or move to the 11 o'clock to 12 o'clock position.
2. Ask the patient to turn the head slightly toward you.
3. Retract the tongue with the mirror.
4. Establish a fulcrum on the lower incisors.

Procedure 18-2

Application of Dental Sealants (Expanded Function)

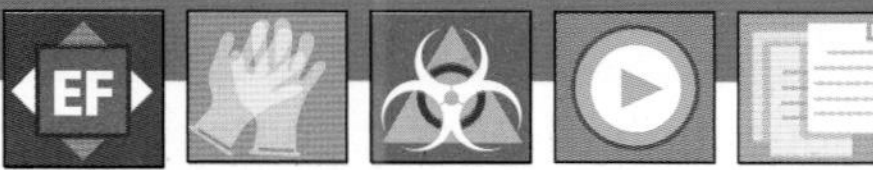

Goal

To apply a light-cured dental sealant according to the manufacturer's instructions and within the scope of responsibilities of the state Dental Practice Act

Equipment and Supplies

- Protective eyewear
- Basic setup
- Cotton rolls or rubber dam setup
- Etching agent (liquid or gel)
- Sealant material
- Applicator syringe or device
- Prophy brush
- Pumice and water
- High-volume evacuator (HVE)
- Curing light and appropriate shield
- Low-speed dental handpiece with contra-angle attachment
- Articulating paper and holder
- Round white stone (latch type)
- Dental floss
- Materials for occlusal adjustments (when using a filled resin product)

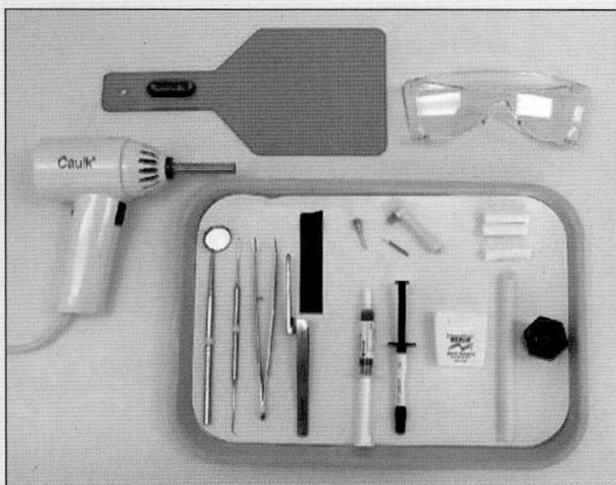

Procedural Steps

1. Select the teeth. The teeth must have deep pits and fissures and be sufficiently erupted so that a dry field can be maintained.

Purpose: The teeth must be sufficiently erupted for sealant placement.

2. Check the air-water syringe. Blow a jet of air from the syringe onto a mirror or glove. If small droplets are visible, then the syringe must be adjusted so that only air is expressed.

Purpose: Any moisture contamination during certain steps of this procedure can cause the retention of the sealant to fail.

3. Clean the enamel. Thoroughly clean the teeth with pumice and water to remove plaque and debris from the occlusal surface. Thoroughly rinse with water.

Note: Do not use any cleaning agents that contain oils. Check the manufacturer's instructions to see whether a fluoride-containing prophy paste is contraindicated for cleaning the enamel. If you use an air polish device that uses sodium bicarbonate for cleaning, then the etching step should be repeated for a second time, or 3% hydrogen peroxide should be applied to the surface for 10 seconds to neutralize the sodium bicarbonate. Thoroughly rinse the tooth with water before the etch is applied.

4. Isolate and dry the teeth. The rubber dam provides the best isolation; however, cotton rolls are acceptable. Use a saliva ejector or HVE.

Purpose: Excess saliva is uncomfortable for the patient and may contaminate the tooth to be sealed.

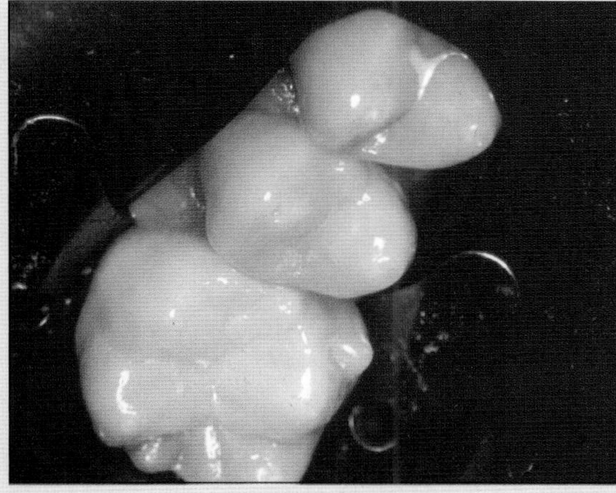

5. Etch the enamel. Use the syringe tip, or device, to apply a generous amount of etchant to all enamel surfaces to be sealed, slightly extending beyond the anticipated margin of the sealant. Etch for a minimum of 15 seconds but no longer than 60 seconds.

Purpose: The sealant will not adhere to surfaces not thoroughly etched.

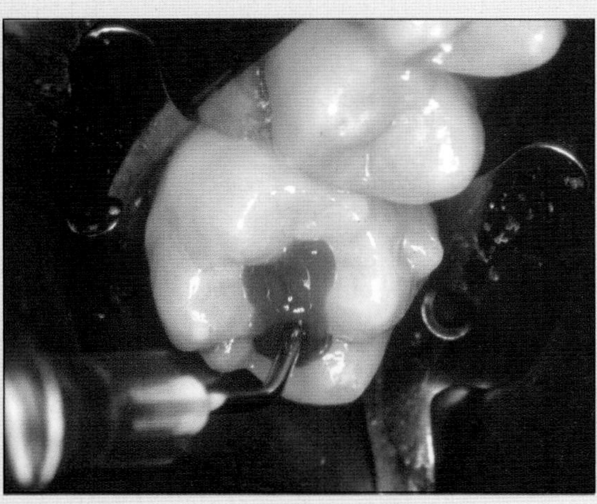

Continued

Procedure 18-2

Application of Dental Sealants (Expanded Function)—cont'd

6. Rinse the etched enamel. Thoroughly rinse the teeth with the air-water syringe to remove the etchant. Remove the rinse water with suction. Do not allow the patient to swallow or rinse.

Note: If saliva contacts the etched surfaces, then re-etch for 5 seconds and rinse again.

Purpose: Saliva will contaminate the etched surface, and the sealant will not properly adhere to the enamel.

7. Dry the etched enamel. Thoroughly dry the etched surfaces using the air-water syringe. The air from the syringe should be dry and free from oil and water. The dry etched surfaces should appear as a matte frosty white. If not, then repeat steps 5 and 6. Do not allow the etched surface to be contaminated.

Purpose: Moisture contamination of etched surfaces is the primary cause of failure of pit and fissure sealants.

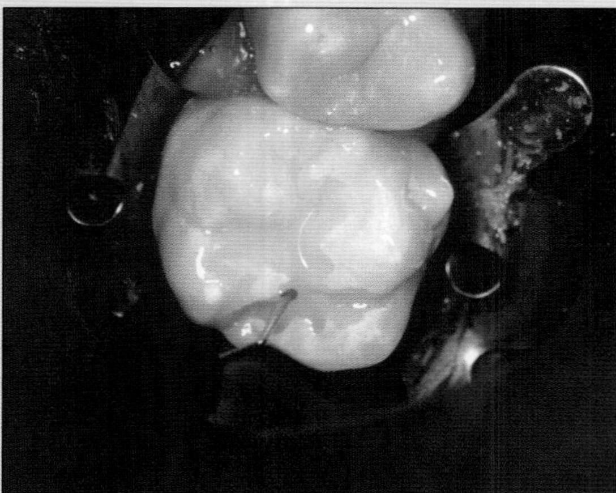

8. Apply the sealant. Using the syringe tip or a brush, slowly introduce the sealant into the pits and fissures. Do not allow the sealant to flow beyond the etched surfaces. Stirring the sealant with the syringe tip or brush during or after placement will help eliminate any possible bubbles and will increase the flow into pits and fissures. An explorer may also be used. Remember to check the manufacturer's recommendations for the most effective technique for sealant placement.
9. Cure the sealant. Hold the tip of the light as close as possible to the sealant without actually touching the sealant. A 20-second exposure is needed for each surface.

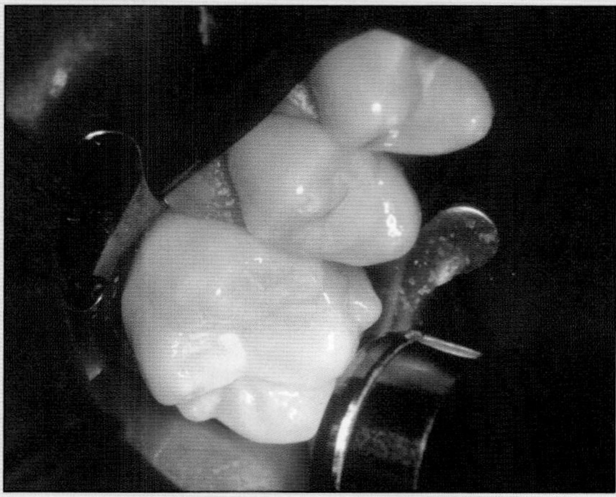

10. Evaluate the sealant. Carefully inspect the sealant for complete coverage and voids. If the surface has not been contaminated, then additional sealant material may be placed. If contamination has occurred, then re-etch and dry before placing more sealant material. Check the interproximal areas using dental floss to ensure that no sealant material is in the contact area.

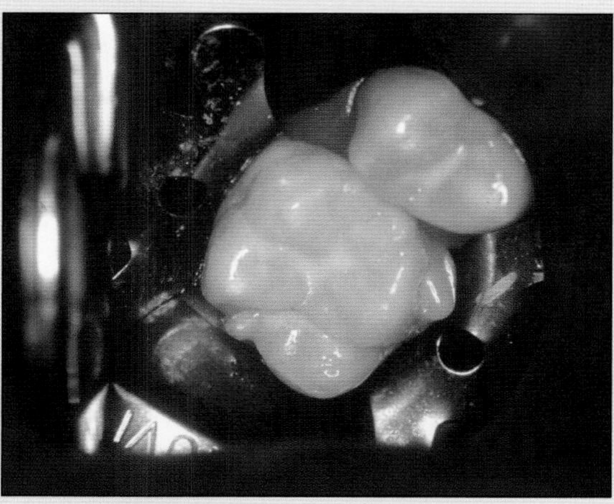

11. To complete the procedure, wipe the sealant with a cotton applicator to remove the thin, sticky film on the surface. Check occlusion using the articulating paper, and adjust if required.
12. Document the procedure in the patient's chart.

DATE	CHARTING NOTES	SIGNATURE
5/10/16	Application of sealants to teeth #3, #14, #19, #30	PJL

Chapter Exercises

Multiple Choice

Circle the letter next to the correct answer.

1. When is a coronal polishing procedure indicated?
- **a.** Before a prophylaxis
- **b.** Before dental dam placement
- **c.** To polish demineralized areas
- **d.** a, b, and c

2. Which of the following influence the rate of abrasion of a polishing agent?
- **a.** Amount of abrasive material used
- **b.** Amount of pressure applied during polishing
- **c.** Rotation speed of the polishing cup
- **d.** All of the above

3. The prophy angle is held in a __________ grasp.
- **a.** palm
- **b.** palm-thumb
- **c.** pen

4. Tetracycline is an example of an __________ stain.
- **a.** extrinsic
- **b.** intrinsic

5. A bristle brush should not be used on cementum or dentin because the surface is __________.
- **a.** stained by the abrasive
- **b.** soft and easily grooved
- **c.** a and b

6. For coronal polishing, the recommended speed of the low-speed handpiece is __________ rpm.
- **a.** 10,000
- **b.** 20,000
- **c.** 100,000
- **d.** 200,000

7. Plaque and stain are removed from the interproximal areas with a(n) __________.
- **a.** abrasive
- **b.** dental floss
- **c.** rubber cup
- **d.** a and b

8. In preparation for a coronal polishing procedure, the patient should be covered with __________.
- **a.** a patient towel
- **b.** a lead apron
- **c.** protective eyewear
- **d.** a and c

9. Which members of the dental team are allowed to scale teeth?
- **a.** Dentist
- **b.** Dental hygienist
- **c.** Dental assistant
- **d.** a and b

10. To prevent injury to the gingival tissue, the rubber-cup stroke should be directed __________.
- **a.** away from the gingival tissue
- **b.** parallel to the gingival tissue
- **c.** toward the gingival tissue

11. When moving the rubber polishing cup from one area to another, what type of motion should be used?
- **a.** Patting
- **b.** Wiping
- **c.** Rubbing
- **d.** a and b

12. The occlusal surfaces of the teeth are polished using a __________.
- **a.** bristle brush
- **b.** rubber cup
- **c.** either of the above

13. When polishing the lingual aspect of the maxillary anterior sextant, the operator is seated at the __________ o'clock position.
- **a.** 6
- **b.** 8 to 9
- **c.** 10

14. The most common extrinsic stain found in children is __________.
- **a.** black line
- **b.** green
- **c.** orange

15. Saliva contamination of the tooth surface during sealant placement will interfere with the retention of the sealant on the tooth.
- **a.** True
- **b.** False

16. When placing dental sealants, protective eyewear should be worn by the __________.
- **a.** dental assistant
- **b.** patient
- **c.** a and b

17. Which of the following is a contraindication to the placement of a dental sealant?
- **a.** Deep pits and fissures
- **b.** Recently erupted tooth
- **c.** Decay on the proximal surface
- **d.** All of the above

18. Which of the following types of sealant materials do NOT require mixing?
- **a.** Self-cured
- **b.** Light-cured

19. All states allow dental assistants to place dental sealants.
- **a.** True
- **b.** False

20. Another term for *conditioning* the tooth before the placement of sealants is __________.
- **a.** abrasion
- **b.** etching
- **c.** polishing
- **d.** drying

Apply Your Knowledge

1. Before performing a coronal polish on 16-year-old Sydnie, the dental assistant noticed in the health history that Sydnie had been given the drug tetracycline as a very young child. Sydnie stated that she repeatedly took the drug over a period of several months. What, if any, conditions might the dental assistant expect to see on Sydnie's teeth?
2. Mrs. Hansen telephones the dental office to notify the dentist that one of the dental sealants recently placed "just fell off of Pamela's tooth." The dental assistant recalls that Pamela was a very uncooperative child with a very plentiful flow of saliva, and moisture control during the procedure had been difficult. What could be the reason that the sealant did not stay in place?
3. Dr. Steiner advised Mr. Woolley that his 6-year-old daughter, Beth, should have dental sealants placed on her first permanent molars. However, the insurance company does not provide coverage for dental sealants, and Mr. Woolley asks the dental assistant to explain again why the sealants are necessary. If you were that dental assistant, how would you respond?
4. Dr. Mackler asks the dental assistant to perform a coronal polish on a patient who is going to have some orthodontic brackets placed. The dental assistant notices some light calculus formation on the lingual surface of the mandibular anterior teeth. Because the calculus is very light, the dental assistant thinks she can easily remove it before beginning the coronal polish. What would you do in this situation?

CHAPTER 19

Instruments, Handpieces, and Accessories

http://evolve.elsevier.com/Robinson/essentials/

LEARNING OBJECTIVES

1. Pronounce, define, and spell the key terms.
2. State the three parts of a hand instrument design, and define the function of each.
3. Identify hand instruments used for the examination of a tooth, and state their use.
4. Identify hand instruments used for the preparation of a tooth, and state their use.
5. Identify hand instruments used for the restoration of a tooth, and state their use.
6. Identify accessory instruments and items and state their use.
7. Discuss the purpose of rotary instruments and their importance in restorative dentistry.
8. Identify dental handpieces by speed and/or type and state their use.
9. Identify dental burs by their basic shapes, materials, and number series.

KEY TERMS

burs
friction-grip
handpieces
instruments
latch-type
manipulated
rotary
torque

This chapter is designed to provide you with an overview of the dental hand **instruments**, handpieces, and accessories frequently used in restorative dentistry. Identifying and knowing the use of this equipment will allow the dental assistant to prepare tray setups for a specific procedure, anticipate the transfer of instruments, and maintain an inventory.

Hand Instruments

Dental hand instruments are so named because they are held and manipulated by the hand. (**Manipulated** is the method in which an instrument is managed and skillfully used.) Each hand instrument has a specific purpose and is used for a specific technique. As you learn to identify new instruments, it is important to understand that manufacturers of instruments will design several styles of the same instrument to accommodate personal preferences.

Hand Instrument Design

Each hand instrument is made up of three parts: (1) handle, (2) shank, and (3) working end (Table 19-1).

Types of Hand Instruments

Hand instruments are designed for and used in all types of dental procedures. The instruments discussed in this chapter are used for restorative procedures and are used in the setup for amalgam and composite resin procedures.

Restorative instruments can be assigned to one of four categories.

1. **Examination instruments** allow the dentist to examine the health status of the teeth and oral cavity (Table 19-2).

   See Procedure 19-1: Identifying Examination Instruments.
2. **Hand (manual) cutting instruments** allow the dentist to remove decay manually and to smooth, finish, and prepare the tooth structure to be restored to its normal

TABLE 19-1
Hand Instrument Design

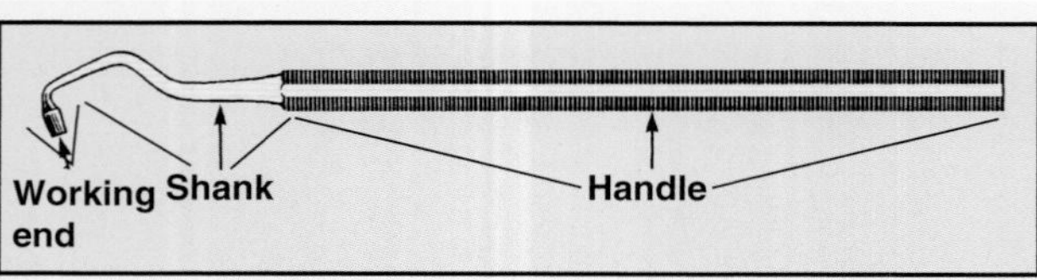

Parts	Function
Handle	Portion of the instrument where the operator grasps or holds the instrument. The handle is designed in various shapes, sizes, and textures to accommodate handling the instrument.
Shank	Portion of the instrument that connects the handle and the working end. The shank may contain bends and angles to allow the operator better accessibility.
Working end	Portion of the instrument with a specific function. The working end can have a point, blade, or nib for use on the tooth structure or soft tissue.

function in preparation for receiving a temporary or permanent restoration (Table 19-3).

See Procedure 19-2: Identifying Hand (Manual) Cutting Instruments.

3. **Restorative instruments** allow the dentist to place, condense, and carve a temporary or permanent restorative material to the original anatomy of the tooth structure (Table 19-4).

   See Procedure 19-3: Identifying Restorative Instruments.

4. **Accessory instruments** are the multipurpose instruments added to the setup of many procedures. These types of instrument are used in preparing the setup, in carrying things to the mouth, or in the application or placement of a dental material (Table 19-5).

   See Procedure 19-4: Identifying Accessory Instruments and Items.

Instrument Setup and Care

Having the supplies, instruments, and dental materials readied before a procedure helps save time and creates a team approach to the procedure. Instruments must be handled with care and organized according to the procedure and their uses.

A procedure tray is set up in a sequential order from left to right, starting with examination instruments and followed

TABLE 19-2
Examination Instruments

Instrument	Use
	The **mouth mirror** is designed to have a straight handle, a slight angle to the shank, and a working end, with a round metal disc and a mirror on one side. The mirror can have a flat or a concave (indented) surface. Mouth mirrors are used for a variety of purposes.
1 2 3	**Explorers** are multifunctional instruments that are included in the setup for every procedure. Explorers are available in many shapes, but all explorers have a thin, flexible, wirelike working end with a sharp point at the tip. Common types of explorers are the *pig tail (1), Shepherd's hook (2),* and *right angle (3).* The thin tip enables the operator to use **tactile** sensitivity to distinguish areas of calculus or decay from discrepancies on the surfaces of teeth.

TABLE 19-2
Examination Instruments—cont'd

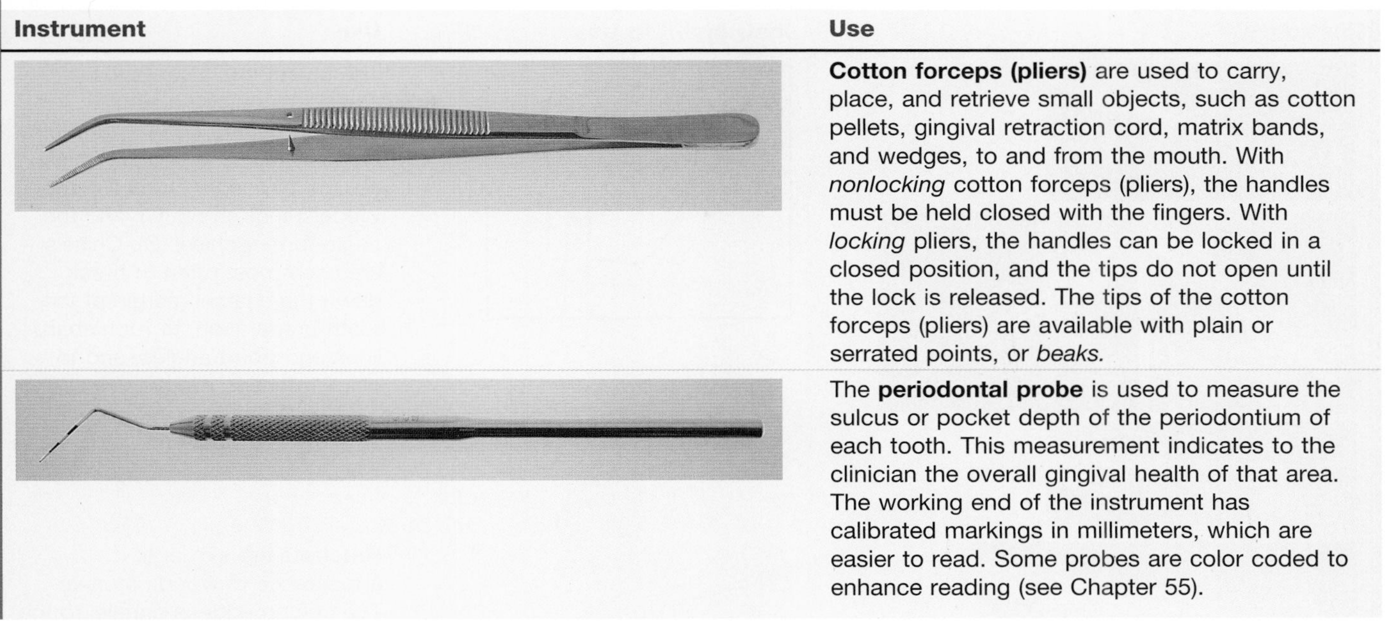

Instrument	Use
	Cotton forceps (pliers) are used to carry, place, and retrieve small objects, such as cotton pellets, gingival retraction cord, matrix bands, and wedges, to and from the mouth. With *nonlocking* cotton forceps (pliers), the handles must be held closed with the fingers. With *locking* pliers, the handles can be locked in a closed position, and the tips do not open until the lock is released. The tips of the cotton forceps (pliers) are available with plain or serrated points, or *beaks.*
	The **periodontal probe** is used to measure the sulcus or pocket depth of the periodontium of each tooth. This measurement indicates to the clinician the overall gingival health of that area. The working end of the instrument has calibrated markings in millimeters, which are easier to read. Some probes are color coded to enhance reading (see Chapter 55).

Content from Bird DL, Robinson DS: *Modern dental assisting,* ed 11, St. Louis, 2015, Saunders. Photos from Boyd LRB: *Dental instruments: a pocket guide,* ed 5, St. Louis, 2015, Saunders.

TABLE 19-3
Tooth Preparation Instruments

Instrument	Instrument in Use	Use
(1) (2)		The **excavator** is one of the most versatile instruments on the tray setup. Excavators have a working end that is circular or elongated. The two most commonly used excavators are the spoon excavator and the black spoon. The *spoon excavator (1)* is used for removal of soft dentin, debris, and decay from the tooth; the *black spoon (2)* has a flat appearance but is used for the same purposes.
		The **hoe** is similar in appearance to the garden tool. The blade is almost perpendicular to the handle. The *hoe* is used to prepare the tooth and to **plane** the walls and floors of the tooth preparation with a push-pull action.

Continued

TABLE 19-3
Tooth Preparation Instruments—cont'd

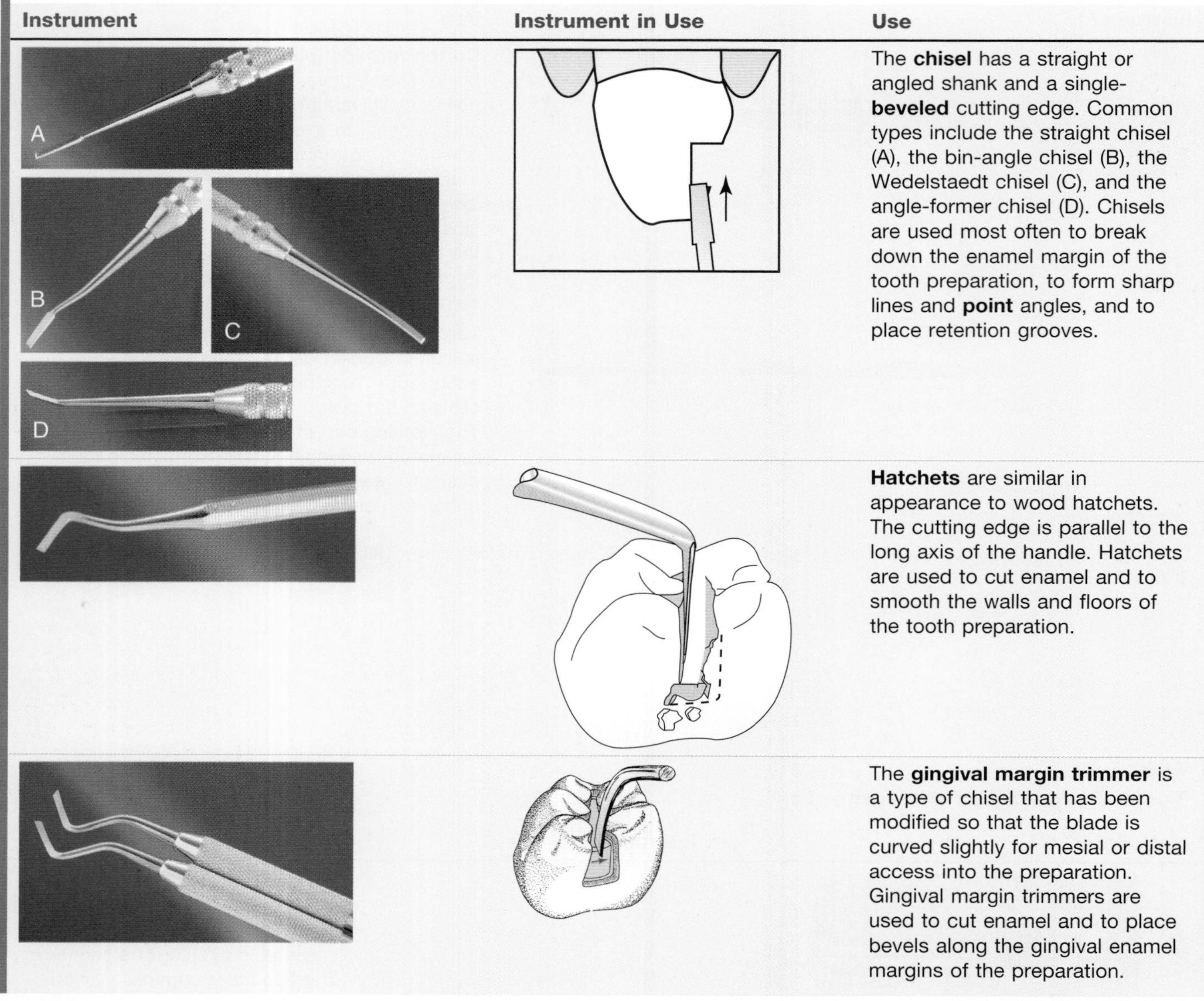

Instrument	Instrument in Use	Use
		The **chisel** has a straight or angled shank and a single-**beveled** cutting edge. Common types include the straight chisel (A), the bin-angle chisel (B), the Wedelstaedt chisel (C), and the angle-former chisel (D). Chisels are used most often to break down the enamel margin of the tooth preparation, to form sharp lines and **point** angles, and to place retention grooves.
		Hatchets are similar in appearance to wood hatchets. The cutting edge is parallel to the long axis of the handle. Hatchets are used to cut enamel and to smooth the walls and floors of the tooth preparation.
		The **gingival margin trimmer** is a type of chisel that has been modified so that the blade is curved slightly for mesial or distal access into the preparation. Gingival margin trimmers are used to cut enamel and to place bevels along the gingival enamel margins of the preparation.

Photos from Boyd LRB: *Dental instruments: a pocket guide,* ed 4, St. Louis, 2012, Saunders. Drawings from Baum L, Phillips RW, Lund MR: *Textbook of operative dentistry,* ed 3, Philadelphia, 1995, Saunders. Content from Bird DL, Robinson DS: *Modern dental assisting,* ed 11, St. Louis, 2015, Saunders.

by hand-cutting instruments, restorative instruments, and, finally, accessory instruments and items. The rationale for this sequencing is based on how instruments are transferred and used throughout a dental procedure. Remember, as the clinical assistant, you will be using the left hand for the transfer of instruments. Therefore the most frequently used instruments will be closer to the dentist for ready availability (Figure 19-1).

Rotary Instruments

Rotary instruments are an essential part of restorative dentistry. The setup includes the dental handpiece and revolving mechanisms, which include cutting and finishing **burs**, polishing tips and points, and abrasive discs and stones that fit into the handpiece. The combination of the handpiece and mechanisms is a miniature representation of a power tool. Although many patients identify the **handpiece** as "the drill," it's important to educate your patients by making it sound less threatening.

The handpiece provides power and rotary motion, whereas the dental bur, which is securely held in the handpiece, does the actual cutting or polishing. Handpieces and burs have a variety of uses in restorative dentistry. The two most commonly used handpieces are the low-speed handpiece and the high-speed handpiece.

Low-Speed Handpiece

The **low-speed handpiece**, often referred to as the **straight handpiece** because of its straight-line design, is the most

Steps to Instrument Setup and Care

Before Procedure

- Instruments are sterilized and remain wrapped until use.
- Complete setup of instruments should be organized and set up from left to right.
- Instruments should be placed in the order of their use.
- Instruments and accessory items should be already assembled, if necessary.

During Procedure

- Keep instruments in order of use.
- Transfer instruments in the transfer zone and for the proper grasp.
- Wipe off each instrument after its use using sterile 2 × 2 gauze.
- Disassemble an instrument or accessory after use. (This saves time when preparing the instruments for sterilization.)

After Procedure

- Discard sharps in a sharps container before taking the instruments to the sterilization center.
- Do not throw or toss instruments into a tub because of possible breakage, chips, and cracks.
- Place the instruments in a holding solution if not able to sterilize immediately.

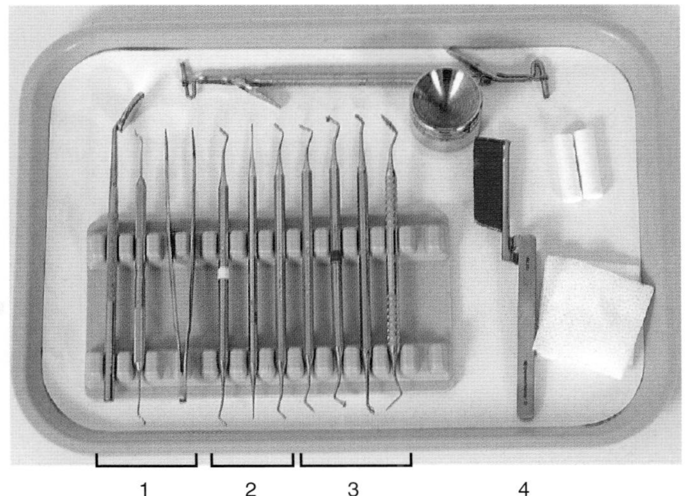

FIGURE 19-1 Tray setup showing appropriate sequence of instruments. (From Bird DL, Robinson DS: *Modern dental assisting,* ed 11, St. Louis, 2015, Saunders.)

TABLE 19-4
Restorative Instruments

Instrument	Use
	Amalgam carrier is a double-ended instrument designed with wells on either end that is used to pack freshly mixed amalgam and carry it to the prepared tooth. Most amalgam carriers are designed to hold a large increment of amalgam at one end and a smaller increment at the opposite end. The dental assistant uses the amalgam carrier to carry an increment of amalgam, then transfers the carrier to the dentist or directly places the amalgam into the prepared tooth.
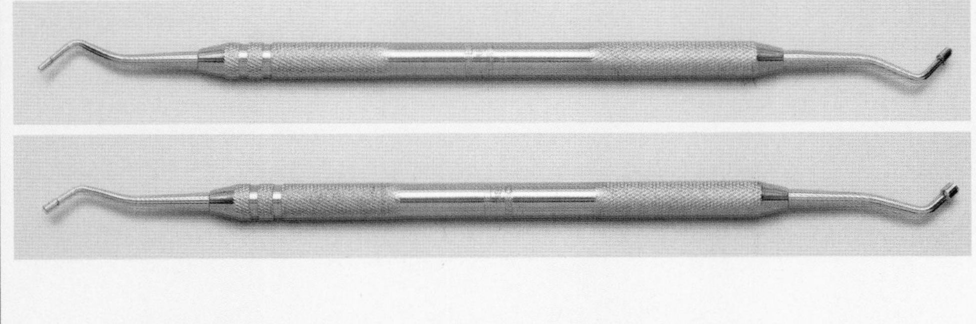	**Condensers** have a flat working end that can be smooth or serrated; they come in varying sizes to accommodate the size of the preparation. To enable the operator to reach all areas of the preparation, the shank of the instrument is angled. The amalgam condenser, also known as a *plugger*, is used to condense (pack down) freshly placed amalgam into the preparation.

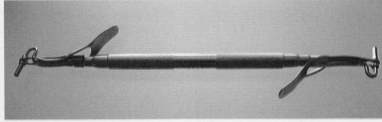

Continued

TABLE 19-4
Restorative Instruments—cont'd

Instrument	Use
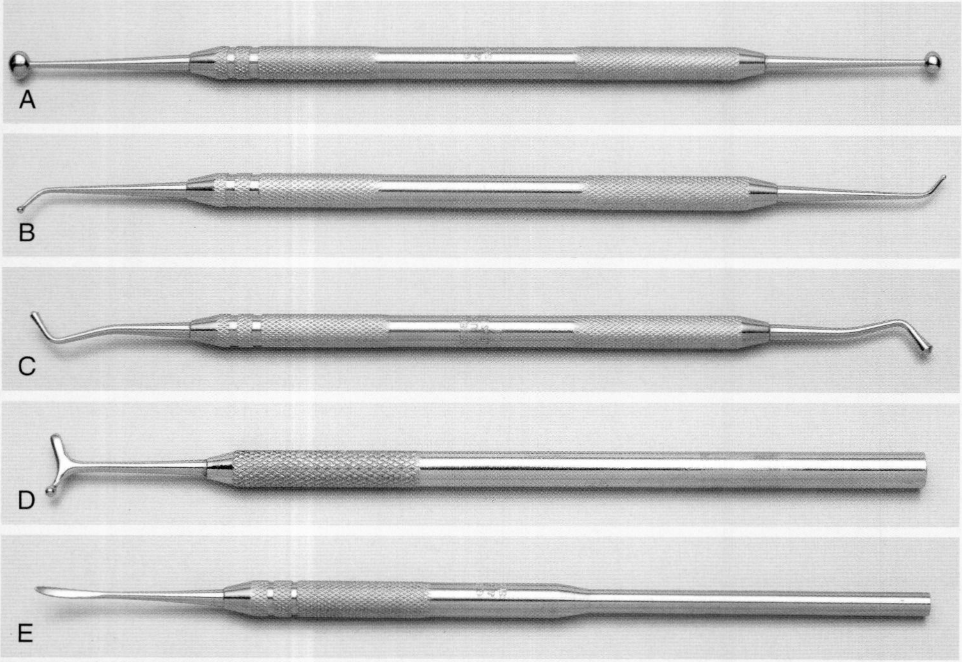 A, B, C, D, E	A **burnisher** is an instrument with a smooth working end. The rounded working end is available in many shapes to accomplish different tasks. Common types include the A. Football B. Ball C. Acorn D. T-ball E. Beavertail Routinely used to smooth the surface of a freshly placed amalgam restoration.
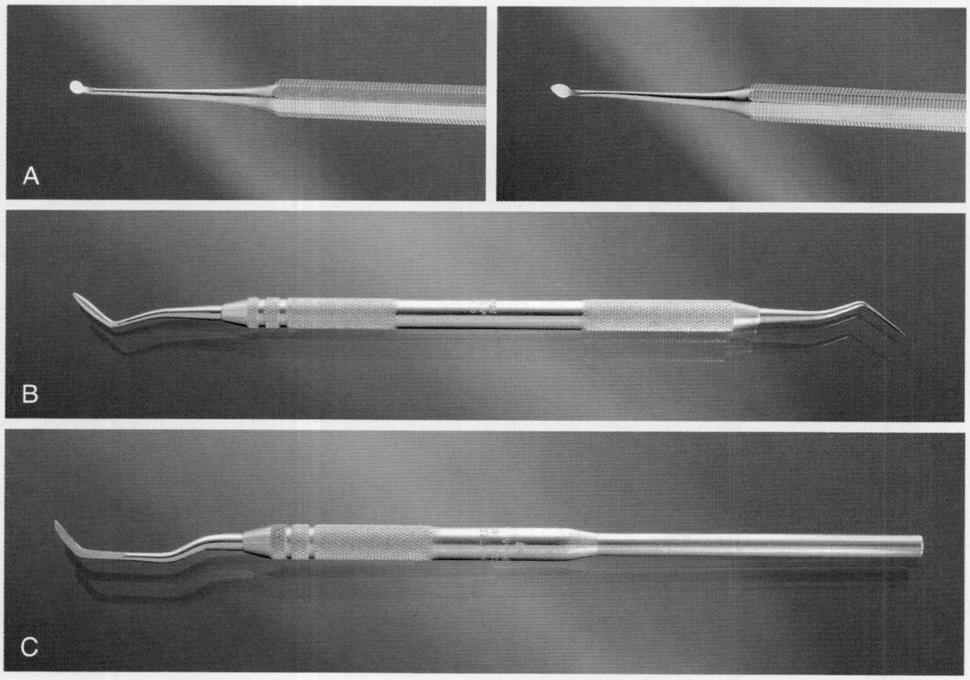 A, B, C	**Carvers** are designed with a sharp edge on the working end to remove excess material, to contour surfaces, and to carve anatomy back into the amalgam or intermediate restoration before it hardens. Various styles of carvers are available: **A, discoid-cleoid carver** is especially useful for carving of the occlusal surfaces. **B, Hollenback carver** is used to contour or remove excess material interproximally. **C, amalgam knife** is designed with a sharp edge for the removal of excess restorative material along the margin where the material and the tooth structure meet. The knife has several angles in the shank and working end that enable the operator to reach specific areas of a tooth, most often interproximal areas.

TABLE 19-4
Restorative Instruments—cont'd

Instrument	Use
1, 2	**Composite placement instrument** is designed specifically for the placement of composite restorative materials. Composite placement instruments are made from anodized aluminum or Teflon. These materials prevent the composite material from being scratched. The instruments do not discolor the composite material, as do stainless steel instruments. *1,* Teflon composite instrument. *2,* Aluminum composite instrument.
1, 2	**Woodson (FP-1)** is a double-ended instrument that is made from hard plastic or stainless steel. *2,* One end is a "paddle" that is used for carrying dental materials to the prepared tooth structure. *1,* The other end is a **nib**, which resembles a condenser.

Photos from Boyd LRB: *Dental instruments: a pocket guide,* ed 5, St. Louis, 2015, Saunders.

TABLE 19-5
Accessory Instruments

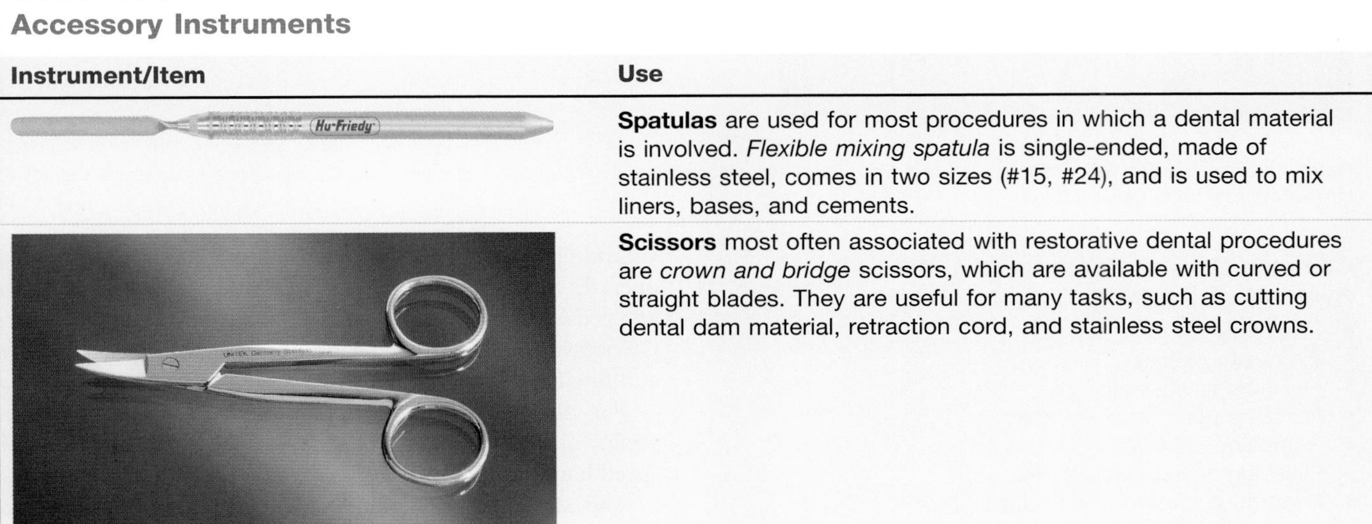

Instrument/Item	Use
	Spatulas are used for most procedures in which a dental material is involved. *Flexible mixing spatula* is single-ended, made of stainless steel, comes in two sizes (#15, #24), and is used to mix liners, bases, and cements.
	Scissors most often associated with restorative dental procedures are *crown and bridge* scissors, which are available with curved or straight blades. They are useful for many tasks, such as cutting dental dam material, retraction cord, and stainless steel crowns.

Continued

TABLE 19-5
Accessory Instruments—cont'd

Instrument/Item	Use
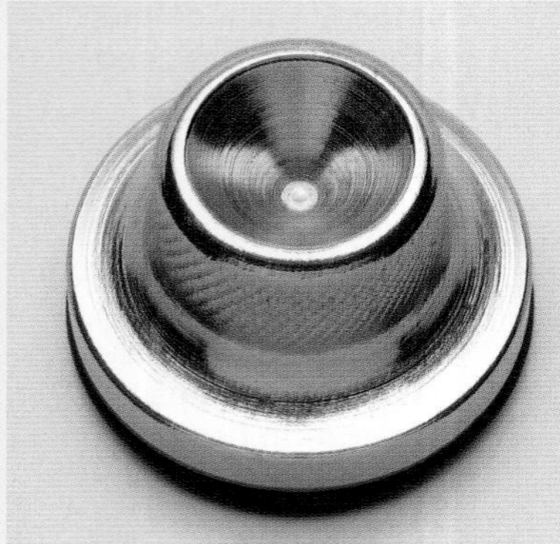	**Amalgam well** is made of metal and is weighted with a nonskid base. The newly mixed amalgam is placed in the well; it is then picked up in the carrier for transfer to the dentist.
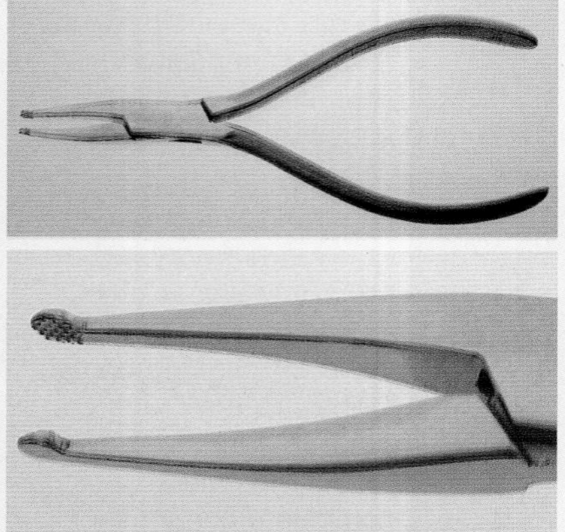	**Howe pliers**, also referred to as **110 pliers**, are versatile pliers that can be used in many procedures for many tasks. Their design is straight and includes beaks that have a flat rounded end, making them useful for holding items. Howe pliers are useful for carrying cotton products to and from the oral cavity, for removing the matrix band, and for placing and removing the wedge.
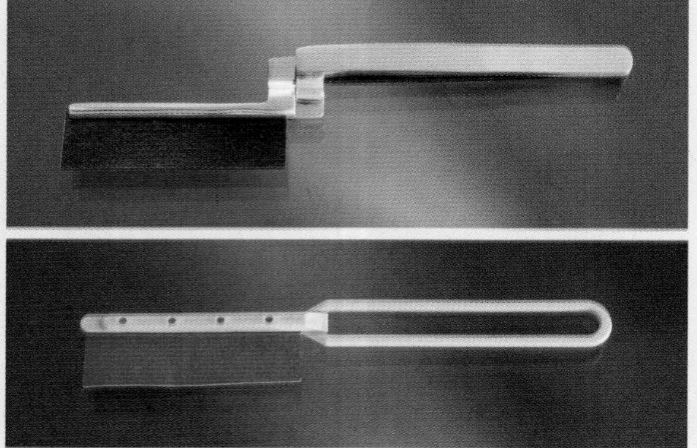	**Articulating paper holder** is used to hold and carry articulating paper to the mouth. This carbon paper material varies in thickness and color and is used to check a patient's "bite" following placement of a new restoration, crown, bridge, or denture. This mark must appear equal in distribution across the occlusal surface of the tooth. If one area appears lighter or darker, the patient's bite is incorrect and will need to be adjusted.

Photos of scissors, amalgam well, and Howe pliers from Boyd LRB: *Dental instruments: a pocket guide,* ed 5, St. Louis, 2015, Saunders. Photo of the spatula courtesy Hu-Friedy Manufacturing, Chicago, Illinois.

Common Uses of Handpieces and Burs in Restorative Dentistry

- Preparing the tooth
- Excavating decay
- Finishing cavity walls
- Finishing restoration surfaces
- Removing old fillings
- Finishing crown preparations
- Separating crowns and bridges
- Adjusting and correcting acrylic temporary crowns

versatile handpiece in dentistry (Figure 19-2). This handpiece operates at speeds up to 25,000 revolutions per minute (rpm) and is used for finishing, polishing, and contouring procedures. On occasion, the low-speed handpiece is used for decay removal and fine finishing of the cavity preparation.

For this handpiece to be used for various procedures, a variety of attachments (sleeves) are adapted to fit onto the low-speed handpiece motor.

The straight-line attachment slides onto the slow-speed motor and is locked into place (Figure 19-3). This handpiece is designed to hold larger burs for procedures completed outside

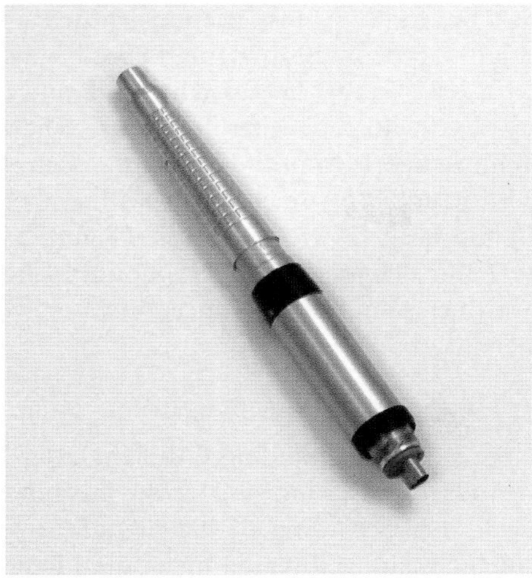

FIGURE 19-2 Low-speed handpiece.

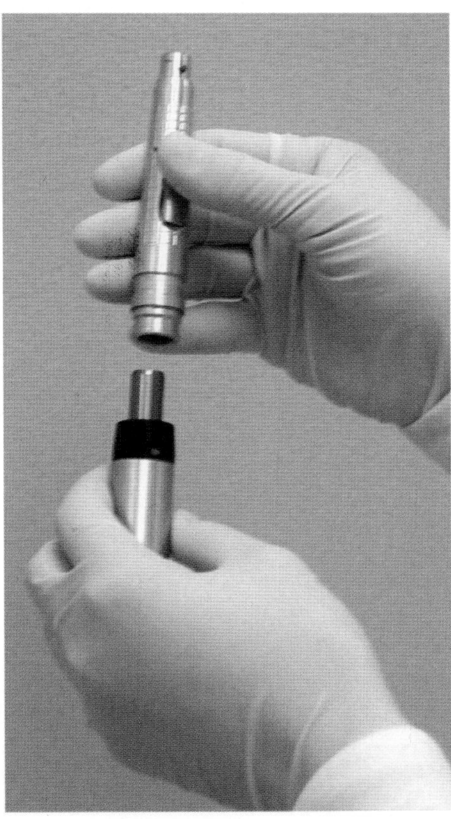

FIGURE 19-3 A straight attachment slides onto the low-speed motor.

of the mouth, such as denture adjustments and preparation of temporary crowns.

Contra-angle attachments are available in both the latch-type and friction-grip varieties. The difference between these types is demonstrated in the method in which burs are held in the contra-angle handpiece. The latch-type angle mechanically holds the bur in place by grasping a small notch on the end of the shank of the bur. The friction-grip angle holds the bur in place by grasping the shank of the bur with a friction chuck in the head of the contra-angle attachment (Figure 19-4).

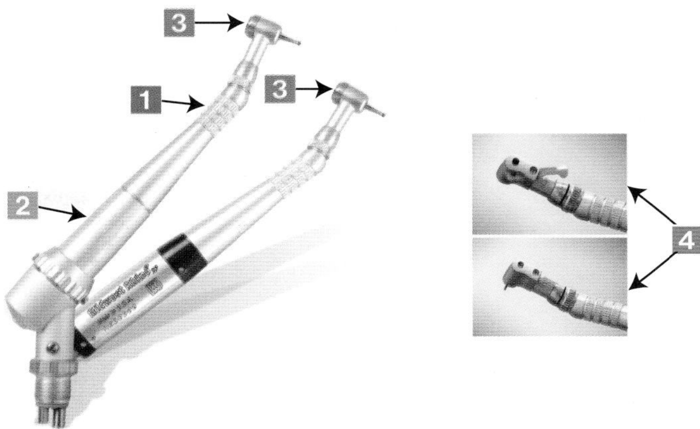

FIGURE 19-4 Contra-angle attachment, showing both the friction-grip and the latch-type devices. 1. The contra-angle attachment, 2. Slow speed motor, 3. Push button to secure bur when using a friction grip bur, 4. Latch type closure. (Left photo courtesy DENTSPLY International, York, PA. Right photo from Boyd LRB: *Dental instruments: a pocket guide,* ed 5, St. Louis, 2015, Saunders.)

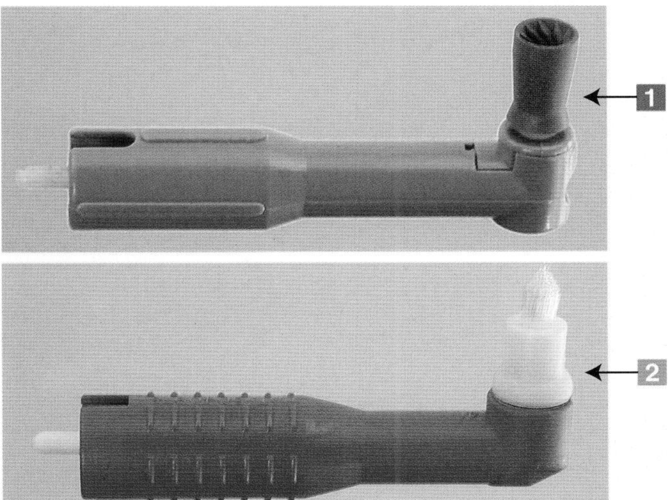

FIGURE 19-5 Disposable prophy cup *(1)* and brush *(2)*. (From Boyd LRB: *Dental instruments: a pocket guide,* ed 5, St. Louis, 2015, Saunders.)

Prophy angles, also referred to as *prophylaxis angles,* are used to hold polishing cups and brushes (Figure 19-5). The most common type of prophy angle is the plastic **disposable prophy angle**, which is discarded after a single use. These angles are available with rubber cup attachments or bristle brushes already in place. The **snap-on** type holds the polishing device in place by snapping over a smooth button.

High-Speed Handpiece

The **high-speed handpiece** operates on air pressure and reaches speeds of 450,000 rpm (Figure 19-6). During restorative procedures, the bulk of the tooth structure is removed using the high-speed handpiece. Refinement of the preparation and removal of decay are accomplished with both the high-speed handpiece and hand-cutting instruments.

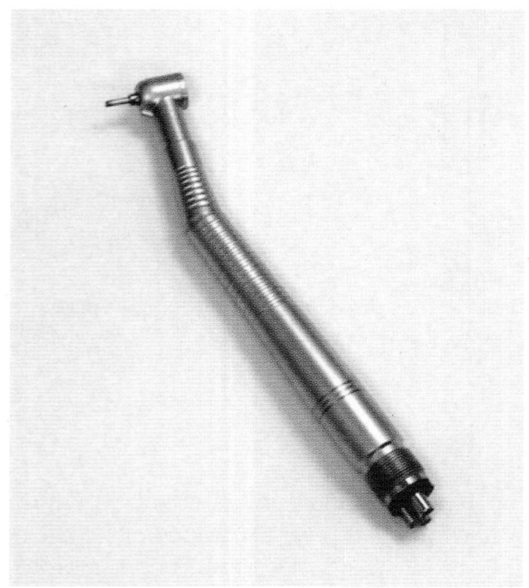

FIGURE 19-6 High-speed handpiece.

To protect the tooth against frictional heat caused by the extremely high speed of the bur, high-speed handpieces are equipped with water-spray devices. The tooth and the bur are constantly sprayed with cool water during use. The water spray also helps remove debris from the cavity preparation.

High-speed handpieces are equipped with a fiberoptic light mounted in the head of the handpiece (Figure 19-7). Light ports near the bur deliver the proper amount of light directly onto the site, which significantly reduces operator eyestrain and improves visibility.

Changing Burs in the Handpiece

With the large variety of handpiece designs available on the market, methods of inserting and removing burs from the handpiece will vary according to the manufacturer's design. Regardless of the manufacturer, all high-speed handpieces use friction-grip burs, diamond stones, and polishing devices.

The locking of burs for high-speed handpieces operates with a friction-grip mechanism, which is different than the locking mechanism for a slow-speed handpiece. Depending on the manufacturer, different styles for securing the bur are available, but they all operate on the same theory (Figure 19-8).

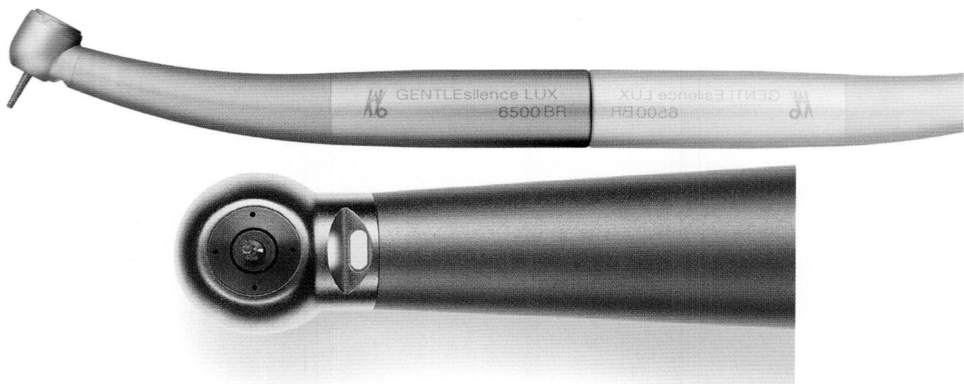

FIGURE 19-7 Fiberoptic light handpiece. (Courtesy KaVo Dental Corporation, Charlotte, North Carolina.)

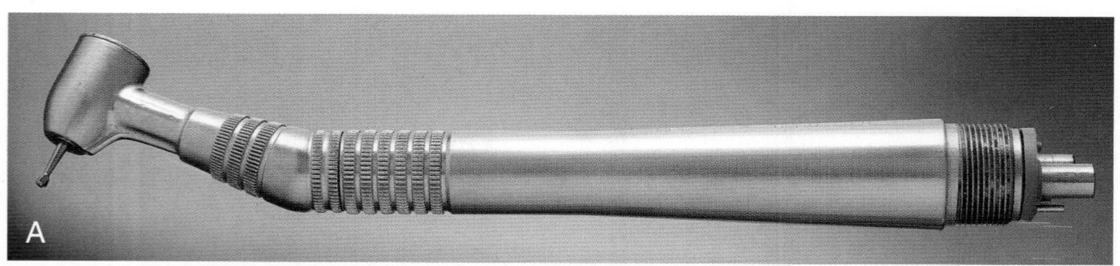

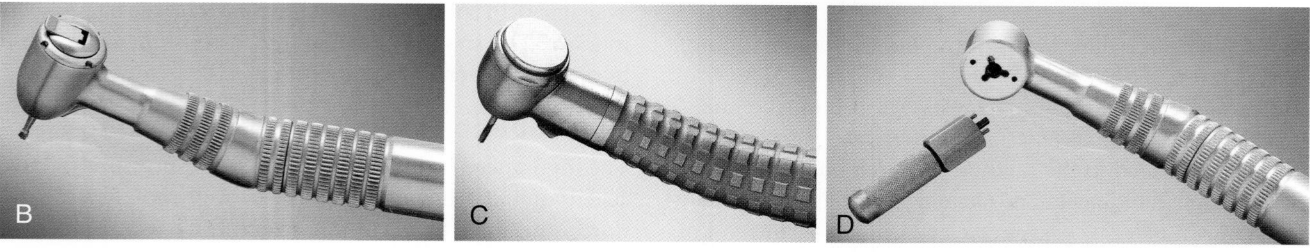

FIGURE 19-8 Locking mechanisms for high-speed handpiece. Assembled handpiece **(A)**, lever **(B)**, push button **(C)**, and conventional chuck **(D)**. (From Boyd LRB: *Dental instruments: a pocket guide,* ed 5, St. Louis, 2015, Saunders.)

Laboratory Handpiece

The **laboratory handpiece** is designed for the dental laboratory and not for the mouth. This type of handpiece operates at speeds up to 20,000 rpm and uses laboratory burs of various shapes and sizes.

The laboratory handpiece provides greater torque than the intraoral handpiece. (Torque is the turning power of the instrument when pressure is applied during the cutting procedure.) Increased torque is better suited to the heavier pressure required during laboratory grinding and polishing procedures.

Ultrasonic Handpiece

The **ultrasonic handpiece** works by converting high-frequency electrical current into mechanical vibrations for the removal of calculus from the tooth surface. Vibrations at the tip of an ultrasonic scaler range from 29,000 to 40,000 cycles per second. Water is needed to cool the friction created between the tip and the tooth surface. (The ultrasonic handpiece is a separate piece of equipment that is not connected to the dental unit; Figure 19-9.)

Air Abrasion Handpiece

An **air abrasion handpiece** is a small version of a sandblaster and is most effective when used for sealant preparation, stain removal, class I and VI preparations, endodontic access, preparation of crown margins, and preparation of a tooth surface for cementation of a cast restoration. The air abrasion technique allows high-pressure delivery of aluminum oxide particles through a small probe to abrade the tooth surface (Figure 19-10).

Laser Handpiece

The **laser handpiece** uses a laser light beam instead of a rotary instrument (Figure 19-11). The introduction of lasers into dentistry is expanding from soft tissue procedures to removal of decay from tooth structure. This pain-free technique represents a promising addition to dental treatment.

See Procedure 19-5: Identifying and Attaching the Dental Handpiece.

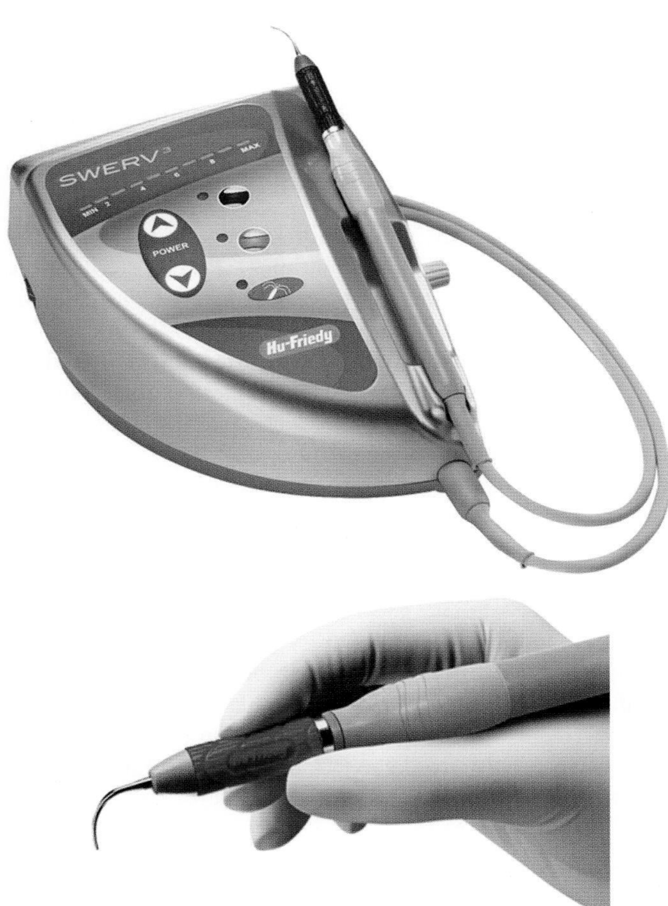

FIGURE 19-9 The Swerv3 Ultrasonic Scaling Unit. (Courtesy Hu-Friedy Manufacturing, Chicago, Illinois.)

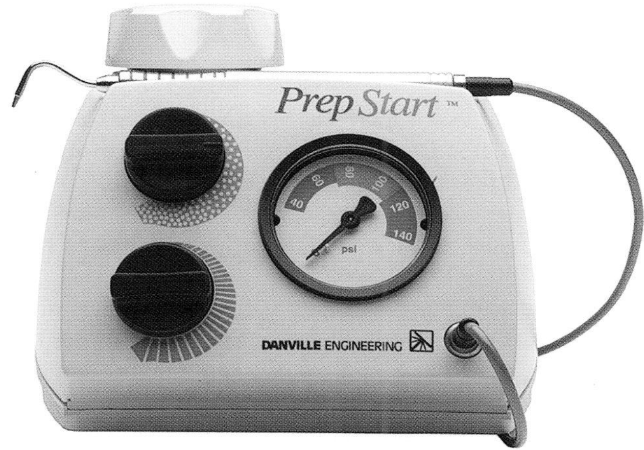

FIGURE 19-10 Air abrasion handpiece. (Courtesy Danville Materials, San Ramen, California.)

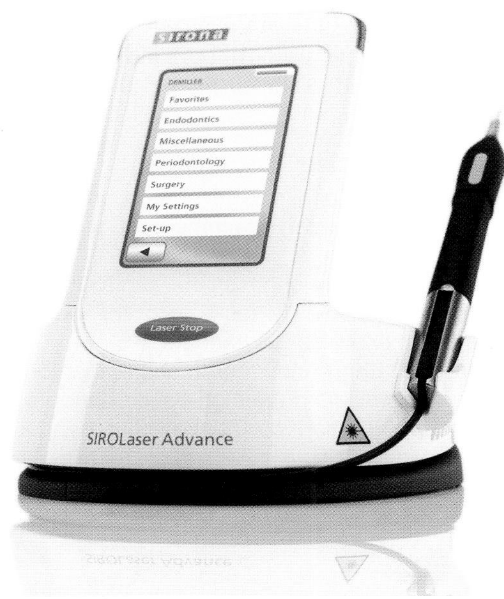

FIGURE 19-11 Soft tissue diode laser unit. (Courtesy Sirona Dental Systems, Charlotte, North Carolina.)

Handpiece Maintenance

Problems with dental handpieces most often result from improper cleaning, sterilization, and lubrication.

Inadequate cleaning of the handpiece before sterilization can result in the collection of debris in the internal parts of the handpiece, which creates wear similar to sludge within an automobile engine. If inappropriate cleaning solutions or techniques are used, then the working life of the handpiece is significantly shortened.

Some types of handpieces require lubrication before sterilization, some require lubrication after sterilization, and others require lubrication both before and after sterilization. Excessive lubrication can be as damaging as inadequate lubrication. Handpieces with ceramic bearings or heads require no lubrication at all.

Following the manufacturer's directions for the maintenance of each handpiece is imperative. Failure to do so can result in voiding of the handpiece warranty.

Handpiece Sterilization

The dental handpiece is a critical instrument (one that comes in contact with blood, saliva, and tissue). Because of its use, it must be sterilized before reuse. Dental handpieces require special considerations for sterilization because blood and saliva can be sucked back into the internal portions of the handpiece.

Before the handpiece is removed from the dental unit, it should run for a minimum of 20 to 30 seconds to discharge water and air, which aids in physically flushing out bioburden that may have entered the turbine and air or water lines. Take care not to spread spray, spatter, and aerosols during this process. (**Bioburden** is visible organic debris; in dentistry, it is most often blood or saliva.)

Dental Burs

Many types of dental burs are available, and each shape is designed for very specific uses. All burs have three basic parts: (1) shank, (2) neck, and (3) head (Figure 19-12).

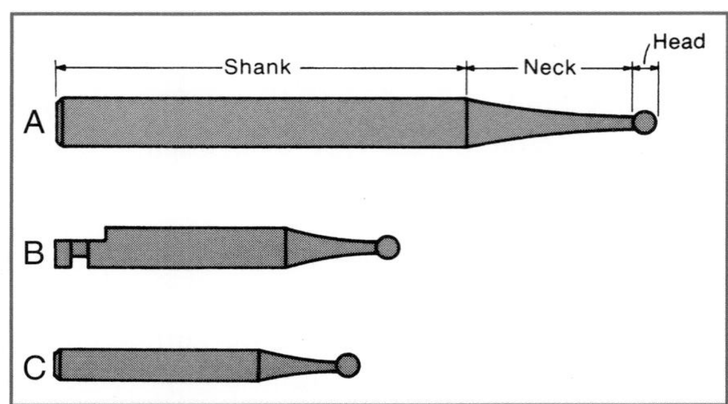

FIGURE 19-12 Bur parts and basic designs. **A,** Long-shank friction bur. **B,** Latch-type bur. **C,** Regular friction–type bur.

Parts of a Dental Bur

Shank **Straight.** Long, straight shank portion of the bur that fits into the straight attachment of the low-speed handpiece

Latch type. Medium-length shank with a small notch at the end that mechanically locks into the contra-angle attachment of the low-speed handpiece

Friction grip. Short and smooth shank that locks by a friction mechanism within the high-speed handpiece

Neck Narrow portion of the bur that connects the shank to the head

Head Cutting, polishing, or finishing part of the bur

Bur Shapes

Burs are made from a strong durable carbide material and are manufactured in a variety of shapes and sizes. A number is assigned to a certain bur shape, and a sequence of numbers designates the size of a specific shape. Table 19-6 provides shapes, numbers associated with shapes, and uses of common bur shapes.

Bur Care

Burs that become dull or worn are discarded in the sharps container. Burs must be sterilized before reuse. To minimize handling of contaminated burs, they should be placed in a bur block or holder before cleaning. This important step also prevents damage to the blades from rubbing or vibrating against each other or against any hard surface during cleaning.

Diamond Accessories

Diamond accessories, also referred to as **diamond burs** or **diamond stones,** have bits of industrial diamonds incorporated into their working surfaces. Many dentists use diamond accessories as an important part of restorative dentistry because of their cutting ability, which shortens preparation time and increases productivity. With multiple uses and sterilization, debonding of the diamond particles occurs, which decreases the cutting efficiency of the bur.

To ensure that the diamond bur or stone is always working at its maximum cutting rate, single-use disposable diamond burs or stones are available prepackaged, sterile, and ready for use, and discarded after a single use.

The shapes of diamond burs are very similar to those of carbide steel burs, and burs of most shapes are available in the diamond bur classification.

Trimming and Finishing Burs

Trimming and finishing burs are very similar in appearance to carbide burs, but the blades or bevels on the burs are significantly sharper and closer together. These instruments are preferred for finishing a composite-resin restoration. They are available only in the XF (super finisher) designation (Figure 19-13).

Abrasive Rotary Instruments

Abrasive rotary instruments are the most varied of the rotary instruments (Figure 19-14). **Polishing discs** and **wheels** are abrasives on a metal or paper backing. Used during finishing

TABLE 19-6
Burs for Restorative Dentistry

Type of Bur	Series of Numbers	Uses	Example
Round 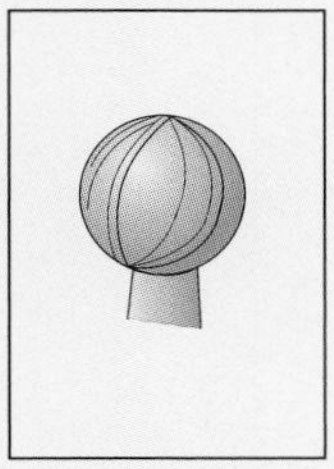	¼, ½, 1-8, 10	Makes the initial entry into the tooth structure. Extends the preparation. Provides retention. Removes decay.	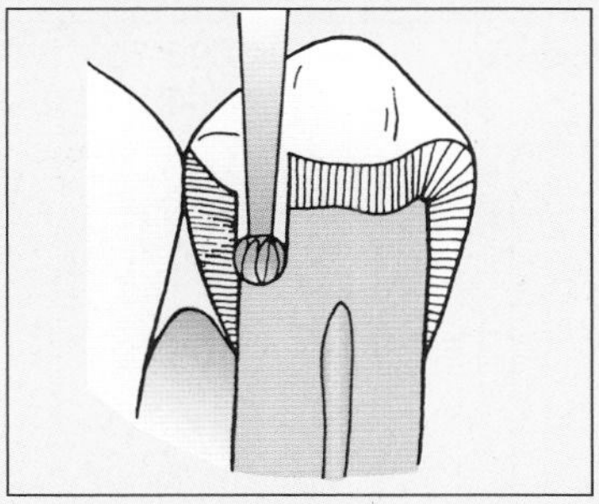
Inverted cone 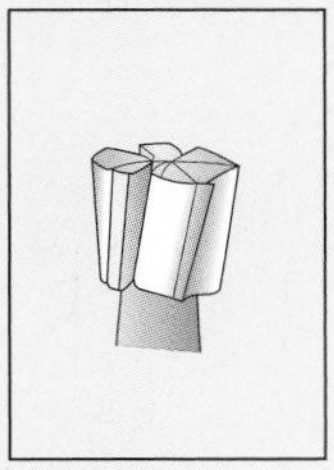	33½, 34-39, 36L, 37L	Removes decay. Establishes retentive grooves.	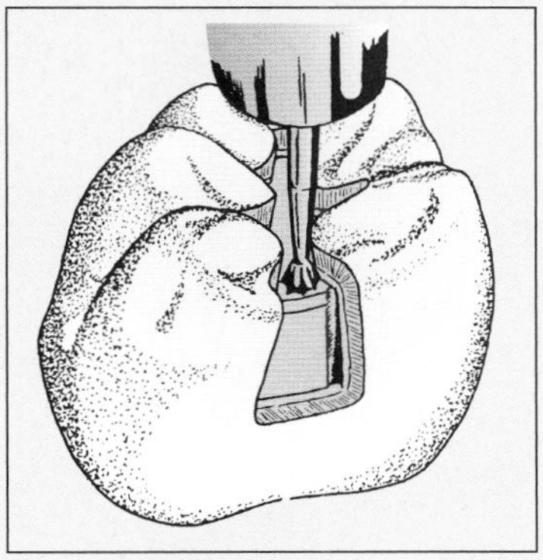
Straight fissure plain cut 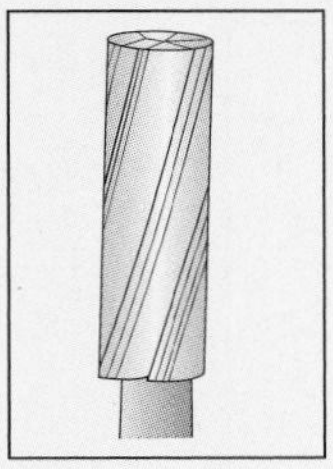	55-60, 57L, 58L	Makes the initial entry into the tooth. Forms the internal walls of the preparation.	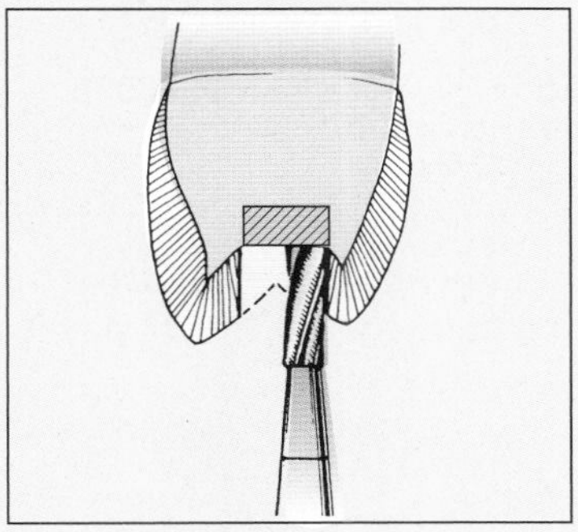
Straight fissure cross-cut 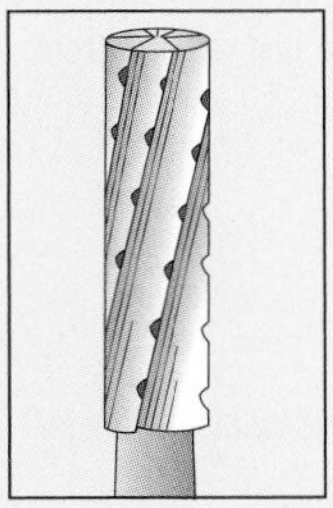	556-560, 567L, 568L	Forms the internal walls of the preparation.	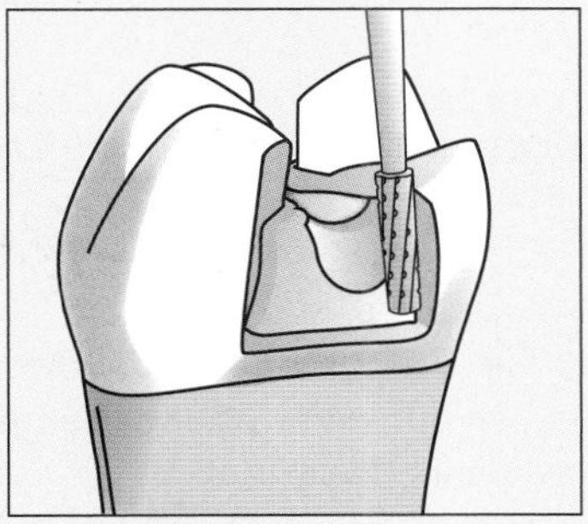
Tapered fissure plain-cut 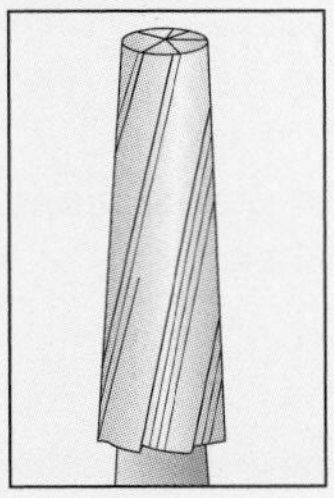	169-172, 169L, 170L, 171L	Provides angles to the walls of the prepared tooth.	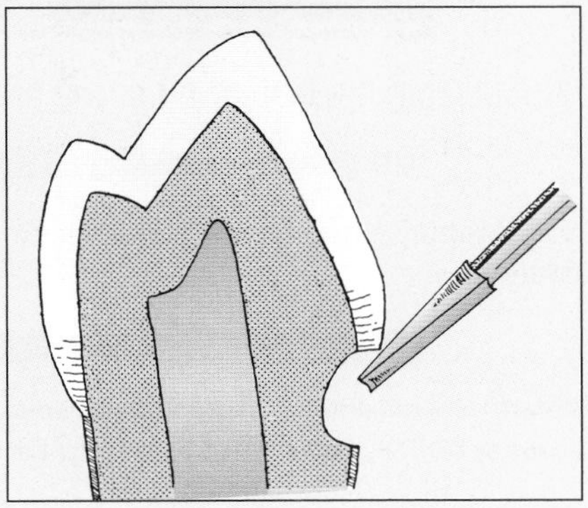

Continued

TABLE 19-6
Burs for Restorative Dentistry—cont'd

Type of Bur	Series of Numbers	Uses	Example
Tapered fissure cross-cut	699-703, 699L, 700L, 701L	Provides angles to the walls of the prepared tooth.	
Pear	330-333, 331L	Makes the initial entry into the tooth structure. Extends the preparation.	
End cutting	957, 958	Makes the initial entry into the tooth structure. Creates a shoulder for the margin of a crown preparation.	

Illustrations in the first column from Finkbeiner BL, Johnson CS: *Mosby's comprehensive dental assisting,* St. Louis, 1995, Mosby. Illustrations in the last column from Baum L, Phillips RW, Lund MR: *Textbook of operative dentistry,* ed 3, Philadelphia, 1995, Saunders.

Indications for Using Diamond Burs

Round-end taper bur removes tooth structure and makes mechanical retention grooves.

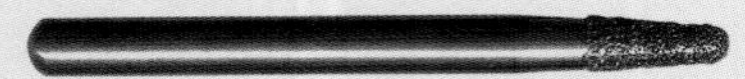

Flat-end taper bur is used for crown preparation.

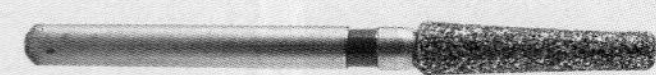

Cylinder bur smooths and finishes the walls in tooth preparations.

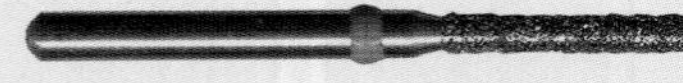

Flame-shaped bur makes bevels in crown preparations.

Round bur provides access to the pulp chamber for endodontic treatment and is used to adjust and shape occlusal surfaces.

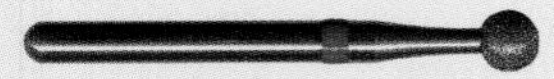

Wheel-shaped bur is used for anterior crown preparations and can be used to adjust and shape occlusal surfaces.

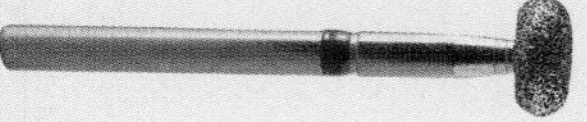

Images courtesy DENTSPLY International, York, Pennsylvania.

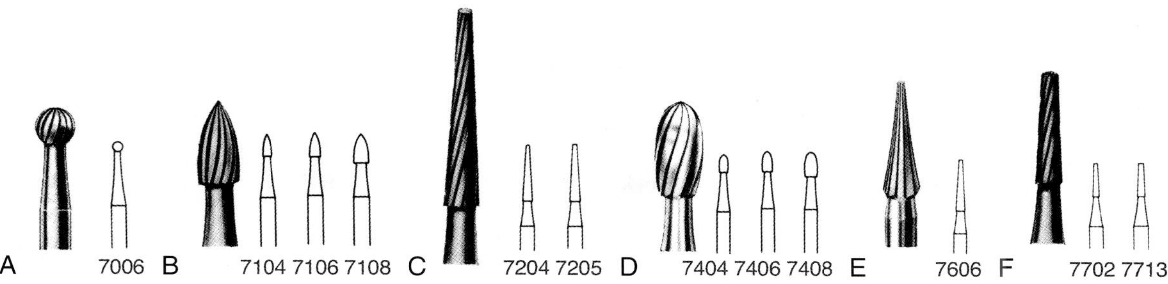

FIGURE 19-13 Trimming and finishing burs. **A,** Round. **B,** flame. **C,** Tapered fissure plain-cut. **D,** Pear. **E,** Tapered fissure cross-cut. **F,** End-cutting. (Courtesy Integra Miltex, York, Pennsylvania.)

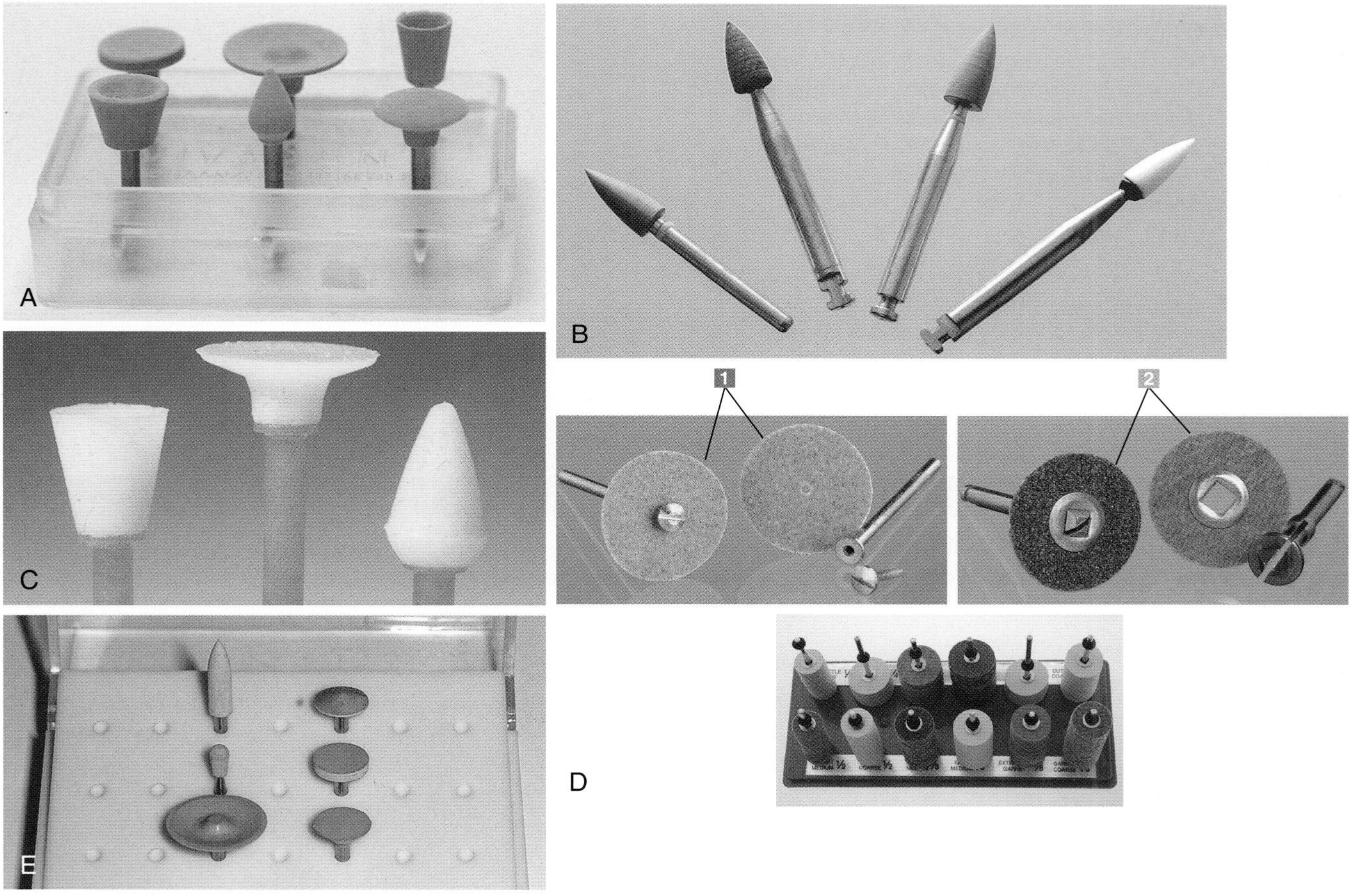

FIGURE 19-14 Accessory abrasive attachments for rotary instruments. **A,** Silicon carbide produces a moderately rough surface and is available in wheels, points, and stones. The color varies from gray-green to black. Silicon carbide is used for polishing metal restorations. **B,** Rubber points come in varying colors, depending on their abrasiveness. The brown is the most abrasive, with green having less abrasiveness; white is a polishing point. **C,** Cuttlebone is most often adhered to discs and points and is used for final finishing and polishing of the restoration. **D,** Sandpaper discs refer to sand particles adhered to flexible paper discs or strips as a medium abrasive. They are used for finishing and polishing a restoration. Sandpaper discs snap on *(1)* or screw on *(2)* a metal center. **E,** Carborundum particles adhered to the disc. As with carborundum on burs, the bur is used to cut or separate one structure from another. (**B** and **D** from Boyd LRB: *Dental instruments: a pocket guide,* ed 5, St. Louis, 2015, Saunders.)

of a restoration, polishing discs are available in four grits: coarse, medium, fine, and super fine. Coarser discs are used to remove excess filling material from the margins of a restoration. Finer discs are used to smooth and polish the completed restoration.

Abrasive discs and wheels are attached to a **mandrel** (metal shaft; Figure 19-15). Mandrels are used to attach these accessories to the dental handpiece.

Stones are used when maximum abrasion is needed during a procedure, as for adjusting the occlusion on an amalgam restoration or a gold crown.

Rubber points are embossed with a polishing agent and are used to polish the anatomic grooves of metallic restorations.

See Procedure 19-6: Identifying and Attaching Burs for Rotary Cutting Instruments.

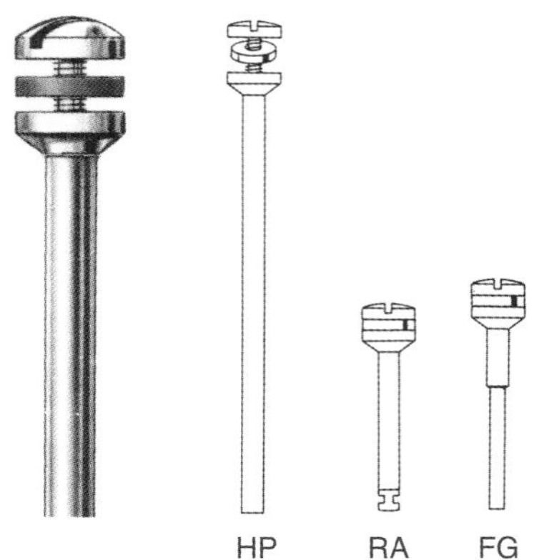

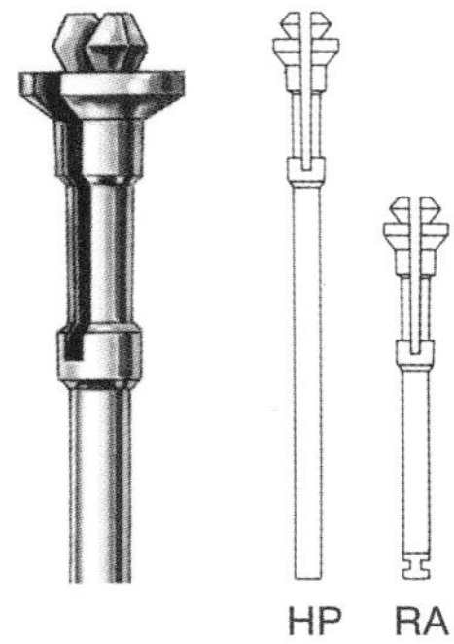

FIGURE 19-15 Types of mandrels. (Courtesy Integra Miltex, York, Pennsylvania.)

Ethical Implications

The care that you take in packaging, sterilizing, storing, and using dental instruments will demonstrate your professional responsibility. The steps you take to decrease the risk that a patient may be injured or may acquire a disease because of a lack of sterilization methods will protect your office from a malpractice lawsuit.

Procedure 19-1
Identifying Examination Instruments

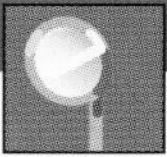

Equipment and Supplies

- Mouth mirror
- Explorer
- Cotton pliers
- Periodontal probe

Procedural Steps

1. Carefully examine each instrument.
2. Consider the general classification of each instrument.
3. Write the complete name of each instrument or item, correctly spell each name, and give the uses for each instrument.

Procedure 19-2
Identifying Hand (Manual) Cutting Instruments

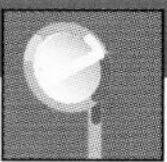

Equipment and Supplies

- Excavators
- Hoe
- Chisels
- Hatchets
- Gingival margin trimmer

Procedural Steps

1. Carefully examine each instrument.
2. Consider the general classification of each instrument.
3. Write the complete name of each instrument or item, correctly spell each name, and give the uses for each instrument.

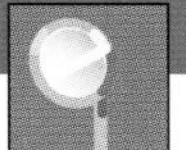

Procedure 19-3
Identifying Restorative Instruments

Equipment and Supplies
- Amalgam carrier
- Condensers
- Burnishers
- Carvers
- Amalgam knife
- Composite placement instruments
- Plastic instrument

Procedural Steps
1. Carefully examine each instrument.
2. Consider the general classification of each instrument.
3. Write the complete name of each instrument or item, correctly spell each name, and give the uses for each instrument.

Procedure 19-4
Identifying Accessory Instruments and Items

Equipment and Supplies
- Cement spatulas
- Impression spatulas
- Scissors
- Dappen dish
- Amalgam well
- Howe pliers

Procedural Steps
1. Carefully examine each instrument.
2. Consider the general classification of each instrument.
3. Write the complete name of each instrument or item, correctly spell each name, and give the uses for each instrument.

Procedure 19-5
Identifying and Attaching the Dental Handpiece

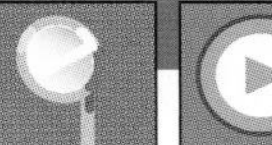

Equipment and Supplies
- Low-speed handpiece
- Straight attachment
- Contra-angle attachment
- Prophylaxis attachment
- High-speed handpiece

Procedural Steps
1. Identify and attach the low-speed handpiece to the dental unit, ensuring that the receptors are aligned and the handpiece correctly fits onto the correct line.

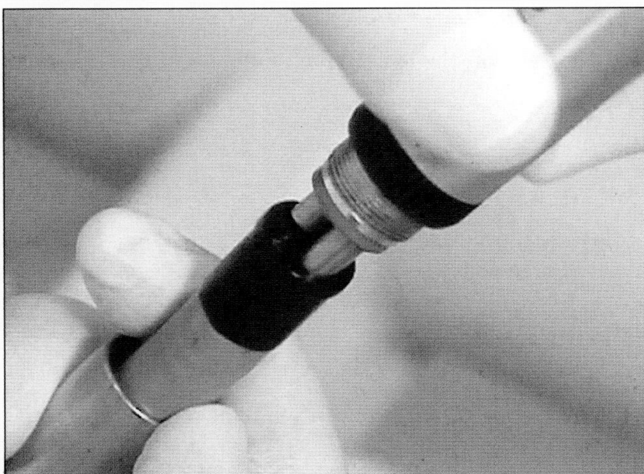

2. Identify and attach the contra-angle attachment onto the straight attachment of the low-speed handpiece, ensuring that the attachment is locked.

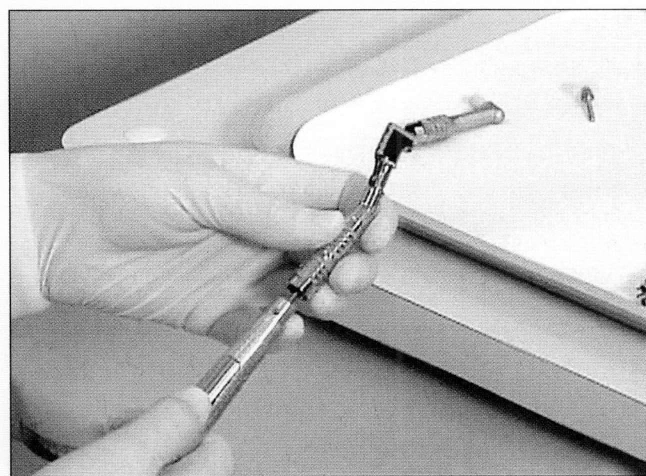

Continued

Procedure 19-5

Identifying and Attaching the Dental Handpiece—cont'd

3. Identify and attach the prophylaxis-angle attachment onto the straight attachment of the low-speed handpiece, ensuring that the attachment is locked.

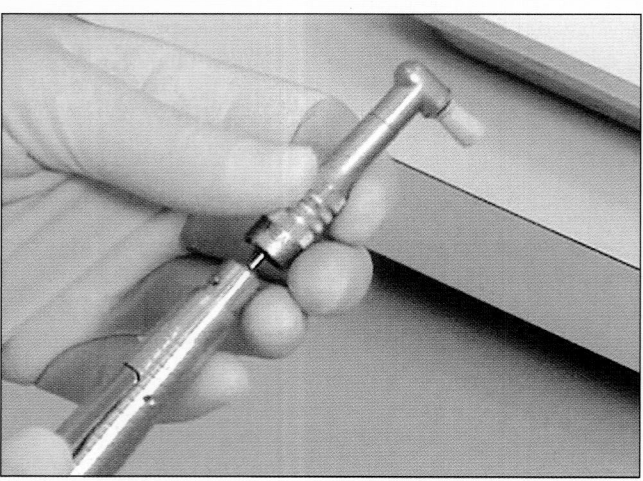

4. Identify and attach the high-speed handpiece to the dental unit, ensuring that the receptors are aligned and that the handpiece correctly fits onto the correct line.

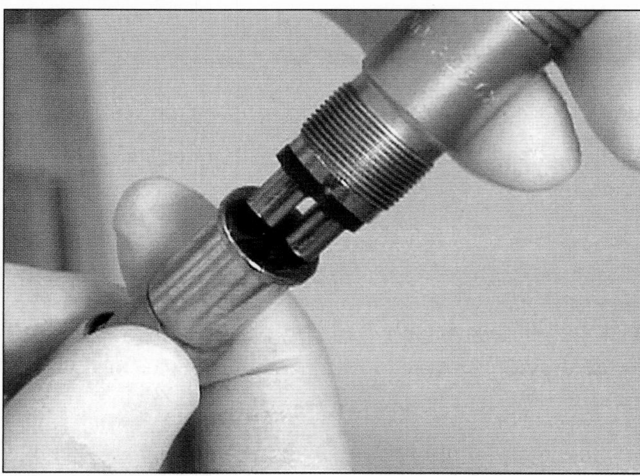

5. Identify and attach the ultrasonic handpiece to the dental unit, ensuring that the receptors are aligned and that the handpiece correctly fits onto the correct line.

Procedure 19-6

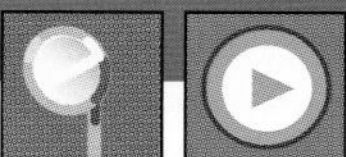

Identifying and Attaching Burs for Rotary Cutting Instruments

Equipment and Supplies

- Various types of dental rotary instruments, including carbide, diamond, finishing, abrasives, and laboratory burs
- Low-speed handpiece
- High-speed handpiece
- Contra-angle attachment
- Mandrel

Procedural Steps

1. Identify specific dental burs, such as carbide, diamond, finishing, and abrasion burs, by their name and number sequence.
2. Attach latch-type burs to the contra-angle attachment on the low-speed handpiece, ensuring that the bur is locked in place.
3. Attach friction-grip burs to the high-speed handpiece, ensuring that the bur is locked in place.
4. Correctly attach abrasive discs to the mandrel by screwing to tighten or by positioning the metal opening onto the mandrel, ensuring that the disc is securely locked.

Chapter Exercises

Multiple Choice

Circle the letter next to the correct answer.

1. A discoid-cleoid is a double-ended variety of this type of instrument __________.
   a. condenser
   b. excavator
   c. gingival margin trimmer
   d. carver
2. During a prophylaxis, what type of handpiece is an addition to but not a substitute for manual scaling and instrumentation in the removal of calculus?
   a. High-speed
   b. Laser
   c. Ultrasonic
   d. b and c
3. What type of instrument is primarily used for the removal of decay and soft dentin?
   a. Explorer
   b. Hatchet
   c. Hoe
   d. Spoon excavator
4. A prophy angle attaches to the __________ handpiece.
   a. Straight slow-speed
   b. high-speed
   c. laser
   d. air abrasion
5. The high-speed handpiece uses what type of mechanism when inserting and locking the bur?
   a. Friction-grip
   b. Latch-type
   c. Mandrel
   d. Snap-on
6. The most commonly used sizes of round burs are __________.
   a. ¼ to 8
   b. 33 to 37
   c. 169 to 171
   d. 556 to 558
7. Inverted cone burs are designed to __________.
   a. open the pulp chamber during endodontic treatment
   b. place retention grooves
   c. remove tooth structure
   d. b and c
8. A mandrel is a device used for __________.
   a. attaching finishing and polishing devices to the handpiece
   b. carving the occlusal surface of a restoration
   c. etching the interproximal surface of a preparation
   d. b and c
9. What type of hand instrument is designed to contour the composite resin to its normal anatomy while the resin is still soft?
   a. Burnisher
   b. Carver
   c. Plastic instrument
   d. Condenser
10. A low-speed handpiece operates at speeds up to __________ rpm.
    a. 7,000
    b. 25,000
    c. 200,000
    d. 450,000

Apply Your Knowledge

1. You are assisting with an amalgam procedure, and Dr. Campbell has just completed the removal of the diseased tooth structure with the high-speed handpiece. She asks for a spoon excavator, but you cannot locate it on the tray. Discuss how this could have been prevented and what you would do at this point.
2. Dr. Campbell has just completed the restorative procedure and is ready to adjust the patient's lower partial. What handpiece is used to adjust a partial outside of the mouth? How would you prepare the handpiece, and what type of bur would be inserted?
3. While you are setting up for a procedure, you notice that the handpiece from the previous procedure is still attached to the dental unit. To save time, can you disinfect the handpiece and place a new sterile bur in the handpiece?

CHAPTER 20

Restorative and Esthetic Dental Materials

http://evolve.elsevier.com/Robinson/essentials/

LEARNING OBJECTIVES

1. Pronounce, define, and spell the key terms.
2. Complete the following as related to dental materials used in restorative dentistry:
   - List the types of dental materials commonly used in restorative dentistry.
   - Discuss the criteria that must be met before a dental material is brought onto the market.
   - Describe the basic properties required of dental materials to be used within the environment of the oral cavity.
3. Describe amalgam and its importance in dentistry, and demonstrate how to mix and transfer dental amalgam.
4. Describe composite resins and their importance in dentistry, and demonstrate how to prepare composite resin materials.
5. Complete the following as related to dental liners:
   - Describe dental liners and their importance in dentistry.
   - List the three commonly placed types of liners.
   - Demonstrate the application of calcium hydroxide and cavity varnish.
6. Complete the following as related to etching systems, bonding systems, and temporary restorative materials:
   - Discuss etching systems and demonstrate how to apply an etchant material.
   - Discuss bonding systems and demonstrate how to apply a bonding system.
   - Discuss temporary restorative materials and demonstrate how to mix intermediate restorative material.
7. Complete the following as related to cements used for restorative dentistry:
   - Discuss the three methods that are used for preparation of a cement product.
   - List the types of dental cements.
   - Demonstrate how to mix zinc oxide-eugenol (ZOE) for a base, temporary cementation, and permanent cementation.
   - Demonstrate how to mix glass ionomer for permanent cementation.
   - Demonstrate how to mix zinc phosphate for a base and permanent cementation.
   - Demonstrate how to mix polycarboxylate for a base and permanent cementation.
8. Describe the use of tooth-whitening products in the esthetic aspect of restorative dentistry.

KEY TERMS

alloy
amalgam
amalgamator
bonding
cements
composite resins
curing
etching
exothermic
force
galvanic
pestle
polymerization
retention
strain
stress
tooth whitening
trituration

Restorative is a term in dentistry that describes the ability to remove decay or disease and bring back the proper function of a tooth. This can be accomplished by a direct restoration or by the insertion of an indirect restoration (further discussed in Chapter 23). **Esthetic** is a term that refers to restoring the tooth or teeth with an artistically attractive appearance.

The types of dental materials used by the general dentist for these types of procedures include: (1) **amalgam**, which is the clinical name for silver fillings (this restorative material was first introduced in 1826 and was perfected by G.V. Black in 1895); (2) **composite resins**, which are the most widely accepted material of choice by dentists and patients because of their natural and esthetic appearance and new advances in their strength; and (3) **tooth-whitening** products, which provide one of the fastest and most cost-effective ways of restoring the esthetic appearance of teeth.

Supplemental materials that are integrated in dental procedures to contribute in the restorative process include: (1) **dental liners**, **bases**, **etchants**, and **bonding agents**—a variety of added materials incorporated in a restorative and esthetic procedure based on the design and need in the restoration process; (2) **temporary restorative materials**—materials selected for a temporary restoration; and (3) **cements**—a group of dental materials that provide a temporary or permanent adhesion for temporary inlays and onlays, as well as crowns and bridges directly to tooth structure.

Characteristics of Dental Materials

When a dental material is introduced to the profession, the product must meet strict guidelines before it can be marketed for use. The Council of Dental Materials, Instruments, and Equipment, a subcommittee of and formed by the American Dental Association (ADA), provides these standards and specifications.

Criteria That Must be Met Before a Dental Material Is Brought Onto the Market

A dental material must:

- Not be poisonous or harmful to the body.
- Not be harmful or irritating to the tissue of the oral cavity.
- Help protect the tooth and oral tissue of the oral cavity.
- Resemble the natural dentition as closely as possible so as to be esthetically pleasing.
- Be easily formed and placed in the mouth to restore natural contours.
- Be able to conform and function, despite limited access, wet conditions and poor visibility.

Properties Affecting a Dental Material

The oral cavity presents every possible challenge to the dentist when selecting a dental material suitable for the mouth. Table 20-1 provides the basic properties required of dental materials, taking into account their limitations within the environment of the oral cavity.

Amalgam

Dental amalgam is a safe, affordable, and durable material predominantly used to restore premolars and molars. Amalgam is

TABLE 20-1
Properties of Dental Materials

Property	Description
Mechanical	Involves the biting and chewing in the posterior area of the mouth. Mechanical properties include **force**, which is the push or pull on matter; **stress**, the reaction within the dental material that can cause distortion; and **strain**, which is any change produced within the dental material as the result of stress.
Ductility and malleability	Involves the measure a metal's capability to withstand permanent deformation by either tensile or compressive forces.
Thermal change	Involves the emperature changes in the mouth. Thermal changes can cause a dental material to contract and expand, resulting in microleakage of fluid, debris, and microorganisms when the dental material pulls away from the tooth structure.
Electrical	Involves the **galvanic** current, which can take place with the condition of metals interacting with saliva.
Corrosive	Invoves the corrosive reaction within a metal when it comes into contact with corrosive products. Certain foods and beverages can corrode or discolor metals.
Hardness	Involves the resistance or wearability of an alloy or metal to scratching or abrasion.
Solubility	Involves the degree to which a substance will dissolve in a wet environment.
Application	Involves the four specific steps in the application process: (1) flow of material, (2) adhesion of the material to the tooth, (3) **retention** to the tooth; and (4) **curing** of the material.

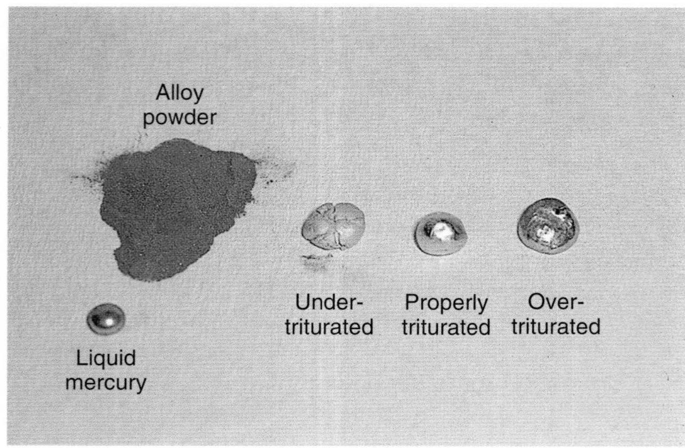

FIGURE 20-1 The mercury and alloy powder are in their purest forms before trituration. (From Hatrick CD, Eakle WS: *Dental materials: clinical applications for dental assistants and dental hygienists,* ed 3, St. Louis, 2016, Saunders.)

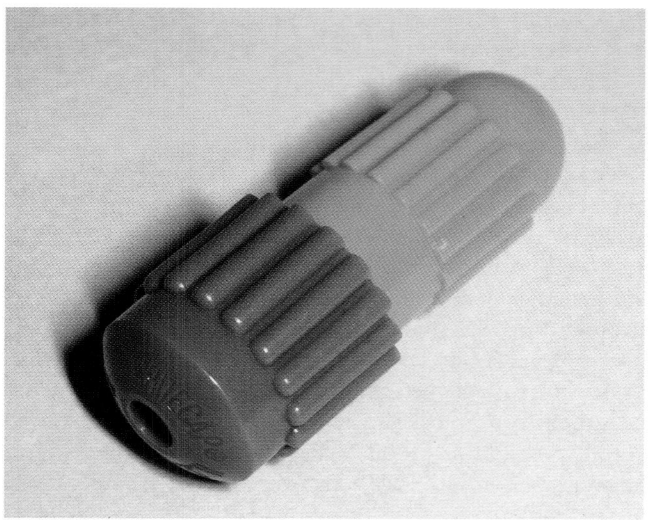

FIGURE 20-2 Precapsulated amalgam.

the end result of mixing approximately equal parts of mercury (43% to 54%) and an amalgam **alloy** powder (57% to 46%), which includes silver, tin, copper, and zinc (Figure 20-1).

Composition of Amalgam Alloy Powder

Silver—gives it strength
Tin—gives it workability and strength
Copper—gives it strength and low corrosion
Zinc—suppresses oxidation

Application of the Dental Amalgam

Amalgam is supplied by the manufacturer in sealed single-use capsules with the proper ratio of alloy powder in one side of the capsule and mercury in the other side and separated by a thin membrane. The single-use capsule ensures an accurate ratio of alloy powder and mercury and reduces the possibility of exposure to any of the materials. Immediately after use, the capsule is reassembled and discarded with nonregulated waste.

Capsules are available in 600 mg of alloy, which is the appropriate amount of material for a small or single-surface restoration, or 800 mg of alloy, which is used for a larger restoration (Figure 20-2). If more amalgam is required, then additional capsules are placed with the setup and triturated as needed.

Trituration is the process by which mercury and alloy powders are mixed together to form the mass of amalgam needed to restore the tooth. The preloaded capsule of amalgam alloy and mercury contains a **pestle**, which aids in the mixing process. Before the capsule is placed into the **amalgamator**, many types of capsules require the use of an activator, which breaks the separating membrane. The activated capsule is placed in the amalgamator, and the cover is closed to prevent mercury vapors from escaping during trituration. The amalgamator is set to operate for the length of time specified in the manufacturer's directions. Amalgam should appear soft, pliable, and easily shaped when first triturated.

The amalgam is carried to the tooth by the amalgam carrier and is placed in increments into the prepared tooth, with each increment immediately condensed with the use of an amalgam condenser. The purpose of condensation is to pack the amalgam tightly into all areas of the prepared cavity and to aid in removing any excess mercury from the amalgam mix.

With the use of hand-carving instruments, the dentist is able to carve back the amalgam material to the tooth's normal anatomy, which was removed during cavity preparation.

See Procedure 20-1: Mixing and Transferring Dental Amalgam.

Amalgam Disposal

Dentistry is committed to recycling dental amalgam. To help in that endeavor, the ADA developed "Best Management Practices for Amalgam Waste," a series of amalgam waste handling and disposal practices. The protocol includes the following practices:

- Use amalgam capsules.
- Have disposable chair-side traps.
- Install amalgam separators that are compliant.
- Use vacuum pump filters.
- Inspect and clean traps.
- Collect and recycle amalgam.

Composite Resins

Composite resin is a tooth-colored dental material that is the most widely used material by dentists and the most requested by patients (Figure 20-3). Early in its use, this material had a composition that made it esthetically pleasing, but it was not able to withstand some of the properties discussed earlier in this chapter. Today, this tooth-colored material is able to (1) withstand the environments of the oral cavity; (2) be easily shaped to the anatomy of a tooth; (3) match the natural tooth color; and (4) be directly bonded to tooth surfaces for strength. The composition of composite resins includes the resin matrix, inorganic fillers, and a coupling agent.

Composition of Composite Resins

- **Resin matrix** (bisphenol A–glycidyl methacrylate; also known as BIS-GMA)—fluidlike material used to make synthetic resins
- **Inorganic fillers**—quartz, glass, silica, and colorants to add the strength and characteristics necessary for a restorative material
- **Coupling agent**—to strengthen and chemically bond the filler to the resin matrix
- **Pigments**—to give it color

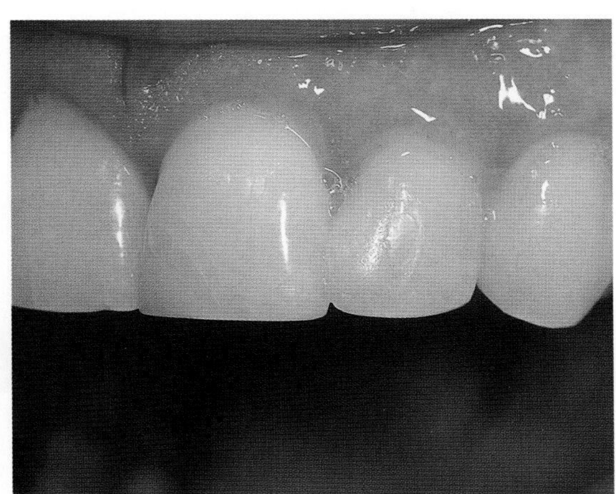

FIGURE 20-3 Class III composite restoration on the mesial surface of tooth #10. (Courtesy Premier Dental Products, Plymouth Meeting, Pennsylvania.)

The inorganic fillers within composite materials are classified by particle size as *megafill, macrofill, midfill, minifill, microfill, and nanofill.* Some of the newer composites today include a combination of particle sizes which are termed *hybrid* (Figure 20-4).

Shade Selection

Color matching is one of the most critical aspects when working with composite resins. If the correct shade is not selected, then the difference will be apparent to the patient after the restoration is in place. The composite kit may include its own shade guide; most manufacturers cross-reference their shades with those of the VITA Shade Guide, which is a universally adopted shade guide (Figure 20-5).

Application of Composite Resins

Composite resins are supplied in lightproof syringes, as a paste, or in capsules (Figure 20-6). Light-cured resins do not require mixing and are directly applied from the syringe with the addition of a syringe tip. The paste contains both the photo initiator and the amine activator and will not polymerize until it is exposed to the curing light. The material is supplied in a kit that includes varying shades of the composite resin, along with an etching and bonding system that specifically works for the application process of that material.

Polymerization is the process by which resin material is changed from a pliable state (in which it can be molded or shaped) into a hardened restoration. Polymerization occurs through an auto-curing or a light-curing process.

The **light-curing process** uses a high-intensity blue light source that provides an effective curing of resins. The blue light

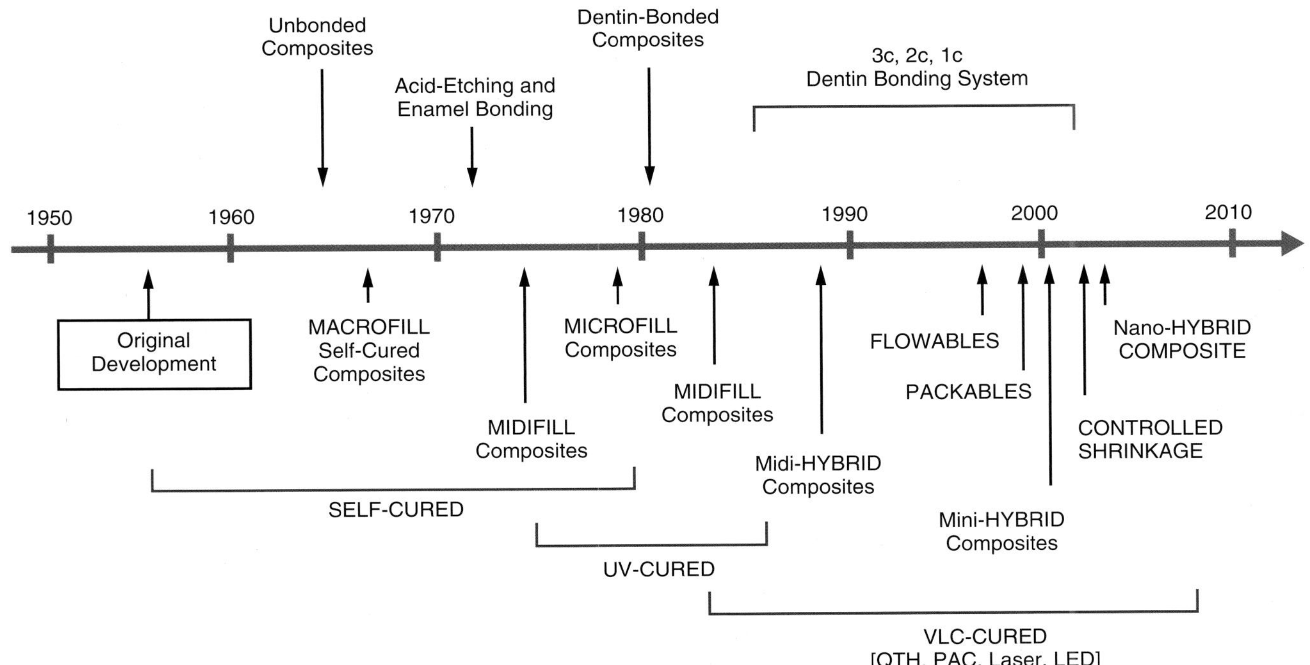

FIGURE 20-4 Summary of the historical evolution of dental composites, curing methods, and accompanying bonding systems. (Courtesy SC Bayne. From Heymann HO, Swift EJ, Ritter AV: *Sturdevant's art and science of operative dentistry,* ed 6, St. Louis, 2013, Mosby.)

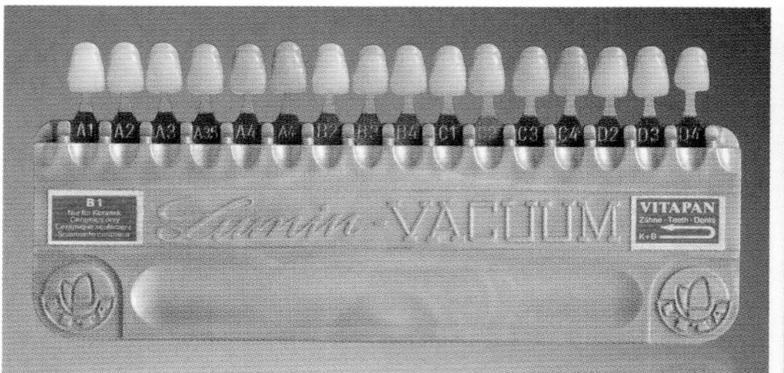

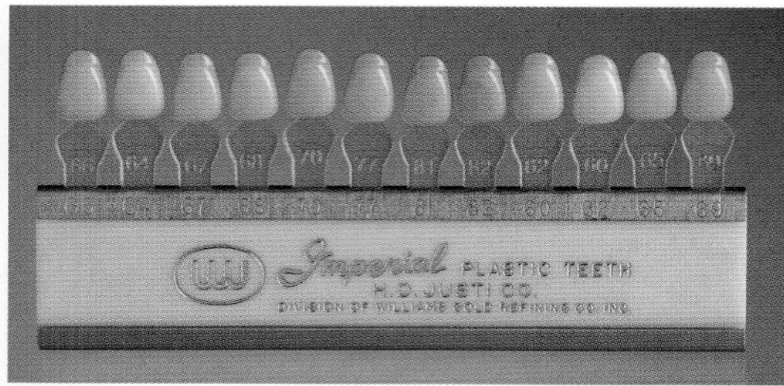

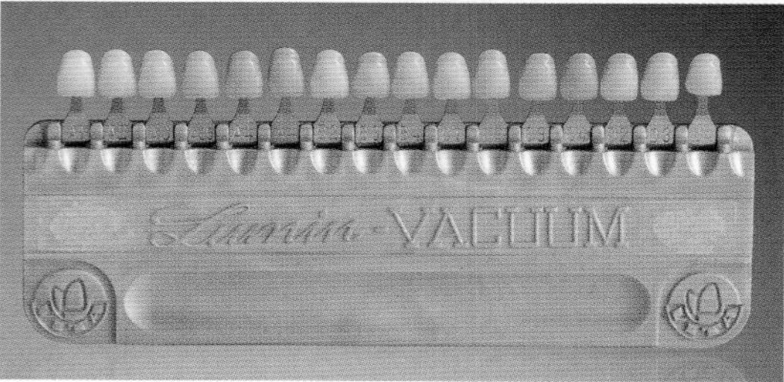

FIGURE 20-5 Types of shade guides. (From Boyd LRB: *Dental instruments: a pocket guide,* ed 5, St. Louis, 2015, Saunders.)

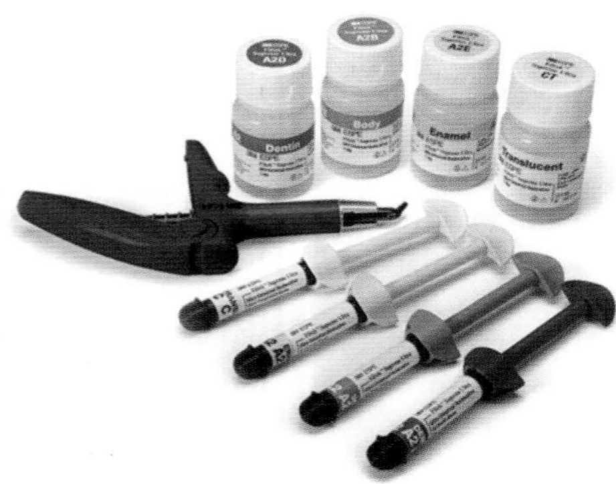

FIGURE 20-6 Composite resin kit. Filtek™ Supreme Ultra Universal Restorative is a visible light-activated composite designed for use in anterior and posterior restorations. A dental adhesive, such as those manufactured by 3M, is used to permanently bond the restoration to the tooth structure. The restorative is available in a wide variety of Dentin, Body, Enamel and Translucent shades. It is offered in both syringes and single-dose capsules. (Photo courtesy of 3M, St. Paul, Minnesota.)

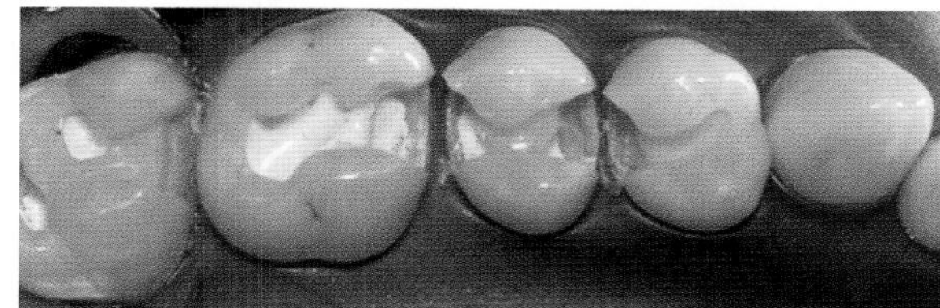

FIGURE 20-7 Placement of a liner.

source is a combination of tungsten and a halogen lighting system. The exact curing time depends on the following:

- Composite manufacturer's instructions (most often 20 to 60 seconds)
- Thickness and size of the restoration (When larger quantities of the material are being placed, each increment is cured before the next is placed.)
- Shade of the restorative material used (The darker the shade, the longer the required curing time.)

Finishing and Polishing

The finishing and polishing of composite resins are significantly different from the completion steps in an amalgam procedure. Because composite materials go from a soft pliable state to being completely hardened by polymerization, the dentist is not able to carve or make adjustments with hand instruments. Finishing burs and abrasive materials are used to contour and polish a finished composite resin.

See Procedure 20-2: Preparing Composite Resin Materials.

Dental Liners

As their name implies, a dental liner is a material that is placed to line the deepest portion of the cavity preparation. Their function is to provide pulpal protection or dentinal regeneration. The health of the tooth and the type of restorative material selected will determine what type of liner should be placed. The three most commonly placed types of liner are calcium hydroxide, dentin sealer, and cavity varnish.

Calcium Hydroxide

Calcium hydroxide is a frequently selected cavity liner because of its unique characteristics. Calcium hydroxide (1) helps protect the pulp from chemical irritation, (2) has the ability to stimulate reparative dentin, and (3) is compatible with all types of restorative materials. Calcium hydroxide is supplied as a paste or in a syringe (Figure 20-7).

See Procedure 20-3: Application of Calcium Hydroxide (Expanded Function).

Cavity Varnish

Cavity varnish is a liquid material that consists of one or more natural resins in an organic solvent. Application of a varnish accomplishes the following:

- Seals the dentinal tubules.
- Reduces microleakage around a restoration.
- Protects the tooth from highly acidic cements such as zinc phosphate.

Cavity varnish is contraindicated with composite resins and glass ionomer restorations because of interference with the materials.

Fluoride varnish is a highly effective cavity varnish and desensitizer. This gel-like material is designed to release fluoride on enamel, root structure, and dentin structure.

See Procedure 20-4: Application of Cavity Varnish (Expanded Function).

Dental Bases

When a tooth preparation becomes moderately deep to deep, placement of a base is necessary before placing the final restoration. This additional layer helps protect the pulp. A base can provide pulpal protection in three ways: as a protective base, as an insulating base, and as a sedative base.

Many of the dental cements that are discussed later in the chapter are used as a base by altering the measurements to the proper consistency.

Etching Systems

Acid etching, also referred to as a tooth conditioner, is a technique applied to a prepared tooth surface before using many permanent restorative materials. This system was first designed for the preparation of the enamel structure for composite materials and sealants, but research has found that etching a surface of enamel or dentin allows the dental material to have better retention to the tooth surface.

The primary ingredient in an etchant material is a phosphoric or maleic acid. This liquid or gel substance is applied to the enamel or dentin surface for a specified period to prepare the tooth for the bonding material.

See Procedure 20-5: Applying an Etchant Material (Expanded Function).

Bonding Systems

Bonding systems are liquid materials that flow into an etched surface of a tooth, creating a **micromechanical retention**. This self-cured or light-cured material improves the adherence between the tooth and the permanent restoration.

Enamel bonding allows the placement of sealants, orthodontic brackets, resin-bonded bridges, and bonded veneers. **Dentin bonding** allows the adhesion of another permanent material to the etched tooth structure. A major success associated with bonding to dentin is the removal of the smear layer through the etching process. The smear layer is a thin layer of debris that consists of fluids and tooth components that have remained on the dentin after cavity preparation; the smear layer needs to be removed.

See Procedure 20-6: Applying a Bonding System (Expanded Function).

Temporary Restorative Materials

A temporary restoration is a short-term restoration that is placed for a short period. This type of restoration is selected instead of a permanent restoration (1) when the condition of the tooth may be questionable, (2) when the patient's health may not permit more extensive dental treatment, and (3) for financial reasons.

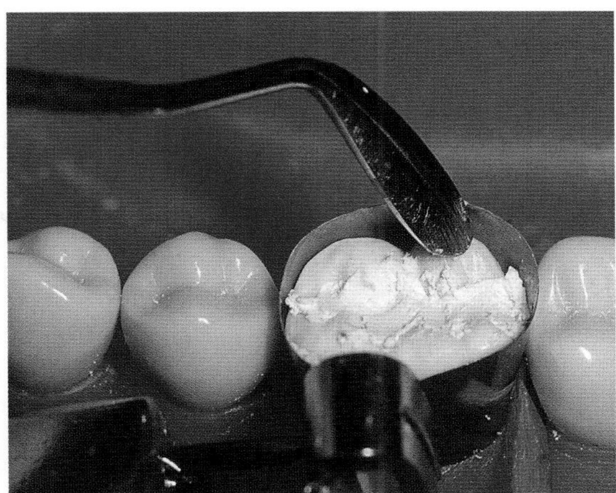

FIGURE 20-8 Placement of intermediate restorative material into a class II prepared molar.

The type of temporary restorative material selected depends on the location and amount of tooth structure that needs to be restored. The dental material most often used for a temporary restoration is **intermediate restorative material**, also referred to as **IRM**. IRM is a reinforced zinc oxide–eugenol material. The eugenol in this material has a sedative effect on the pulp, and fillers are added to improve the strength and durability of the material (Figure 20-8).

See Procedure 20-7: Mixing Intermediate Restorative Material.

Dental Cements

Dental cements represent a category of dental materials that is routinely used when working with indirect restorations (refer to Chapter 23 for types of casting). Depending on the dental procedure and the specific cement, there are three methods that are used for the preparation of a cement product.

1. A **luting agent** is used to permanently cement a casting to the tooth. This material should be fluid in its consistency to enable its application to the casting in a very thin layer.
2. A **temporary cement** holds two things together for a period. The consistency of the material should be slightly thicker than that of a luting agent. Most temporary cements have a healing agent in the material that is soothing to the pulp.
3. A **base** is placed on the pulpal floor of a prepared tooth before the placement of the permanent restoration. Some permanent cements have protective and insulating effects to soothe the pulp. The consistency of the material should resemble that of putty.

Mixing Dental Cements

Dental cements are supplied in various forms: liquid-powder mixes, capsules, and syringes. If using a liquid-powder method, then each type is mixed in a methodical manner. The differences include how the liquid and powder are dispensed, as well as the ratios of liquid to powder. When learning a new material, make sure to:

- Carefully read and follow the manufacturer's instructions.
- Determine the use, and then measure the powder and liquid according to the manufacturer's instructions.
- Place the powder toward one end of the glass slab or paper pad and the liquid toward the opposite end. (The space in the middle is for mixing.)
- Divide the powder into increments. Each manufacturer uses a slightly different system for sectioning the powder. Some divide it into equal parts; others divide the powder into progressively smaller increments. When increment sizes vary, the smaller increments are brought into the liquid first.
- Incorporate each powder increment into the liquid, and then thoroughly mix. (The mixing time per increment varies.)

Types of Cements

Zinc Oxide–Eugenol Cement

Zinc oxide–eugenol cement is one of the most versatile cements available.

Type I zinc oxide–eugenol (TempBond) is supplied as a two-paste system and is a temporary cement. The material is supplied either in a syringe or as two pastes that are dispensed in equal lengths on a paper pad and then mixed according to the manufacturer's directions.

Type II zinc oxide–eugenol is used as a base for permanent cementation of cast restorations or appliances. With a pH level of approximately 7.0, which is less acidic than most other cements, this cement material is known to be one of the least irritating of all dental cements.

Ortho-ethoxybenzoic acid is a stronger type of zinc oxide–eugenol cement and is also referred to as *reinforced*, *modified*, or *improved* zinc oxide–eugenol.

See Procedure 20-8: Mixing Zinc Oxide–Eugenol for a Base, Temporary Cementation, and Permanent Cementation.

Glass Ionomer Cements

Glass ionomer cement bonds to enamel, dentin, and metallic materials.

Type I glass ionomer cement is a luting cement used for metal and ceramic restorations and for direct bonding of orthodontic brackets. This cement is available in powder or liquid form and offers many advantages.

Advantages of Type I Glass Ionomer Cement

Type I glass ionomer:

- Is an acid-soluble calcium fluoroaluminosilicate glass; the slow release of fluoride from this powder inhibits recurrent decay.
- Causes less trauma to the pulp than many other types of cement.
- Has low solubility in the mouth.
- Slightly adheres to moist tooth surfaces.
- Has a very thin film thickness for excellent ease of seating.

Type II glass ionomer cement is designed for restoring areas of erosion near the gingival.

Type III glass ionomer cement is used as a liner and dentin bonding agent.

During preparation for glass ionomer cementation, the tooth should never be overdried, which can increase postoperative sensitivity. Glass ionomers are available in self-curing and light-cured formulas. They are supplied in powder and liquid, which are manually mixed, or in premeasured capsules, which are triturated. The capsules have the advantages of (1) being more convenient to use, (2) requiring less mixing time, and (3) producing consistent mixes because of the controlled powder-to-liquid ratio.

See Procedure 20-9: Mixing Glass Ionomer for Permanent Cementation.

Zinc Phosphate Cement

Zinc phosphate, one of the oldest dental cements in use, can be classified as follows:

Type I (fine-grain) zinc phosphate cement is used for the permanent cementation of cast restorations.

Type II (medium-grain) zinc phosphate cement is recommended for use as an insulating base for deep cavity preparations.

Zinc phosphate cement is exothermic in action. (**Exothermic** means giving off heat.) To dissipate heat before placing in the casting or in the cavity preparation, the cement must be spatulated over a wide area of a cool, dry, thick glass slab.

The temperature of the glass slab is an important variable in the mixing of zinc phosphate cement. The ideal temperature for the slab is 68° F (20° C). A warmer slab will shorten the setting time of the cement, and a colder slab will increase the setting time. Colder temperatures can cause condensation on the slab, and the moisture can weaken the material.

See Procedure 20-10: Mixing Zinc Phosphate for a Base and Permanent Cementation.

Polycarboxylate Cement

Polycarboxylate cement, also known as *polyacrylic cement,* is used as a luting agent for cast restorations and cementation of orthodontic bands. The material is supplied as a powder and a liquid. The composition of the powder is similar to that of zinc phosphate cement. The liquid is made up of polyacrylic acid and water. The liquid has a limited shelf life because it thickens over time when the water evaporates. If evaporation occurs, then the liquid should be discarded.

See Procedure 20-11: Mixing Polycarboxylate for a Base and Permanent Cementation.

Tooth-Whitening Materials

Tooth-whitening products are available in everyday items, such as toothpaste, floss, mouth rinses, and even chewing gum. Most tooth-whitening products are made from a peroxide-based ingredient and are supplied in different concentrations (10%, 16%, and 22%). The peroxide-based whitening product works deep within the enamel to remove staining and discoloration that have come from years of accumulated stain and aging

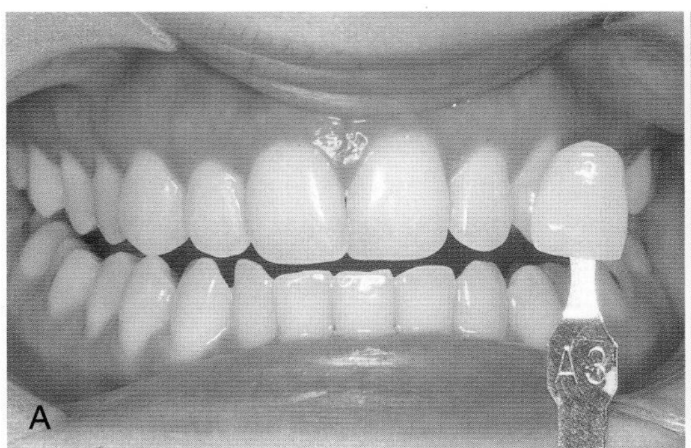

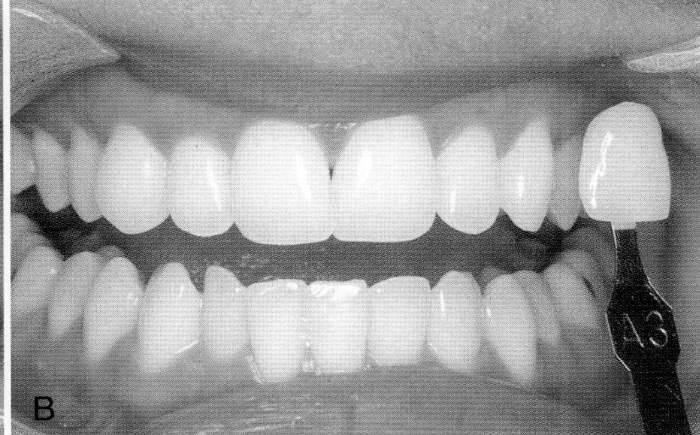

FIGURE 20-9 Before **(A)** and after **(B)** using a whitening product.

(Figure 20-9). When the peroxide-based product contacts the teeth, it allows oxygen to enter the enamel and then whitens the colored substances.

Methods of Tooth Whitening

Patients can choose from two distinct options when wanting to whiten their teeth: (1) in-office or (2) at-home **tooth whitening**.

Most in-office whitening procedures is power or light-accelerated bleaching, also referred to as laser bleaching. This technique uses light energy to speed the process of bleaching. Different types of energy can be used in this procedure, with the most common being the halogen light. A power bleaching treatment typically involves the isolation of soft tissue with a resin-based, light-curable barrier; the application of a professional dental-grade hydrogen-peroxide whitening gel (25% to 38% hydrogen peroxide); and exposure to the light source for 6 to 15 minutes. Most power teeth-whitening treatments can be performed in approximately 30 minutes to 1 hour, during a single visit.

For at-home whitening systems, a patient has custom trays fabricated, and a prescribed amount of bleaching agent is prescribed on a daily use. The bleaching gel typically contains between 10% and 30% carbamide peroxide (15% is recommended), which is roughly equivalent to a 3% to 10% hydrogen-peroxide concentration.

Ethical Implications

Preparing and mixing restorative materials must be precise and exact. The dentist expects the clinical assistant to be knowledgeable and experienced with the materials used in the dental office. The dental team is responsible for educating patients about what to expect with a newly placed restoration and how they should feel and care for that restoration.

Procedure 20-1

Mixing and Transferring Dental Amalgam

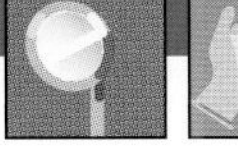
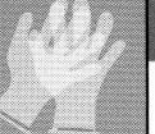
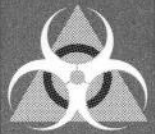
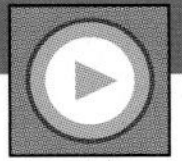

Equipment and Supplies

- Amalgam capsule
- Capsule activator
- Amalgamator
- Amalgam well or cloth
- Amalgam carrier

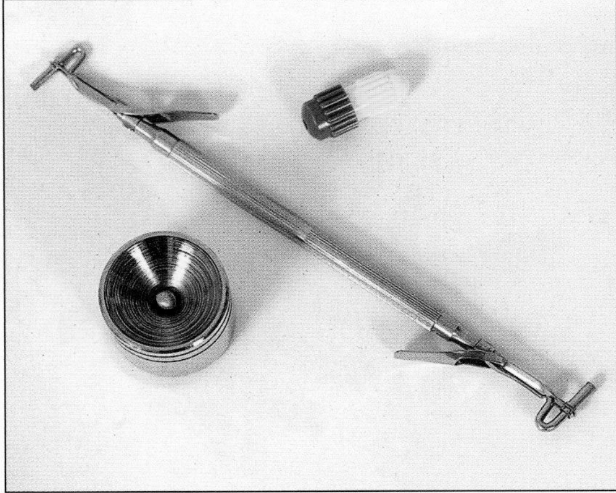

Procedural Steps

1. Activate the capsule using the activator, if required, for the type of amalgam.

Purpose: The activator breaks the separating membrane to allow the mercury and alloy powder to mix.

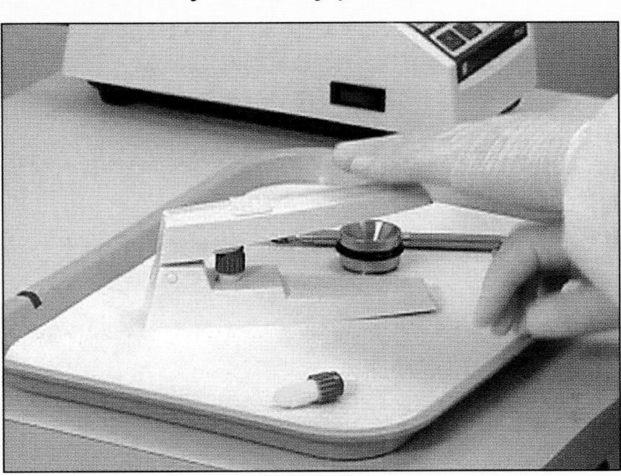

Continued

Procedure 20-1

Mixing and Transferring Dental Amalgam—cont'd

2. Place the capsule in the amalgamator.

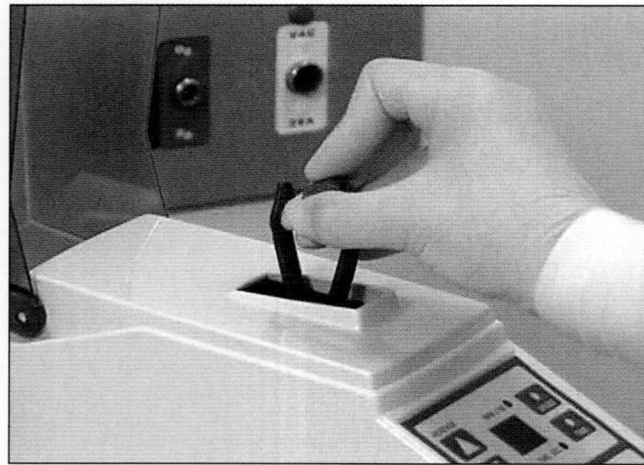

3. Adjust the settings on the amalgamator.
4. Close the cover on the amalgamator, and begin trituration.
5. Remove the capsule, twist it open, and dispense amalgam in the well or amalgam cloth.

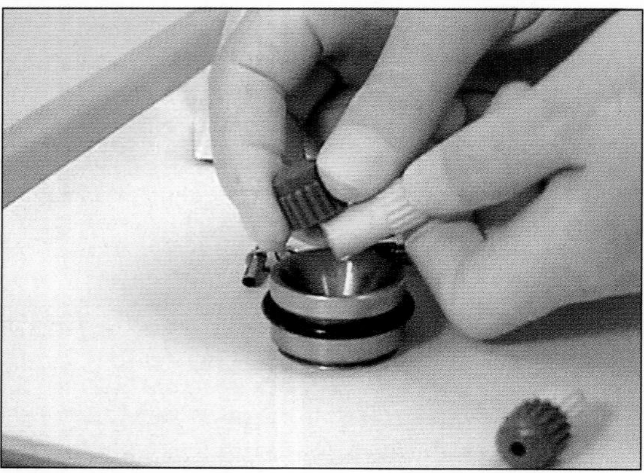

6. Fill the small end of the carrier first; then transfer the carrier, making sure that the end of the carrier is directed toward the preparation.

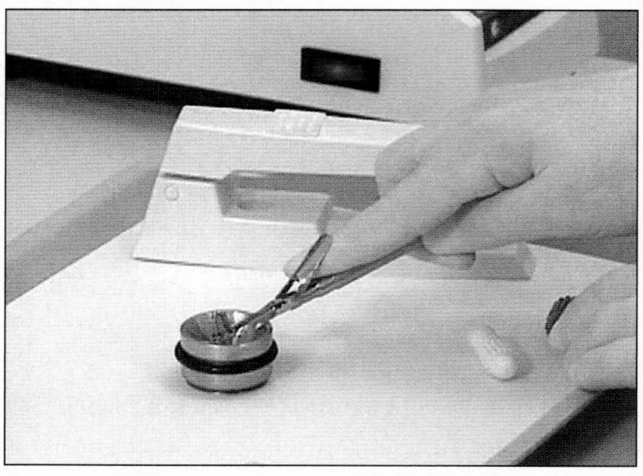

7. Transfer the carrier to the operator with the small end facing toward the tooth to be filled.

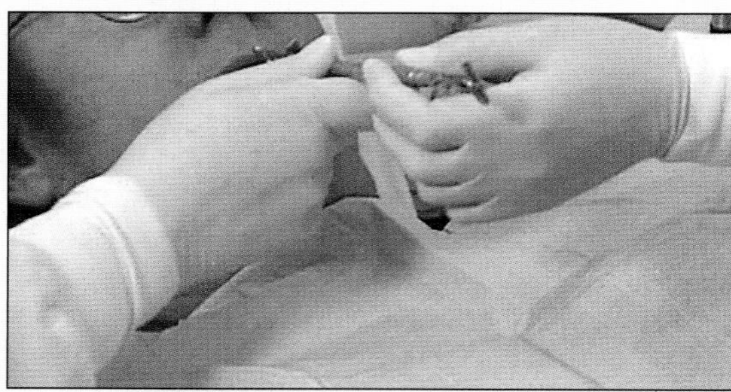

8. Continue this process until the preparation is overfilled.

Procedure 20-2

Preparing Composite Resin Materials

Equipment and Supplies

- Shade guide
- Composite resin material
- Treated paper pad or material dispenser
- Composite instrument
- 2 × 2-inch alcohol gauze pads
- Curing light

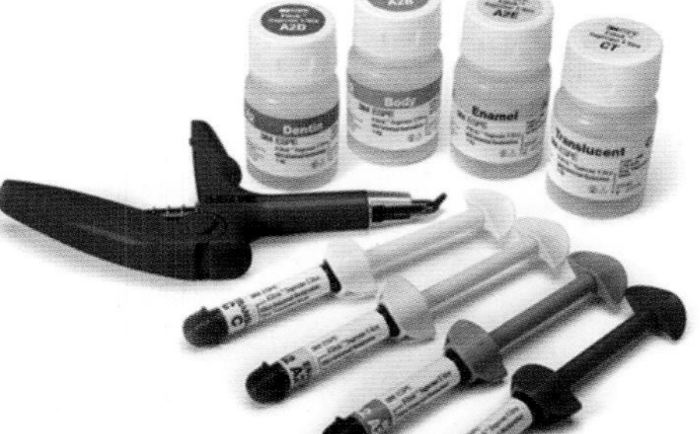

(Courtesy 3M ESPE, St. Paul, Minnesota.)

Procedure 20-2

Preparing Composite Resin Materials—cont'd

Procedural Steps

1. Select the shade of the tooth.

Purpose: Composites are supplied in varying shades. With the use of a shade guide, select the shade that most closely resembles the patient's natural tooth color.

Note: Use natural lighting for making this decision. Fluorescent lighting can alter the natural tooth color.

2. Once the shade is selected, prepare the composite syringe or express the amount for the restoration onto the treated pad or in the light-protected well.

Note: Most often, you will need a very small amount; therefore do not waste the material.

3. Transfer the composite instrument and material to the transfer zone for the dentist.
4. The dentist may ask for the liquid bonding resin or alcohol gauze to be available during the placement of material increments.

Purpose: These will aid in the flow of material.

5. Have the curing light ready during the placement of the material. The best time to light-cure the material is as the increments are placed.

Purpose: This step completes the final setting of the material.

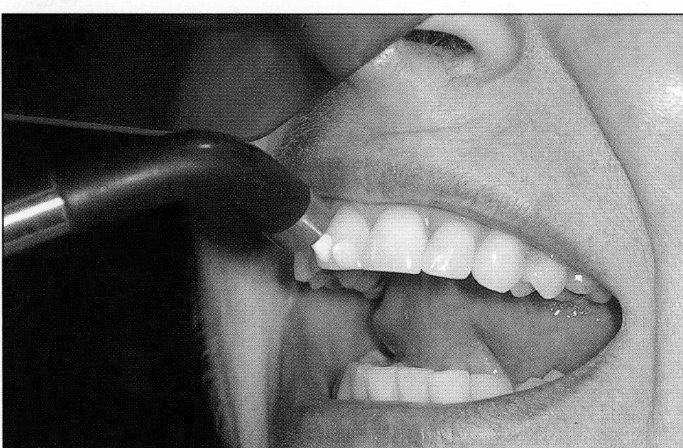

Procedure 20-3

Application of Calcium Hydroxide (Expanded Function)

Equipment and Supplies

- Small paper mixing pad
- Small spatula
- Calcium hydroxide applicator
- Calcium hydroxide base and catalyst paste (from the same manufacturer)
- 2 × 2-inch gauze pads

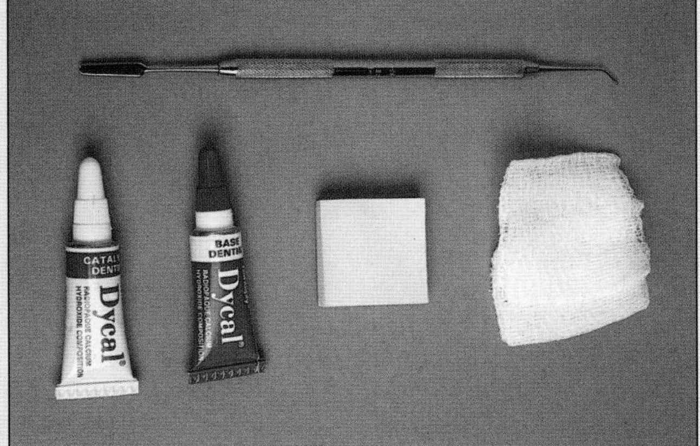

Procedural Steps

1. Dispense small, equal amounts of the catalyst and base pastes onto the paper mixing pad.

Purpose: The area to be covered will be 0.5 to 1 mm, depending on the size of the cavity preparation.

2. Using a circular motion, quickly mix (10 to 15 seconds) the material over a small area of the paper pad with the spatula.

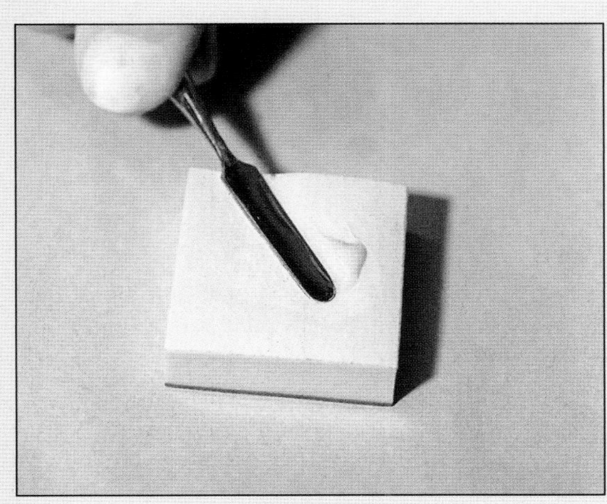

Continued

Procedure 20-3

Application of Calcium Hydroxide (Expanded Function)—cont'd

3. Use gauze to clean the spatula.
4. With the tip of the applicator, pick up a small amount of the material, and apply a thin layer at the deepest area of the preparation.
5. Use an explorer to remove any material from the enamel before drying.
6. Clean and disinfect the equipment.

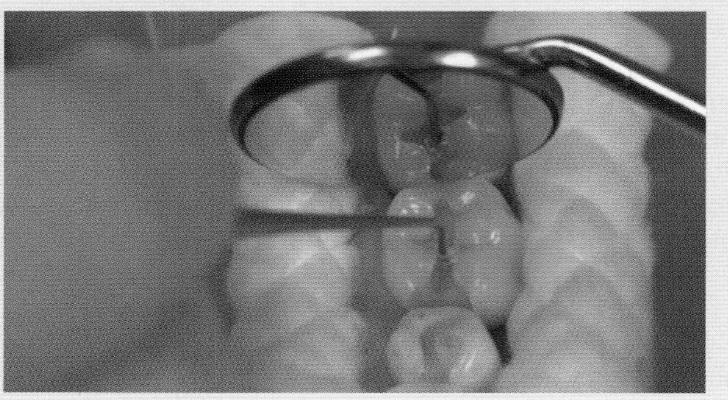

Procedure 20-4

Application of Dental Varnish (Expanded Function)

EF

Equipment and Supplies

- Microbrush applicators (2)
- Cotton pliers and cotton pellets (2)
- Dental varnish

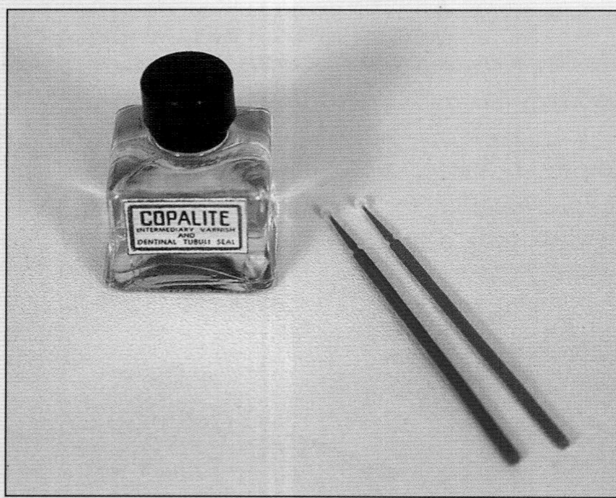

Procedural Steps

1. Retrieve a new applicator or cotton pellets in cotton pliers.
2. Open the bottle of varnish, and place the tip of the applicator or cotton pellet into the liquid.
3. Immediately replace the cap on the bottle.

Purpose: When varnish is exposed to the air, evaporation causes this liquid to thicken. If it becomes too thick, then a thinning agent must be added.

4. Place a thin coating of varnish on the walls, floor, and margin of the cavity preparation. Allow it to air-dry.
5. Apply a second coat, and repeat steps 1 through 4.

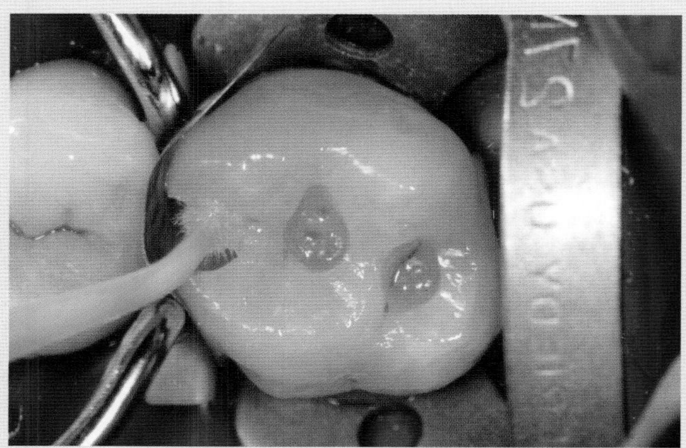

(From Heymann HO, Swift EJ, Ritter AV: *Sturdevant's art and science of operative dentistry,* ed 6, St. Louis, 2013, Mosby.)

Procedure 20-5

Applying an Etchant Material (Expanded Function)

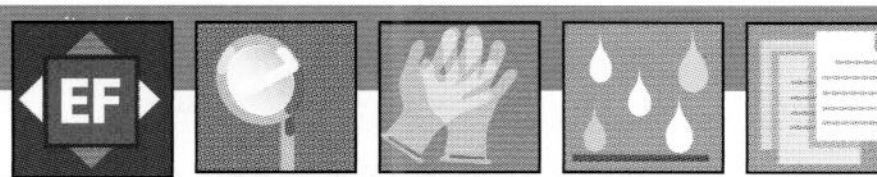

Equipment and Supplies

- Basic setup
- Cotton rolls and/or dental dam for isolation
- Applicator (cotton pellets for liquid etchant and syringe tip for gel)
- Etchant material
- High-velocity evacuator
- Air-water syringe
- Timer

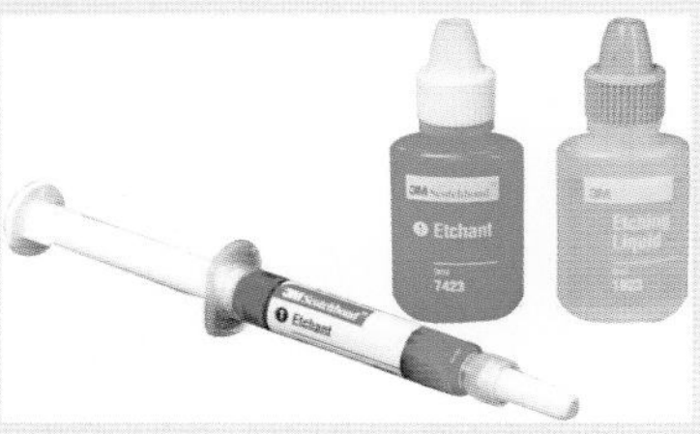

(Courtesy 3M ESPE, St. Paul, MN.)

Procedural Steps

1. The prepared tooth must be isolated from contamination. A dental dam or cotton rolls are placed before the etching process begins.

Purpose: Saliva must not contaminate the preparation.

2. The surface of the tooth structure must be clean and free of any debris, plaque, or calculus before etching.

Purpose: Debris on the surface may interfere with the etching process.

3. After cleaning, the surface is carefully dried but is not desiccated.

Purpose: Too much drying of the tooth structure will harm the tooth.

4. The etchant material is selected. Most manufacturers supply a gel etchant in a syringe that can be applied to enamel or dentin.

Purpose: The gel allows the etchant to be carefully placed only where needed.

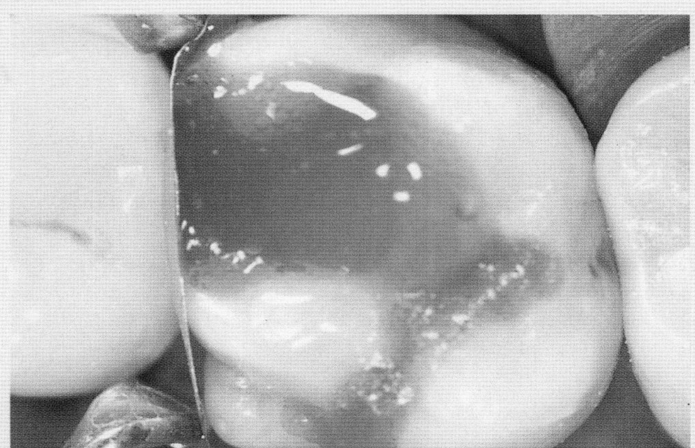

(Courtesy Dr. William Libenberg. From Hatrick CD, Eakle WS, Bird WF: *Dental materials: clinical applications for dental assistants and dental hygienists,* ed 2, St. Louis, 2011, Saunders.)

5. The tooth structure is etched for the time recommended by the manufacturer, usually ranging from 15 to 30 seconds.

Purpose: The exact time depends on the material and its use. For example, etching time for placing sealants is not the same as etching time for bonding orthodontic brackets.

6. After etching, the surface is thoroughly rinsed and dried for 15 to 30 seconds.
7. An etched surface has a frosty-white appearance. If the surface does not have this appearance or has been contaminated with moisture, then repeat the etching process.

Procedure 20-6

Applying a Bonding System (Expanded Function)

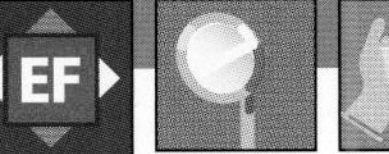

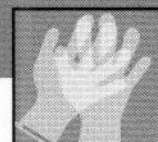
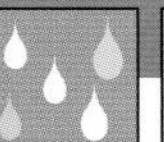
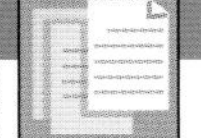

Equipment and Supplies

- Bonding agent
- Applicator device or brush
- Air-water syringe
- Oral evacuation system
- 2 × 2-inch gauze pads

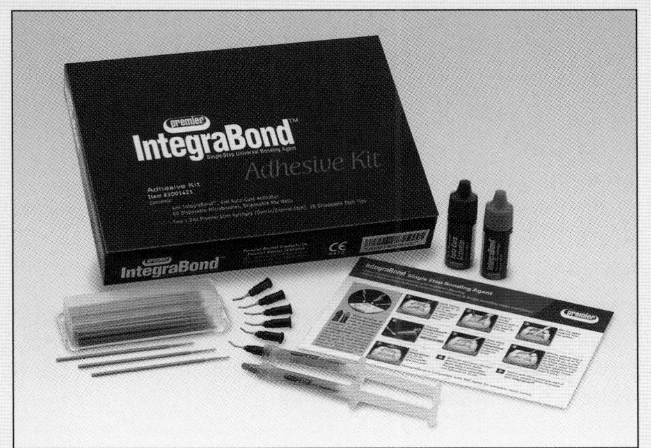

Continued

Procedure 20-6

Applying a Bonding System (Expanded Function)—cont'd

Procedural Steps

1. If a metal matrix band is used, then the band is prepared with cavity varnish or wax before placing it around the tooth.

Purpose: This step prevents the bonding resin and amalgam from adhering to the surface (see Chapter 21 for the application of a matrix).

2. The cavity preparation and the enamel margins should be etched according to the manufacturer's directions.
3. A primer is applied to the entire preparation in one or multiple coats, depending on the manufacturer's directions.
4. The dual-cured adhesive resin is placed in the entire cavity preparation and is lightly air-thinned. The resin should appear unset or partially set.

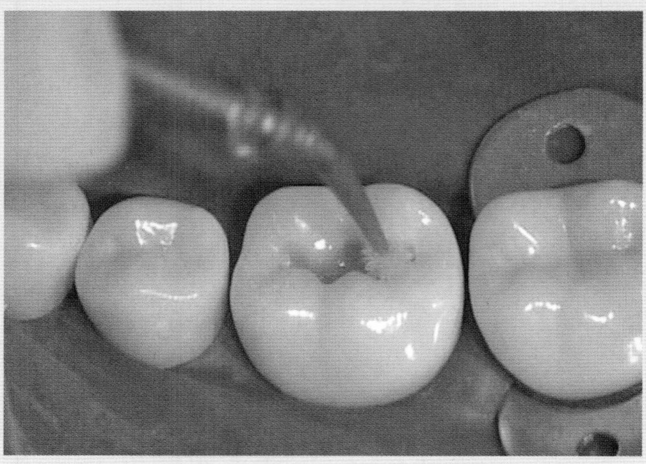

5. The restorative material is mixed and then readied for placement into the cavity preparation.

Purpose: This step integrates the restorative material and bonding material at the preparation walls before the resin has had time to polymerize (set).

Procedure 20-7

Mixing Intermediate Restorative Material

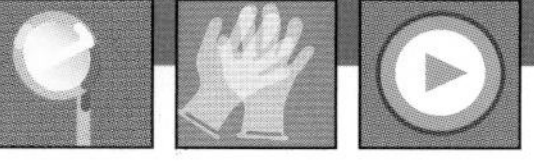

Equipment and Supplies

- Treated paper pad
- Spatula (flexible stainless steel)
- Intermediate restorative materials (IRMs)—powder and dispenser
- IRM liquid and dropper
- 2 × 2-inch alcohol gauze

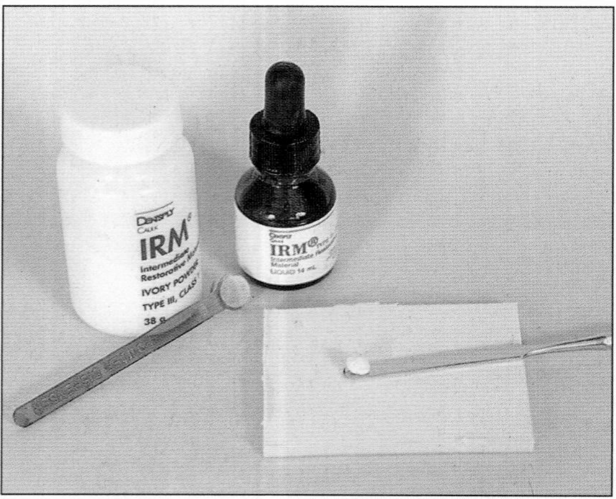

Procedural Steps

1. Shake the powder before dispensing, and then measure the powder onto the mixing pad.

Purpose: When the powder is fluffed, it will not be as packed, thus creating a drier mix.

2. IRM is dispensed in equal ratios, meaning one scoop of powder to one drop of liquid. Make a well in one half of the powder, and then dispense the liquid into the mix. Recap the containers.
3. Incorporate the remaining powder into the mixture in two or three increments, and thoroughly mix with the spatula. The mix will be quite stiff at this stage.
4. Wipe the mix back and forth on the mixing pad for 5 to 10 seconds. The resulting mix should be smooth and adaptable. The mix must be completed within 1 minute.
5. Immediately clean and disinfect the equipment.

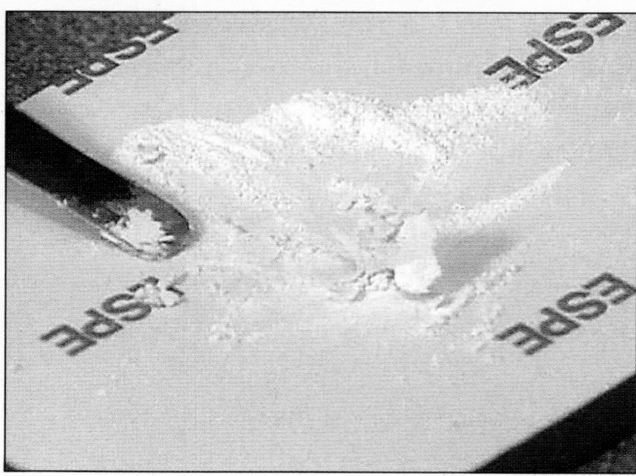

Procedure 20-8

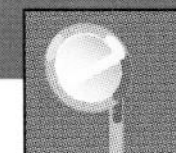
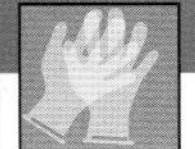

Mixing Zinc Oxide–Eugenol for a Base, Temporary Cementation, and Permanent Cementation

Equipment and Supplies

- Treated paper pad or glass slab
- Spatula (flexible stainless steel)
- Zinc oxide powder and dispenser
- Eugenol liquid and dropper
- 2 × 2-inch gauze pads

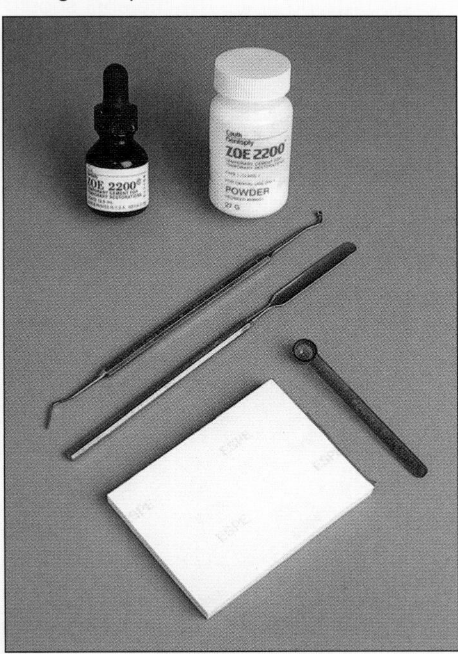

(From Bird DL, Robinson DS: *Modern dental assisting,* ed 11, St. Louis, 2015, Saunders.)

Zinc Oxide–Eugenol (ZOE) as a Base

Procedural Steps

1. Measure the powder onto the mixing pad. Immediately replace the cap.
2. Dispense the liquid near the powder on the mixing pad. Immediately replace the cap.
3. Incorporate one half of the powder into the liquid, and mix with the spatula for 20 to 30 seconds.
4. Incorporate the remaining portion into the mixture. Continue mixing for an additional 20 to 30 seconds. The material should be thick and have a puttylike appearance.

ZOE as Permanent Cement

Procedural Steps

1. Measure the powder, and place it onto the mixing pad or glass slab. Immediately replace the cap on the powder.
2. Dispense the liquid near the powder. Immediately replace the cap on the liquid container.
3. Incorporate the powder and liquid all at once, and then mix with the spatula for 30 seconds.
4. Initially, the mix is puttylike; with additional mixing for 30 seconds, however, the mix will become more fluid for loading into the casting.
5. Immediately clean and disinfect the equipment.

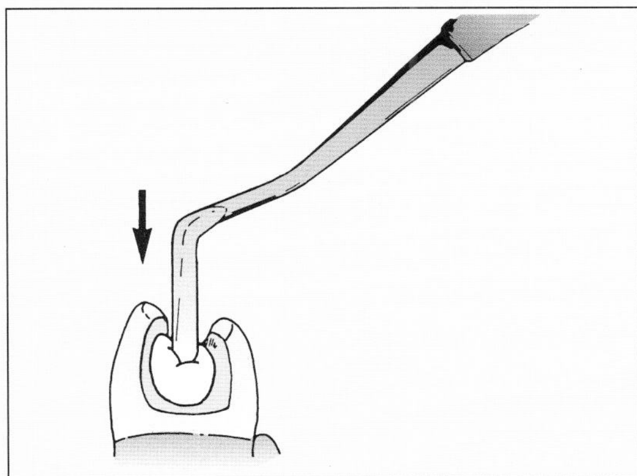

(From Baum L, Phillips RW, Lund MR: *Textbook of operative dentistry,* ed 3, Philadelphia, 1995, Saunders.)

Procedure 20-9

Mixing Glass Ionomer for Permanent Cementation

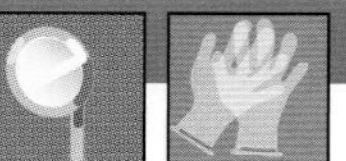

Equipment and Supplies

- Paper mixing pad
- Spatula (flexible stainless steel)
- Glass ionomer powder and dispenser
- Glass ionomer liquid and dropper
- 2 × 2-inch gauze pads

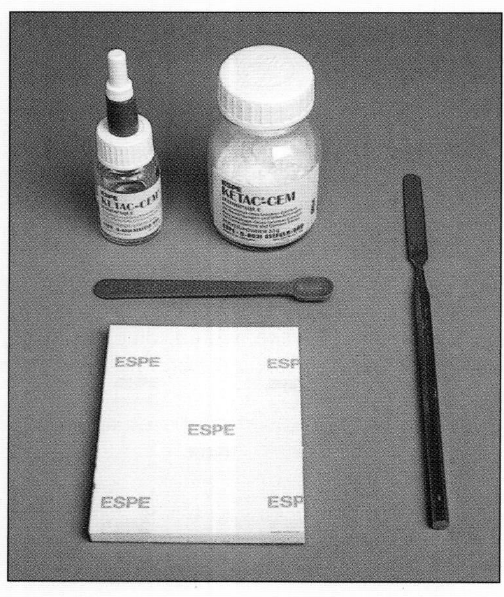

Procedural Steps

1. Dispense the manufacturer's recommended proportion of the liquid on one half of the paper pad.
2. Dispense the manufacturer's recommended proportion of the powder on the other half of the pad; the powder is usually divided into two or three increments.
3. Incorporate the powder and the liquid, following the recommended mixing time. The material should have a glossy appearance.
4. Immediately clean and disinfect the equipment.

Procedure 20-10

Mixing Zinc Phosphate for a Base and Permanent Cementation

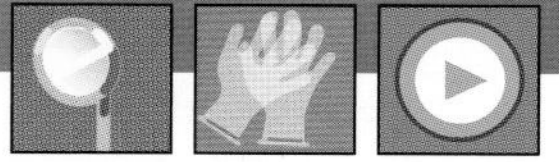

Equipment and Supplies

- Glass slab (cool)
- Spatula (flexible stainless steel)
- Zinc phosphate powder and dispenser
- Zinc phosphate liquid and dropper
- 2 × 2-inch gauze pads

Zinc Phosphate for a Base

Procedural Steps

1. Dispense the powder and liquid onto the pad.

Note: When used for a base, the liquid portion is decreased to make a thicker consistency.

2. Incorporate all the powder into the liquid; the total mixing time should not exceed 45 seconds.
3. Form the completed mix into a small ball.

Zinc Phosphate for Permanent Cementation

Procedural Steps

Preparing the Mix

1. Dispense the powder toward one end of the slab and the liquid at the opposite end.
2. Recap the containers.

Purpose: These materials are damaged by prolonged exposure to air and humidity.

3. Divide the powder into small increments as directed by the manufacturer.
4. Incorporate each powder increment into the liquid.

Note: When increment sizes vary, the smaller increments are used first. Mixing time per increment also varies; the time is approximately 15 to 20 seconds.

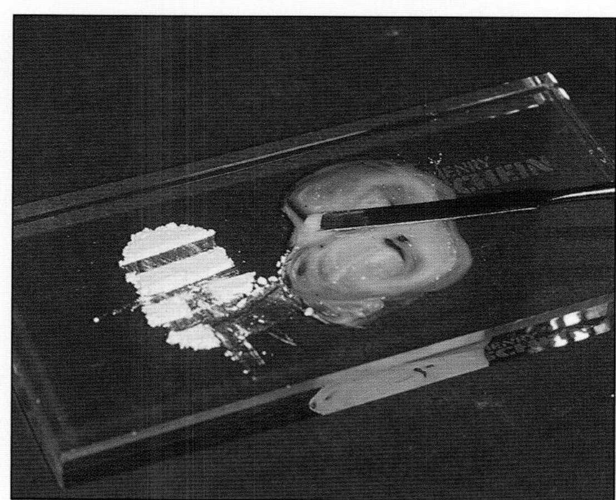

Procedure 20-10

Mixing Zinc Phosphate for a Base and Permanent Cementation—cont'd

5. Thoroughly spatulate the mix, using broad strokes or a figure-eight movement over a large area of the slab.

Purpose: This step helps dissipate the heat that is generated during mixing.

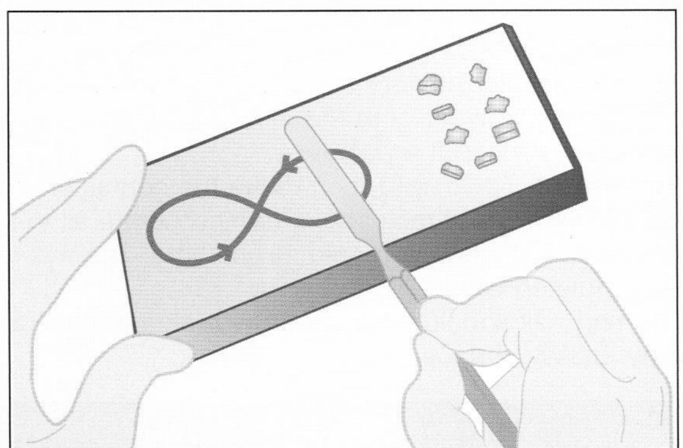

6. Test the material for appropriate cementation consistency. The cement should string up and break approximately 1 inch from the slab. Total mixing time is approximately 1 to 2 minutes.

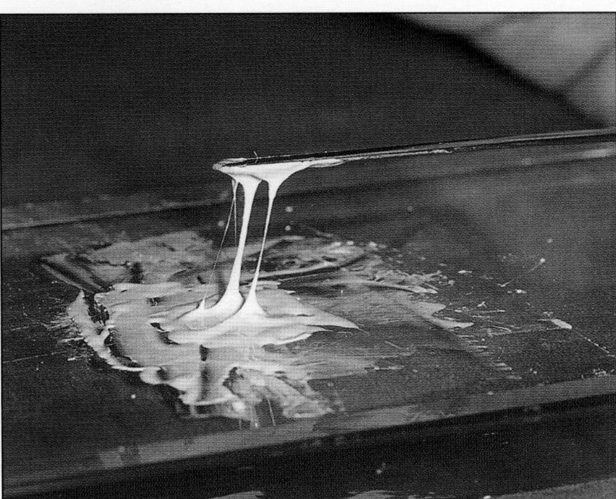

Placing Cement in the Casting. In addition to preparing and mixing the material, the assistant will have the important responsibility of placing the cement in the casting.

7. Hold the casting with the inner portion facing upward.
8. Retrieve the cement onto the spatula. Scrape the edge of the spatula along the margin to cause the cement to flow from the spatula into the casting.

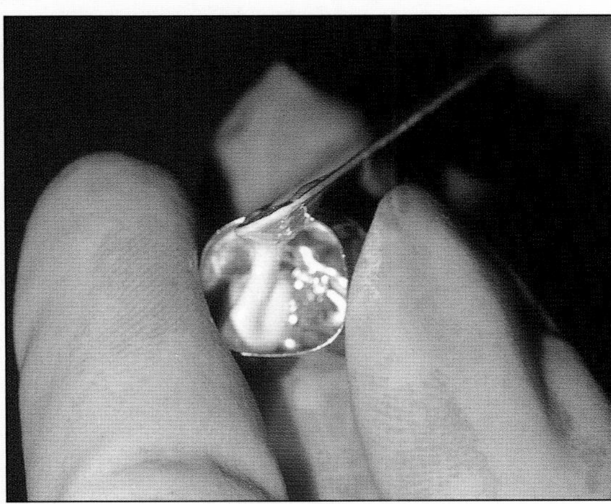

9. Place the tip of the spatula or a black spoon into the bulk of the cement; move the material so that it covers all internal walls with a thin lining of cement.
10. Turn the casting over in your palm, and transfer it to the dentist.

Purpose: By having the outer portion of the casting facing up, the dentist can safely rotate it to obtain a better grasp for seating it.

11. Transfer a cotton roll so that the patient can bite down on it to help seat the crown and displace the excess cement.
12. Immediately clean and disinfect the equipment.

Procedure 20-11

Mixing Polycarboxylate for a Base and Permanent Cementation

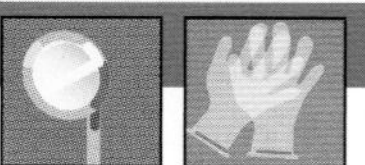

Equipment and Supplies

- Treated paper pad or glass slab
- Spatula (flexible stainless steel)
- Polycarboxylate powder and dispenser
- Polycarboxylate liquid (in plastic squeeze bottle or calibrated syringe)
- 2 × 2-inch gauze pads

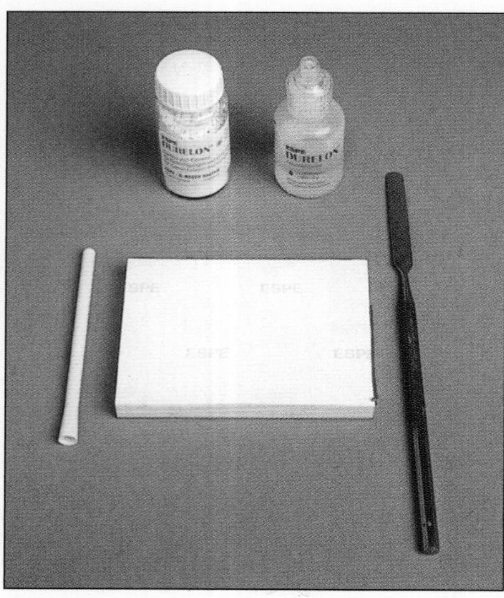

Polycarboxylate for a Base

Procedural Steps

1. Dispense the powder and liquid onto the pad.

Note: When used for a base, the liquid portion is decreased to make a thicker consistency.

2. Incorporate all the powder into the liquid; the total mixing time should not exceed 45 seconds.
3. Form the completed mix into a small ball.

Polycarboxylate for Permanent Cement

Procedural Steps

1. Gently shake the powder to fluff the ingredients. Measure the powder onto the mixing pad, and immediately recap the container.
2. Dispense the liquid, and then recap the container.
3. Use the flat side of the spatula to incorporate all the powder quickly into the liquid at one time. The mix must be completed within 30 seconds.
4. A correct mix should be somewhat thick and have a shiny, glossy surface.

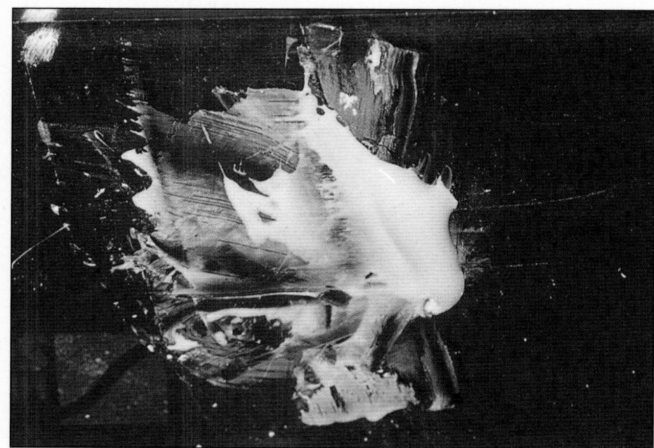

5. Immediately clean and disinfect the equipment.

Chapter Exercises

Multiple Choice

Circle the letter next to the correct answer.

1. Dental cements are versatile in their use. How is dental cement used in a restorative procedure?
   - **a.** As a liner
   - **b.** As an insulating base
   - **c.** For permanent cementation
   - **d.** b and c
2. When two metals touch in the mouth, a small shock is created. This shock is known as a __________.
   - **a.** deformation
   - **b.** galvanic action
   - **c.** microleakage
   - **d.** thermal conduction
3. Glass ionomer cement is unique because it can be used as a __________.
   - **a.** base
   - **b.** luting agent
   - **c.** restorative material
   - **d.** a, b, and c
4. Before dentin bonding, the smear layer is removed from the prepared tooth surface by the process of __________.
   - **a.** drying
   - **b.** etching
   - **c.** sealing
   - **d.** varnish
5. The completed mix of polycarboxylate cement should appear __________.
   - **a.** dull
   - **b.** glossy
   - **c.** puttylike
   - **d.** stringy
6. The slow release of fluoride in __________ cements is capable of inhibiting recurrent decay.
   - **a.** zinc oxide–eugenol
   - **b.** IRM
   - **c.** zinc phosphate
   - **d.** glass ionomer
7. When working with light-cured composite resins, the darker the shade of the material, the __________ the curing time required.
   - **a.** longer
   - **b.** shorter
8. A(n) __________ restoration is expected to last from a few weeks to a few months.
   - **a.** amalgam
   - **b.** composite resin
   - **c.** temporary
   - **d.** sealant
9. An alloy is a __________.
   - **a.** cement used in the adherence of a restoration
   - **b.** tooth-colored material for anterior teeth
   - **c.** mixture of metals
   - **d.** base material placed for insulating effects
10. Zinc phosphate cement should be mixed __________.
    - **a.** on a paper pad
    - **b.** on a cool, thick glass slab
    - **c.** on a treated paper pad
    - **d.** in an amalgamator

Apply Your Knowledge

1. You are preparing to mix zinc phosphate material for a permanent cementation of a crown. You notice that after you have incorporated half of the powder, the cement is starting to thicken. What could have happened? Should you (1) stop mixing and use the mix at this point, (2) keep incorporating all of the powder, or (3) start over?
2. A patient comes in for an emergency appointment because of losing a "filling" and describes discomfort in the tooth. The tooth involved is tooth #4. What would be your protocol for the emergency situation with this patient?
3. The patient from the emergency appointment comes back to have a new amalgam restoration placed in tooth #4. Dr. Smith explains that the decay is very close to the pulp and that some sensitivity may be felt in the area. What material would the dentist possibly recommend to decrease the sensitivity for the patient?

CHAPTER 21

Restorative Procedures

http://evolve.elsevier.com/Robinson/essentials/

LEARNING OBJECTIVES

1. Pronounce, define, and spell the key terms.
2. Define *restorative dentistry* and *esthetic dentistry* and discuss dental conditions requiring both types of treatment.
3. Describe the process and principles of tooth preparation.
4. Give the importance of the matrix system for Class II, III, and IV restorations, and demonstrate the following procedures:
   - Assemble a matrix band and universal retainer.
   - Place a plastic matrix for a Class III or Class IV restoration.
   - Place and remove a matrix band and wedge for a Class II restoration.
5. Discuss permanent and complex restorations, and describe the procedures of both an amalgam and a composite restoration.
6. Describe veneers.
7. Describe vital bleaching.

KEY TERMS

cavity
esthetic dentistry
matrix
operative dentistry
preparation
restorations
restorative dentistry
veneer
vital bleaching
wedge

Restorative dentistry, also referred to as **operative dentistry**, is an integral part of the general dental practice. This chapter introduces the background knowledge and describes the techniques necessary for the clinical dental assistant to be better prepared when assisting with restorative procedures in a general dental practice.

Responsibilities of the Dental Assistant in a Restorative Dental Procedure

- Preparing the tray setup, paper products, and dental materials
- Knowing and understanding the sequence of a specific procedure
- Having the ability to anticipate the dentist's needs
- Assisting in the examination of the tooth or teeth (see Chapter 12)
- Assisting in the administration of local anesthesia (see Chapter 14)
- Assisting in moisture control (see Chapter 10)
- Assisting in the removal of decay (see Chapter 19)
- Assisting in the placement of dental materials (see Chapter 20)
- Maintaining patient comfort and appropriate exposure control precautions
- Performing legally permitted delegated expanded functions

Restorative dentistry is indicated when teeth are to be restored to their original structure with the use of direct and indirect restorative dental materials. The common types of procedures include amalgam **restorations**, composite resin restorations, and complex restorations.

Dental Conditions Requiring Restorative Dental Treatment

- Management and treatment of carious lesions by restoring them with a permanent restoration
- Restoration of defects in tooth structure
- Replacement of failed restorations
- Abrasion or wearing away of tooth structure
- Erosion of tooth structure

Esthetic dentistry is directed on improving the appearance of teeth by restoring imperfections with direct and indirect restorative materials or with the use of whitening techniques. The common types of procedures are composite resin restorations, resin veneer restorations, and tooth whitening.

Dental Conditions Requiring Esthetic Dental Treatment

- Discoloration attributable to extrinsic or intrinsic staining
- Anomalies caused by developmental disturbances
- Abnormal spacing between teeth
- Trauma

Cavity Preparation

Regardless of the type of dental material selected, understanding the steps of a restorative procedure is important. The steps include removal of the decay by the dentist, **preparation** of the tooth **cavity**, placement of dental materials, and finishing the restoration.

The most detailed part in restoring a tooth is the cavity preparation. The purpose of cavity preparation is to remove the decay along with a small amount of healthy tooth structure, which, when completed, provides a solid foundation for the restorative dental material to be placed as a final restoration. To understand the different types of tooth preparations, you can review the types of cavity classifications in Chapter 12.

The dentist will use a high-speed handpiece with a variety of burs and hand instruments to accomplish this preparation step. Once the decay is removed, the dentist will use the high-speed handpiece with a different-shape bur to place retentive grooves in the preparation. These small grooves in the tooth allow the material to flow into the groove area, harden, and create the retentive result.

In the next step, the dentist determines the type of restorative material that will be used. This decision is based on the size, shape, and location of the preparation. With small preparations, an amalgam or composite material can be directly placed over sound dentin. With deeper preparations, a cavity liner, base, and bonding material may be required before the amalgam or composite is placed.

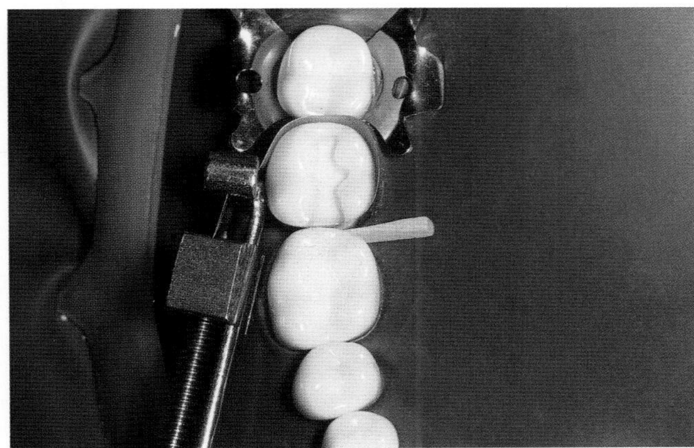

FIGURE 21-1 Matrix and wedge correctly positioned.

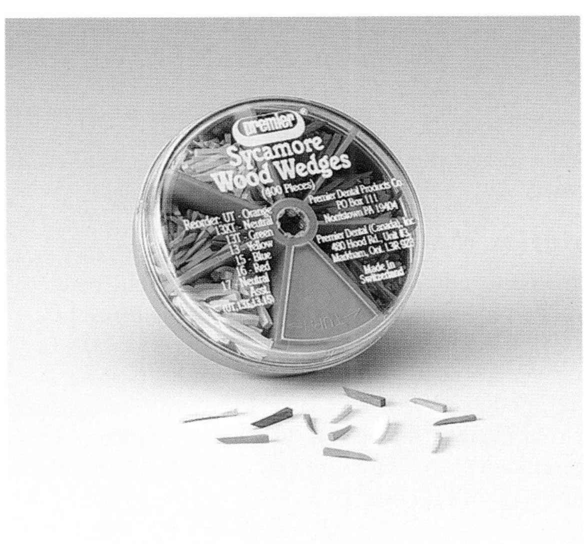

FIGURE 21-2 Assortment of wedges. (Courtesy Premier Dental Products Company, Plymouth Meeting, Pennsylvania.)

Matrix Systems

A tooth that is to receive a Class II, III, or IV restoration will have a minimum of one interproximal wall or surface of the tooth removed during the cavity preparation stage. By including the use of a matrix system, a temporary wall is created, against which the restorative material is placed until the material has set.

The universal retainer and matrix band is the system most commonly used when placing posterior restorations (Figure 21-1). The retainer firmly holds the matrix in place. A **matrix** is a metal or clear plastic band used to replace the missing proximal wall of a tooth during placement of the restorative material. (*Matrix* is singular. The plural form is *matrices.*) Clear plastic matrices are used for anterior composite restorations.

A **wedge** is triangular or round and is supplied in wood or plastic (Figure 21-2). The wedge is available in different sizes, depending on the location and space between the teeth. By

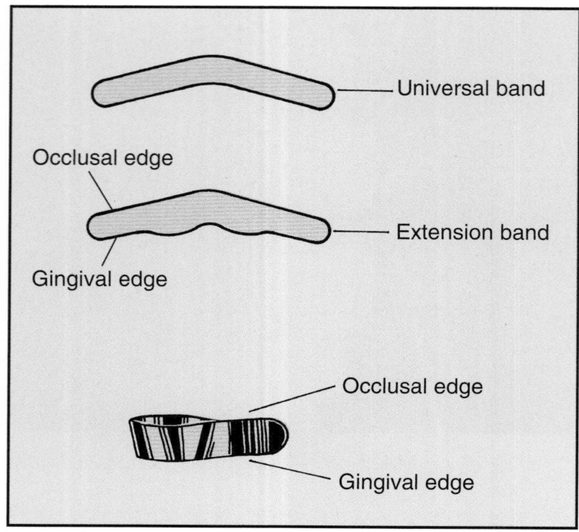

FIGURE 21-3 Assorted matrix bands.

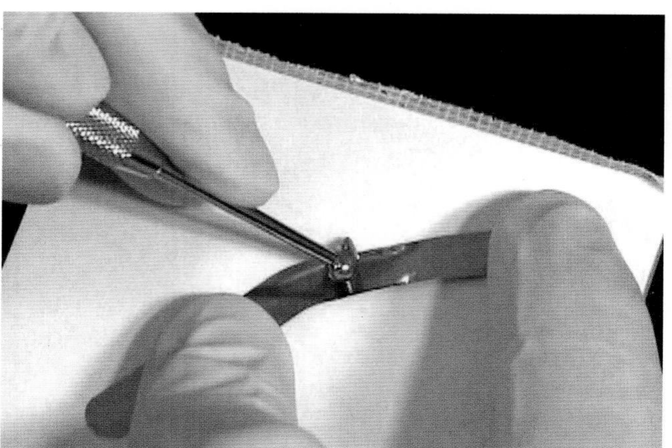
FIGURE 21-4 Burnishing the matrix band will provide a better contour. (From Heymann HO, Swift EJ, Ritter AV: *Sturdevant's art and science of operative dentistry,* ed 6, St. Louis, 2013, Mosby.)

placing a wedge, the proper anatomic contour of a restoration is created.

Posterior Matrix System

The matrix band and universal retainer should be assembled before the procedure to save time during the procedure.

Matrix Bands

Matrix bands selected for Class II posterior restorations are made of a flexible stainless steel and are available in **universal** and **extension** sizes. The band wraps around the tooth, creating a temporary wall (Figure 21-3).

Before the band and the retainer are assembled, the band should be **contoured** in the proximal area so the tooth can make proper contact with the adjacent tooth (Figure 21-4). To contour the band, place the band on a paper pad, using a burnisher or handle end of cotton pliers. Rub the inner surface of the band until the ends begin to curl. This thins the band and provides a normal curvature of the band to fit around the tooth.

Universal Retainer

The universal retainer, also referred to as Tofflemire retainer, is a device that holds the matrix band in position. The components of the universal retainer are described in the box titled "Components of a Universal Retainer."

See Procedure 21-1: Assembling a Matrix Band and Universal Retainer.

Components of a Universal Retainer

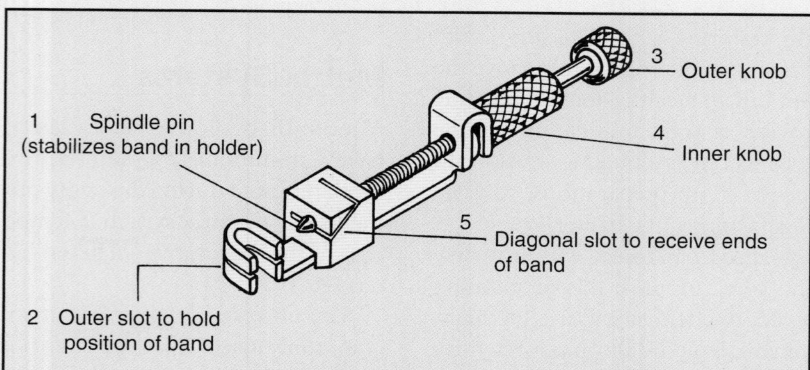

1. **Spindle:** This internal screwlike pin fits into the diagonal slot to hold the ends of the matrix band. When the retainer is assembled, the spindle point must be clear of the slot while the band is slid into the slot and then tightened.
2. **Outer guide slots:** Also known as guide channels, these slots are located at the end of the retainer and serve as channels to guide the loop of the matrix band. The channel selected is determined according to the quadrant that is being treated.
3. **Outer knob:** The outer knob is used to tighten or loosen the spindle within the diagonal slot and to hold the matrix band securely in the retainer. To tighten the

Components of a Universal Retainer—cont'd

spindle, turn the outer knob away from you. To loosen the spindle, turn the outer knob toward you. Be careful not to turn it too far, or the diagonal slot vise will fall off the spindle. If this happens, then insert the end of the spindle into the diagonal slot vise, and turn the outer knob away from you.

4. **Inner knob:** The inner knob is used to increase or decrease the size of the matrix band loop. The size of the loop formed by the band depends on the tooth to be restored. When the band is placed over the tooth, the size of the loop circumference should be larger than the tooth, and the band should be tightened after placement.
5. **Diagonal slot:** This slot is within the boxlike structure and is used to position the ends of the matrix band into the vise; the retainer is always positioned in the mouth with the diagonal slot facing toward the gingiva.

From Bird DL, Robinson DS: *Modern dental assisting,* ed 11, St. Louis, 2015, Saunders.

Anterior Matrix System

A clear plastic matrix strip is the matrix of choice for Class III and IV anterior restorations. Composite resins have inorganic filler particles that could be scratched or marked if a stainless steel matrix system were used.

The plastic matrix strip is supplied already contoured or as a clear flat strip that is contoured (rounded) to adapt to the shape of the tooth. To contour the strip, pull it lengthwise over the handle of a mouth mirror (Figure 21-5). The strip is placed interproximally (between the teeth) before etching the tooth and before the placement of the restorative material. The strip is then tightly pulled around the tooth to adapt the composite to the natural contour of the tooth. The matrix is held in place by hand or with a retainer clip until the composite is hardened from the light-cured process.

See Procedure 21-2: Placing a Plastic Matrix for a Class III or Class IV Restoration (Expanded Function).

Wedges

Wedges are used for all Class II, III, and IV matrix systems. A wedge is placed into the embrasure to hold the matrix band firmly against the gingival margin of the preparation (Figure 21-6). This placement allows the dentist to carve the restorative dental material back to the original normal contour with proximal contacts of the tooth. If the contact is not there, then the tooth could slightly drift, allowing food to impact the area, creating problems for the patient.

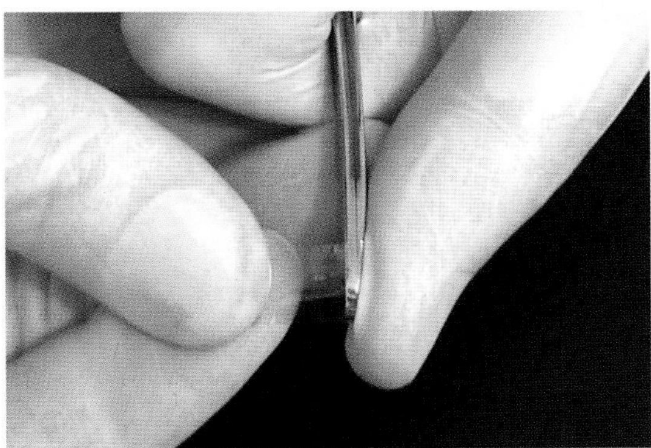

FIGURE 21-5 Contouring a plastic matrix band. (From Heymann HO, Swift EJ, Ritter AV: *Sturdevant's art and science of operative dentistry,* ed 6, St. Louis, 2013, Mosby.)

Cotton pliers or Howe pliers are used to place the wedge firmly into the embrasure. If a universal retainer is used, then the retainer is situated from the buccal side of the tooth and the wedge is inserted from the lingual side.

See Procedure 21-3: Placing and Removing a Matrix Band and Wedge for a Class II Restoration (Expanded Function).

Permanent Restoration

A permanent restoration can range from a small Class I restoration to an extensive Class II multisurface foundation. With the exception of steps added to the procedure by using supplementary accessories and dental materials, a restorative procedure will follow a standardized format.

- The assistant will communicate with the patient about the procedure and what to expect during treatment.
- The assistant will correctly position the patient for the dentist and specific area of the mouth.

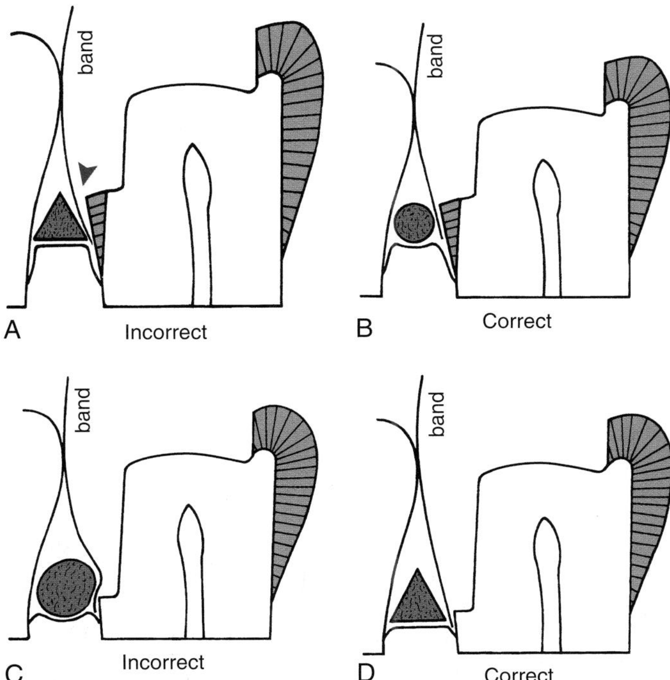

FIGURE 21-6 Proper placement of wedges. (From Heymann HO, Swift EJ, Ritter AV: *Sturdevant's art and science of operative dentistry,* ed 6, St. Louis, 2013, Mosby.)

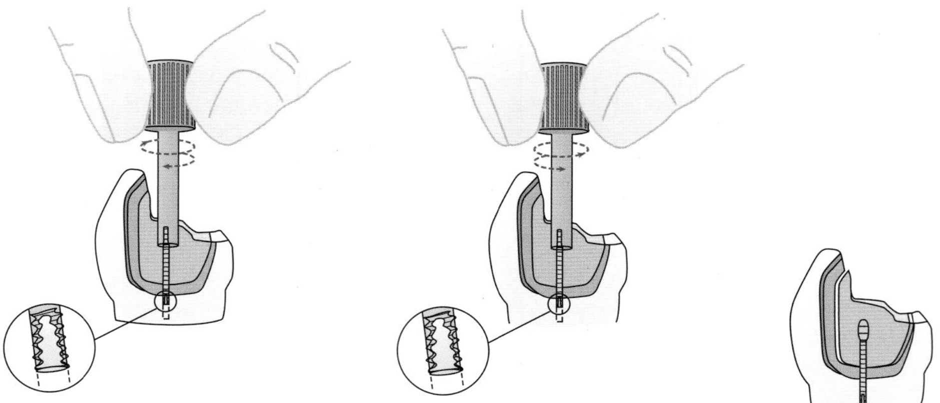

FIGURE 21-7 Placement of a retention pin for added internal strength.

- The dentist will evaluate the tooth to be restored.
- The dentist will administer local anesthesia (see Chapter 14).
- The assistant will prepare and assist in the type of moisture control (cotton roll, dry angles, dental dam) to be used for the procedure (see Chapter 10).
- The dentist will prepare the tooth, including using dental hand instruments and dental handpieces with rotary instruments (see Chapter 19).
- The dentist will specify which dental materials are to be used (see Chapter 20).
- The assistant will prepare and assist in the placement of the dental materials.
- The assistant will prepare and assist in checking the occlusion.
- The dentist will finish and polish the restoration.

See Procedure 21-4: Assisting in a Class II Amalgam Restoration, and Procedure 21-5: Assisting in a Class III or IV Composite Restoration.

Complex Restorations

If the loss of tooth structure is greater than the remaining natural tooth, then the dentist must decide whether to (1) move ahead and restore the tooth with an amalgam or a composite material, or (2) change the treatment plan and replace the tooth structure with a cast restoration. Bonding techniques and retention pins are best suited for use in teeth that require very large restorations with little tooth structure remaining to provide strength and retention for the amalgam.

Retention pins provide internal strength to the placed material (Figure 21-7). These pins are available in a variety of diameters (widths) and styles to fit all sizes of teeth. Because all retention pins are very small (approximately one half the size of a bur) and are easily dropped, the dental dam should be indicated for this procedure.

Veneers

A **veneer** is a thin layer of tooth-colored material that can be directly bonded onto the tooth or fabricated in the laboratory using a porcelain material and then cemented to the tooth surface (Figure 21-8).

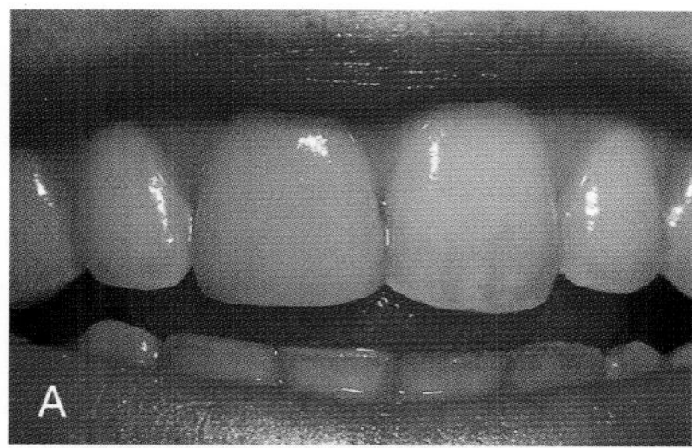

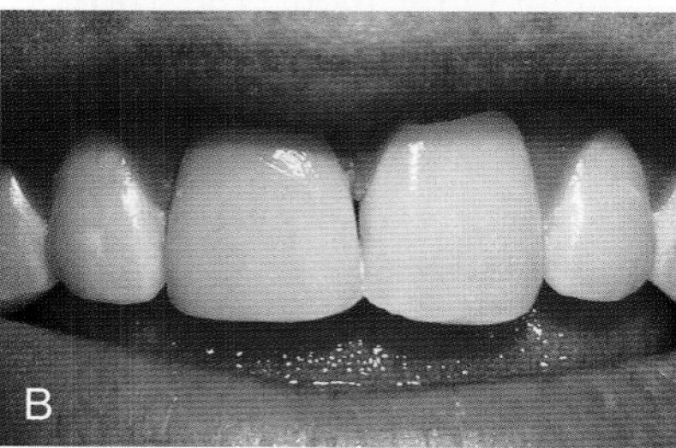

FIGURE 21-8 Veneers placed on teeth #8 and #9 to reduce discoloration and to cover stain. **A,** Before placement. **B,** After placement. (From Heymann HO, Swift EJ, Ritter AV: *Sturdevant's art and science of operative dentistry,* ed 6, St. Louis, 2013, Mosby.)

Veneers are used to improve the appearance of teeth that are slightly abraded, eroded, or discolored from stains or from endodontic treatment. Veneers can also be used to improve the alignment of teeth or to close a diastema.

Vital Bleaching

Vital bleaching, also referred to as tooth whitening, is a technique that involves the whitening of the external surfaces of the teeth. This desired whitening is completed for esthetic purposes, not for restorative purposes (Figure 21-9).

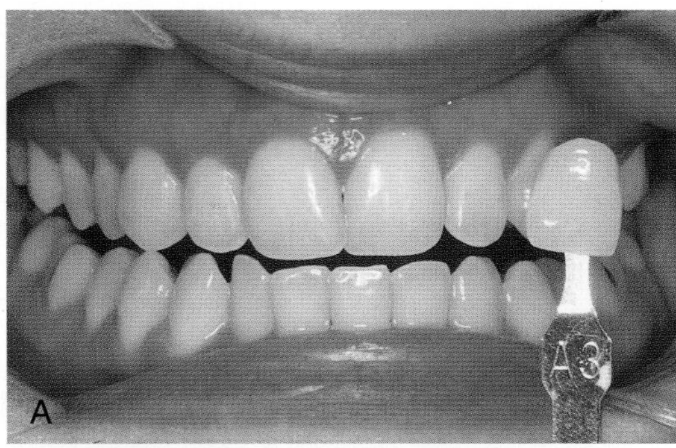

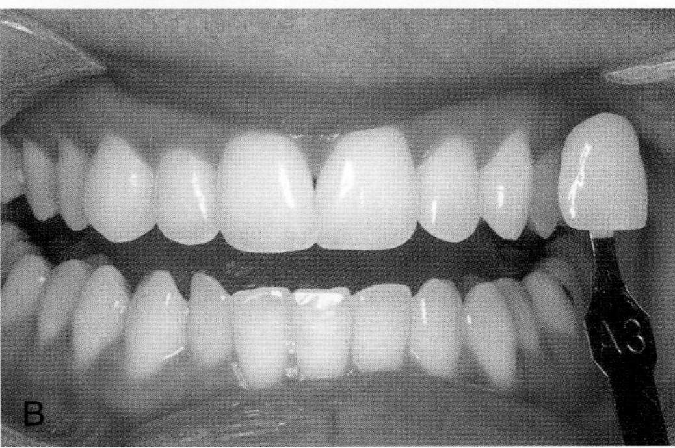

FIGURE 21-9 Tooth whitening used to treat extrinsic stains. **A,** Before placement. **B,** After placement.

Treatment Options

In-office treatment is a professionally applied tooth-whitening procedure that takes place in one appointment by using a whitening agent at a high concentration; a light or laser source is used to enhance the application.

With **at-home treatment**, the patient is under the care of a dentist and is provided a kit, which includes a custom tray and whitening material. The custom tray (see Chapter 22) is worn for a specific amount of time daily. The tray holds the gel-type material made of hydrogen peroxide, carbamide, and a thickening agent. The whitening process can take 2 to 6 weeks, depending on the strength of the gel and the length of time the tray is worn daily.

Over-the-counter whitening options include a variety of tooth-whitening products manufactured by oral health companies. These products are safe, reliable, and effective but will not achieve the dramatic changes that can be attained with the use of dentist-supervised products.

Ethical Implications

One important reason a patient is a part of your dental practice is because of the type of dental treatment he or she receives. The dental team's responsibility to the patient is to restore diseased teeth to a healthy normal state of function, which means providing the most up-to-date restorative care to your patients. The dental team's responsibility and obligation is to continually update their knowledge of procedures and materials.

When a specific intraoral task is delegated by a dentist to a clinical dental assistant, that task is considered an expanded function. To complete the task, two criteria must be met. (1) It must be legal in that specific state for the dental assistant to perform the function, and (2) the dental assistant must have received advanced training and proper credentials. You are placing your patient, yourself, and your dentist at risk by performing functions that you have not been trained to do.

Procedure 21-1

Assembling a Matrix Band and Universal Retainer

Equipment and Supplies

- Basic setup
- Universal retainer
- Matrix band
- Ball burnisher
- Paper pad

Procedural Steps

1. Rinse and dry the preparation.
2. Examine the outline of the cavity preparation using a mirror and explorer.
3. Determine the design of the matrix band to be used for the procedure.

Purpose: The band is selected according to the type of tooth and the depth of the cavity preparation.

4. Place the middle of the band on the paper pad, and burnish this area with a burnisher.

Purpose: This creates a thin, slightly contoured area, where the contact will be located.

5. Hold the retainer with the diagonal slot facing you, and turn the outer knob counterclockwise until the end of the spindle is visible and away from the diagonal slot in the vise.

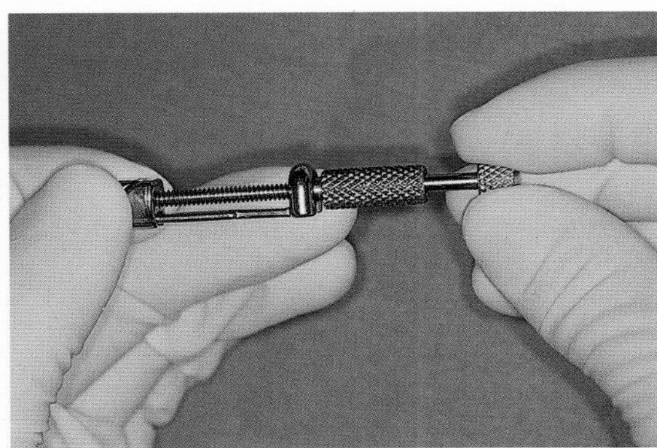

6. Turn the inner knob until the vise moves next to the guide slots.

Purpose: The retainer is ready to receive the matrix band.

Continued

Procedure 21-1

Assembling a Matrix Band and Universal Retainer—cont'd

7. Bring together the ends of the band to identify the occlusal and gingival aspects of the matrix band. The occlusal edge has the larger circumference. The gingival edge has the smaller circumference.

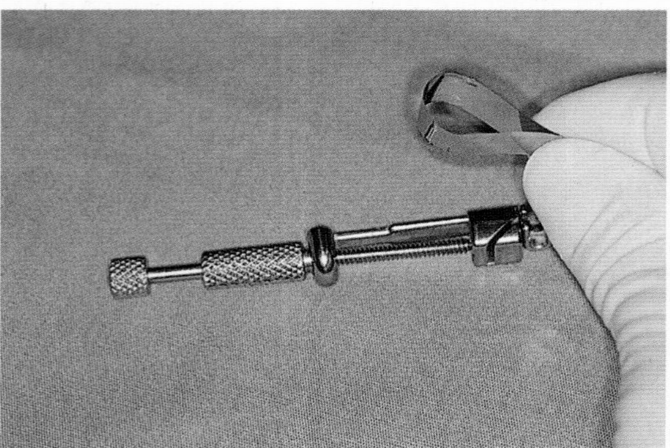

8. With the diagonal slot of the retainer facing toward you, slide the joined ends of the band, *occlusal edge first (wider circumference),* into the diagonal slot on the vise.

9. Guide the band into the correct guide slots.

Purpose: The position of the band loop in the guide slots depends on whether the tooth being restored is maxillary, mandibular, right, or left.

10. Tighten the outer knob on the retainer to secure the band.

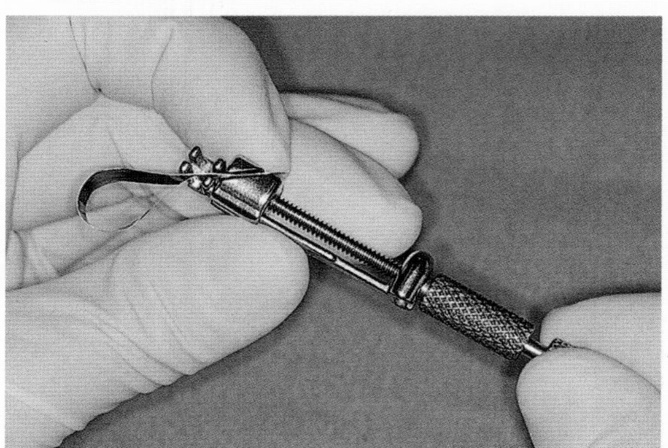

Photos and content from Bird DL, Robinson DS: *Modern dental assisting,* ed 11, St. Louis, 2015, Saunders.

Procedure 21-2

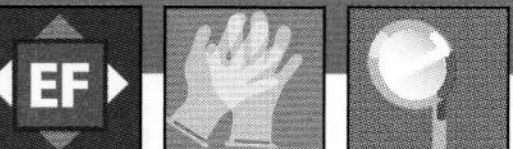

Placing a Plastic Matrix for a Class III or Class IV Restoration (Expanded Function)

Prerequisites for Performing This Procedure

- Mirror skills
- Operator positioning
- Dental anatomy
- Instrumentation

Equipment and Supplies

- Basic setup
- Clear matrix strip
- Wedges
- #110 pliers

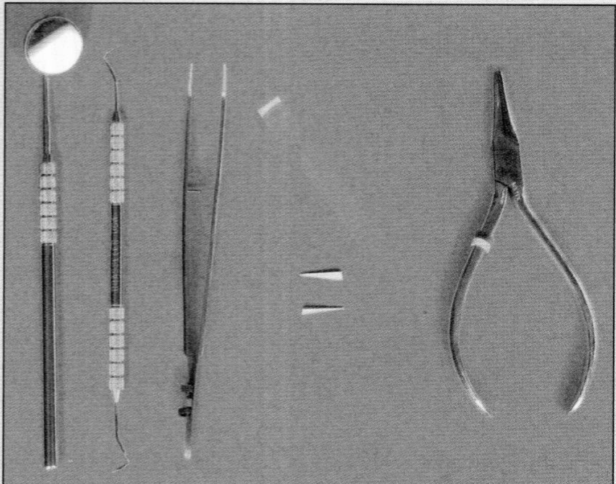

Procedural Steps

1. Examine the contour of the tooth and preparation site, paying special attention to the outline of the preparation.
2. Contour the matrix strip.
3. Slide the matrix interproximally, ensuring that the gingival edge of the matrix extends beyond the preparation.

Purpose: **If the matrix does not completely cover the preparation, the cavity preparation could be filled incorrectly.**

Note: **If a matrix is placed during the etching process, make sure a new matrix is used for placement of the composite resin material.**

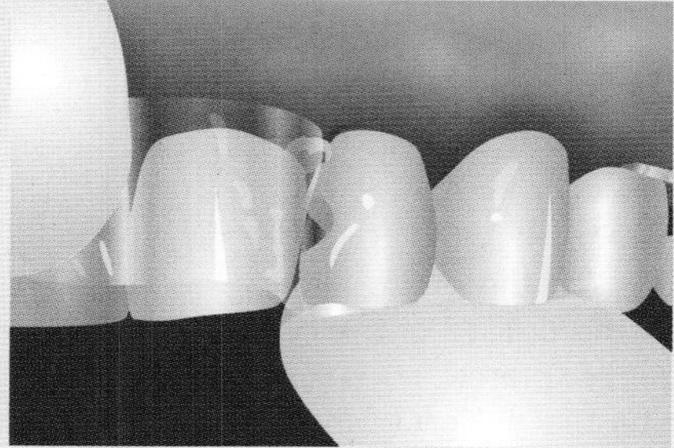

4. Using your thumb and forefinger, pull the band over the prepared tooth on the facial and lingual surfaces.
5. Using pliers, position the wedge within the gingival embrasure.

Note: **The wedge can be positioned from the facial or the lingual side for anterior restorations.**

6. After the preparation has been filled and light-cured, the matrix is removed.

Photos and content from Bird DL, Robinson DS: *Modern dental assisting,* ed 11, St. Louis, 2015, Saunders.

Procedure 21-3

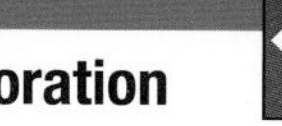

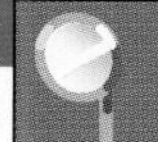

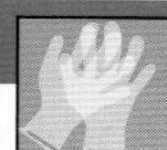

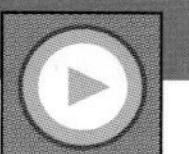

Placing and Removing a Matrix Band and Wedge for a Class II Restoration (Expanded Function)

Prerequisites for Performing This Procedure

- Mirror skills
- Operator positioning
- Dental anatomy
- Instrumentation

Equipment and Supplies

- Basic setup
- Prepared matrix band and retainer
- Wedge for each proximal space involved
- No. 110 pliers

Procedural Steps

Preparing the Band Size

1. If necessary, use the handle end of the mouth mirror to open the loop of the band.

Purpose: The band can become flattened or bent during placement in the retainer and may not easily slide onto the tooth preparation.

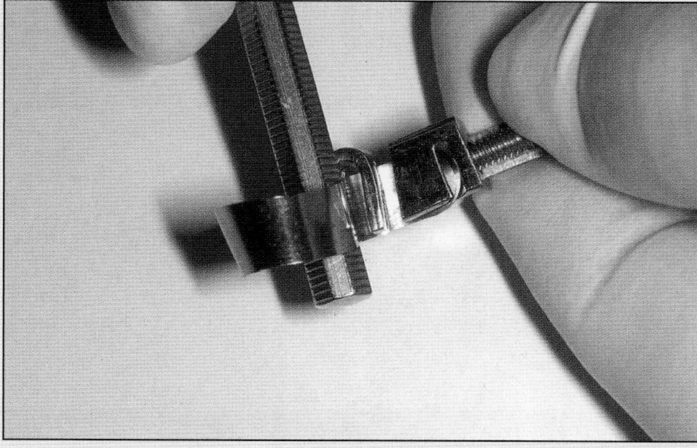

2. If necessary, adjust the size (diameter) of the loop to fit over the tooth by turning the inner knob.

Placing the Matrix Band and Universal Retainer

1. Position and seat the loop of the band over the occlusal surface, with the retainer parallel to the buccal surface of the tooth. Ensure that the band remains beyond the occlusal edge by approximately 1.0 to 1.5 mm.

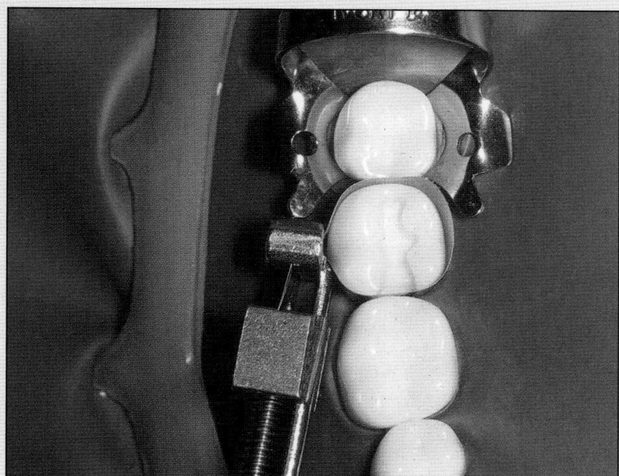

2. Securely hold the band in place by applying finger pressure over its occlusal surface. Slowly turn the inner knob clockwise to tighten the band around the tooth.
3. Use the explorer to examine the adaptation of the band.

Purpose: Gingival tissue or dental dam material can become trapped between the band and the proximal box of the cavity preparation.

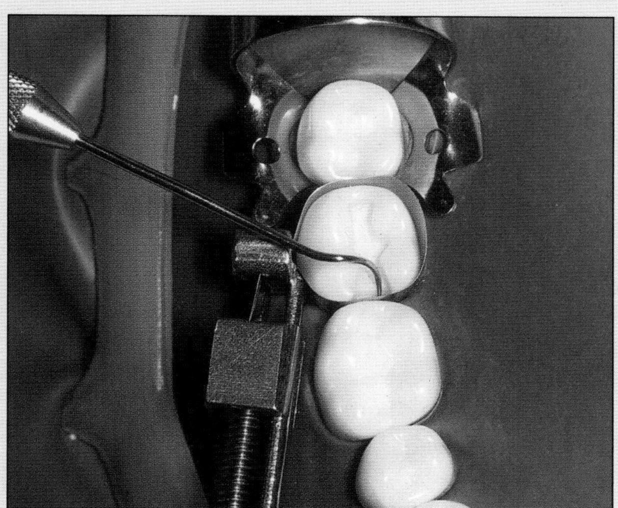

4. Use a burnisher to contour the band at the contact area, creating a slightly concave area.

Continued

Procedure 21-3

Placing and Removing a Matrix Band and Wedge for a Class II Restoration (Expanded Function)—cont'd

Placing the Wedge

1. Select the proper wedge size and shape.

Purpose: The size of the embrasure will determine the size and shape of the wedge for complete closure of the band and cavity preparation.

2. Place the wedge in the pliers so that the flat, wider side of the wedge is toward the gingiva.

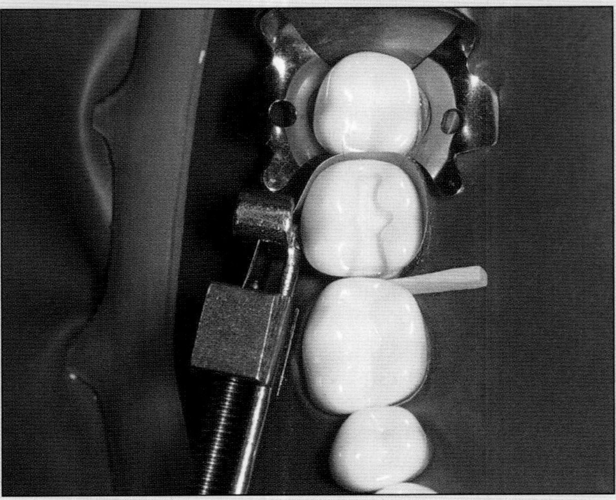

3. Insert the wedge into the lingual embrasure next to the preparation and the band.

Note: If both proximal surfaces (mesial and distal) are being restored, then a wedge is inserted for each open contact.

4. Check the proximal contact to ensure that the seal at the gingival margin of the preparation is closed.

Removing the Universal Retainer, Matrix Band, and Wedge

1. After the dentist completes the initial carving of the restorative material, loosen the retainer from the band by placing a finger over the occlusal surface and slowly turning the outer knob of the retainer.
2. Carefully slide the retainer toward the occlusal surface while leaving the band around the tooth.
3. Gently lift the matrix band in an occlusal direction, using a seesaw motion.

Purpose: This step helps avoid fracturing the newly placed material.

4. Discard the matrix band into the sharps container.
5. Using No. 110 pliers, grasp the base of the wedge to remove it from the lingual embrasure.

Purpose: The wedge remains in place to help prevent a fracture of the restoration when the matrix band is removed.

6. The restoration is now ready for the final carving steps.

Photos from Bird DL, Robinson DS: *Modern dental assisting,* ed 11, St. Louis, 2015, Saunders.

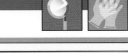

Procedure 21-4

Assisting in a Class II Amalgam Restoration

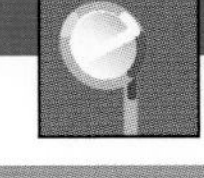
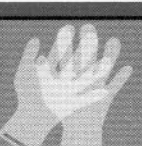
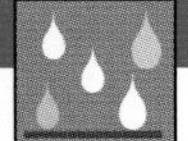

Equipment and Supplies

- Restorative tray (basic setup, hand-cutting instruments, amalgam carrier, condensers, burnishers, carvers, articulating paper holder)
- Local anesthetic setup
- Dental dam setup
- High-volume oral evacuator (HVE) tip
- Saliva ejector
- High-speed and low-speed handpieces
- Assorted burs (dentist's choice)
- Matrix setup
- Dental liners, base, sealers, and bonding agents
- Premeasured amalgam capsules
- Dental floss
- Articulating paper
- Cotton pellets, cotton rolls, 2 × 2-inch gauze
- Dental floss

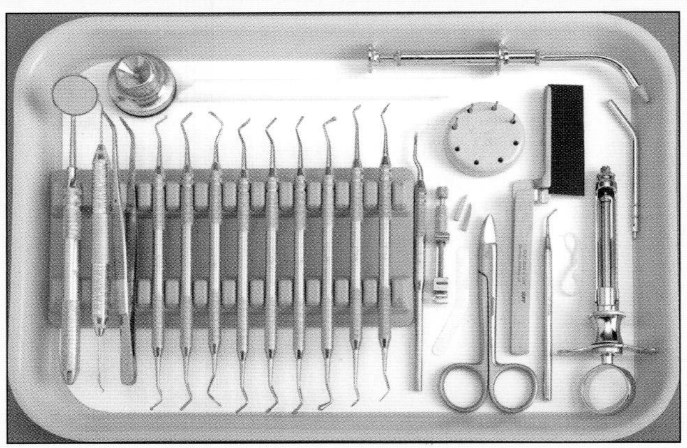

(From Boyd LRB: *Dental instruments: a pocket guide,* ed 5, St. Louis, 2015, Saunders.)

Procedure 21-4

Assisting in a Class II Amalgam Restoration—cont'd

Procedural Steps

Preparing the Tooth

1. Transfer the mouth mirror and explorer to the dentist.

Purpose: The dentist examines the tooth to be prepared.

2. Assist in the administration of the local anesthetic agent.
3. Place and secure moisture control techniques (cotton roll, dental dam).

Preparing the Cavity

1. Transfer the mirror and the high-speed handpiece with cutting bur to the dentist.
2. During cavity preparation, use the HVE and air-water syringe, adjust the light, and retract the patient's cheek as necessary to maintain a clear field of vision for the dentist.

Purpose: With efficient placement and use of the HVE and air-water syringe, the dentist will maintain a clear operating field with comfort to the patient.

3. Transfer the explorer, excavators, and hand-cutting instruments as needed throughout the cavity preparation.

Placing the Base and Cavity Liner (Expanded Function)

1. After the examination, rinse and dry the preparation. Mix and place any necessary cavity liners and the base.

Placing the Matrix Band and Wedge (Expanded Function)

1. Assist in placing the preassembled universal (Tofflemire) retainer and matrix.
2. Assist in placing the wedge or wedges in the proximal box using cotton pliers or No. 110 pliers.

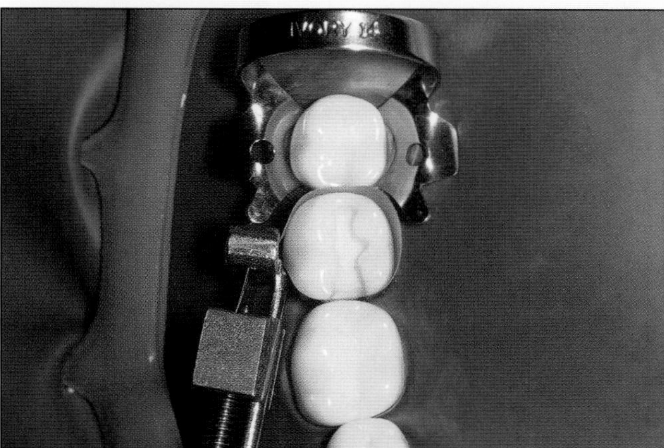

Placing the Bonding Agent (Expanded Function)

1. After the tooth is etched and primed, assist the dentist in preparing and placing the bonding material.

Mixing the Amalgam

1. Activate the capsule, place it in the amalgamator, close the cover, and set the timer for the time recommended by the manufacturer.
2. At the signal from the dentist, start the amalgamator.
3. Open the capsule, and remove the pestle with cotton pliers. Drop the amalgam into the amalgam well.
4. Reassemble and discard the capsule.

Purpose: This step prevents mercury vapor from escaping into the air.

Placing and Condensing the Amalgam

1. Fill the smaller end of the amalgam carrier, and transfer the carrier to the dentist.
2. Assist when necessary as the dentist exchanges the carrier for a condenser and begins to condense the first increments of amalgam with the smaller end of the condenser.

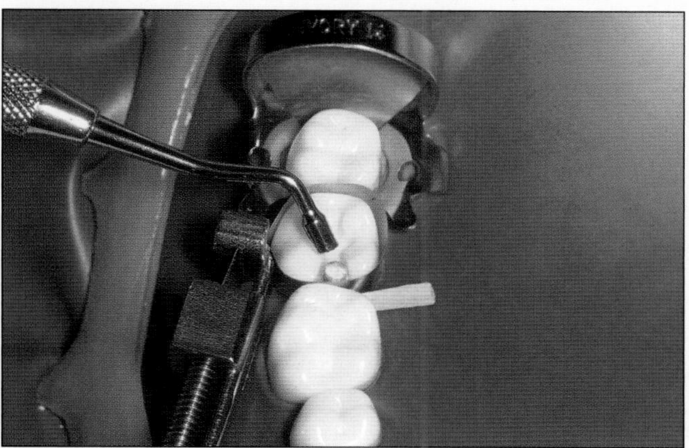

3. Assist as the process of placing and condensing the amalgam is repeated until the cavity is slightly overfilled.
4. When the cavity preparation is slightly overfilled, exchange the condenser for the burnisher so that the dentist can burnish the surface and margins of the restoration.

Purpose: This step strengthens the filled restoration by burnishing the excess mercury to the surface.

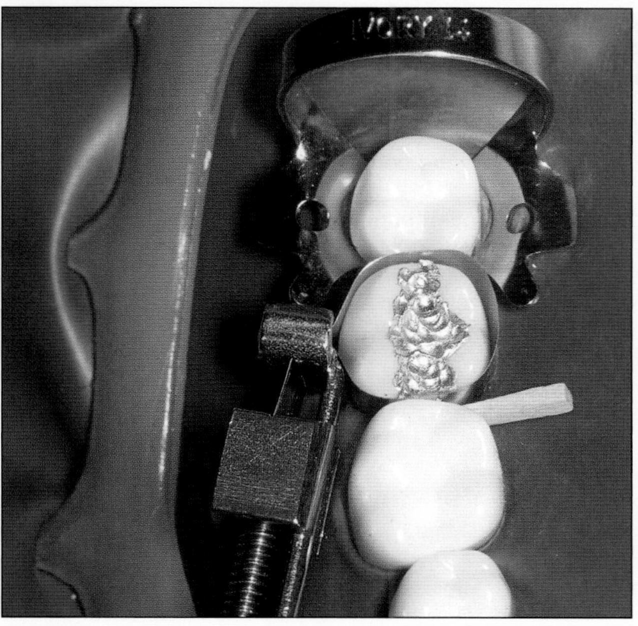

Continued

Procedure 21-4

Assisting in a Class II Amalgam Restoration—cont'd

Initial Carving

1. Assist while the dentist uses an explorer and a discoid-cleoid carver to remove excess amalgam on the occlusal surface from between the matrix band and the marginal ridge of the tooth.

Purpose: This step prevents the restoration from fracturing during the removal of the matrix band.

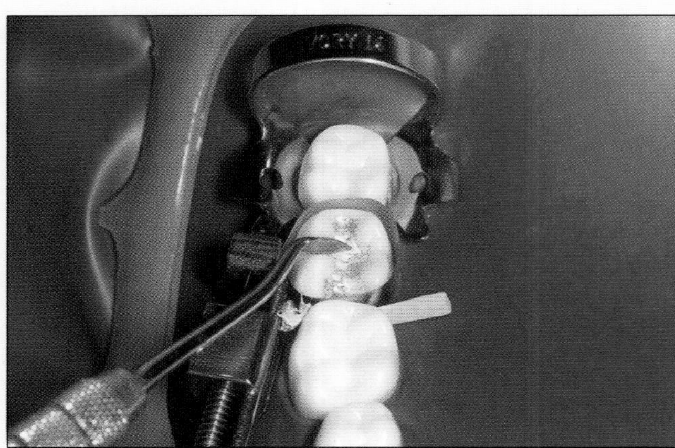

2. Assist in removing the universal retainer, matrix band, and wedge.

Final Carving

1. Transfer the amalgam carvers until the carving is complete.
2. Keep the tip of the HVE close to the restoration during the carving process.

Purpose: All amalgam particles are removed as soon as possible.

Note: This step is especially important when a dental dam is not used.

Occlusal Adjustment

1. Remove moisture control materials (cotton rolls, dental dam).
2. Place articulating paper on the teeth to be checked, and instruct the patient to close the teeth together very gently.

Note: Heavy blue marks will appear on any high spots on the new restoration. If the patient bites too hard, then the restoration may fracture.

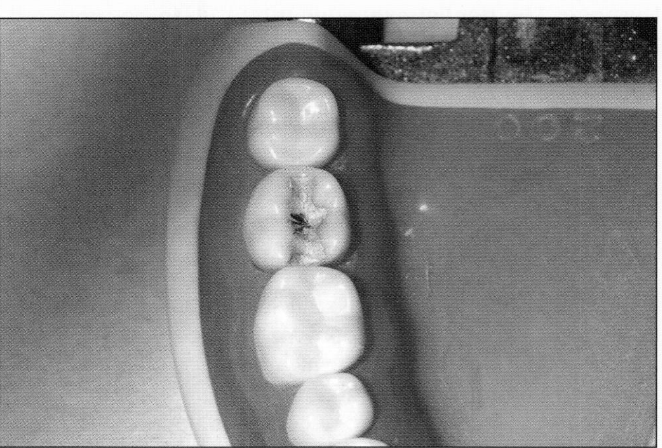

3. Assist with transfers as the dentist uses an amalgam carver to remove any remaining high spots.

Note: This step is repeated as often as necessary to bring the new restoration into proper occlusion.

4. Transfer a moist cotton pellet in cotton pliers to rub the surface of the amalgam gently.

Purpose: Any remaining small surface irregularities are removed.

Postoperative Instructions

1. Caution the patient not to chew on the new restoration for a few hours.

Purpose: Amalgam takes several hours to reach its maximum strength, and biting on it could cause the restoration to fracture.

DATE	TOOTH	SURFACE	CHARTING NOTES
7/20/17	31	MO	1 carpule Xylocaine w/o epinephrine, dam isolation, liner/bonding/ Sybraloy. Pt tolerated procedure fine. T. Clark, CDA L. Stewart, DDS

Procedure 21-5

Assisting in a Class III or IV Composite Restoration

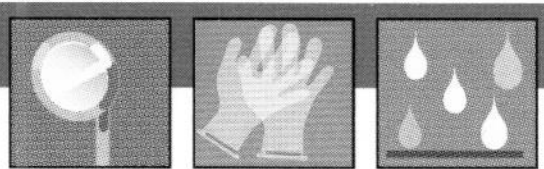

Equipment and Supplies

- Restorative tray (basic setup, hand-cutting instruments, composite placement instrument, carvers, and articulating paper holder)
- Composite shade guide
- Local anesthetic setup
- Dental dam setup
- High-volume oral evacuator (HVE) tip
- Saliva ejector
- High-speed and low-speed handpieces
- Assorted burs (dentist's choice)
- Mylar matrix setup
- Dental liners, base, sealers, and bonding agents
- Composite material
- Curing light with protective shield
- Finishing burs and diamonds
- Dental floss
- Articulating paper
- Cotton pellets, cotton rolls, 2 × 2-inch gauze
- Dental floss
- Abrasive strips
- Articulating paper
- Polishing kit (disc and mandrel)
- Polishing paste

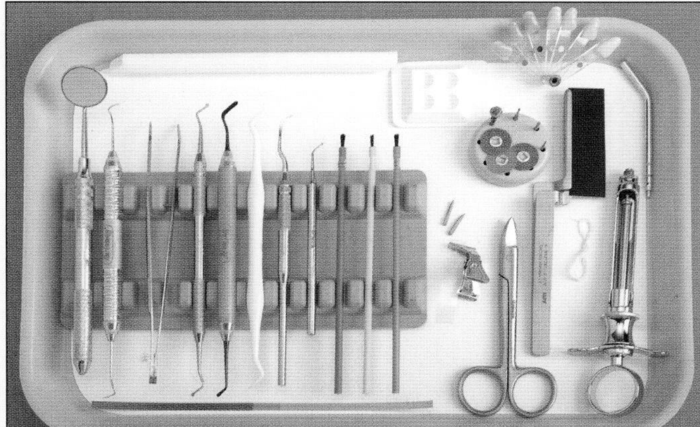

(From Boyd LRB: *Dental instruments: a pocket guide,* ed 5, St. Louis, 2015, Saunders.)

Procedural Steps

Preparing the Tooth

1. Transfer the mouth mirror and explorer to the dentist.

Purpose: The dentist examines the tooth to be prepared.

2. Assist in the administration of the local anesthetic.
3. Assist in selecting of the shade of the composite material.
4. Place and secure moisture control techniques (cotton roll, dental dam).

Preparing the Cavity

1. Transfer the high-speed handpiece and hand-cutting instruments so that the dentist can remove the decayed tooth structure. Use the HVE to maintain a clear operating field.
2. Rinse and dry the tooth throughout the procedure. If indicated, place a cavity liner.

Etching, Bonding, and Composite Placement

1. After the preparation is etched, rinse and dry according to the manufacturer's instructions.
2. Assist in placing the matrix strip. If indicated, then a wedge can also be placed.
3. Assist in the application of the primer and bonding resin, which are light-cured in accordance with the manufacturer's instructions.

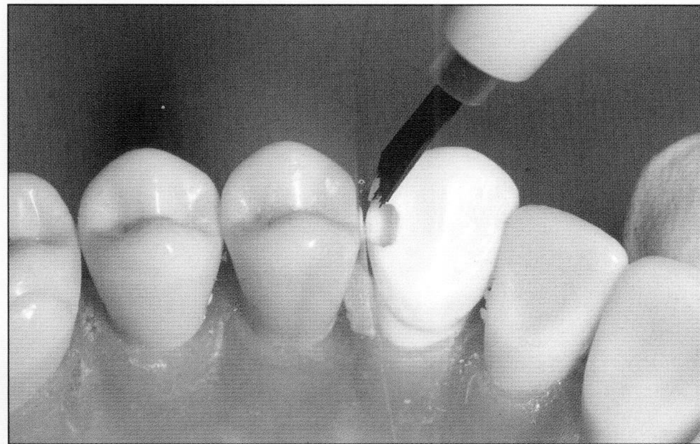

(From Bird DL, Robinson DS: *Modern dental assisting,* ed 11, St. Louis, 2015, Saunders.)

4. Dispense the composite material on a paper pad, or insert the capsule into a composite syringe, and transfer it along with the composite instrument to be placed into the preparation.

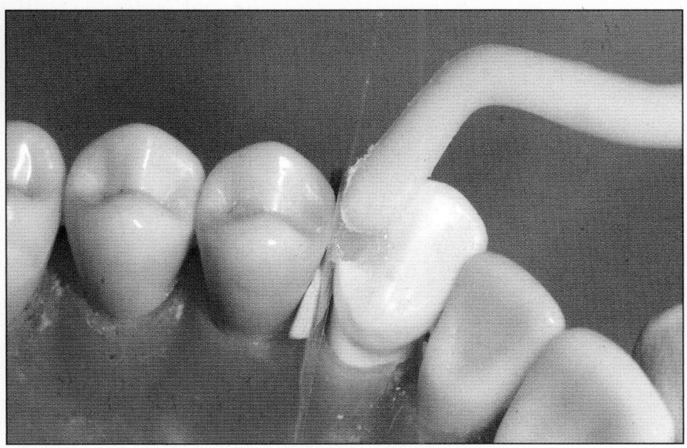

(From Bird DL, Robinson DS: *Modern dental assisting,* ed 11, St. Louis, 2015, Saunders.)

5. Assist as the matrix is pulled and tightly held around the tooth while the composite material is light-cured from the lingual and facial surfaces.

Continued

Procedure 21-5

Assisting in a Class III or IV Composite Restoration—cont'd

Finishing the Restoration

1. Remove the matrix strip and wedge.
2. Assist with transfers as the dentist uses finishing burs or diamonds in the high-speed handpiece to contour the restoration.
3. If indicated, then transfer the finishing strips for smoothing the interproximal surface.
4. Remove the moisture control technique, and use articulating paper to check the occlusion. Adjustments are made as necessary.
5. Assist while the dentist uses polishing discs, points, and cups in the low-speed handpiece to polish the restoration.

(From Bird DL, Robinson DS: *Modern dental assisting,* ed 11, St. Louis, 2015, Saunders.)

DATE	TOOTH	SURFACE	CHARTING NOTES
7/20/17	6	MI	1 carpule Xylocaine w/o epinephrine, cotton roll isolation, etching/bonding/Silux shade YL. Pt tolerated procedure fine. T. Clark, CDA L. Stewart, DDS

Chapter Exercises

Multiple Choice

Circle the letter next to the correct answer.

1. The __________ circumference of the universal matrix band is placed toward the gingiva.
  a. wider
  b. narrow

2. For a complex restoration, the dentist may have to place a __________ in the cavity preparation of a tooth for internal strength.
  a. wedge
  b. liner
  c. veneer
  d. retentive pin

3. A __________ is a metal or plastic strip used to replace the missing interproximal wall of a tooth during the placement of the restorative dental material.
  a. wedge
  b. matrix
  c. retainer
  d. retentive pin

4. Which instrument would not be placed on the tray setup for a Class IV restorative procedure for tooth #6?
  a. Explorer
  b. Spoon excavator
  c. Articulating paper holder
  d. Amalgam carrier

5. In the placement of a matrix for a Class II amalgam restoration, the wedge would be positioned in the interproximal space from the __________ surface.
  a. buccal
  b. distal
  c. lingual
  d. mesial

6. Which restorative classification would require a clear plastic matrix system?
  a. Class I
  b. Class II
  c. Class III
  d. Class V

7. Tooth-whitening systems are esthetic procedures indicated for __________.
  a. endodontically treated teeth
  b. internal stains
  c. lightening the color of the external surfaces of teeth
  d. a and c

8. When the matrix band is assembled in the universal retainer, the diagonal slot should be facing __________.
  a. away from you
  b. toward you

9. To achieve the proper interproximal contour and contact of a restoration, a __________ must be inserted into the embrasure to restore proper contact.
  a. retentive pin
  b. wedge
  c. universal retainer
  d. matrix band

10. Which instrument would not be placed on the tray setup for an amalgam restorative procedure?
  a. Cotton pliers
  b. Wedge
  c. Shade guide
  d. Articulating paper holder

Apply Your Knowledge

1. You are assisting in a Class III restoration. (1) What tooth surfaces are involved in a Class III restoration? (2) What type of moisture control isolation would best suit this procedure? (3) What type of matrix should be readied? (4) What restorative material should be set out?

2. While reviewing a new patient's health history form, you notice that the patient does not like the color of her teeth. After talking with her more about this, you find that she drinks a lot of coffee, which seems to be staining her teeth. What technique could the dentist recommend to the patient to alter the color of her teeth? How would you explain this procedure to the patient?

3. You are assisting in the restoration of tooth #29. The tooth is charted to receive a mesio-occluso-distal (MOD) amalgam. (1) What type of matrix system will be used? (2) Describe the assembly of the matrix and any additional items needed to restore the proper contour of the tooth.

4. Dr. Smith is running behind and asks you to complete the etching, place the primer, and begin adding increments of the composite resin to the small Class I pit. Are there any steps that you should not do?

CHAPTER 22

Impression Materials and Laboratory Procedures

http://evolve.elsevier.com/Robinson/essentials/

LEARNING OBJECTIVES

1. Pronounce, define, and spell the key terms.
2. Complete the following related to impressions and impression trays:
   - List the three types of impressions obtained.
   - Describe the types of impression trays and their characteristics of use.
3. Discuss various impression materials and their properties, uses, mixing techniques, and applications, and perform the following associated procedures:
   - Mix alginate impression material.
   - Take a mandibular preliminary impression.
   - Take a maxillary preliminary impression.
   - Mix a two-paste final impression material.
   - Prepare an automix final impression material.
4. Describe the importance of a bite registration and its uses in a procedure.
5. List the uses of a diagnostic cast, and perform the following procedures:
   - Mix dental plaster.
   - Pour dental models using the inverted-pour method.
   - Trim and finish dental models.

KEY TERMS

alginate
automix
centric
diagnostic cast
extrude
impression
irreversible hydrocolloid
model trimmer
plaster
polyether
polysulfide
registration
silicone
stone
viscosity

Many dental procedures will require an **impression** to be taken of the patient's teeth and surrounding oral tissues. Three types of impressions can be obtained:

1. **Preliminary impression**—Is used for making (a) diagnostic models, (b) custom trays, (c) provisional coverage, (d) dental and orthodontic appliances, and (e) pretreatment and post-treatment records (Figure 22-1).
2. **Final impression**—Shows accurate detail of the tissue and tooth structure for the laboratory technician to make a cast restoration (inlay, onlay, veneer, crown, or bridge) (Figure 22-2).
3. **Occlusal (bite) registration**—Reproduces the occlusal relationship of the maxillary and mandibular teeth when occluded (Figure 22-3).

Because of the many uses of an impression, many types of impression trays and impression materials are available. The dental assistant is responsible for knowing the different types of trays and impression materials to set up for the procedure, how the tray is prepared, and how the material is mixed. Then the dental assistant either assists in the procedure or is delegated to take the impression.

Impression Trays

Impression **trays** are designed for obtaining an accurate impression of the area required. The type of tray selected for a procedure will depend on (1) the dentist's preference and (2) the type of tray that will provide the most accurate result for the type of impression material being used.

Impression trays are supplied as **quadrant trays**, which cover one half of the arch; **section trays**, which are suited for the

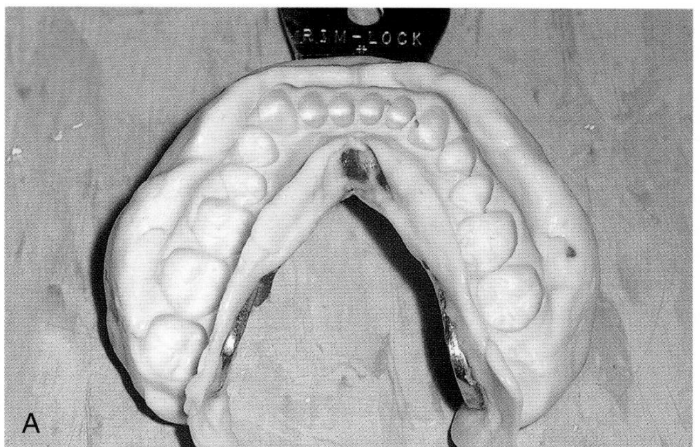

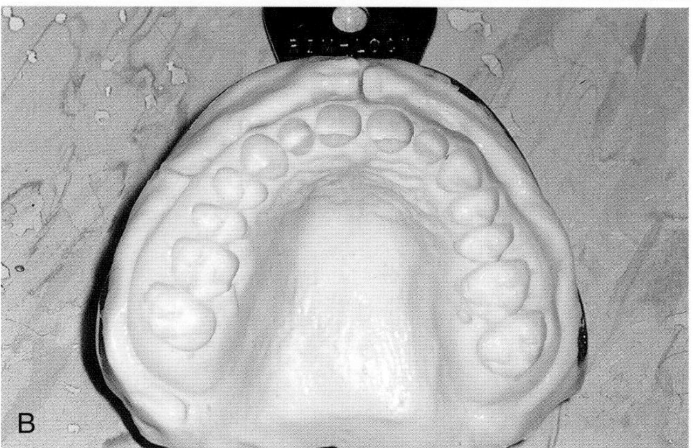

FIGURE 22-1 Example of a preliminary impression.

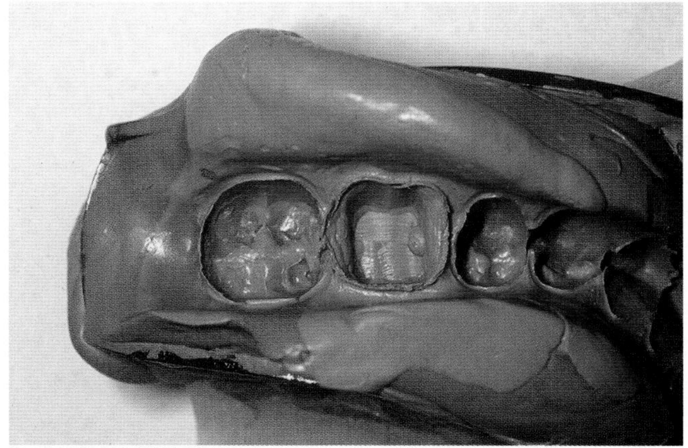

FIGURE 22-2 Example of a final impression. (From Hatrick CD, Eakle WS: *Dental materials: clinical applications for dental assistants and dental hygienists,* ed 3, St Louis, 2016, Saunders.)

anterior teeth; and **full-arch trays**, which cover the complete arch. Table 22-1 reviews the different types of trays.

Impression Materials

Impression materials are selected because of their unique qualities that allow the dentist to obtain the most accurate

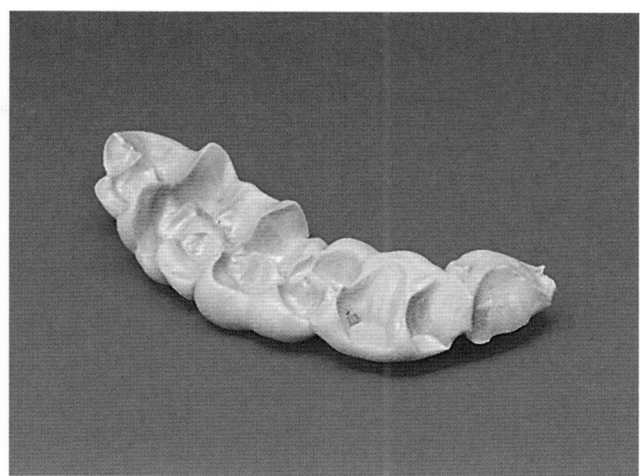

FIGURE 22-3 Example of a bite registration. (Courtesy 3M Dental Products, St Paul, Minnesota.)

reproduction. An impression material is classified according to specific properties:

- **Mechanical property**—Indicates the flexibility of a material. The two types of material are inelastic and elastic. *Inelastic* material is rigid and will fracture when deformed. This type includes impression compounds, impression plaster, and zinc oxide–eugenol (ZOE) impression paste. *Elastic* materials can be deformed and returned to their natural appearance. This type includes alginate, elastomers, and agar.
- **Setting property**—*Irreversible* material indicates that a chemical reaction has occurred and that the material cannot go back to its original state. This type includes alginate, elastomeric impression materials, ZOE impression paste, and impression plaster. A *reversible* material can be altered by temperature and includes agar and impression compounds.

Types of Impression Materials

Alginate

Alginate is an **irreversible hydrocolloid** (*hydro* means *water*, and *colloid* means a *gelatinous* substance) and is the material of choice when taking preliminary impressions. Alginate consists of potassium alginate, which is derived from seaweed, calcium sulfate, trisodium phosphate, diatomaceous earth, zinc oxide, and potassium titanium fluoride. Alginate goes through two physical phases during the setting process: a **sol** (solution) phase, during which the material is in a liquid or semiliquid form, and a **gel** (solid) phase, during which the material becomes semisolid.

Alginate is available in two settings: **normal set**, which has a working time of 2 minutes and a setting time of up to 4½ minutes, and **fast set**, which has a working time of 1¼ minutes and a setting time of 1 to 2 minutes.

Alginate is supplied as a powder and is packaged in premeasured packages or in bulk canisters. A plastic scoop is provided for dispensing the powder, and a plastic cylinder is supplied for measuring the water (Figure 22-4). The water-to-powder ratio for mixing alginate is 1 scoop of powder to 1 *measure line* of water. When mixing the material for a mandibular impression, generally 2 scoops of powder and 2 measure lines of water are

TABLE 22-1
Types of Impression Trays

Type	Characteristics	Use
Perforated tray 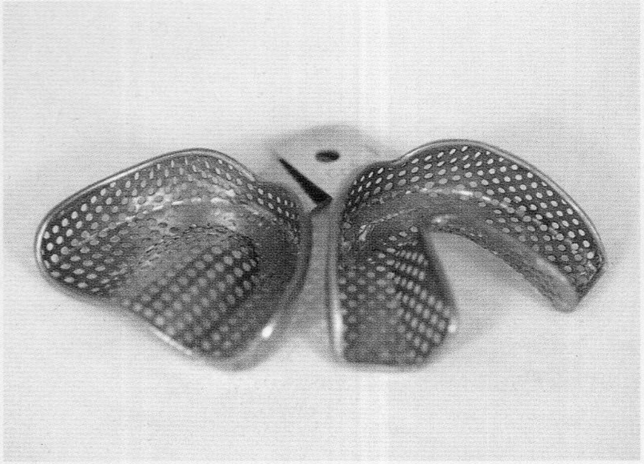 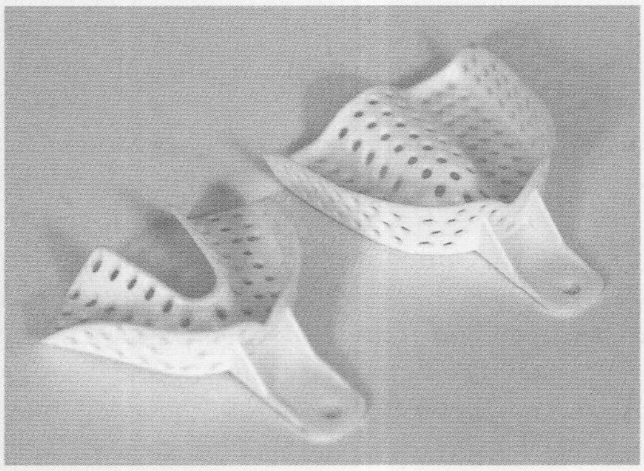	Is a preformed tray made from metal or hard plastic and is supplied in standard sizes for children through adult. Allows the impression material to form a mechanical lock with the tray.	Preliminary impression
Plastic sooth tray	Is supplied in standard sizes. Requires an adhesive to be applied to hold the impression material securely in the tray.	Final impression
Gauze tray 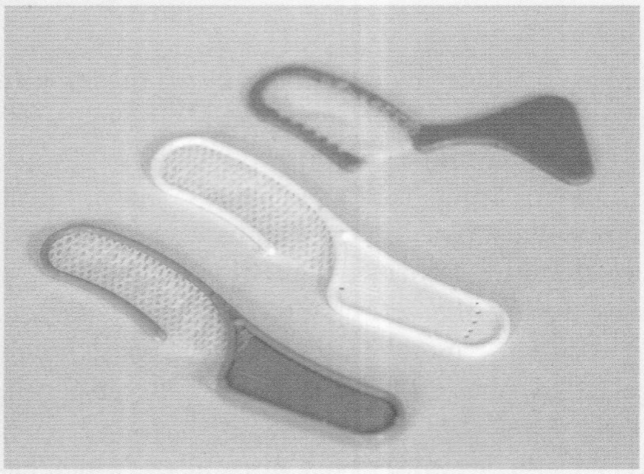	Is a thin meshlike material that allows the patient to bite normally.	Bite registration

TABLE 22-1
Types of Impression Trays—cont'd

Type	Characteristics	Use
Triple tray (From Boyd LRB: *Dental instruments: a pocket guide,* ed 5, St Louis, 2015, Saunders.)	Is designed to eliminate steps by taking the final impression and bite registration at the same time.	Final impression and bite registration
Custom tray (From Heymann HO, Swift EJ Jr., Ritter AV: Sturdevant's art and science of operative dentistry, ed 6, St Louis, 2013, Mosby.)	Is customized to fit a patient's mouth and made from light-cured resin, acrylic resin, or thermoplastic resin.	Final impression
Water-coolant tray (Courtesy Dux Dental, Oxnard, California.)	Is a metal tray that is used with reversible hydrocolloid impression material.	Final Impression

required. For a maxillary impression, 3 scoops of powder and 3 measure lines of water are necessary.

Most alginate impression materials must be *poured up* within 1 hour of taking the impression—a requirement dictated by the environment. Because much of the material is derived from water, a slight change in its environment can distort the impression and cause **dimensional** change.

An alginate impression is sensitive to its environment; if too much water was introduced, then it could cause the alginate to absorb and expand, causing a condition called **imbibition.** If an alginate impression were to remain in the open air, then moisture will evaporate from the material, causing it to shrink and distort, which is a condition called **syneresis.** Before pouring an alginate impression, the disinfected impression is stored in a plastic biohazard bag and covered with a slightly moistened towel, which will provide an atmosphere close to 100% relative humidity, which causes the least amount of distortion.

See Procedure 22-1: Mixing Alginate Impression Material.

Taking alginate impressions Preliminary impressions are used to create a negative reproduction of the teeth and their surrounding tissues and structures. When an impression is poured up in stone or plaster to make a model, it is then creating a positive reproduction of the teeth and their surrounding structures. The term model can also referred to as a **cast**.

It is important for the clinical assistant to be ready to mix the alginate, load the tray, and help maintain comfort for the patient while taking the impression. If this procedure is a legal function in the state in which the dental assistant works, then he or she would proceed with taking the impression. Before taking the impression, the procedure should be explained to the patient to ensure his or her comfort. The patient should be informed that:

- The material will feel cold, have no unpleasant taste, and will quickly set.
- He or she should breathe deeply through the nose, which will help him or her relax and be more comfortable.
- He or she should not talk after the tray has been placed; if the need to communicate arises, then he or she should do so through hand gestures.

See Procedure 22-2: Taking a Mandibular Preliminary Impression (Expanded Function) and Procedure 22-3: Taking a Maxillary Preliminary Impression (Expanded Function).

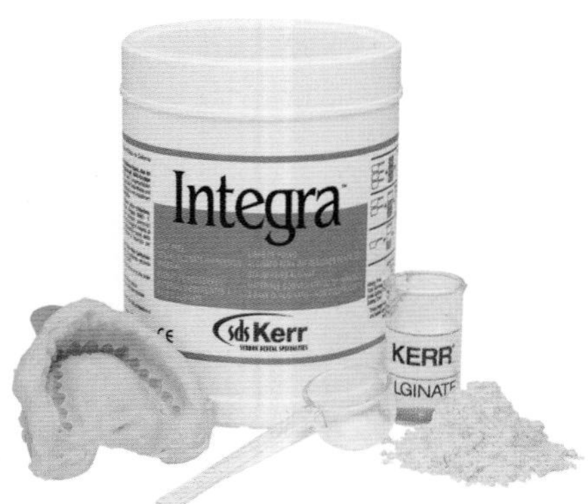

FIGURE 22-4 Packaging of alginate material. (Courtesy of Kerr Corporation, Orange, California.)

Elastomeric Impression Materials

Elastomeric impression materials have an elastic or rubberlike quality after setting. These materials are supplied as a **base** and **catalyst** and are self-curing. The types of elastomeric materials commonly used in dental practice are polysulfide, polyether, **condensation** silicone, and **addition silicone**. Each type of material has different properties and characteristics. Table 22-2 provides a summary of the comparative properties of these materials.

Final impression materials are supplied in three forms or viscosities (viscosity is the ability of the material to flow):

1. **Light body** is the easiest-flowing material of the three forms. This material is expressed from a syringe around the tooth and into the sulcus of the prepared tooth or teeth, which provides the detail of the margin that was created by the dentist.
2. **Regular body** is slightly thicker than the light body form. This material is used as a tray material but has the ability to flow easily, thus requiring improved control from the tray.
3. **Heavy body** is the thickest of the three forms. This material is used as a tray material and has the ability to force the light-bodied material into close contact with the prepared tooth and surrounding tissue to ensure a more accurate impression.

TABLE 22-2
Properties of Final Impression Materials

Type	Characteristics	Working Abilities
Polysulfide	A paste material is supplied in two tubes. A strong odor and taste is associated with the material. The stiffness and stability of the material are poor.	Harder material to mix Longer mixing time of 60 seconds Longer setting time of 10-20 minutes
Polyether	A paste material is supplied in tubes or cartridges. Has an acceptable odor and taste. The stiffness and stability of the material are very good.	An easy material to mix Short mixing time of 30-45 seconds Fast setting time of 6-7 minutes
Condensation silicone	The material is supplied as a paste and a liquid. Has an acceptable odor and taste. The stiffness and stability are average.	Easy material to mix Average mixing time of 30-60 seconds Average setting time of 6-10 minutes
Addition silicone (also referred to as vinyl polysiloxane)	A paste material is supplied as a two-paste system, as a putty material or cartridges. Has an acceptable odor and taste. The stiffness and stability are excellent.	Easy material to mix Short mixing time of 30-45 seconds Average setting time of 6-8 minutes

Mixing Impression Materials

Impression materials are packaged several ways to accommodate preferences of use:

- **Paste system.** The material is supplied in tubes and involves the use of a spatula and paper pad. The catalyst is picked up and spatulated into the base until the material is uniform in appearance. The material is then gathered onto the spatula and loaded into the tray (Figure 22-5).
- Automix **system.** Provides a homogeneous mix with the appropriate amount of material without waste. The extruder is used to mix and dispense elastomeric impression materials automatically (Figure 22-6).
- **Table-top or wall-mounted mixing unit.** This unit saves time and mechanically mixes the material and expresses it into the tray (Figure 22-7).
- **Putty impression material.** Provides the benefits of true putty, including a dense consistency and insertion force than observed with heavy-bodied materials. Because the material is kneaded in the palms, the material is already warm when it is seated in the mouth (Figure 22-8).

Sequence of use is an important process to understand when assisting in a final impression procedure. The most common steps include light- and heavy-bodied materials in this sequence:

1. The material is selected by the dentist as determined by the type of procedure.
2. The tooth is isolated using a retraction system (refer to Chapter 23), and the teeth are rinsed and carefully dried.
3. The light-bodied material (most commonly used in a cartridge system with a syringe tip) is placed in the sulcus, and the material is displaced around and over the prepared tooth and onto the surrounding tissue.
4. The impression tray is loaded with the heavy-bodied material and then is seated over the light-bodied material.
5. When the impression materials have reached final set, the impression is removed and inspected for accuracy.
6. The impression is disinfected, placed in a biohazard container or bag, and taken to the laboratory.

See Procedure 22-4: Mixing a Two-Paste Final Impression Material, and Procedure 22-5: Preparing an Automix Final Impression Material.

Bite Registration

In addition to having an accurate impression of the prepared teeth, the dentist and the laboratory technician will require an accurate bite registration of the normal centric relationship of

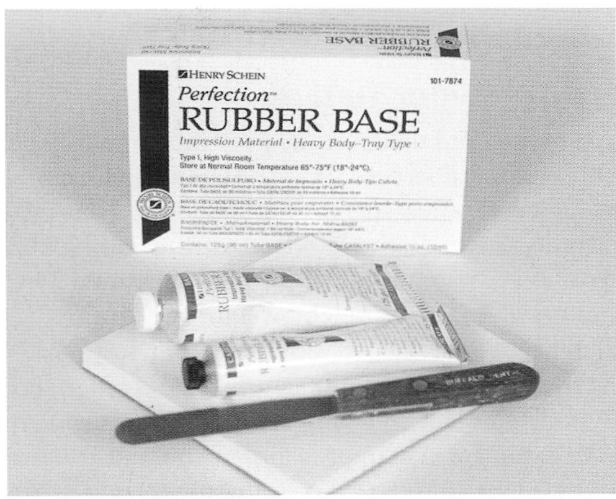

FIGURE 22-5 Final impression paste system.

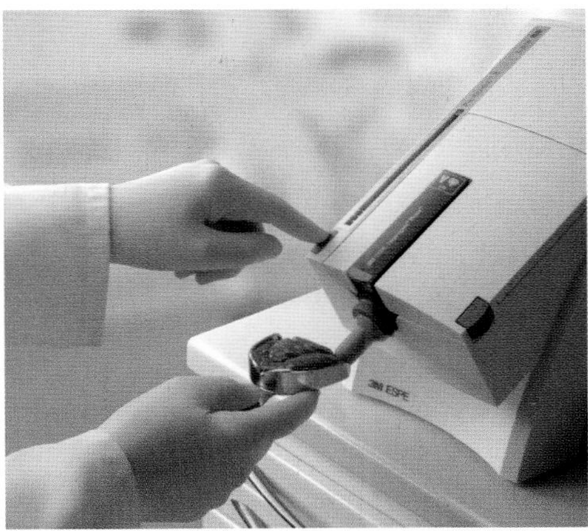

FIGURE 22-7 Tabletop impression system. (Courtesy Y-W Chen, University of Washington Department of Restorative Dentistry, Seattle, WA.)

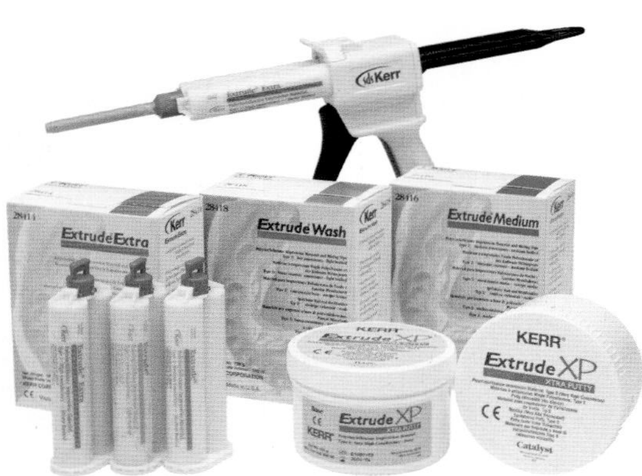

FIGURE 22-6 Automix impression paste system. (Courtesy Kerr Corporation, Orange, California.)

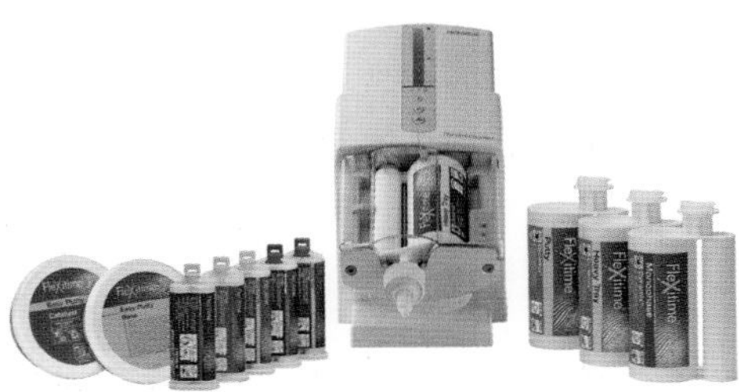
FIGURE 22-8 Putty impression material. (Courtesy Heraeus Kulzer, South Bend, Indiana.)

the maxillary and mandibular arches. (Centric is when the jaws are closed in a position that produces maximal stable contact between the occluding surfaces of the maxillary and mandibular teeth.)

This relationship is recorded as the **occlusal registration** or **bite registration.** When the casts of the upper and lower jaws are mounted on the articulator, this bite registration is used to establish the proper centric relationship. (An articulator is a device that simulates the movements of the jaws and the temporomandibular joint.)

Bite Registration Materials

Materials used for bite registration have a low flow ability, which allows the material to remain where it is placed. A wax bite or a bite gauze tray can be used, or the material can be directly placed on the occlusal surface of the teeth.

Wax Bite Registration

A wax bite registration is used to show the occlusal relationship of the maxillary and mandibular teeth (Figure 22-9). A baseplate wax is softened for this procedure. When taking a wax bite registration, you should:

- Instruct the patient to practice opening and closing their mouth normally.
- Use a heat source to soften the wax.
- Place the softened wax against the biting surfaces of the teeth.
- Instruct the patient to bite gently and naturally into the wax.
- Allow the wax to cool.
- Carefully remove the wax bite registration to prevent distortion.
- Store with impressions or casts.

Bite Registration Paste

Bite registration materials have gained popularity in taking a bite registration because the material:

- Is fast setting.
- Is convenient to use.
- Is supplied as a two-paste system or in cartridges.
- Can be directly applied to the arch or to a gauze tray into which the patient is instructed to bite.

In addition, the paste has:

- No resistance to biting forces.
- No odor or taste.

Laboratory Procedures

The dental laboratory is a separate area of the dental office (away from the patient treatment area) where the dentist and the clinical staff pour up the preliminary impressions and trim and finish the diagnostic models. When working in the laboratory, safety is the first concern. Following safety precautions and infection control procedures is essential.

Diagnostic Casts

A diagnostic cast is the model made from the impression. The materials most commonly used to create diagnostic casts are model plaster and dental stone.

Model plaster, which is a derivative of plaster of Paris, is used when strength is not essential and dimensional accuracy is not critical. Model plaster is easy to trim and is excellent for diagnostic casts because of its clean appearance (Figure 22-10).

Dental stone, which is a form of gypsum, is stronger than model plaster and is commonly used when a more durable diagnostic cast is required, for example, when used as a working model to make a retainer, a custom tray, or a casting by the laboratory technician (Figure 22-11).

Water-to-Powder Ratios

Although plaster and dental stone have the same chemical formulas, their physical structures are different, and using specific water-to-powder ratios for each is necessary. The water-to-powder ratio has a dramatic effect on the setting time and strength of any gypsum product. Water is measured by **volume (ml)**, and powder is measured by **weight (g)**.

Each type of cast has an optimal water-to-powder ratio, which is specified by the manufacturer. These ratios should be carefully followed. The following are the recommended water-to-powder ratios for one impression, including the base:

- **Model plaster:** 45 to 50 ml of water to 100 g of powder
- **Dental stone:** 30 to 32 ml of water to 100 g of powder

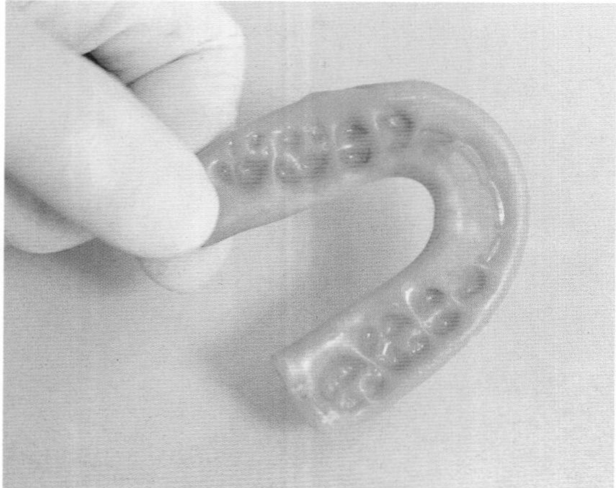

FIGURE 22-9 Wax bite registration.

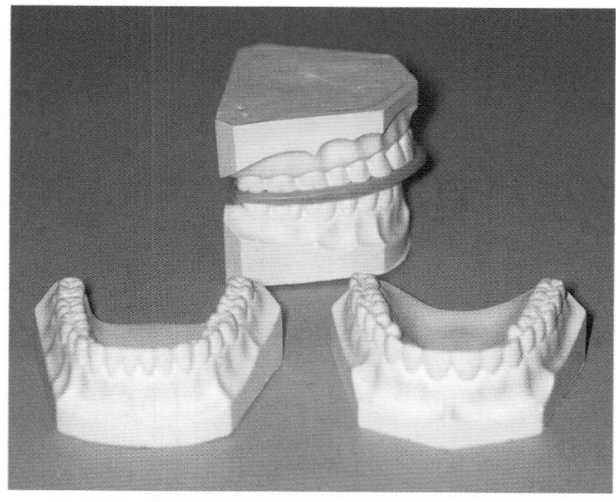

FIGURE 22-10 Dental casts made from plaster.

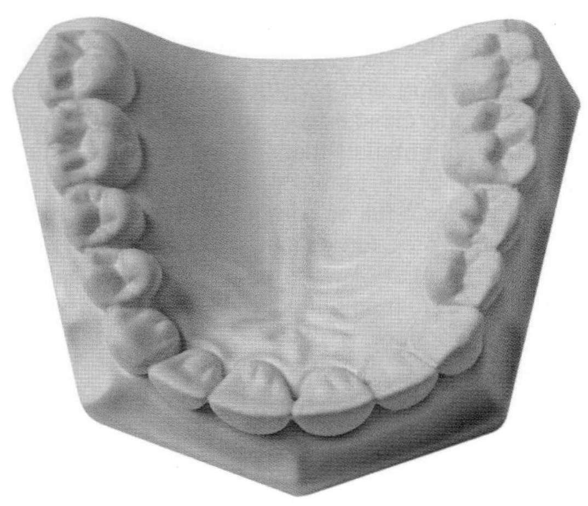

FIGURE 22-11 Dental cast made from stone. (Courtesy Whip Mix Corporation, Louisville, Kentucky.)

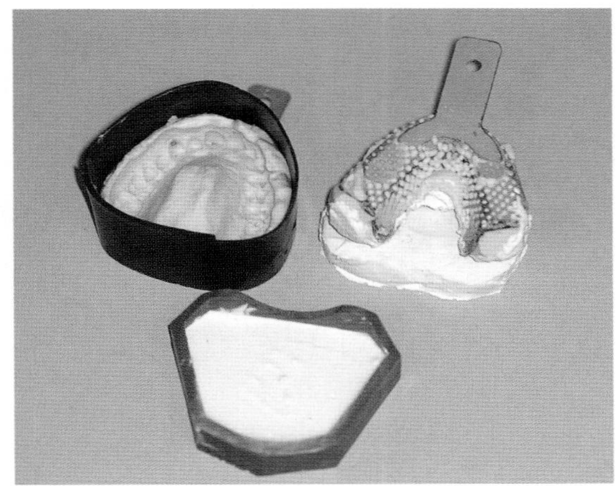

FIGURE 22-12 Examples of pouring methods. Boxed *(upper left)*; inverted *(upper right)*; double pour *(lower)*.

TABLE 22-3
Factors Influencing the Setting of Gypsum

Factors	Action and Reaction
Type of gypsum	Model plaster sets faster than dental stone.
Water-to-powder ratio	The less water that is used, the faster the set.
Mixing	The longer and faster the mixing, the faster the set.
Temperature of water	For best results, water should be at room temperature and no warmer than 70° F (21.1° C). The warmer the water, the faster the set.
Humidity	On a humid day, the gypsum can absorb the moisture in the air, which will slow the set.

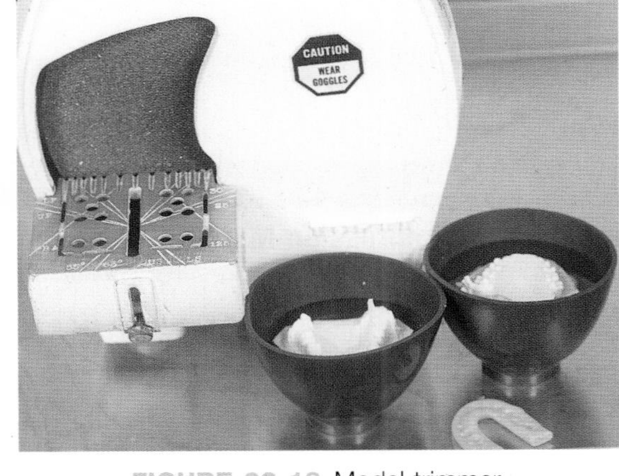

FIGURE 22-13 Model trimmer.

- **High-strength stone:** 19 to 24 ml of water to 100 g of powder

Influences on Setting Time

Having adequate working time to mix the material and to place it into the impression is important. The setting time is the length of time it takes for the mixture of stone or plaster to turn into a rigid solid. The setting time of gypsum products is influenced by the factors described in Table 22-3.

See Procedure 22-6: Mixing Dental Plaster.

Pouring Diagnostic Casts

Three methods are commonly used for pouring diagnostic casts: (1) **double-pour** method, (2) **box-and-pour** method, and (3) **inverted-pour** method. These methods differ only in the way the base portion is formed (Figure 22-12).

See Procedure 22-7: Pouring Dental Models Using the Inverted-Pour Method.

Trimming and Finishing Diagnostic Casts

When diagnostic casts are to be used for a case presentation or as part of the patient's permanent record, they should have an esthetic appearance. This is accomplished by trimming the casts to a geometric standard.

Casts are trimmed by using a **model trimmer** (Figure 22-13). A model trimmer is a device that is set up in the laboratory. The trimmer has a circular abrasive wheel that is set at 90 degrees to the cast. The wax bite **registration** is used to articulate the casts during the trimming process.

The cast consists of anatomic and art portions (Figure 22-14).

The **anatomic portion** includes the teeth, oral mucosa, and muscle attachments. This portion should make up two thirds of the overall cast.

The **art portion** forms the base. This section should be no more than ½ inch thick and should make up one third of the overall cast.

See Procedure 22-8: Trimming and Finishing Dental Models.

Maxillary model

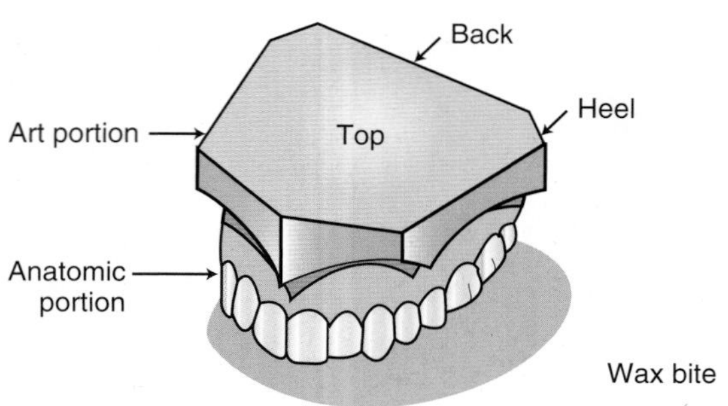

Mandibular model

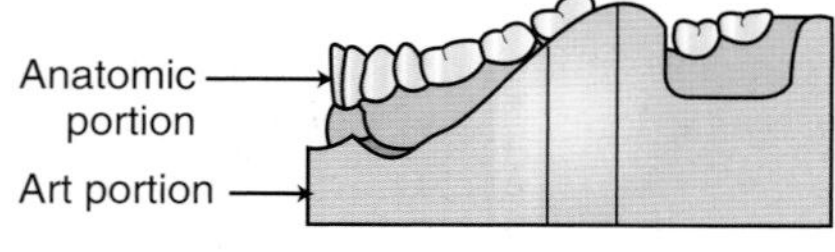

FIGURE 22-14 Anatomic and art portions of a dental cast.

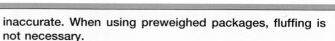

Ethical Implications

The timing of mixing and taking impressions is of utmost importance for the clinical assistant and the dentist. Most of the impression materials that you will mix will be for direct use by the laboratory technician when designing a cast crown, a bridge, or a full or partial denture. Remember that your role in these procedures is to mix impression materials and assist the dentist. Always check to see whether it is legal for you to obtain specified impressions in the state in which you are working.

Procedure 22-1

Mixing Alginate Impression Material

Equipment and Supplies

- Alginate
- Powder measure
- Water measure
- Medium-size rubber bowl
- Beavertail-shaped, wide-blade spatula

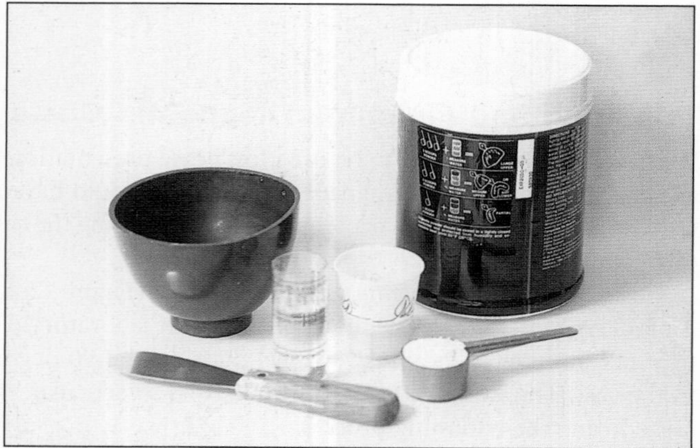

Procedural Steps

1. Place the appropriate amount of water in the bowl.
2. Shake the can of alginate to *fluff* the contents. After fluffing, carefully lift off the lid to prevent the particles from flying into the air.

Purpose: Alginate is fluffed because the material tends to settle and pack down in the can, making the measurement inaccurate. When using preweighed packages, fluffing is not necessary.

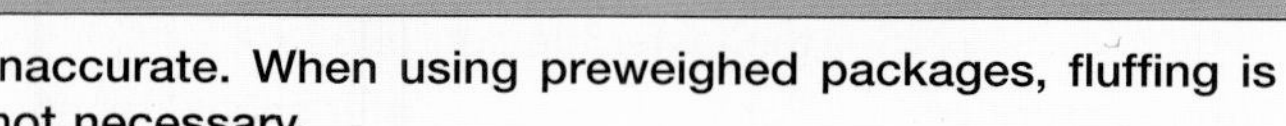

3. Sift the powder into the water, and use the spatula to mix with a stirring action to wet the powder until it has all been moistened.
4. Firmly spread the alginate between the spatula and the side of the rubber bowl.

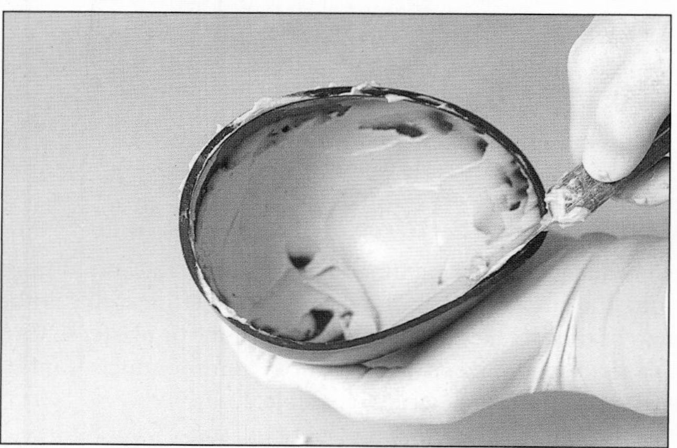

5. Mix with the spatula for the appropriate time. The mixture should appear smooth and creamy.

Purpose: Inadequate mixing of alginate causes the mix to contain air bubbles and a grainy texture, which may produce an unsatisfactory impression.

6. Wipe the alginate mix into one mass on the inside edge of the bowl.

Procedure 22-2

Taking a Mandibular Preliminary Impression (Expanded Function)

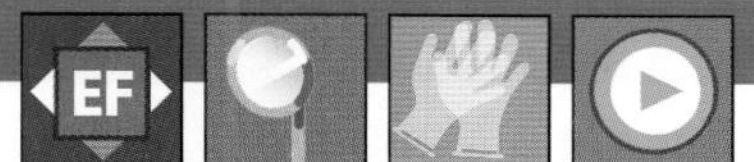

Equipment and Supplies

- Alginate powder
- Alginate measure scoop (provided by the manufacturer)
- Water measure (provided by the manufacturer)
- Room-temperature water (Cold water can increase the setting and warm water decrease the setting time.)
- Rubber bowl
- Wide-blade spatula
- Sterile impression trays
- Tray adhesive (used on nonperforated trays)
- Utility wax (if the tray needs to be extended)
- Saliva ejector
- Precaution (biohazard) bag

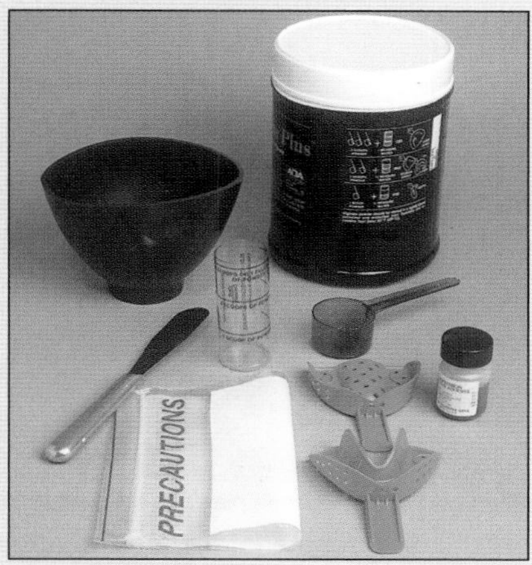

Preparation

1. Gather all necessary supplies.
2. Seat and prepare the patient.
3. Explain the procedure to the patient.
4. Select and prepare the mandibular impression tray.
5. Take 2 measures of room-temperature water with 2 scoops of alginate. Mix as specified in Procedure 22-1.

Loading the Mandibular Impression Tray

1. Gather half of the alginate in the bowl onto the spatula, then wipe alginate into one side of the tray from the lingual side. Quickly press the material down to the base of the tray.

Purpose: This step removes any air bubbles trapped in the tray.

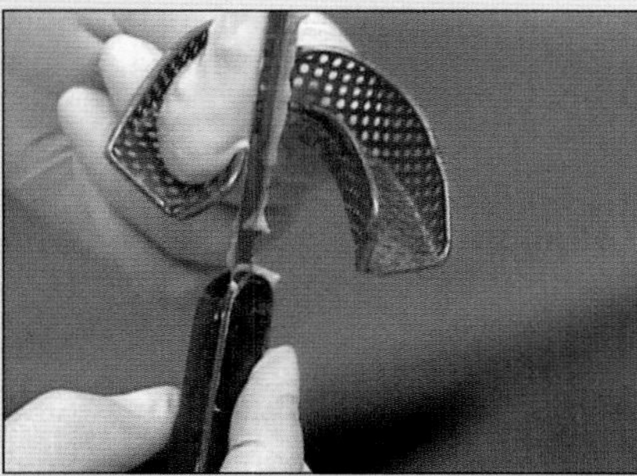

2. Gather the remaining half of the alginate in the bowl onto the spatula; then load the other side of the tray in the same way.
3. Smooth the surface of the alginate by wiping a moistened finger along the surface.

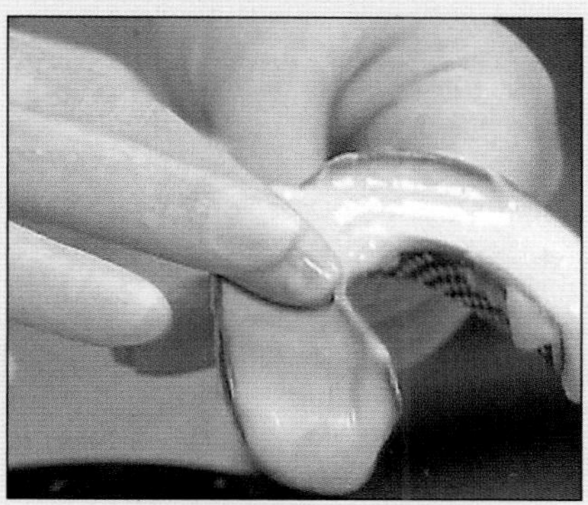

Seating the Mandibular Impression Tray

1. Place additional material over the occlusal surfaces of the mandibular teeth.

Purpose: This step places any extra material in the fissures and interproximal surfaces to create less discrepancy in the anatomy of the impression.

2. Retract the patient's cheek with the index finger.
3. Slightly turn the tray sideways when placing it into the mouth.
4. Center the tray over the teeth.

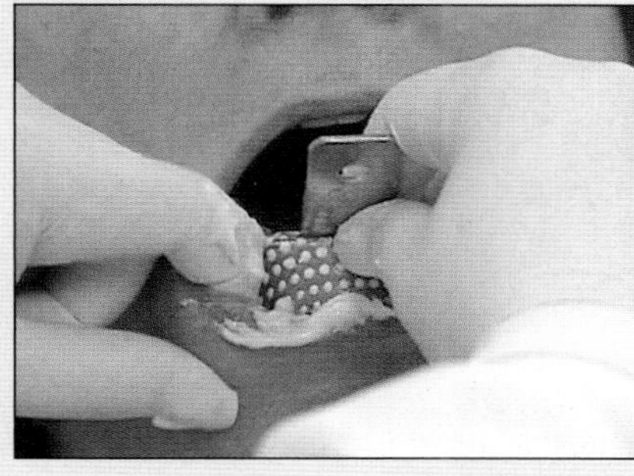

5. First, gently press down the posterior border of the tray.

Purpose: This step forms a seal.

6. Push down the anterior portion of the tray, and ask the patient to lift the tongue to the roof of the mouth and then to relax it.

Purpose: This step allows the alginate to form an impression of the lingual aspect of the alveolar process.

7. Instruct the patient to breathe normally while the tray is in place.
8. Observe the alginate around the tray to determine when the material has set.

Note: When set, the material should not register a dent when pressed with a finger.

Continued

Procedure 22-2

Taking a Mandibular Preliminary Impression (Expanded Function)—cont'd

Removing the Mandibular Impression

1. First, place your fingers on the top of the impression tray.

Purpose: This step protects the maxillary teeth from damage during the removal of the mandibular tray.

2. Gently break the seal between the impression and the peripheral tissue by moving the inside of the patient's cheeks or lips with your finger.
3. Grasping the handle of the tray with your thumb and index finger, use a firm lifting motion to break the seal.
4. Snap up the tray and impression from the dentition.
5. Instruct the patient to rinse with water to remove any excess alginate material.
6. Evaluate the impression for accuracy.
7. Rinse, disinfect, wrap the impression in a slightly moistened towel, and place it in the appropriate precaution bag before pouring up.

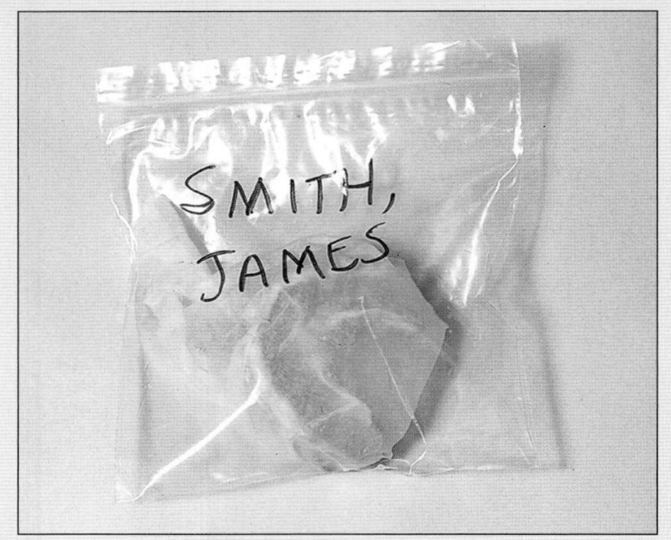

Procedure 22-3

Taking a Maxillary Preliminary Impression (Expanded Function)

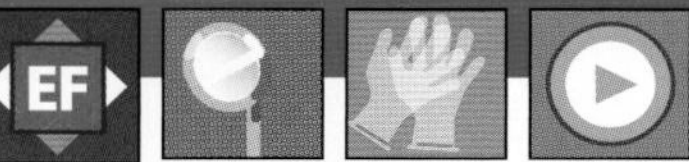

Equipment and Supplies

- Maxillary tray
- Other equipment and supplies are the same as assembled for a mandibular impression (see Procedure 22-2). If the same bowl and spatula are reused, then make certain they are clean and dry before beginning the next mix. For a maxillary impression, 3 measures of water are mixed with 3 scoops of powder.

Preparation

1. The preparation of the material is the same as performed in Procedure 22-2.

Loading the Maxillary Impression Tray

1. Load the maxillary tray in one large increment, using a wiping motion to fill the tray from the posterior end.

Purpose: This step helps prevent the formation of air bubbles in the material.

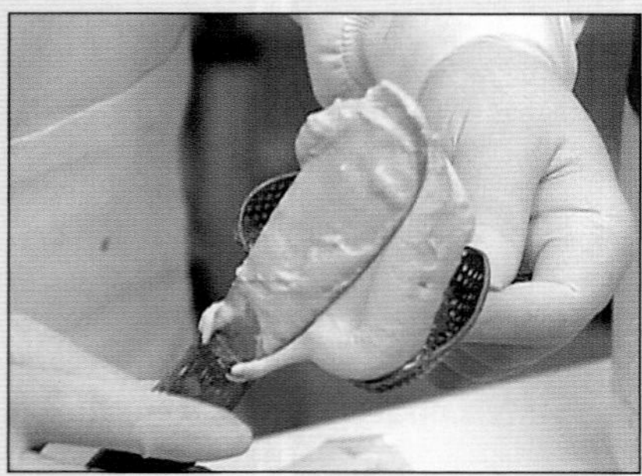

2. Place the bulk of the material toward the anterior palatal area of the tray.

Purpose: This step prevents the alginate from flowing beyond the tray and into the patient's throat during tray placement.

3. Moisten your fingertips with tap water, and smooth the surface of the alginate.

Seating the Maxillary Impression Tray

1. Use your index finger to retract the patient's cheek.
2. Slightly turn the tray sideways to position the tray into the mouth.

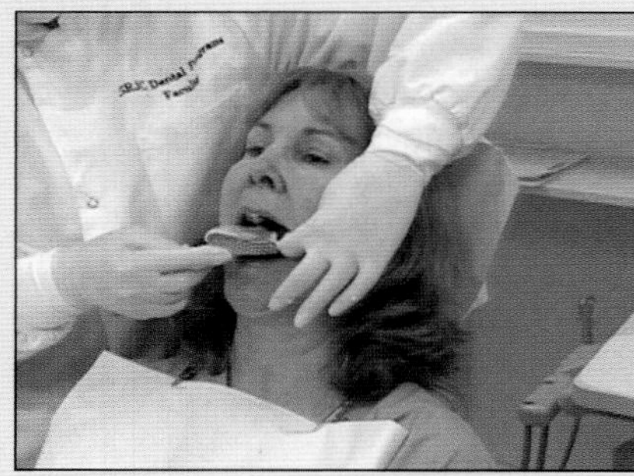

3. Center the tray over the patient's teeth.
4. Seat the posterior border (back) of the tray up against the posterior border of the hard palate to form a seal.

Purpose: This step prevents the excess material from going toward the back of the mouth.

Procedure 22-3

Taking a Maxillary Preliminary Impression (Expanded Function)—cont'd

5. Direct the anterior portion of the tray upward over the teeth.
6. Gently lift the patient's lips out of the way as the tray is seated.

Purpose: Retraction of the lips allows the material to flow into the vestibular areas.

7. Check the posterior border of the tray to ensure that no material is flowing into the patient's throat. If necessary, wipe excess material away with a cotton-tip applicator.

Purpose: This technique helps prevent triggering the gag reflex when the material touches the soft palate area.

8. Firmly hold the tray in place while the alginate sets.

Removing the Maxillary Impression

1. To avoid injury to the impression and to the patient's teeth, place a finger along the lateral borders of the tray to push down and break the palatal seal.
2. Use a straight, downward snapping motion to remove the tray from the teeth.
3. Instruct the patient to rinse with water to remove any excess alginate impression material.

Caring for Alginate Impressions

1. Gently rinse the impressions under cold tap water to remove any blood or saliva.

Purpose: Bioburden will interfere with the setting of gypsum products.

2. Spray the impression with an approved disinfectant.
3. If the impression must be stored before pouring, then wrap it in a damp paper towel and store the impression in a covered container or plastic bag labeled with the patient's name.

Before Dismissing the Patient

1. Examine the patient's mouth for any remaining fragments of alginate, and remove them using an explorer and dental floss.
2. Use a moist facial tissue to remove any alginate from the patient's face and lips.

Procedure 22-4

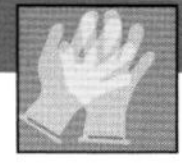

Mixing a Two-Paste Final Impression Material

Equipment and Supplies

- Stock custom tray with appropriate adhesive
- Large, stiff, tapered spatulas (2)
- Large paper pads (2)
- Light-bodied base and catalyst
- Heavy-bodied base and catalyst
- Impression syringe with sterile tip
- 2 × 2-inch gauze pads

Procedural Steps

Preparing Light-Bodied Syringe Material

1. Dispense approximately 1½ to 2 inches of equal lengths of the base and catalyst of the light-bodied material onto the top one third of the pad, making sure that the materials are not too close to each other.

Purpose: Some paste materials tend to start spreading on the pad, and preventing a premature reaction is important.

2. Wipe the tube openings clean with gauze, and immediately recap.

Purpose: Cleaning the top of the tube and the threads prevents the cap from becoming messy and sticking.

3. Place the tip of the spatula blade into the catalyst and base. Mix in a swirling direction for approximately 5 seconds.
4. Gather the material onto the flat portion of the spatula. Place it on a clean area of the pad, preferably in the center.

Purpose: By beginning the mix on a clean area of the pad, a more homogeneous mix will be obtained.

5. Smoothly spatulate, wiping back and forth and trying to use only one side of the spatula during the mixing process.

Purpose: Material is lost by using both sides of the blade.

6. To obtain a more homogeneous mix, pick the material up by the spatula blade and wipe it onto the pad.

Purpose: The material is pulled from the bottom to the top of the mix.

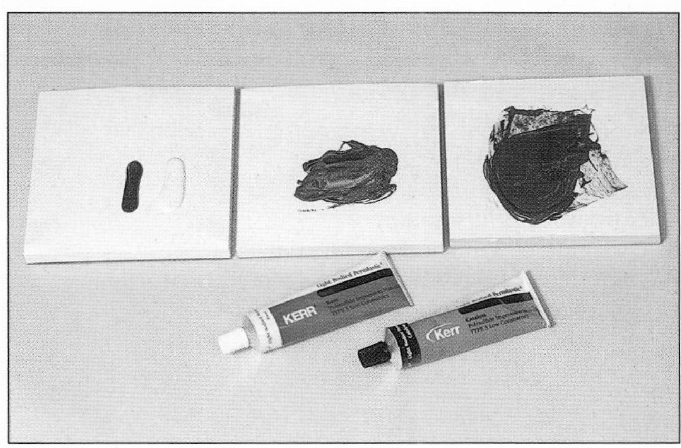

7. Gather the material together, and take the syringe tube and begin *cookie cutting* the material into the syringe.

Continued

Procedure 22-4

Mixing a Two-Paste Final Impression Material—cont'd

Insert the plunger, and express a small amount of the material to make sure it is in working order.

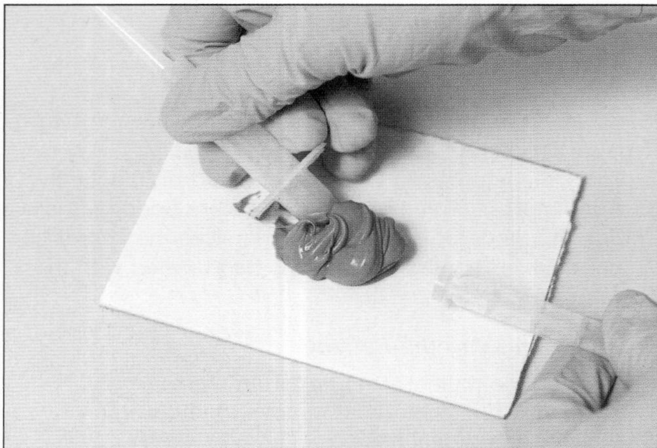

8. Transfer the syringe to the dentist, making sure the tip of the syringe is directed toward the tooth.

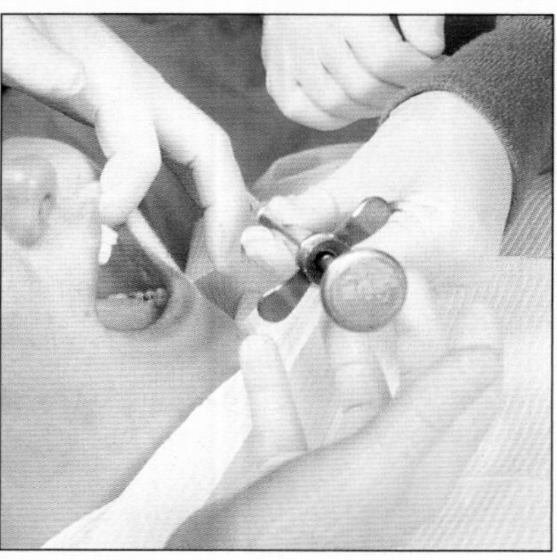

Preparing Heavy-Bodied Tray Material

1. Dispense approximately 3 to 4 inches of equal lengths of the base and catalyst of the heavy-bodied material on the top third of the pad for a quadrant tray.

Note: The amount of material placed depends on whether you are using a quadrant tray or a full-arch tray.

2. Place the tip of the spatula blade into the catalyst and base. Mix in a swirling direction for approximately 5 seconds.
3. Gather the material onto the flat portion of the spatula, and place it on a clean area of the pad, preferably in the center.

Purpose: Starting the mix on a clean area of the pad results in a more homogeneous mix.

4. Smoothly spatulate, wiping back and forth and trying to use only one side of the spatula during the mixing process.

Purpose: Material is lost by using both sides of the blade.

5. To obtain a more homogeneous mix, pick up the material by the spatula blade and wipe it on the pad.

Purpose: The material is pulled from the bottom to the top of the mix.

6. Gather the bulk of the material with the spatula, and load it into the tray. The best way to complete this step without incorporating air is to use the flat side of the spatula and to follow around the outside rim of the tray, *wiping* the material into the tray.
7. Using the tip of the spatula, evenly spread the material from one end of the tray to the other without picking up the material.

Purpose: When the material is pulled in an upward direction, air is incorporated into the mixture.

8. Retrieve the syringe from the dentist, and transfer the tray, making sure the dentist is able to grasp the handle of the tray properly.

Procedure 22-5

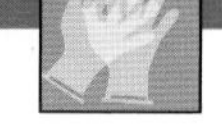

Preparing an Automix Final Impression Material

Equipment and Supplies

- Stock or custom tray with appropriate adhesive
- Extruder units (2)
- Extruder mixing tips (2)
- Light-bodied mixing tip
- Cartridge of light-bodied material
- Cartridge of heavy-bodied material
- 2 × 2-inch gauze pads

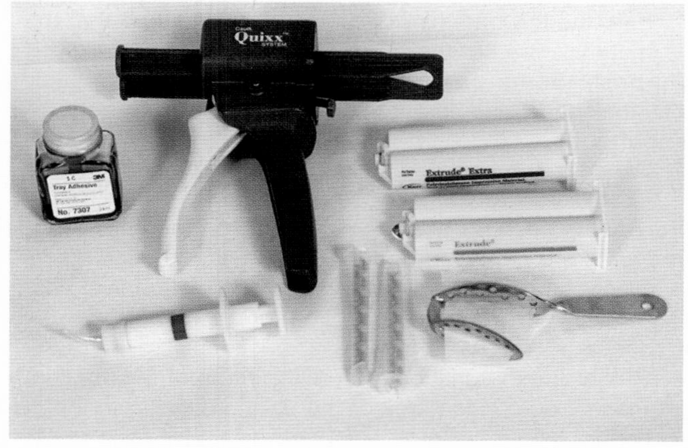

(From Hatrick CD, Eakle WS: Dental materials: clinical applications for dental assistants and dental hygienists, ed 3, St Louis, 2016, Saunders.)

Procedure 22-5

Preparing an Automix Final Impression Material—cont'd

Procedural Steps

1. Load the extruder with dual cartridges of the base and the catalyst of light-bodied material.
2. Remove the caps from the tube, and **extrude** (force or push out) a small amount of unmixed material onto the gauze pad.

Purpose: This step ensures that no air bubbles are in the mix and removes any hardened material that might remain.

3. Attach a mixing tip on the extruder along with a syringe tip for the light-bodied application by the dentist.

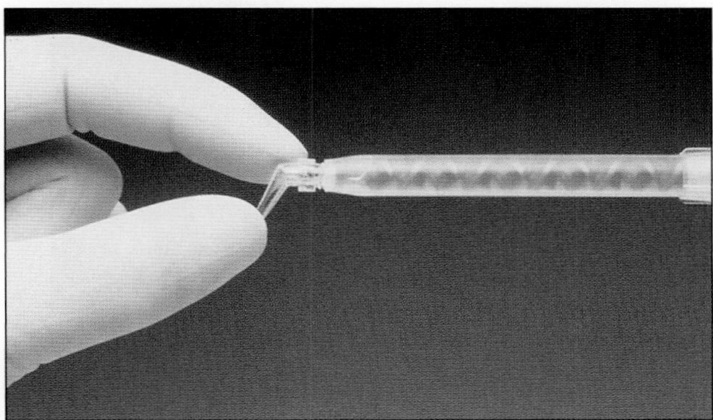

(Courtesy 3M ESPE, St Paul, Minnesota.)

4. When the dentist signals readiness, begin squeezing the trigger until the material has reached the tip.
5. Transfer the extruder to the dentist, ensuring that the tip is directed toward the area of the impression.
6. The dentist places the light-bodied material over and around the prepared teeth and onto the surrounding tissue.

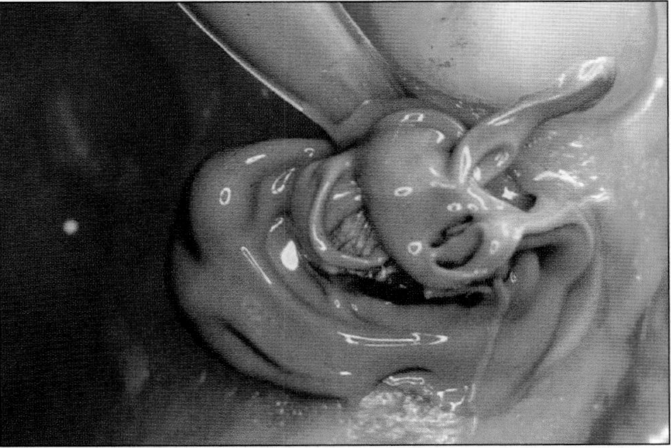

(Courtesy 3M ESPE, St Paul, Minnesota.)

7. Place the heavy-bodied cartridges in the extruder, making sure to express a small amount (the same as with the light-bodied material). Attach the mixing tip to the cartridge.
8. When the dentist signals readiness, begin squeezing the trigger, mixing the heavy-bodied material.
9. Load the impression tray with the heavy-bodied material, making sure not to trap air in the material.

Note: Begin expressing the material at one end of the tray, and follow through to the other end without taking the tip out of the material.

10. Transfer the tray, making sure the dentist is able to grasp the handle of the tray.
11. When the impression materials have reached final set, the impression is removed and is inspected for accuracy by the dentist.

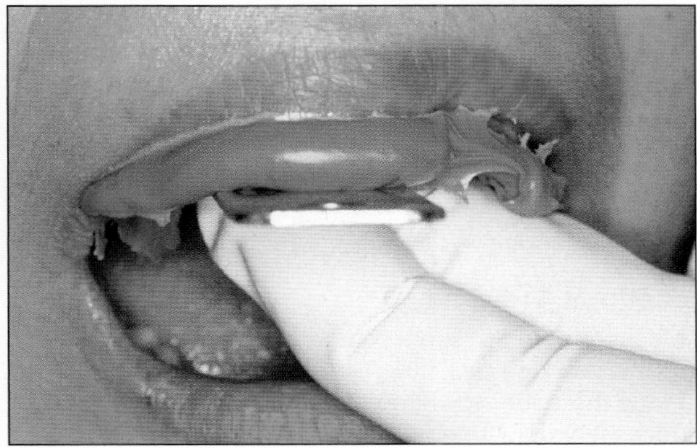

(Courtesy 3M ESPE, St Paul, Minnesota.)

12. The impression is disinfected, placed in a precaution bag, labeled with the patient's name, and taken to the laboratory.

Procedure 22-6

Mixing Dental Plaster

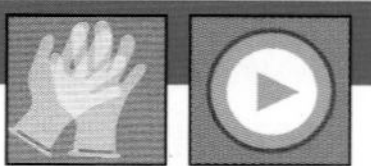

Equipment and Supplies

- Flexible rubber mixing bowl (clean and dry)
- Metal spatula (stiff blade with a rounded end)
- Scale
- Plaster (100 g)
- Water-measuring device
- Room-temperature water (70° F)
- Vibrator with a disposable cover

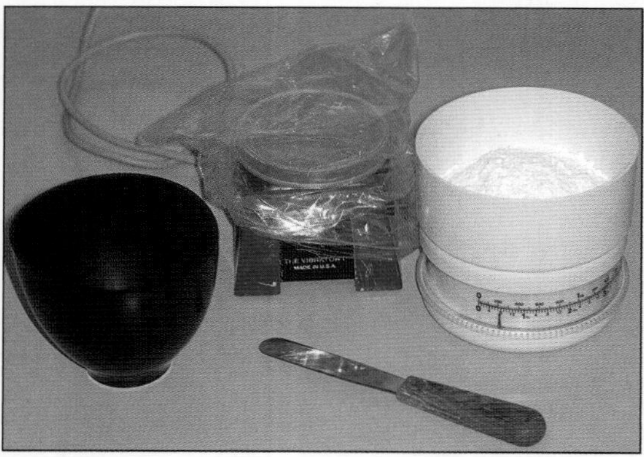

Procedural Steps

1. Measure 45 ml of room-temperature water into a clean rubber mixing bowl.
2. Place the paper towel on the scale, and make necessary adjustments.
3. Weigh out 100 g of dental plaster.
4. Add the powder to the water in steady increments. Allow the powder to settle into the water for approximately 30 seconds.

Purpose: This step prevents the trapping of air bubbles.

5. Use the spatula to incorporate the powder slowly into the water. A smooth and creamy mix should be achieved in approximately 20 seconds.

Purpose: This step helps avoid spilling the powder.

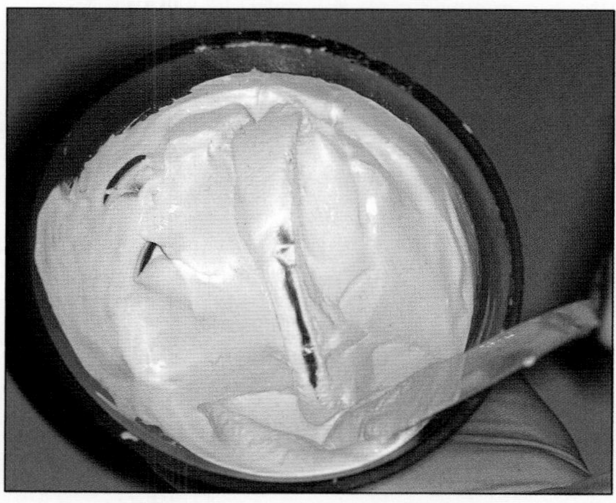

6. Turn the vibrator to low or medium speed, and place the bowl of plaster mix on the vibrator platform.

Purpose: This step helps reduce the air in the mix.

7. Lightly press and rotate the bowl on the vibrator. Air bubbles will rise to the surface.
8. Complete mixing and vibration of the plaster for no longer than 2 minutes.

Procedure 22-7

Pouring Dental Models Using the Inverted-Pour Method

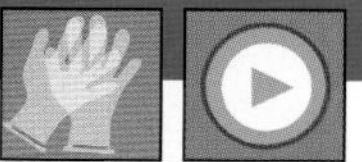

Equipment and Supplies

- Maxillary and mandibular impressions
- Glass slab or tile
- Laboratory spatula
- Laboratory knife and cutters
- 150 g of plaster (additional plaster is needed for the base)
- 60 ml of water (additional water needed for the base)
- Flexible rubber bowl
- Vibrator

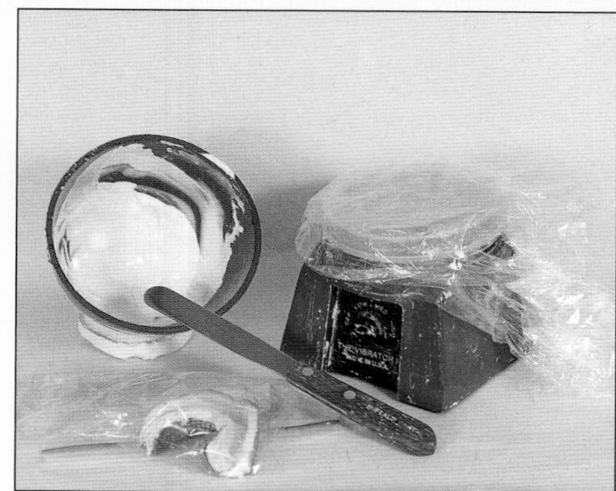

Procedure 22-7

Pouring Dental Models Using the Inverted-Pour Method—cont'd

Procedural Steps

Preparing the Impression

1. Use a gentle stream of air to remove excess moisture from the impression. Be careful not to dry out the impression.

Purpose: Overdrying can cause distortion of the material.

2. Use your laboratory knife or laboratory cutters to remove any excess impression material that will interfere with the pouring of the model.

Pouring the Mandibular Model and Base

1. Mix the plaster, and then set the vibrator at low to medium speed.

Note: A separate mix is made for each impression.

2. Hold the impression tray by the handle, and place the edge of the base of the handle on the vibrator.
3. Dip the spatula into the plaster mix, picking up a small increment (approximately ½ teaspoon).
4. Place the small increment in the impression near the most posterior tooth. Guide the material as it flows lingually.

Purpose: The flowing action pushes out the air ahead of it and eliminates air bubbles.

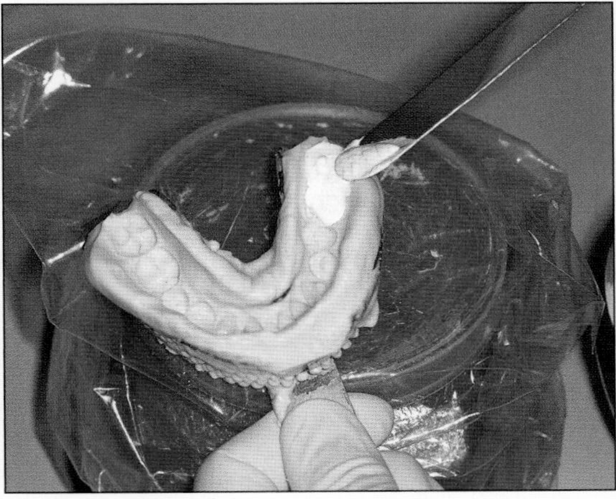

5. Continue to place small increments in the same area as the first increment, and allow the plaster to flow toward the anterior teeth.
6. Turn the tray on its side to provide the continuous flow of material forward into each tooth impression.
7. Once all of the teeth in the impression are covered, begin to add larger increments until the entire impression is filled.

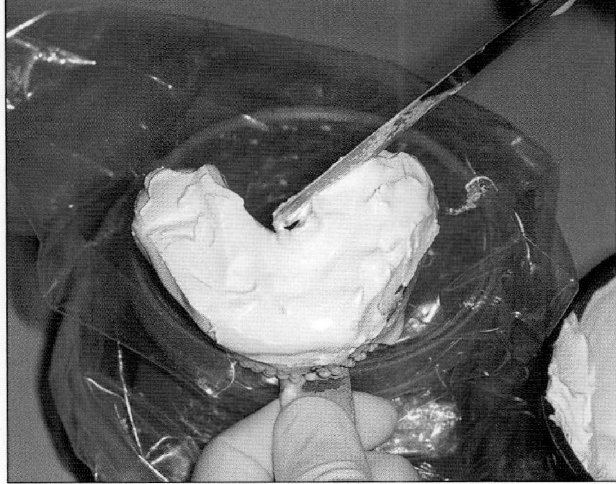

8. Place the additional material onto a glass slab (or tile); shape the base to approximately 2 × 2 inches by 1 inch thick.

Note: Commercial rubber molds are available for making bases. These molds provide symmetry to the cast and reduce the need for trimming.

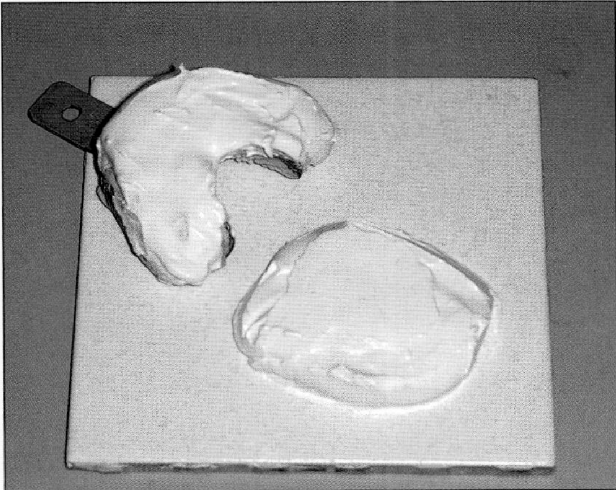

9. Invert the impression onto the new mix. Do not push the impression into the base.

Purpose: When the poured impression is inverted onto the new mix, the fresh material tends to flow excessively, which can result in a base that is too large and too thin.

10. Holding the tray steady, use a spatula to smooth the plaster base mix up onto the margins of the initial pour. Be careful not to cover the impression tray with

Continued

Procedure 22-7
Pouring Dental Models Using the Inverted-Pour Method—cont'd

material; otherwise, removing the cast from the impression will be difficult.

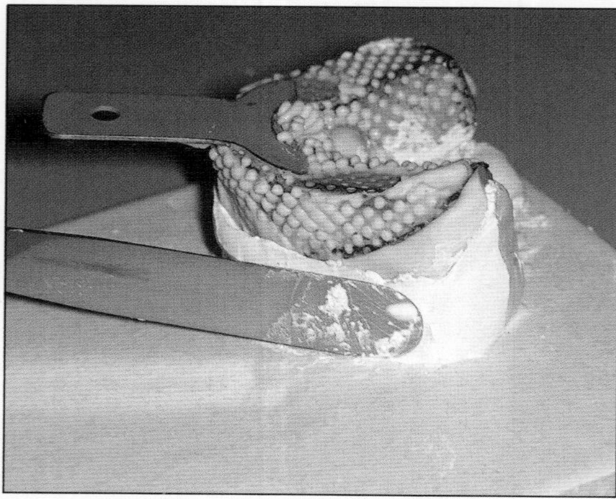

Pouring the Maxillary Cast

1. Repeat steps 3 through 5, using clean equipment for the fresh mix of stone.
2. Place the small increment of plaster in the posterior area of the impression. Guide the material as it flows down into the impression of the most posterior tooth.
3. Continue to place small increments in the same area as the first increment, and allow the plaster to flow toward the anterior teeth.
4. Rotate the tray on its side to provide the continuous flow of material into each tooth impression.
5. Once all the teeth in the impression are covered, begin to add larger increments until the entire impression is filled.
6. Place the mix onto a glass slab (or tile), and shape the base to approximately 2 × 2 inches by 1 inch thick.

Note: Commercial rubber molds are available for making bases. These molds provide symmetry to the cast and reduce the need for trimming.

7. Invert the impression onto the new mix. Do not push the impression into the base.

Purpose: When the poured impression is inverted onto the new mix, the fresh material tends to flow excessively, which can result in a base that is too large and too thin.

8. Holding the tray steady, use a spatula to smooth the stone base mix onto the margins of the initial pour. Be careful not to cover the impression tray with plaster; otherwise, removing the cast from the impression will be difficult.
9. Place the impression tray on the base so that the handle and the occlusal plane of the teeth on the cast are parallel with the surface of the glass slab (or tile).

Purpose: This step helps form a base with uniform thickness.

Separating the Cast From the Impression

1. Wait 45 to 60 minutes after the base has been poured before separating the impression from the model.

Purpose: The material needs to complete its initial setting stage, or teeth could fracture while removing the impression.

2. Use the laboratory knife to separate the margins of the tray gently.
3. Apply firm, straight, and upward pressure on the handle of the tray to remove the impression.
4. If the tray does not easily separate, then check to see where the tray is still attached to the impression. Again, use the laboratory knife to free the tray from the model.
5. Pull the tray handle straight up from the model.

Note: Never wiggle the impression tray from side to side while it is on the cast. This movement can cause the teeth on the cast to fracture.

6. The models are ready for trimming and polishing.

Procedure 22-8
Trimming and Finishing Dental Models

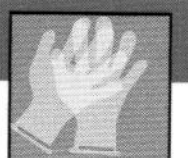

Equipment and Supplies

- Poured stone maxillary and mandibular dental model
- Wax bite registration
- Pencil
- Ruler
- Laboratory knife
- Model trimmer

Procedural Steps

Preparing the Model

1. Soak the art portion of the model in a bowl of water for at least 5 minutes.

Purpose: Soaking the art portion makes the trimming easier.

Procedure 22-8

Trimming and Finishing Dental Models—cont'd

Trimming the Maxillary Model

1. Place the maxillary model on a flat countertop with the teeth setting on the table. Use your pencil to measure up 1¼ inches from the counter, and draw a line around the model.

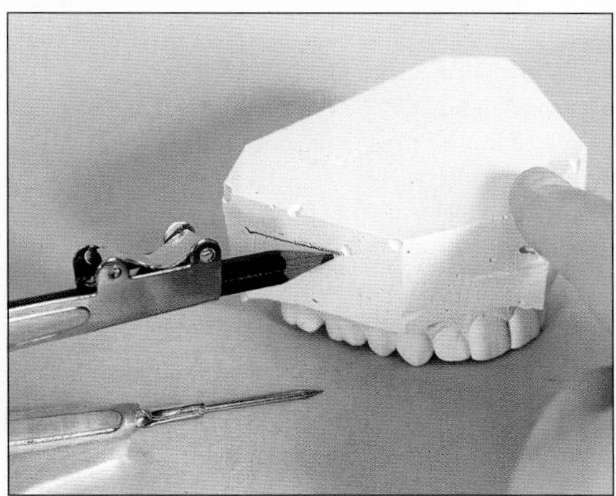

2. Turn on the trimmer. Firmly hold the model against the trimmer, and trim the bottom of the base to the drawn line.
3. Draw a line ¼ inch behind the maxillary tuberosities. With the base flat on the trimmer, remove excess plaster in the posterior area of the model to the marked line.
4. To trim the sides of the model, draw a line through the center of the occlusal ridges on one side of the model. Measure out ¼ inch from this line, and draw a line parallel to the previous drawn line.

Note: If you need to measure beyond ¼ inch to ensure that the mucobuccal fold is not trimmed away, do so.

5. Repeat these measurements on the other side of the model.
6. Trim the sides of the cast to the lines drawn.

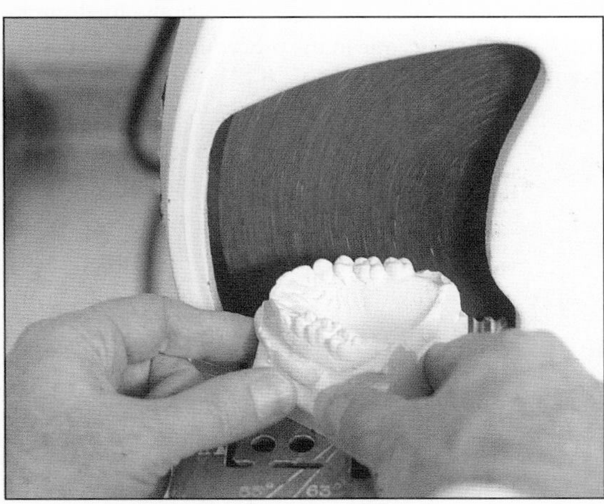

7. Draw a line behind the tuberosity that is perpendicular to the opposite canine, and trim to the drawn line. This steps completes the maxillary heel cuts.
8. The final cut is made by drawing a line from the canine to the midline at an angle. Complete this on both sides, and trim to the drawn line.

Trimming the Mandibular Model

1. Occlude the mandibular model with the maxillary model using the wax bite.
2. With the mandibular base on the trimmer, trim the posterior portion of the mandibular model until it is even with the maxillary model.
3. Place the models upside down (maxillary base on the table), measure 3 inches from the surface up, and mark a line around the base of the mandibular model.
4. Trim the mandibular model base to the drawn line.

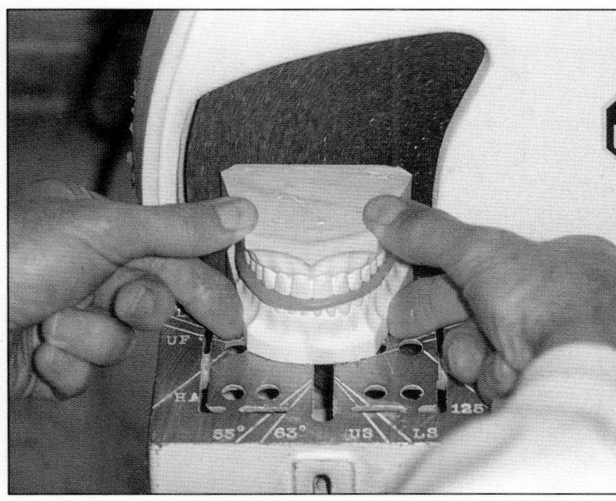

5. With the models in occlusion with the wax bite, place the mandibular model on the trimmer, and trim the lateral cuts to match the maxillary lateral cuts.
6. Trim the back and heel cuts to match the maxillary heel cuts.
7. Check that the mandibular anterior cut is rounded from the mandibular right canine to the mandibular left canine.
8. The models are now ready to be finished.

Finishing the Model

1. Mix a slurry of gypsum and water, and fill in any voids.
2. Using a laboratory knife, remove any extra gypsum that occurs as beads on the occlusion or model.

Chapter Exercises

Multiple Choice

Circle the letter next to the correct answer.

1. A maxillary alginate impression routinely requires __________ scoops of powder.
   - a. 1
   - b. 2
   - c. 3
   - d. 4
2. Diagnostic casts can be used by the dentist and the laboratory technician for __________ cases.
   - a. orthodontic
   - b. endodontic
   - c. prosthodontic
   - d. a and c
3. The light-bodied final impression material is most commonly applied to the prepared tooth using a __________.
   - a. tray
   - b. syringe
   - c. crown form
   - d. spatula
4. The dentist will be taking a final impression specifically for tooth #24. The __________ tray design would be selected for this procedure.
   - a. quadrant
   - b. section
   - c. full-arch
   - d. b or c
5. When an extruder unit is used, the impression material is actually mixed __________.
   - a. on a paper pad first
   - b. within the cartridges
   - c. in the mixing tip
   - d. in the tray
6. An acceptable diagnostic cast should be trimmed for a case presentation. The best way to trim the cast is to use __________.
   - a. a slow-speed handpiece with a laboratory bur
   - b. hand instruments
   - c. sandpaper discs
   - d. a laboratory model trimmer
7. The water-to-powder ratio for plaster for a single cast and its base is 100 g of powder to __________ ml of water.
   - a. 45 to 50
   - b. 55 to 65
   - c. 65 to 75
   - d. 75 to 80
8. Before diagnostic casts are trimmed, the casts should be __________.
   - a. set in a warm environment
   - b. soaked in water
   - c. placed in the refrigerator
   - d. blown dry
9. A procedure that is used to replicate a patient's occlusion is a(n) __________.
   - a. wax bite
   - b. alginate
   - c. bite registration
   - d. a and c
10. When mixing a final impression paste material on a pad, incorporate the __________ into the __________.
    - a. base; catalyst
    - b. catalyst; base
    - c. paste; liquid
    - d. alginate; water

Apply Your Knowledge

1. You are assisting the dentist in taking a final impression of the upper-right quadrant for a single crown. You are using an automix system of impression material. While loading the tray, you notice that the cartridge has run out of material. What should you do?
2. Your dentist has asked you to take an impression on the patient in the next room and to pour the models for an orthodontic consultation. Which type of impression can you legally take, and what material will you use to pour the impression?
3. The dentist is running behind schedule and has to get to the next patient. He asks you to go ahead and take the final impression on tooth #5. Is this your role in the procedure? If so, what steps do you take? If not, how do you handle this situation?

CHAPTER 23

Prosthodontics and Dental Implants

http://evolve.elsevier.com/Robinson/essentials/

LEARNING OBJECTIVES

1. Pronounce, define, and spell the key terms.
2. Complete the following related to fixed prosthodontics:
   - Discuss the specific types of fixed prosthetics.
   - List the indications and contraindications to prescribing fixed prosthodontics.
   - Describe the differences among a full crown, inlay, onlay, and veneer.
   - List the types of provisional coverage.
   - Describe the procedures related to fixed prosthodontics.
3. Identify and state the functions and components of a removable partial denture.
4. Identify and state the functions and components of a complete denture.
5. Describe how to reline a complete partial denture and discuss when immediate dentures are used.
6. Identify the types of dental implants, and describe the surgical procedures for implantation.
7. Describe home care instructions for fixed and removable prosthodontics and dental implants.

KEY TERMS

abutment
articulator
bridge
core
crown
edentulous
endosteal
fixed bridge
flange
framework
gingival retraction
implants
inlay
onlay
osseointegration
pontic
post
provisional coverage
rests
retainers
saddle
subperiosteal
transosteal
unit

Prosthodontics is comprised of two specialty areas in dentistry: **fixed prosthodontics**, which is the replacement of missing teeth with a cast prosthesis that is cemented in place and cannot be removed by the patient, and **removable prosthodontics**, which is the replacement of missing teeth with a prosthesis that the patient can freely take in and out of the mouth.

Dental implants provide a natural-looking and functional replacement for missing teeth that incorporates the principles from fixed and removable prosthodontics with the use of a bone-anchored implant. Dental implants are now considered the standard of care in the replacement of a single tooth or multiple teeth.

Fixed Prosthodontics

Fixed prosthodontics, also referred to as **crown** or **bridge**, is often the dentist's preferred choice if more than three fourths of a tooth structure requires restoration. Table 23-1 illustrates the different types of fixed prosthetics that can be used for a specific need.

TABLE 23-1
Types of Fixed Prosthodontics

Name	Description
Inlay 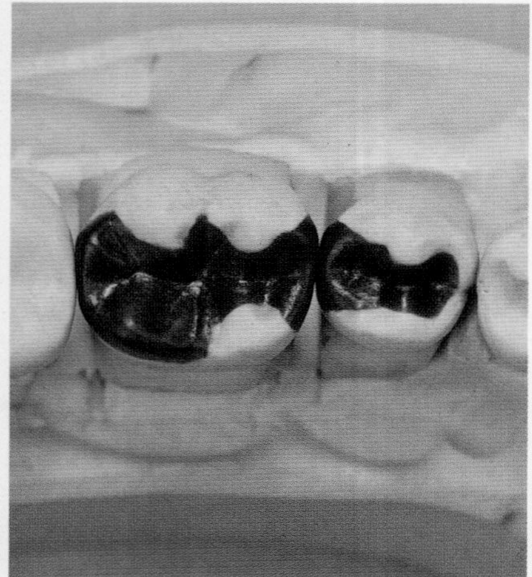 (From Heymann HO, Swift EJ, Ritter AV: *Sturdevant's art and science of operative dentistry,* ed 6, St Louis, 2013, Mosby.)	An inlay cast restoration is made from either porcelain or gold, which is created to fit into a Class II preparation. The inlay restoration involves the occlusal surface and one or more proximal surfaces.
Onlay 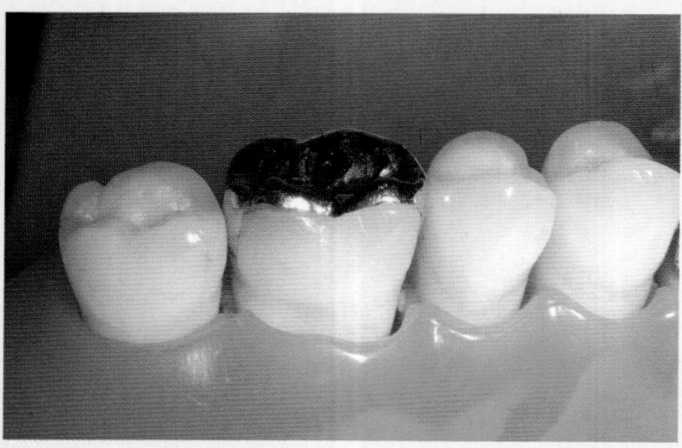	An onlay cast restoration is made from either porcelain or gold. The onlay restoration involves multiple surfaces, covering all of the occlusal and a portion of the proximal surfaces.
Crown 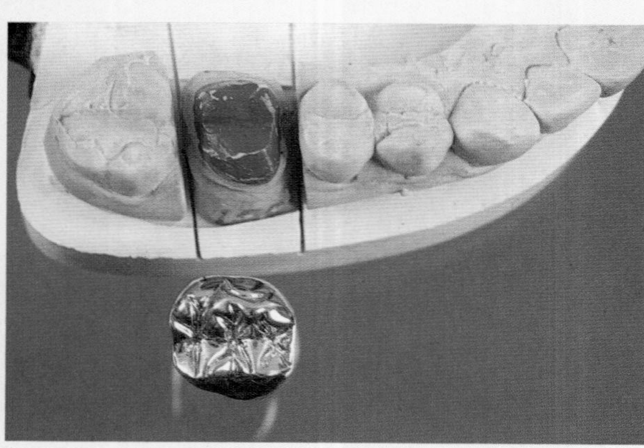	A crown is a single cast restoration that completely covers the anatomic portion of a tooth. The materials used to make crowns are porcelain fused to metal (PFM), porcelain, or gold. PFM castings allow the esthetics of porcelain to be placed on the facial side of the crown or bridge and the strength of the metals on the occlusal, lingual, and proximal surfaces to provide strength for occlusion.

TABLE 23-1
Types of Fixed Prosthodontics—cont'd

Name	Description
Fixed bridge 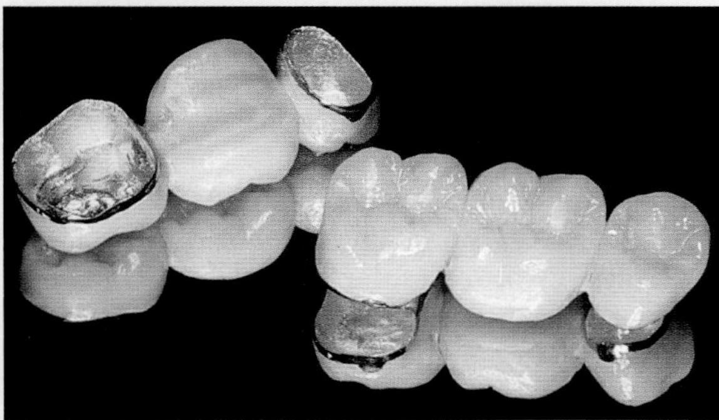 (Courtesy Captek, The Argen Corporation, San Diego, California.)	The fixed bridge replaces one or more missing teeth adjacent to each other in the same arch. A bridge can be fabricated from PFM, porcelain, or gold. Because more than one tooth is involved, the parts of the bridge are as follows: • A unit indicates the number of teeth involved in the bridge (e.g., three teeth involved would be a three-unit bridge). • A **pontic** is the artificial tooth that it replaces in the bridge. • Abutments are the natural teeth involved in the bridge that support the pontics. At least one abutment is required.
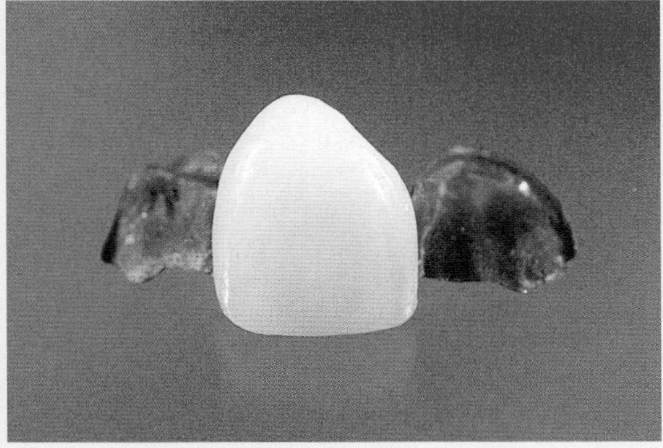	Also referred to as a Maryland bridge, a fixed bridge consists of a pontic that is made of porcelain with a winglike extension framework that is bonded into place on the lingual sides of the adjacent teeth.

Considerations for Prescribing Fixed Prosthodontics

Indications

- One or two adjacent teeth are missing in the same arch.
- Supportive tissues are healthy.
- Suitable abutment teeth are present.
- Patient is in good health and wants to have the prosthesis placed.
- Patient has the skills and motivation to maintain good oral hygiene.

Contraindications

- Supportive tissues are diseased or missing.
- Suitable abutment teeth are not present.
- Patient is in poor health or is not motivated to have the prosthesis placed.
- Patient has poor oral hygiene habits.
- Patient cannot afford the treatment.

Crown and Bridge Procedural Steps

Shade Selection

If the inlay, onlay, crown, or bridge is to be cast to match adjacent teeth with porcelain or porcelain fused to metal **(PFM)**, then matching the shade is completed at the first appointment, before the procedure is started. A **shade guide**, which contains samples of all available shades, is used to match the natural tooth color (Figure 23-1).

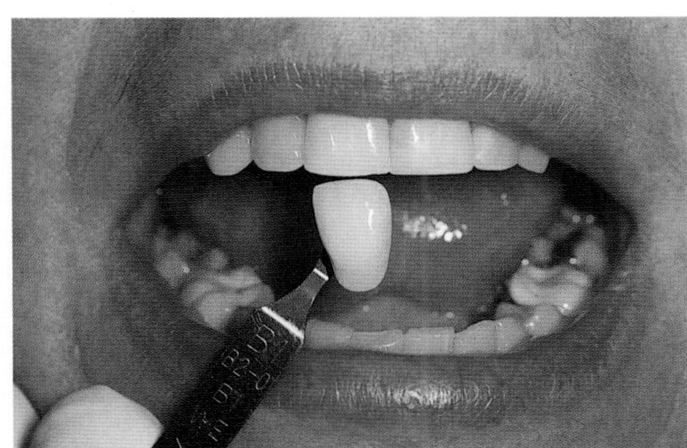

FIGURE 23-1 Shade guide used to match the exact color of teeth. (From Hatrick CD, Eakle WS: *Dental materials: clinical applications for dental assistants and dental hygienists,* ed 3, St Louis, 2016, Saunders.)

To ensure an exact match, using natural light is best. The shade selected is identified by a number from the shade guide and is noted on the patient's record and on the laboratory prescription. The shade guide is a semicritical item that cannot withstand the heat of sterilization. After use, it must be disinfected.

Preparation

The creation of a single **unit** cast restoration (**inlay**, **onlay**, or crown) or a multiple unit (**fixed bridge**) cast restoration requires a minimum of two appointments. The first appointment is scheduled for taking preliminary impressions, preparing the tooth structure, taking final impressions, and the placement of a temporary restoration. The second appointment is for the *try-in* of the casting, adjustments, and final cementation of the completed restoration.

Tooth Preparation

During tooth preparation, the height and contour of the natural tooth or teeth are reduced to remove any diseased tooth structure and to prepare the tooth for the casting. The prepared tooth is shaped so that the cast restoration can fit down over the preparation to resemble its natural tooth (Figure 23-2).

If the coronal portion of the tooth is extensively decayed, fractured, or worn, then providing additional support for the crown may be necessary.

Core buildups A **core** buildup uses amalgam or core material to add onto the prepared natural tooth when there is not enough natural structure to hold a fixed restoration (Figure 23-3). If an amalgam restoration is already in place, then this may be shaped and prepared for use as the core.

Pin retention Pin retention may be necessary to add strength to the core buildup for the crown. When pins are used, they are directly incorporated into the buildup material (Figure 23-4).

Post and core If a tooth has been endodontically treated, then a **post** is placed into the pulp canal. The core is then built up around the post to provide additional strength and stability for the crown (Figure 23-5).

Gingival Retraction

For the laboratory technician to create an accurate fitting cast, a final impression is taken to prepare the working cast. As stated in Chapter 22, the final impression includes details of the preparation that extend slightly below the finish line of the preparation. The best way to achieve this detail and not harm the tissue is with the use of the **gingival retraction cord.**

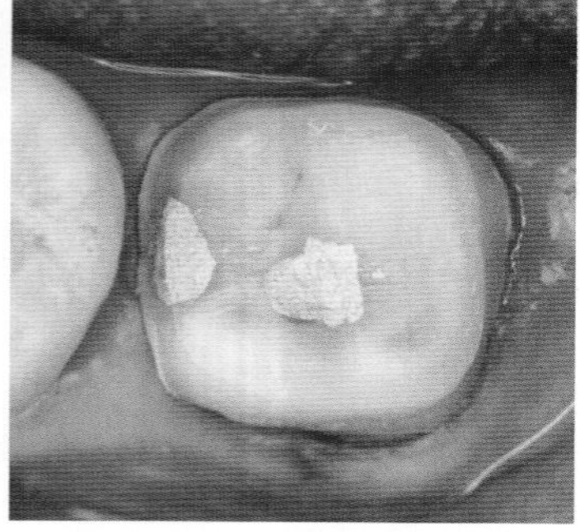

FIGURE 23-2 A crown preparation reduces the height and contour of the tooth. (From Rosenstiel SF, Land MF, Fujimoto J: *Contemporary fixed prosthodontics,* ed 5, St Louis, 2016, Elsevier.)

The gingival retraction cord temporarily pushes the gingival tissue away from the tooth and widens the sulcus, which allows the impression material to flow around all parts of the preparation (Figure 23-6).

Retraction cords are available as untwisted, twisted, or braided. For easy application, the cord is moistened in water or in a vasoconstrictor solution, and is then twisted just before placement. Once placed, the cord will expand and open the sulcus, ready to receive the impression material.

To control hemorrhage from the preparation procedure, the retraction cord can be impregnated (saturated) with an astringent and a **vasoconstrictor** solution, which controls bleeding and short-term constriction of the tissue. Special caution must be taken if the patient is taking a blood thinner because of a cardiovascular condition; the patient should not receive a retraction cord prepared with a vasoconstrictor solution.

See Procedure 23-1: Placing and Removing the Gingival Retraction Cord (Expanded Function).

Final Impression

After the prescribed time that the gingival retraction cord is within the sulcus, the retraction cord is removed, the sulcus is rinsed and dried, and the final impression is taken of the prepared tooth and surrounding tissue. (Refer to Chapter 22 on the procedure for taking final impressions.)

Provisional

A **provisional**, also known as a temporary, is a protective material that is temporarily placed for any type of preparation from an inlay, onlay, or a single crown or for the **abutment** teeth for a bridge.

A provisional remains until the cast restoration or bridge is returned from the dental laboratory and readied for permanent cementation. This period may take from several days to a few weeks.

Specific Objectives for Provisional Coverage

- To reduce sensitivity and discomfort of the prepared tooth
- To maintain function and esthetics of the tooth
- To protect the margins of the prepared tooth
- To prevent shifting of adjacent or opposing teeth

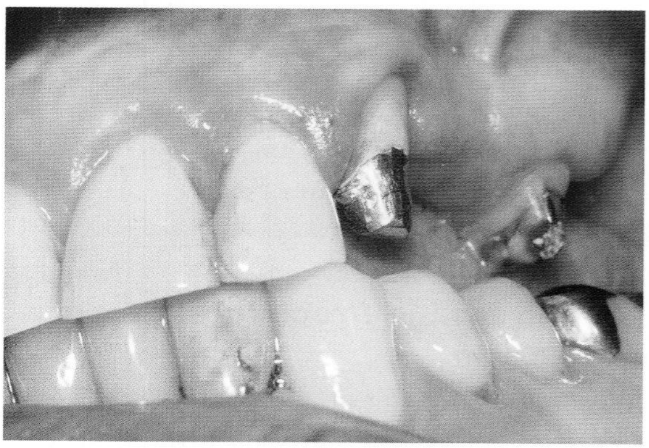

FIGURE 23-3 Core buildup on tooth #11.

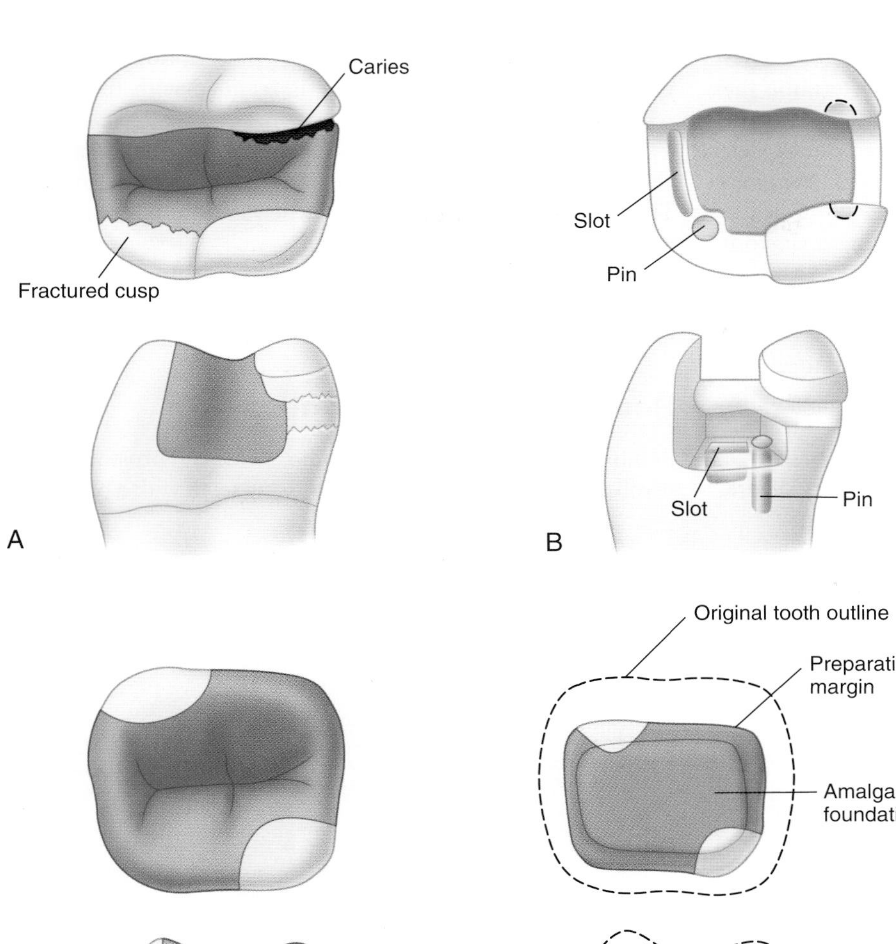

FIGURE 23-4 Pin retention. (From Heymann HO, Swift EJ Jr., Ritter AV: *Sturdevant's art and science of operative dentistry,* ed 6, St Louis, 2013, Mosby.)

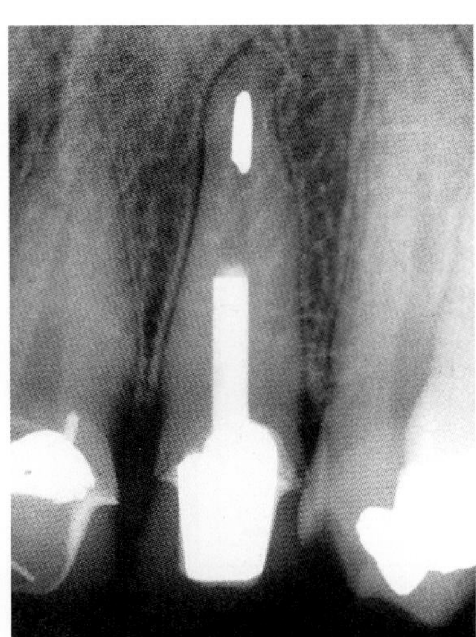

FIGURE 23-5 Post and core. (From Chong BS, Ed: *Harty's endodontics in clinical practice,* ed 6, Edinburgh, 2010, Churchill Livingstone.)

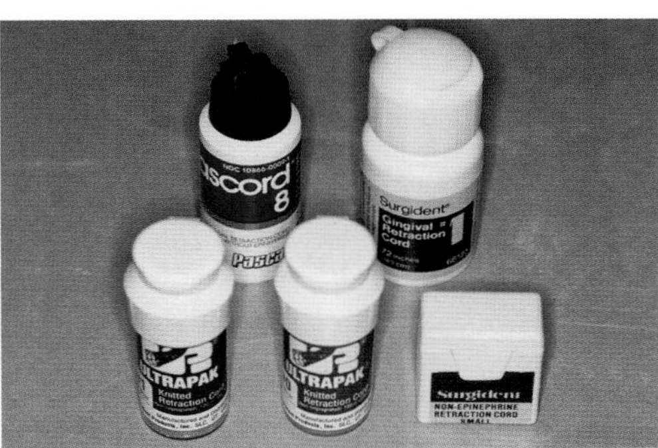

FIGURE 23-6 Types of gingival retraction cords. (From Rosenstiel SF, Land MF, Fujimoto J: *Contemporary fixed prosthodontics,* ed 5, St Louis, 2016, Elsevier.)

Types of provisional coverage Several types of provisional coverage are available. The dentist will determine the type of temporary based on the needs of the patient. The construction and cementation of temporary coverage can be delegated to the expanded function dental assistant (EFDA) or to a registered dental assistant (RDA) (Table 23-2).

See Procedure 23-2: Fabricating and Cementing a Custom Acrylic Provisional Crown.

Laboratory Prescription

At the completion of the first appointment, a laboratory prescription is completed and sent to the laboratory along with the final impression and bite registration. The laboratory technician can fabricate a single crown or a bridge on the basis of a written prescription from the dentist. Also known as a work order or requisition, one copy of the prescription is included with the case, and another copy is retained with the patient record (Figure 23-7).

Laboratory working days The laboratory requires a specific number of working days to complete the cast restoration. This time must be a consideration when scheduling the patient's return visit.

See Procedure 23-3: Assisting in a Crown and Bridge Restoration, and Procedure 23-4: Assisting in the Delivery and Cementation of a Cast Restoration.

Removable Prosthodontics

Removable prosthodontics is the field of prosthodontics involved with the replacement of missing teeth with a prosthesis

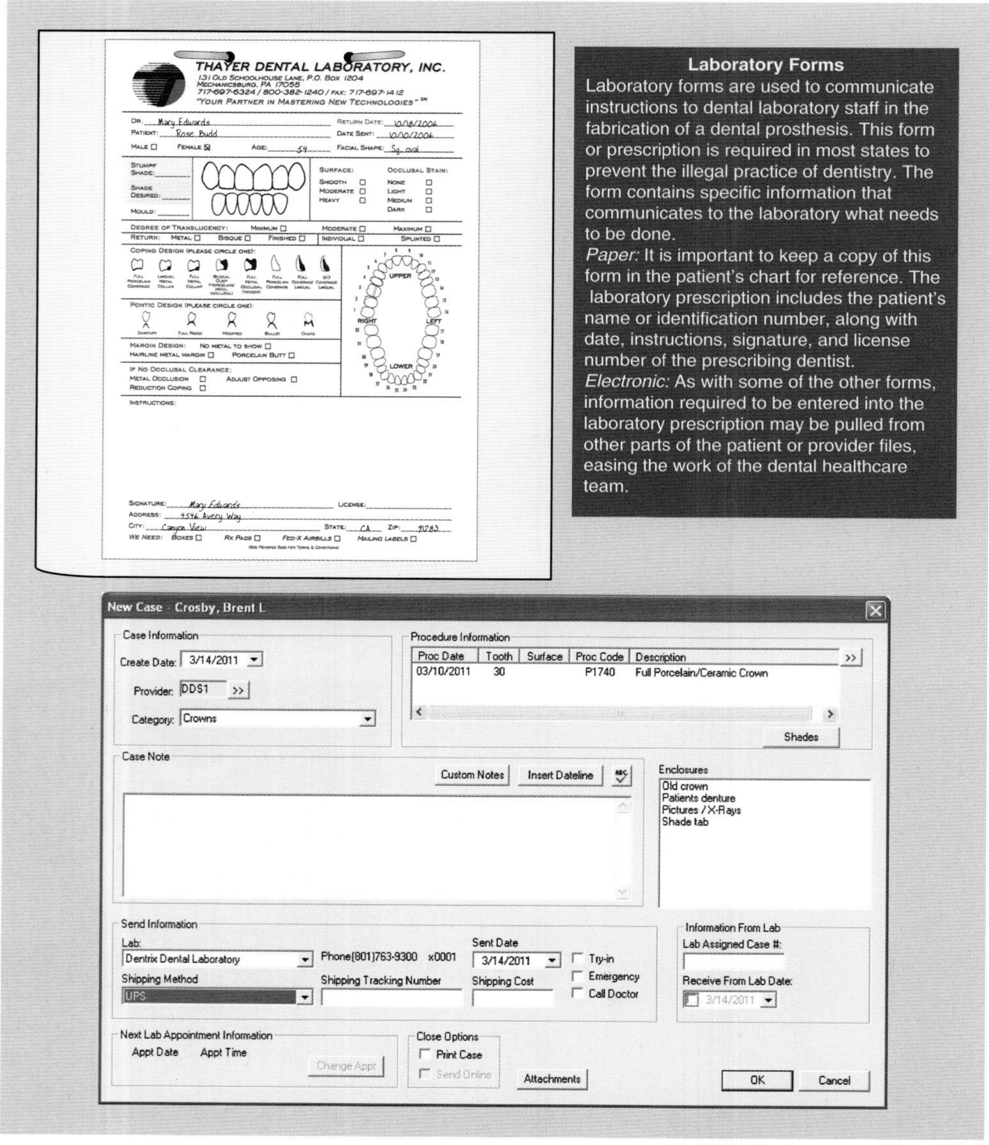

FIGURE 23-7 Laboratory prescription. (Form courtesy The Dental Record, Wisconsin Dental Associations, Milwaukee, Wisconsin. Dentrix screen shot courtesy Henry Schein Practice Solutions, American Fork, Utah. From Gaylor LJ: *The administrative dental assistant,* ed 3, St Louis, 2012, Saunders.)

TABLE 23-2
Types of Provisional Materials

Types	Description
Intermediate restorative material (IRM) 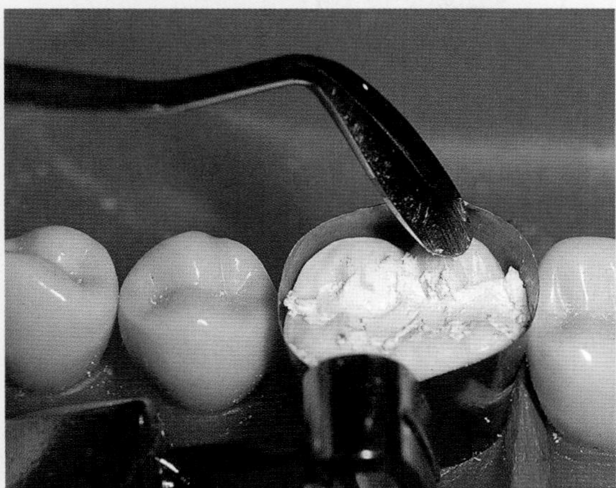	An IRM is used as provisional for an inlay or onlay preparation. This material is adapted to the prepared area using condensers and carvers to bring about normal anatomy. It is then allowed to harden.
Preformed polymer crown 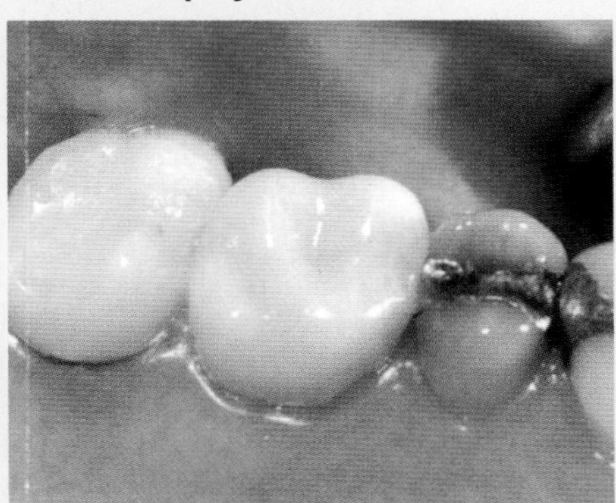	These shell-like crowns are available for posterior single crowns and for bridgework. The prostheses are supplied with a hybrid composite resin that bonds with the preformed crown.
Preformed polycarbonate crown 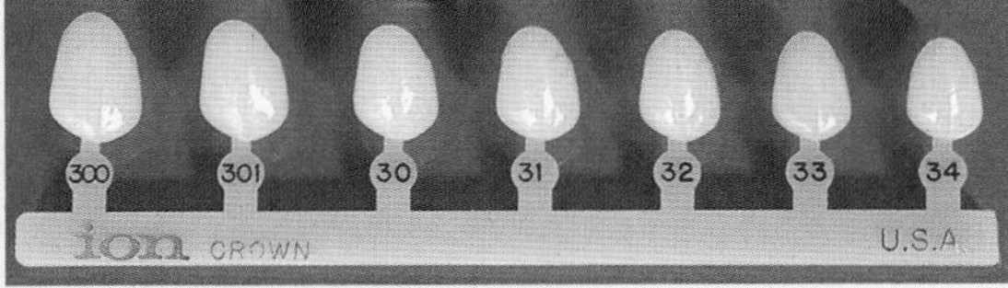	Made from a strong acrylic resin, the preformed polycarbonate crown is manufactured in a variety of sizes for anterior teeth where appearance is important. The crown is adapted to fit the prepared tooth using an acrylic laboratory bur and a Burlew wheel. It is then cemented.
Custom acrylic temporary 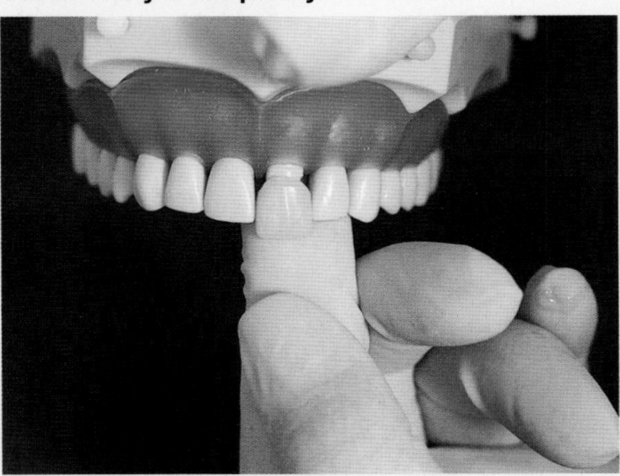	Made from a tooth-colored acrylic resin, the material is loaded in a vacuum-formed custom tray or alginate impression, seated onto the prepared area, allowed to set, removed from the tray, and finished using acrylic burs and finishing stones. It is then cemented to provide temporary coverage of a single crown or bridge.

(From Hatrick CD, Eakle WS: *Dental materials: clinical applications for dental assistants and dental hygienists,* ed 3, St Louis, 2016, Saunders.)

that the patient is able to take in and out of the mouth. The two major types of removable prosthodontics are (1) removable partial dentures and (2) removable full dentures.

A **removable partial denture**, commonly referred to as a partial, replaces one or more teeth that are missing in a specific quadrant or arch (Figure 23-8).

A **removable full denture**, commonly referred to as a denture, replaces all of the teeth that are missing in one arch (Figure 23-9).

The laboratory technician plays an important role in the construction of these types of prostheses. The technician follows the dentist's written prescription and works in close cooperation with the dentist in the fabrication of the prosthesis.

Partial Dentures

A removable partial denture receives its support and retention from the underlying tissue and from the remaining teeth that serve as abutments. The prosthesis is designed to distribute the forces of mastication between the abutments and the supporting tissue.

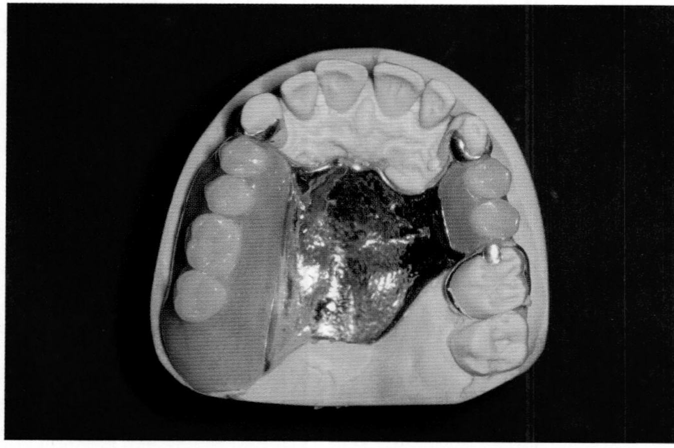

FIGURE 23-8 Removable partial denture. (From Hatrick CD, Eakle WS: *Dental materials: clinical applications for dental assistants and dental hygienists,* ed 3, St Louis, 2016, Saunders.)

Considerations for Prescribing a Partial Denture

Indications

- Aids in eating and in maintaining good health.
- Improves appearance, confidence, and smile. This improvement is achieved by restoring the natural contours of the lips, cheeks, and face. The denture prevents the development of premature aging lines and wrinkles around the mouth.
- Corrects the effect of speech caused by the loss of teeth by closing the spaces left by the lost teeth.
- Corrects the positioning of the jaws necessary to prevent jaw joint problems.
- Protects the health of remaining oral tissues.
- Prevents other teeth from drifting into the gaps left by extractions.

Contraindications

- Lack of suitable teeth in the arch to support, stabilize, and retain the removable prosthesis
- Rampant caries and/or severe periodontal conditions that threaten the remaining teeth in the arch
- Lack of patient acceptance and/or chronic poor oral hygiene

Components of a Partial Denture

The basic components of a removable partial denture are described in Table 23-3.

Abutment Teeth

A partial denture is primarily supported and stabilized by the abutment teeth. Abutments can be remaining natural teeth or surgical implants.

Selection of Abutment Teeth

Because of the stress placed on them, abutment teeth must have strong roots and strong bone support. Canines and molars, which have strong roots, are the teeth best suited for this purpose. Because of their relatively weak root structure,

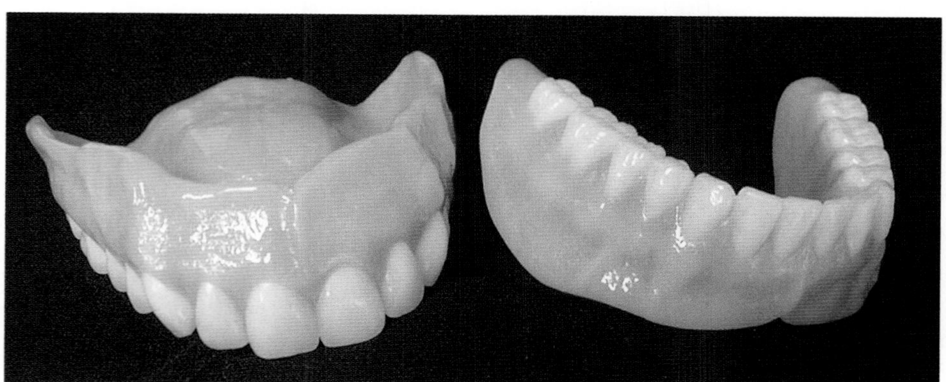

FIGURE 23-9 Full denture. (Courtesy Ivoclar Williams, Amherst, New York.)

TABLE 23-3
Components of a Partial Denture

Framework	The framework is the cast metal skeleton that provides support for the saddle and the connectors of the partial denture.
Major connector	The major connector, also known as a bar, is the piece of rigid metal that joins the right and left quadrant framework of the partial denture.
Saddle	The saddle is a metal mesh extension of the connector that is covered with acrylic. The saddle rests on the oral mucosa covering the alveolar ridge, holds the artificial teeth, and provides some support for the prosthesis.
Retainers	A retainer, also known as a clasp, is the portion of the framework that directly supports and provides stability to the partial denture by partially circling an abutment tooth.
Rests	A rest is a metal projection on or near the clasp that is designed to control the extent of seating of the prosthesis.
Artificial teeth	Artificial teeth are constructed from acrylic or porcelain.

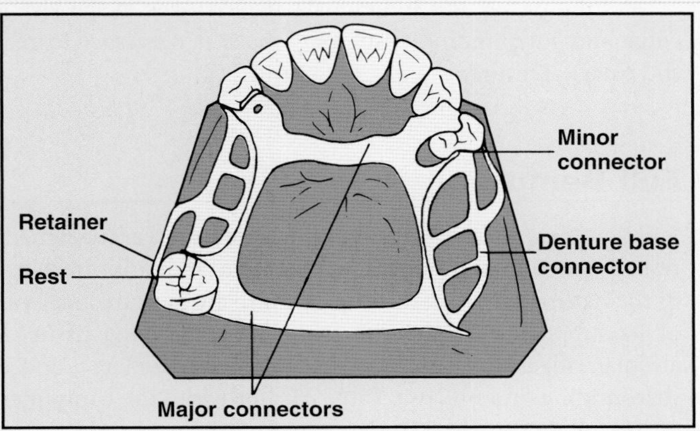

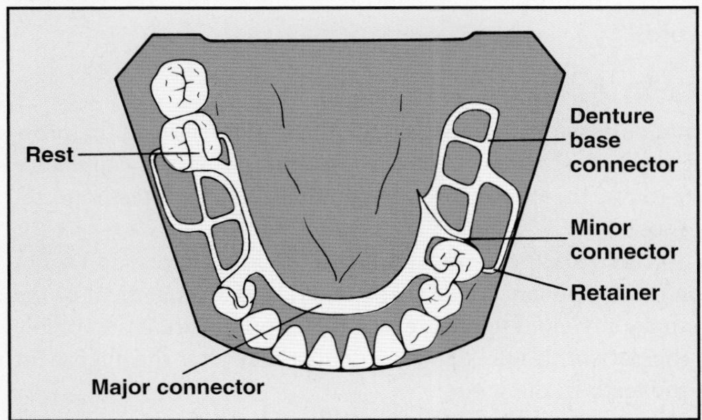

(Modified from Kratochvil FJ: *Partial removable prosthodontics,* Philadelphia, 1988, Saunders.)

individual maxillary and mandibular anterior incisors are least acceptable for use as abutments.

Preparation of Abutment Teeth

Abutment teeth are prepared according to the type of rest selected (see Table 23-3). Preparation may involve one of the following options:

- Slight modification of the tooth itself
- Modification of an amalgam restoration, if present
- Placement of a cast metal restoration with a recessed area to receive the rest or precision attachment

Final Impressions

A **final impression** is required for creating the **working casts** used by the laboratory technician during the construction of the partial denture.

Because this impression must be exact, a custom tray is made and an elastomeric impression material is used. The dentist chooses the type of tray, the material, and the impression technique to be used (see Chapter 22).

Although accuracy is extremely important, the use of gingival retraction is not required for a removable prosthesis; the teeth are not prepared below the gingival margin.

In addition to the final impression, taking an impression of the opposing arch and obtaining an occlusal registration is necessary. Most commonly, this is an occlusal registration; the technique is described in Chapter 22.

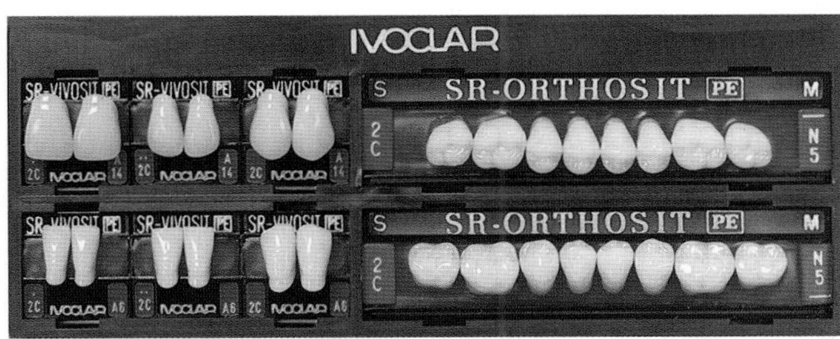

FIGURE 23-10 Artificial teeth. (Courtesy Ivoclar Vivadent, Amherst, New York.)

Selecting the Artificial Teeth

The **shade** (color) and **mold** (shape) of the teeth are determined. The manufacturer of the artificial teeth provides a shade guide. To identify the teeth, the mold and shade numbers are imprinted by the manufacturer on the back of each tooth in the shade guide (Figure 23-10).

When choosing the tooth shade and shape, the dentist considers the age and body size of the patient, the length of the lip, and the space to be occupied by the artificial tooth or teeth. The goal is to match the color, size, and shape of the patient's natural teeth as closely as possible.

The shade of the artificial teeth is examined using natural light for accuracy. When the selection has been made, the shape and shade of the artificial teeth are written in the patient's record.

This information, plus the name of the manufacturer and the material of the teeth, is also noted on the laboratory prescription to ensure that the technician will select the correct artificial teeth.

Laboratory Prescription

Before a case is sent to the laboratory, the dentist prepares a written prescription that includes all of the details concerning the construction of the prosthesis. The dentist must sign this prescription, and a copy is retained with the patient's records.

Try-In Appointment

An appointment is scheduled for the initial *try-in* of the prosthesis in the patient's mouth. At this point, the appliance consists of the cast framework, and the artificial teeth are set in wax.

At this visit, the dentist evaluates the fit, comfort, and function of the appliance. The shade, mold, and arrangement of the teeth are reviewed to ensure that their appearance is acceptable to the patient. If necessary, the dentist may alter the alignment of the teeth in the wax.

When the appliance is acceptable, another bite registration may be required to reflect any changes made during the try-in appointment. Any changes in the partial denture design are noted on the laboratory prescription. The wax-up and bite registration are disinfected and returned to the dental laboratory technician along with the prescription.

The laboratory technician finishes the partial denture as prescribed by the dentist. The completed prosthesis is delivered to the dental office in a sealed, moist container. (The acrylic saddle must be kept moist at all times to prevent warping.)

The appliance is disinfected and rinsed before the try-in of the appliance in the patient's mouth.

Delivery of the Partial Denture

A 20- to 30-minute appointment is usually adequate for the delivery of the partial denture. The day before the appointment, the assistant verifies that the case has been returned from the laboratory. See Procedure 23-5: Assisting in the Delivery of a Partial Denture.

Home Care Instructions to the Patient with a Partial Denture

- Maintain good oral hygiene.
- After meals, remove the partial and brush or rinse it to clean the retainers, rests, and saddles.
- Carefully brush and floss the abutment teeth and the remaining natural teeth to keep them free of food debris and plaque.
- When not wearing the partial, store the prosthesis in water or in a moist, airtight container. If the partial denture is allowed to get dry or too hot, the acrylic portion can warp.

Postdelivery Check

The patient is scheduled for a 10- to 20-minute postdelivery appointment within a few days after the delivery of the partial denture.

At this time, the dentist checks the mucosa for pressure areas and sore spots. If necessary, minor adjustments are made to the partial denture using a laboratory bur and a polishing lathe. When the dentist and patient are satisfied that the prosthesis is correctly functioning, the patient is given a recall appointment for several months later.

It is important that the patient regularly return for recall visits. The recall appointment should include dental prophylaxis and the evaluation of the function and fit of the prosthesis.

As time passes and individuals age, changes in the alveolar ridge and surrounding tissue may make it necessary to reline the partial denture.

Full Dentures

Full dentures, also known as complete dentures, are designed to restore function and esthetics of the natural dentition when all of the natural teeth are missing. A complete denture receives all of its support and retention from the underlying tissue, the alveolar ridges, the hard and soft palates (maxillary), and the surrounding oral mucosa. Table 23-4 provides the components of the full denture and its description.

Considerations for Prescribing a Complete Denture

Indications

- The patient is edentulous in at least one arch.
- The remaining teeth cannot be saved.
- The remaining teeth cannot support a removable partial denture, and no available alternatives are acceptable.
- The patient refuses alternative treatment recommendations.

Contraindications

- When any other acceptable alternative is available and teeth can be saved or implants are completed
- Physical or mental illness affecting the patient's ability to cooperate during fabrication of the denture and to accept and/or wear the denture
- Hypersensitivity to denture materials (A hypoallergenic denture material may be indicated for these patients.)
- Patient not interested in replacing missing teeth

Denture Retention

Retention of a Maxillary Denture

Retention of a maxillary denture primarily depends on the suction seal known as the **post dam** or the posterior palatal seal, which is formed at the junction of the tissue and the posterior border of the denture.

TABLE 23-4
Components of a Full Denture

Name	Description
Base	The base covers the entire hard palate and fits over the residual alveolar ridge and surrounding gingival area. The base is usually constructed from denture acrylic; however, to provide additional strength, it may be reinforced with a metal mesh embedded in the acrylic.
Post dam	The post dam extends across the entire posterior of the denture from one buccal space across the back of the palate behind the maxillary tuberosity to the opposite buccal space.
Flange	The flange is an extension beyond the residual ridge and over the attached mucosa to the tuberosities and the junction of the hard and soft palates.
Artificial teeth	Denture teeth are made of acrylic or porcelain. Third molars are not included on dentures because of the need to provide space in the posterior region to allow the patient to close, chew, swallow, and speak normally.

Retention of a Mandibular Denture

Achieving good retention of a mandibular denture can be difficult. It lacks the broad suction area found in a maxillary denture, and the constant action of the tongue can dislodge it. Retention for a mandibular denture depends on the support of the remaining alveolar ridge and the suction that can be achieved between the prosthesis and the tissue covering the ridge.

The **base** and flange of a mandibular denture extend over the residual ridge and attached mucosa, down to the oblique ridge and mylohyoid ridges, and over the genial tubercles and retromolar pads.

Impressions for Diagnostic Casts of Edentulous Arches

Taking an alginate impression of an edentulous arch differs from taking other alginate impressions in three ways: (1) the height of the teeth is eliminated, (2) including more extensive tissue details is important, and (3) an edentulous tray is used to take this impression.

An edentulous tray is not as deep as other trays used for alginate impressions because the space required for the teeth is not needed. In addition, soft beading wax or rope wax should be attached to the edges of the tray to modify the borders for a custom fit.

This modification allows **border molding**, also known as muscle trimming, to achieve closer adaptation of the edges of the impression of the tissue in the mucobuccal fold. Border molding is performed after the impression tray is in place. The dentist uses his or her fingers to gently massage the area of the face over these borders. Border molding shapes the wax-covered edges of the tray so these edges more closely approximate the tissue.

Final Impressions for Complete Dentures

Because accuracy is essential, an elastomeric impression material is selected for the final impressions for the making of working casts (Figure 23-11). Because of the shape of the edentulous arch, custom trays are required for the final impression. The edges of the custom tray for an edentulous arch are modified with beading wax to allow for border molding. The edges of the completed tray should extend to 2 mm short of the mucobuccal fold.

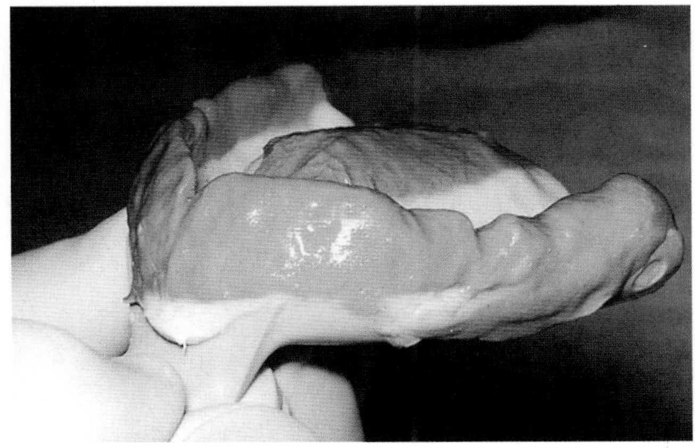

FIGURE 23-11 Completed maxillary edentulous impressions. (Courtesy Ivoclar Vivadent, Amherst, New York.)

Try-In of the Baseplate–Occlusal Rim Assembly

The **baseplate** is made of a semirigid material, such as self-curing or heat-cured resins. The **occlusal rims** are built of wax on the alveolar crest of the baseplate and are high and wide enough to occupy the space of the missing teeth.

The baseplate–occlusal rim assembly is used while (1) bite relationship records are made, (2) the casts are articulated, (3) the artificial teeth are arranged, and (4) the prosthesis is tried in the mouth.

The baseplate–occlusal rim assembly is returned to the dental office.

Before the try-in of the baseplate–occlusal rim assembly in the patient's mouth, it is removed from the articulator, disinfected, and rinsed. On the occlusal rims, the dentist records the:

- Vertical dimensions of the arches (i.e., the space occupied by the height of the teeth, which is considered normal occlusion)

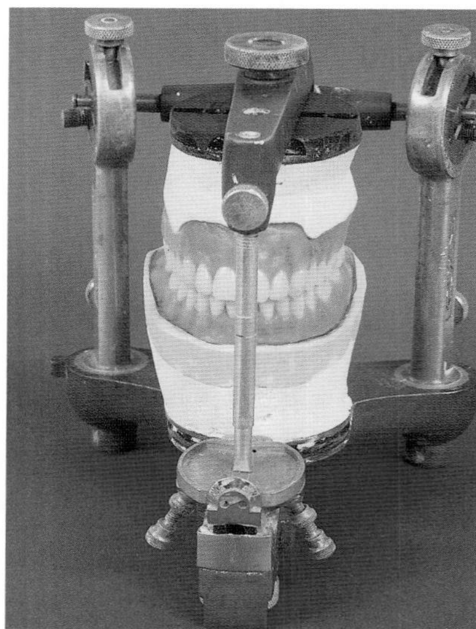
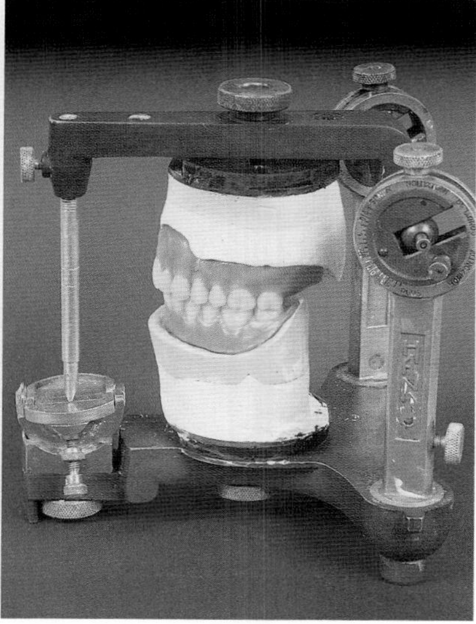

FIGURE 23-12 Wax-up of a complete denture on an articulator.

- Occlusal relationships (e.g., centric, protrusive, retrusive, and lateral excursion movements) of the arches
- Smile line (i.e., number of teeth that normally show when the patient is smiling)
- Canine eminence (i.e., vertical line that indicates the location of the canines)

Selecting the Artificial Teeth

At this appointment, the dentist will select the shape, shade, and material of the artificial teeth to be placed in the denture. These factors are determined in the same way as the teeth of a partial denture.

When placing the teeth in the denture, the laboratory technician is able to modify the arrangement as requested to produce a more natural appearance for the patient, for example, slightly overlapping the mesial incisal margin of the maxillary lateral over the distal margin of the central incisor.

Occlusal Registration

During the construction of a complete denture, the laboratory technician must have an accurate and extensive record of the patient's occlusion. The technician uses this information to articulate the casts so that the completed prosthesis will replicate these normal motions.

The measurements most frequently used are the patient's bite registered in the following positions:

- **Centric relation** with the jaws closed, relaxed, and comfortably positioned
- **Protrusion** with the mandible placed as far forward as possible from the centric position
- **Retrusion** with the mandible placed as far posterior as possible from the centric position
- **Lateral excursion**, which is the sliding of the mandible to the left or right of the centric position

These exaggerated motions simulate the actual movements of the mandible as it functions in the acts of mastication, biting, yawning, and speaking. Various devices are used to obtain these measurements.

Wax Setup Try-In Appointment

The **wax setup** consists of the baseplate with the artificial teeth set in wax, which resembles gingival tissue. Shaping of the wax to simulate normal tissue contours, grooves, and eminence is known as **festooning**.

The complete denture try-in, which has been fabricated in wax by the laboratory technician on an articulator, is returned to the dental office before the patient's appointment. An **articulator**, as shown in Figure 23-12, is a laboratory device that simulates the movements of the mandible and the temporomandibular joint. The wax setup is removed from the articulator and disinfected before it is tried in the patient's mouth.

See Procedure 23-6: Assisting in the Delivery of a Full Denture.

Home Care Instructions to the Patient with a Partial and Full Denture

The patient should be provided written home care instructions to reinforce the following verbal instructions for daily care:

- With the denture removed, thoroughly rinse the oral tissues at least once daily.
- On removal, thoroughly clean all surfaces with a special denture brush and a nonabrasive denture cleanser. During cleaning, carefully hold the prosthesis over a sink with water to protect from accidental dropping.
- Do not soak in hot water or a strong solution.
- When not in the mouth, store dentures in a moist, airtight container to prevent drying and warping.
- Do not wear during sleep. It is important for the gingival tissues to be free from constant compression.

Relining of a Partial or Complete Denture

The purpose of relining a denture is to accommodate changes in the supporting tissue to ensure that the prosthesis properly fits. Relining is accomplished by placing a new layer of denture resin over the tissue surface of the appliance.

Impression for Laboratory Relining

- At the preliminary appointment, when it is agreed that relining is necessary, the patient is instructed that he or she will be without a denture for at least 8 to 24 hours while it is being processed in the laboratory.
- The impression is taken using the present (loose) denture as the impression tray. The dentist will use a zinc oxide–eugenol impression paste or elastomeric impression material. The material is allowed to flow into the tissue side of the denture.
- The denture is reseated in the mouth, and the patient is instructed to close in normal occlusion to hold the denture in place until the impression paste reaches a final set. The denture is removed and disinfected.
- The denture and written prescription are sent to the laboratory technician for relining.

Delivery of a Laboratory Relined Denture

- When the relined denture is returned from the laboratory, it is disinfected and rinsed before returning to the patient's mouth.
- If necessary, minor trimming may be accomplished with an acrylic bur in a straight handpiece. Minor polishing may be completed on the laboratory lathe with a sterile rag wheel with pumice paste. Note that the tissue-bearing surfaces are never polished; polishing will alter the fit of the appliance.
- The patient is dismissed and advised to return for a checkup of the tissue and adaptation of the prosthesis within a time specified by the dentist.

Immediate Dentures

An immediate denture is one that is immediately placed after extraction of the patient's teeth. During the healing process, the denture serves as a compress and bandage to protect the surgical area. The sterilized denture is rinsed with saline solution and positioned in the mouth. The patient returns in 24 hours for a postoperative checkup. During this time, the denture is to be continuously worn except when removed for cleaning. Daily visits continue until initial healing has started and the sutures are removed, which commonly occurs 48 to 72 hours after surgery. During each visit, the area is irrigated with a mild antiseptic solution, and the soft tissue is checked for pressure points. After the sutures have been removed and the dentist and patient are satisfied with the prosthesis, the patient is scheduled for another appointment within a few months.

Dental Implants

Dental **implants** are used to attach artificial teeth to anchors (similar to posts) that have been surgically embedded into the bone. The implantation process involves several steps and can take from 3 to 9 months to complete. Depending on the type of implant, the steps will vary.

The placement of dental implants involves both surgery and the placement of the prosthesis. Several specialists, including an oral and maxillofacial surgeon, periodontist, prosthodontist, and or *implantologist* (general dentist with specialized training), may perform the procedure.

Considerations for Prescribing a Dental Implant

Indications

- To replace one or more teeth as single units without affecting adjoining teeth
- To support a bridge and to eliminate the need for a removable partial denture
- To provide support for a denture, making it more secure and comfortable
- To prevent bone loss and gum recession that often accompany bridgework and dentures
- To enhance the patient's confidence in smiling and speaking
- To improve the patient's overall psychologic health
- To improve the esthetic appearance of the patient's teeth and mouth

Contraindications

- The financial investment is greater than that for a conventional bridge or denture.
- Treatment can take several months or longer to complete.
- As with any surgical procedure, implants convey a risk of infection and other complications.
- An implant may loosen, requiring replacement.
- Emotionally, the implant procedure may be challenging for some patients.
- *Bruxism* is a significant component of failed implants.

Types of Dental Implants

Endosteal Implant

Endosteal implants, also known as *osseointegrated* implants, are the most common type of dental implant. The implant is surgically placed into the maxilla or mandible. Each implant holds one or more prosthetic teeth. This type of implant is generally used as an alternative for patients that would be prescribed a crown, bridge, or partial denture.

Implants and abutment screws are commonly made from the metal **titanium** because of its compatibility with bone and oral tissues. Titanium implants can be coated with **hydroxyapatite**, a ceramic substance that rapidly osseointegrates the implant to the bone.

Components of Endosteal Implants

Endosteal implants have three components:

1. The *titanium implant* is surgically embedded into the bone during stage I surgery and is supplied as either a blade form, a cylinder form, or a screw form (Figure 23-13).
2. The *titanium abutment screw* is screwed into the implant after osseointegration of the implant during stage II surgery.
3. The *abutment post* or *cylinder* attaches to the artificial tooth or denture.

Osseointegration (*osseo-* meaning bone) is the process by which the living cells of the bone naturally grow around the implanted dental supports. It refers to a bond that develops between living bone and the surface of an implant fixture. Osseointegrated implants are used to support, stabilize, and retain removable dentures, fixed bridges, and single-tooth implants.

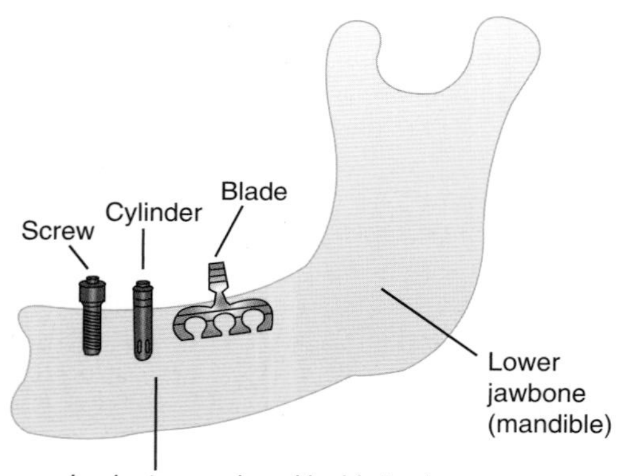

FIGURE 23-13 Diagram showing the types of endosteal implants. (From Darby ML, Walsh MM: *Dental hygiene, theory and practice,* ed 3, St Louis, 2010, Saunders.)

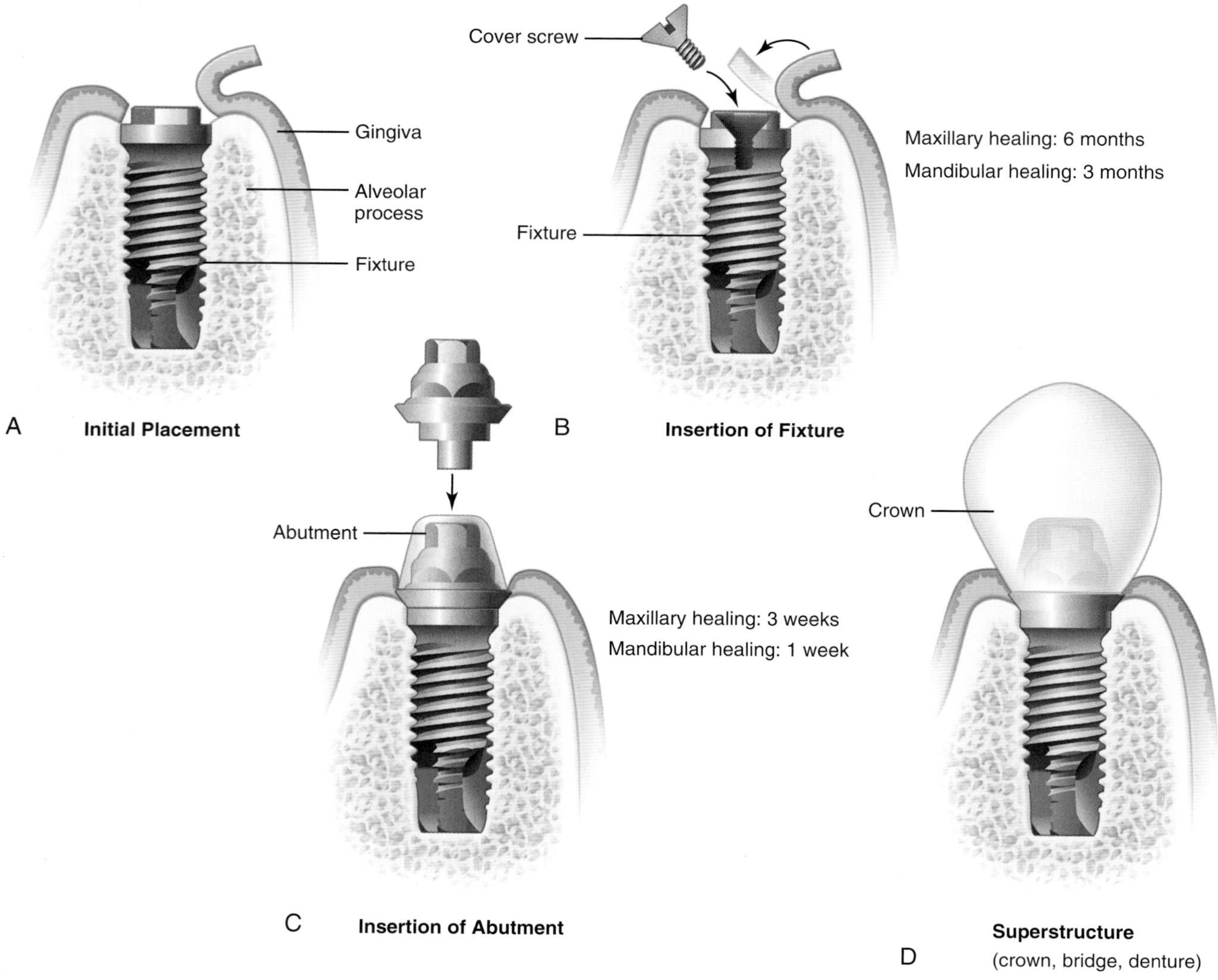

For this type of implant, three appointments are required to complete the procedure. At the *first surgery,* implant fixtures are placed within receptor sites in the jawbone at predetermined locations. The mucosa is sutured over the fixtures. After a 1- to 2-week healing period, the existing prosthesis (when applicable) may be removed and relined to adapt to the healed ridge.

A period of 3 to 6 months, the *osseointegration period,* is required to permit the fixture to osseointegrate or bond to the bone. Care must be taken during this healing period to avoid trauma to the mucosa overlying the implant sites.

At the *second surgery,* the endosteal implant fixture is exposed, and the abutment screw is connected to the anchor. This portion protrudes through the mucosa and connects the fixture to the prosthesis.

After both surgeries have been completed and tissues have healed, the patient begins the *restorative phase,* during which the final crown, bridge, partial denture, or full denture is fabricated. The entire implant process can require 3 to 9 months to reach completion (Figure 23-14).

Gingiva
Alveolar process
Fixture
A **Initial Placement**

Cover screw
Fixture
Maxillary healing: 6 months
Mandibular healing: 3 months
B **Insertion of Fixture**

Abutment
Maxillary healing: 3 weeks
Mandibular healing: 1 week
C **Insertion of Abutment**

Crown
D **Superstructure** (crown, bridge, denture)

FIGURE 23-14 Dental implant.

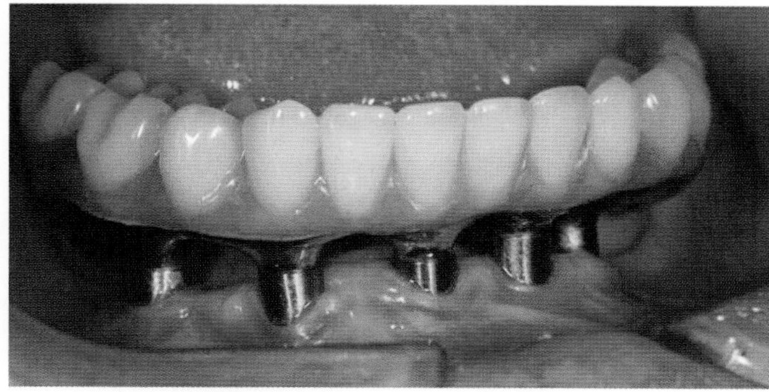

FIGURE 23-15 Subperiosteal implant with full-arch denture prosthesis. (From Newman M, Takei T, Klokkevold P, Carranza F, editors: *Carranza's clinical periodontology,* ed 11, St Louis, 2012, Saunders.)

See Procedure 23-7: Assisting in an Endosteal Implant Surgery.

Subperiosteal Implant

A **subperiosteal** implant is a metal frame that is placed under the periosteum and *on top* of the bone. In contrast to an endosteal implant, a subperiosteal implant is *not* placed into the bone.

Subperiosteal implants are indicated for patients who do not have sufficient alveolar ridge remaining to support the endosteal-type implant. This type of implant is most frequently used to support a mandibular complete denture (Figure 23-15).

Two surgical procedures are required for this type of implant. During the *first surgery,* the alveolar ridge is exposed and impressions are taken of the alveolar ridge. After the impressions are taken, the tissue is repositioned over the ridge and is sutured back into place. The impression is sent to a dental laboratory, where a metal frame with posts is fabricated.

After the frame has been fabricated, the *second surgery* is performed. The alveolar ridge is again surgically exposed, and the metal frame is placed over the ridge. When the frame is in place, the tissues are repositioned and sutured into place.

Transosteal Implant

The **transosteal** implant is inserted through the inferior border of the mandible and into the edentulous area. The most common type is the *transmandibular staple implant,* or fixed mandibular implant. These implants are primarily used in patients with severely resorbed ridges and only when no other options exist.

Maintenance of Dental Implants

Long-term maintenance is an integral part of treatment for patients with dental implants. Maintenance includes home care by the patient and periodic maintenance visits to the dental office.

The health of the peri-implant tissue is a critical factor in the success of dental implants. This tissue is similar to the gingival sulcus that surrounds a natural tooth. Peri-implant tissue responds to bacterial plaque with inflammation and bleeding, similarly to gingival tissues around a normal tooth.

Recall Visits

Recall visits are essential for the long-term success of implants. It is important that patients understand the need to maintain optimal plaque control with home care and frequent professional recalls. Patients should be scheduled at regular intervals for examination, radiography, prophylaxis, removal of fixed components, replacement of components, and relines and remakes as recommended.

Ethical Implications

Prosthodontics is an area of dentistry that relies on knowledge, technique, and communication with the patient and laboratory technician. Understanding the process of prosthodontics is important for the dental assistant.

The procedures of placing the retraction cord and the fabrication of a provisional crown or bridge may be legal for the CDA or RDA in the state in which you are working. Before you assume an additional responsibility within the clinical setting, always confirm that it is legal.

Procedure 23-1

Placing and Removing the Gingival Retraction Cord (Expanded Function)

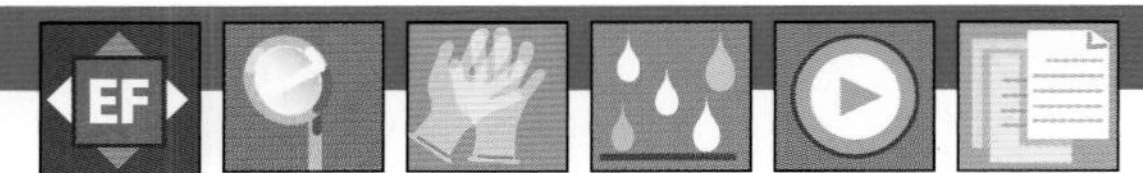

Equipment and Supplies

- Basic setup
- Cotton rolls
- Cord-packing instrument
- Gingival retraction cord
- Dappen dish
- Scissors

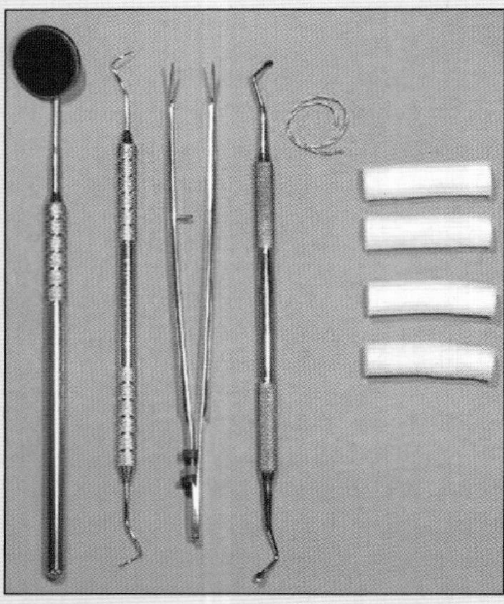

Procedural Steps

Preparation

1. Rinse and gently dry the prepared tooth. Isolate the quadrant with cotton rolls.

Purpose: Dry tissue makes it easier to see the details of the gingival tissue and to place the retraction cord.

2. Cut a piece of retraction cord 1 to 1½ inches in length, depending on the size and type of the tooth being prepared.

Note: The length is determined by the circumference of the prepared tooth and the placement technique to be used.

3. Use cotton pliers to form a loose loop of the cord.

Purpose: A loose loop makes it easy to slip the cord over the tooth, but the loop is not tied or knotted.

Placement

1. Make a loop in the retraction cord, slip it over the tooth, and position the loop in the sulcus around the prepared tooth.

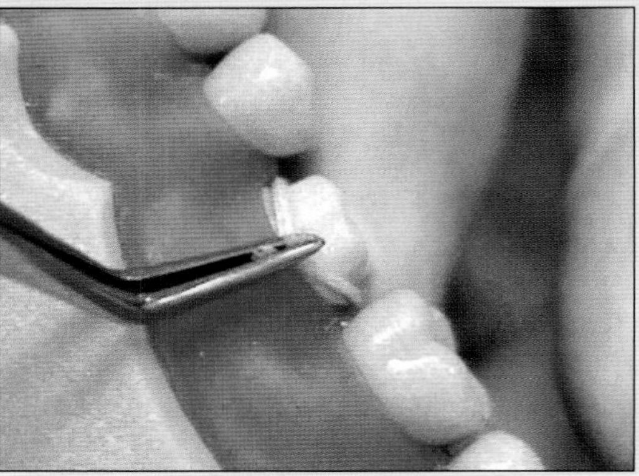

2. Using the cord-packing instrument and working in a clockwise direction, gently pack the cord into the sulcus surrounding the prepared tooth with the ends on the facial aspect.

Purpose: The ends in this position are easier to reach for removal of the cord.

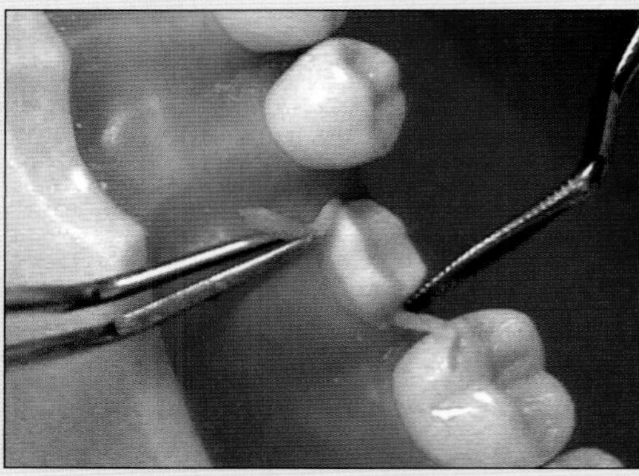

3. Pack the cord into the sulcus by gently rocking the instrument slightly backward as the instrument is moved forward to the next loose section of the retraction cord. Repeat this action until the length of cord is packed in place.
4. Overlap the cord where it meets the first end of the cord. The ends may be tucked into the sulcus on the facial aspect.

Note: An alternative is to leave a short length of the cord sticking out of the sulcus, which makes it easier to grasp and quickly remove the cord.

5. *Optional:* When a wider and deeper sulcus is required, two retraction cords may be placed with one on top of the other. Before the impression material is taken, remove the top cord. After the impression is completed, remove the second retraction cord.
6. The cord should be left in place for a maximum of 5 to 7 minutes. Instruct the patient to remain still to keep the area dry.

Procedure 23-1

Placing and Removing the Gingival Retraction Cord (Expanded Function)—cont'd

Purpose: The time allows the cord to push the tissue away from the tooth and to stay in this position.
Note: The exact time depends on the type of chemical retraction used.

Removal

1. Grasp the end of the retraction cord with cotton pliers, and remove it in a counterclockwise direction (the reverse of the method that was used in packing the cord).
2. Remove the retraction cord just before the impression material is placed.

Note: Usually the operator removes the cord while the assistant prepares the syringe type of impression material.

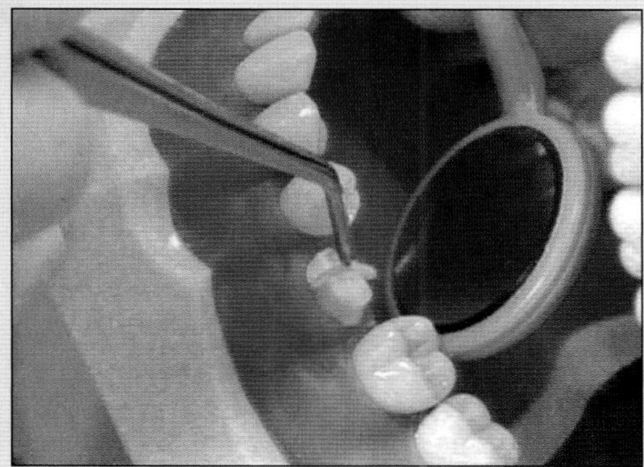

3. Gently dry the area, and apply fresh cotton rolls.

Note: The impression is immediately taken.

Procedure 23-2

Fabricating and Cementing a Custom Acrylic Provisional Crown

Equipment and Supplies

- Basic setup
- Spoon excavator
- Alginate impression (obtained before preparation of the teeth)
- Separating medium
- Cotton rolls
- Self-curing acrylic resin (liquid and powder)
- Spatula (small, cement type)
- Mixing container or dappen dish
- Scissors
- Surgical knife (optional)
- Burnisher (beaver tail or ball)
- Straight handpiece and mandrel
- Finishing diamond, discs, or burs
- Polishing discs or burs
- Articulating paper
- Pumice paste
- Lathe and sterile white rag wheel
- Provisional cementation setup

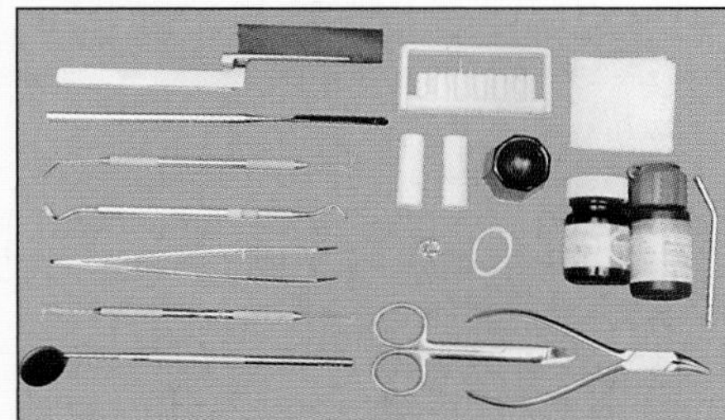

Procedural Steps

1. Obtain an alginate impression of the arch before the teeth are prepared.

Purpose: The provisional coverage should be a replica of the tooth or teeth before the dentist prepares them.

2. Check the impression to ensure that it is free of debris and tears in the area selected for construction of the provisional crown or bridge covering.
3. Rinse and disinfect the impression, and keep it moist until needed.

Purpose: If the impression is allowed to dry, then it will be distorted, and the provisional coverage will not fit.

4. Isolate the prepared tooth with cotton rolls to maintain moisture control.
5. Lightly apply petroleum jelly or a liquid medium to the prepared tooth to facilitate separating the acrylic dough from the preparations.
6. Unwrap the alginate impression, and gently dry the area of the teeth to receive provisional coverage.
7. Directly express the acrylic resin from a cartridge into the impression.
8. Place the acrylic-loaded impression back into the patient's mouth on the prepared tooth or teeth.
9. Allow the material to reach an initial set, approximately 3 minutes, and then remove the tray from the patient's mouth.
10. Carefully remove the provisional coverage from the alginate impression, and place it onto the patient's teeth.

Purpose: This step helps prevent excess shrinkage during the final curing stage.

Continued

Procedure 23-2

Fabricating and Cementing a Custom Acrylic Provisional Crown—cont'd

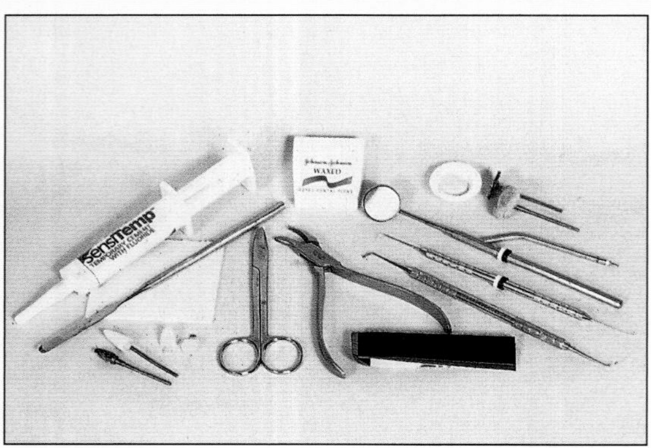

11. Mark the marginal border and contact points of the provisional coverage with a pencil to provide better visualization of the markings.

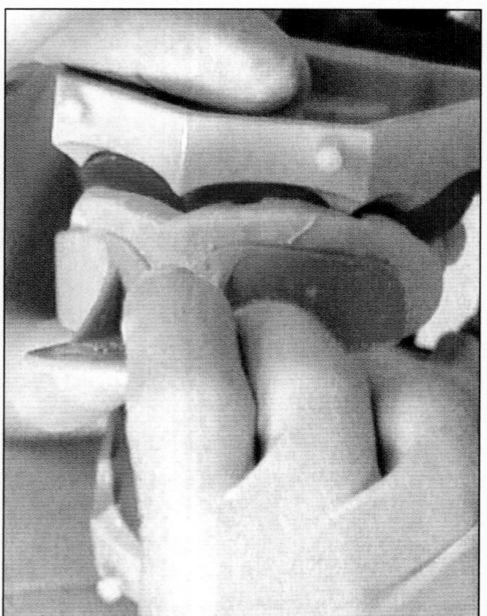

12. Trim the acrylic resin to within 1 mm of the gingival shoulder of the prepared tooth with an acrylic bur or stone.

Note: Any trimming completed by the expanded function dental assistant (EFDA) must be completed outside the mouth with the low-speed handpiece and acrylic burs.

13. Check the occlusion, accuracy, and completeness of the provisional coverage, and adjust as necessary. Remove the provisional coverage from the prepared tooth, and complete the trimming with an acrylic bur.
14. Remove the provisional coverage and take it to the laboratory to be polished with a sterile white rag wheel and pumice on the laboratory lathe.

***Caution:* Safety goggles must be worn throughout the trimming and polishing procedure. In addition, be aware that the rag wheel could remove a large bulk of acrylic or could overheat and cause distortion of the provisional coverage.**

15. Temporarily cement the provisional coverage with provisional cement, such as zinc oxide–eugenol (TempBond) or intermediate restorative material.
16. Check the occlusion with articulating paper. If any reduction is required, then the dentist will use an acrylic-trimming bur.

Procedure 23-3

Assisting in a Crown and Bridge Restoration

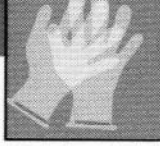
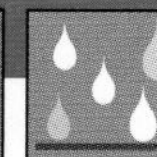
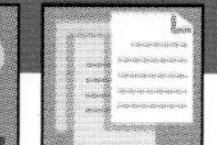

Equipment and Supplies

- Local anesthetic agent setup
- Alginate impression setup
- Shade guide (for tooth-colored restoration)
- Large spoon excavator
- Additional hand instruments (dentist's choice)
- Burs, diamond stones, and discs (dentist's choice)
- Gingival retraction setup
- Cotton rolls and gauze sponges
- High-volume evacuator (HVE) tip

At this visit, setups are also required for the following:

- Elastomeric impressions, which may include a custom tray
- Occlusal (bite) registration
- Provisional coverage fabrication, adjustment, and cementation supplies

Procedure 23-3

Assisting in a Crown and Bridge Restoration—cont'd

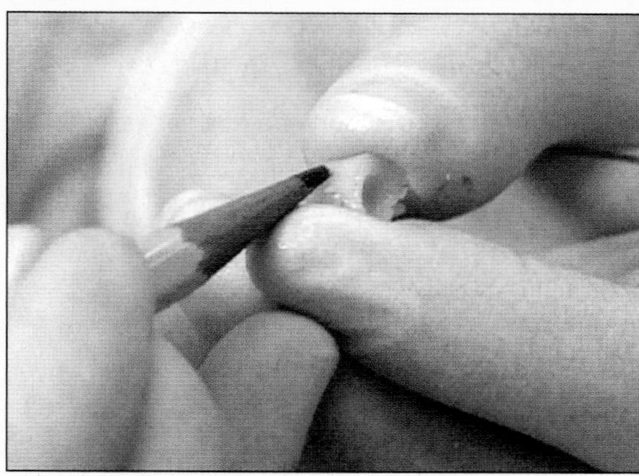

Procedural Steps

Preliminary Steps

1. Assist in administering the local anesthetic agent.
2. If an alginate impression is needed to fabricate the provisional coverage, then the impression is obtained at this time. In addition, an occlusal registration is taken (see Chapter 22).
3. If a silicone two-step impression method is used, then the first impression is obtained at this time.
4. If this procedure involves a tooth-colored restoration, then the shade is selected at this time.

Tooth Preparation

1. Throughout the preparation, maintain a clear operating field by using the HVE to retract the lips and tongue and to remove water and debris.
2. The dentist uses diamond stones in the high-speed handpiece to remove all decay and fractured portions of the tooth.

Purpose: Diamond stones are used during crown preparation because they can rapidly remove tooth structure.

3. Assist in bur changes as necessary while the dentist reduces tooth bulk and completes the preparation using burs of different shapes.
4. When the preparation is complete, the gingival retraction cord is placed.
5. Assist in readying the final impression material.
6. Before transferring the light-bodied material, transfer the cotton pliers to the dentist for the removal of the gingival retraction cord.

Note: The dentist may want to rinse and dry the sulcus before applying the light-bodied material.

7. While the dentist is applying the light-bodied material, ready the tray with heavy-bodied material.
8. Have the air-water syringe available for the dentist to blow air around the preparation.

Purpose: This step thins out the material, allowing it to flow better in the sulcus and around the margins.

9. Retrieve the light-bodied material syringe from the dentist, and transfer the tray, ensuring that the dentist can properly grasp the handle and insert the tray.
10. After the recommended time for the material to set, the dentist will remove the tray.
11. The occlusal registration is obtained.
12. Provisional coverage is fabricated and temporarily cemented to protect the prepared teeth.
13. The patient is scheduled for a cementation appointment and dismissed.

Note: Ensure that the laboratory has sufficient time to fabricate the crown before scheduling the patient for another appointment.

14. After the dentist writes the laboratory prescription, prepare the case and send it to the laboratory.

DATE	TOOTH	SURFACE	CHARTING NOTES
8/15/17	4	PFM	Crown prep, 2 carpules Xylocaine w/ epinephrine, final impression, temporary made and cemented with TempBond, shade C2 for porcelain. Pt tolerated procedure well. Reschedule in 2 weeks for cementation. T. Clark, CDA/L. Stewart, DDS

Procedure 23-4

Assisting in the Delivery and Cementation of a Cast Restoration

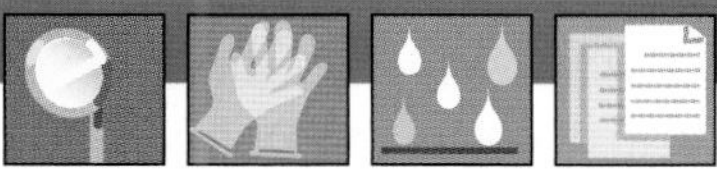

Equipment and Supplies

- Local anesthetic agent setup (if needed)
- Cast restoration
- Backhaus towel forceps (to remove provisional coverage)
- Large spoon excavator
- Cavity varnish and sealer with applicator (optional)
- Bonding supplies (dentist's choice)
- Cementation supplies (dentist's choice)
- Cotton rolls
- Saliva ejector
- Bite stick
- Articulating paper and holder
- Polishing points and stones (dentist's choice)
- Scaler (to remove excess cement)
- Dental floss

Continued

Procedure 23-4

Assisting in the Delivery and Cementation of a Cast Restoration—cont'd

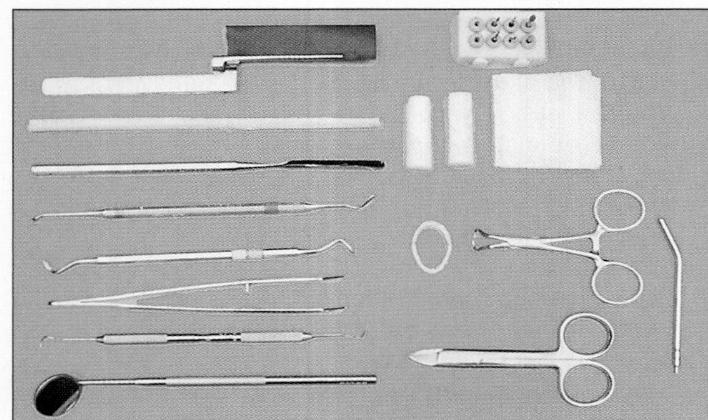

Procedural Steps

1. Transfer the cast restoration to the dentist to try on for fit. Transfer mirror and explorer.
2. When the dentist signals, mix the prepared cement.
3. Quickly apply the mixed cement to the internal surface of the casting, and transfer the prepared crown to the dentist.
4. The dentist places the crown on the prepared tooth, seating it into place, and then asks the patient to bite down on a wooden bite stick or Burlew wheel to seat the restoration completely.

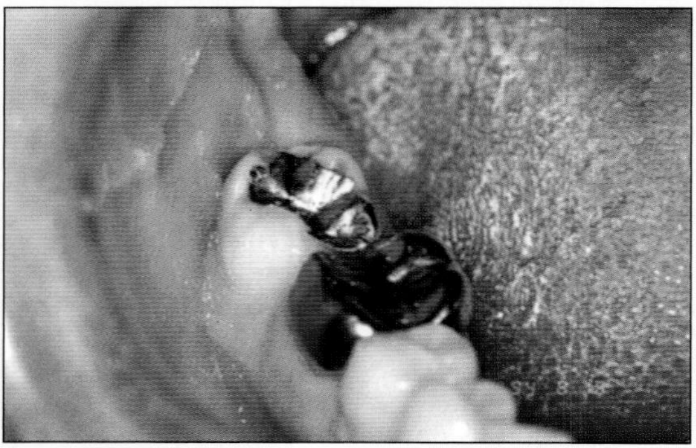

5. Instruct the patient to continue this biting pressure until the cement reaches the initial set, approximately 8 to 10 minutes.
6. *Optional:* Once the casting is firmly seated, a saliva ejector may be placed in the floor of the patient's mouth.
7. After the cement has set, remove the cotton rolls.
8. An explorer is used to remove the excess cement carefully from the crowns of the teeth.

Note: This step is completed very carefully so as not to scratch the newly placed crown or injure the gingiva.

9. A firm fulcrum is necessary for the hand that is holding the instrument.

Purpose: The fulcrum prevents the instrument from slipping and, consequently, injuring the gingiva.

10. The tip of the instrument is placed at the gingival edge of the cement, and overlapping vertical strokes are used to remove the bulk of the cement.
11. Slight lateral pressure is applied (toward the tooth surface) to remove the remaining cement.
12. Dental floss with tied knots is passed between the teeth to remove excess cement from the interproximal areas.

Purpose: The knots provide added bulk in removing the cement.

13. After the excess cement has been removed, the dentist may polish by using polishing points in the low-speed handpiece.

DATE	TOOTH	SURFACE	CHARTING NOTES
9/03/17	4	—	Crown delivered, cemented with glass ionomer. Pt pleased with crown's fitting and appearance. T. Clark, CDA/L. Stewart, DDS

Procedure 23-5

Assisting in the Delivery of a Partial Denture

Equipment and Supplies

- Basic setup
- Articulating paper and holder
- Pressure indicator paste
- Low-speed and high-speed handpieces
- Acrylic burs
- Finishing burs
- Three-prong pliers

Procedural Steps

1. Seat the patient.
2. The dentist places the new partial denture in the patient's mouth, and the patient is instructed to close his or her teeth together.

Important: Before the prosthesis is placed in the patient's mouth, it must be disinfected and rinsed with water.

3. To check the occlusion, assist in placing articulating paper on the occlusal surface of the mandibular teeth,

Procedure 23-5

Assisting in the Delivery of a Partial Denture—cont'd

and ask the patient to simulate chewing motions. If the occlusion is too high, then the dentist reduces the artificial teeth with a small, round carbide bur.

4. To detect pressure points (high spots) that could cause discomfort to the patient, apply pressure-indicator paste on the tissue surface of the prosthesis. The prosthesis is placed in the patient's mouth. As necessary, these high spots on the prosthesis are adjusted.
5. The retainers are checked for tension on the natural abutment teeth. The dentist very carefully uses pliers to adjust the tension on the retainers.
6. After adjustments are made, the partial denture is polished on the laboratory lathe, using appropriate pastes and sterile buffing wheels.
7. Scrub the partial denture with soap, water, and a brush; disinfect and rinse; and return it to the treatment room for delivery to the patient.
8. Instruct the patient on the placement, removal, and care of the partial denture.

DATE	TOOTH	SURFACE	CHARTING NOTES
8/20/17	—	—	Deliver maxillary partial, minor adjustments made. Pt pleased with appearance. Reschedule pt in 3 days for postdelivery check. T. Clark, CDA/L. Stewart, DDS

Procedure 23-6

Assisting in the Delivery of a Full Denture

Equipment and Supplies

- Basic setup
- Dentures
- Hand mirror
- Articulating paper and holder
- High-speed and low-speed handpieces
- Finishing burs
- Acrylic burs

Procedural Steps

1. Seat the patient.
2. The try-in of the new denture in the patient's mouth is accomplished, and the shade and mold of the artificial teeth are checked for natural appearance.
3. Ask the patient to perform the facial expressions and actions of swallowing, chewing, and speaking, using *s* and *th* sounds.

Note: These sounds also are appropriate exercises to help the patient learn to speak normally with the new denture.

4. Occlusion is checked with the use of articulating paper.

Purpose: Cusps that are too high in contact will be marked with the color of the articulating paper.

5. If the cusps are too high, then the denture is removed from the mouth and adjusted with a stone mounted on a straight handpiece by the dentist.
6. The denture is replaced in the mouth, and the procedure is repeated until the cusps appear to be in occlusion with the opposing arch.

Note: If the denture must be taken into the laboratory for adjustment, then it must be disinfected again before it is returned to the patient.

7. When the patient is pleased with the appearance, function, and comfort of the denture, another appointment is scheduled for the postdelivery checkup.
8. Before dismissal, the patient is informed that learning to wear a new denture will take several days or weeks.

DATE	TOOTH	SURFACE	CHARTING NOTES
8/28/17	—	—	Delivery of maxillary full denture. Pt pleased with change of canines. Teeth and shading good. Pt pleased with fit and appearance. Reschedule in 3 days for postdelivery check. T. Clark, CDA/L. Stewart, DDS

Procedure 23-7

Assisting in an Endosteal Implant Surgery

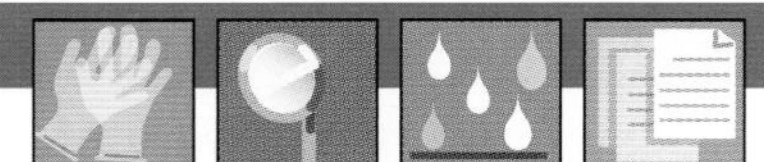

Equipment and Supplies

- Basic setup
- Local anesthetic
- Sterile surgical gloves
- Sterile surgical drilling unit
- Surgical irrigation tip
- Scalpel
- Periosteal elevator
- Implant instrument kit
- Implant kit
- Sterile saline solution
- Low-speed handpiece with contra-angle attachment
- Inserting mallet
- Suture setup
- Electrosurgical unit and tips (or tissue punch)
- 3% hydrogen peroxide with syringe
- Sterile cotton pellets
- Sterile 2 × 2–inch gauze sponges

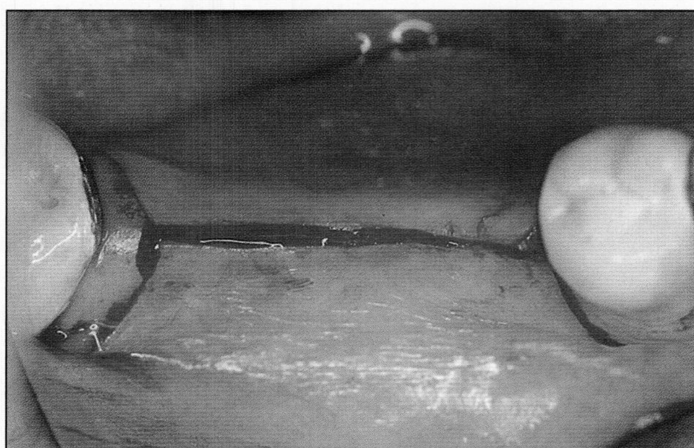

(From Newman M, Takei T, Klokkevold P, Carranza F, editors: *Carranza's clinical periodontology,* ed 12, St Louis, 2015, Saunders.)

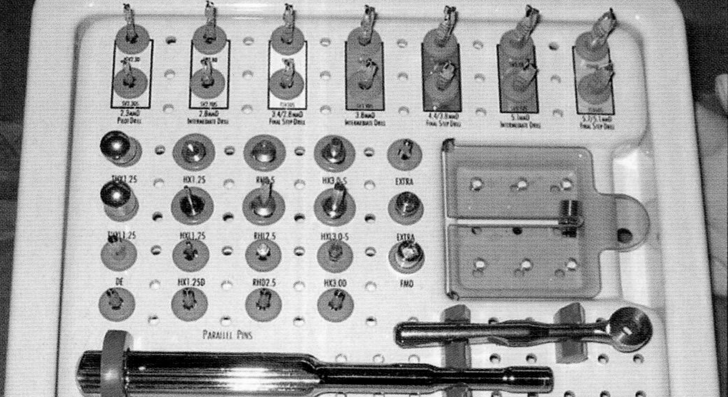

(From Bird DL, Robinson DS: *Modern dental assisting,* ed 11, St Louis, 2015, Saunders.)

Procedural Steps

Stage I Surgery: Implant Placement

1. The surgical stent (template) is placed in position in the patient's mouth.
2. After achieving adequate anesthesia, the surgeon uses a *pilot drill* (similar to a Pesso bur) to drill through the stent and into the soft tissue on the ridge, creating a target point on the bone for the implant site.

Note: All drilling of the bone is accomplished with generous amounts of sterile saline irrigation.

3. The surgeon removes the surgical stent and makes the incision at the implant site.
4. The mucoperiosteal tissues are reflected.

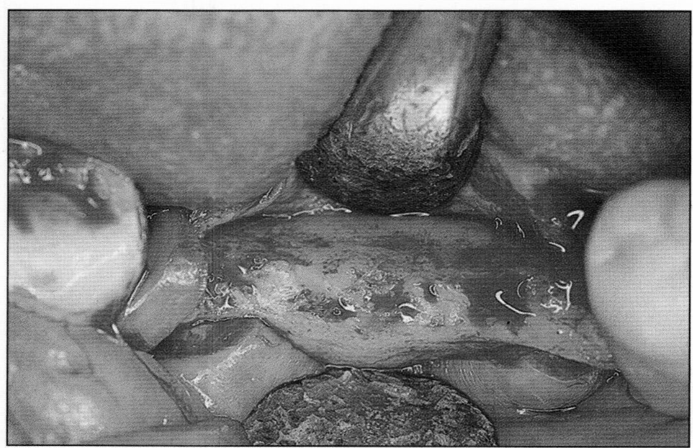

(From Newman M, Takei T, Klokkevold P, Carranza F, editors: *Carranza's clinical periodontology,* ed 12, St Louis, 2015, Saunders.)

5. The surgeon smooths any sharp edges on the crest of the ridge. The crest should be at least 2 mm wider than the implant that is being used.
6. A variety of drill tips (similar to burs) are used to prepare the osseous receptor site.
7. The implant cylinder (with a plastic cap over the top of it) is partially inserted into the osseous receptor site.
8. The plastic cap is removed, and the implant is tapped into its final position with the inserting mallet.
9. The sterile sealing screw (also called a *healing collar*) is placed into the implant cylinder with the contra-angle screwdriver. Final tightening of the sealing screw is accomplished with the handheld screwdriver.

Procedure 23-7

Assisting in an Endosteal Implant Surgery—cont'd

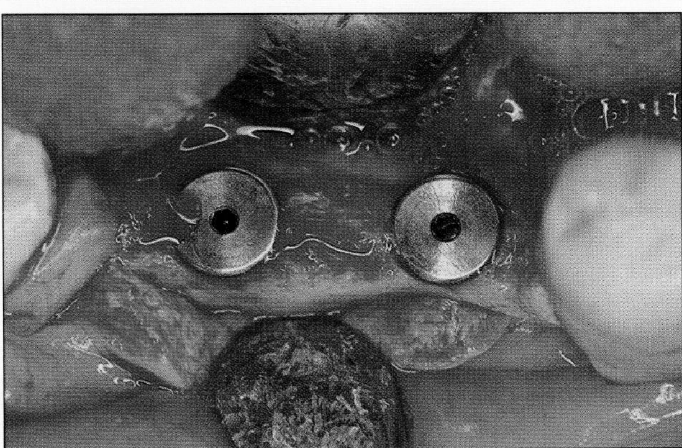

(From Newman M, Takei T, Klokkevold P, Carranza F, editors: *Carranza's clinical periodontology,* ed 12, St Louis, 2015, Saunders.)

10. The retraction suture is removed, and the mucoperiosteal flaps are repositioned and sutured in place. The implant receptor is now covered by the tissue and is not visible in the mouth.

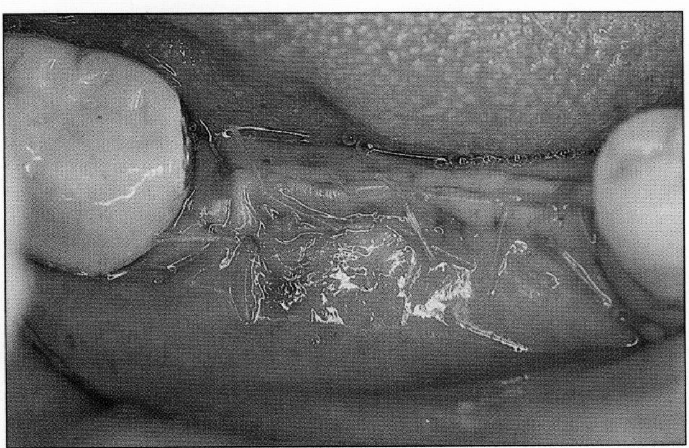

(From Newman M, Takei T, Klokkevold P, Carranza F, editors: *Carranza's clinical periodontology,* ed 12, St Louis, 2015, Saunders.)

Osseointegration Period

1. A period of 3 to 6 months is required to permit the fixture or fixtures to osseointegrate or bond to the bone. During this period, the existing denture or provisional coverage can be adapted to the healed alveolar ridge for temporary use—a procedure usually performed by the *restorative dentist.* The goal of the restorative dentist is to provide patients with beautiful teeth and a beautiful smile, so they can continue their normal activities without delay.

Stage II Surgery: Implant Exposure

1. After local anesthesia is administered, the surgical stent (template) is repositioned.
2. A sharp instrument such as a periodontal probe is lowered through the opening in the stent to make bleeding points.

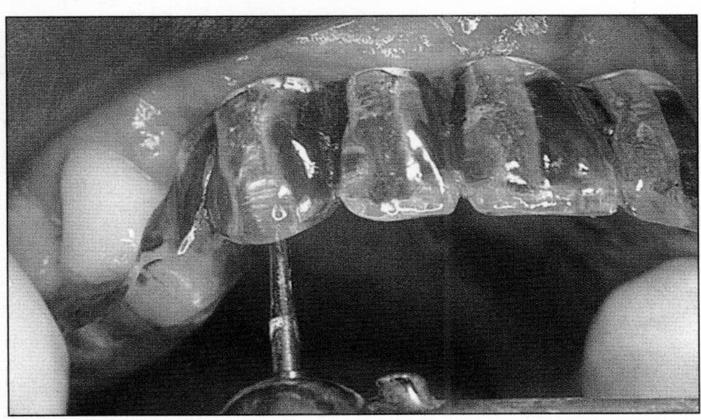

(From Bird DL, Robinson DS: *Modern dental assisting,* ed 11, St Louis, 2015, Saunders.)

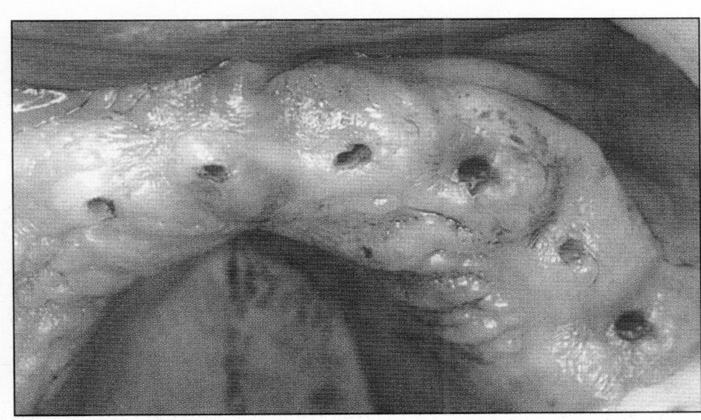

(From Bird DL, Robinson DS: *Modern dental assisting,* ed 11, St Louis, 2015, Saunders.)

3. The stent is removed, and the mark on the soft tissue shows the position of the previously placed implant.
4. An electrosurgical loop is used to remove the soft tissue over the implant site by peeling it back one layer at a time until the titanium sealing screw is located. A special tissue punch can be used to remove the tissue from over the implant.
5. The implant is uncovered, and the sealing screw is removed.

Continued

Procedure 23-7

Assisting in an Endosteal Implant Surgery—cont'd

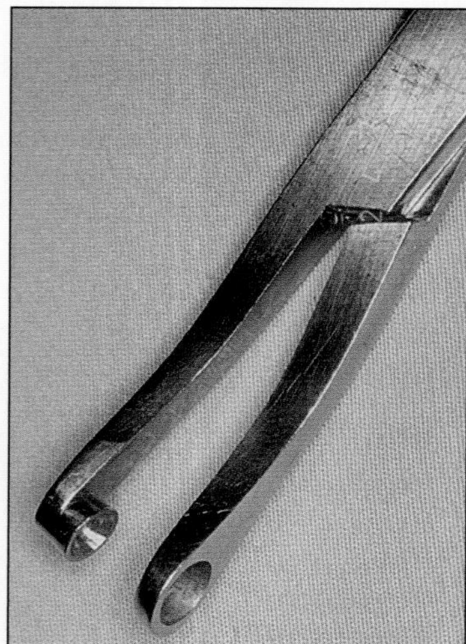

(From Bird DL, Robinson DS: *Modern dental assisting,* ed 11, St Louis, 2015, Saunders.)

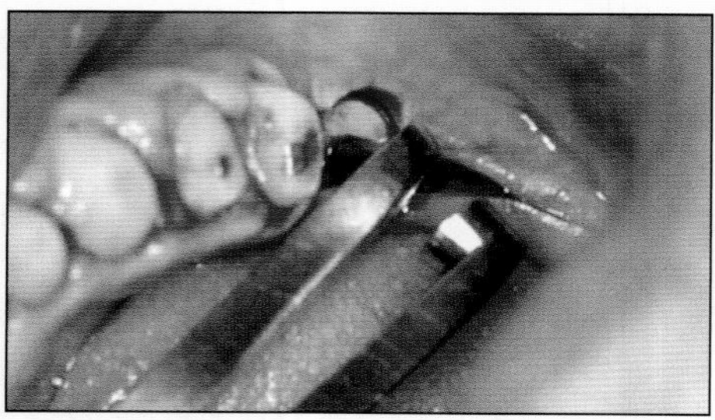

(From Bird DL, Robinson DS: *Modern dental assisting,* ed 11, St Louis, 2015, Saunders.)

6. The inside of the implant cylinder is cleaned with sterile cotton soaked in hydrogen peroxide.
7. A healing collar is screwed into the implant. This attachment will now extend above the mucosa.

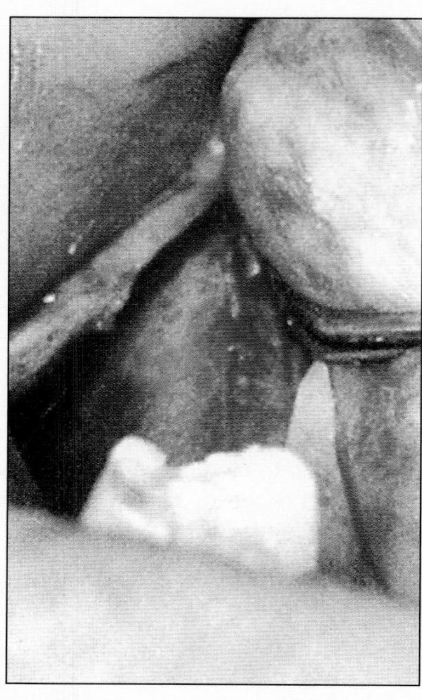

(From Bird DL, Robinson DS: *Modern dental assisting,* ed 11, St Louis, 2015, Saunders.)

8. The soft tissues are allowed to heal for 10 to 14 days before a permanent crown is fabricated.

Procedure from Bird DL, Robinson DS: *Modern dental assisting,* ed 11, St Louis, 2015, Saunders.

Chapter Exercises

Multiple Choice

Circle the letter next to the correct answer.

1. The portion of a fixed bridge that replaces the natural tooth is termed the ______________.
   a. abutment
   b. clasp
   c. pontic
   d. retainer
2. A cast restoration that covers the proximal surfaces and most of the occlusal surface is called a(n) ______________.
   a. inlay
   b. bridge
   c. onlay
   d. partial denture
3. The screw portion of the dental implant is commonly fabricated from what material?
   a. Bone graft
   b. Porcelain
   c. Titanium
   d. Enamel
4. A post and core is used to strengthen a restoration and improve retention in a(n) ______________.
   a. badly decayed tooth
   b. fractured anterior tooth
   c. endodontically treated tooth
   d. implant
5. When a fixed bridge is created, there must be at least ______________ of the bridge.
   a. one abutment
   b. one pontic
   c. two or more pontics
   d. two or more retainers
6. The use of a gingival retraction cord with epinephrine ______________ recommended for a patient with cardiovascular disease.
   a. is
   b. is not
7. Provisional coverage can remain on a prepared tooth or teeth for a few days to ______________.
   a. a few hours
   b. a few weeks
   c. a few months
   d. indefinitely
8. The saddle of a removable partial denture ______________.
   a. holds the artificial teeth
   b. provides some support for the prosthesis
   c. rests on the oral mucosa covering the alveolar ridge
   d. attaches to the abutment teeth
9. Retention of the maxillary denture primarily depends on the ______________.
   a. support of the alveolar ridge
   b. abutment teeth
   c. occlusion
   d. suction seal of the post dam
10. Osseo means the ___________.
    a. occlusal portion of an implant
    b. gingival tissues surrounding the implant
    c. stent used in implant placement
    d. bone in which the implant is imbedded

Apply Your Knowledge

1. A patient calls the office and is having discomfort in her jaw on the same side that her crown was placed last week. You remember assisting in the cementation of this crown and that the crown fit great. What could be wrong?
2. You have been instructed to make an acrylic temporary crown for a patient who is having a crown fabricated for tooth #14. When you try on the temporary after the material has set, you notice that the margins of the temporary are short. What is your plan of action to finish the temporary crown? Remake it, add on to the existing temporary, or go ahead and temporarily cement it?
3. Why would infection control be so important during the preparation and procedure steps of a dental implant?

PART NINE Specialized Dentistry

CHAPTER 24

Periodontics

http://evolve.elsevier.com/Robinson/essentials/

LEARNING OBJECTIVES

1. Pronounce, define, and spell the key terms.
2. Describe the characteristics of periodontal disease, as well as risk factors, signs, and symptoms.
3. Complete the following related to the periodontal examination:
   - Explain the procedures necessary for a comprehensive periodontal examination.
   - Explain why vertical bitewing radiographs are useful in periodontics.
   - Describe the mobility of teeth.
   - Identify the instruments used in the periodontal examination and explain the indications for their use.
4. Discuss instruments used in periodontal surgery.
5. Name and describe the types of periodontal surgeries.
6. Describe the benefits and contraindications for the ultrasonic scaler.
7. Explain the purpose of scaling, root planing, and gingival curettage.
8. Complete the following related to periodontal treatment and surgery:
   - Discuss the purpose of antimicrobial and antibiotic agents in periodontal treatment.
   - List the five main reasons for periodontal surgery.
   - Demonstrate how to assist with gingivectomy and gingivoplasty.
   - Describe postperiodontal surgery instructions.
   - Explain the purposes of periodontal surgical dressings and demonstrate the technique for proper placement.

KEY TERMS

gingival graft
gingivectomy
gingivitis
gingivoplasty
mobility
ostectomy
osteoplasty
periodontal dressing
periodontal flap surgery
periodontal pocket
periodontist
periodontitis
periodontium
root planing
scaling
sulcus
supragingival/subgingival calculus
supragingival calculus
ultrasonic scaler
vertical bite-wing radiographs

Periodontal diseases are the leading cause of tooth loss in adults. Fortunately, with early detection and treatment of periodontal disease, it is now possible for most people to keep their teeth for a lifetime. The **periodontist** (a dentist with advanced training in the specialty of periodontics) deals with the causes, prevention, and treatment of diseases of the tissue of the periodontium. The **periodontium** consists of the tissue that surrounds and supports the teeth (Figure 24-1 and Table 24-1).

Periodontal Diseases

Most periodontal diseases begin as an inflammation caused by an accumulation of bacterial biofilm (see Chapter 17 for a discussion of biofilm plaque and calculus formation) adhering to the teeth, to calculus, and to fixed and removable restorations. Periodontal diseases and dental caries are infectious diseases caused by pathogenic (disease-causing) microorganisms found in microbial biofilm. Calculus is mineralized microbial biofilm.

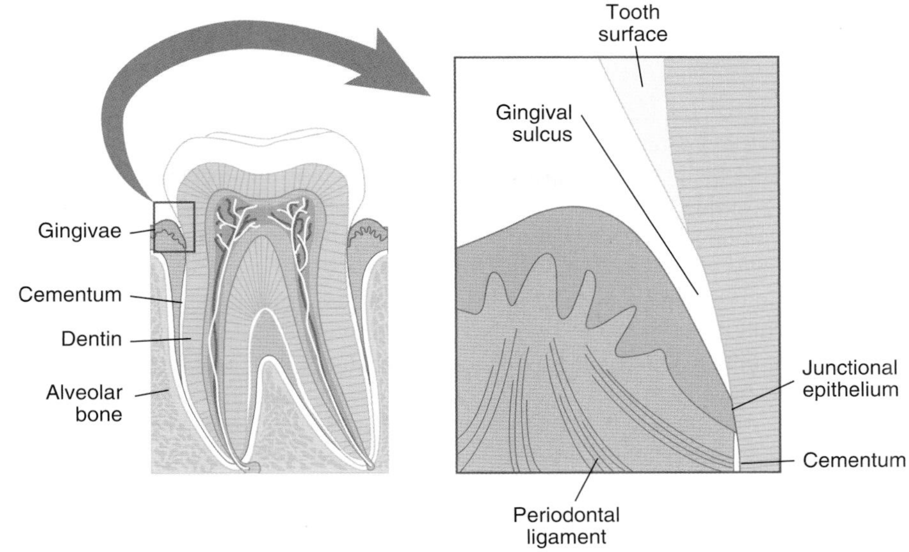

FIGURE 24-1 Structures of the periodontium, junctional epithelium, gingival sulcus, periodontal ligaments, and cementum.

TABLE 24-1
Structures of the Periodontium

Name	Description
Gingivae	Commonly referred to as *gums*, this mucosa covers the alveolar process of the jaws and surrounds the necks of the teeth.
Epithelial attachment	This tissue is at the base of the sulcus where the gingiva attaches to the tooth.
Gingival sulcus	The sulcus is the space between the tooth and the free gingiva.
Periodontal ligaments	These tense connective fibers connect the cementum covering the root of the tooth with the alveolar bone of the socket wall.
Cementum	The cementum covers the root of the tooth; its primary function is to anchor the tooth to the bony socket with the attachments of the periodontal ligaments.
Alveolar bone	Alveolar bone supports the tooth in its position within the jaw. The alveolar socket is the cavity in the bone that surrounds the tooth.

General oral health depends on the daily removal of bacterial biofilm deposits.

Other conditions in the mouth and systemic conditions, such as hormonal disturbances, may also cause periodontal diseases (Table 24-2 and Box 24-1).

Description of Periodontal Disease

Periodontal disease is described in terms of the severity of the disease and how much of the mouth is affected:

- If less than 30% of sites in the mouth are affected, then the disease is considered localized.
- If more than 30% of sites in the mouth are affected, then the disease is considered generalized.

The severity of the disease is determined by the amount of lost attachment as follows:

- Slight or early
- Moderate
- Severe or advanced

The American Academy of Periodontology has identified seven basic case types of periodontal disease, based on the severity of the disease and the amount of tissue destruction that has occurred at the time of examination.

Signs and Symptoms

The following signs and symptoms are observed most often in patients with periodontal disease:

- Red, swollen, or tender gingiva
- Bleeding gingiva while brushing or flossing
- Loose or separating teeth
- Pain or pressure when chewing
- Pus around the teeth or gingival tissue

Gingivitis

Gingivitis is inflammation of the *gingival tissue* (Figure 24-2) and is perhaps the most common human disease and is among the easiest to treat and control. The gingivae appear red and

TABLE 24-2
Common Risk Factors for Periodontal Disease

Risk Factor	Rationale
Smoking	Smokers have a greater loss of attachment, bone loss, periodontal pocket depths, calculus formation, and tooth loss. Periodontal treatments are less effective in smokers than in nonsmokers.
Diabetes mellitus	Diabetes is a strong risk factor for periodontal disease. Individuals with diabetes are three times more likely to have attachment and bone loss. Persons who have diabetes under control have less attachment and bone loss than those with poor control.
Poor oral hygiene	Lack of good oral hygiene increases the risk of periodontal disease in all age groups. Excellent oral hygiene greatly reduces the risk of severe periodontal disease.
Osteoporosis	An association between alveolar bone loss and osteoporosis has been noted. Women with osteoporosis have increased alveolar bone resorption, attachment loss, and tooth loss, compared with women without osteoporosis. Estrogen deficiency has been linked to decreases in alveolar bone.
HIV or AIDS	Gingival inflammation is increased around the margins of all teeth. Often patients with HIV or AIDS will develop necrotizing ulcerative periodontitis (NUP).
Stress	Psychologic stress is associated with depression of the immune system, and studies show a link between stress and periodontal attachment loss. Research is ongoing to determine the link between psychologic stress and periodontal disease.
Medications	Some medications, such as tetracycline and nonsteroidal antiinflammatory drugs (NSAIDs), have a beneficial effect on the periodontium, and others have a negative effect. More than 400 medications, including diuretic, antihistamine, antipsychotic, antihypertension, and analgesic agents, can cause a decrease in salivary flow (xerostomia). Antiseizure drugs and hormones such as estrogen and progesterone can cause gingival enlargement.
Local factors	Overhanging restorations, subgingival placement of crown margins, orthodontic appliances, and removable partial dentures also may contribute to the progression of periodontal disease.

HIV, Human immunodeficiency virus; *AIDS,* acquired immunodeficiency syndrome.

BOX 24-1 Characteristics of Periodontitis

I. Chronic periodontitis*
- The onset of chronic periodontitis can occur at any age, but it is most prevalent in adults. Chronic periodontitis is characterized by inflammation of the supporting structures of the teeth, loss of clinical attachment attributable to the destruction of the periodontal ligament, and loss of adjacent bone. Prevalence and severity increase with age. The following levels of chronic periodontal classifications have been identified:
  - *Slight or early periodontitis:* Gingival inflammation progresses into the alveolar bone crest, and early bone loss results in a slight attachment loss of 1 to 2 mm with periodontal probing depths of 3 to 4 mm.
  - *Moderate periodontitis:* This more advanced state of the previous condition exhibits increased destruction of periodontal structures, clinical attachment loss of up to 4 mm, moderate-to-deep pockets (5 to 7 mm), moderate bone loss, tooth mobility, and furcation involvement not exceeding Class I in molars.
  - *Severe or advanced periodontitis:* Further progression of periodontitis characterizes this state with severe destruction of periodontal structures, clinical attachment loss greater than 5 mm, increased bone loss, increased pocket depth (usually 7 mm or deeper), increased tooth mobility, and furcation involvement greater than Class I in molars.

II. Aggressive periodontitis†
- The onset of aggressive periodontitis occurs before 35 years of age and is associated with a rapid rate of progression of tissue destruction, host defense defects, and composition of subgingival flora. The following subclassifications have been identified:
  - *Prepubertal periodontitis:* Onset occurs between the eruption of the primary teeth and puberty. It occurs in localized forms, is usually not associated with a systemic disease, and its generalized forms are usually accompanied by an alteration of neutrophil functioning. This classification clinically exhibits attachment loss around the primary and/or permanent teeth.
  - *Juvenile periodontitis:* This classification has both localized and generalized forms. Generalized juvenile periodontitis (GJP) occurs late in the teenage years with a variable microbial cause that may include *Actinobacillus actinomycetemcomitans* (Aa) and *Porphyromonas gingivalis* (Pg). GJP affects most teeth. Localized juvenile periodontitis (LJP) is associated with less acute clinical signs of

BOX 24-1 Characteristics of Periodontitis—cont'd

inflammation than would be expected, based on the severity of destruction. LJP is associated with bone and attachment loss primarily confined to permanent first molars
and/or incisors. Age of onset is at or around puberty and is associated with Aa and neutrophil dysfunction.

III. Necrotizing periodontal diseases[‡]

- *Necrotizing ulcerative gingivitis (NUG):* This gingival infection has a complex origin (e.g., biofilm, temporary depression of polymorphonuclear neutrophil [PMN] functioning, stress, poor diet) and is characterized by the sudden onset of pain, necrosis of the tips of the gingival papillae (punched-out appearance), and bleeding. Secondary features include fetid breath and a pseudomembrane covering. Fusiform bacteria, *Prevetella intermedia,* and spirochetes have been associated with gingival lesions.
- *Necrotizing ulcerative periodontitis (NUP):* Necrosis of gingival tissues, periodontal ligament, and alveolar bone characterize this disease. NUP is associated with immune disorders such as HIV infection and with immunosuppressive therapies; characteristics include severe and rapid periodontal destruction. Extensive necrosis of the soft tissue simultaneously occurs with alveolar bone loss, resulting in a lack of deep pocket formation.

From Darby M, Walsh M: *Dental hygiene theory and practice,* ed 4, St. Louis, 2015, Saunders.
*Slavkin HC: Building a better mousetrap: toward an understanding of osteoporosis, *J Am Dent Assoc* 150:1632, 1999.
[‡]Armitage G: Development of a classification system for periodontal diseases and conditions, *Ann Periodontol* 4:1, 1999.
[†]Fedi P, Vernino A, Gray J: *The periodontic syllabus,* Philadelphia, 2000, Lippincott Williams & Wilkins.

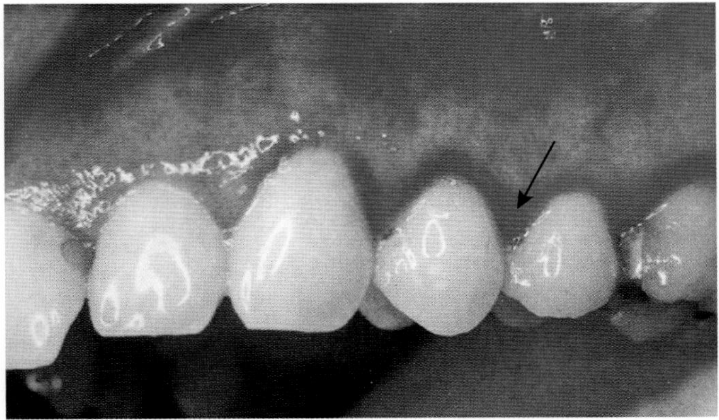

FIGURE 24-2 Gingivitis *(arrow).*

swollen and have a tendency to bleed easily. Gingivitis is *directly related* to the presence of bacterial biofilm on the tooth surface and the amount of time that the biofilm is allowed to remain undisturbed. (Biofilm plaque is discussed in Chapter 17.)

Periodontitis

Periodontitis occurs as the infection from the gingivae progresses into the *alveolar bone.*

Periodontitis is divided into case types according to the severity of the disease and the amount of tissue destruction that has occurred at the time of the examination. Periodontitis usually occurs in older individuals and is often referred to as adult-onset periodontitis. However, periodontitis is also found in children.

Periodontal Examination

In addition to a thorough dental examination as described in Chapter 12, specialized procedures are necessary to diagnose and plan appropriate treatment for periodontal disease. A periodontal examination includes medical and dental histories, radiographic evaluations, examination of the teeth, examination of the gingivae and supporting structures, and periodontal charting, which consists of pocket readings and taking note of furcations, tooth mobility, exudate (pus), and gingival recession (Figure 24-3).

Radiographs

Radiographs are a valuable aid for evaluating periodontal disease. The accuracy of the radiographs is critical in the diagnosis of periodontal disease because a distortion can result in a diagnostic error. **Vertical bite-wing radiographs** (Figure 24-4) are frequently taken during a periodontal examination because they show generalized horizontal bone loss on both arches better than the traditional horizontal bite-wing radiographs.

Examination of the Teeth

The examination of the teeth focuses on indications of periodontal disease or factors that could contribute to periodontal disease (Table 24-3).

Mobility

All teeth have a slight normal **mobility** (tooth movement in the socket) because of the function of the periodontal membrane. Excessive mobility, however, can be an important sign of periodontal disease (Figure 24-5). The following scale is used to record the degree of mobility.

0 = Normal
1 = Slight mobility
2 = Moderate mobility
3 = Severe mobility

Examination of the Gingivae and Supporting Structures

The periodontal examination includes an assessment of the amounts of biofilm and calculus and of changes in gingival health, as well as an assessment of bleeding at the bone level

Perio Chart (Partial Exam - 09/21/2010) - Smith, John (11)

Maxillary

	1	2	3	4	5	6	7	8	9	10	11	12	13	14	15	16
ATTACH		1 2 1	4 4 3	4 2 3	3 3 3	3 3 2	4 2 1	2 2 2	5 2 2	1 1 4	4 1 3	1 2 2	5 2 2	2 0 2	4 4 1	
POCKET		0 1 0	2 1 0	2 1 0	1 2 0	1 0 1	2 2 0	2 1 0	2 1 0	1 0 2	1 0 1	0 2 1	2 1 0	1 0 1	2 1 0	
FGM		1 1 1	2 3 3	2 1 3	2 1 3	2 3 1	2 0 1	0 1 2	3 1 2	0 1 2	3 1 2	1 0 1	3 1 2	1 0 1	2 3 1	
CALC																
SUPP																
BLEED																
MOBIL																

Facial

M

Lingual

M

	1	2	3	4	5	6	7	8	9	10	11	12	13	14	15	16
ATTACH		3 1 2	2 2 5	2 0 4	2 0 3	1 1 1	1 2 2	1 1 2	2 2 2	3 3 3	3 1 2	2 3 2	0 3 3	3 2 2	2 5 2	
POCKET		0 0 2	1 2 3	1 0 2	1 0 2	1 0 1	0 2 1	1 0 2	1 0 2	1 2 3	1 0 2	1 3 1	0 1 2	3 1 2	1 3 2	
FGM		3 1 0	1 0 2	1 0 2	1 0 1	0 1 0	1 0 1	0 1 0	1 2 0	2 1 0	2 1 0	1 0 1	0 2 1	0 1 0	1 2 0	
CALC																
SUPP																
BLEED																

A

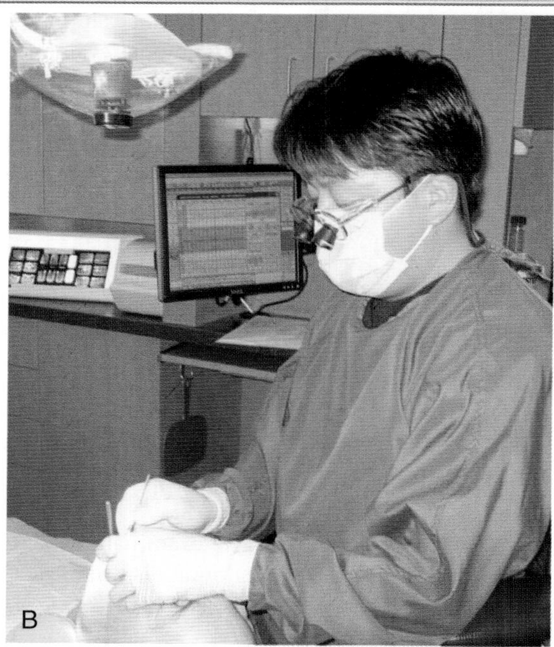

FIGURE 24-3 **A,** Screen shot of Axium 2 Perio Charting. **B,** Periodontal chart on a computer screen. This periodontist can easily refer to the chart as he treats the patient. (**A,** Courtesy Exan Enterprises, Las Vegas, Nevada. **B,** From Bird DL, Robinson DS: *Modern dental assisting,* ed 11, St. Louis, 2015, Saunders.)

and detection of periodontal pockets (Figure 24-6). A **periodontal pocket** occurs when disease causes the normal gingival **sulcus** to become deeper than normal (a normal sulcus measures 3 mm or less; Table 24-4).

Probing Periodontal Pockets

The depth of the periodontal pocket is measured by using a periodontal probe (Figure 24-7). The dentist or dental hygienist will take six measurements for each tooth (Figure 24-8). The dental assistant records the deepest measurement on each surface on the patient's periodontal chart. The surfaces measured are:

- Mesiofacial
- Facial
- Distofacial
- Mesiolingual
- Lingual
- Distolingual

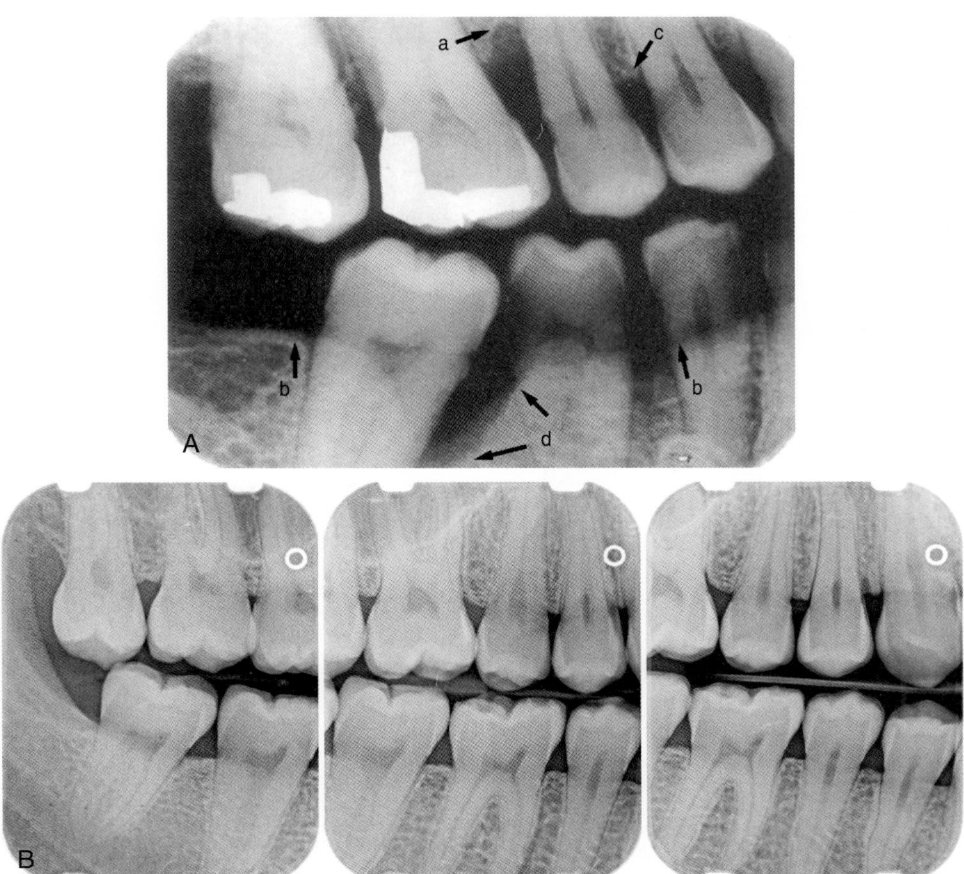

FIGURE 24-4 **A,** The *arrows* indicate varying amounts of bone loss attributable to periodontal disease. **B,** Vertical bite-wing films can be used to cover a larger area of the alveolar bone. (**A,** From Miles DA, Van Dis ML, Williamson GF, Jensen CW: *Radiographic imaging for the dental team,* ed 4, St. Louis, 2009, Saunders. **B,** From Newman M, Takei T, Klokkevold P, Carranza F, editors: *Carranza's clinical periodontology,* ed 12, St. Louis, 2015, Saunders.)

TABLE 24-3
Dental Conditions That Contribute to Periodontal Disease

Condition	Description
Pathologic migration	Loss of periodontal support can cause a shift in the position of the teeth.
Clenching or grinding (bruxism)	These oral habits place excessive biting forces on the teeth and may accelerate bone loss.
Defective restorations or bridge work	Defective restorations or bridge work may retain biofilm plaque and increase the risk of periodontal disease.
Mobility	Mobility is movement of a tooth within its socket. Although all teeth have a very small degree of natural mobility (see Figure 24-5), excessive mobility can be an important sign of periodontal disease. Mobility is recorded with the following scale: 0, normal; 1, slight mobility; 2, moderate mobility; 3, extreme mobility.
Occlusal interferences	Areas on a tooth that prevent the teeth from properly occluding do not directly cause periodontal disease but can contribute to mobility, tooth migration, and temporomandibular joint pain.

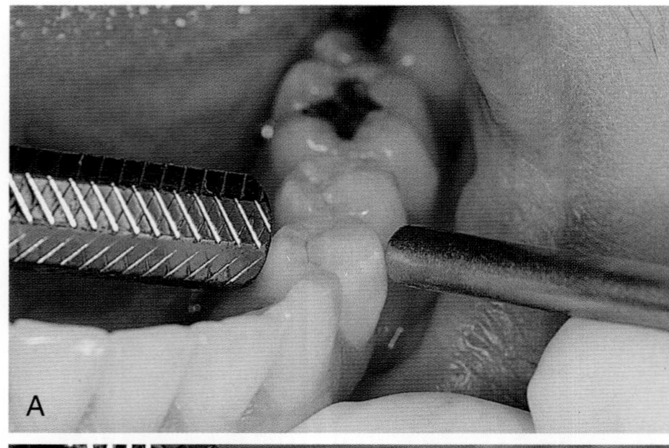

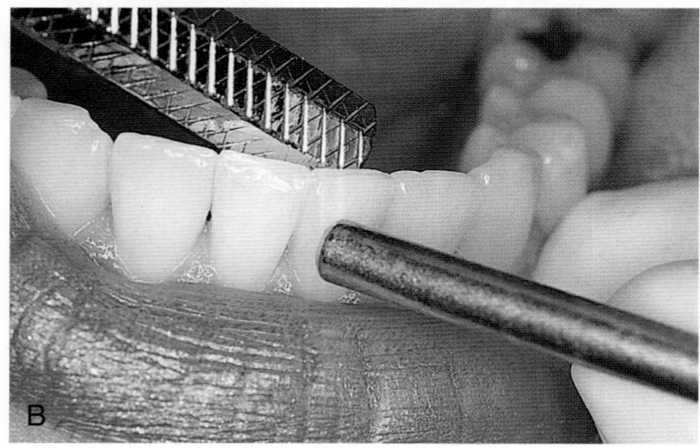

FIGURE 24-5 Mobility is detected with the blunt ends of two instruments. (From Daniel SA, Harfst SA: *Mosby's dental hygiene concepts, cases, and competencies,* ed 2, St. Louis, 2008, Mosby.)

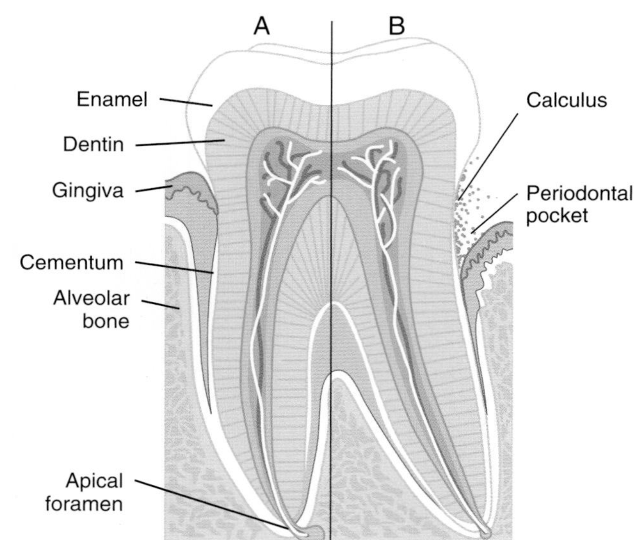

FIGURE 24-6 Cross-section of a tooth and associated anatomic structures. **A,** Illustrates the depth of a normal gingival sulcus. **B,** Illustrates a periodontal pocket.

TABLE 24-4
Examination of the Gingivae and Supporting Tissue

Assessment	Description
Biofilm	Biofilm is the primary cause of gingival inflammation and most other forms of periodontal disease.
Calculus	Calculus is hard mineralized biofilm. Calculus may be supragingival (above the gingivae) or subgingival (below the gingivae) and adheres to the surfaces of natural teeth, crowns, bridges, and dentures. Calculus is a contributing factor in periodontal disease because it is always covered with biofilm.
Gingival recession	As disease progresses, the gingivae may recede, leaving portions of the roots of the teeth exposed below the cementoenamel junction. Gingival recession levels can be visualized on the chart by drawing a dotted or color line to indicate the gingival margin (see Figure 24-3).
Bleeding index	The severity of gingival inflammation is measured by the amount of bleeding observed during probing. Several different indices can be used to measure bleeding. Each system is based on the principle that healthy gingivae do not bleed.
Measurement of periodontal pockets	A periodontal pocket occurs when the disease causes the normal gingival sulcus to become deeper than normal. (A normal sulcus measures 3 mm or less.)
Assessment of bone level	Radiographs and probing measurements are used to assess the patient's bone level. These may also be visualized on the chart by drawing a color line to indicate the bone level (see Figure 24-3).
Radiographs	Radiographs are used to: • Detect interproximal bone loss. • Show changes in bone as periodontitis progresses. • Locate furcation involvements. • Measure the crown-to-root ratio (the length of the clinical crown compared with the length of the root of the tooth). • Show signs of traumatic occlusion.

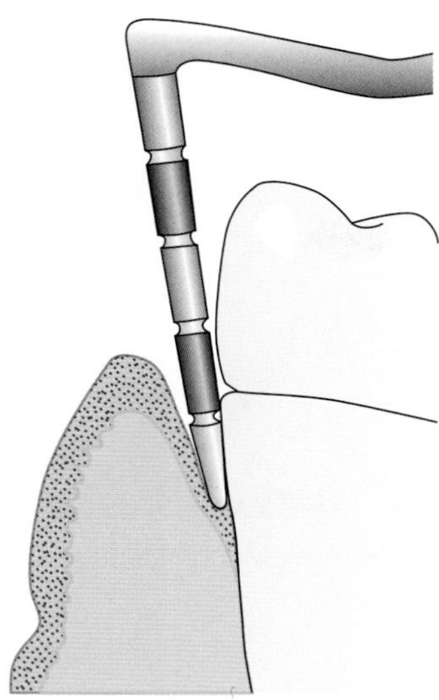

FIGURE 24-7 Diagram showing probing of the periodontal pocket depth. The millimeter measurement indicates the distance from the gingival margin to the base of the pocket. (From Perry D, Beemsterboer P, Essex G: *Periodontology for the dental hygienist,* ed 4, St. Louis, 2014, Saunders.)

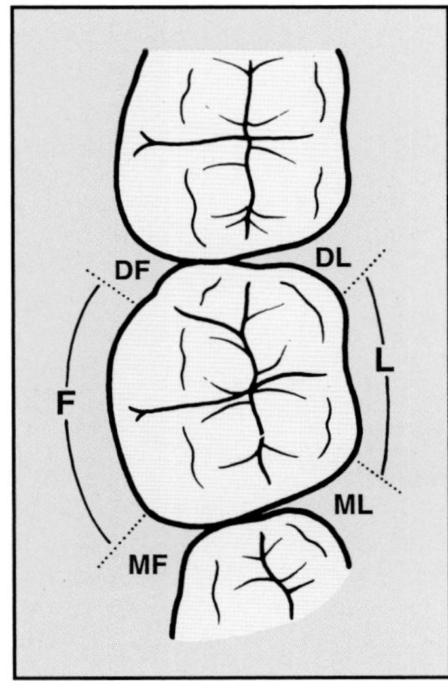

FIGURE 24-8 Six probing depths are taken for each tooth. *DF,* Distofacial; *DL,* distolingual; *F,* facial; *L,* lingual; *MF,* mesiofacial; *ML,* mesiolingual. (Modified from Perry DA, Beemsterboer P, Carranza FA: *Techniques and theory of periodontal instrumentation,* Philadelphia, 1990, Saunders.)

Instruments Used in the Periodontal Examination

Periodontal Probes

Periodontal probes, which are calibrated in millimeters, are used to locate and measure the depth of periodontal pockets (Figure 24-9). On some periodontal probes, the tip is color-coded to make the measurements easier to read.

The manual probe is tapered to fit into the gingival sulcus and has a blunt or rounded tip. This probe is available in many designs, and selection depends on the personal preferences of the operator.

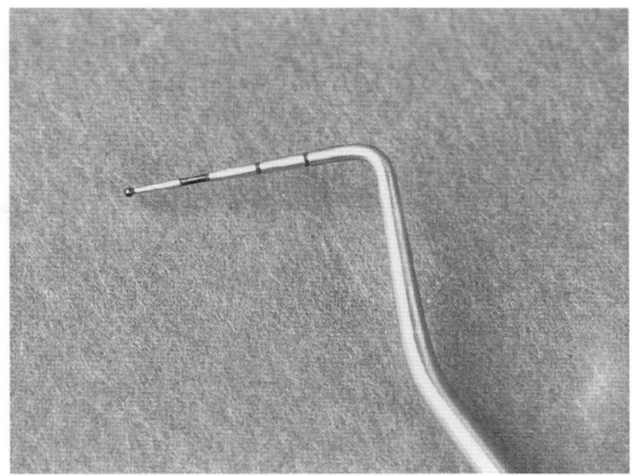

FIGURE 24-9 Working end of a periodontal probe.

Automated computerized probes are extremely accurate electronic devices used to measure the depth of periodontal pockets. With the probe, a thin wirelike device is inserted into the sulcus, and data are recorded by a microcomputer. Voice-activated recording systems are becoming popular in periodontal assessment. The operator will speak the measurement, and the computer will automatically enter the information.

Explorers

Explorers are used in periodontics to locate calculus deposits and provide tactile information to the operator about the roughness or smoothness of the root surfaces. Many styles of explorers are used in periodontal treatment, and they are longer and more curved than explorers used for caries detection. (Explorers are discussed in Chapter 12.)

The working ends of periodontal explorers are thin and fine, enabling them to be easily adapted around tooth surfaces. They are also long enough to reach the base of deep pockets and furcations. A furcation is the point at which the roots of a multirooted tooth diverge (Figure 24-10). Furcations are noted on the patient's periodontal record.

Scalers

Sickle scalers are primarily used to remove large deposits of **supragingival calculus** (above the gumline). A sickle scaler with a long straight shank is used to remove calculus from the anterior areas of the oral cavity (Figure 24-11). A contra-angle sickle scaler, which is angled at the shank, is designed to remove calculus from the posterior teeth.

Chisel scalers are used to remove supragingival calculus in the contact area of the anterior teeth. The blade on the chisel scaler is slightly curved to adapt to the tooth surfaces (Figure 24-12).

Hoe scalers are used to remove heavy supragingival calculus. Hoes are most effective when used on buccal and lingual surfaces of the posterior teeth.

Files are used to crush or fracture very heavy calculus. The fractured calculus is then removed from the tooth surface with a curette (Figure 24-13).

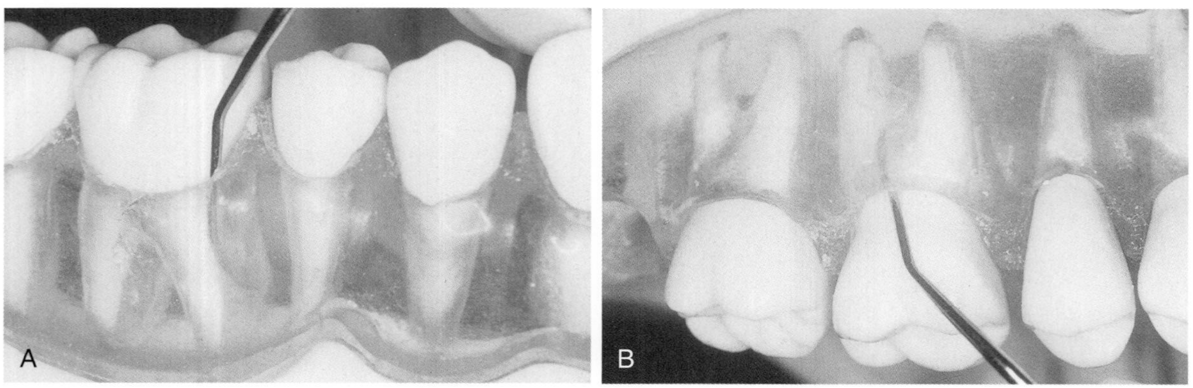

FIGURE 24-10 Various styles of periodontal explorers. (Courtesy Hu-Friedy Manufacturing, Chicago, Illinois.)

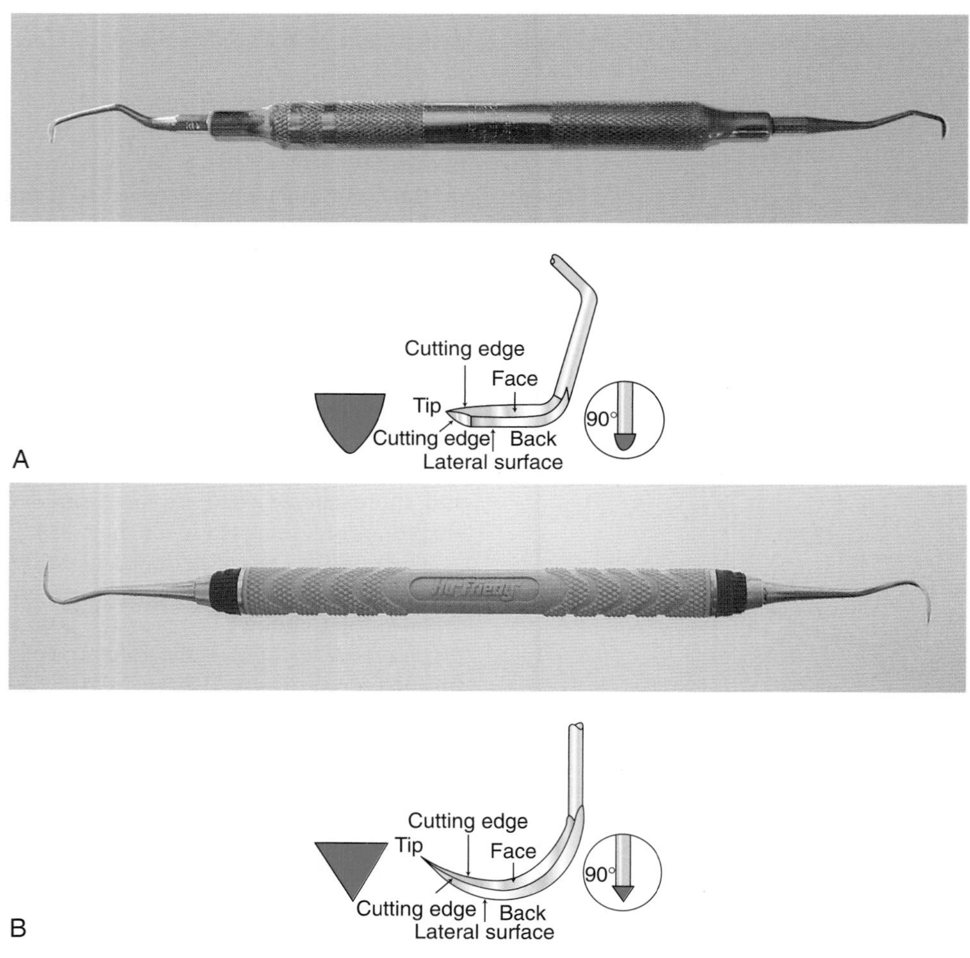

FIGURE 24-11 **A,** Straight sickle scaler. **B,** Curved sickle scaler. (From Boyd LRB: *Dental instruments: a pocket guide,* ed 5, St Louis, 2015, Saunders.)

Curettes

Curettes can be used to remove **supragingival** (above the gumline) and **subgingival calculus** (below the gumline), to smooth rough root surfaces (root planing), and to remove the diseased soft tissue lining of the periodontal pocket (soft tissue curettage). Curettes have a rounded end, unlike a scaler, which has a pointed end (Figure 24-14). Two basic designs of curettes are available: the universal curette and the Gracey curette.

Universal curettes are designed so that one instrument is able to adapt to all tooth surfaces, thus the name *universal.* Two cutting edges are found on each side of the blade. Universal curettes resemble the spoon excavators used in restorative dentistry (Figure 24-15).

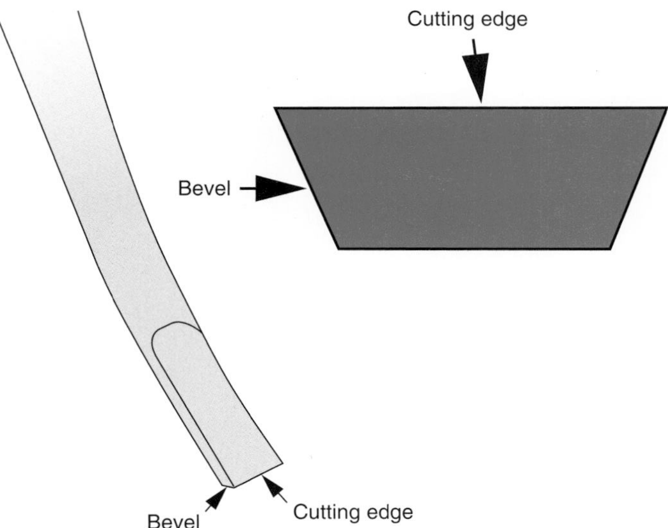

FIGURE 24-12 The chisel has a single blade with a firm shank. The cutting edge is at the end of the instrument so that when it is pushed against a deposit, the leading edge engages the calculus. (From Daniel SA, Harfst SA: *Mosby's dental hygiene concepts, cases, and competencies,* ed 2, St. Louis, 2008, Mosby.)

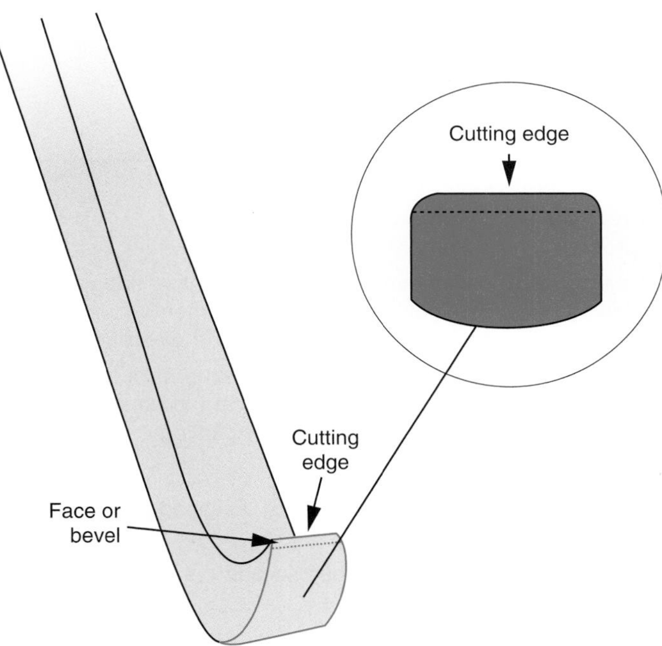

FIGURE 24-13 The hoe has one blade with a firm shank. When placed beneath a ledge of calculus, a vertical stroke is usually successful in removing deposits. As shown, the corners of the blades should be dulled with a sharpening stone. (From Daniel SA, Harfst SA: *Mosby's dental hygiene concepts, cases, and competencies,* ed 2, St. Louis, 2008, Mosby.)

Gracey curettes have one cutting edge and are specific to an area, which means that they are designed to adapt to specific tooth surfaces (mesial or distal). Treatment of the full dentition requires the use of several Gracey curettes (Figure 24-16).

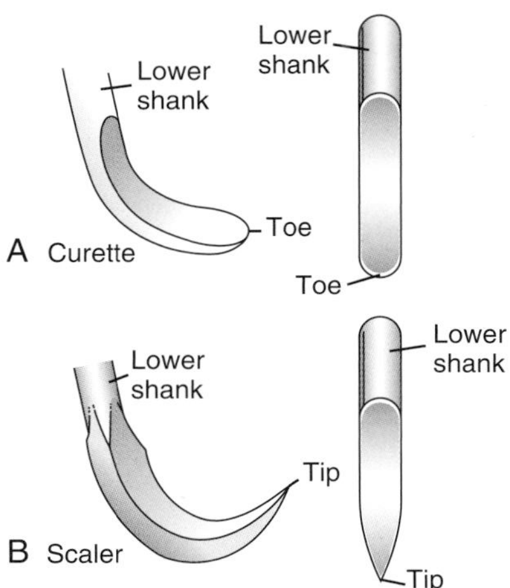

FIGURE 24-14 Comparison of the end of a scaler (pointed) and the end of a curette (rounded).

Periodontal Surgical Instruments

Periodontal Knives

Kirkland knives are one of the most common type of knives used in periodontal surgery. These instruments are usually double-ended with kidney-shaped blades.

Orban knives are used to remove tissue from the interdental areas. These knives are shaped similar to spears and have cutting edges on both sides of the blades (Figure 24-17).

Pocket Markers

Pocket markers are similar in appearance to cotton pliers: however, one tip is smooth and straight, and the other tip is sharp and bent at a right angle. The smooth tip of the pocket marker is inserted into the base of the pocket. When the instrument is pressed together, the sharp tip makes small perforations in the gingivae, which are referred to as *bleeding points* and are used to outline the area for a gingivectomy.

Periodontal Treatment Procedures

The realm of periodontal treatment ranges from the basic dental prophylaxis to the most sophisticated periodontal surgeries involving tissue grafts and implants of bone (Table 24-5).

The method of treatment depends on the severity of the disease and the amount of tissue destruction that has occurred. Many general dentists provide basic periodontal services, such as scaling and root planing, and refer more complex cases involving surgery to the periodontist. Regardless of the treatment plan, ongoing good daily oral hygiene is essential for the success of any type of periodontal therapy.

Dental Prophylaxis

A dental prophylaxis, commonly referred to as a *prophy,* is the complete removal of calculus, soft deposits, biofilm, and stains from all supragingival and unattached subgingival tooth surfaces. The dentist and the dental hygienist are the only members of the dental team licensed to perform this procedure.

See Procedure 24-1: Assisting With a Dental Prophylaxis.

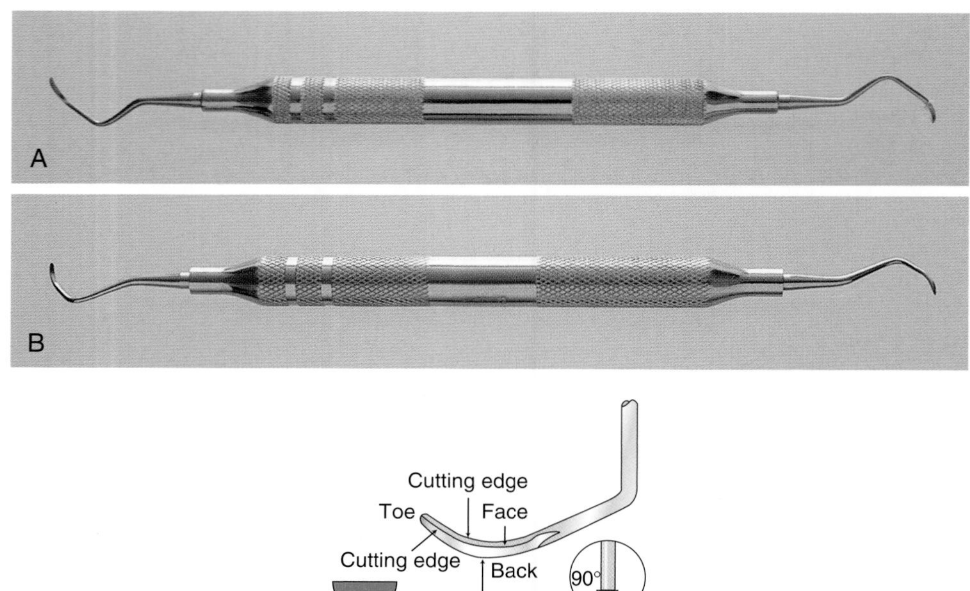

FIGURE 24-15 The universal curettes. **A,** Barnhart ½. **B,** Ratcliff ¾. **C,** The arrows indicate the cutting edges on a universal curette. (From Boyd LRB: *Dental instruments: a pocket guide,* ed 5, St. Louis, 2015, Saunders.)

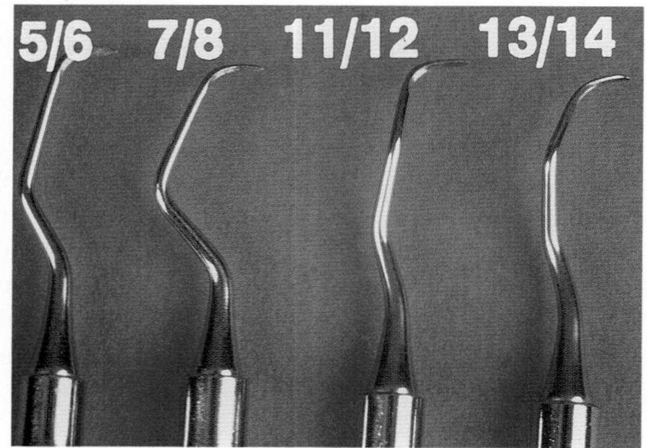

FIGURE 24-16 Assorted Gracey curettes. (Courtesy Hu-Friedy Manufacturing, Chicago, Illinois.)

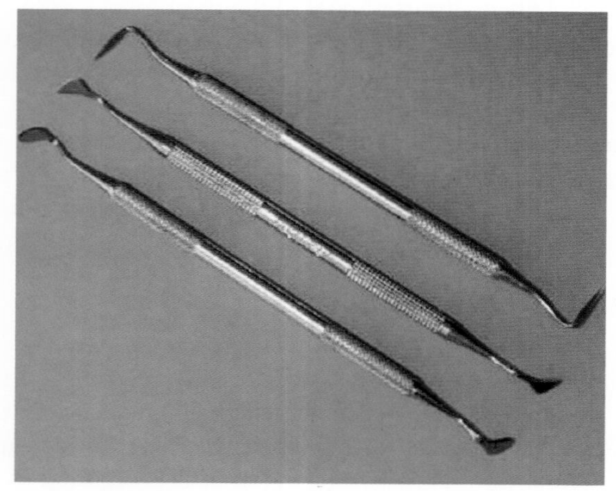

FIGURE 24-17 Kirkland and Orban interdental knives.

TABLE 24-5
Types of Periodontal Treatment

Procedure	Purpose
Primary	
Prophylaxis (prophy)	Primary preventive measure Primary treatment for gingivitis
Scaling, root planing	Removal of supragingival and subgingival calculus and necrotic cementum, leaving root surfaces smooth and glasslike
Curettage	Removal of necrotic tissue from the wall of the periodontal pocket in conjunction with scaling and root planing
Surgical	
Gingivectomy	Surgical removal of diseased gingival tissue
Gingivoplasty	Surgical reshaping and contouring of gingival tissue
Periodontal flap	Gaining surgical access to and visibility of bone and tooth roots
Gingival grafting	Removal of oral tissue from one site for placement on another
Osteoplasty	Surgical recontouring and reshaping of bone (may include adding bone)
Ostectomy	Surgical removal of bone

BOX 24-2 Indications for Using the Ultrasonic Scaler

- Removal of supragingival calculus and difficult stains
- Subgingival periodontal removal of calculus, attached biofilm, and endotoxins from the root surface
- Cleaning of furcation areas
- Removal of deposits before surgery
- Removal of orthodontic cement, debonding
- Removal of overhanging margins of restorations

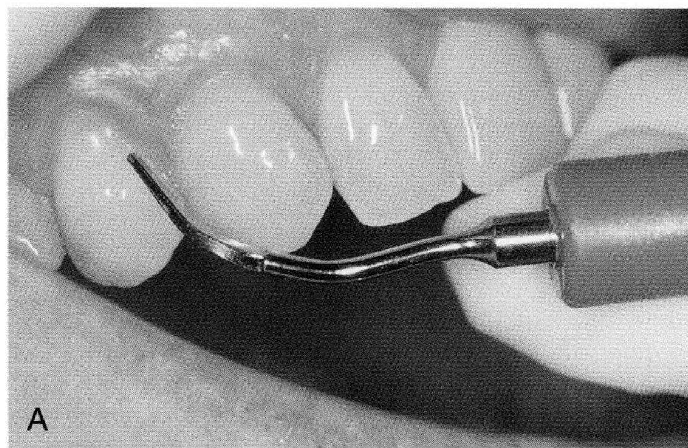

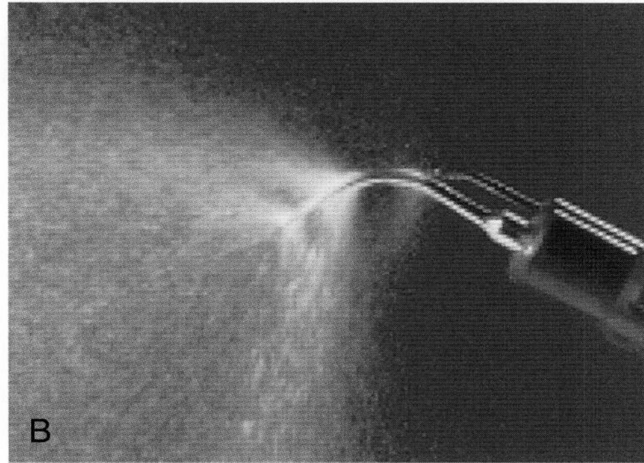

FIGURE 24-18 **A,** Positioning of the ultrasonic scaler. **B,** Ultrasonic scaler with water source turned on. (Courtesy Hu-Friedy Manufacturing, Chicago, Illinois.)

A dental prophylaxis is indicated for patients with healthy gingivae as a preventive measure and is most commonly performed during recall appointments. A dental prophylaxis is also the primary treatment for gingivitis.

Ultrasonic Scaler

The ultrasonic scaler rapidly removes calculus and significantly reduces hand fatigue for the operator. Newer styles and slimmer instrument tips have been designed to allow better access to subgingival pockets. The use of these devices has increased (Box 24-2).

The ultrasonic scaler converts very-high-frequency sound waves into mechanical energy in the form of very rapid vibrations (20,000 to 40,000 cycles per second) at the tip of the instrument. A spray of water at the tip prevents the buildup of heat and provides a continuous flush of debris and bacteria from the base of the pocket (Figure 24-18 and Table 24-6).

TABLE 24-6
Ultrasonic Instrumentation

Advantages	Disadvantages
Slender tip provides greater access with less tissue distention.	Some handpieces cannot be sterilized.
Provides healing advantages from water lavage and sulcus irrigation.	Is not as portable as hand instruments.
Results in less operator fatigue.	Requires water evacuation.
Does not require resharpening.	Produces a contaminated aerosol.
Provides a washed field for greater visibility.	Poses a possible risk to patients with pacemakers.
Has a possible bactericidal effect.	Effect of noise and vibrations on operator is yet to be determined.

Modified from Hu-Friedy, Chicago, Illinois.

BOX 24-3 Contraindications and Precautions of the Ultrasonic Scaler: Ultrasonic Scaling and Children

- Tissue in young patients is very sensitive to ultrasonic vibrations.
- Vibrations and heat may damage the pulp tissue of primary and newly erupted permanent teeth, which have large pulp chambers.

Contraindications and precautions must be considered for pediatric patients and for people with certain medical and oral conditions (Boxes 24-3 through 24-5).

Scaling, Root Planing, and Gingival Curettage

Scaling and root planing are indicated as the initial treatment before periodontal surgery. In some cases, gingival curettage is also indicated (Figure 24-19).

Scaling

During scaling, scalers are used to remove supragingival calculus from the tooth surface, and curettes are used to remove subgingival calculus. Some areas on the root surface may remain rough after calculus removal. This roughness occurs because the cementum has become necrotic (dead) or because the scaling has produced grooves and scratches.

Root Planing

Root planing follows scaling procedures to remove any remaining particles of calculus and necrotic cementum embedded in the root. After root planing, the surfaces of the root are smooth and glasslike. Smooth root surfaces resist new calculus formation and are easier for the patient to keep clean.

BOX 24-4 Contraindications and Precautions of the Ultrasonic Scaler: General Health Considerations

- *Communicable disease:* A patient can transmit a disease, such as tuberculosis, by aerosols.
- *Susceptibility to infection:* A compromised patient is open to infection. Examples of patients with a compromised health status include the patient in chemotherapy or a patient with human immunodeficiency virus (HIV) infection, uncontrolled diabetes, debilitation, and kidney or other organ transplants.
- *Respiratory problems:* Materials can be aspirated into the lungs of patients with respiratory problems. Examples of respiratory conditions include chronic pulmonary disease, asthma, emphysema, cystic fibrosis, or other breathing problems.
- *Swallowing difficulty:* An ultrasonic scaler can stimulate the gag reflex in the patient who has a swallowing problem. Examples of such a condition include muscular dystrophy, multiple sclerosis, paralysis, or amyotrophic lateral sclerosis.
- *Cardiac pacemaker:* Consultation with the patient's cardiologist is necessary because, theoretically, an ultrasonic scaler can possibly disrupt a pacemaker (although no cases have been reported). The newer models of scalers have protective coatings.

BOX 24-5 Contraindications and Precautions of the Ultrasonic Scaler: Oral Conditions

- *Demineralized areas:* The vibrations of the ultrasonic scaler tip can remove the areas of remineralization that begin to cover the demineralization.
- *Exposed dentinal surfaces:* Removed tooth structures can cause tooth sensitivity.
- *Restorative materials:* Some restorative materials, such as porcelain, amalgam, composite resins, and laminate veneers, can be damaged by an ultrasonic scaler.
- *Titanium implant abutments:* Unless a special plastic sheath is used to cover the tip, the ultrasonic scaler will damage titanium surfaces.
- *Narrow periodontal pockets:* The tip of the ultrasonic scaler will not fit into very narrow subgingival pockets without interfering with proper angulation and limiting visibility.

Gingival Curettage

In addition to scaling and root planing, some areas in the mouth may require a procedure called *gingival curettage.* (*Curettage* means scraping or cleaning with a curette.) Gingival curettage, also referred to as *subgingival curettage,* consists of scraping the gingival wall of a periodontal pocket to remove necrotic tissue from the pocket wall.

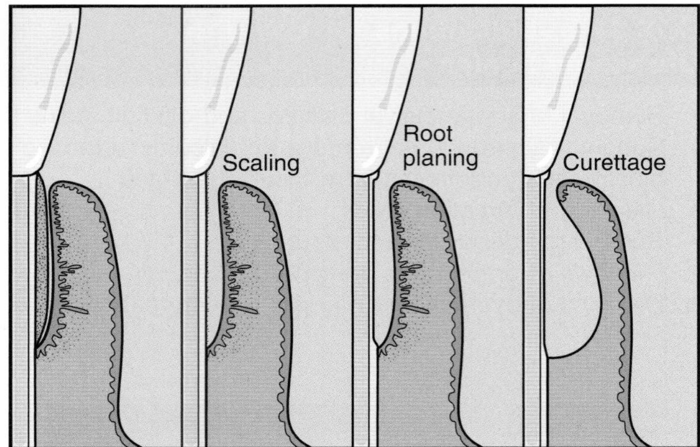

FIGURE 24-19 Scaling, root planing, and curettage. (From Perry DA, Beemsterboer P, Carranza FA: *Technique and theory of periodontal instrumentation,* Philadelphia, 1990, Saunders.)

Postoperative Instruction after Scaling and Curettage

Most patients appreciate the dental assistant explaining postoperative instructions to them so that they have the opportunity to ask questions. Postoperative instructions are an important legal consideration; therefore providing written postoperative instructions for the patient to take home is wise.

Discomfort Mild discomfort may be noted for a few hours after the local anesthetic agent has worn off. Usually a mild analgesic drug, such as acetaminophen (Tylenol) or ibuprofen (Advil), is adequate for relieving this discomfort.

Diet A normal diet is recommended; however, avoiding very spicy foods, citrus fruits, and alcoholic beverages is recommended.

The patient is also advised not to smoke. Smoking irritates the tissue and delays healing.

Home care Good home care is essential for the success of scaling and curettage. Normal home care should be resumed the following day.

Antimicrobial and Antibiotic Agents

The dentist may prescribe antimicrobial and/or antibiotic agents for use in conjunction with periodontal treatment.

Tetracycline is an antibiotic used for the treatment of periodontitis, juvenile periodontitis, and rapidly destructive periodontitis.

Chlorhexidine rinse twice daily is the most effective agent available to reduce biofilm and gingivitis. However, chlorhexidine can cause some temporary brown staining of the teeth, tongue, and resin restorations.

Metronidazole is used in treating rapidly progressing periodontitis. It is not prescribed to treat juvenile periodontitis because metronidazole is not effective against the type of bacteria found in this disease.

Fluoride mouth rinses have been shown to reduce bleeding by delaying bacterial growth in the periodontal pockets.

Periodontal Surgery

Periodontal surgery may be recommended for five primary reasons (Box 24-6 and Figure 24-20).

Gingivectomy

A **gingivectomy** is the surgical removal of diseased gingival tissue. This procedure is performed when reducing the depth of the periodontal pocket and removing fibrous gingival tissue are necessary.

This surgical procedure involves making bleeding points with pocket markers and removing the gingival tissue with periodontal knives and surgical scissors. After healing, cleaning the area when the pockets have been reduced is easier for the patient.

Gingivoplasty

A **gingivoplasty** involves surgical reshaping and contouring of the gingival tissue. The presence of deep periodontal pockets with fibrous tissue is the primary indication for both the gingivectomy and the gingivoplasty. Often, the two procedures are simultaneously performed. During the gingivoplasty procedure, the gingivae are recontoured using periodontal knives, rotary diamond burs, curettes, and surgical scissors. Gingival margins are thinned and given a scalloped edge.

See Procedure 24-2: Assisting With Gingivectomy and Gingivoplasty.

BOX 24-6 Reasons for Periodontal Surgery

1. To reduce or eliminate periodontal pockets
2. To create or improve access to the root surface
3. To treat osseous (bone) defects
4. To correct mucogingival defects
5. To create new tissue attachment

Periodontal Flap Surgery

Periodontal flap surgery involves separating the gingivae from the underlying tooth roots and alveolar bone, similar to the flap of an envelope. When the flap is elevated (lifted up), the dentist has excellent visibility and may perform one or more of the following procedures:

- Thorough scaling and root planing of exposed root surfaces
- Moving the flap laterally (to the side) to cover the root surfaces of an adjacent tooth that does not have adequate tissue coverage (this procedure is called a *laterally sliding flap.*)
- Recontouring (reshaping) of the underlying bone
- Closing the flap and suturing it into place after the surgery is completed (Figure 24-21; a periodontal pack is usually placed after flap surgery.)

Gingival Grafting

Some patients may benefit from a **gingival graft**, a procedure during which tissue is taken from one site in the patient's mouth and placed on another. The palate is frequently used as the

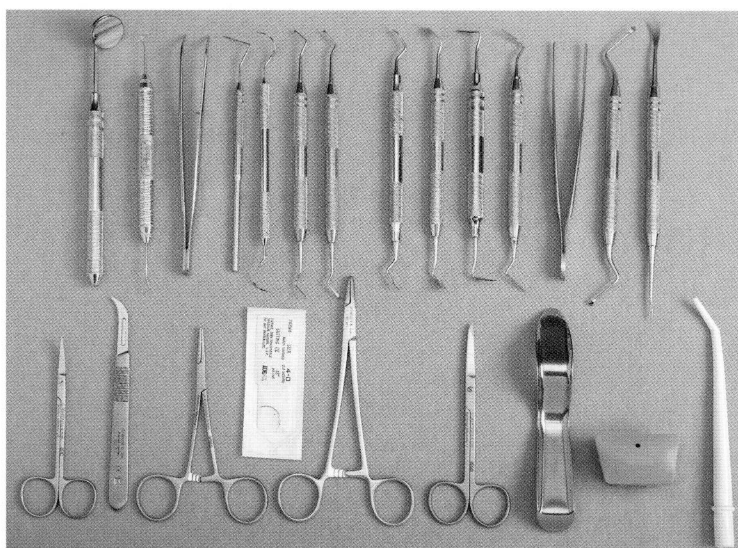

FIGURE 24-20 Periodontal surgical tray. *Top row, left to right:* Mouth mirror, explorer, cotton forceps (pliers), periodontal probe, furcation probe, mesial-distal hoe, buccal-lingual hoe, back-action hoe, kidney-shape periodontal knife, interproximal knife, bone file, tissue forceps, surgical curette, periosteal elevator. *Bottom row, left to right:* Tissue scissors, scalpel with #12 blade, hemostat, silk sutures with needle, needle holder, suture scissors, cheek and tongue retractor (Minnesota) mouth prop, disposable high-volume surgical evacuation tip. (From Boyd LRB: *Dental instruments: a pocket guide,* ed 5, St. Louis, 2015, Saunders.)

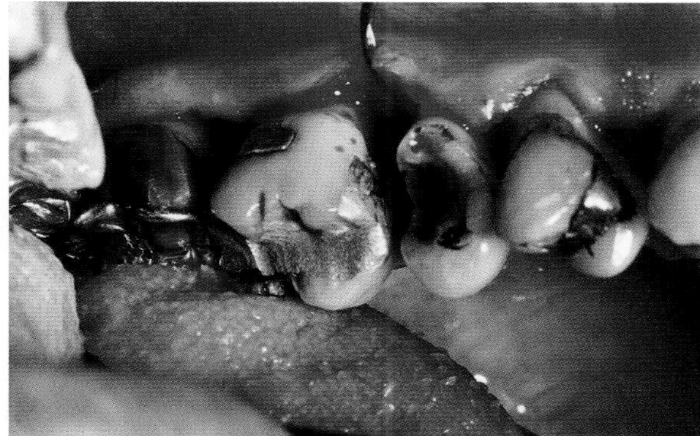

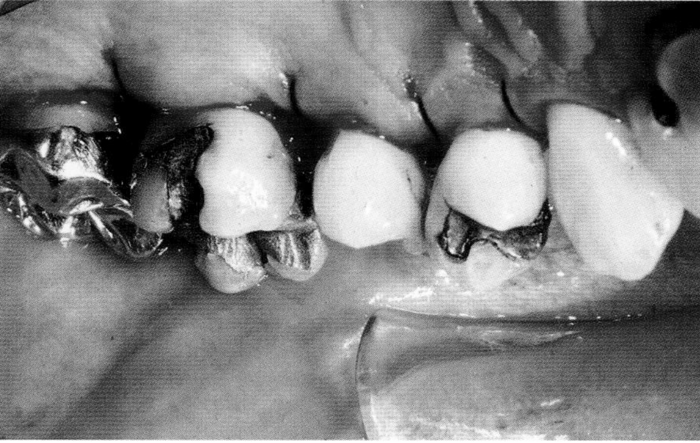

FIGURE 24-21 Periodontal flap procedure. (Courtesy James F. Coggan, DDS.)

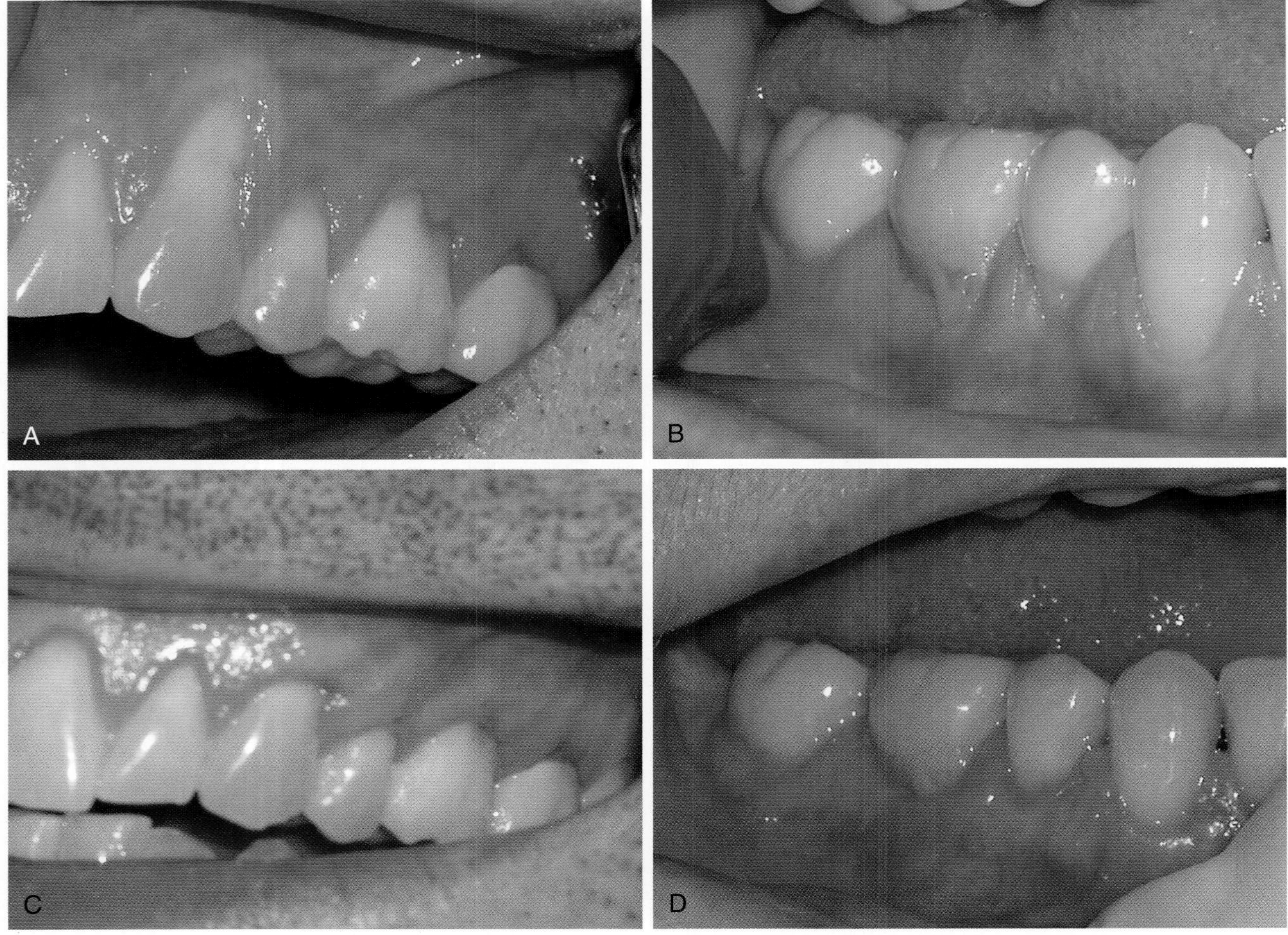

FIGURE 24-22 **A** and **B,** Presurgical recession of gingival tissues. **C** and **D,** Healed tissues after gingival graft surgery. (Courtesy Dr. Christine Ford, Santa Rosa, California.)

donor site. A section of tissue is removed and then carefully positioned and sutured into the recipient area. The donor site on the palate is usually covered with a periodontal dressing until it has healed (Figure 24-22).

Osseous Surgery

Osseous (bone) surgery is performed to remove defects and to restore normal contours in the bone. Two types of bone surgeries are the *osteoplasty* and the *ostectomy*. Each one requires surgically exposing the bone and recontouring it with a rotary diamond stone or bone chisel (Figure 24-23).

Osteoplasty

In the **osteoplasty**, or additive surgery, bone is contoured and reshaped. In addition, bone may be *added* through bone grafting (taking bone from one area and placing it in another), or substitute materials may be placed. This procedure is useful for some patients with bone defects caused by periodontal disease.

Ostectomy

In the **ostectomy**, or subtractive surgery, bone is removed. This type of procedure is necessary when the patient has large exostoses (bony growths). For example, an ostectomy is performed if a patient needs a denture and the bony growth would interfere with the comfort and fit of the denture.

Postperiodontal Surgery

Instructions

Postoperative instructions should be given to the patient in written form. These instructions should include information about discomfort, periodontal dressing, rinsing the mouth, diet, activity, home care, and postoperative visits.

Discomfort

Mild-to-moderate discomfort can be expected, especially during the first 24 hours. If indicated, pain medication is prescribed.

Periodontal Dressing

If bleeding is present under the dressing, then the patient is instructed to call the dental office immediately. Small pieces of the periodontal dressing may break off. If no pain or bleeding occurs, then the dressing does not usually have to be replaced.

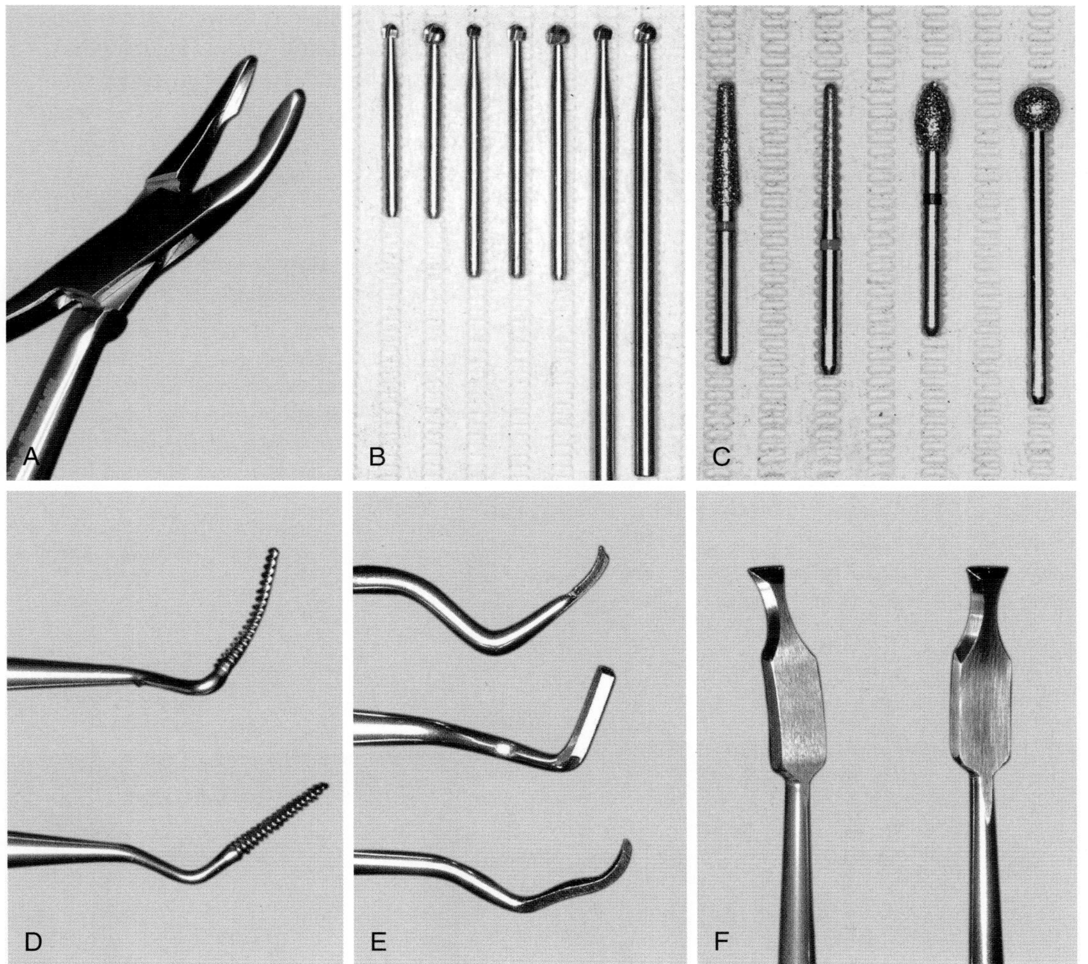

FIGURE 24-23 Instruments often used in osseous surgery. **A,** Rongeur. **B,** Carbide round burs. *Left to right,* Friction grip, surgical-length friction grip, and slow-speed handpiece. **C,** Diamond burs. **D,** Schluger and Sugarman interproximal files. **E,** Back-action chisels. **F,** Ochsenbein chisels. (From Newman M, Takei T, Klokkevold P, Carranza F, editors: *Carranza's clinical periodontology,* ed 12, St. Louis, 2015, Saunders.)

Rinsing

The patient should not rinse his or her mouth for the first 24 hours. After 24 hours, a warm salt-water rinse (1 tsp of salt in 8 oz of warm water) is indicated.

Diet

A normal diet is recommended. Avoiding hard foods, alcoholic beverages, citrus fruit, and spicy foods is recommended.

Activity

Avoid excessive exercise for the first few days, which allows a firm clot to form in the surgical area.

Home Care

The areas of the mouth that were not involved in the surgery should be brushed and flossed normally. The areas of the periodontal dressing should be gently cleaned using a soft toothbrush.

Postoperative Visit

Approximately 1 week after surgery, the dressing will be removed for a postoperative check. Usually after the dressing is removed, it is not necessary to replace it.

Periodontal Dressing

A **periodontal dressing** is similar to a bandage over a surgical site. Periodontal dressings (periopacks) are used to:

- Hold the flaps in place
- Protect the newly forming tissue
- Minimize postoperative pain, infection, and hemorrhage
- Protect the surgical site from trauma during eating and drinking
- Support mobile teeth during the healing process

Types of Periodontal Dressings

A variety of materials are used for periodontal dressings. The most commonly used materials are the zinc oxide–eugenol and noneugenol types.

Zinc oxide–eugenol dressing Zinc oxide–eugenol dressings are supplied as a powder and liquid that are mixed before using. The material may be mixed ahead of time, wrapped in wax paper, and frozen for future use (Figure 24-24). This type of dressing has a slow set, which allows for longer working time. It sets to a firm and heavy consistency and provides good support and protection for tissues and flaps.

Some patients are allergic to the eugenol and experience redness and burning pain in the area of the dressing.

Noneugenol dressing Noneugenol dressing is the most widely used type of periodontal dressing. The material is supplied in two tubs—one contains the base material and the other contains the accelerator.

The material is easy to mix and to place; it has a smooth surface for patient comfort. Noneugenol dressing has a rapid setting time if exposed to warm temperatures and cannot be mixed in advance and stored (Figure 24-25).

See Procedure 24-3: Preparing and Placing Noneugenol Periodontal Dressing, and Procedure 24-4: Removing a Periodontal Dressing.

Ethical Implications

Failure to diagnose periodontal disease at an early stage is a leading complaint in malpractice lawsuits. Ethically, it is incumbent upon the dental professional to educate and instruct patients about periodontal care. Careful documentation related to issues of patient education, compliance with home care advice, and referrals to periodontists must be prepared.

From an ethical and a legal standpoint, including a periodontal evaluation as part of every dental examination is important.

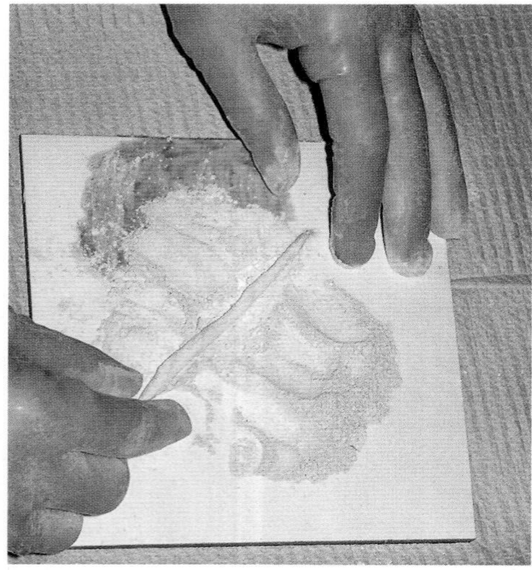

FIGURE 24-24 Zinc oxide powder and liquid eugenol are mixed in advance.

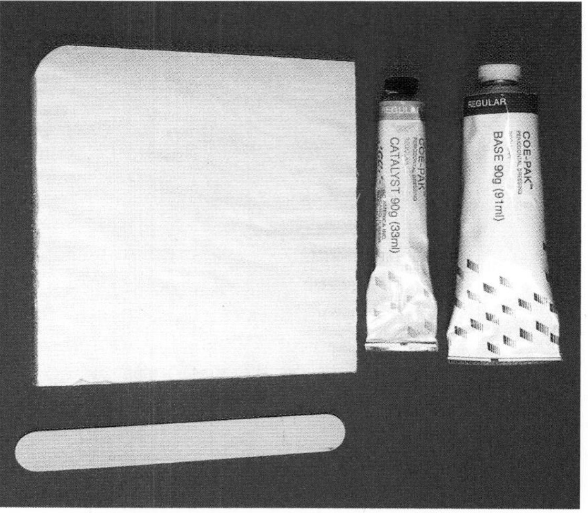

FIGURE 24-25 Paste for noneugenol dressing is ready to be mixed.

Procedure 24-1

Assisting with a Dental Prophylaxis

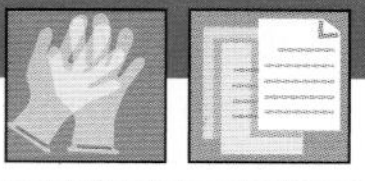

Goal

To assist competently with a dental prophylaxis procedure.

Equipment and Supplies

- High-volume evacuator (HVE) tip or saliva ejector
- Basic instrument setup
- Scalers, universal curette
- Prophy angle
- Rubber polishing cup and brushes
- Polishing agent
- Dental floss and/or tape
- Preprocedural mouth rinse

Procedure 24-1

Assisting with a Dental Prophylaxis—cont'd

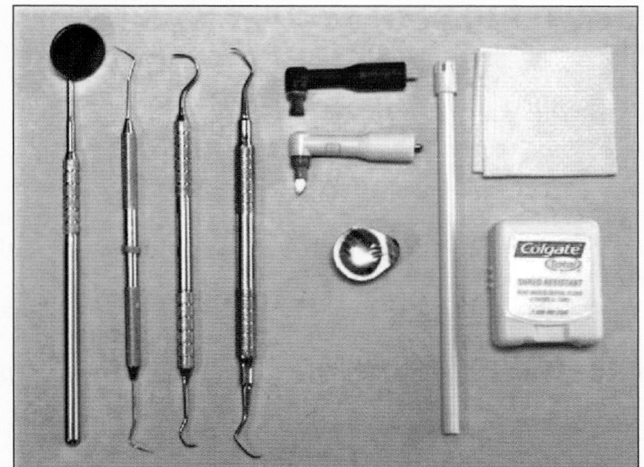

(From Bird DL, Robinson DS: *Modern dental assisting,* ed 11, St. Louis, 2015, Saunders.)

Procedural Steps

1. Assist with the transfers as the operator uses an explorer to locate interproximal and subgingival calculus.

Note: The operator must have good access and visibility during this procedure.

2. Use the HVE as necessary, and retract the lips, tongue, and cheeks to improve visibility and access as the operator uses scalers and curettes to remove all calculus and biofilm.
3. The operator checks for and removes any remaining calculus.
4. The operator polishes the teeth using polishing paste, a rubber cup, and bristle brushes.
5. The operator removes any remaining interproximal debris with dental floss or tape.
6. Provide oral hygiene instructions appropriate to the individual needs of the patient.

Procedure 24-2

Assisting with Gingivectomy and Gingivoplasty

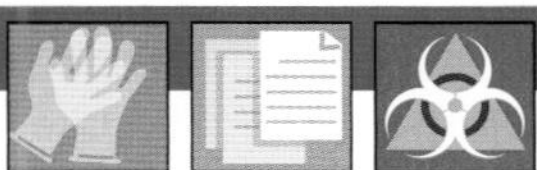

Goal

To assist the dentist competently in performing gingivectomy and gingivoplasty periodontal procedures

Equipment and Supplies

- High-volume evacuator (HVE) tip and surgical aspirating tip
- Local anesthetic setup
- Scalpel and blades
- Surgical periodontal knives
- Surgical tissue retraction forceps
- Periodontal pocket marker
- Tissue tweezers
- Scalers and curettes
- Diamond burs and sterile stones
- Suture needle and sutures
- Hemostat and surgical scissors
- Periodontal surgical dressing materials
- Sterile gauze sponges
- Sterile irrigation solution (water or saline)

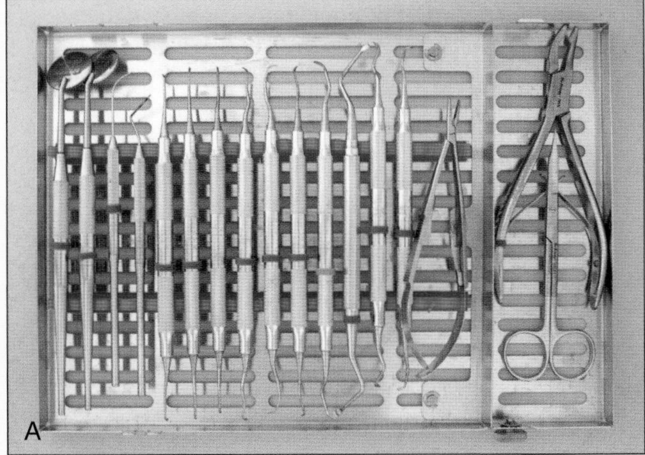

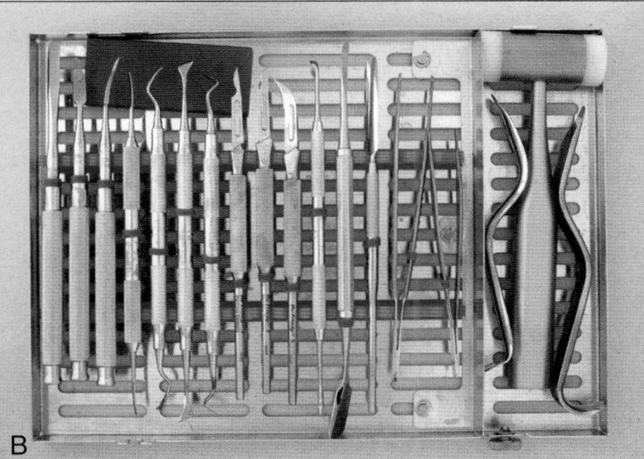

Typical series of periodontal surgical instruments, divided into two cassettes. **A,** *From left,* Mirrors, explorer, probe, series of curettes, needle holder, rongeur instrument, and scissors. **B,** *From left,* Series of chisels, Kirkland knife, Orban knife, scalpel handles with surgical blades (#15C, #15, #12D), periosteal elevators, spatula, tissue forceps, cheek retractors, mallet, and sharpening stone. (Courtesy Hu-Friedy Mfg. Co., LLC, Chicago, Illinois.)

Continued

Procedure 24-2

Assisting with Gingivectomy and Gingivoplasty—cont'd

Procedural Steps

Role of the Dental Assistant

1. Set out the patient's health history, radiographs, and periodontal chart.

Purpose: The dentist needs to review the case before surgery.

2. Assist in the administration of the local anesthetic agent.
3. Anticipate the dentist's needs, and be prepared to transfer and retrieve surgical instruments when needed.

Purpose: This step saves time and makes the procedure less stressful.

4. Have gauze ready to remove tissue from the instruments as necessary.

Purpose: Periodontal surgery can generate heavy bleeding.

5. Provide oral evacuation and retraction.

Purpose: Good access and visibility are critical for the dentist, and the patient will be more comfortable.

6. Irrigate with sterile saline.

Purpose: Irrigation keeps the surgical site clean and free of debris.

7. If sutures are used, then prepare the suture needle and suture material and position them in a hemostat or needle holder. Transfer them to the dentist when requested.

Purpose: This step simplifies the procedure for the dentist and increases patient comfort.

8. Place, or assist with the placement of, the periodontal dressing.

Purpose: The dressing acts as a bandage to protect the surgical site.

Note: Check your state's Dental Practice Act before placing a periodontal dressing without assistance.

9. Wipe any blood or debris from the patient's face. Provide postoperative instructions to the patient.

Purpose: This step ensures that the patient clearly understands the postoperative instructions as necessary for personal well-being and to address legal considerations.

Role of the Dentist

1. The dentist administers the local anesthetic agent.

Purpose: In addition to pain control, local anesthesia aids visibility by constricting blood vessels and reducing the amount of blood at the surgical site.

2. The dentist marks the pockets on the facial and lingual gingivae by using the periodontal pocket marker.

Purpose: The bleeding points indicate the pocket depth and thus the point for the initial incision.

3. The dentist uses a scalpel or a periodontal knife to incise the gingiva at a 45-degree angle, following along the bleeding points. The incision is beveled to create a normally contoured, free gingival margin.
4. The dentist removes the gingival tissue along the incision line using surgical knives.
5. The dentist tapers the gingival margins and creates a scalloped marginal outline.

Purpose: This marginal outline creates an attractive and healthy appearance.

6. The dentist shapes the interdental papillae using interdental knives.

Purpose: This step contours the interdental grooves.

7. The dentist performs scaling and root planing of the root surfaces.

Purpose: This step removes any residual calculus that was inaccessible before surgery.

8. The dentist places sutures if needed.
9. The dentist irrigates the surgical site and then covers it with a periodontal dressing.

Purpose: Periodontal dressing protects the surgical site.

Note: In some states, the placement and removal of the periodontal dressing are delegated to the dental assistant (expanded function).

Procedure 24-3

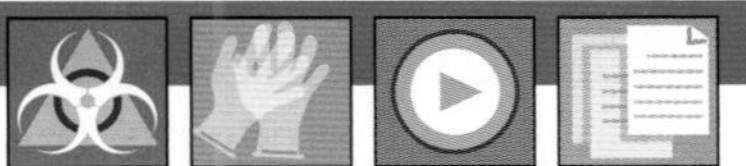

Preparing and Placing Noneugenol Periodontal Dressing

Goal

To prepare and assist the dentist in placing a noneugenol periodontal dressing

Equipment and Supplies

- Paper mixing pad (supplied by the manufacturer)
- Wooden tongue depressor
- Noneugenol dressing (base and accelerator)
- Paper cup filled with room-temperature water
- Saline solution
- Plastic type of filling instrument

Procedural Steps

Mixing the Material

1. Extrude equal lengths of the two pastes on the paper pad.
2. Mix the pastes with a wooden tongue depressor until a uniform color has been obtained (2 to 3 minutes).
3. When the paste loses its tackiness, place it in the paper cup filled with room-temperature water.
4. Lubricate gloved fingers with saline solution.

Purpose: This step prevents the material from sticking to the gloves.

5. Roll the paste into strips approximately the length of the surgical site.

Placing the Dressing

1. Press small triangle-shaped pieces of dressing into the interproximal spaces.

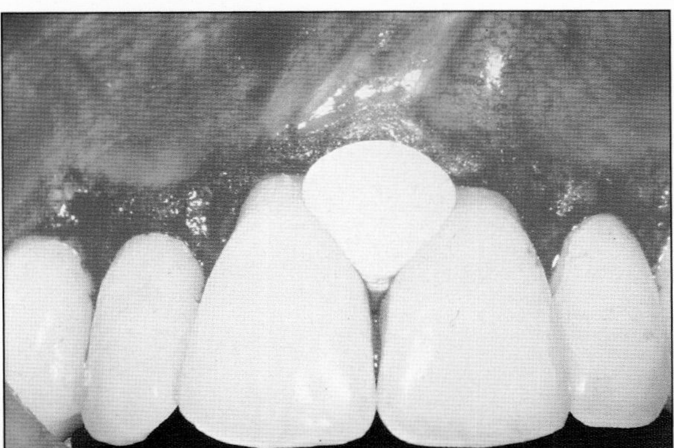

2. Adapt one end of the strip around the distal surface of the last tooth in the surgical site.
3. Bring the remainder of the strip forward along the facial surface, and gently press the strip along the incised gingival margin.
4. Gently press the strip into the interproximal areas.

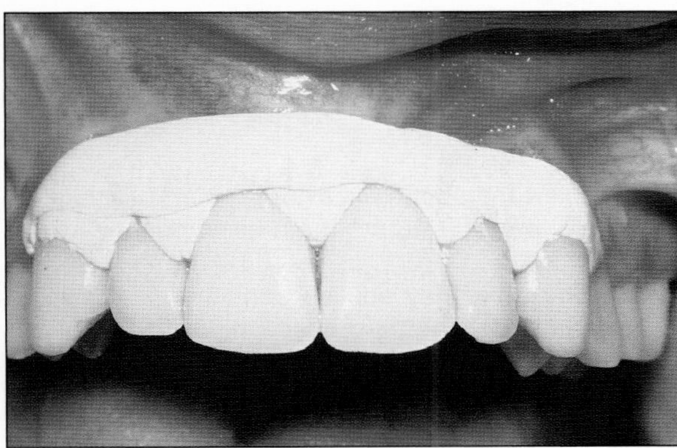

5. Apply the second strip in the same manner from the lingual side.
6. Join the facial and lingual strips at the distal surface of the last tooth at both ends of the surgical site.
7. Apply gentle pressure on the facial and lingual surfaces.
8. Check the dressing for overextension and interference with occlusion.

Purpose: Excess packing irritates the mucobuccal fold and floor of the mouth.

9. Remove any excess dressing, and adjust the new margins to remove any roughness.

Purpose: If the pack is not properly adapted, it can break off.

Procedure 24-4

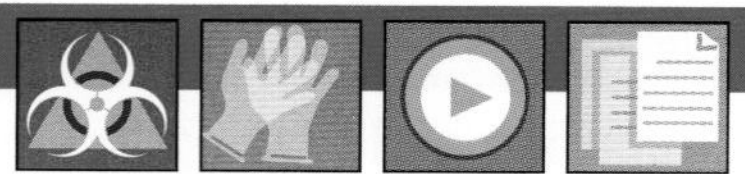

Removing a Periodontal Dressing

Goal

To remove a periodontal dressing

Equipment and Supplies

- Spoon excavator
- Suture scissors (if sutures are present)
- Dental floss
- Warm saline solution
- Irrigating solution
- High-volume evacuator (HVE) tip or saliva ejector

Procedural Steps

1. Gently insert the spoon excavator under the margin.
2. Use lateral pressure to pry the dressing gently away from the tissue.

Purpose: The area may still be sensitive, and the newly healed tissue is delicate and easily injured.

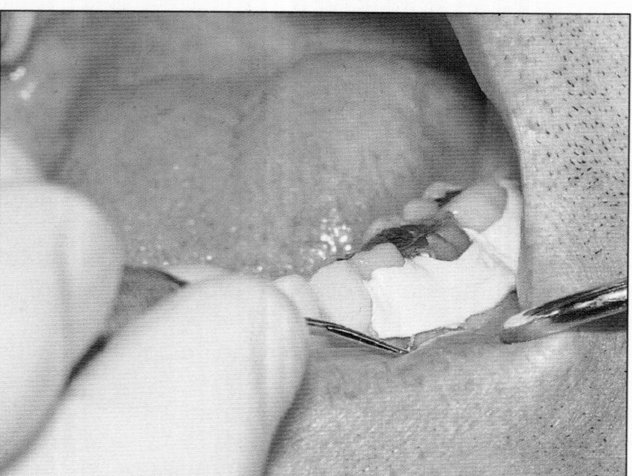

3. If sutures are embedded in the dressing material, cut the suture material free. Gently remove the sutures from the tissue.

Purpose: Accidentally pulling the sutures could be painful for the patient and might open the wound.

4. Gently use dental floss to remove all fragments of dressing material from the interproximal surfaces.

Purpose: Remaining fragments could cause discomfort for the patient and result in tissue irritation.

5. Gently irrigate the entire area with warm saline solution to remove superficial debris.

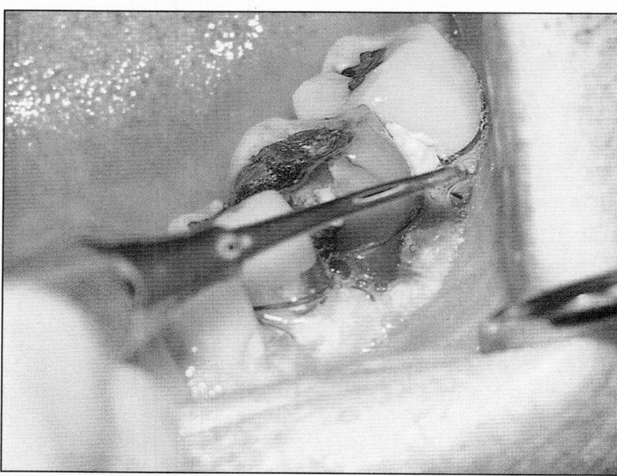

6. Use the HVE tip or saliva ejector to remove fluid from the patient's mouth.

Chapter Exercises

Multiple Choice

Circle the letter next to the correct answer.

1. The leading cause of tooth loss in adults is __________.
   a. periodontal disease
   b. root caries
   c. occlusal trauma
   d. root abscess
2. The most common periodontal disease and the easiest one to treat is __________.
   a. gingivitis
   b. early periodontitis
   c. advanced periodontitis
   d. refractory periodontitis
3. How many periodontal probing measurements are taken for each tooth?
   a. 4
   b. 6
   c. 8
4. Curettes that are designed with two cutting edges are called __________.
   a. universal curettes
   b. Gracey curettes
5. The procedure in which the gingival wall of the pocket is scraped is called a __________.
   a. gingival curettage
   b. gingivectomy
   c. gingivoplasty
6. A periodontal examination and diagnosis includes __________.
   a. evaluation of radiographs
   b. medical and dental histories
   c. periodontal probing
   d. all of the above
7. The primary cause of gingivitis and most forms of periodontal disease is __________.
   a. calculus
   b. defective restorations
   c. food debris
   d. dental biofilm
8. The depth of a periodontal pocket is measured with a(n) __________.
   a. curette
   b. explorer
   c. periodontal probe
   d. pocket marker
9. Which dental professional(s) is (are) licensed to perform a dental prophylaxis?
   a. Dental assistant
   b. Dentist
   c. Dental hygienist
   d. b and c
10. What surgical procedure is required to reshape the bone to remove defects and to restore normal contour?
    a. Gingivectomy
    b. Gingivoplasty
    c. Osteoplasty
    d. Root planing
11. The procedure that removes calculus, soft deposits, and stains from all unattached tooth surfaces is known as __________.
    a. dental prophylaxis
    b. curettage
    c. root planing
    d. scaling
12. To locate calculus deposits, a(n) __________ is used.
    a. explorer
    b. curette
    c. periodontal probe
13. In charting mobility, moderate mobility is recorded as __________.
    a. 0
    b. 1
    c. 2
    d. 3
14. Which of the following instruments is used to outline the area for a gingivectomy?
    a. Periodontal knife
    b. Periodontal probe
    c. Pocket marker
15. During the first 24 hours after a gingivectomy, the patient can expect __________.
    a. bleeding from under the dressing
    b. mild-to-moderate pain
    c. severe pain
    d. a and c

Apply Your Knowledge

1. Jimmie, a 9-year-old, is brought into your dental office for a checkup. The dentist notes that Jimmie has gingivitis around the lingual surfaces of his mandibular molars. What do you think is the likely cause of this localized gingivitis?
2. Mrs. Georgette Pecqueux is a very pleasant woman in her mid-60s. Her periodontal charting shows generalized pocketing between 6 and 8 mm. In addition, the mobility for most teeth is recorded as 2. Based on her records, Mrs. Pecqueux is what case type of periodontitis?
3. The dentist has asked you to give Mr. Michael Matthews postoperative instructions after a gingivectomy. What would you include in your instructions to Mr. Matthews?
4. You are responsible for setting up new periodontal instrument cassettes. At first glance, what is the distinguishing characteristic between a scaler and a curette? Then, how will you distinguish between a universal curette and a Gracey curette?

CHAPTER 25

Endodontics

http://evolve.elsevier.com/Robinson/essentials/

LEARNING OBJECTIVES

1. Pronounce, define, and spell the key terms.
2. Describe the subjective and objective portions of the endodontic diagnosis.
3. Describe the role and use of radiographs in endodontics.
4. Describe how an endodontic diagnosis is presented to the patient.
5. Demonstrate the assistant's role in the application of an electric pulp vitality test.
6. Identify the specialized instruments used in endodontic treatment, including the use of the operating microscope.
7. List the procedures of pulp therapy.
8. Describe the assistant's role in preparing and assisting in the placement of medications or materials in endodontics.
9. Discuss the dental assistant's role in an endodontic procedure.
10. Discuss surgical endodontic techniques.

KEY TERMS

apicoectomy	hemisection	pulpectomy
control tooth	indirect pulp cap	pulpotomy
debridement	irreversible pulpitis	retrograde restoration
direct pulp cap	necrotic	reversible pulpitis
endodontist	nonvital	root amputation
gutta-percha	obturation	sealer

Endodontics is the specialty in dentistry involved in the prevention, diagnosis, and treatment of diseases of the dental pulp. Endodontic treatment, which is often referred to as *root canal therapy,* provides an effective means of saving a tooth that might otherwise require extraction.

The general dentist is trained to care for simple endodontic cases; however, most dentists will refer a patient in need of pulp therapy to an **endodontist**, who specializes in this area of dentistry. Endodontic treatment does not include the placement of a final restoration after root canal therapy. Once endodontic treatment has been completed, the patient returns to his or her general dentist for the placement of a permanent fixed restoration.

Endodontic Diagnosis

The endodontic diagnosis is made through an examination that has both subjective and objective components.

The **subjective** portion of the **examination** includes the evaluation of symptoms or problems described by the patient. These include the patient's description of the *location*, *intensity*, and *duration* of the pain. Specific questions to ask a patient include:

- Is there pain when you bite down or chew?
- Do you experience any sensitivity to hot or cold?
- Have you noticed any swelling?

The **objective examination** includes the patient's medical and dental histories, radiographs, clinical examination, and pulp vitality tests. Table 25-1 describes the types of tests completed to determine a tooth's vitality.

The **medical history** may provide information about conditions that could contribute to the pain the patient is experiencing. An example is a patient with severe allergies may be experiencing unexplained dental pain in the maxillary anterior region.

The **dental history** may provide information concerning injury to a tooth or recent dental treatment that might help explain the pain the patient is experiencing.

A **control tooth** is used during each type of pulp testing procedure, providing the dentist with a comparison of a healthy

TABLE 25-1
Diagnostic Testing of Vital Teeth

Diagnostic Test	Description
Percussion test	Tapping on the incisal or occlusal surface with a mouth mirror handle provides the dentist with the ability to determine whether the inflammation process has extended into the periapical tissue.
Palpation test	Firm pressure is applied to the mucosa above the apex of the root. This pressure helps the dentist determine whether the inflammation process has extended into the periapical tissue.
Cold test	Ice, dry ice, or ethyl chloride is used to determine the pulp response to a cold temperature.
Heat test	A small piece of heated gutta-percha or the end of an instrument is heated and placed on the occlusal or incisal surface of the tooth to determine the pulp response.
Electric pulp test	A small electrical stimulus is delivered to the pulp. A small quantity of toothpaste is used to establish an adequate contact to conduct the current from the pulp tester to the tooth.

tooth with an infected tooth in terms of level of sensitivity. A healthy tooth (of the same type) in the opposite quadrant is selected as a control tooth. For example, if the maxillary right first premolar (tooth #5) is the suspected tooth, then the control tooth will then be the maxillary left first premolar (tooth #12).

See Procedure 25-1: Assisting in Electric Pulp Vitality Testing.

Use of Radiographic Imaging in Endodontics

Radiographic images are a necessity in endodontics. The endodontist will request a **periapical image** to expose the full length of the tooth and the periapical tissue immediately surrounding the tooth in question.

A minimum of four images are exposed throughout an endodontic procedure. The following list describes when a radiograph is required and at what stage of treatment:

1. **Initial radiographic image:** A periapical image of the tooth in question is exposed and completed at the diagnostic stage (Figure 25-1).
2. **Working length radiograph:** A periapical image is exposed to determine the length of the canal. Detecting the canal length is easier with the file remaining in the tooth.

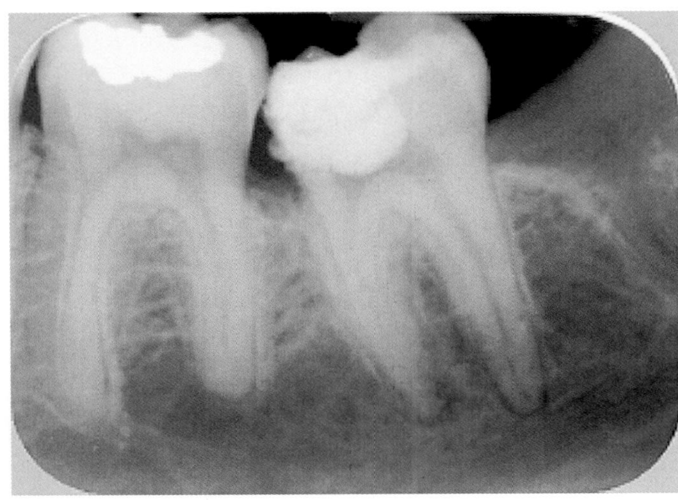

FIGURE 25-1 Initial radiograph showing the second molar in question. (From Johnson W: *Color atlas of endodontics,* Philadelphia, 2002, Saunders.)

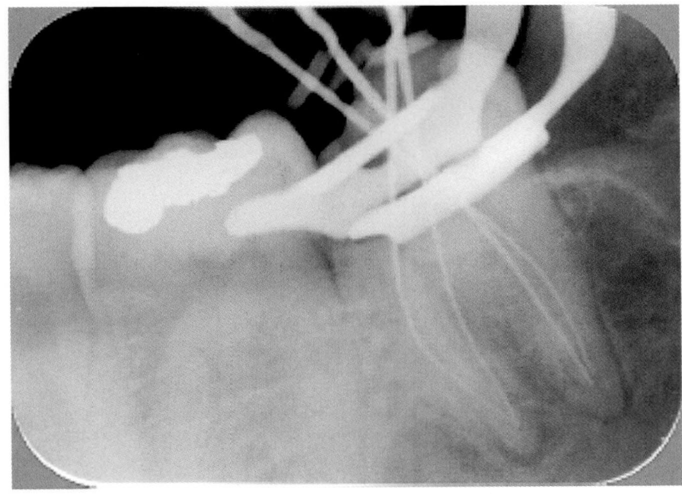

FIGURE 25-2 Final instrumentation radiograph. (From Johnson W: *Color atlas of endodontics,* Philadelphia, 2002, Saunders.)

3. **Final instrumentation radiograph:** A periapical image of the tooth is taken with the final size of the file in all canals involved (Figure 25-2).
4. **Root canal completion radiograph:** A final periapical image is exposed of the completed canal that has been filled and temporized with an intermediate restorative material (Figure 25-3).

Diagnostic Conclusions

Once the subjective and objective tests have been completed, a diagnosis is presented to the patient.

Normal pulp indicates no subjective symptoms or objective signs. The tooth responded normally to sensory stimuli, and a healthy layer of dentin surrounds the pulp. **Necrosis,** also referred to as necrotic or nonvital, is determined if the tooth does not respond to sensory stimulus.

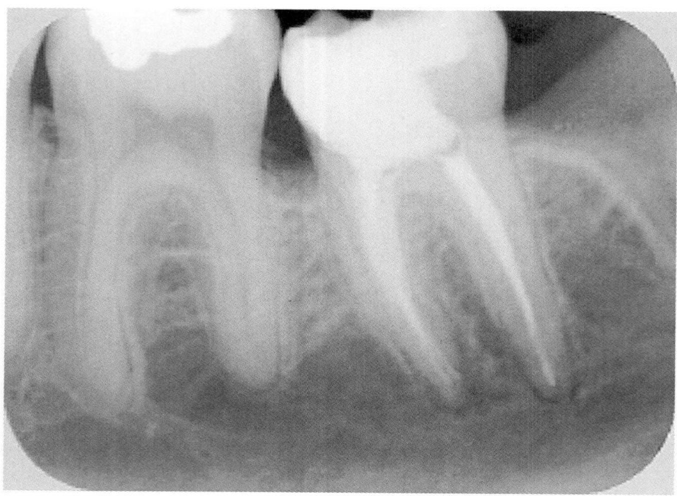

FIGURE 25-3 Completion radiograph. (From Johnson W: *Color atlas of endodontics,* Philadelphia, 2002, Saunders.)

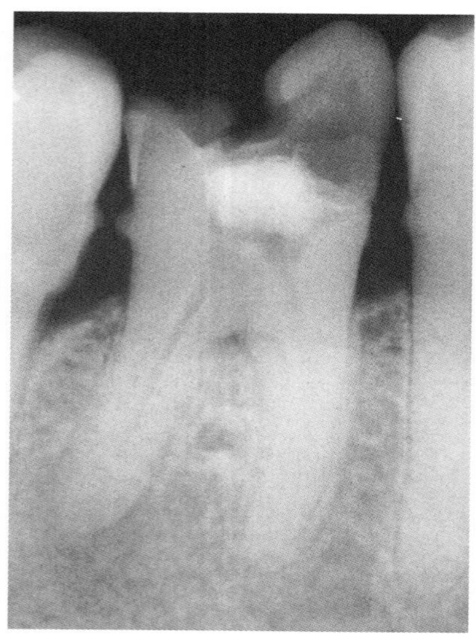

FIGURE 25-4 Radiograph showing extensive decay into the pulp. (From Johnson W*: Color atlas of endodontics,* Philadelphia, 2002, Saunders.)

Pulpitis indicates that pulpal tissues have become inflamed. Pulpitis can be clinically described as follows: **reversible pulpitis** occurs when the pulp is irritated from decay or moisture, and the patient is experiencing pain to thermal stimuli. By eliminating the irritant and placing a sedative material, the pulp may be saved. **Irreversible pulpitis** shows symptoms of lingering pain. Clinical diagnostic findings show that the pulp is incapable of healing, which would indicate the need for root canal therapy or extraction (Figure 25-4).

Periradicular abscess is an inflammatory reaction to pulpal infection (Figure 25-5). The lesion can be chronic, which would be asymptomatic with little or no discomfort, or acute, which would be associated with pain, tenderness, pus formation, and swelling.

Periodontal abscess is an inflammatory reaction caused by bacteria entrapped in the periodontal sulcus. Most often, a

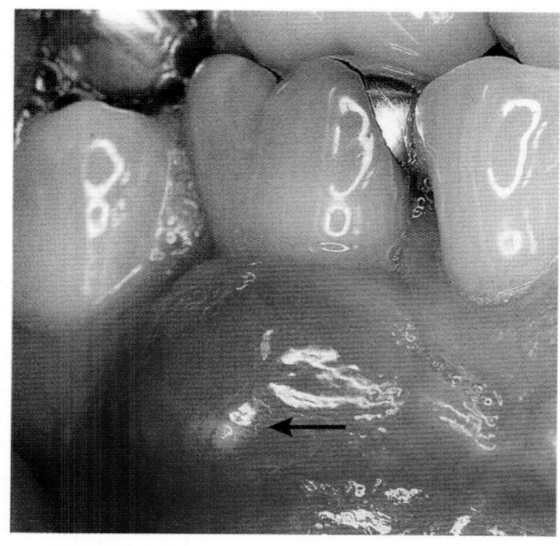

FIGURE 25-5 Abscess *(arrow)* associated with mandibular first molar, resulting from extensive decay into the pulp. (From Darby ML, Walsh MM: *Dental hygiene: theory and practice,* ed 4, St. Louis, 2015, Saunders.)

patient will experience rapid onset, pain, tenderness to pressure, pus formation, and swelling.

A periradicular cyst develops at or near the root of a necrotic tooth. This type of cyst occurs as an inflammatory response to pulpal infection and necrosis of the pulp.

Instruments in Endodontics

Endodontic instruments and accessories are designed to be flexible and to fit into the pulpal canal. To provide uniformity between manufacturers, the American Dental Association (ADA) has standardized the numbering and color-coded system used for files.

Files are supplied in different diameters, ranging from size 08 (the smallest) to size 140 (the largest). Files are available in various diameters and designs, based on their specific function. See Table 25-2 for images and descriptions of the hand and rotary instruments most commonly used in the practice of endodontics.

Microscopic Endodontics

The development of the operating microscope in the field of endodontics has essentially changed the practice of endodontics, resulting in a more efficient, effective, and patient-friendly endodontic procedure. Operating microscopes are beneficial from diagnosis to the location of canals or missed canals, for cleaning and shaping the canal, and for filling the canal. Endodontic procedures can be completed in less time because of the greater visibility of the root canal anatomy, with the final product reducing procedural errors (Figure 25-6).

The operating microscope accomplishes three objectives:

1. Magnification—Acts similar to binoculars, allowing the endodontist to view the pulpal canal in a magnification mode.
2. Illumination—The light from a 100-watt halogen bulb illuminates the canal; the light intensity is controlled by a rheostat and cooled by a fan.

TABLE 25-2
Instruments and Armamentarium Used for Endodontic Procedures

Name	Description
Endodontic explorer	The endodontic explorer is a double-ended instrument with the working ends at an angle. The working end is long enough to enter and locate canal openings.
Endodontic spoon excavator 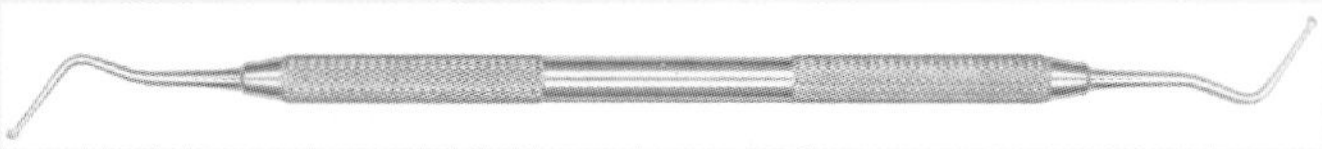	The endodontic spoon excavator is a double-ended instrument similar to other spoon excavators except that the shank is long, allowing the instrument to reach into the tooth and canal.
Endodontic K-type file 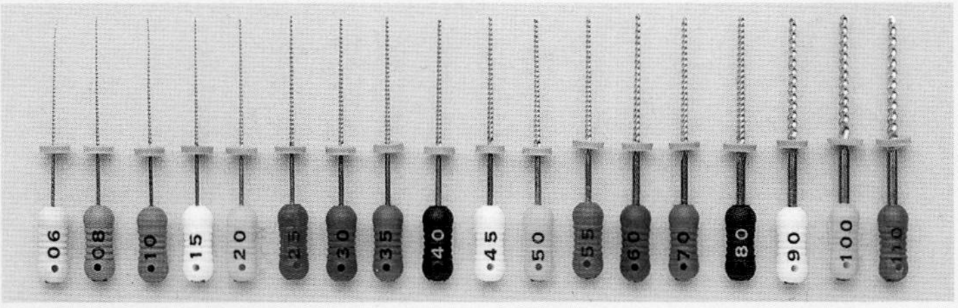 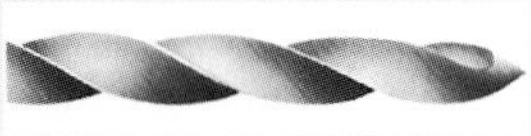	The endodontic K-type file has a twisted design and is used in the initial debridement (cleaning) of the canal and during the later stages of shaping and contouring the canal.
Hedström file 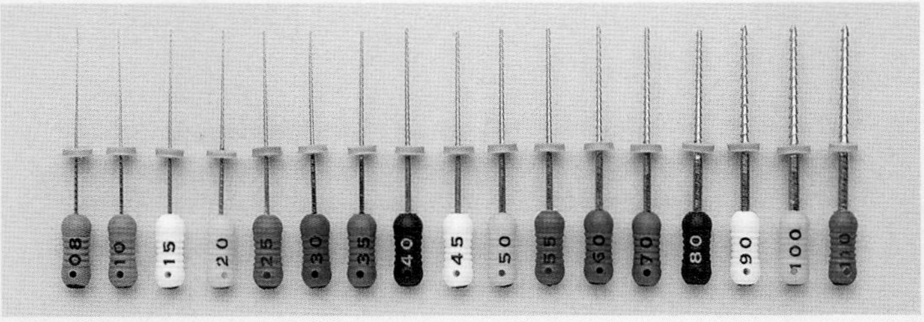 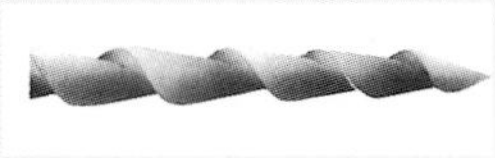	The Hedström file provides cutting efficiency because of the design and is used for final enlargement of the canal.
Reamer file 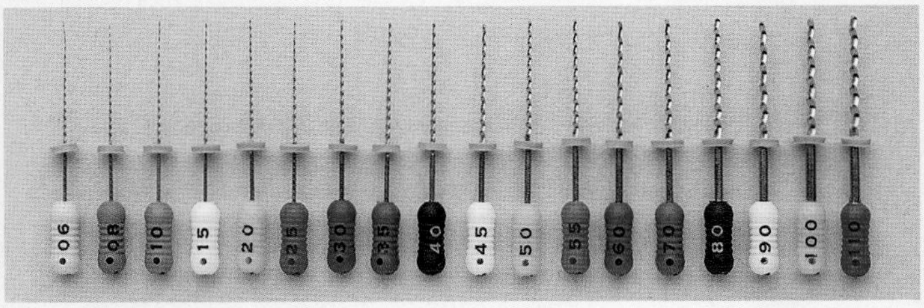 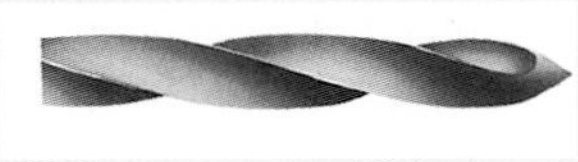	The reamer file is similar in design to the K-type file but with cutting edges farther apart. Its functions are to remove dentin structure and to smooth and increase the size of the canal.

Continued

TABLE 25-2
Instruments and Armamentarium Used for Endodontic Procedures—cont'd

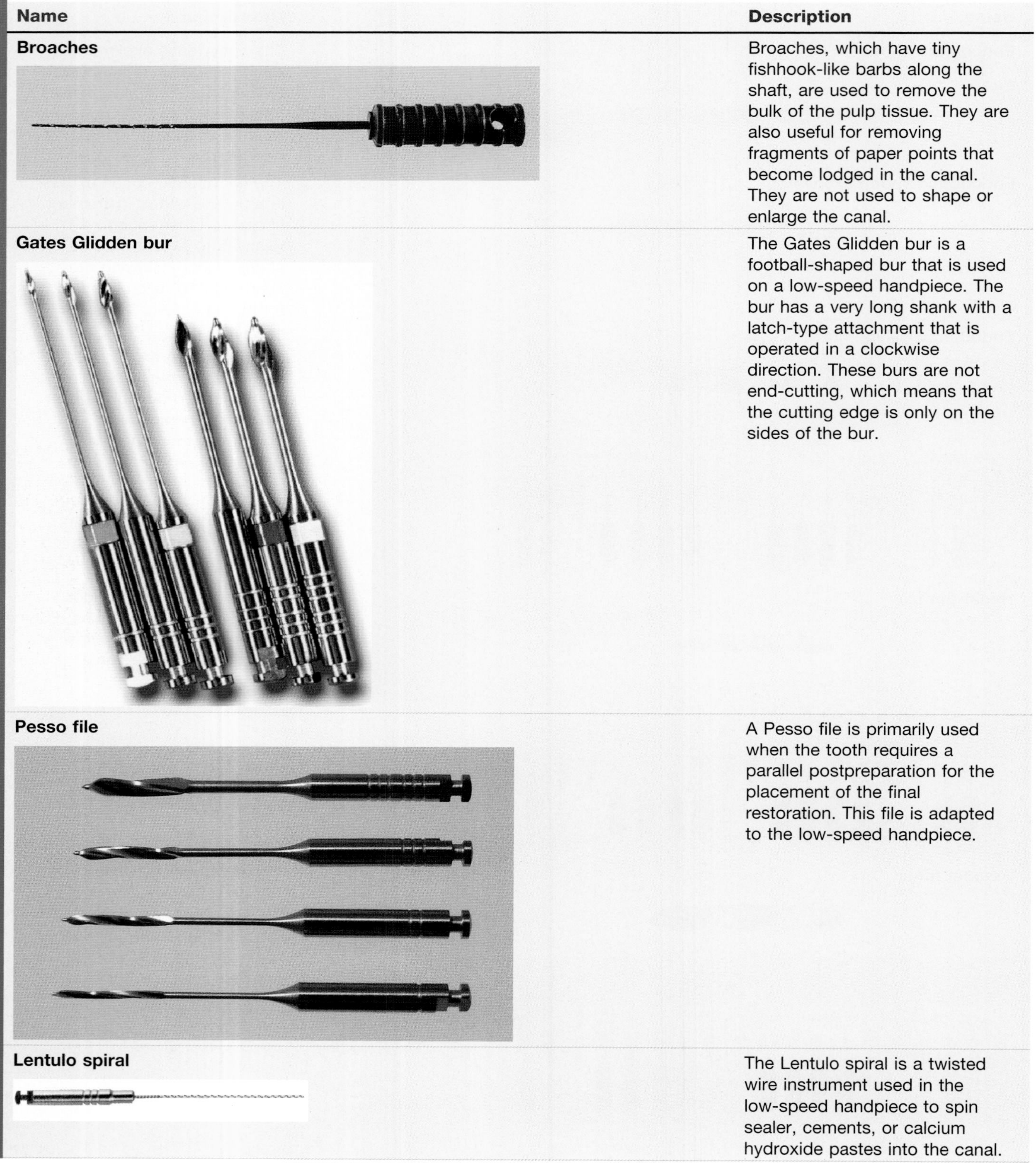

Name	Description
Broaches	Broaches, which have tiny fishhook-like barbs along the shaft, are used to remove the bulk of the pulp tissue. They are also useful for removing fragments of paper points that become lodged in the canal. They are not used to shape or enlarge the canal.
Gates Glidden bur	The Gates Glidden bur is a football-shaped bur that is used on a low-speed handpiece. The bur has a very long shank with a latch-type attachment that is operated in a clockwise direction. These burs are not end-cutting, which means that the cutting edge is only on the sides of the bur.
Pesso file	A Pesso file is primarily used when the tooth requires a parallel postpreparation for the placement of the final restoration. This file is adapted to the low-speed handpiece.
Lentulo spiral	The Lentulo spiral is a twisted wire instrument used in the low-speed handpiece to spin sealer, cements, or calcium hydroxide pastes into the canal.

TABLE 25-2
Instruments and Armamentarium Used for Endodontic Procedures—cont'd

Name	Description
Double-ended Glick no. 1 instrument 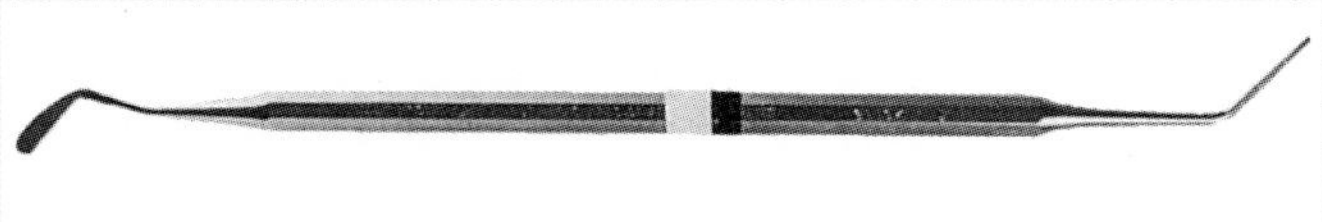	The paddle-shaped end of the double-ended Glick no. 1 instrument is designed for the placement of temporary restorations, and the rod-shaped plugger at the opposite end is ideal for the removal of excess gutta-percha. The plugger end is graduated at 5-mm increments and can be heated for the placement or removal of gutta-percha.
Endodontic spreader 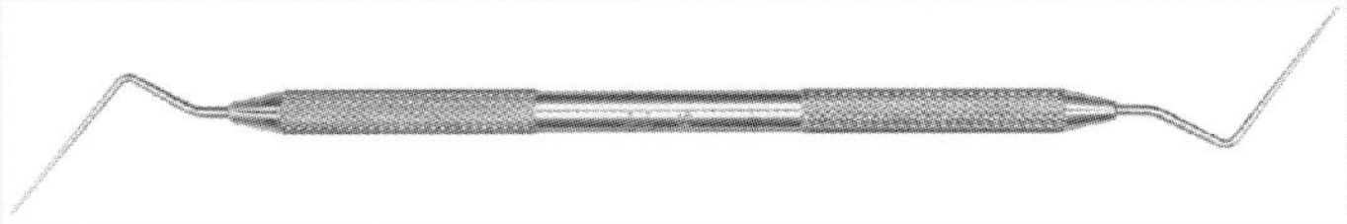	The endodontic spreader is a long, pointed working tip instrument. The dentist uses this instrument to obturate (fill) the canal by spreading the gutta-percha points in a lateral direction.
Endodontic plugger 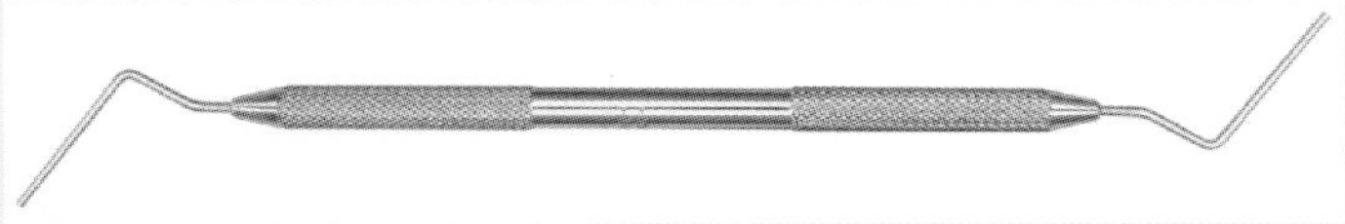	The endodontic plugger is a long, flat-ended working tip instrument. The dentist uses this instrument to condense and adapt the gutta-percha points to the canal in a lateral direction.
Millimeter ruler 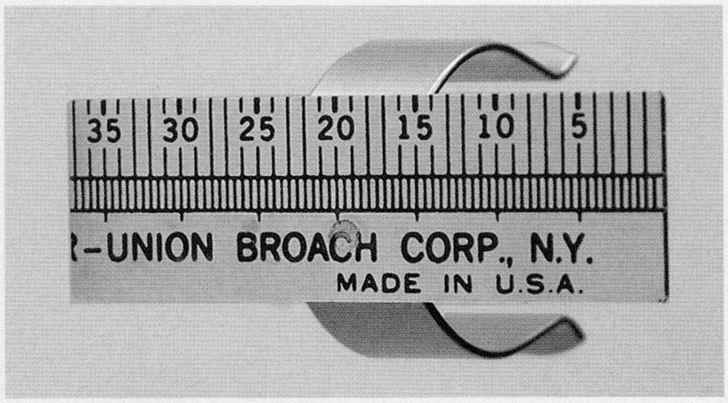	A millimeter ruler is a small ruler that accurately measures files and instruments used in the pulpal canal.
Rubber stop(s) 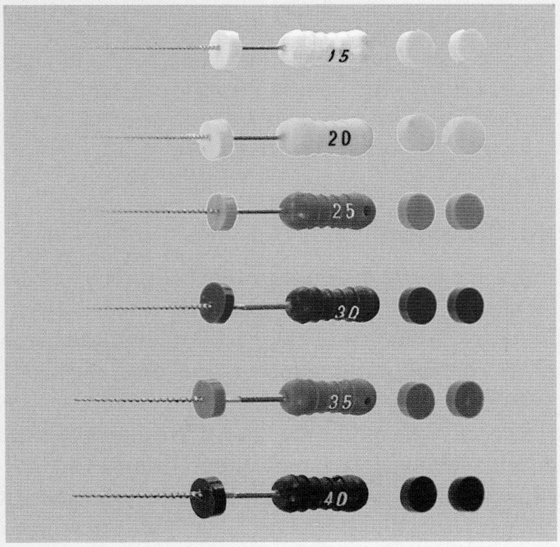	Rubber stops are small, round pieces of rubber or plastic that prevent the files from perforating the apex of the tooth during instrumentation. The dentist uses a precise radiograph and a millimeter ruler to measure the length of the canal. The rubber stop is precisely placed at the predetermined working length of the canal on the file.

Continued

TABLE 25-2
Instruments and Armamentarium Used for Endodontic Procedures—cont'd

Name	Description
Paper points	Paper points are made of absorbent paper rolled into long, narrow points. A paper point is held with locking pliers and inserted into the canal to absorb the irrigating solution and to dry the canal.

Figures of the endodontic explorer, endodontic spoon excavator, endodontic spreader, and endodontic plugger courtesy Hu-Friedy Manufacturing Company, Chicago, Illinois. Figures of the K-type file, Hedström file, and reamer file courtesy Premier Dental, Plymouth Meeting, Pennsylvania. Figures of the broach, Pesso file, double-ended Glick no. 1 instrument, millimeter ruler, rubber stops, and paper points from Boyd LRB: *Dental instruments: a pocket guide,* ed 5, St. Louis, 2015, Saunders. Figure of the Gates Glidden bur from Johnson W: *Color atlas of endodontics,* Philadelphia, 2002, Saunders. Figure of the Lentulo spiral instrument from Walton RE, Torabinejad M: *Principles and practice of endodontics,* Philadelphia, 1989, Saunders.

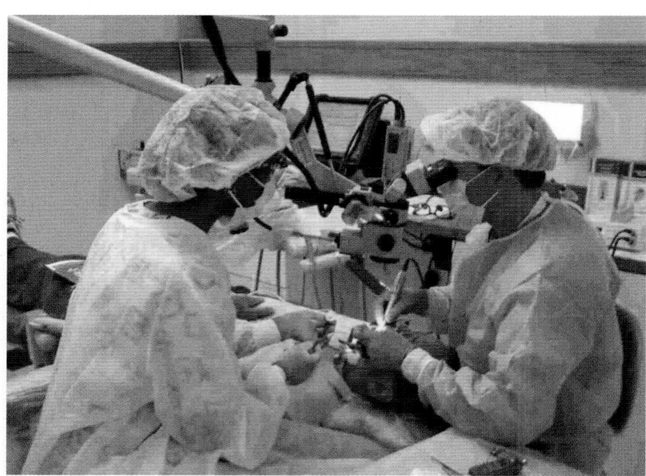

FIGURE 25-6 Operating endodontic microscopic. (From Hargreaves KM, Berman LH, Rotstein I: *Cohen's Pathways of the Pulp,* ed 11, St Louis, 2016, Elsevier.)

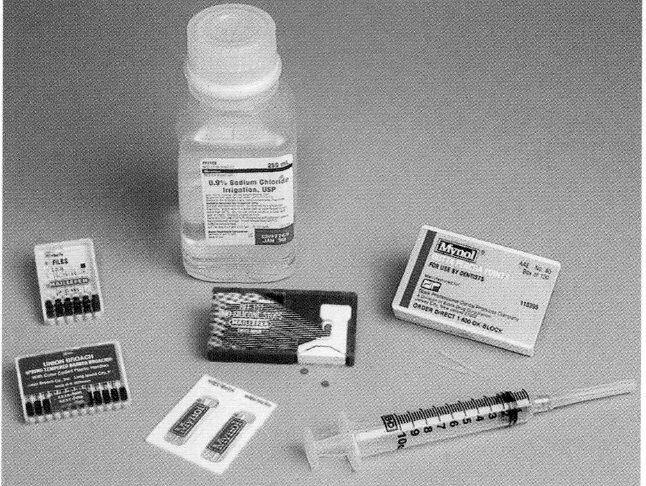

FIGURE 25-7 Materials needed for the preparation and obturation of the pulpal canal. *Top,* Sterile irrigating solution. *Bottom,* Sterile paper points and syringe used with irrigating solution. *Left and center,* Files. *Right,* Gutta-percha points.

3. Addition of accessories—A liquid crystal display (LCD) monitor and video camera provide visualization and documentation.

Medication and Filling Materials in Endodontics

In treating an endodontically affected tooth, the dental assistant will be asked to prepare and assist in the placement of medications or materials for the pulpal canal (Figure 25-7).

Irrigation Solution

In endodontics, irrigating the pulpal canal helps remove bacteria, tooth structure, and materials from the canal, as well as provides tissue dissolution, bleaching, deodorizing, and hemorrhage control. The following solutions are used during this process:

- *Sodium hypochlorite,* commonly known as *household bleach,* is diluted with equal parts of sterile water for use as an irrigation solution. A 5- to 6-ml disposable plastic syringe with a special 27-gauge needle is used for irrigation. This solution

has a solvent action on necrotic pulp tissue and organic debris and provides an antimicrobial agent. Sodium hypochlorite must be used with caution because a bleach solution causes skin irritation, and drips or splashes can ruin the patient's clothing.
- *Hydrogen peroxide* is a clear, colorless liquid with disinfectant and bleaching properties for endodontics.
- *Parachlorophenol (PCP)* is a colorless, crystalline toxic phenol compound that is used as an antimicrobial agent for disinfecting the pulp canal.

Root Canal–Filling Materials

Gutta-percha points are a natural rubber material made from the Palaquium gutta tree. They are used to **obturate** the pulpal canal after treatment has been completed. Gutta-percha is an organic substance that is solid at room temperature and becomes soft and pliable when heated. This radiopaque material is supplied in various sizes and is followed by a sealer (Figure 25-8).

Root Canal Sealers

A root canal sealer is a cement type of material that seals out unfilled voids during the obturation process. Several cements, including calcium hydroxide, zinc oxide–eugenol, and glass ionomer, can be used as a sealer for root canal therapy. These materials are designed to have very little shrinkage and are easy to place, radiopaque for detection in a radiograph, nonstaining to the teeth, bacteriostatic, gentle on the periapical tissue that surrounds them, and able to resist moisture.

Formocresol is a mixture of formaldehyde and cresol in a water-glycerin base. This type of solution is used as a sealer for pulpotomy of deciduous teeth and as an intracanal medicament for permanent teeth during root canal therapy.

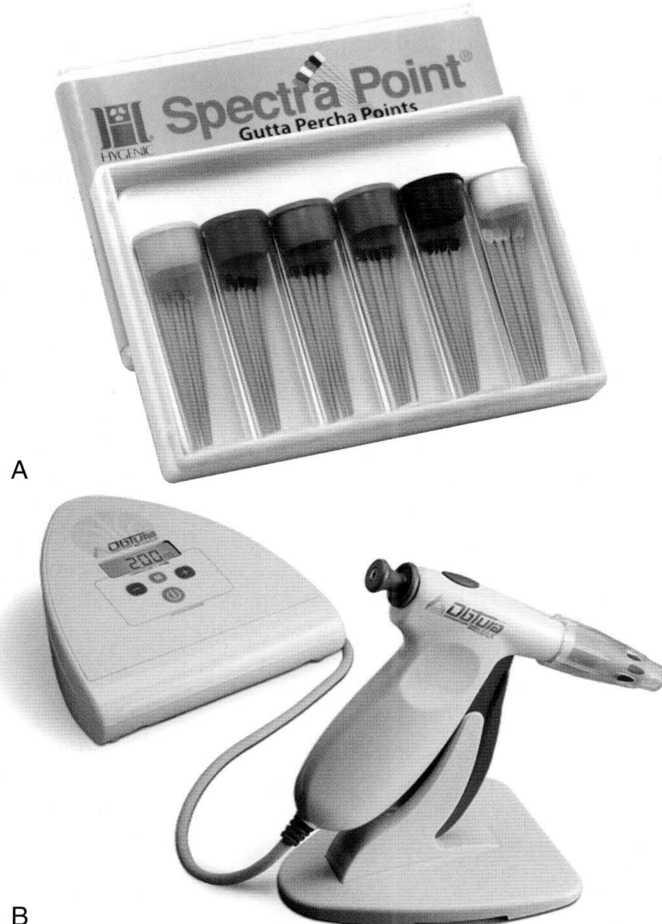

FIGURE 25-8 **A,** Gutta-percha is the most widely-used obturation material. It has benefits of being biocompatible, radiopague and easy to manipulate. Various obturation techniques with gutta-percha are currently practiced including warm vertical compaction and lateral compaction. Since many root canal systems are quite complex, use of a cold filling system minimalize the risk of voids due to shrinkage. **B,** The Obtura Max is a heated gutta-percha delivery system used to deliver warm gutta-percha to the root canal system for obturation. (**A,** Courtesy Coltene/Whaledent, Cuyahoga Falls, Ohio. **B,** Courtesy Obtura Spartan Endodontics, Algonquin, Illinois.)

Pulp Therapy

The choice of endodontic treatment depends on the diagnosis. The first line of treatment in pulpal therapy is an attempt to stimulate pulpal regeneration and save the pulp. When pulpal therapy is not effective, the endodontist will move to a more extreme measure, including root canal therapy or surgery.

Pulp Capping

In an attempt to save the pulp, a covering of calcium hydroxide is placed over an exposed or nearly exposed pulp to encourage the formation of secondary dentin at the site of injury.

An indirect pulp cap is indicated when a thin partition of dentin is still intact. The pulp has not yet been exposed, but the pulp may become exposed when decay that is near the pulp is removed. The goals are (1) to promote pulpal healing by removing most of the decay, and (2) to stimulate the production of reparative dentin through the placement of calcium hydroxide.

A direct pulp cap is indicated when the pulp has been slightly exposed. With a direct pulp cap, the tooth is still vital; however, it may become infected, requiring additional treatment, or it may become necrotic and require root canal therapy. When a direct pulp cap is performed, it is necessary to inform the patient that problems may develop later and that periodic monitoring is essential.

Pulpotomy

A pulpotomy involves the removal of the coronal portion of an exposed vital pulp. This procedure is completed to preserve the vitality of the remaining portion of the pulp within the root of the tooth. Pulpotomy is often indicated for vital primary teeth, teeth with deep carious lesions, and emergency situations.

Pulpectomy

A pulpectomy, also referred to as *root canal therapy,* involves the complete removal of the dental pulp.

Overview of Root Canal Therapy

Root canal therapy consist of five steps of treatment: (1) anesthesia and pain control, (2) isolation and disinfection of the operating field, (3) access preparation, (4) debridement and shaping of the canal, and (5) obturation.

Anesthesia and Pain Control

The anesthetic techniques of choice for endodontic treatment are infiltration (supraperiosteal injection) for maxillary teeth and nerve blocks for mandibular teeth (see Chapter 14). A local anesthetic agent is administered any time vitality (life) remains in the tooth to be treated. If the tooth is nonvital, then the endodontist may advise the patient that a local anesthetic agent is not necessary.

After the pulp has been removed, a local anesthetic agent may or may not be administered during subsequent visits, depending on the patient's preference. Inflamed and infected tissues are difficult to anesthetize. Because endodontic procedures generally involve inflamed pulp or periapical tissues or both, obtaining an adequate level of anesthesia can be a problem. Injecting an additional local anesthetic solution directly into the pulp may be necessary. In addition, sedatives (oral or inhalation) may be used for patients who are apprehensive about the procedure.

Isolation and Disinfection of the Operating Field

The standard of care established by the ADA for endodontic treatment requires the use of a dental dam. Once the dam is placed, disinfecting the tooth, the dental dam clamp, and the surrounding dental dam material with an iodine solution or a sodium hypochlorite solution is necessary.

Access Preparation

During access preparation, the dentist uses a high-speed handpiece and a round bur to create an opening in the coronal portion of the tooth for the instrumentation to reach the root canals. Access is gained through the occlusal surfaces of the posterior teeth and the lingual surfaces of the anterior teeth.

Estimated Working Length

The dentist must know the length of the completed canal preparation and root canal filling. Problems that result from inaccurate measurement of length include (1) perforation of the apex, (2) overinstrumentation or underinstrumentation of the canal length, (3) overfilling or underfilling of the canal, and (4) postoperative pain.

Because exact apex locations vary and are not always visible on radiographs, the working length is estimated and is termed the *estimated working length.* The estimated working length is determined by selecting a reference point on the tooth, usually the highest point on the incisal or occlusal surface. On a periapical radiograph, a millimeter endodontic ruler is used to measure the distance from the reference point to the apex of the tooth. From this measurement, all files are measured to the exact length, and rubber stops are used for placement. It is extremely important that the tooth length as represented on the radiograph be accurate and not distorted.

An electronic apex locator is a supplemental technique that can be used to facilitate the identification in the apex of the root canal (Figure 25-9). The use of an electronic apex locator as an aid to endodontic therapy can reduce the number of diagnostic radiographs required for determining the estimated working length.

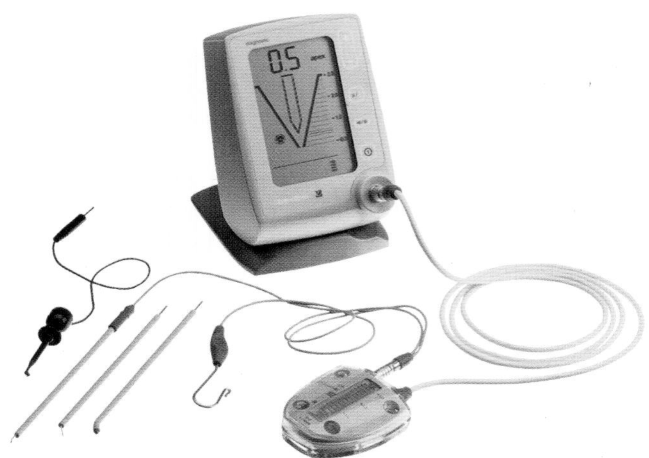

FIGURE 25-9 Electronic apex locator. (Courtesy Kerr Corporation, Orange, California.)

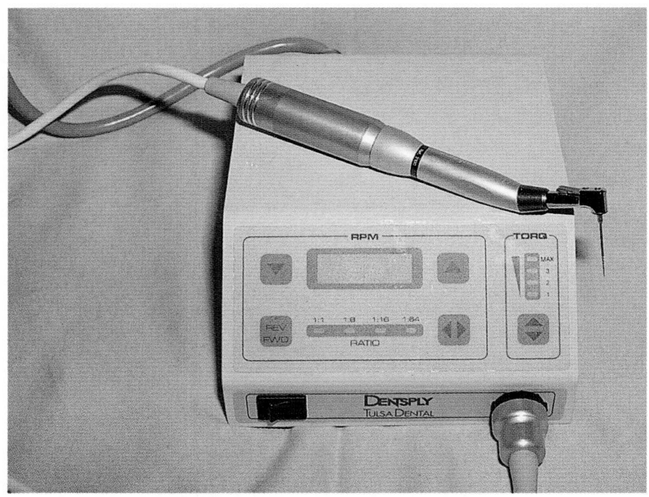

FIGURE 25-10 Rotary handpiece used for endodontics. (From Johnson W: *Color atlas of endodontics,* Philadelphia, 2002, Saunders.)

Debridement and Shaping of the Canal

The purposes of **debridement** and shaping of the canal are the use of specific shaped files to (1) remove bacteria, necrotic tissue, and organic debris from the root canal and (2) smooth and shape the canal so that the filling material can be completely adapted to the walls of the canal.

Rotary files are similar to hand files but are latch-type files placed in a high-torque, low-rpm handpiece designed for nickel-titanium (NiTi) rotary instruments (Figure 25-10). These groups of instruments are becoming more popular than traditional hand instruments because of their makeup, ease in use, and efficiency.

Obturation

After the canal has been debrided to the desired size and shape, it is dried; the canal is now ready to be obturated or filled by the endodontist using gutta-percha. If the tooth has more than one canal, then each canal is individually filled, and each canal requires a properly fitted and sealed gutta-percha point.

See Procedure 25-2: Assisting in Root Canal Therapy.

Surgical Endodontics

Root canal therapy is successful approximately 90% to 95% of the time. In exceptional situations, however, surgical endodontic techniques must be used to save a tooth from extraction.

Apicoectomy involves the surgical removal of the apical portion of the root with the use of a tapered fissure bur in a high-speed handpiece.

Retrograde restoration, also referred to as root end filling, is completed when the apical seal is not adequate.

Root amputation is a surgical procedure that is used to remove one or more roots of a multirooted tooth without removing the crown.

Hemisection is a procedure during which the root and the crown are cut lengthwise and removed.

Ethical Implications

Endodontic therapy is an area of dentistry in which the dental team is almost always working with a patient who is in pain. It is important that the patient understand the steps involved in determining the origin of the pain. Communicating to the patient about what to expect throughout the procedure is the dental team's responsibility.

For a root canal to be effectively completed, remembering that accuracy is the number-one criterion when exposing diagnostic and working radiographs and when measuring and preparing endodontic files is important.

Procedure 25-1

Assisting in Electric Pulp Vitality Testing

Equipment and Supplies

- Electric pulp tester
- Toothpaste
- Electric pulp testing kit

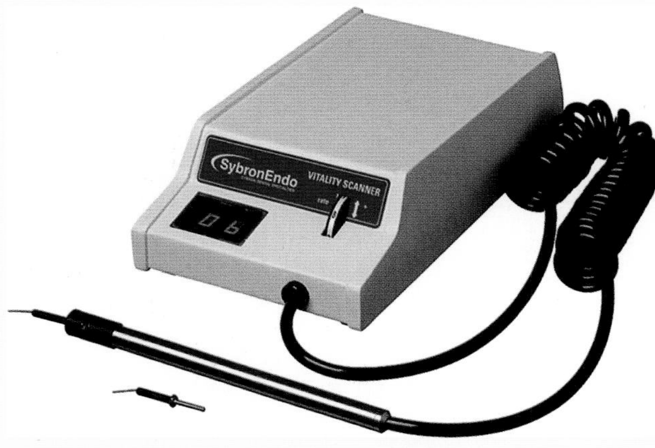

(Courtesy SybronEndo, Orange, California.)

Procedural Steps

1. Describe the procedure to the patient, and explain that the patient may feel a tingling or warm sensation.
2. Identify the teeth to be tested (the suspect tooth and the control tooth), and then isolate these teeth and thoroughly dry them.

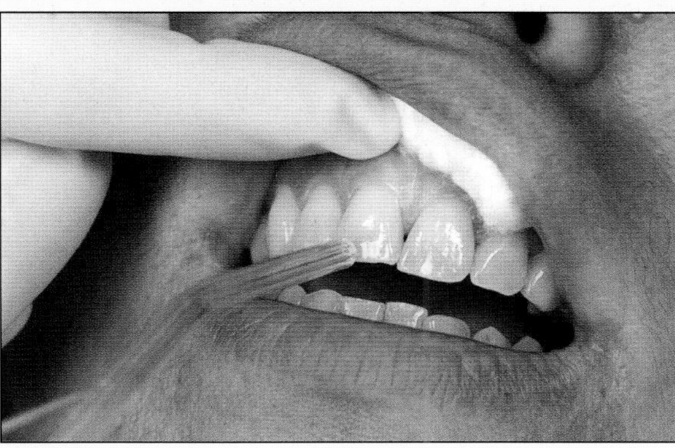

3. Set the dial (current level) at zero.
4. Place a thin layer of toothpaste on the tip of the pulp tester electrode.

Purpose: The toothpaste provides adequate contact to conduct a current from the pulp tester to the tooth.

5. Test the control tooth first.

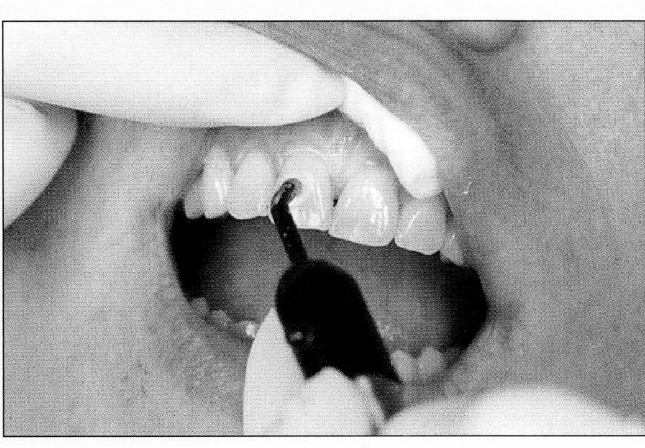

Continued

Procedure 25-1
Assisting in Electric Pulp Vitality Testing—cont'd

6. Place the tip of the electrode on the facial surface of the tooth at the cervical third.
7. Gradually increase the level of the current until the patient feels a sensation. Document the level at which the response occurred in the patient's record.
8. Repeat the procedure on the suspect tooth.

DATE	TOOTH	SURFACE	CHARTING NOTES
8/12/17	7	—	Pt complained of pain. Tooth #10 used as control tooth. Vitality test showed tooth still responding to sensation. T. Clark, CDA/L. Stewart, DDS

Procedure 25-2
Assisting in Root Canal Therapy

Equipment and Supplies

- Basic setup
- Local anesthetic agent setup (optional)
- Dental dam setup
- High-speed handpiece with burs (dentist's choice)
- Low-speed handpiece with latch attachment
- 5- to 6-ml syringe with 27-gauge needle
- Broaches and Hedström and K-type files (assorted sizes and lengths)
- Rubber instrument stops
- Paper points
- Gutta-percha points
- Endodontic sealer supplies
- Endodontic spoon excavator
- Endodontic explorer
- Double-ended Glick no. 1 instrument
- Lentulo spiral instrument
- Millimeter ruler
- Locking cotton pliers
- Sodium hypochlorite solution
- Hemostat
- High-volume evacuator (HVE) tip

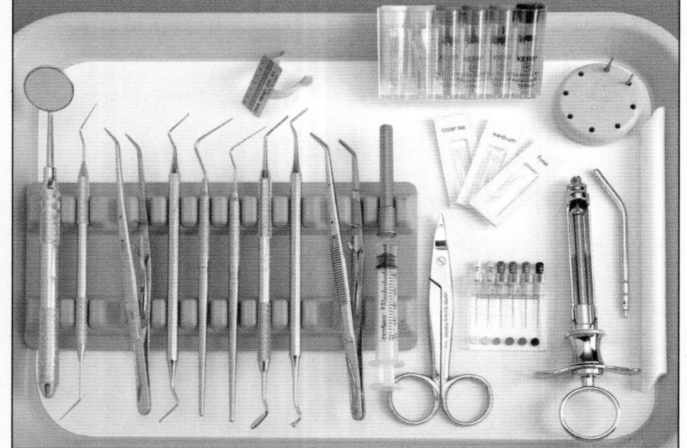

(From Boyd LRB: *Dental instruments: a pocket guide,* ed 5, St. Louis, 2015, Saunders.)

Procedural Steps

Preparing the Field of Operation

1. Assist in the administration of the local anesthetic agent (if applicable).
2. Assist with the preparation and placement of the dental dam.

Note: Expose only the tooth being treated.

3. Swab the antiseptic solution over the exposed tooth, the clamp, and the surrounding dental dam.

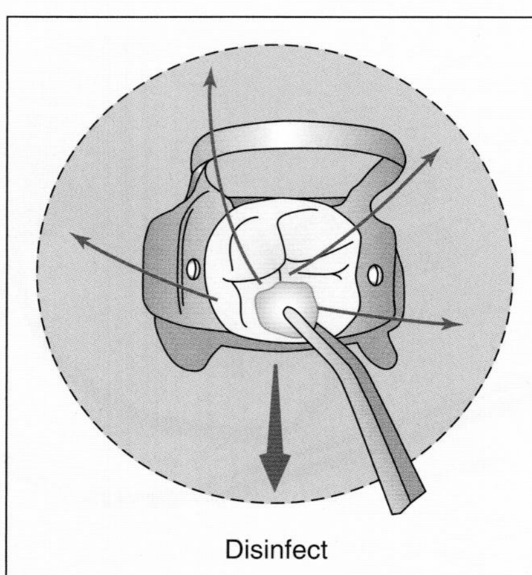

Removing the Pulp

1. The dentist enters the coronal portion of the tooth with a carbide bur and removes the decay and infected tooth structure.

Procedure 25-2

Assisting in Root Canal Therapy—cont'd

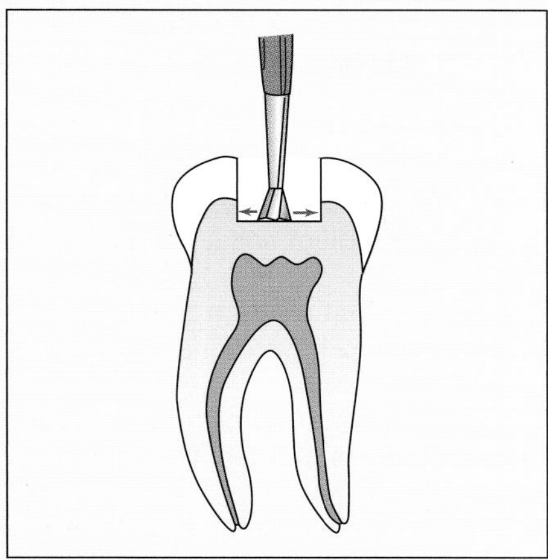

2. Once the canals are located with the endodontic explorer, the pulp tissue is removed with intracanal instruments.

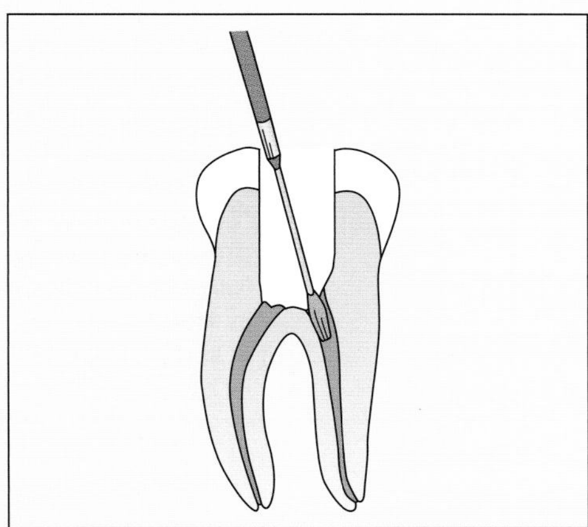

3. The canals are gently irrigated with the sodium hypochlorite solution. Excess solution is removed with the HVE tip.
4. The dentist uses a small endodontic file to rub the irrigation solution against the walls of the canal and pulp chamber.

Purpose: The solution acts as a disinfectant to destroy bacteria in the canal and to wash away debris. This step is called *biochemical cleaning.*

Cleaning and Shaping the Canal

1. The dentist inserts files into the canal and moves them up and down with short strokes.

Purpose: During this motion, the cutting edges of the files will remove dentin and debris from the walls of the canal.

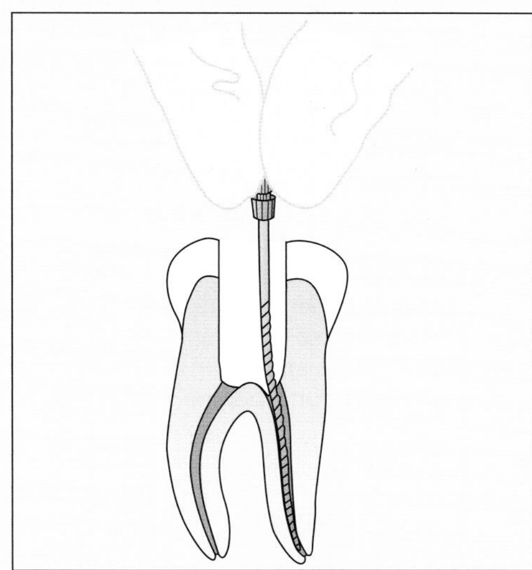

2. Transfer larger files to the dentist to clean and shape the canals.

Purpose: The increase in the size of the files is used to enlarge the diameter of the canal.

3. The rubber stop must be placed on the file at the desired working length for each canal.
4. Thoroughly irrigate the canals at frequent intervals during this shaping and cleaning process.

Purpose: Irrigation prevents the dentin shavings from clogging the cutting edges of the instruments.

5. Transfer paper points for insertion into the canals until the points come out dry.

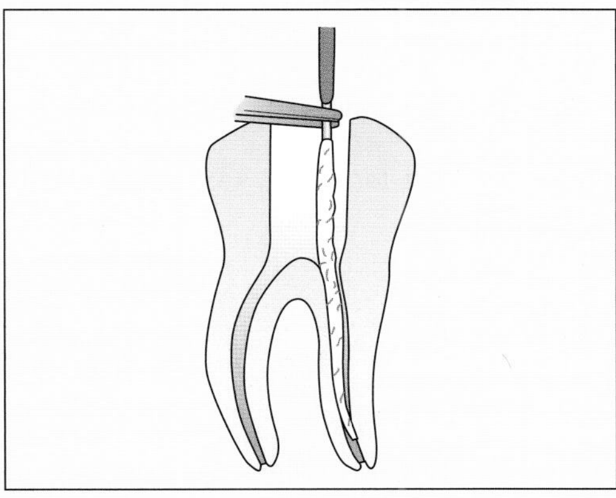

Preparing to Fill the Canal

1. Select an appropriately sized gutta-percha point, and cut it to the predetermined length. This length is called the *trial point.*
2. Take a periapical radiograph of the tooth with the trial point in the canal; this is the working length radiograph.
3. If the radiograph does not show the tip of the trial point within 1 mm of the apex of the root, then the point is repositioned and another radiograph is taken.

Continued

Procedure 25-2

Assisting in Root Canal Therapy—cont'd

4. At the signal from the dentist, prepare a thin mix of sealer on a sterile glass slab.

Purpose: The sealer is used to ensure a perfect seal at the apical foramen.

Filling the Canal

1. The master cone is removed from the canal, coated with sealer, and reinserted by the dentist.
2. The dentist inserts the finger spreader into the canal within 1 mm of the working length. The spreader is rotated counterclockwise to spread the sealer around the canal and to create space for the other cones.
3. Continue transferring gutta-percha points to fill the canal.

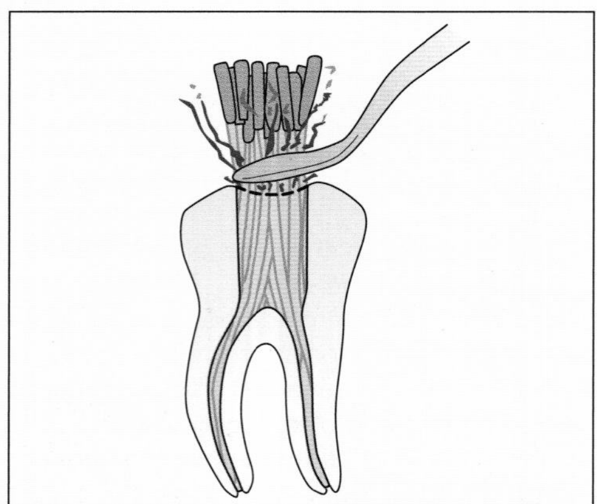

4. Transfer the Glick no. 1 instrument, heated at the working end, to remove the excess ends of the gutta-percha points.
5. Transfer the plugger for the dentist to compact vertically.
6. Continue step 2 through 5 until the canal is completely filled.
7. The dentist places a temporary restoration.

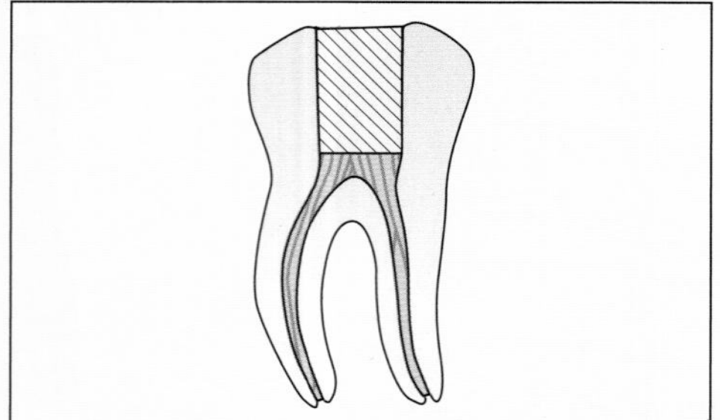

8. Expose a posttreatment radiograph.
9. The dentist checks the occlusion and adjusts as needed.

Posttreatment Instructions and Follow-up

1. Instruct the patient to call the practice immediately if indications of a problem arise, such as swelling or pain.
2. Remind the patient that a return to his or her regular dentist is necessary to have a final restoration placed.
3. Request that the patient return to the endodontist for follow-up examinations at intervals ranging from 3 to 6 months.

Purpose: Follow-up appointments enable the endodontist to ensure that the treatment is successful and that no complications have developed.

DATE	TOOTH	SURFACE	CHARTING NOTES
8/14/18	30	—	Root canal therapy, 2 carp. Xylocaine w/ epinephrine, dam isolation, tooth opened, maximum file used #70, working length 24 mm, Formocresol pellet, gutta-percha working/ posttreatment radiographs. Pt tolerated procedure well. Return for postoperative check in 1 week. T. Clark, CDA/L. Stewart, DDS

Chapter Exercises

Multiple Choice

Circle the letter next to the correct answer.

1. Before treatment, the patient seeking endodontic treatment should be informed that __________.
   a. all root canal treatments are successful and no further treatment will be required
   b. he or she will need to complete the restorative phase of the procedure with his or her general dentist
   c. patients never experience postoperative pain
   d. the chance exists that the tooth may still need to be extracted
2. Root canal therapy is not recommended when the __________.
   a. diagnosis is reversible pulpitis
   b. patient has a medical condition that precludes any dental treatment
   c. tooth has severe periodontal involvement
   d. all of the above
3. After the irrigation of a pulpal canal, the canals are dried with __________.
   a. cotton pellets
   b. paper points
   c. quick blasts of air
   d. gutta-percha
4. To place the sealer and cement into the pulpal canal, a __________ is inserted into a low-speed handpiece.
   a. flexible K-type file
   b. Gates Glidden bur
   c. Lentulo spiral
   d. Pesso file
5. After the placement of the dental dam, the tooth should be wiped with __________.
   a. an alcohol wipe
   b. an antiseptic
   c. hydrogen peroxide
   d. sodium hypochlorite
6. __________ have tiny fishhook-like barbs along the shaft and are used to remove the bulk of the pulpal tissue.
   a. Broaches
   b. Endodontic explorers
   c. Hedström files
   d. Pesso files
7. The pulpal canal is filled with what final dental material?
   a. Amalgam
   b. Calcium hydroxide
   c. Composite resin
   d. Gutta-percha
8. During endodontic treatment, the canals should be irrigated with __________.
   a. 2% glutaraldehyde
   b. alcohol
   c. iodine
   d. diluted sodium hypochlorite
9. During pulp testing, if the suspected tooth is #4, then the control tooth should be tooth #_____.
   a. 5
   b. 13
   c. 20
   d. 29
10. A __________ is a football-shaped, rotary instrument with its cutting edge on the sides rather than at the end.
    a. K-type file
    b. broach
    c. Pesso file
    d. Gates Glidden bur

Apply Your Knowledge

1. You are assisting the endodontist with root canal therapy on tooth #3. The dentist indicates that all roots are to be treated today. How many roots are in the maxillary right first molar? How would these roots appear on a radiographic image?
2. A patient calls the office in reference to experiencing severe pain in the lower right jaw. What specific questions could be asked of the patient to help identify what kind of pain the patient is having and which teeth could possibly be affected?
3. You are a clinical dental assistant in a pediatric dental office, and the child has extensive decay in a primary molar. The decay has not affected the pulp at this point. What would you suspect the diagnostic conclusion to be? What procedure will the dentist complete at this stage in the child's treatment?

CHAPTER 26

Oral and Maxillofacial Surgery

http://evolve.elsevier.com/Robinson/essentials/

LEARNING OBJECTIVES

1. Pronounce, define, and spell the key terms.
2. Define the specialty of oral and maxillofacial surgery and describe oral and maxillofacial procedures.
3. Discuss the surgical environment, and identify and describe the function of instruments used for surgical procedures.
4. Describe the importance of the chain of asepsis throughout a surgical procedure and describe the surgical assistant's role in oral surgery.
5. Describe the surgical procedures (e.g., forceps extraction, multiple extractions, alveoloplasty, removal of teeth, suture placement and removal) commonly performed in a general dental practice.
6. Describe the types of postoperative care provided after a surgical procedure.

KEY TERMS

alveolitis
alveoloplasty
asepsis
extraction
impaction
luxate
oral and maxillofacial surgery (OMFS)
sutures

Oral and maxillofacial surgery (OMFS) is the specialty of dentistry that provides the diagnosis and surgical treatment of diseases and repairs injuries and defects of hard and soft tissues of the oral and maxillofacial regions.

The general dentist is trained in basic surgical procedures, and many perform single tooth extractions in their practice. For more complicated procedures, however, dentists will refer their patient to an oral and maxillofacial surgeon.

Description of Oral and Maxillofacial Procedures

- Extraction of decayed teeth that cannot be restored
- Surgical removal of impacted teeth
- Extraction of nonvital teeth
- Preprosthesis surgery to smooth and contour the alveolar ridge
- Removal of teeth for orthodontic treatment
- Removal of root fragments
- Reconstructive surgery
- Removal of cysts and tumors
- Biopsy of a questionable area
- Treatment of fractures of the bones of the face and jaws
- Surgery to alter the size or shape of a facial bone
- Surgery of the temporomandibular joint
- Surgical implants
- Reconstructive surgery
- Surgical repair of cleft lip and cleft palate
- Salivary gland surgery

Surgical Environment

Oral surgery, even when performed in the general dental office, is just as much a surgical procedure as one performed in a hospital surgical unit. It is imperative for the dental team to have the patient's clinical record, emergency equipment, anesthetic supplies, and surgical instruments readied before seeing the patient for a surgical procedure.

Patient Record

The dentist must have a complete patient record, which includes a current medical history, radiographs showing the area to be treated, recorded vital signs, appropriate charting of treatment, and the type of pain control methods that are prescribed before, during, and after surgery.

Signed Consent

Once the procedure has been reviewed with the patient or legal guardian, it is important that the responsible party sign a release form indicating that he or she understands the procedure to be performed and any possible complications that may occur.

Oral Surgery Instruments

Oral surgery instruments have specific uses and are designed to separate the tooth from the socket, to retract surrounding tissue, to loosen and elevate the tooth within the socket, and to remove the tooth from the socket. The oral surgery instruments most commonly used in surgical procedures are discussed in this chapter. All surgical instruments are classified as critical instruments and must be sterilized after each use (Table 26-1).

Extraction Forceps

Extraction forceps are available in many different shapes and designs to accommodate the dentist's needs in grasping teeth with different crown shapes, root configurations, and locations within the mouth. The goal is to remove the tooth in one piece with the crown and root intact.

Forceps are used to remove teeth from the alveolar bone after they have been slightly loosened in the socket by the application of elevators. The handles, which are held firmly in a palm grasp, provide the dentist the necessary leverage to luxate and remove the tooth (**luxate** means to rock back and forth) (Figure 26-1).

Surgical Asepsis

Establishing and maintaining the chain of asepsis in a surgical procedure means that the instruments, surgical drapes, and gloves worn by the dental team must be sterile from setup to completion of the procedure. (**Asepsis** means the absence of pathogenic microorganisms.) Contact with anything that is not sterile will break the chain of asepsis and contaminate the surgical area.

See Procedure 26-1: Performing a Surgical Scrub, and Procedure 26-2: Performing Sterile Gloving.

Surgical Procedures

When preparing for a surgical procedure, specific criteria must be met for a smooth, efficient performance of the procedural steps. Every surgical procedure requires preparation and advance planning by the dental team.

TABLE 26-1
Oral Surgery Instruments

Name of Instrument	Description of Use
Periosteal elevator	A periosteal elevator separates and retracts the periosteum from the bone that is holding the tooth in its socket.
Straight elevator	A straight elevator is used to apply leverage against the tooth to loosen it from the periodontal ligament and to ease the extraction.
Root tip picks	Root tip picks are used to remove root tips, tooth fragments, or debris that may have broken away from the tooth during the extraction.
Surgical curette	A surgical curette resembles a large spoon excavator and is used after an extraction to clean the interior of the socket or to remove diseased tissue.
Rongeur	A rongeur is a scissors-shaped instrument with short blades used to trim alveolar bone. The rongeur instrument is commonly used after multiple extractions to remove sharp projections and to shape the edentulous ridge.
Bone file	The bone file is a flat working instrument with large cutting grooves. The bone file is used with a push-pull motion to smooth the surface of the bone after using the rongeur instrument or to smooth the rough margins of the alveolus.

Continued

TABLE 26-1
Oral Surgery Instruments—cont'd

Name of Instrument	Description of Use
Scalpel	A scalpel is a surgical knife used to make a precise incision into soft tissue. Scalpel blades are available in many sizes and styles. A one-piece disposable instrument consisting of a scalpel blade and handle is supplied in a sterile sealed package. Bard-Parker single-use blades are available to attach to a reusable metal handle. Common sizes of surgical blades are #12 and #15.
Hemostat	A hemostat has beaks with serrations or grooves and a locking mechanism on the handle, which makes it useful for grasping and holding an object or tissue.
Needle holder	The needle holder resembles the hemostat, but the beaks are straight with fine serrations to grasp a suture needle firmly.
Surgical scissors	Surgical scissors are available in fine straight or curved blades and are used to trim soft tissue.
Tissue retractors	Tissue retractors are used to grasp and hold soft tissue during surgical procedures. Extreme care must be taken when retracting tissue to prevent trauma or damage to the tissue.
Surgical chisel and mallet	A surgical chisel and mallet are used to split a tooth for easy removal by tapping the mallet on the chisel, which helps in the removal of a tooth or to reshape bone.
Surgical aspirating tip	A surgical aspirating tip is used in a surgical procedure. The smaller tip easily fits into the socket or surgical site.

All images courtesy Hu-Friedy, Chicago, Illinois.

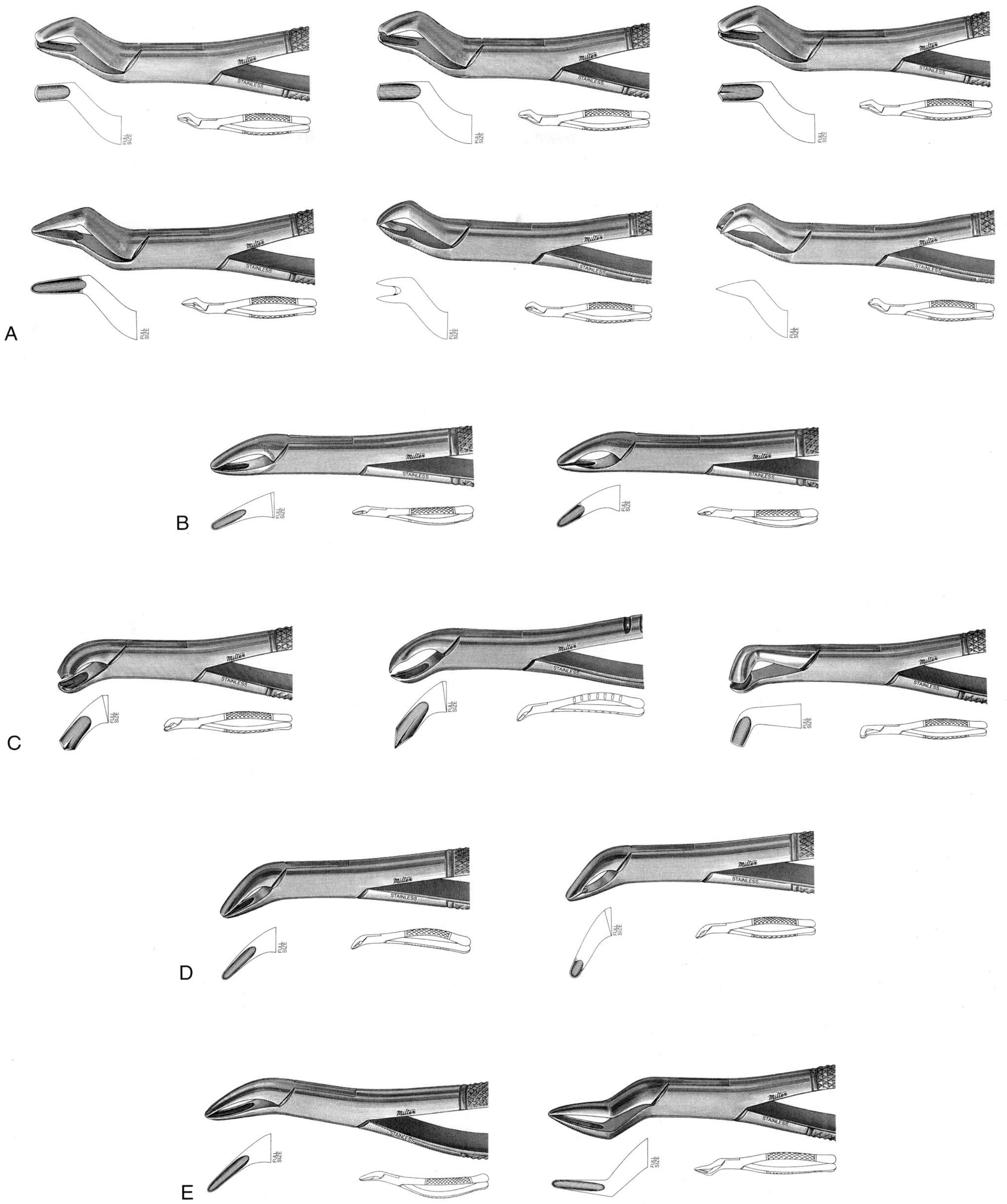

FIGURE 26-1 Types of extraction forceps. **A,** Maxillary molar extraction forceps. **B,** Maxillary anterior extraction forceps. **C,** Mandibular molar extraction forceps. **D,** Mandibular anterior extraction forceps. **E,** Root tip extraction forceps. (Courtesy Miltex, Inc., York, Pennsylvania.)

Surgical Assistant's Role in Oral Surgery

Advance Preparation

- Review the patient record, and prepare radiographic images.
- Confirm that the consent forms are signed and available for review.
- Verify that any information requested from the patient's physician has been received.
- If a prosthesis will be delivered to the patient, then determine whether the dental laboratory has returned it.
- Verify that the appropriate surgical setup has been prepared and sterilized.
- Contact the patient, and provide preoperative instructions for taking any premedication and instructions for eating or drinking after midnight.
- Instruct the patient to have someone drive him or her and to stay during the procedure.

Treatment Room Preparation

- Prepare the treatment room by placing protective barriers on anything that may be touched during the procedure.
- Keep surgical instruments in their sterile wraps until ready for use. If a surgical tray has been set out, then open it and place a sterile towel over the instruments.
- Have the appropriate pain control medications (e.g., local anesthesia, nitrous oxide–oxygen inhalation, intravenous sedation) ready for administration.
- Have the necessary postoperative instructions ready to provide to the patient.

Patient Preparation

- Update the patient's medical history and all laboratory reports.
- Check that the patient has taken his or her prescribed premedication. If not, the surgeon should be immediately alerted.
- Illuminate radiographic images.
- Take the patient's vital signs to determine a baseline, and record the signs in the patient's record.
- Prepare any additional monitoring equipment to be applied.
- Seat and drape the patient. (To protect the patient's clothing, a large drape is often used, in addition to a patient towel.)
- Adjust the chair into a comfortable reclining position. If general anesthesia is to be administered, then place the patient in a supine position.

During Surgery

- Maintain the chain of asepsis.
- Assist in the administration of local anesthetic medications.
- Monitor the administration of nitrous oxide and intravenous sedation (refer to Chapter 14 for a description of these procedures).
- Transfer and receive instruments.
- Aspirate and retract as needed.
- Maintain a clear surgical field with adequate light.
- Monitor the patient's vital signs, oximetry, and electrocardiogram (ECG; refer to Chapter 11 for a description of these procedures).
- Steady the patient's head and mandible if necessary during the use of a mallet and chisel.
- Observe the patient's condition, and anticipate the surgeon's needs.

After Surgery

- Stay with the patient until he or she has sufficiently recovered to leave the office.
- Give verbal and written postoperative instructions to the patient and to the responsible person who has accompanied the patient.
- Confirm a postoperative visit as directed by the dentist.
- Update the patient's treatment records, including a copy of any new prescription given to the patient.
- Return the patient's records to the business assistant.
- Break down and disinfect the treatment area.
- Transport all contaminated items to the sterilization center.

Types of Surgical Procedures

Forceps Extraction

Forceps extraction is often described as a *routine* or *simple* **extraction**. These terms are misleading because all extractions are considered surgical procedures. Using these terms implies that the extraction can be completed without extensive instrumentation.

A forceps extraction is performed on a tooth that is fully erupted, has a solid intact crown, and can be firmly grasped with the forceps. Most routine forceps extractions will not require the placement of **sutures**.

See Procedure 26-3: Assisting in a Forceps Extraction.

Multiple Extractions

When several teeth are to be extracted at the same time, the forceps extraction procedure is essentially the same. However, if the teeth being extracted are proximal to one another, then the alveolar socket will have bony projections where the teeth have been removed. The dentist must then complete an **alveoloplasty**. Alveoloplasty involves surgically contouring and smoothing the remaining bone to provide a properly contoured ridge for proper healing and also for a bridge, partial, or denture, if one is to be placed.

See Procedure 26-4: Assisting in Multiple Extraction and Alveoloplasty.

Removal of Impacted Teeth

The term **complex extraction** is used when conditions exist that require additional skill, effort, and instrumentation to remove a tooth. The extraction of an impacted mandibular third molar is an example of a complex extraction. (An **impacted tooth** is one that has not erupted normally. It may be partially or totally covered by tissue and/or bone.)

In the case of a tissue impaction, a scalpel would be used to expose the unerupted tooth. For a bony impaction, the dentist would first use the scalpel. Then, with the use of a surgical bur, the dentist would go through bone to gain access to the tooth for removal. As a rule, if a scalpel has been used to expose tissue, then sutures will be placed for proper healing.

See Procedure 26-5: Assisting in the Removal of an Impacted Tooth.

Suture Placement

Sutures provide several functions for the healing process of a surgical site. They (1) help control bleeding, (2) promote healing, and (3) assist in creating an even attachment of tissue. Therefore when a scalpel is added to the tray setup, suture equipment is also added.

The suture needle is circular in shape and held in a hemostat or a needle holder. Suture needles are supplied already threaded and in a sterile pack. The surgeon uses a technique that will use the least amount of suture material but will still promote the healing process.

Sutures are available in both **absorbable** and **nonabsorbable** varieties. Absorbable suture materials include plain catgut, chromic catgut, and polydioxanone. These sutures are readily absorbed by the body and do not have to be removed.

Nonabsorbable suture materials include silk, polyester fiber, and nylon. Black silk suture material is popular because it is strong, durable, and easy to manipulate. Nonabsorbable sutures, as a rule, are removed 5 to 7 days after surgery.

See Procedure 26-6: Assisting in Suture Placement, and Procedure 26-7: Performing Suture Removal (Expanded Function).

Immediate Postoperative Care

In addition to directions from the dentist, the assistant will provide postoperative instructions to the patient and to the individual accompanying the patient. Instructions for home care should be provided in both written and verbal forms.

Control of Bleeding

The patient is given the following instructions regarding the control of bleeding:

1. Avoid rinsing or spitting during the first 12 hours.
2. A pressure pack made of folded sterile gauze has been placed over the socket to control bleeding and to encourage clot formation.
3. Keep the pack in place for a minimum of 30 minutes. If the pack is removed too soon, then clot formation may be disturbed and increased bleeding may occur.
4. If bleeding increases or does not stop, then call the dental office.
5. Do not disturb the clot with your tongue or by vigorously rinsing your mouth.
6. Strenuous work or physical activity should be restricted for a few days.

Control of Swelling

The patient is given the following instructions regarding the control of swelling:

1. The dentist may recommend the use of a nonsteroidal anti-inflammatory drug (NSAID) such as ibuprofen before and after surgery. (An NSAID is helpful in preventing and controlling swelling, and it also relieves pain.)
2. During the first 24 hours, a cold pack is placed in a cycle of 20 minutes on and 20 minutes off.
3. After the first 24 hours, external heat may be applied to the area of the face to enhance circulation and to promote healing.
4. After the first 24 hours, the patient can gently rinse the oral cavity with warm saline solution (1 tsp of salt to 8 oz of warm water) every 2 hours to promote healing.

Alveolitis (Dry Socket)

After a tooth is extracted, healing immediately begins with blood filling the socket and forming a clot. An open wound such as this will heal itself from the inside first. The clot is important in this process because it protects the wound and is later replaced by granulation tissue and, ultimately, by bone.

Failure of the process can result in alveolitis, also known as *dry socket.* This very painful condition commonly occurs 2 to 4 days after the extraction of a tooth.

Treatment for alveolitis is to have the patient immediately come in, irrigate the socket with warm saline solution, and pack the socket with medicated gauze (**iodoform**), which contains a topical antiseptic medication that soothes the nerves and covers the exposed bone to allow the healing process to begin.

Ethical Implications

The specialty area of oral and maxillofacial surgery is one that requires the dental team to be prepared at all times for the care of a patient. Developing a surgical conscience is especially important for the surgical assistant. Most surgical procedures are invasive, and the assistant must always preserve the integrity of the sterile field, monitor the patient's vital signs throughout the procedure, be ready to assist, and be alert to the needs of the surgeon and the patient. Oral surgery can be a traumatic experience for a patient, and it takes the entire dental team to be empathetic, supportive, and, most of all, in control of the procedure and the patient.

Procedure 26-1

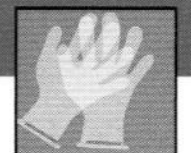

Performing a Surgical Scrub

Equipment and Supplies

- Orange stick
- Antimicrobial soap, such as chlorhexidine gluconate
- Sterile surgical scrub brush
- Sterile disposable towels

Procedural Steps

1. Remove all jewelry.
2. Cover your hair, and put on protective eyewear and mask before performing a surgical scrub.

Purpose: Once your hands are scrubbed, they should not touch anything.

3. With water running, use the orange stick to clean under your nails. Discard the stick, and rinse your hands without touching the faucet or the inside of the sink.

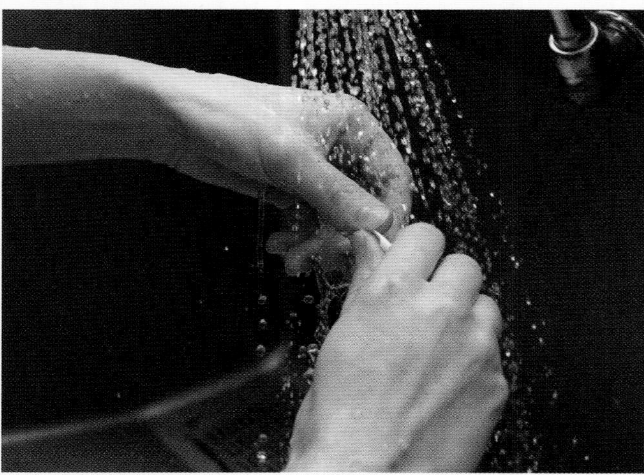

4. Wet hands and forearms up to the elbows with warm water, and then dispense approximately 5 ml of antimicrobial soap into cupped hands.

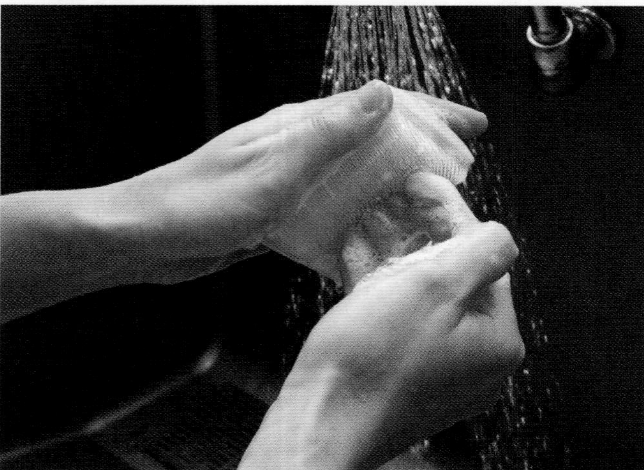

5. Use the surgical scrub brush to scrub the hands and forearms for 7 minutes.

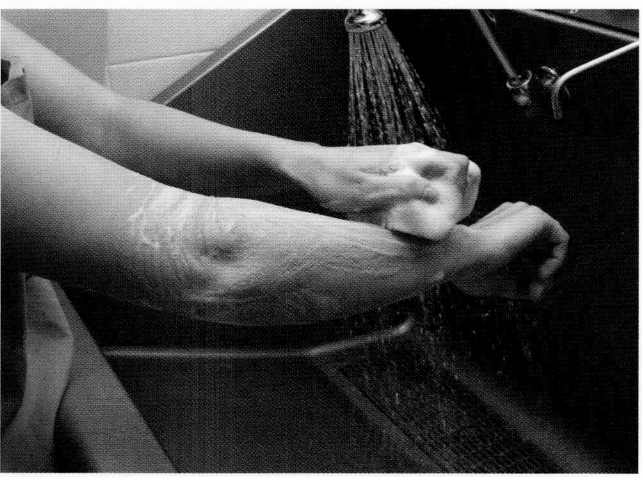

6. Thoroughly rinse the hands and forearms with warm water. Keep your hands up and above waist level.

Purpose: Keeping your hands above the waist allows the water to run toward the elbows, keeping the hands clean.

7. Dispense another 5 ml of antimicrobial soap, and repeat the scrub.
8. Wash for an additional 7 minutes without using a brush. Rinse so the contaminated water runs down the arms and off the elbows.
9. Dry hands and arms with a sterile towel. Use a patting motion, and continue up the forearms
10. Keep your hands above your waist before donning your sterile gown.

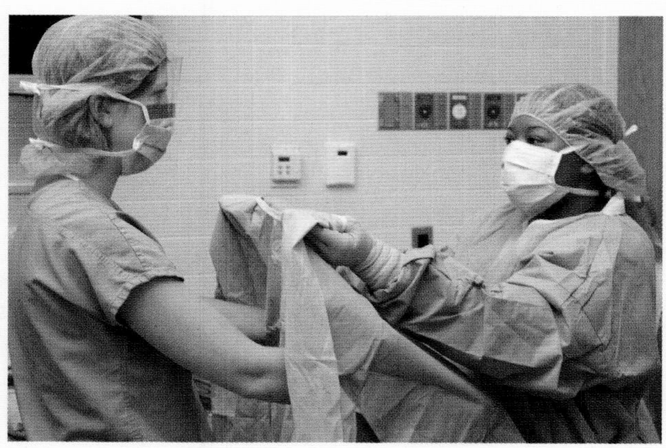

Photos from Hupp JR, Ellis E III, Tucker M: *Contemporary oral and maxillofacial surgery,* ed 6, St Louis, 2014, Mosby.

Procedure 26-2

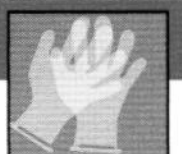

Performing Sterile Gloving

Procedural Steps

1. The glove package should already be opened before the surgical scrub. Be sure to touch only the inside of the package at this point.

Note: The open glove pack is a sterile field.

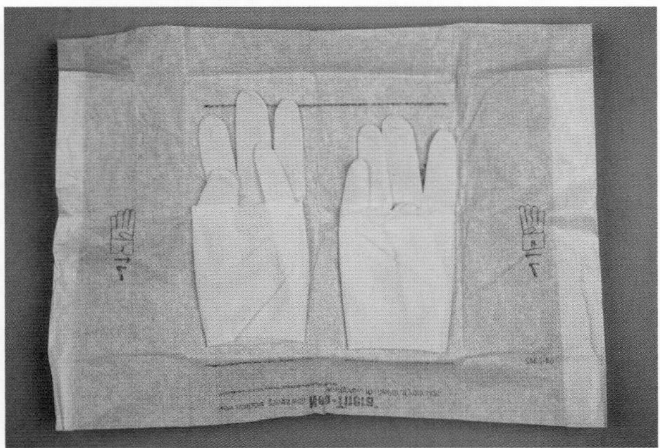

2. Glove your dominant hand first.

Purpose: Applying the second glove is more difficult, and you will have greater dexterity with your dominant hand.

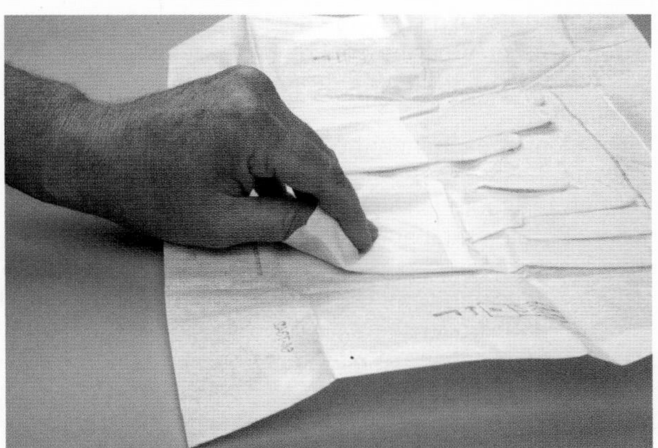

3. Pull the glove over the hand, touching only the folded cuff.

Purpose: Remember to touch only the inside of the glove.

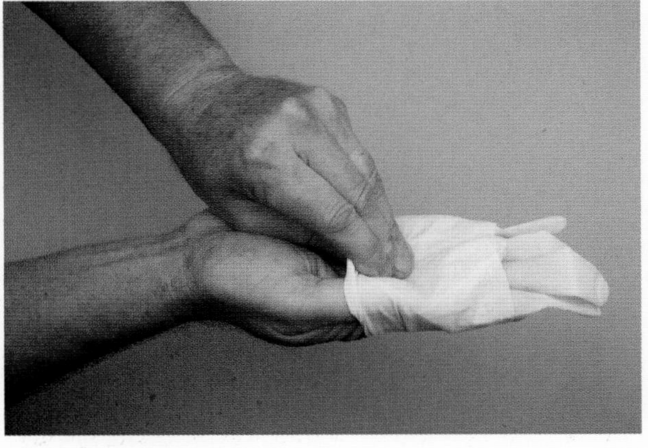

4. With your dominant hand gloved, slide your forefingers under the cuff of the other glove.

Purpose: You can touch the sterile portion of the glove only with your dominant hand.

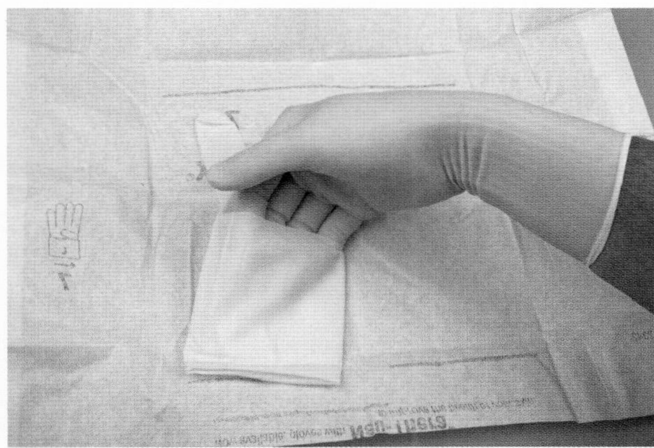

5. Pull the glove up over your other hand.

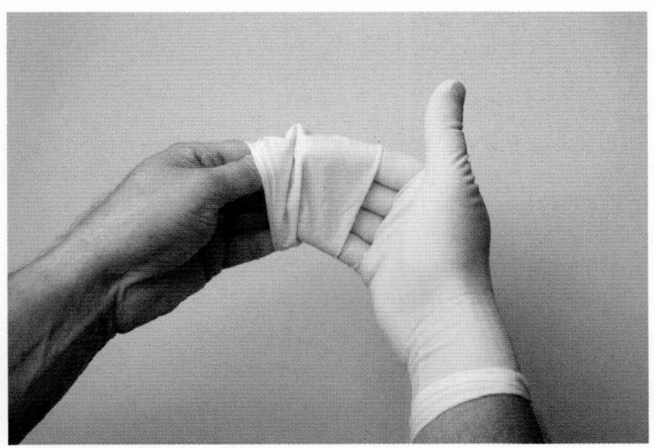

6. Unroll the cuff from your gloves.

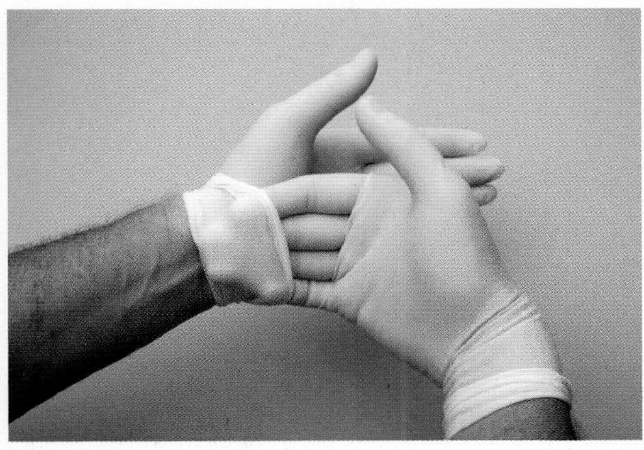

All photos from Hupp JR, Ellis E III, Tucker M: *Contemporary oral and maxillofacial surgery,* ed 6, St Louis, 2014, Mosby.

Procedure 26-3

Assisting in a Forceps Extraction

Equipment and Supplies

- Local anesthetic agent setup
- Basic setup
- Periosteal elevator
- Elevator (dentist's choice)
- Forceps (dentist's choice)
- Surgical curette
- Sterile gauze sponge
- Surgical aspirator tip

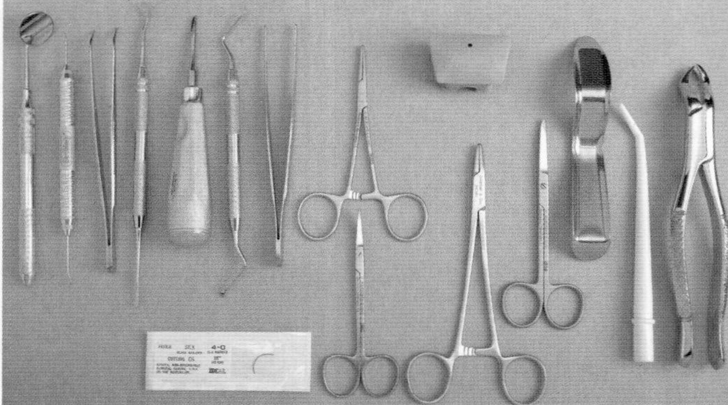

(From Boyd LRB: *Dental instruments: a pocket guide,* ed 5, St Louis, 2015, Saunders.)

Procedural Steps

1. Assist in the administration of a local anesthetic agent.
2. Transfer the explorer for the dentist to probe the area to determine the level of anesthesia.
3. Transfer the periosteal elevator for the dentist to loosen the gingival tissue gently and to compress the alveolar bone surrounding the neck of the tooth.

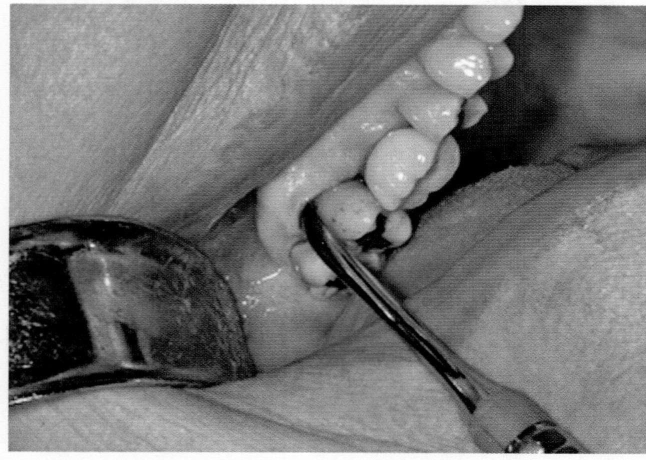

(Courtesy Dr. Edward Ellis III.)

4. Transfer an elevator (most often straight) as requested by the dentist to loosen the tooth.
5. The dentist places the beaks of the forceps on the tooth and firmly grasps the tooth around and below the cementoenamel junction.

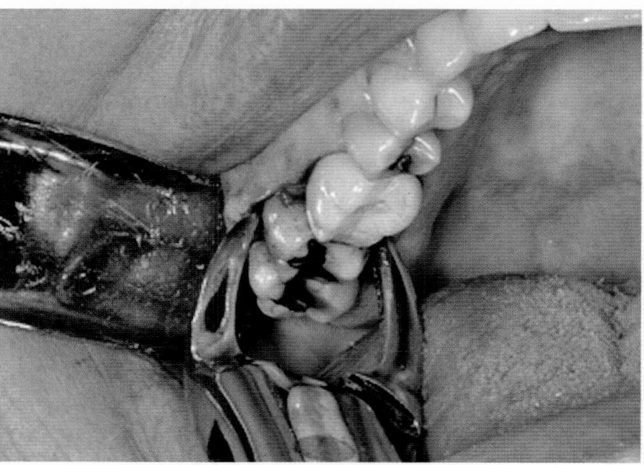

(Courtesy Dr. Edward Ellis III.)

6. The tooth is luxated in the socket to compress the bone and enlarge the socket. When luxation is complete, the tooth can be freely lifted from the socket.
7. The dentist examines the tooth to ensure that the root is intact.
8. When the tooth is removed, use the aspirating tip to debride the surgical site.
9. Fold several sterile gauze sponges into a tight pad to form a pressure pack. Retract the cheek, and place the folded gauze over the extraction site.
10. Instruct the patient to bite firmly on the pack for at least 30 minutes.

Purpose: This pressure aids in controlling bleeding and in blood clotting.

11. Slowly move the dental chair to an upright position.
12. Provide the patient with postoperative instructions.

DATE	TOOTH	SURFACE	CHARTING NOTES
8/26/18	4	—	Extraction, 2 carpules Xylocaine 1/50,000. Pt tolerated procedure well. Postoperative instructions given. T. Clark, CDA/L. Stewart, DDS

Procedure 26-4

Assisting in Multiple Extraction and Alveoloplasty

Equipment and Supplies

- Forceps extraction setup
- Additional elevators and forceps (dentist's choice)
- Rongeur
- Curettes
- Bone file
- Scalpel
- Suture material and needle
- Needle holder or hemostat
- Suture scissors
- Sterile saline solution

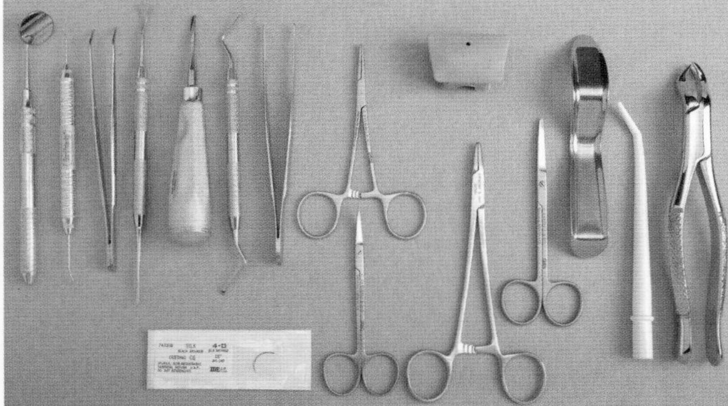

(From Boyd LRB: *Dental instruments: a pocket guide,* ed 5, St Louis, 2015, Saunders.)

Procedural Steps

1. Follow steps 1 through 9 in Assisting in Forceps Extraction (see Procedure 26-3) until all the teeth have been extracted.
2. After the teeth have been extracted, the dentist uses the rongeur to trim the alveolus. After each cut with the rongeur, have a sterile gauze available to remove debris from the cutting ends carefully.

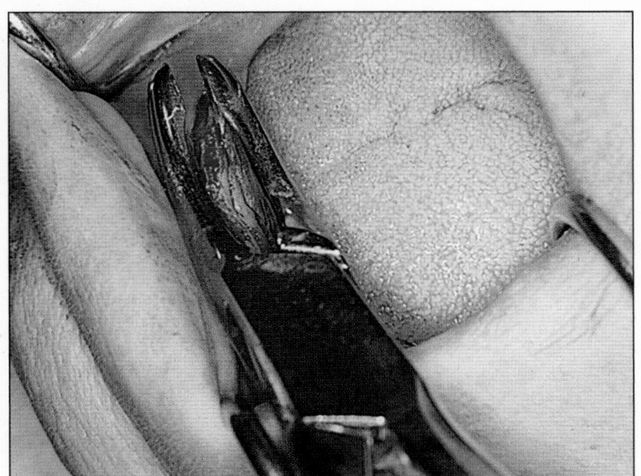

(From Boyd LRB: *Dental instruments: a pocket guide,* ed 5, St Louis, 2015, Saunders.)

3. After the rongeur is used, transfer the bone file to the dentist to finish smoothing any rough margins. After each stroke with the file, use a clean sterile gauze square to remove debris from the grooves.

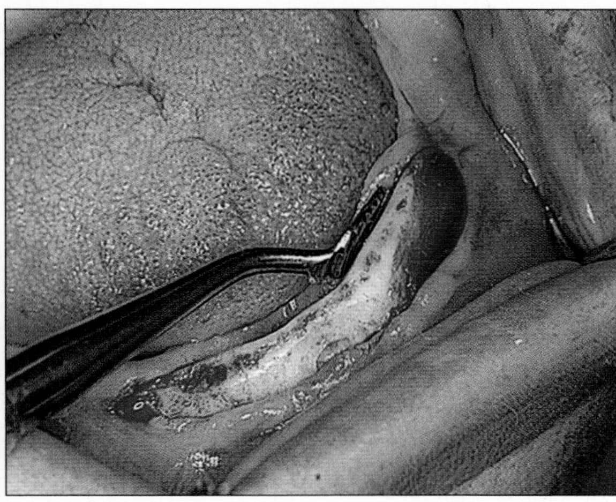

(From Boyd LRB: *Dental instruments: a pocket guide,* ed 5, St Louis, 2015, Saunders.)

4. Irrigate and aspirate the surgical site with sterile saline solution to remove bone fragments. The dentist repositions the mucosa over the ridge and sutures it into place.

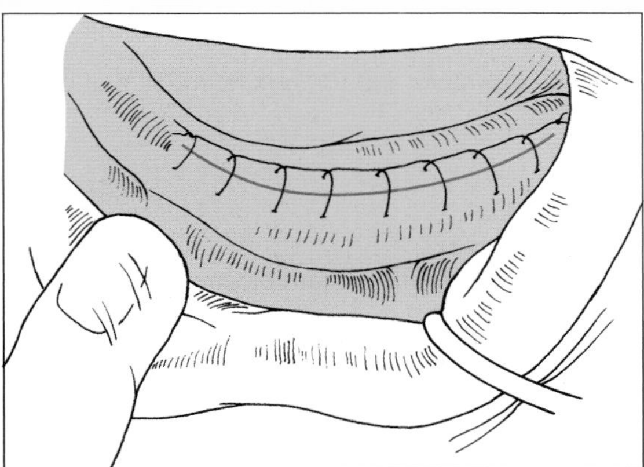

(From Peterson LJ, Ellis III E, Hupp JR, et al: *Contemporary oral and maxillofacial surgery,* ed 4, St Louis, 2003, Mosby.)

Continued

Procedure 26-4

Assisting in Multiple Extraction and Alveoloplasty—cont'd

5. Place pressure packs made of sterile gauze sponges as needed. Provide the patient with postoperative instructions, both verbal and written, and complete the patient's dismissal.

DATE	TOOTH	SURFACE	CHARTING NOTES
8/26/18	22-27	—	Vitals: P 90 bpm, BP 140/90 mm Hg. Extractions, 3 carpules Xylocaine 1:20,000, alveoloplasty, 8 nylon sutures placed. Pt tolerated procedure well. Postoperative instructions provided. Prescription for Tylenol w/ Codeine, and Penicillin 500 VK. Pt to return in 1 wk for suture removal and check. T. Clark, CDA/L. Stewart, DDS

Procedure 26-5

Assisting in the Removal of an Impacted Tooth

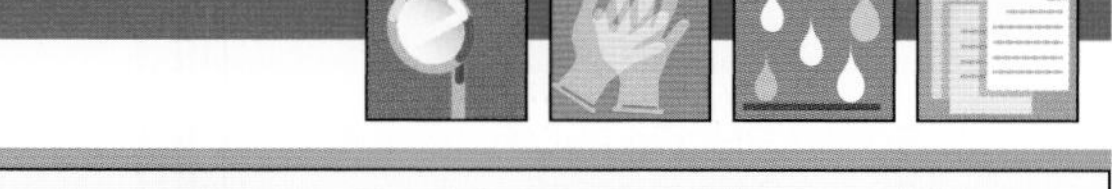

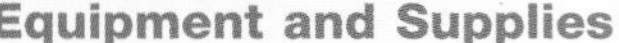

Equipment and Supplies

- Forceps extraction setup
- Scalpel, #15 blade and handle
- Additional elevators and forceps (surgeon's choice)
- Rongeur
- Bone file
- Curettes
- Root tip picks
- Surgical scissors
- Conventional high-speed handpiece with surgical bur or mallet and chisel
- Irrigating syringe
- Sterile saline solution
- Sterile suture material and needle
- Needle holder or hemostat
- Suture scissors
- Sterile gauze sponges

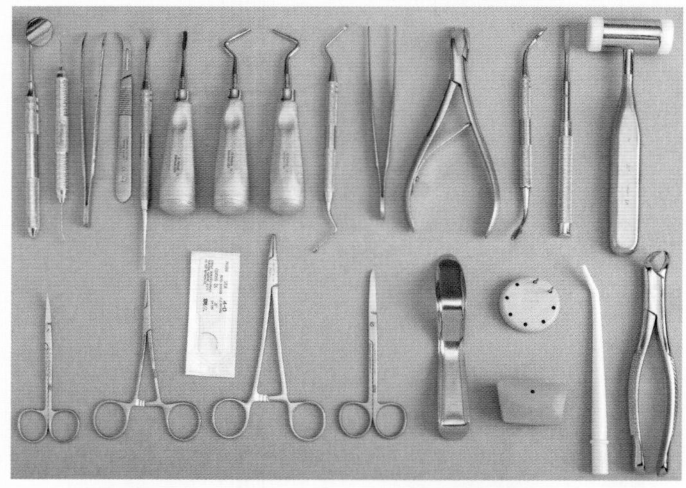

(From Boyd LRB: *Dental instruments: a pocket guide,* ed 5, St Louis, 2015, Saunders.)

Procedure 26-5

Assisting in the Removal of an Impacted Tooth—cont'd

Procedural Steps

Surgical Preparation

1. The surgeon determines that adequate anesthesia has been achieved.
2. Transfer the scalpel for the surgeon to make the initial incision along the ridge through both the gingival mucosa and the periosteum.

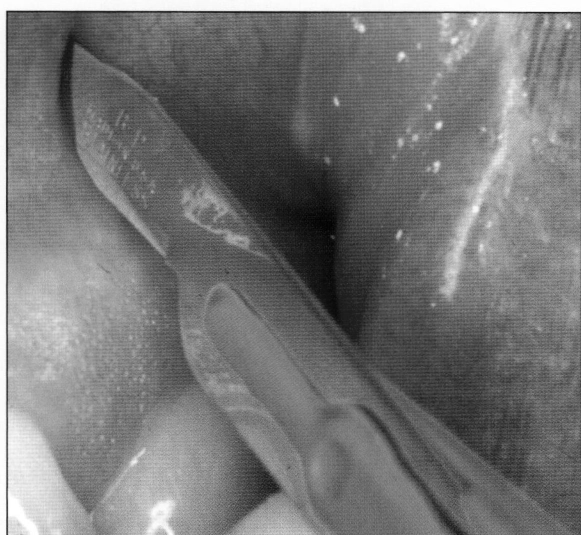

(From Boyd LRB: *Dental instruments: a pocket guide,* ed 5, St Louis, 2015, Saunders.)

3. The periosteal elevator is used to retract the tissue from the bone.
4. Once the incision is made, continuously evacuate blood, debris, and saliva from the surgical site.
5. A surgical mallet and chisel or a surgical handpiece with surgical burs will be used to remove the bony covering from the impacted tooth.

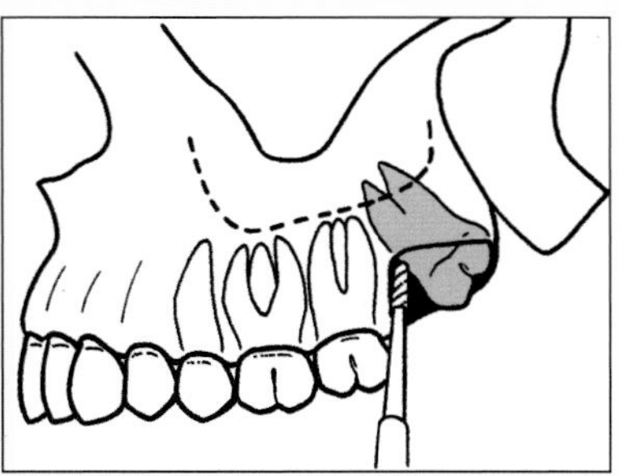

Removing the Impacted Tooth

1. When the surgeon has uncovered the impacted tooth, it can be luxated and lifted from the alveolus with an elevator or extraction forceps.

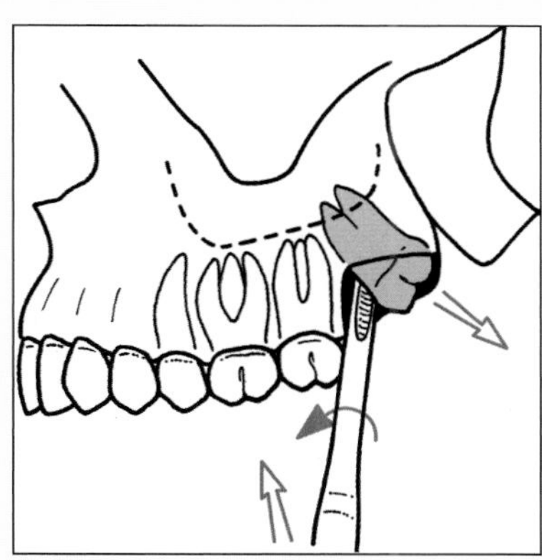

2. In some cases, the tooth is lodged between bone and another tooth. This position may necessitate sectioning the crown of the impacted tooth with the mallet and chisel or a surgical bur.
3. After the tooth has been removed, the surgical site is curetted, irrigated, and evacuated to remove all debris and infectious material.
4. After a thorough debridement, the surgeon returns the mucoperiosteal flap to its normal position over the wound and sutures it into place.
5. Slowly return the patient to an upright position.
6. Provide the patient with postoperative instructions.

DATE	TOOTH	SURFACE	CHARTING NOTES
8/26/18	18	—	Vitals: P 80 bpm, BP 130/82 mm Hg. Extraction, N_2O sedation, 2 carpules Xylocaine 1:20,000; incision using #12 blade, tooth removed in sections; 2 gut sutures placed. Pt tolerated procedure well. Prescription for Tylenol w/ Codeine, and Penicillin 500 VK Postoperative instructions Provided. Pt to return in 1 wk. T. Clark, CDA/ L. Stewart, DDS

Procedure 26-6

Assisting in Suture Placement

Equipment and Supplies

- Suture material
- Hemostat
- Needle holder
- Suture scissors
- Sterile gauze sponges

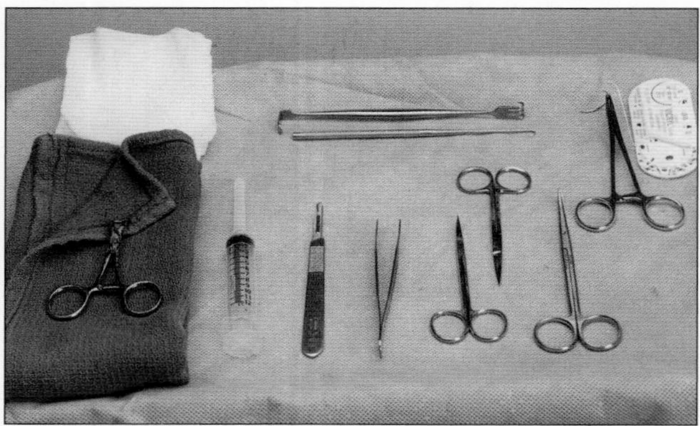

Procedural Steps

1. Remove the suture material from its sterile package.
2. Using the needle holder, clamp the suture needle at the upper third.

Purpose: If you clamp too close to the thread, then you may cause the suture to detach from the needle; if you clamp too close to the needle end, then you may damage the needle point.

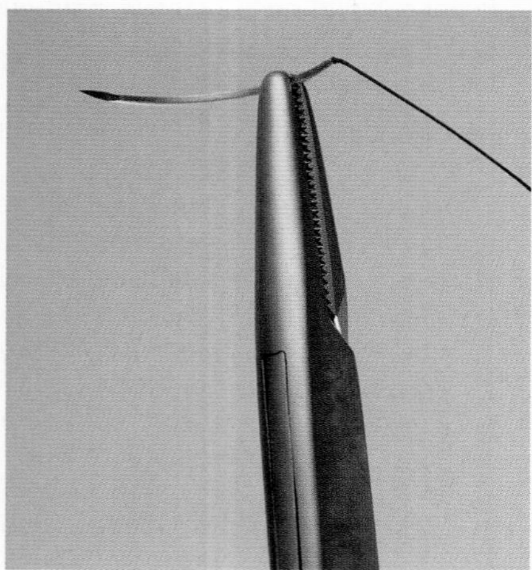

(From Hupp JR, Ellis E III, Tucker M: *Contemporary oral and maxillofacial surgery,* ed 6, St Louis, 2014, Mosby.)

3. Transfer the needle holder to the surgeon while grasping the hinge, which allows the surgeon to grasp the handle of the instrument.
4. Retract the tongue or cheek to provide a clear line of vision for the surgeon as the sutures are placed.

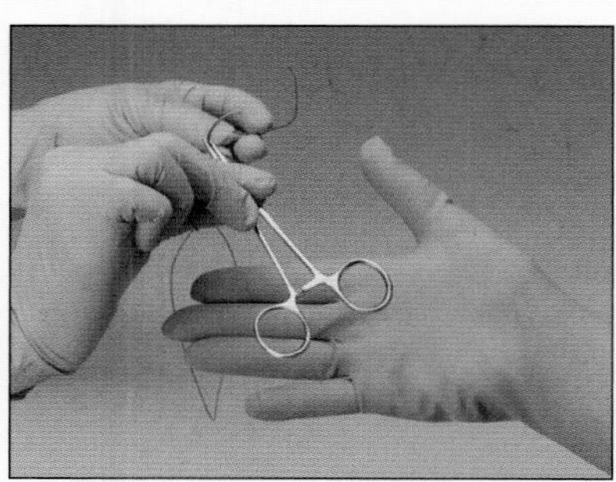

(Young AP, Kennedy DB: *Kinn's the medical assistant: an applied learning approach,* ed 9, St Louis, 2003, Saunders.)

5. After tying each suture and if directed by the surgeon, use the suture scissors to cut the sutures, leaving approximately 2 to 3 mm of suture material beyond the knot.
6. Retrieve the suturing supplies from the surgeon, and replace them on the surgical tray.
7. Record the numbers and types of sutures placed in the patient's record.

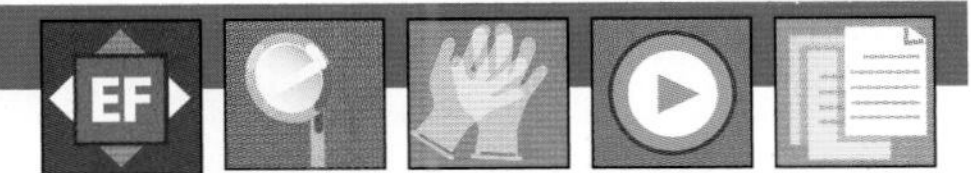

Procedure 26-7

Performing Suture Removal (Expanded Function)

Equipment and Supplies

- Basic setup
- Suture scissors
- Sterile cotton gauze
- Cotton-tip applicator

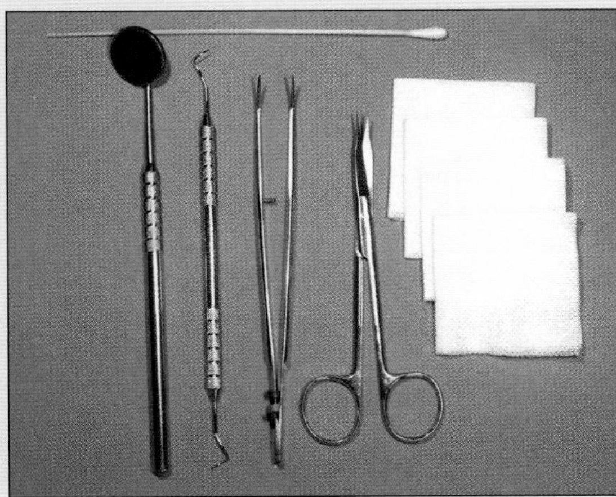

Procedural Steps

1. The surgeon examines the surgical site to evaluate healing. If healing is satisfactory, then the sutures may be removed.
2. Swab the site with an antiseptic agent to remove any debris.
3. Use cotton pliers to hold the suture gently away from the tissue to expose the attachment of the knot. Gently slip one blade of the suture scissors under the suture. Cut near the tissue.

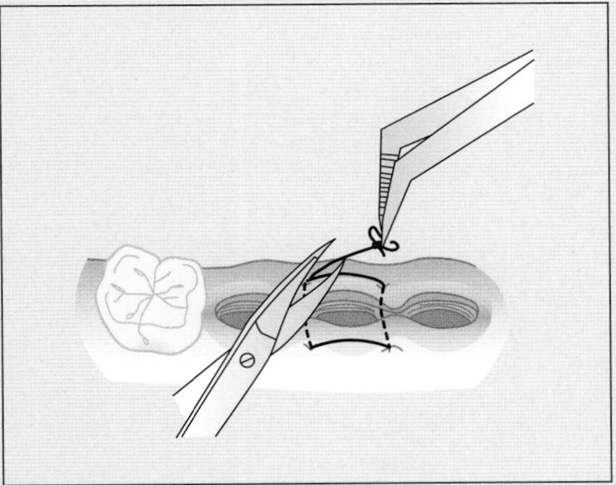

4. Use the cotton pliers to grasp the knot, and gently tug it so that the suture slides through the tissue.

Note: Never pull ("yank") the knot through the tissue.

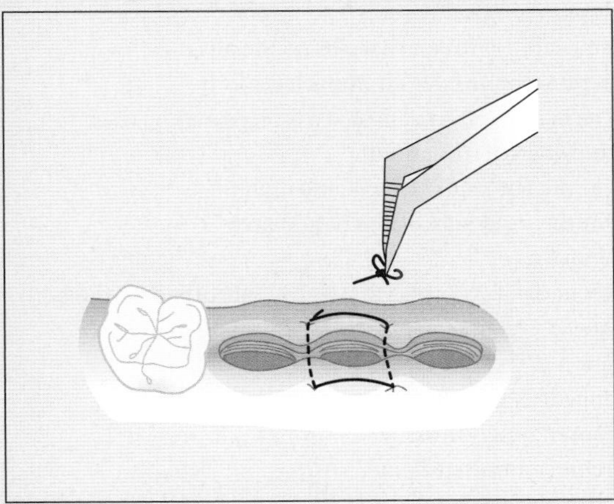

5. If bleeding occurs, then irrigate the surgical site with an antiseptic solution or warm saline solution. Briefly apply a compress to the surgical site to promote clotting.
6. Count the sutures that have been removed, and compare this number with the number indicated in the patient's record.

DATE	TOOTH	SURFACE	CHARTING NOTES
9/3/18	—	—	Suture removal, 3 nylon sutures removed. Pt. healing well, with no complications. T. Clark, CDA/L. Stewart, DDS

Chapter Exercises

Multiple Choice

Circle the letter next to the correct answer.

1. A bone file is used to __________.
   - a. debride the socket
   - b. loosen gingival tissue
   - c. smooth the rough margins of the alveolus
   - d. remove bone over an impacted tooth
2. The term *universal* means that a forceps may be used __________.
   - a. anywhere in the mouth
   - b. on the left side of the dental arch
   - c. on the right side of the dental arch
   - d. b and c
3. Nylon and silk sutures __________ absorbed by the body.
   - a. are
   - b. are not
4. A rongeur is used to __________.
   - a. loosen gingival tissue
   - b. remove infected tissue
   - c. trim alveolar bone
   - d. retrieve root fragments
5. The common term for alveolitis is __________.
   - a. dry socket
   - b. impaction
   - c. excessive bleeding
   - d. extraction
6. During a surgical procedure, __________ are to be worn.
   - a. examination gloves
   - b. overgloves
   - c. sterile gloves
   - d. utility gloves
7. A(n) __________ is used to control immediate postoperative bleeding.
   - a. gauze pressure pack
   - b. heating pad
   - c. ice pack
   - d. moistened tea bag
8. Periosteal elevators are used to __________.
   - a. remove clots and debris from the socket after the extraction
   - b. remove the tooth from the socket
   - c. separate the periosteum from the surface of the bone
   - d. remove gauze from the surgical site
9. The surgical reshaping of the alveolar ridge is known as a(n) __________.
   - a. alveolitis
   - b. alveoloplasty
   - c. gingivectomy
   - d. impaction
10. Sutures that are not resorbed by the body are commonly removed in __________ days.
    - a. 1 to 2
    - b. 3 to 4
    - c. 5 to 7
    - d. 10 to 14

Apply Your Knowledge

1. You are assisting in a forceps extraction on tooth #4. List the surgical instruments that would be set up for this procedure.
2. A patient calls the office after hours describing extreme pain 2 days after having her wisdom teeth extracted. You remember the patient because the procedure took longer than expected because the teeth were impacted. What might this patient be experiencing?
3. You have identified the problem in the previous question. How do you instruct this patient to relieve her pain and discomfort?

CHAPTER 27

Pediatric Dentistry

http://evolve.elsevier.com/Robinson/essentials/

LEARNING OBJECTIVES

1. Pronounce, define, and spell the key terms.
2. Complete the following related to the pediatric dental office:
   - Describe the appearance and setting of a pediatric dental office.
   - Describe the behavioral management techniques for pediatric patients.
   - Describe guidelines for child behavior.
   - Describe how to handle a challenging patient.
   - Discuss pediatric patients with special needs.
3. Describe the steps of an examination of the pediatric patient.
4. Complete the following related to pediatric procedures:
   - Discuss the importance of preventive dentistry in pediatrics.
   - Describe the types of procedures commonly provided in a pediatric dental practice.
   - Discuss preventative orthodontics, sports safety, restorative procedures, pulp therapy, and stainless steel crowns as they relate to pediatric patients.
   - Demonstrate how to assist in pulpotomy of a primary tooth.
   - Demonstrate how to assist in the placement of a stainless steel crown.
5. Describe the types of traumatic injuries that can be commonly seen in a pediatric practice.

KEY TERMS

autonomy
avulsed
cross-bite
fluoride
rapport
space maintainer
stainless steel crowns

Pediatric dentistry is a specialized area of dentistry that is focused on providing oral health care for the needs of infants, children, adolescents, and individuals with special needs. The emphasis of the pediatric dental practice is to focus on developmental guidance, early detection, prevention, and treatment of dental diseases.

Clinical Procedures Provided for a Pediatric Patient

- Preventive care
- Restorative procedures
- Pulp therapy
- Surgical procedures
- Space maintenance
- Interceptive orthodontics

Pediatric Dental Office

The design of a pediatric dental office should portray a cheerful, pleasant, and nonthreatening atmosphere to a child. Many pediatric dental offices are designed with several dental chairs arranged in one large treatment area or bay (Figure 27-1). This design provides reassurance from one child to another when they can see other children being treated. An open-bay design can be psychologically effective because children are often hesitant to express fear or to misbehave in the presence of other children.

The pediatric office will also have a "quiet room." This treatment area is separate from the open area and is used for children whose behavior may upset other children.

Behavioral Management Techniques

Children are treated differently from adult patients, and the techniques used in managing a child's behavior will depend on the age of the child. (See Table 27-1 for the stages of behavior.) Members of the dental team in a pediatric office will make modifications in the way they practice dentistry for several reasons: age, size, and how the child is behaving (Figure 27-2).

Guidelines for Child Behavior

The development of trust between the parent and child and the dentist serves as the basis for a productive, effective means of

TABLE 27-1
Stages of Behavior

Age Range	Behavioral Characteristics
Birth through 2 years of age	Children may act friendly toward strangers but then become afraid of them. They may experience fear of separation from a parent. Toddlers are too young to be expected to cooperate with dental treatment. If the parent is with the child, then the initial examination is easier.
3 through 5 years of age	Children are learning to follow simple instructions at this age. They want **autonomy**. Allow children at this age to make choices (e.g., ask him or her to choose the flavor of fluoride).
6 through 11 years of age	Children in this age group are in the period of socialization. They want to learn the rules. They have overcome most of their fears.
12 through 20 years of age	Through this age, young people have acquired self-certainty and a sexual identity. They will seek leadership and will develop their own ideals.

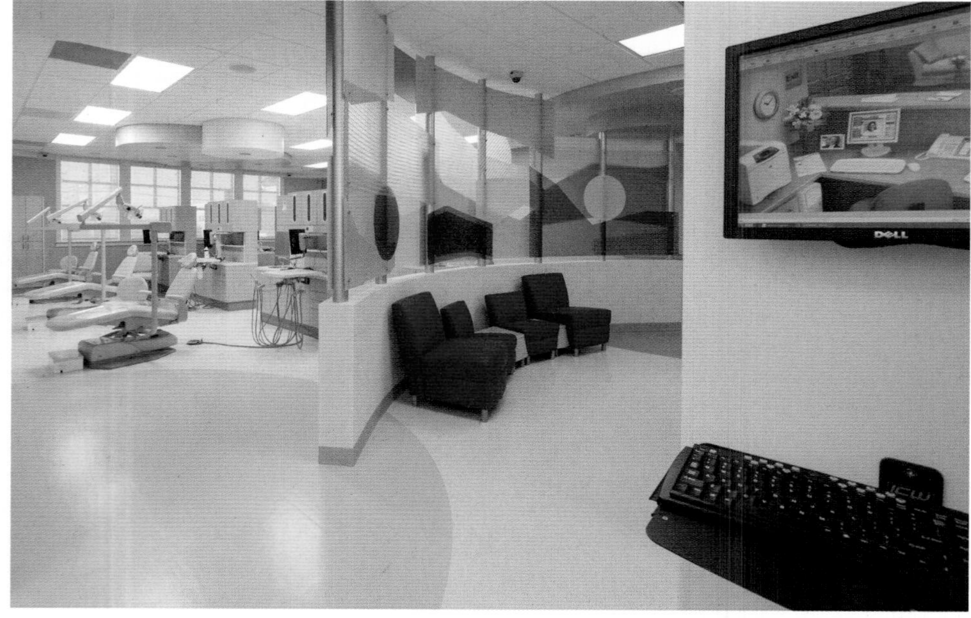

FIGURE 27-1 Example of a pediatric dental office. (Courtesy Patterson Dental, St. Paul, Minnesota.)

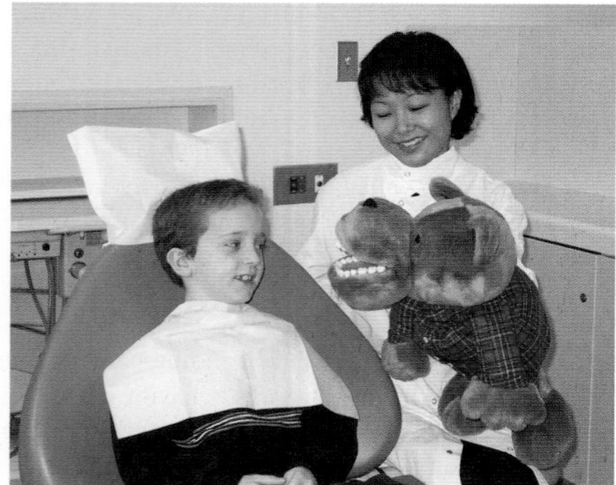

FIGURE 27-2 Patient at a pediatric dental office.

providing dental health care. Dental procedures can be accomplished for patients of all ages if the dental team practices the following procedural guidelines:

- Be honest with the child.
- Consider the child's point of view.
- Always "tell, show, and do."
- Give positive reinforcement.

Challenging Patient

Treating an anxious, fearful, or uncooperative child can be challenging for the dentist, assistant, parents, and especially for the child. In some situations, a child will remain uncooperative, despite the fact that the dental team has used every possible approach to provide a positive dental experience. Occasionally, a child's behavior during treatment requires a more assertive management style to be used to protect him or her from possible injury. Voice control (speaking calmly but firmly) will usually prevent the need for additional steps.

In certain cases, some form of restraint may be required for the patient's protection. A **restraint** can be pharmacologic or physical. If the dentist knows that restraint will be needed, then a premedication can be prescribed to calm and ease the patient before treatment. Mild sedation, such as nitrous oxide–oxygen or a sedative, may benefit an anxious child. A **papoose board**, which is a temporary stabilization wrap for a child, can also be used. This device gently *hugs* or wraps around the child's arms, legs, and middle section during a procedure to help keep a patient's movement or activity to a minimum.

Patients With Special Needs

Physical and mental challenges can slow or challenge a child's physiologic and social growth. Intellectual challenges such as Down syndrome and cerebral palsy can influence how individuals are able to care for themselves. Parents and caregivers may be required to take on more responsibilities for maintaining daily physical and oral health needs.

The pediatric dentist receives extensive education and training to care for patients with special needs. The severity of each individual patient's disorder dictates whether treatment is provided in the pediatric dental office or in the hospital setting. An evaluation of a patient's medical and social history will help determine necessary modifications to the treatment plan.

Examination of the Pediatric Patient

According to the American Academy of Pediatric Dentistry, the first dental appointment for a child should take place around his or her first birthday. This initial examination is often the first dental experience for a child. The rapport that is developed with the child during this initial examination can establish a positive attitude toward dental health that will last for the child's lifetime. (**Rapport** means a feeling of ease or comfort.)

The child's parent or legal guardian must provide consent (permission) before any dental treatment is provided for a child younger than 18 years of age.

Medical and Dental Histories

The parent or guardian completes the **medical history form**, which includes information about the child's general health background. If medical problems are noted, then the dentist may choose to contact the child's pediatrician to obtain a more complete medical background.

The **dental history** includes information about the eruption pattern of the teeth, past dental problems and care, **fluoride** intake, and current oral hygiene habits.

General Appraisal and Behavioral Assessment

A general appraisal addresses physical conditions and developmental levels. It also includes vital signs and baseline health data for emergency situations.

A behavioral assessment is used to evaluate the communication skills of the patient and to determine whether behavioral management techniques are necessary.

Intraoral Examination

The intraoral examination requires the use of a mouth mirror, an explorer, and gauze squares. Very young children may be uncooperative and may allow only fingers in their mouths. Other young children may allow only a mirror.

Ideally, each of the 20 primary teeth should be examined. In addition to charting the erupted teeth, the occlusion is analyzed to determine spacing and crowding and the presence or absence of teeth.

Radiographic Examination

A radiographic examination is necessary for the dentist to make a complete diagnosis. However, young children often have difficulty with the radiographic procedure, and the radiographic examination may have to be deferred until the child can comprehend the need to remain still and follow directions. When radiographs are possible, techniques are available that can be helpful when introducing the procedure to the child.

Techniques for Introducing a Child to Radiographs

- Use a "big camera" comparison to explain the procedure. This works only if the child is old enough to understand the concept.
- Use the "tell-show-do" introduction. By "practicing" the position of the film or sensor and the x-ray machine, you can determine whether the child will sit for the exposure, which helps prevent an unproductive exposure to radiation.
- Match the size of the film to the level of comfort for the child. In some cases, bending the anterior corners helps in bite-wing placement.
- Perform the easiest procedures first. Usually, occlusal projections are the most comfortable for the child.
- If the parent is accompanying the child to stabilize film or sensor placement, then both the parent and the child must be adequately shielded with a lead apron.
- *Important:* The assistant never holds the film or sensor in a patient's mouth during a radiographic exposure.

Pediatric Procedures

The procedures described in this chapter are introduced to help maintain the health of the primary, mixed, and permanent dentition through early adult years.

Preventive Dentistry

Prevention is one of the most encompassing areas for a pediatric dental practice. It not only involves the complete dental team in educating the patient and parents, but it also reaches to the community and local school systems. The role of the pediatric dentist is to communicate preventive dental health in such areas as oral hygiene, fluoride use, nutrition, and preventive and protective procedures.

Oral Hygiene

Oral hygiene instructions are geared toward improving a child's brushing and flossing techniques. Eventually, this learning process is intended to lead to cleaner teeth and healthier gums.

When children are encouraged to develop the habit of effectively brushing twice a day with fluoride toothpaste and flossing once a day, they will maintain proper oral habits throughout their lives (see Chapter 17).

Nutrition

A diet that is healthy is balanced and naturally supplies all the nutrients a child needs to grow. Chapter 17 describes the types of foods that children should eat for normal growth and identifies foods that can increase decay.

Topical Fluorides

Fluorides have played a primary role in bringing about the decline in dental caries; however, for many children, decay is still a major dental problem. Often these children are those who have not had the benefits of fluoride from birth. Professional topical application of fluoride is very important in controlling caries in children. (Fluorides are discussed in Chapter 17.)

Sealants

Sealants are a common preventive tool provided in a pediatric office. Sealants protect the grooves and pitted surfaces of teeth, especially the chewing surfaces of molars and premolars, where most decay is detected. Sealants are made of a clear or tooth-colored composite resin and are applied to the pits and fissures to help keep them cavity free. (See Chapter 18 for further discussion.)

Preventive Orthodontics

It is never too early to start evaluating a child's oral and facial (orofacial) development. The pediatric dentist is the first to identify malocclusion, crowded or crooked teeth, and habits that can affect the dentition. The pediatric dentist can actively intervene or can refer the patient to an orthodontist to guide the teeth as they emerge in the mouth. Early preventive and interceptive orthodontic treatment can prevent more extensive treatment later.

Preventive orthodontics can prevent or eliminate irregularities and malpositions in the developing dentofacial region. Preventive orthodontics includes the following:

- Control of decay to prevent the premature loss of primary teeth, which may result in loss of space for the eruption of permanent teeth
- Use of a space maintainer to save space for the eruption of permanent teeth (Figure 27-3) (Space maintainers most often are cemented in place and retained until the permanent tooth erupts.)
- Use of appliances cemented in place to correct oral habits, such as thumb sucking, that can affect the permanent dentition (Figure 27-4)
- Early detection of genetic and congenital anomalies that may influence dental development
- Supervision of the natural exfoliation (shedding) of the primary teeth (If retained for too long, the primary teeth may cause the permanent teeth to erupt out of alignment or to be impacted.)

Interceptive orthodontics allows the dentist to intercede or correct problems as they develop. For example, a cross-bite occurs when one or both sides of the maxillary teeth are positioned lingual to the mandibular teeth. Interceptive orthodontics includes the following:

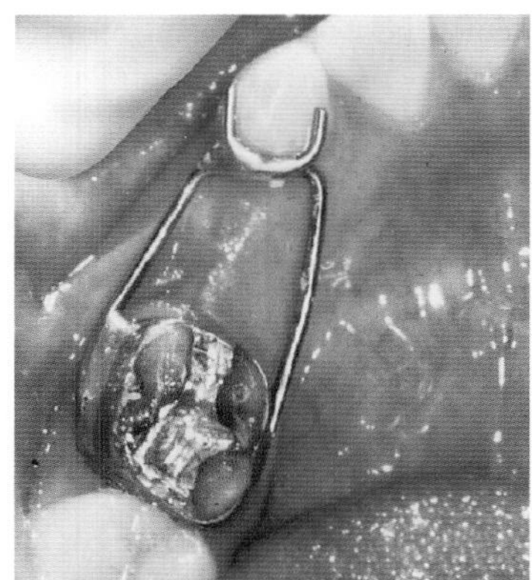

FIGURE 27-3 Space maintainer is used to reserve the space until the permanent tooth erupts.

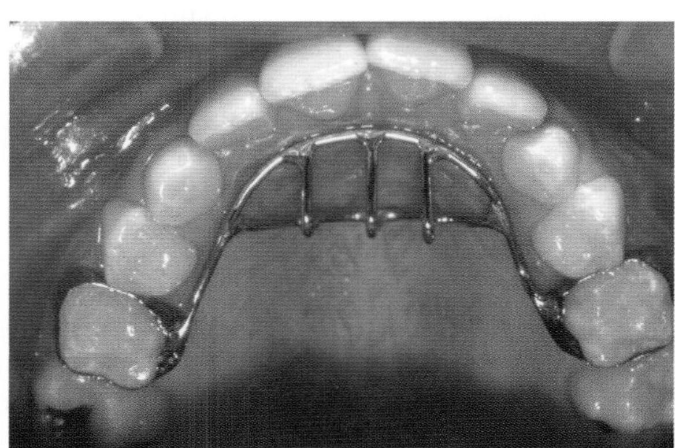

FIGURE 27-4 Example of a fixed appliance to discourage thumb sucking. (Courtesy Dr. Frank Hodges.)

- Extraction of primary teeth that can contribute to malalignment of the permanent dentition
- Correction of a cross-bite through the use of a removable or fixed appliance (Figure 27-5)
- Correction of a jaw size discrepancy through the use of a removable or fixed appliance (Figure 27-6)
- Extraction of primary or permanent teeth to correct overcrowding

Sports Safety

The fields of sports medicine and dentistry have documented the benefits of wearing protective face equipment during recreational sports that might injure the mouth area. Many states have regulations that require athletes in school contact sports to wear protective mouth guards to help prevent traumatic injuries to the teeth.

Commercial or custom mouth guards may be used. Commercial mouth guards are supplied as kits. The material is heated in warm water, placed in the individual's mouth, and molded to fit the arch.

Custom mouth guards are created in the dental office. An alginate impression is obtained of the player's maxillary arch,

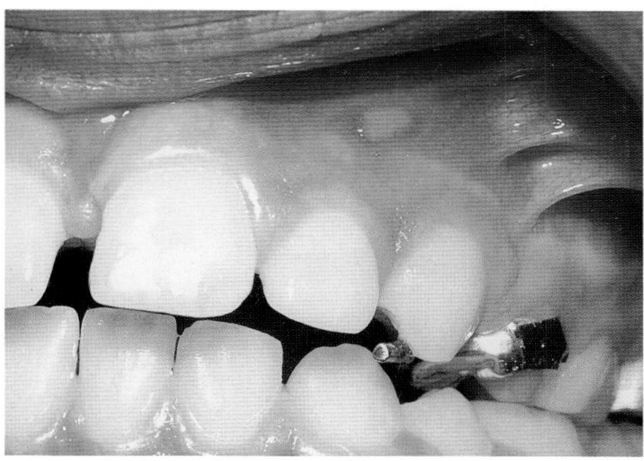

FIGURE 27-5 Example of a fixed appliance to correct crossbite. (Courtesy Dr. Frank Hodges.)

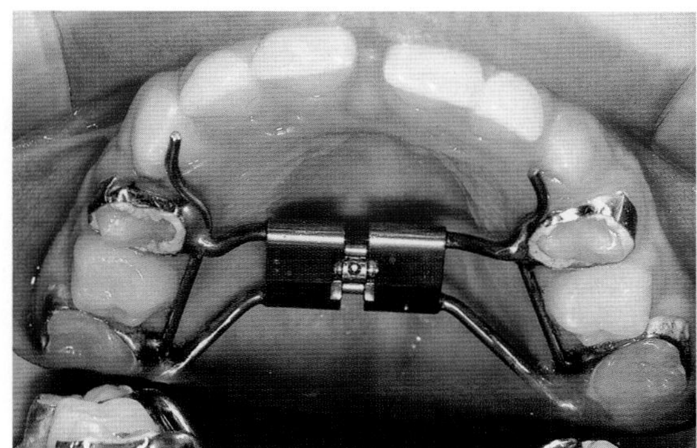

FIGURE 27-6 Palatal expansion appliance used to widen the maxillary arch. (Courtesy Dr. Frank Hodges.)

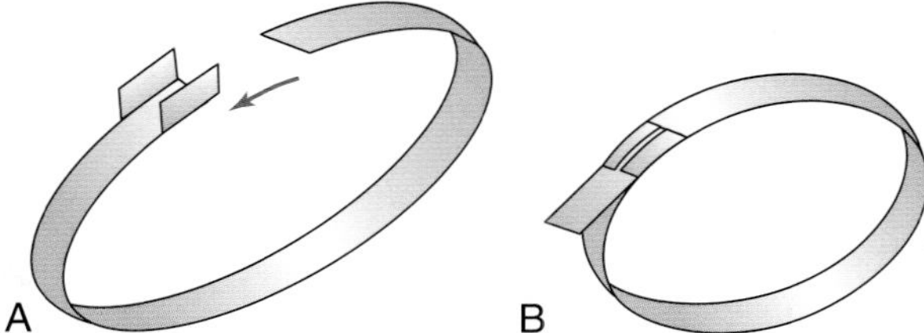

FIGURE 27-7 Copper T-band used for primary molars. **A,** In preparation for closing the band. **B,** End of band held in place by closing tabs.

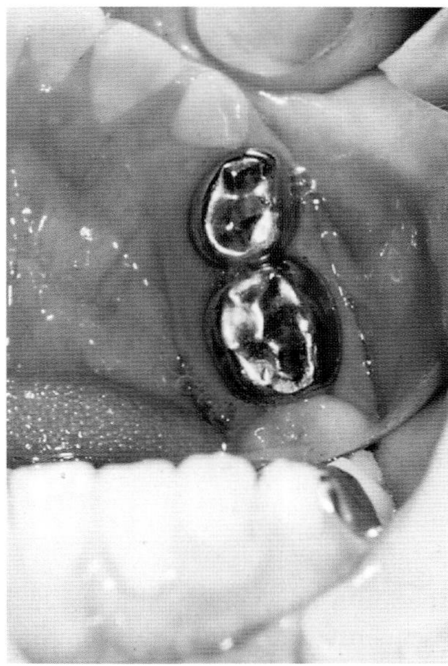

FIGURE 27-8 Stainless steel crowns are trimmed and contoured to fit properly.

and a diagnostic cast is created. The mouth guard is vacuum-formed on this cast.

Restorative Procedures

Restorative procedures, described in Chapter 21, are also performed on primary teeth. The dentist follows many of the same restorative principles as with permanent teeth. The major difference is the size and shape of the teeth. When preparing the dental dam, isolating the tooth receiving a restoration is best, and the tooth behind or distal receives the dental clamp.

Matrix Systems for Primary Teeth

The two matrix systems most commonly used on primary teeth are the (1) T-band, which is a small, copper T-shaped band that, when the top portion of the T is bent, provides an adjustable band to fit around the circumference of a primary molar (Figure 27-7); and (2) spot-welded band, which is form-fitted around the tooth using No. 110 pliers. The band is then removed and placed in a smaller form of a welder that fuses the metal together to make a custom band.

Pulp Therapy

The primary objective of pulp therapy in a pediatric setting is to stimulate and preserve pulpal regeneration of a primary tooth. The two most common factors that affect the pulpal health of primary teeth are deep decay and traumatic injury. Decay is more likely to affect the posterior teeth, and trauma is more likely to affect the anterior teeth.

Indirect and direct pulp capping is indicated for a young permanent tooth to promote pulpal healing and to stimulate the production of reparative dentin.

Pulpotomy

Pulpotomy is the complete removal of the coronal portion of the dental pulp. The goal of this procedure is to remove the portion of the pulp that is inflamed while maintaining the healthy vital pulp tissue in the canals of the primary tooth.

See Procedure 27-1: Assisting in Pulpotomy of a Primary Tooth.

Stainless Steel Crowns

Stainless steel crowns are used in the treatment of posterior primary and permanent teeth. This type of crown is considered the treatment of choice over large multisurface amalgam restorations in a child (Figure 27-8). Stainless steel crowns are available in a variety of sizes.

Indications for Use of Stainless Steel Crowns

- Restoration of primary or permanent teeth with extensive decay
- Restoration of primary teeth after pulpotomy or pulpectomy procedures (See discussion of the pulpotomyse procedure earlier in this chapter.)
- Permanent restoration after accidental fracture of a tooth
- Temporary restoration of a fractured tooth
- Restorations for patients who have difficulty maintaining good oral hygiene, such as disabled children

Types of Stainless Steel Crowns

Two types of stainless steel crowns are commonly used in pediatric dentistry.

Pretrimmed crowns have straight sides but are festooned to follow a line parallel to the gingival crest. They must be trimmed and contoured to fit the tooth. (*Festooned* means trimmed. *Contoured* means shaped to fit.)

Precontoured crowns are already festooned and contoured. Some additional trimming and contouring may be necessary but usually only minimally.

See Procedure 27-2: Assisting in the Placement of a Stainless Steel Crown.

Traumatic Injury

An injury to the tooth of a young child can have serious and long-term consequences, including discoloration and possible loss of the tooth. Many injuries to primary teeth commonly occur at 1½ to 2½ years of age—the toddler stage. The teeth most frequently injured in the primary dentition are the maxillary central incisors (Figure 27-9). These types of injuries can have damaging effects on permanent teeth forming directly below the roots of the primary teeth.

Common causes of dental injury to children include falling, bicycle accidents, sports injuries, and possible child abuse (Figure 27-10).

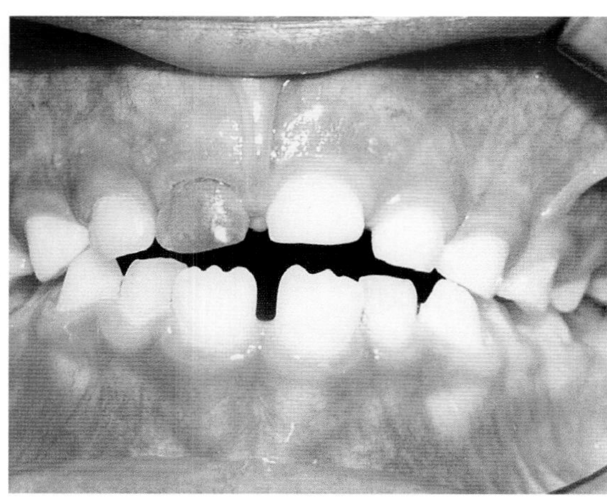

FIGURE 27-9 Traumatized maxillary incisor. (Courtesy Dr. Frank Hodges.)

Fractured Anterior Teeth

Fractures of anterior teeth are common emergencies in a pediatric dental practice.

The business assistant should instruct the parents of a child with a fractured tooth to come to the office immediately. Complete documentation of the accident, clinical examination, vitality testing, and radiographs are almost always part of the emergency visit (Figure 27-11).

The plan of treatment is to delay restorative treatment for 3 to 6 weeks to prevent further trauma to the pulp of an injured tooth. This delay gives the pulp a greater opportunity to recover without additional injury.

In the meantime, the dentist provides temporary relief by covering all exposed dentin with calcium hydroxide to prevent thermal sensitivity and places an interim covering of resin material. Radiographs and vitality tests are taken at subsequent appointments to determine the status of the injured tooth.

If the pulp shows vitality, then a definitive restorative procedure can be performed on the injured tooth.

Avulsed Teeth

Permanent teeth that have been avulsed, which means that the tooth has come completely out of the tooth socket, can be replanted with varying degrees of success (Figure 27-12). Primary teeth are not usually replanted. (**Avulsed** means torn away or removed by force.)

The more quickly a tooth can be repositioned, the greater the chance for success. The highest success rate occurs when the permanent tooth is replanted within 30 minutes of the accident.

Ethical Implications

The provision of dental care to children is a responsibility of the dental team. The image and memories that a child has of his or her dental experiences will be carried with him or her throughout life. Use words and terminology that are age appropriate and creates a nonthreatening experience when you explain a procedure as you speak to a child. Allow children to ask questions, but be ready to answer questions in a nonthreatening manner. Many expanded functions can be completed by the certified dental assistant in the pediatric office. Make certain that you have the current knowledge and skill required for these procedures.

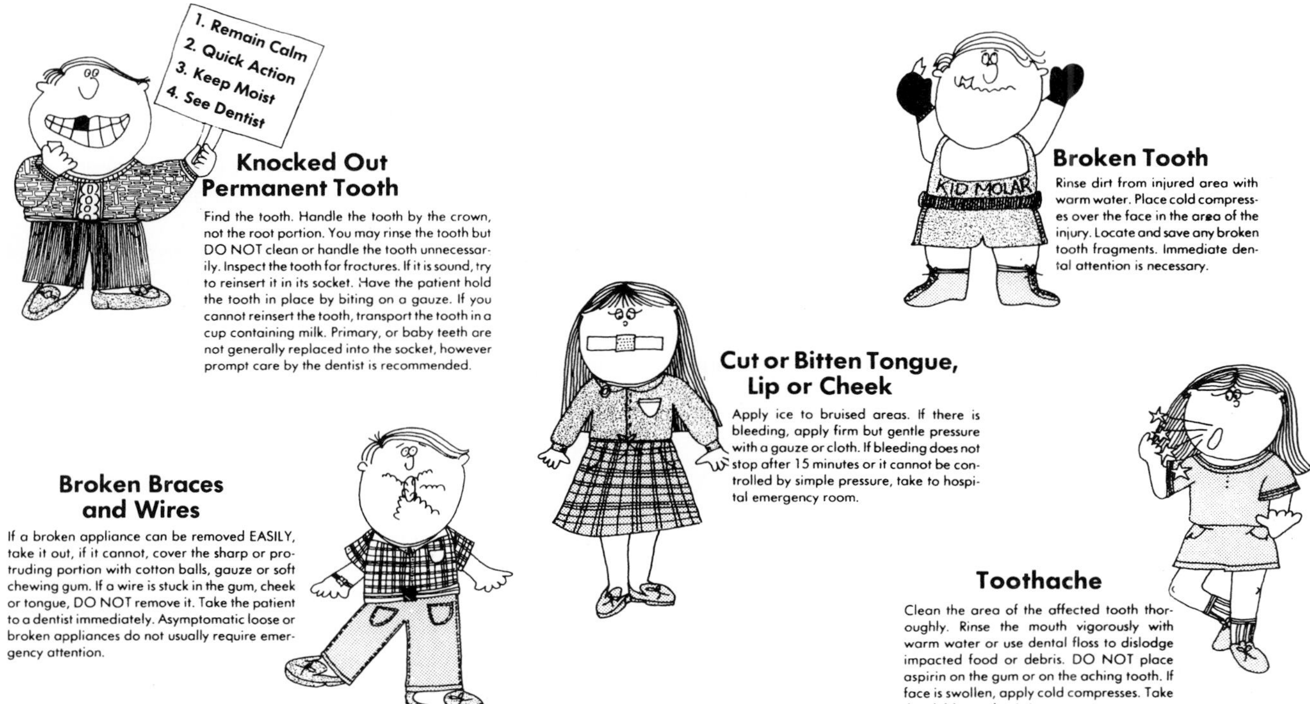
First Aid for Dental Emergencies
1. Remain Calm
2. Quick Action
3. Keep Moist
4. See Dentist
Knocked Out Permanent Tooth
Find the tooth. Handle the tooth by the crown, not the root portion. You may rinse the tooth but DO NOT clean or handle the tooth unnecessarily. Inspect the tooth for fractures. If it is sound, try to reinsert it in its socket. Have the patient hold the tooth in place by biting on a gauze. If you cannot reinsert the tooth, transport the tooth in a cup containing milk. Primary, or baby teeth are not generally replaced into the socket, however prompt care by the dentist is recommended.
KID MOLAR
Broken Tooth
Rinse dirt from injured area with warm water. Place cold compresses over the face in the area of the injury. Locate and save any broken tooth fragments. Immediate dental attention is necessary.
Cut or Bitten Tongue, Lip or Cheek
Apply ice to bruised areas. If there is bleeding, apply firm but gentle pressure with a gauze or cloth. If bleeding does not stop after 15 minutes or it cannot be controlled by simple pressure, take to hospital emergency room.
Broken Braces and Wires
If a broken appliance can be removed EASILY, take it out, if it cannot, cover the sharp or protruding portion with cotton balls, gauze or soft chewing gum. If a wire is stuck in the gum, cheek or tongue, DO NOT remove it. Take the patient to a dentist immediately. Asymptomatic loose or broken appliances do not usually require emergency attention.
Toothache
Clean the area of the affected tooth thoroughly. Rinse the mouth vigorously with warm water or use dental floss to dislodge impacted food or debris. DO NOT place aspirin on the gum or on the aching tooth. If face is swollen, apply cold compresses. Take the child to a dentist!

FIGURE 27-10 Flyer on actions to take in a dental emergency distributed to school personnel. (Courtesy Dr. John Christensen.)

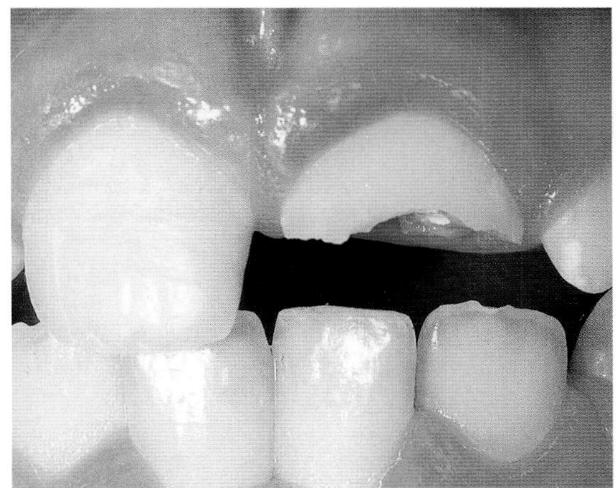

FIGURE 27-11 Fracture of an anterior tooth. (Courtesy Dr. Frank Hodges.)

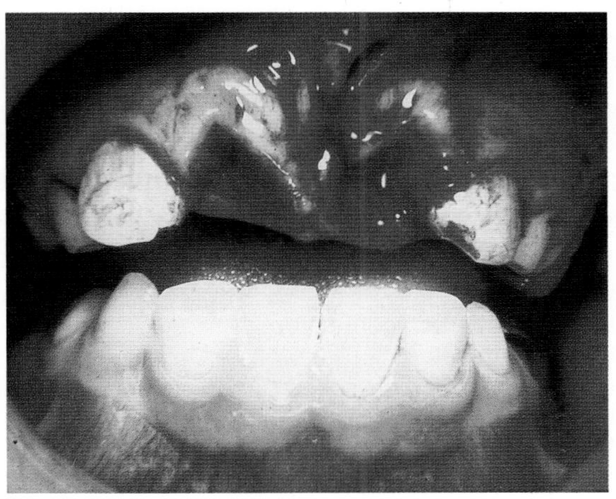

FIGURE 27-12 Avulsion of maxillary central incisors. (Courtesy Dr. Frank Hodges.)

Procedure 27-1

Assisting in Pulpotomy of a Primary Tooth

Equipment and Supplies

- Local anesthetic agent setup
- Basic setup
- Dental dam setup
- Low-speed handpiece
- Round burs
- Spoon excavators (various sizes)
- Sterile cotton pellets
- Formocresol
- Zinc oxide–eugenol (ZOE) base
- Final restorative material and instruments for placement

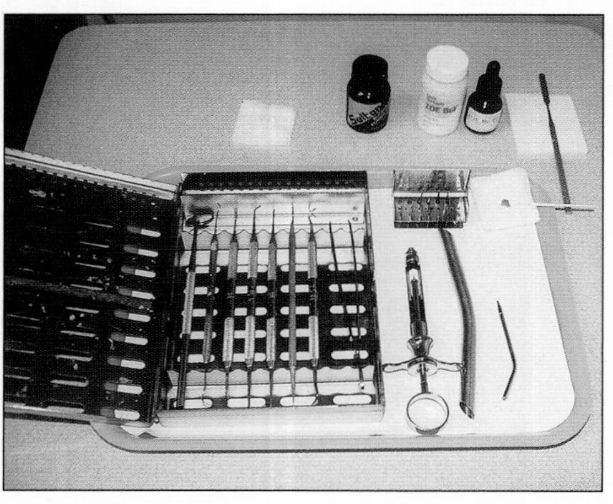

Procedural Steps

1. The local anesthetic agent is administered.
2. The dental dam is placed.
3. The dentist will use a round bur in the low-speed handpiece to remove the caries and expose the pulp chamber.
4. Transfer a spoon excavator for the dentist to remove all pulp tissue inside the coronal chamber.
5. Transfer a sterile cotton pellet moistened with formocresol for the dentist to place in the pulp chamber for approximately 5 minutes to control hemorrhaging.
6. Once bleeding is controlled, the pulp chamber is filled with ZOE paste, to which a drop of formocresol has been added.
7. The ZOE base and the final restoration are placed.

DATE	TOOTH	SURFACE	CHARTING NOTES
9/4/18	C	—	Pulpotomy, 1 carpule Xylocaine, 1:100,000 w/o epinephrine. Dam isolation, tooth opened, formocresol placed. ZOE base, amalgam. Pt tolerated procedure well. T. Clark, CDA/L. Stewart, DDS

Procedure 27-2

Assisting in the Placement of a Stainless Steel Crown

Equipment and Supplies

- Basic setup
- Local anesthetic agent setup
- Dental dam setup
- Low-speed and high-speed handpieces
- High-volume evacuator (HVE) tip
- Friction grip burs (dentist's choice of diamond or carbide)
- Spoon excavator
- Selection of stainless steel crowns
- Crown and bridge scissors
- Contouring and crimping pliers
- Mandrel
- Finishing and polishing discs
- Mounted green stones
- Cotton rolls
- Cementation setup
- Dental floss
- Articulating paper and holder

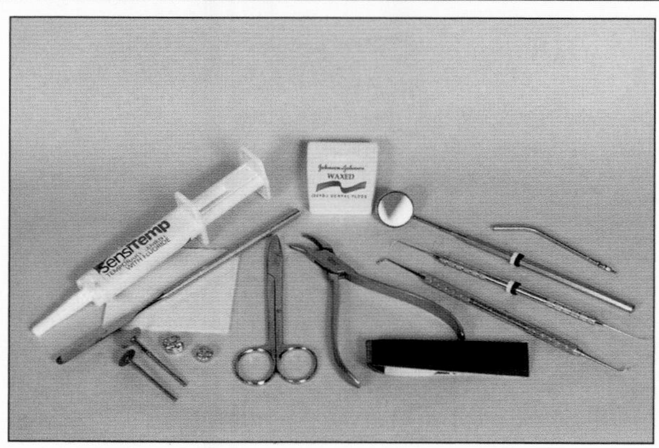

Hatrick CD, Eakle WS: *Dental materials: clinical applications for dental assistants and dental hygienists,* ed 3, St Louis, 2016, Saunders.

Procedure 27-2

Assisting in the Placement of a Stainless Steel Crown—cont'd

Procedural Steps

Preparing the Tooth

1. After the local anesthetic agent has been administered and has taken effect, the dental dam is applied.
2. The dentist will use the high-speed handpiece and a tapered diamond or carbide bur to prepare the tooth by a method similar to that used for a cast crown (see Chapter 23).
3. The dentist reduces the entire circumference of the tooth and the height of the tooth.
4. All dental caries are removed with hand instruments and burs.

Selecting and Sizing the Stainless Steel Crown

1. The crown is selected and tried on the prepared tooth for fit.
2. The stainless steel crown is properly sized when it fits snugly on the prepared tooth and has both mesial and distal contact.
3. Clean and sterilize any crowns that were tried in the mouth but not used; then return them to storage.

Trimming and Contouring the Crown

1. The dentist will use a crown and bridge scissors to reduce the height of the crown until it is approximately the same height as the adjacent teeth.

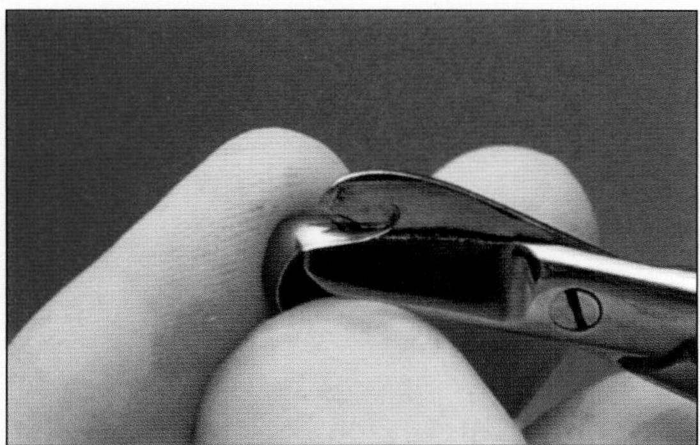

(From Duggal MS, Curzon MEJ, Fayle SA, et al: *Restorative techniques in pediatric dentistry,* Philadelphia, 1995, Saunders.)

2. The dentist may use a green stone to smooth the rough edges of the crown along the cervical margin.
3. The cervical margin of the crown may be polished with a rubber abrasive wheel.
4. The occlusion is checked and adjusted as needed.
5. The dentist uses contouring pliers to crimp the cervical margins of the crown toward the tooth to obtain a tight fit and a proper cervical contour.

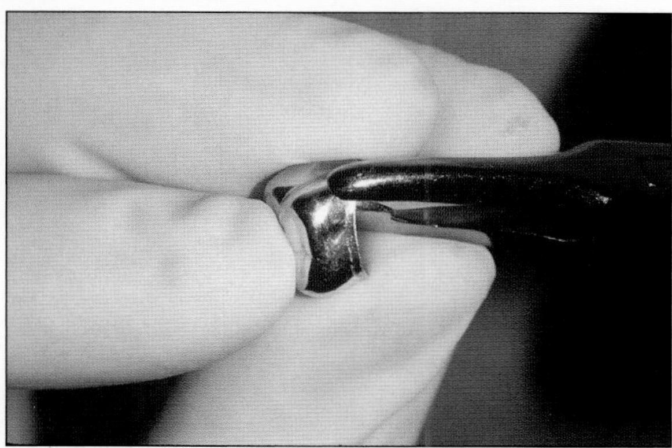

(From Hatrick CS, Eakle WS: *Dental materials: clinical applications for dental assistants and dental hygienists,* ed 3, St. Louis, 2016, Saunders.)

Cementation

1. Thoroughly rinse and dry the tooth. Place cotton rolls to maintain dry conditions.
2. Mix the permanent cement (polycarboxylate is often selected).
3. Line the crown with the cement, and transfer to the dentist for placement.

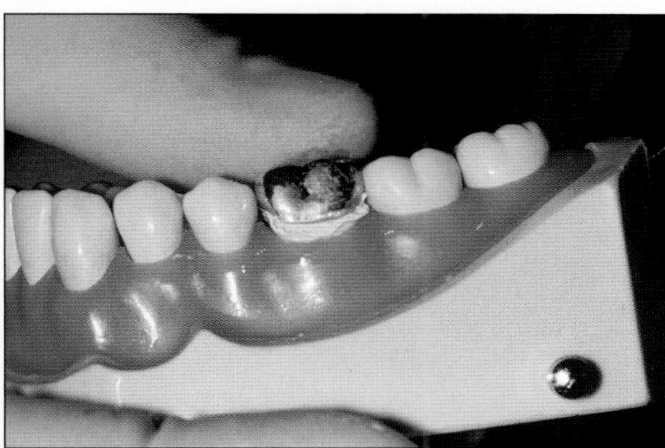

(From Hatrick CS, Eakle WS: *Dental materials: clinical applications for dental assistants and dental hygienists*, ed 3, St. Louis, 2016, Saunders.)

4. Transfer an explorer to the dentist to remove the excess cement from around the tooth.
5. Use dental floss to remove any remaining cement from the interproximal areas.

Continued

Procedure 27-2

Assisting in the Placement of a Stainless Steel Crown—cont'd

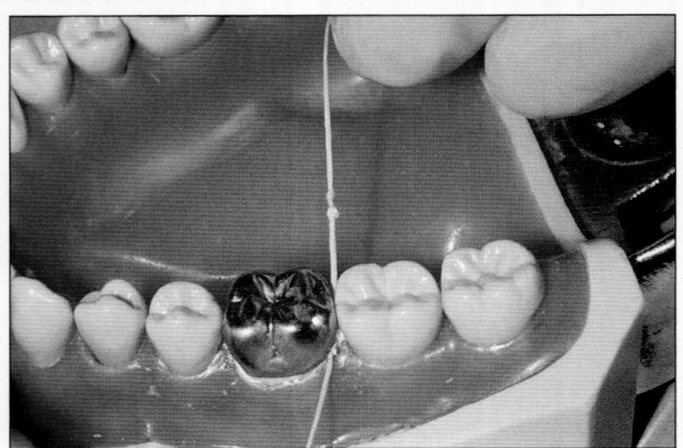

(From Hatrick CS, Eakle WS: *Dental materials: clinical applications for dental assistants and dental hygienists,* ed 3, St. Louis, 2016, Saunders.)

6. Use the air-water syringe and HVE tip to rinse the patient's mouth before dismissal.

DATE	TOOTH	SURFACE	CHARTING NOTES
9/5/18	L	—	Placement of Stainless steel crown, 1 carpule Xylocaine1:100,000 w/o epinephrine. Cotton roll isolation, cemented crown w/Duralon. Pt tolerated procedure well. T. Clark, CDA/L. Stewart, DDS

Chapter Exercises

Multiple Choice

Circle the letter next to the correct answer.

1. The types of procedures provided in a pediatric dental office include __________.
   - a. pulp therapy
   - b. restorative procedures
   - c. preventive procedures
   - d. all of the above
2. The age groups served by a pediatric dental practice include __________.
   - a. infancy through 2 years of age
   - b. 3 through 5 years of age
   - c. 13 through 20 years of age
   - d. all of the above
3. What is unique about the treatment areas of a pediatric practice?
   - a. Dental chairs are isolated from each other.
   - b. More than one dentist will use a dental chair.
   - c. Open-bay concept is present.
   - d. Chairs are situated for the parents to sit in the dental treatment area.
4. At what stage of life does a child first want control and structure of his or her environment?
   - a. Birth to 2 years of age
   - b. 3 through 5 years of age
   - c. 6 through 11 years of age
   - d. 12 through 20 years of age
5. At what phase of orthodontics would a pediatric dentist intercede in getting a patient to stop sucking his or her thumb?
   - a. Interceptive
   - b. Preventive
   - c. Corrective
   - d. Elective
6. Stainless steel crowns are __________.
   - a. considered to be permanent restoration for a primary tooth
   - b. indicated when rampant decay is present
   - c. used for primary molars
   - d. all of the above
7. What endodontic procedure is performed on primary teeth?
   - a. Apicoectomy
   - b. Pulpectomy
   - c. Pulpotomy
   - d. Retrograde
8. What type of matrix system is recommended for primary molars?
   - a. Universal metal band
   - b. T-band
   - c. Mylar matrix
   - d. Palodent
9. The teeth most frequently injured by toddlers are the __________.
   - a. mandibular incisors
   - b. mandibular molars
   - c. maxillary incisors
   - d. maxillary molars
10. A tooth that was knocked completely out of its socket is said to be __________.
    - a. avulsed
    - b. extruded
    - c. exfoliated
    - d. luxated

Apply Your Knowledge

1. Your patient is 3 years old, and you are in the reception area ready to escort him to the treatment area, but the patient begins to cling to his mother. What do you do?
2. You are scheduled to apply sealants to the primary molars of a 5-year-old. Your plan is to use cotton rolls as your moisture control method. You notice that this child has a hard time keeping the cotton roll on the lingual side by the tongue. The cotton roll will not stay in place. Any suggestions on how you can maintain a dry field and still complete the procedure?
3. Dr. Stewart has asked you to take a preliminary impression for a space maintainer. As soon as you try-in the impression tray, the child gags. How do you think the child is going to handle the impression material, and how will you get this impression?
4. An emergency patient has just arrived. A 2-year-old patient has fallen and hit her front tooth. You have been asked to take a periapical radiograph of the area. Describe the best technique for obtaining a radiograph on a young child.

CHAPTER 28

Orthodontics

http://evolve.elsevier.com/Robinson/essentials/

LEARNING OBJECTIVES

1. Pronounce, define, and spell the key terms.
2. Identify the classifications of malocclusion and indications for orthodontic treatment.
3. Describe the types of records used by the orthodontist to make a diagnosis and treatment plan.
4. List and describe the four categories of orthodontic treatment.
5. Identify and describe the function of orthodontic instruments.
6. Describe the components of fixed appliances, attachments, auxiliaries, and arch wires, and demonstrate the following procedures:
   - Place and remove elastomeric ring separators.
   - Assist in the fitting and cementation of orthodontic bands.
   - Assist in the direct bonding of orthodontic brackets.
   - Place arch wires.
   - Place and remove ligature ties.
7. Discuss oral hygiene and dietary instructions, as well as adjustment visits and completed treatments for the orthodontic patient.

KEY TERMS

arch wires
auxiliaries
bands
cephalometric
fixed appliances
headgear
malocclusion
removable appliances
retainer
separator
tipping

Orthodontics is the specialty of dentistry that includes the diagnosis, prevention, interception, and treatment of all forms of malocclusion of the teeth and surrounding structures. (**Malocclusion** is an abnormal or a malpositioned relationship of the maxillary teeth to the mandibular teeth when occluded.)

Types of treatment include straightening teeth that are rotated, tilted, improperly aligned, crowded, or unevenly spaced; correcting bite problems; and surgically aligning the upper and lower jaws.

Angle Classifications of Malocclusion

The system developed by Dr. Edward H. Angle is used to describe and classify occlusion and malocclusion. In this system, the key to understanding the relationship of a person's *bite* is identifying the relationship of the permanent first molars when the patient is in centric occlusion. See Figure 28-1 for further clarification.

Indications for Orthodontic Treatment

Orthodontic treatment may be necessary as a result of any combination of the following conditions:

- Psychosocial influences on patients, such as self-esteem, and negative feelings about their appearance attributable to malocclusion and dental facial deformities
- Oral function, such as chewing problems from malocclusion, jaw discrepancies, speech sounds, and temporomandibular joint pain
- Dental disease, such as dental decay, and periodontal disease affected by malocclusion

Class	Model	Photo	Arch Relationships	Descriptions
Normal occlusion	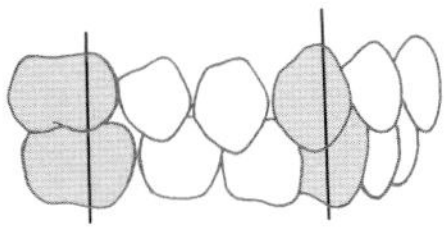	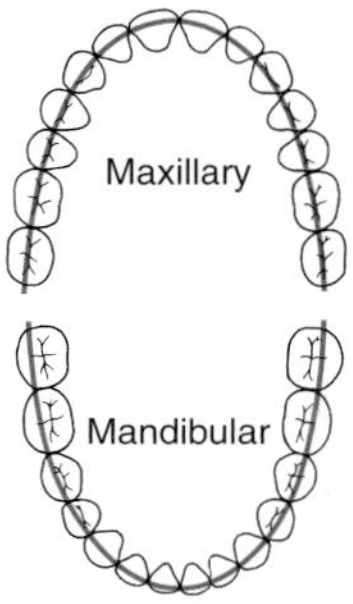 Maxillary Mandibular Line of Occlusion	Molar: MB cusp of the maxillary first molar occludes with the MB groove of the mandibular first molar. Canines: Maxillary canine occludes with the distal half of the mandibular canine and the mesial half of the mandibular first premolar.	No dental malalignments present, such as crowding or spacing.
Class I	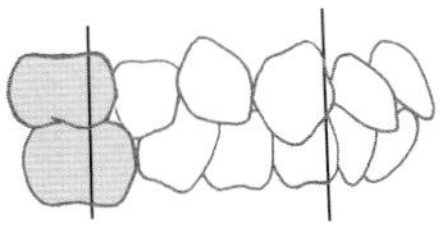	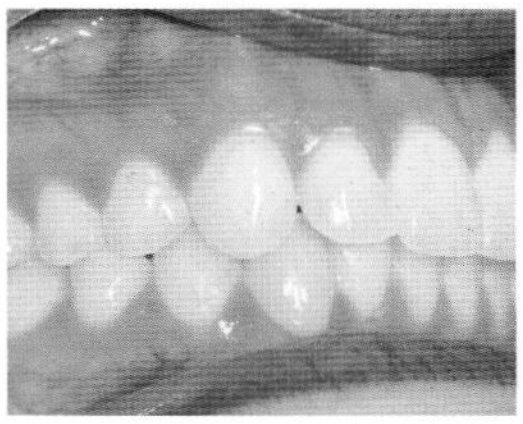	Molar: MB cusp of the maxillary first molar occludes with the MB groove of the mandibular first molar. Canines: Maxillary occludes with the distal half of the mandibular canine and the mesial half of the mandibular first premolar.	If malalignment is present, such as crowding or spacing, this would be referred to as a class I malocclusion.
Class II	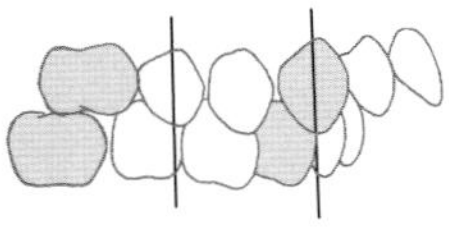 Division 1 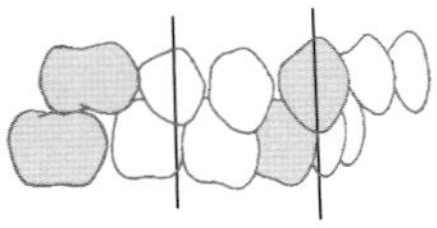 Division 2	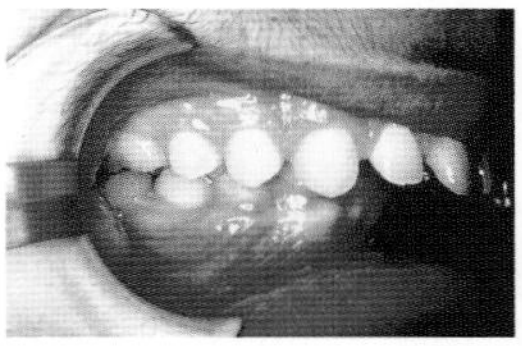	Molar: MB cusp of the maxillary first molar occludes (by more than the width of a premolar) mesial to the MB groove of the mandibular first molar. Canines: Distal surface of the mandibular canine is distal to the mesial surface of the maxillary canine by at least the width of a premolar.	Division 1: Maxillary anteriors protrude facially from the mandibular anteriors, with deep overbite. Retrognathic profile. Division 2: Maxillary central incisors may be upright or retruded, and lateral incisors may be tipped labially or may overlap the central incisors with deep overbite. Mesognathic profile.
Class III	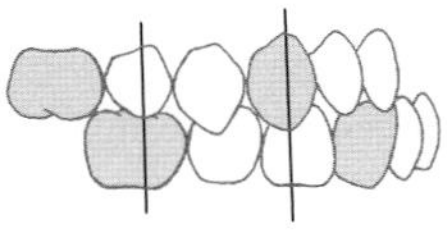	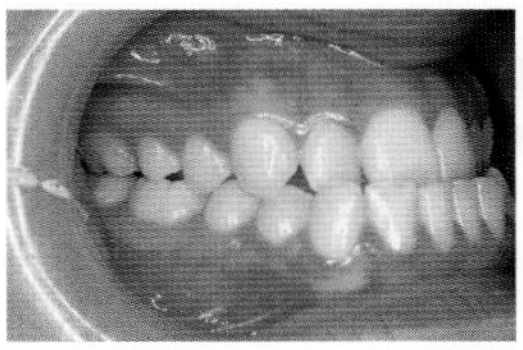	Molar: MB cusp of the maxillary first molar occludes (by more than the width of a premolar) distal to the MB groove of the mandibular first molar. Canines: Distal surface of the mandibular canine is mesial to the mesial surface of the maxillary canine by at least the width of a premolar.	Mandibular incisors in complete cross-bite. Prognathic profile.

MB, Mesiobuccal.
*Note: This system deals with the classification of permanent dentition.

FIGURE 28-1 Angle classification of malocclusion. (Diagrams and format modified from Bath-Balogh M, Fehrenbach MF: *Illustrated dental embryology, histology, and anatomy,* ed 3, St Louis, 2011, Saunders; Darby ML, Walsh MM: *Dental hygiene theory and practice,* ed 4, St Louis, 2015, Saunders; and Bird DL, Robinson DS: *Modern dental assisting,* ed 11, St Louis, 2015, Saunders. Photos from Proffit WR, Fields HW, Sarver DM: *Contemporary orthodontics,* ed 5, St Louis, 2013, Mosby.)

Records Visit and Treatment Planning

The first orthodontic appointment is scheduled to obtain records required by the orthodontist to make a diagnosis and to create a treatment plan. The patient's diagnosis is based on information from three major sources:

1. Interview with the patient and/or the parent or guardian
2. Clinical examination of the patient
3. Evaluation of diagnostic records

Interview Information

Through an interview with the patient and/or the parent or guardian, the orthodontist gathers important information about their desire to improve the appearance and function of their teeth.

Medical and Dental History

A thorough medical and dental history is necessary to provide a comprehensive understanding of the physical condition and to evaluate specific orthodontic-related concerns.

Physical Growth Evaluation

Because orthodontic treatment in children is closely related to growth stages, evaluating the child's physical growth status is necessary. Questions will include how rapidly the child has recently grown, such as a growth spurt, and what signs of sexual maturing are evident.

Social and Behavioral Evaluation

Motivation for seeking treatment is very important. What outcome can the patient and parent or guardian expect as a result of treatment? How cooperative or uncooperative is the patient likely to be? The major motivation for orthodontic treatment for children can be the parent or guardian's desire for treatment; however, the child's willingness and cooperation are essential.

Adults seek orthodontic treatment for themselves for many reasons, including improving personal appearance, correcting the function of their teeth, and also the ability to acquire orthodontic treatment by means of insurance through an employer or self-insurance. Exploring the reasons the patient is seeking treatment at this time is important.

Clinical Examination

The purpose of the orthodontic clinical examination is to document and evaluate the facial aspects, occlusal relationship, and functional characteristics of the jaws. At the records visit, the orthodontist decides which diagnostic records are required for the patient.

Evaluation of Facial Form

Facial form analysis is the visual examination of the face. It provides information that cannot be gathered from dental radiographs and diagnostic casts (Figure 28-2).

Frontal evaluation (from the front)—the orthodontist examines the face to determine:

- Bilateral symmetry
- Size proportions of midline-to-lateral structures
- Vertical proportions

Profile evaluation (from the side)—the orthodontist examines the face in profile to:

- Determine whether the jaws are proportionately positioned
- Evaluate lip protrusion
- Evaluate the vertical facial proportions

Evaluation of Oral Health

A thorough hard and soft tissue examination and an oral hygiene assessment must be completed before orthodontic treatment begins. If problems are detected, then the patient is referred for preventive and restorative treatment before orthodontic treatment is started.

Diagnostic Records

Diagnostic records include photographs, radiographic images, and diagnostic casts that provide data related to tooth angulation, dental crowding, and the presence of unerupted teeth. When possible, having these records available at the time of the clinical examination is best.

Photographs

Photography is useful as an aid in patient identification, treatment planning, case presentation, case documentation, and patient education and instruction.

Extraoral photographs Two standard extraoral photographs are taken: (1) the frontal view, with lips in a relaxed position; and (2) a profile view of the patient's right side, with lips in a relaxed position (Figure 28-3).

Intraoral photographs Three standard intraoral photographs are also required: (1) the full direct view, which includes all teeth in occlusion; (2) the maxillary occlusal view, which includes the palate and all maxillary occlusal surfaces; and (3) the right buccal view, which includes the distal of the canine to the distal of the last molar (Figure 28-4).

Cephalometric Radiographs

A **cephalometric** radiograph is an extraoral radiograph that is exposed from a side view, showing how the major functional skeletal structures of the face are related to each other (Figure 28-5). This type of radiographic image makes it possible for the orthodontist to measure and evaluate dentofacial proportions and to clarify the anatomic basis for a malocclusion.

Diagnostic Casts

Evaluation of the occlusion requires impressions for diagnostic casts and a record of the patient's occlusion, enabling the casts to be articulated. Alginate impressions and diagnostic casts are discussed in further detail in Chapter 22.

For orthodontic purposes, the bases of the diagnostic casts are trimmed to a symmetric shape that is oriented to the midline of the palate, which makes detecting asymmetry within the dental arches easier. The casts are polished to provide a more acceptable case presentation for the patient (Figure 28-6).

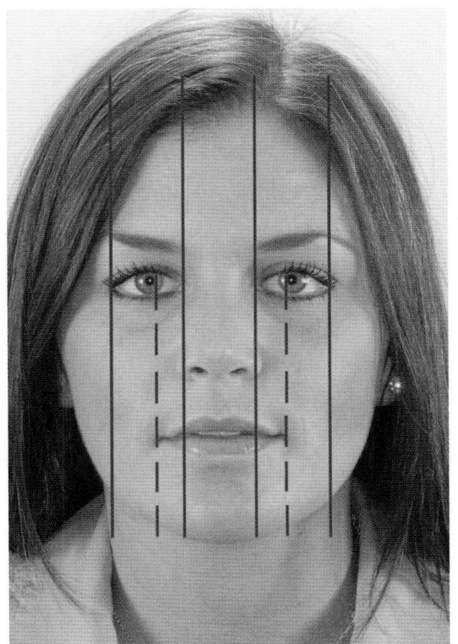

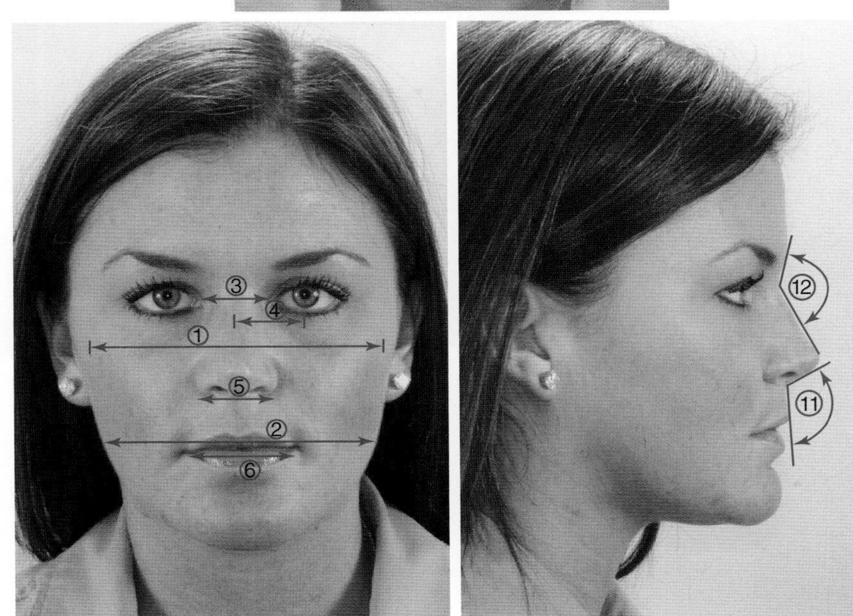

FIGURE 28-2 Facial analysis from frontal and profile views. (From Proffit WR, Fields HW, Sarver DM: *Contemporary orthodontics,* ed 5, St Louis, 2013, Mosby.)

Case Presentation

The orthodontist studies the information gathered and develops a treatment plan and a cost estimate for the patient in preparation for the case presentation.

Approximately 1 hour is reserved for the case presentation visit, and the patient—and parent or responsible adult if the patient is a child—should be present. This presentation includes the approximate length of treatment, the fees involved, and a clear statement of the responsibility of the patient in helping ensure the successful completion of the treatment.

Orthodontic Treatment

Orthodontic treatment can be divided into four broad categories: (1) preventive, (2) limited, (3) interceptive, and (4) comprehensive.

Preventive Orthodontic Treatment

Preventive orthodontic procedures are designed to prevent or minimize the degree of severity of future orthodontic problems. The pediatric or general dentist commonly provides and oversees most of this type of treatment.

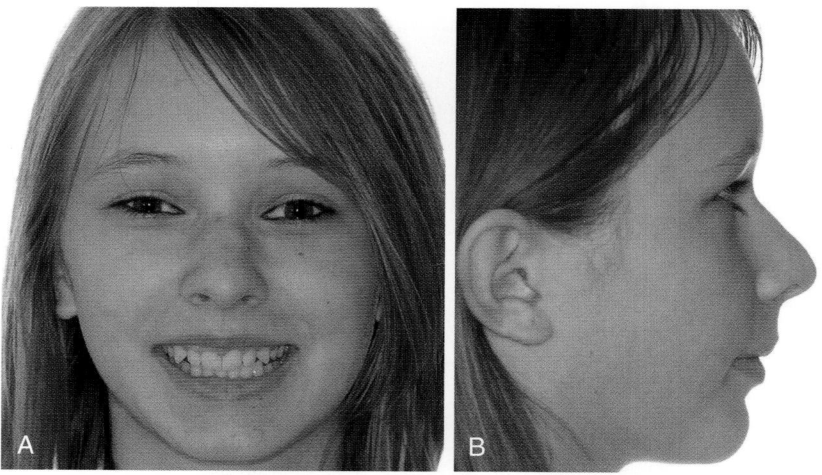

FIGURE 28-3 Extraoral photographs. **A,** Frontal view. **B,** Profile view from the right side. (From Graber LW: *Orthodontics: current principles and techniques,* ed 5, St Louis, 2012, Mosby.)

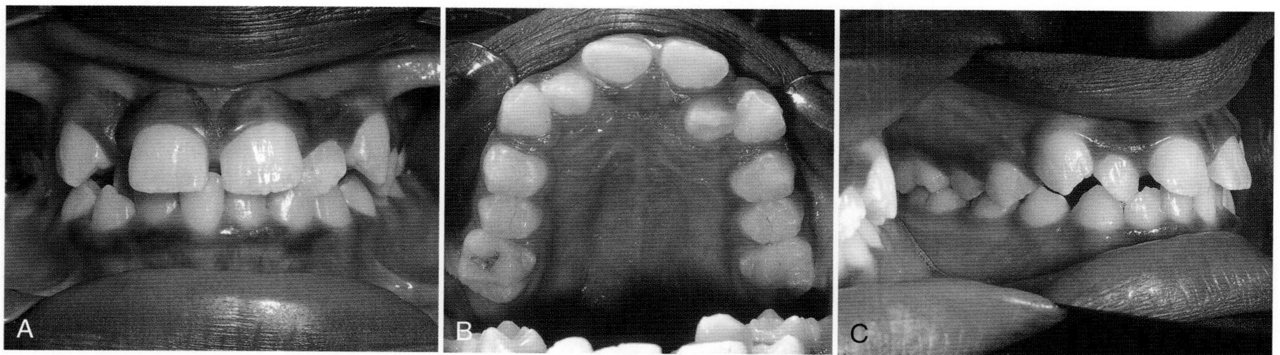

FIGURE 28-4 Intraoral photographs showing a patient's front view in occlusion **(A)**, maxillary occlusal view **(B)**, and right buccal view **(C)**.

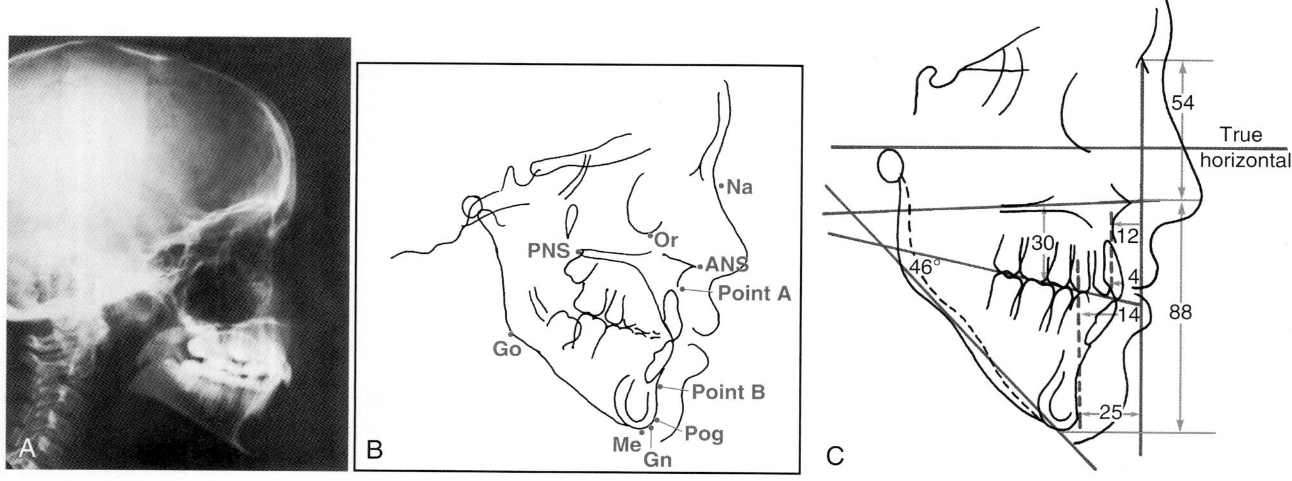

FIGURE 28-5 **A,** Cephalometric radiograph. **B,** Cephalometric landmark and points. *ANS,* Anterior nasal spine; *Gn,* gnathion; *Go,* gonion; *Me,* menton; *Na,* nasion; *Or,* orgitale; *Pog,* pogonion; *Point A,* innermost point on the contour of the premaxilla between the ANS and the incisor; *Point B,* innermost point on the contour of the mandible between the incisor and the bony chin; *PNS,* posterior nasal spine. **C,** Cephalometric analysis. (From Proffit WR, Fields HW, Sarver DM: *Contemporary orthodontics,* ed 5, St Louis, 2013, Mosby.)

Preventive orthodontic treatment includes:

- Care to prevent premature loss of primary teeth
- If a tooth is lost, a space maintainer to save the space for the permanent tooth
- Correction of oral habits, such as thumb sucking, which may affect the development and alignment of the permanent dentition (Thumb sucking is not considered a problem until the permanent teeth are in position.)
- Early detection of developmental factors that may cause malocclusion
- Supervision of the natural exfoliation of the primary teeth (Primary teeth retained too long may cause the permanent teeth to erupt out of alignment or to be impacted.)

Limited Orthodontic Treatment

This category of orthodontic treatment involves an isolated area that would not involve the entire dentition. Examples of this category would be to correct crowding teeth in only one arch, to open a space or to upright a tooth to allow an adjacent tooth to move into the space, and to treat for the closure of one or more spaces.

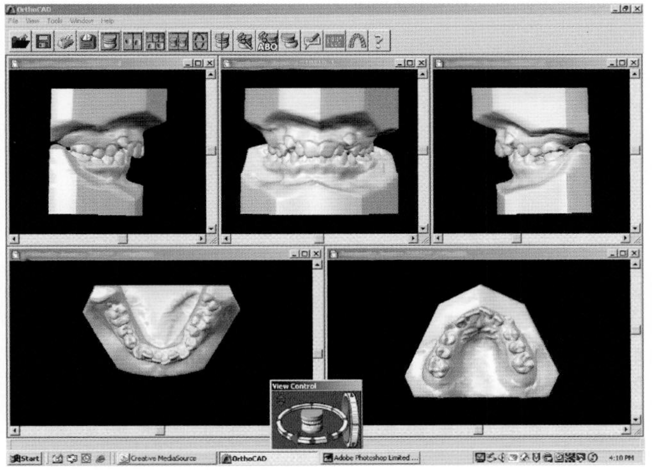

FIGURE 28-6 Diagnostic model. (From Proffit WR, Fields HW, Sarver DM: *Contemporary orthodontics,* ed 5, St Louis, 2013, Mosby.)

Interceptive Orthodontic Treatment

Interceptive treatment is an extension of preventive and/or limited orthodontic treatments but can also include localized tooth movement in an otherwise normal dentition.

Interceptive orthodontic treatment usually occurs in the transitional dentition and may include such procedures as the redirection of a tooth that has erupted out of position, correction of an isolated cross-bite, or recovery of lost space where overall space is not adequate.

Another interceptive step is the serial extraction of primary or permanent teeth to correct critical overcrowding in the arch, which is performed only when more conservative methods of treatment will not be effective. When extractions are required, the orthodontist refers the patient to a general dentist or to an oral and maxillofacial surgeon.

Comprehensive Orthodontic Treatment

Comprehensive orthodontic treatment involves coordinated diagnosis and treatment, leading to an improvement of the patient's craniofacial dysfunction and/or dentofacial deformity, including anatomic, functional, and esthetic relationships. This type of treatment can use fixed or removable orthodontic appliances.

Fixed appliances, commonly known as braces, are bonded to the teeth and assist in tooth movement (Figure 28-7). These appliances are discussed later in this chapter.

Removable appliances, which can be placed and removed by the patient, provide a wide range of uses.

Orthodontic **alignment technique** is an orthodontic **alignment technique** used today for the simple alignment of the teeth. The **Invisalign** is one brand of this technology. The vacuum-formed clear aligner (similar in design and fit to the thermoplastic vacuum–formed tray) is a series of clear *aligners* designed by the computer. The customized aligners are fabricated and worn at 2-week intervals (Figure 28-8). Although not suitable to treat all cases of malocclusion, this alignment system is increasingly the system of choice because of its ease of use.

The other type of removable appliance is the retainer, which is versatile in its use. A retainer is primarily used after comprehensive treatment or in tipping teeth. (**Tipping** is the movement

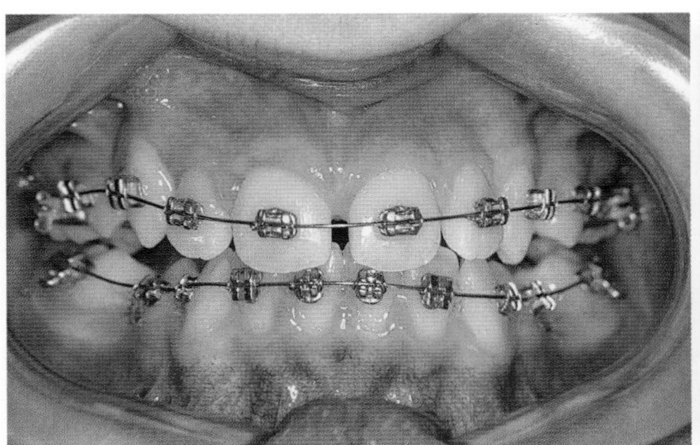

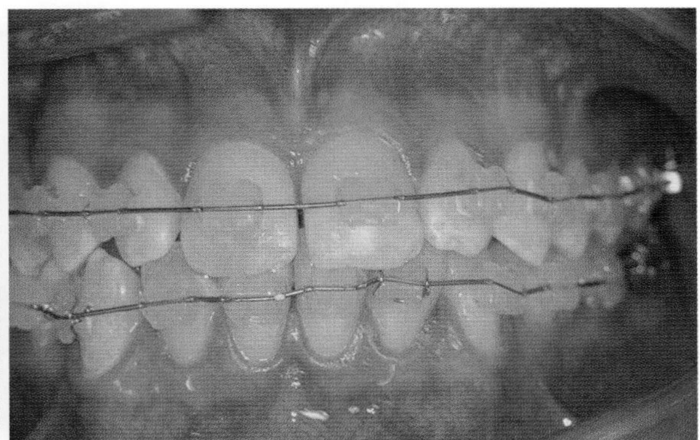

FIGURE 28-7 Full braces. (From Boyd LRB: *Dental instruments: a pocket guide,* ed 5, St Louis, 2015, Saunders.)

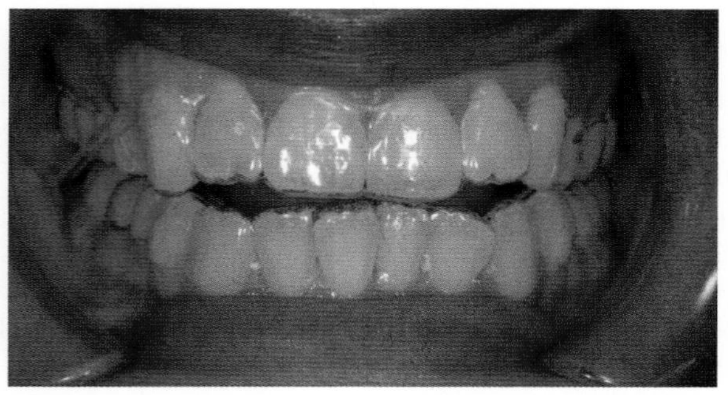

FIGURE 28-8 Invisalign is an alignment system used to correct malocclusion. (From Graber LW: *Orthodontics: current principles and techniques,* ed 5, St Louis, 2012, Mosby.)

of a tooth into a more upright position.) Additional information on retainers is provided later in this chapter.

Instruments for Orthodontics

Orthodontics requires the use of highly specialized instruments. See Table 28-1 for the names of the most common types of orthodontic instruments and their descriptions of use.

Fixed Orthodontic Appliances

Through the use of fixed appliances, a tooth can be moved in six directions: (1) mesially, (2) distally, (3) lingually, (4) facially,

TABLE 28-1
Orthodontic Instruments and Their Uses

Instrument	Description of Use
Orthodontic scaler 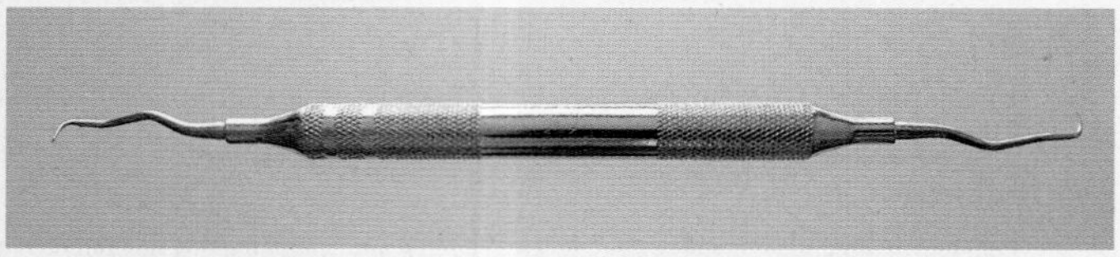 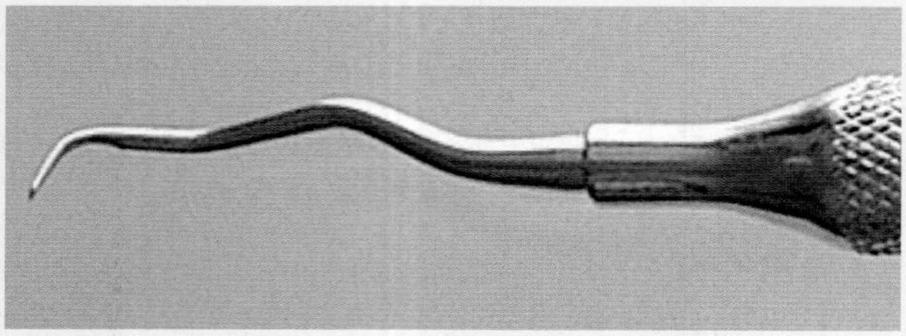	Aids in bracket placement, removal of elastomeric rings, and removal of excess cement or bonding material.
Ligature director 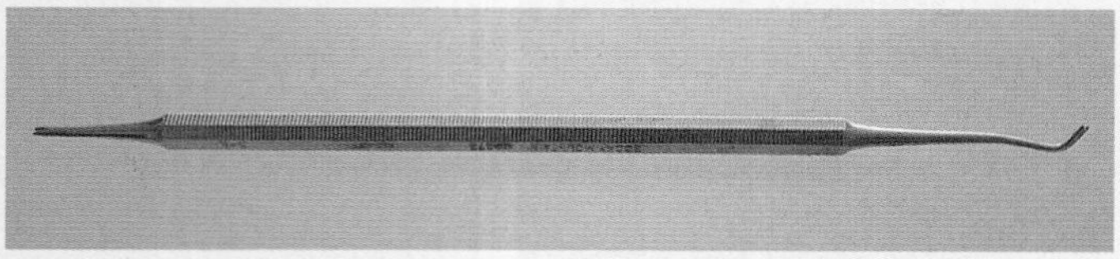 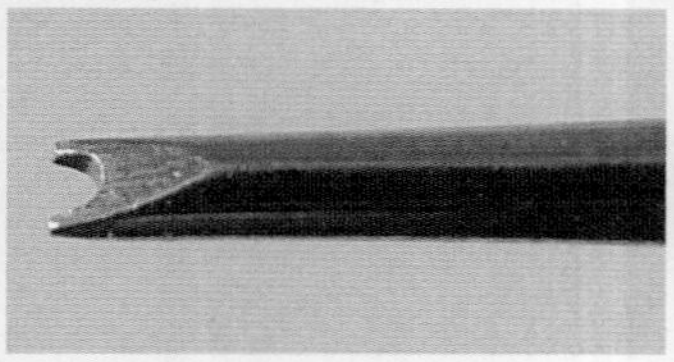 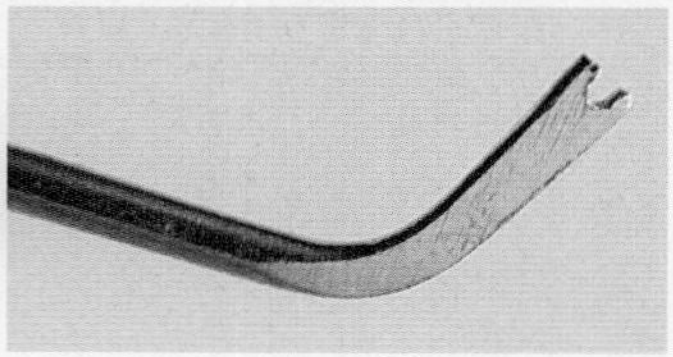	Guides the elastic or wire ligature tie around the bracket. In addition, the operator can guide the cut tie under the arch wire.
Band plugger or pusher 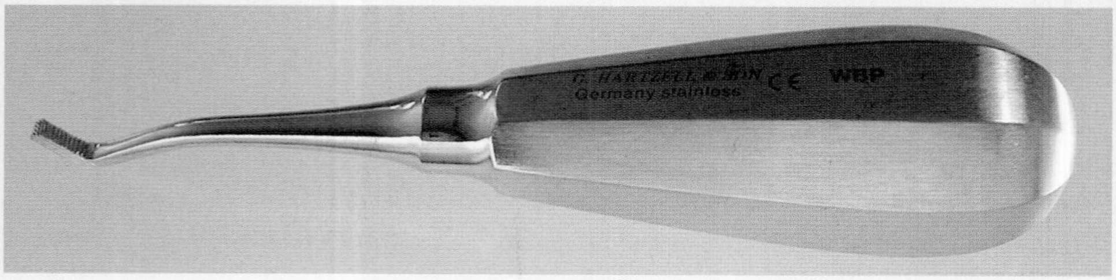	Has a serrated end to help seat maxillary molar bands.

TABLE 28-1
Orthodontic Instruments and Their Uses—cont'd

Instrument	Description of Use
Bite stick 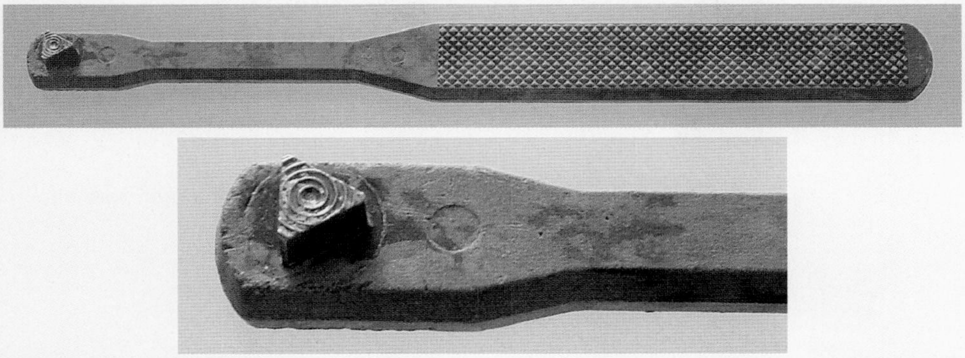	Has a triangular serrated working area to help seat a mandibular molar band.
Bracket placement tweezers 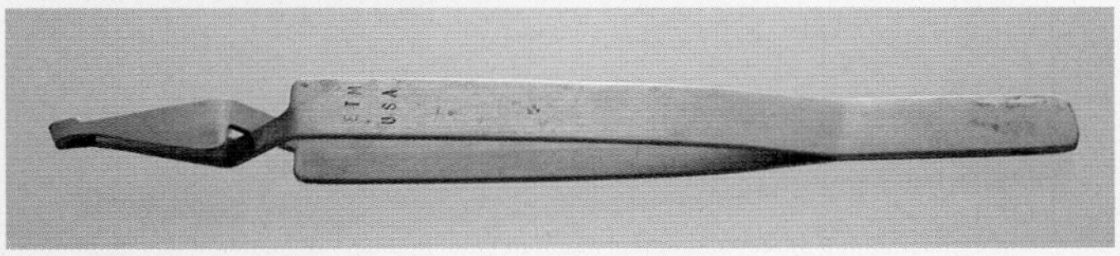	Is a long-tip reverse action tweezers that is used to carry and place the brackets directly on the facial surface of the tooth.
Bird-beak pliers 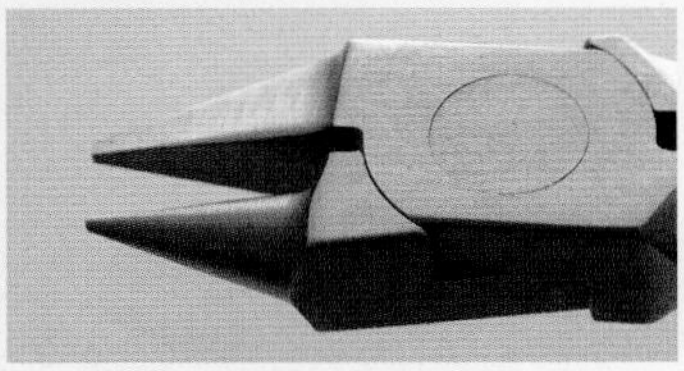	Is useful in forming or bending wires for fixed or removable appliances.
Three-Prong pliers 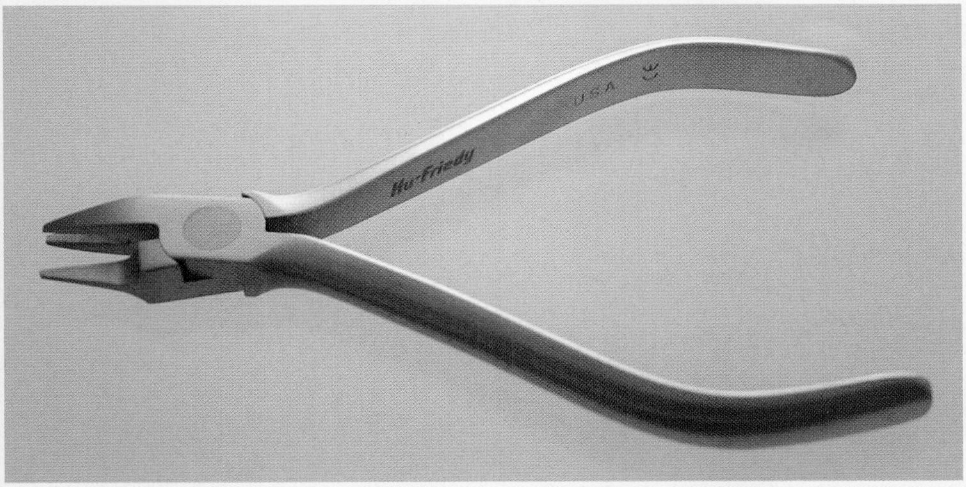	Is used to contour or bend the arch wire for tooth movement.
Distal end cutter 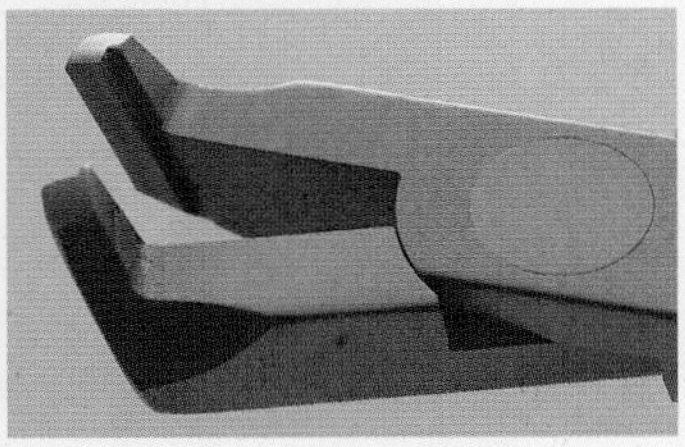	Is used to cut the end of the arch wire once it has been placed in the buccal tube.

Continued

TABLE 28-1
Orthodontic Instruments and Their Uses—cont'd

Instrument	Description of Use
Pin and ligature cutter 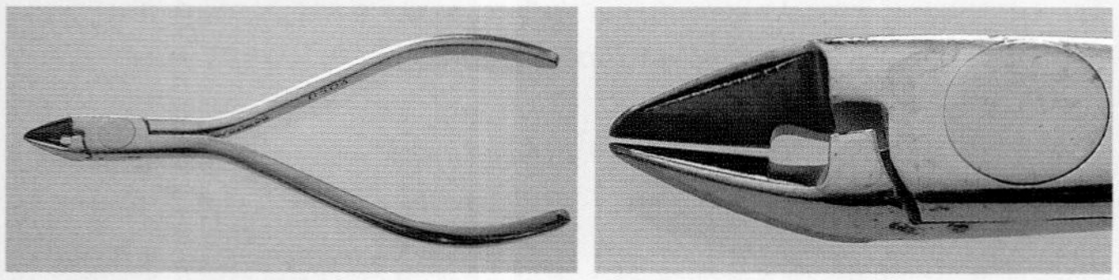	Is used to cut the ligature wire after its placement around the bracket and in the removal of the arch wire.
Weingart utility pliers 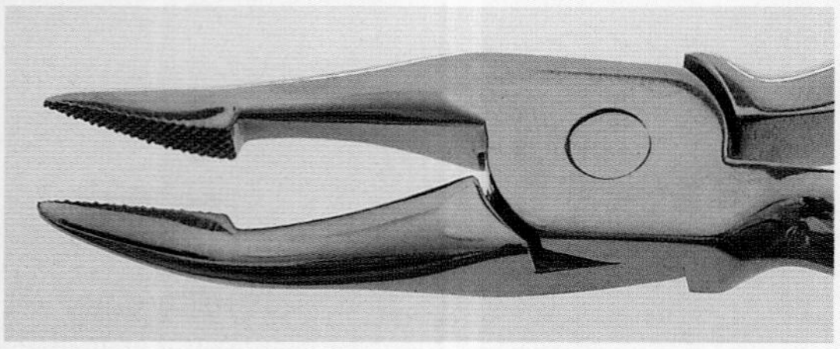	Helps guide the arch wire into the brackets.
Band remover 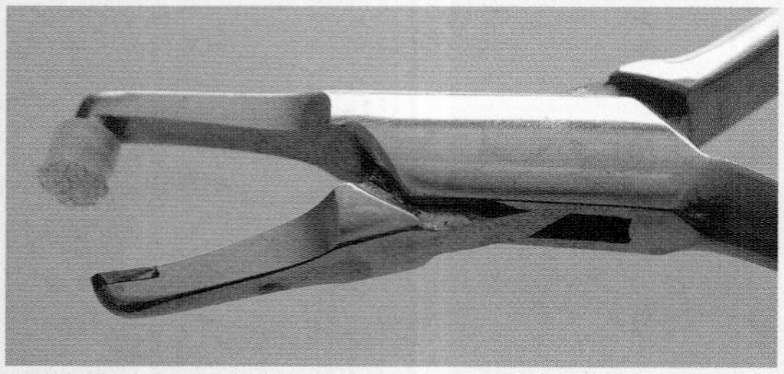	Removes bands without placing stress on the tooth, which would result in discomfort to the patient.
Orthodontic hemostat 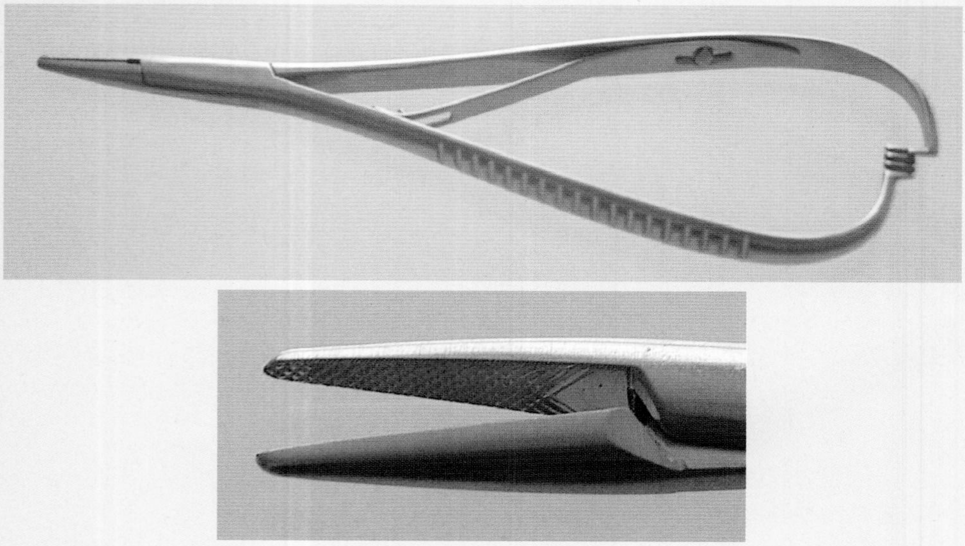	Helps twist the ligature tie around the bracket.

Photographs from Boyd LRB: *Dental instruments: a pocket guide,* ed 5, St Louis, 2015, Saunders.

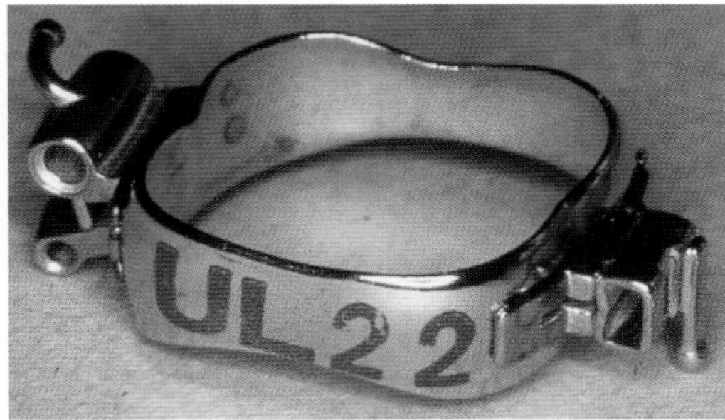

FIGURE 28-9 Molar band showing the attachments of tubes and cleats to hold the arch wire, headgear, and elastics. (From Boyd LRB: *Dental instruments: a pocket guide,* ed 4, St Louis, 2012, Saunders.)

(5) apically, and (6) occlusally. Fixed appliances are also used when rotating (turning) or moving a tooth to the left or right within its socket.

The principle components of fixed appliances are bands, brackets, arch wires, and auxiliaries.

Orthodontic Bands

Bands are preformed stainless steel rings fitted around the teeth and cemented in place. Buttons, tubes, and cleats may also be attached to a band to hold the arch wire and power products. (A **power product** is anything that is elastic and is used to create tooth movement) (Figure 28-9).

Use of Separators Before Banding

Tight interproximal contacts can make it impossible to seat a band properly; therefore the teeth must be separated before fitting and placing the bands. A separator is used for this purpose.

The two items commonly used for separation are steel separating springs and elastomeric separators. Both work on the same principle. A week before the banding appointment, a separator is placed to force the mesial and distal spaces of the tooth slightly apart. By the time of the banding appointment, the required space is present.

See Procedure 28-1: Placing and Removing Elastomeric Ring Separators (Expanded Function).

Selecting Bands

The manufacturer supplies preformed bands of different sizes in a tray. These bands are set up to fit specific teeth (e.g., UL = upper left).

At chairside, bands can be selected by visually inspecting them and by estimating the size of the tooth. The band is removed from the tray with sterile cotton pliers and fitted around the tooth. If a band is tried in the mouth but is not selected, then it must be sterilized before returning it to the tray.

An alternative approach is to select, adapt, and fit the bands on the patient's diagnostic cast. This method eliminates the lengthy process at chairside, and minor alterations can be accomplished at chairside as necessary.

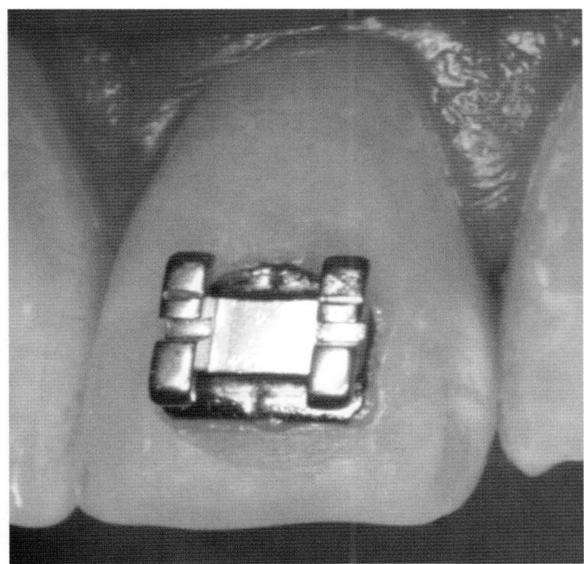

FIGURE 28-10 Example of an edgewise bracket bonded to a central incisor. (From Proffit WR, Fields HW, Sarver DM: *Contemporary orthodontics,* ed 5, St Louis, 2013, Mosby.)

Fitting Maxillary Bands

Initially, a maxillary band is positioned over the tooth using finger pressure on the mesial and distal surfaces. This pressure brings the band down close to the height of the marginal ridges. Then a **band pusher** is used on the mesiobuccal and distolingual edges to push the band into place.

Fitting Mandibular Bands

Initially, a mandibular band is positioned with finger pressure on the proximal surfaces. A **band seater** is placed along the buccal margins, and the patient's biting force is used to seat the band into place.

Cementing Bands

Cementing orthodontic bands is similar to cementing cast restorations; the difference is that the cementation is exclusively to enamel. Glass ionomer or polycarboxylate cement is regularly selected for orthodontic purposes. The consistency of the cement should be slightly thicker than the consistency of the cement for an inlay or a crown, since the escape of excess from the margins of a band is not the same problem as it is from beneath a cast restoration.

See Procedure 28-2: Assisting in the Fitting and Cementation of Orthodontic Bands.

Bonded Brackets

The edgewise bracket is the most universal type of bracket and is attached to a stainless steel backing pad that is bonded to the enamel surface of the tooth. (The term **edgewise** describes a type of bracket.) These brackets are designed with four tie wings; the arch wire is placed in the bracket and ligated (attached) to it (Figure 28-10).

See Procedure 28-3: Assisting in the Direct Bonding of Orthodontic Brackets.

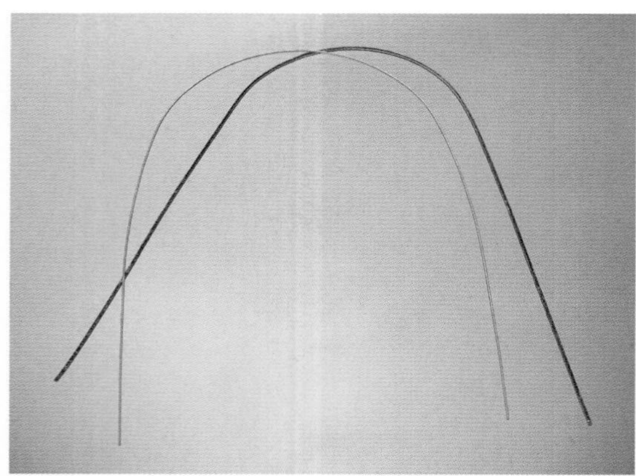

FIGURE 28-11 Example of arch wires. (From Boyd LRB: *Dental instruments: a pocket guide,* ed 5, St Louis, 2015, Saunders.)

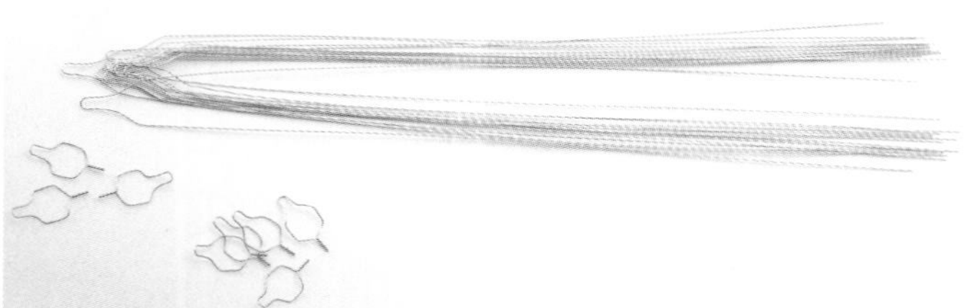

FIGURE 28-12 Ligature wires. (Courtesy DynaFlex, St. Louis, Missouri.)

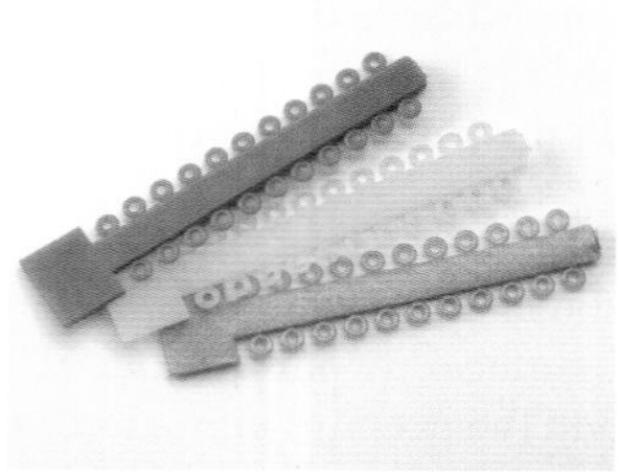

FIGURE 28-13 Elastomeric ties. (Courtesy DynaFlex, St. Louis, Missouri.)

Arch Wires

The arch wire serves as a pattern for correcting the dental arch (Figure 28-11). When the arch wire is attached (ligated), a force is transmitted through the brackets to the teeth. Arch wires are designed to be round, square, or twisted and are available in different gauge sizes. The orthodontist will make the decision regarding which wire to use, based on the stage of treatment and the type of movement required. Bending the arch wire causes the tooth or teeth to move in the desired direction.

See Procedure 28-4: Placing Arch Wires (Expanded Function).

Ligating the Arch Wire

Once the arch wire has been positioned, it must be ligated (tied) to be held in place. The four types of ligature ties are:

1. **Wire ligatures:** Thin wires are twisted around the bracket to hold the arch wire in place (Figure 28-12).
2. **Elastomeric ties:** These ligature ties are made of a plastic or rubberlike material and are available in many colors (Figure 28-13).

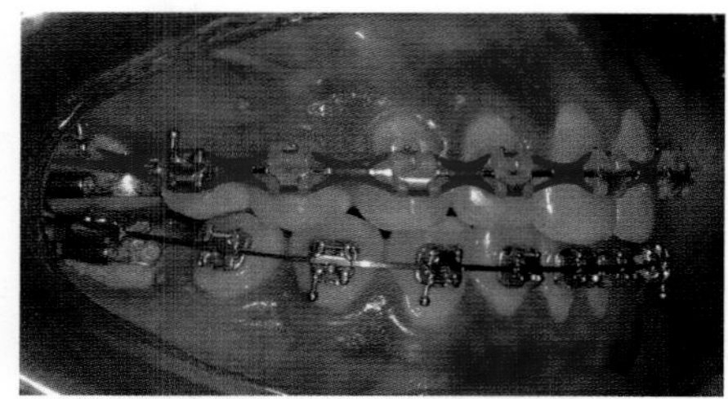

FIGURE 28-14 Elastic chain ties. (From Graber LW: *Orthodontics: current principles and techniques,* ed 5, St Louis, 2012, Mosby.)

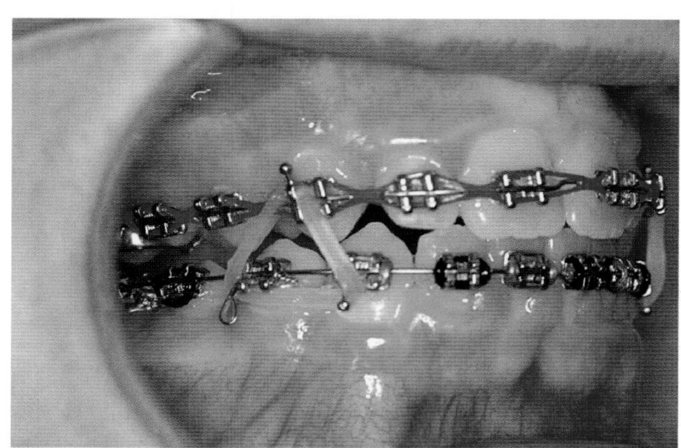

FIGURE 28-15 Elastics. (From Proffit WR, Fields HW, Sarver DM: *Contemporary orthodontics,* ed 5, St Louis, 2013, Mosby.)

3. **Elastic chain ties:** Are continuous, round rings that form a chain. Commonly referred to as Os, elastic chain ties are used to close the space between the teeth or to correct rotated teeth (Figure 28-14).
4. **Continuous wire ties:** Although similar to wire ligatures, continuous wire ties are primarily used to close spaces where two or more teeth are to be ligated (tied) together.

See Procedure 28-5: Placing and Removing Ligature Ties (Expanded Function).

Elastics

Elastics, commonly referred to as rubber bands, are placed between the maxillary and mandibular arches to bring about tooth movement. On the basis of the movement required, the orthodontist determines where and when the elastics are to be placed (Figure 28-15).

The patient is instructed on how to place and remove these elastics and is encouraged to wear them regularly as directed.

Auxiliaries

Auxiliaries are added to the brackets and bands, making it possible to attach the arch wire to the tooth. The combination of these auxiliaries with the arch wire creates the forces required to move the teeth.

Headgear tubes are round tubes commonly placed on maxillary first molar bands. They are used for the insertion of the inner bow of a face-bow appliance.

Edgewise tubes are rectangular tubes gingivally placed to the plane of the main arch wire. These tubes should be present on the facial surfaces of the upper and lower first molars to receive the arch wire.

Labial hooks are hooks located on the facial surfaces of the first and second molar bands for both arches. These hooks hold the interarch elastics.

Lingual arch attachments are cleats or brackets located on the lingual portion of the bands for stabilization of the arch to reinforce anchorage and tooth movement.

Headgear

Another aspect of the treatment phase in fixed appliances is the use of **headgear** to control growth and tooth movement. Headgear is made up of two parts: (1) face bow and (2) traction device (Figure 28-16).

Face Bow

The face bow is used to stabilize or to move the maxillary first molar distally, creating more room in the arch. The intraoral part of the face bow fits into the buccal tubes of the maxillary first molars. The outer part of the bow attaches to the traction device.

Traction Devices

The traction device applies the extraoral force used to achieve the desired treatment results. Four types of traction devices are available: high-pull, cervical, combination, and chin cap.

Oral Hygiene and Dietary Instructions

Oral Hygiene

Orthodontic appliances will harbor areas of food and plaque that can be trapped and hidden, making brushing more difficult. Good oral hygiene during orthodontic treatment is imperative.

If the patient does not properly take care of his or her mouth, then the results can include rampant caries and periodontal disease.

Dietary Instructions

Poor eating habits are an additional concern with patients in orthodontic treatment. The patient should be reminded to use good sense when selecting foods and to avoid those that can weaken or break bands and bonds or bend arch wires.

Examples of foods to be avoided are ice, hard foods such as popcorn and nuts, and sticky foods such as caramel candy and chewing gum.

Adjustment Visits

Throughout active orthodontic treatment, the patient must regularly return for adjustments. At these appointments, the orthodontist reviews the patient's progress and makes adjustments as necessary.

Although these visits are brief, each is extremely important, and the necessity of keeping each appointment should be stressed to the patient.

Checking the Appliance

At each adjustment appointment, the chairside assistant is responsible for examining the patient's appliance and looking for:

- Loose, broken, or missing arch wires or ligature ties
- Loose brackets and bands
- Loose, broken, or missing rubber bands

Bands

Loose bands can result from a break in the cement seal, from poor eating habits, or from the use of elastics, headgear, or other types of power products.

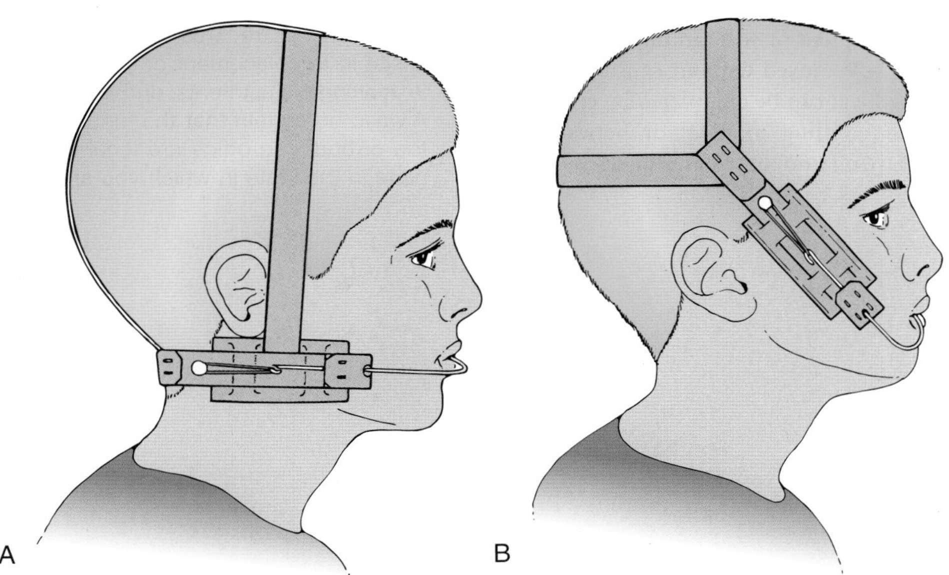

FIGURE 28-16 Headgear. (From Graber LW: *Orthodontics: current principles and techniques,* ed 5, St Louis, 2012, Mosby. Adapted from McNamara, JA Jr., Brudon, WL: *Orthodontics and dentofacial orthopedics.* 2001, Needham Press, Ann Arbor, MI.)

A loose band can be spotted by its appearance. Bands are checked with an explorer or a scaler, and loose bands slide up and down on the tooth. Unless the band has been distorted, it can be cleaned and recemented.

Bonded Brackets

Two primary problems are associated with bonded attachments: (1) an attachment can become loose or come off the surface of the tooth; and (2) on rare occasions, the bracket may break loose from the pad of the bond.

Most bonds are replaced, unless the orthodontist elects to leave the attachment off because it is not necessary for the current phase of treatment.

Arch Wires

Poor eating habits and the patient picking or playing with the appliance can bend the arch wire. Bent or broke wires must be reshaped or replaced.

The patient should be advised to call the office if a problem develops between appointments. The orthodontist should promptly make repairs without waiting for the regular adjustment appointment.

When checking for bends in the arch wire, the assistant also looks for broken wires. Some breaks are hard to see. A tooth that moves out of alignment or a complaint of a sore tooth can be an indication of a problem; it should be investigated.

Completed Treatment

Once the patient has completed the treatment phase of orthodontics, the bands and bonded attachments are removed.

Bands are removed with band-removing pliers. The cushioned tip of the pliers is placed on the distobuccal cusp, and the blade edge of the pliers is used against the buccogingival margin of the band. Then the band is gently lifted upward. If necessary, this process is repeated on the mesial and lingual aspects. Any cement left on the teeth after debanding can be easily removed by scaling with a hand instrument or with an ultrasonic scaler.

Bonded brackets must be removed without causing damage to the enamel surface. Removal can be completed by creating a fracture within the resin bonding material or between the bracket and the resin and then removing the residual resin from the enamel surface.

Retention

Although a patient may believe that his or her treatment is complete when the fixed appliances are removed, an important stage in orthodontic treatment lies ahead. If excellent long-term results are to be achieved, then orthodontic control of tooth position and occlusal relationships must be gradually, not abruptly, withdrawn. Retention is necessary to:

- Allow gingival and periodontal tissues the required time to heal from changes that occurred during treatment.
- Support the teeth that are in an unstable position to ensure that pressure from the cheeks and tongue does not cause a relapse.
- Control changes caused by growth.

The **positioner** is a custom appliance made of rubber or pliable acrylic that fits over the patient's dentition after orthodontic treatment. The positioner is designed to retain the teeth in their desired position and to permit the alveolus to rebuild support around the teeth before the patient wears a retainer.

The **retainer** is the most commonly placed appliance after fixed orthodontics. It is worn to passively retain the teeth in their new position after removal of the orthodontic bands. The retainer also encourages some tooth movement to close band spaces and provides control of the incisors.

Ethical Implications

As a chairside assistant in an orthodontic practice, you must realize the importance of your role in the care of a patient's treatment. You may see one patient on a regular basis for 2 years. The accomplishments of the dental team in the orthodontic office for a patient can change a person's perception of his or her own dental function and dental appearance.

The assistant's role in this specialty is to prepare all of the diagnostic records for the orthodontist, as well as to assist in the placement of fixed orthodontics and to assist in making adjustments during the many visits thereafter. Always be certain that the functions you are performing in the orthodontic office are legal functions for you to complete in the state in which you are practicing.

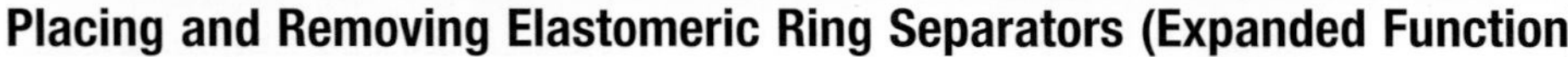

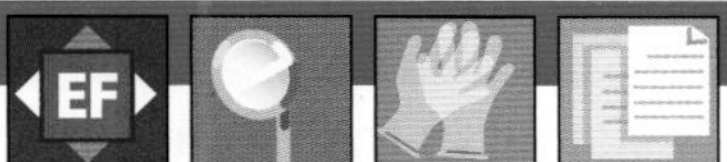

Procedure 28-1

Placing and Removing Elastomeric Ring Separators (Expanded Function)

Equipment and Supplies

- Elastomeric separators
- Separating pliers
- Floss
- Orthodontic scaler

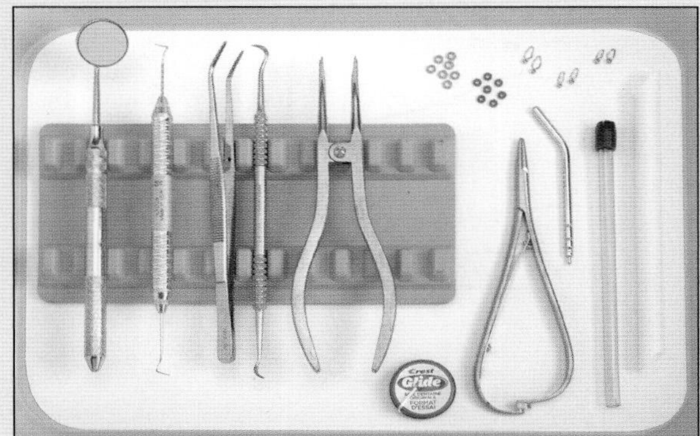

(From Boyd LRB: *Dental instruments: a pocket guide,* ed 5, St Louis, 2015, Saunders.)

Procedural Steps

Placing Elastomeric Ring Separators

1. Place the separator over the beaks of separating pliers.
2. Stretch the ring, and then use a see-saw motion to push it gently through the contact.

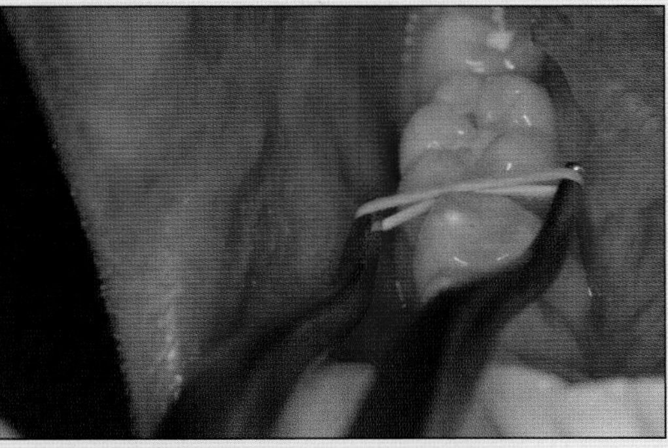

(From Proffit WR, Fields HW, Sarver DM: *Contemporary orthodontics,* ed 5, St Louis, 2013, Mosby.)

3. An alternative method is to use two loops of dental floss to stretch the ring and to guide it into place.

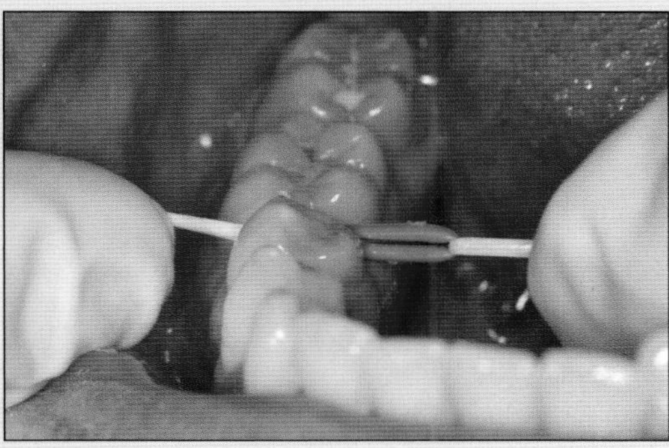

(From Proffit WR, Fields HW, Sarver DM: *Contemporary orthodontics,* ed 5, St Louis, 2013, Mosby.)

4. This type of separator can be left in place for up to 2 weeks.

Removing Elastomeric Ring Separators

1. Slide an orthodontic scaler into the doughnut-shaped separator.
2. Use slight pressure to remove the ring from under the contact.

Procedure 28-2

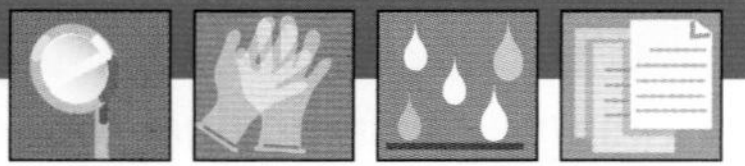

Assisting in the Fitting and Cementation of Orthodontic Bands

Equipment and Supplies

- Basic setup
- Preselected orthodontic bands
- Chilled glass slab
- Spatula (stainless steel)
- Gauze sponges
- Band pusher
- Band seater
- Scaler
- Band remover
- Contouring pliers
- Isopropyl alcohol
- Masking tape
- ChapStick or utility wax
- Selected cement

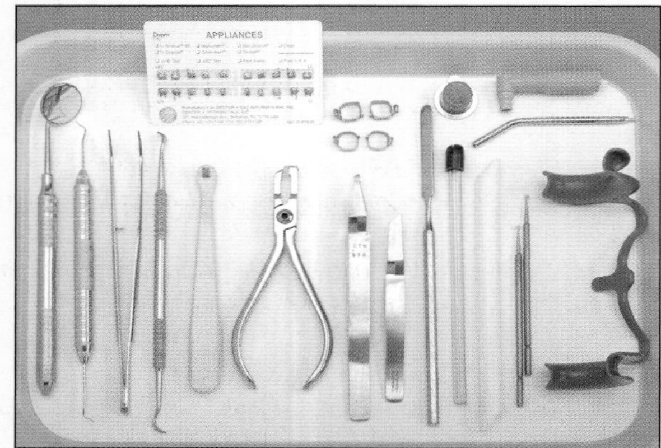

(From Boyd LRB: *Dental instruments: a pocket guide,* ed 5, St Louis, 2015, Saunders.)

Procedural Steps

Preparation

1. Place each preselected orthodontic band on a small square of masking tape with the occlusal surface on the tape and the gingival margin of the band upright.

Purpose: This step keeps the bands in order and prevents the cement from flowing out of the other side.

2. Wipe any buccal tubes or attachments with ChapStick or utility wax.

Purpose: This step prevents the cement from getting into or around these areas.

Mixing and Placing the Cement

1. The teeth are isolated and dried.
2. At a signal from the orthodontist, dispense the cement according to the manufacturer's directions; then quickly mix the cement until it is homogeneous.
3. Hold the band by the margin of the masking tape. The gingival surface is upright, and the cement spatula is placed on the margin of the band.
4. Wipe the spatula over the margin, allowing the cement to flow into the circumference of the band.

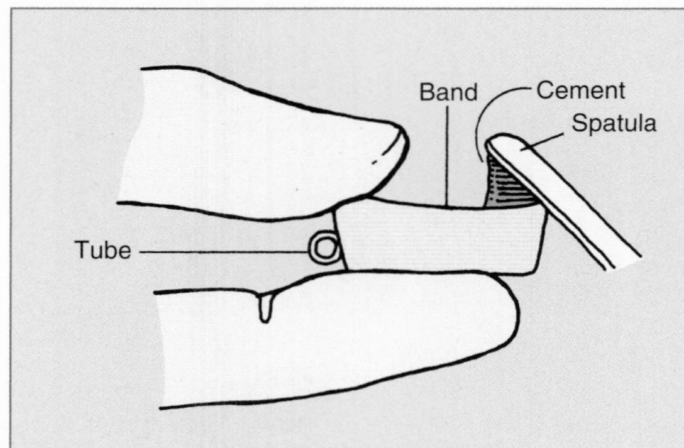

5. Transfer the cement-filled band to the orthodontist, who inverts the band over the tooth.
6. Transfer the band seater. The orthodontist places it on the buccal margin of the band.
7. The patient is instructed to bite gently on the band. This action forces the band down onto approximately the middle third of the tooth crown.
8. Excess cement is forced out from under the gingival and occlusal margins of the bands and is allowed to harden.
9. This process is repeated until all of the bands have been seated.

Removing Excess Cement

1. After the cement has reached its final stage of setting, a scaler or an explorer is used to remove excess cement from the enamel surfaces.
2. The patient's mouth is rinsed, flossed, and checked to ensure that all of the excess cement has been removed.

DATE	TOOTH	SURFACE	CHARTING NOTES
9/6/17	—	—	Upper and lower bands cemented w/glass ionomer on first molars, UR-22, UL-24, LL-21, LR-22. Schedule for bonding. T. Clark, CDA/L. Stewart, DDS

Procedure 28-3

Assisting in the Direct Bonding of Orthodontic Brackets

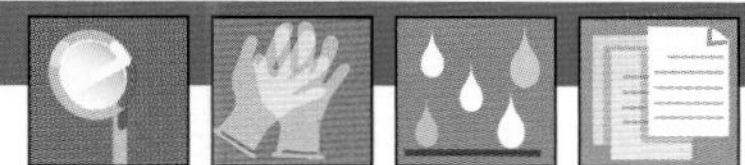

Equipment and Supplies

- Brackets (type specified by the orthodontist)
- Cotton rolls or lip retractors
- Prophy cup
- Pumice
- Bonding setup
- Bracket placement tweezers
- Orthodontic scaler

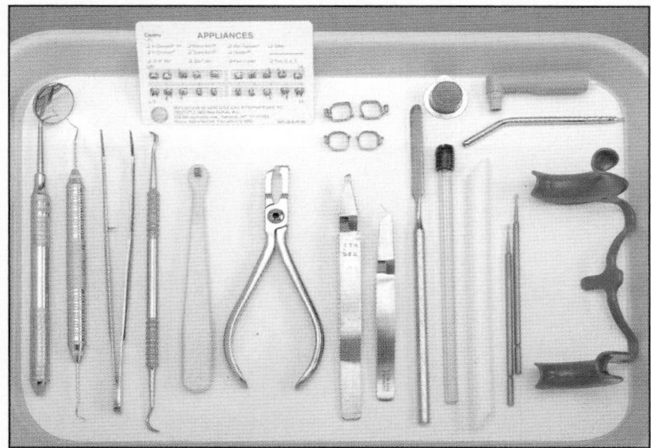

(From Boyd LRB: *Dental instruments: a pocket guide,* ed 5, St Louis, 2015, Saunders.)

Procedural Steps

Preparing the Teeth

1. The tooth surface must be cleaned with a prophy cup and pumice slurry and then rinsed and dried.
2. Use cotton rolls or retractors to isolate the teeth.
3. An etchant gel is placed on the facial area of the tooth that is to receive the bonding agent. This gel remains on the tooth for the manufacturer's specified time and then is rinsed and thoroughly dried.

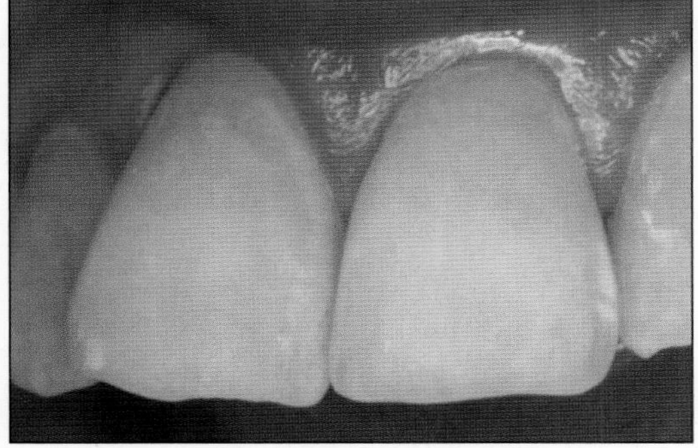

(From Proffit WR, Fields HW, Sarver DM: *Contemporary orthodontics,* ed 5, St Louis, 2013, Mosby.)

Bonding the Brackets

1. The orthodontist applies a liquid sealant, usually the monomer of the bonding agent, to the prepared tooth surface.
2. Mix a small quantity of bonding material, and place it on the back of the bracket. Bracket placement tweezers are used to transfer the bracket to the orthodontist.

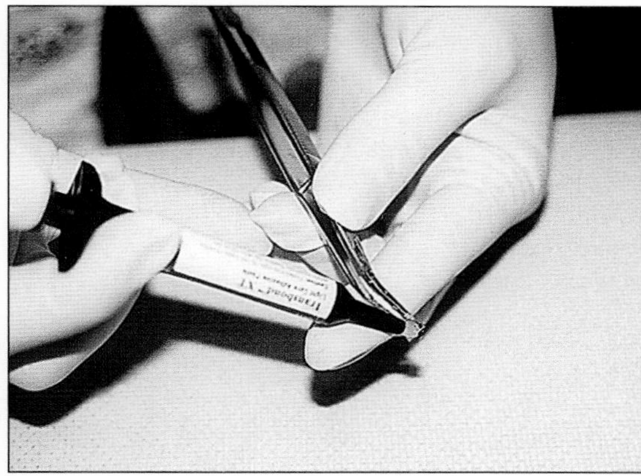

3. Transfer the orthodontic scaler. The orthodontist will place the bracket and move it into its final position with a scaler.
4. The orthodontist uses the scaler to remove the excess bonding material immediately before light-curing the material.

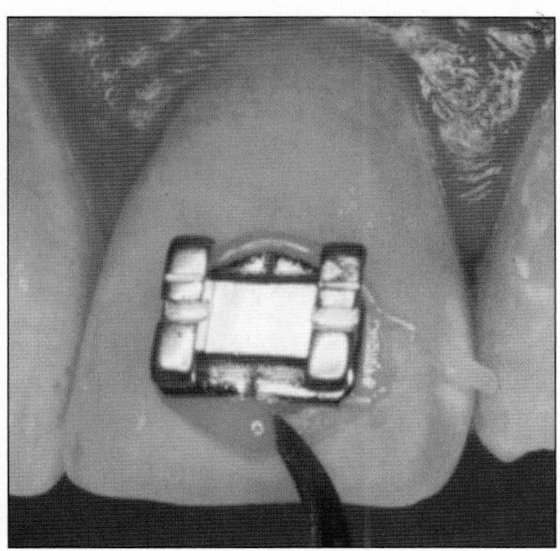

(From Proffit WR, Fields HW, Sarver DM: *Contemporary orthodontics,* ed 5, St Louis, 2013, Mosby.)

DATE	TOOTH	SURFACE	CHARTING NOTES
9/7/17	—	—	Edgewise brackets bonded on maxillary 5-1/1-5 and mandibular 4-1/1-4. Light arch wire placed. T. Clark, CDA/L. Stewart, DDS

Procedure 28-4

Placing Arch Wires (Expanded Function)

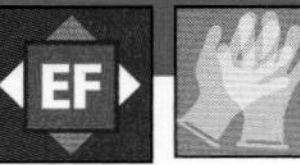

Prerequisites for Performing this Procedure

- Mirror skills
- Operator positioning
- Dental anatomy
- Instrumentation
- Fulcrum

Equipment and Supplies

- Preformed arch wires
- Patient's diagnostic casts (or previously used arch wire)
- Weingart pliers
- Bird-beak pliers
- Torquing pliers
- Distal end cutter

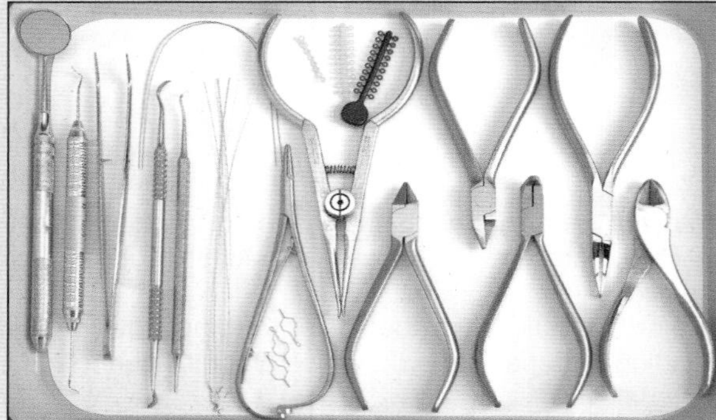

(From Boyd LRB: *Dental instruments: a pocket guide,* ed 5, St Louis, 2015, Saunders.)

Procedural Steps

Measuring the Arch Wire

1. Preformed wires are measured before they are placed in the mouth. The wire should be long enough to extend past the end of the buccal tube on the molar band but not so long that it injures the patient's tissues.
2. Measure the wire by trying it on the patient's diagnostic model or by holding it against the arch wire that is being replaced.
3. If the orthodontist has to place any bends in the wire, then additional wire must be allowed for the length.

Positioning the Arch Wire

1. Locate the mark at the center of the arch wire.

Purpose: This location indicates the midline or the center of the arch form.

2. Position the wire in the mouth with the mark between the central incisors.

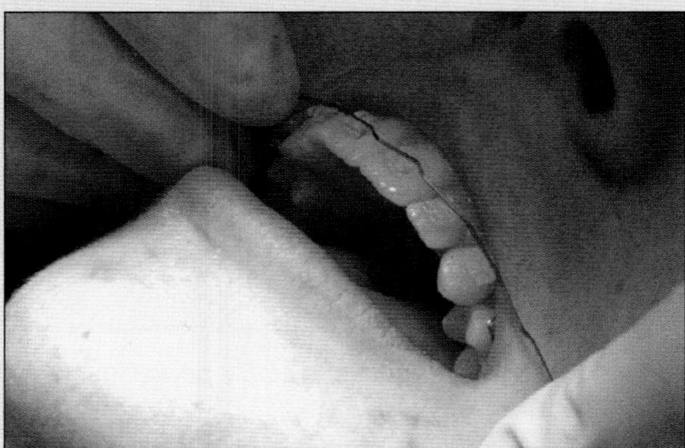

(From Proffit WR, Fields HW, Sarver DM: *Contemporary orthodontics,* ed 5, St Louis, 2013, Mosby.)

3. Place the arch wire in the main arch wire slot of the buccal tube.
4. Use the Weingart pliers to slide the wire in on either side of the arch and to position the wire within the bracket slots.
5. Check the distal ends to determine whether they are securely positioned or are too long or too short.

Procedure 28-5

Placing and Removing Ligature Ties (Expanded Function)

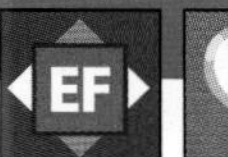

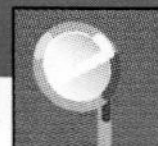
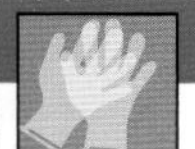

Equipment and Supplies

- Ligature ties
- Ligature director
- Hemostat
- Ligature cutter

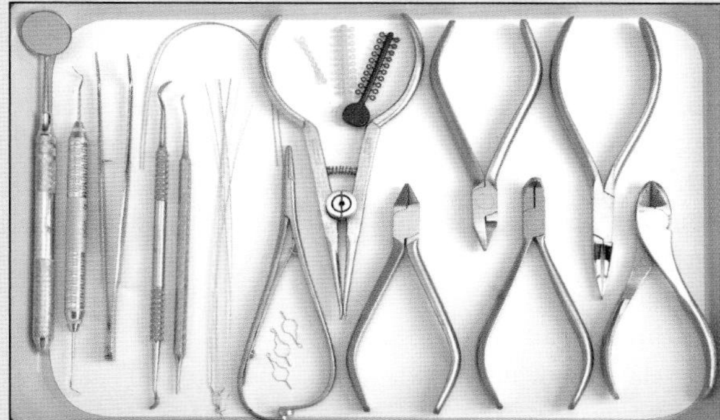

(From Boyd LRB: *Dental instruments: a pocket guide,* ed 5, St Louis, 2015, Saunders.)

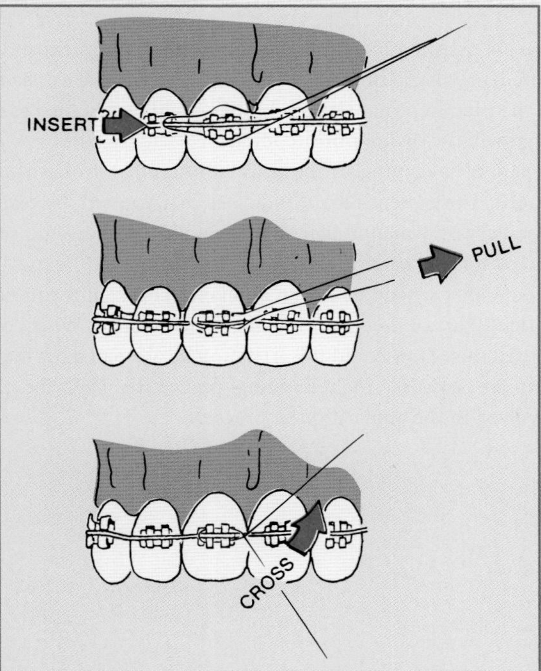

Placing Wire Ligatures

1. Holding the ligature between the thumb and the index finger, slide the wire between these fingers so that only the section that wraps around the bracket is exposed. Make sure to work toward the midline.
2. Slide the ligature around the bracket, using the ligature director to push the wire against the tie wing.
3. Twist together the ends of the ligature. Place the hemostat approximately 3 to 5 mm from the bracket, and snugly twist the wire against the bracket.

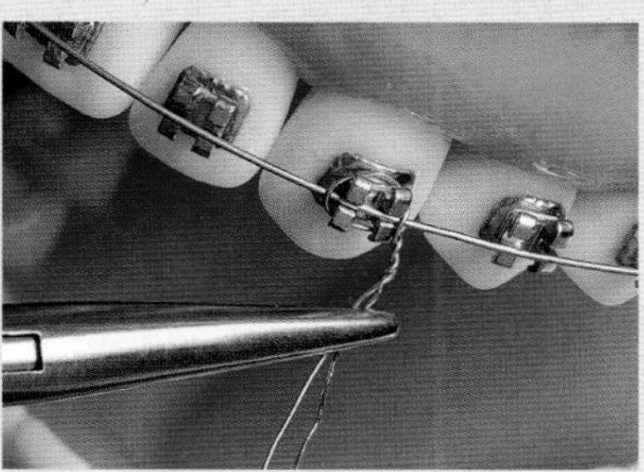

(From Boyd LRB: *Dental instruments: a pocket guide,* ed 5, St Louis, 2015, Saunders.)

4. After all teeth have been ligated, use a ligature cutter to remove the excess wire, leaving a 4- to 5-mm pigtail.

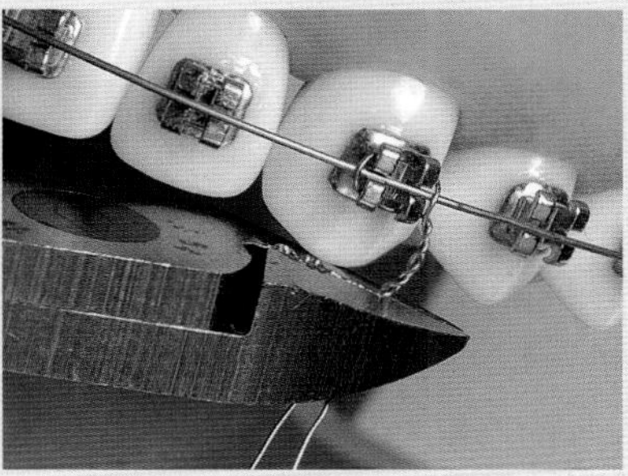

(From Boyd LRB: *Dental instruments: a pocket guide,* ed 5, St Louis, 2015, Saunders.)

5. Use the ligature director to tuck the pigtails under the arch wire toward the gingiva at the interproximal space.

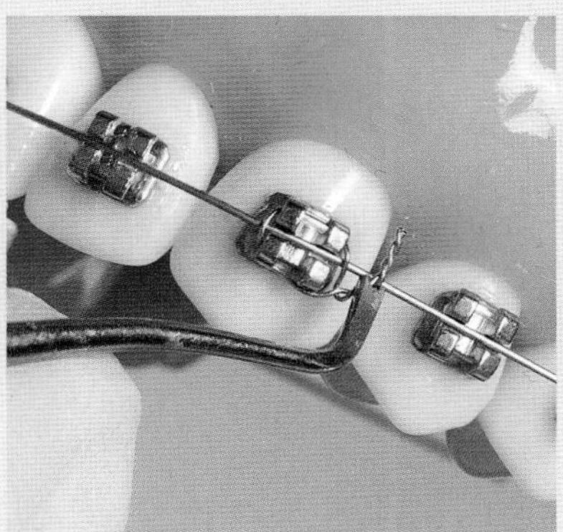

(From Boyd LRB: *Dental instruments: a pocket guide,* ed 5, St Louis, 2015, Saunders.)

6. Repeat this procedure until all ligatures have been cut and tucked away.
7. Run a finger along the arch to ensure that there are no protruding wires that could injure the patient.

Removing Ligature Ties

1. Using the ligature cutter, place the beaks of the pliers at the end of the twisted wire and snip it off; make sure to hold on to the cut portion.
2. Carefully remove a portion of the wire.
3. Do not twist or pull as you cut and remove the ligatures.

Chapter Exercises

Multiple Choice

Circle the letter next to the correct answer.

1. In the definition of Angle classification, a prognathic profile would be viewed in a Class __________ malocclusion.
   - a. I
   - b. II
   - c. III
2. Indications for orthodontic treatment include __________.
   - a. psychosocial influences
   - b. oral function
   - c. dental disease
   - d. all of the above
3. The arch wire serves as a(n) __________.
   - a. pattern that gives the dental arch its shape
   - b. attachment to labial hooks
   - c. item directly bonded to the teeth
   - d. a and b
4. Ligature ties are twisted and tightened around a bracket with the use of a(n) __________.
   - a. bird-beak pliers
   - b. explorer
   - c. hemostat
   - d. scaler
5. Dentofacial proportions are most effectively evaluated on a __________ radiographic image.
   - a. cephalometric
   - b. panoramic
   - c. periapical
6. Using orthodontic separators is necessary for the placement of __________.
   - a. arch wires
   - b. bands
   - c. bonded brackets
   - d. ligatures
7. The patient should be educated on __________ when wearing braces.
   - a. oral hygiene procedures
   - b. speech patterns
   - c. dietary instructions
   - d. a and c
8. To determine the correct length of an arch wire, it can be measured __________.
   - a. on the radiograph
   - b. in the patient's mouth
   - c. on the patient's diagnostic casts
   - d. b or c
9. In preparation of the facial surface of teeth for bonding of the brackets, __________.
   - a. a preliminary impression is taken
   - b. the teeth are isolated using cotton rolls or retractors
   - c. the teeth are cleaned with a prophy cup and pumice
   - d. b and c
10. Buccal tubes on molar bands are designed to hold the __________ securely.
    - a. main arch wire
    - b. brass separators
    - c. elastomeric ligatures
    - d. headgear

Apply Your Knowledge

1. You are assisting in a records appointment. As an expanded function dental assistant (EFDA) or a registered dental assistant (RDA) in the practice, what responsibilities could be assigned to you, and what will the orthodontist complete?
2. A patient is coming to the orthodontic office to have separators placed. The patient record indicates that you will be banding the maxillary and mandibular first molars. Where are the separators placed for this patient?
3. A patient is scheduled for an appliance check, and you notice the patient's buccal mucosa is inflamed and irritated. What could have caused this? How could this irritation be alleviated for the patient?
4. You are assisting in a bonding procedure. Describe the steps involved in the application of brackets.

PART TEN Preparation for Employment

CHAPTER 29

The Job Search

http://evolve.elsevier.com/Robinson/essentials/

LEARNING OBJECTIVES

1. Pronounce, define, and spell the key terms.
2. Determine your personal career goals.
3. Identify the types of employment opportunities for the dental assistant.
4. Complete the following related to the job search:
   - List several sources for employment leads.
   - Name three social media sites.
   - Identify the social media site that is the most used by professionals.
5. Prepare a resume, cover letter, and job application form.
6. Describe techniques for a successful job interview and prepare a follow-up letter.
7. Describe methods of negotiating salaries and benefits.
8. Discuss the steps for terminating employment.

KEY TERMS

career	follow-up letter	resume
cover letter	interview	social media
Facebook	LinkedIn	Twitter

A **career** in dental assisting offers many exciting employment opportunities in a variety of settings. Your knowledge, skills, and credentials enable you to select a position in which you will be recognized as a valuable member of the dental health care team.

Personal and Professional Goals

Before beginning your search for employment, determine your own realistic personal needs and professional goals. Will you be living at home? Will you have roommates? What about transportation? Figure your basic living expenses so that you do not say "yes" to a position and then find yourself in debt. Ask yourself, "What is important to me in a job?" "What type of career do I want?" Then you can establish concrete career goals that focus on your talents and accomplishments (Box 29-1).

Career Opportunities

Private Practice

Private practice in general dentistry or in a specialty practice can provide an opportunity for you to gain experience at chairside, in the business office, and in the dental laboratory. Many dental assistants find great personal pride and fulfillment by joining a private practice. In addition, they enjoy developing a close rapport with the patients and with other members of the dental team.

Insurance Company

If you think you might enjoy a challenging career in business and administration, then consider working for a dental insurance company. Dental insurance companies are continually looking for talented dental assistants with knowledge of the

BOX 29-1 What Is Important to You in a Job

Rank the following job characteristics in order of importance to you, and use them as a guide when you are seeking employment:

- Set working hours
- Flexible working hours
- No need to relocate
- Pleasant coworkers
- Responsibilities
- Attractive office
- Informal work environment
- More formal work environment
- Job security
- Type of practice
- Vacation time
- Sick leave
- Profit sharing
- Child care allowance
- Good salary
- Distance from home
- Medical and dental insurance
- Retirement plan
- Vision plan
- Excellent infection control
- Written job description
- Involvement in planning
- Recognition for your work
- Understanding of personal problems
- Paid continuing education
- Holidays
- Dues to professional organization

processing of insurance claims and customer service. These companies will train you in the specifics of their own operation.

Sales Representative

If you enjoy sales and traveling, then you might find a rewarding career as a representative for a dental manufacturing or supply company. These positions often include travel opportunities, entertaining, commissions, and bonuses. Other opportunities with dental manufacturers involve the areas of research and development.

Public Health and Government Programs

Public health and other government-supported dental facilities function at the federal, state, and local levels. Dental public health programs promote dental health through organized community efforts. Dental assistants may be employed in programs in which dental services are provided at no cost or at a minimal cost to patients who are eligible to receive care. Public health practices almost always involve a team effort with other professionals such as physicians, nurses, social workers, and nutritionists.

Dental Schools

Dental assistants with a business or clinical background can be employed at a dental school. An assistant would be an asset to the faculty and to the dental students in many areas in a school. Employment in a dental school provides the assistant with the stimulation of working in an educational setting with faculty, students, and patients. In addition, opportunities for staff members to attend continuing education courses are offered.

Hospital

Many university-based hospitals have a fully staffed dental clinic. Patients seen in this clinic are generally those who are hospital bound because of an acute or infectious disease and must receive their dental care in a hospital setting.

Teaching

A career in teaching dental assisting might be another consideration. Teaching in a dental assisting program is a challenging and rewarding career. The American Dental Assistants Association (ADAA) accreditation states that a dental assisting instructor must hold certification by the Dental Assisting National Board (DANB) or registration as a dental assistant and should be working toward a bachelor's degree.

If you think you would enjoy teaching, then consider taking college courses on a part-time basis while gaining valuable work experience in the dental office.

Marketing Your Skills

Once you have narrowed your potential areas of interest for employment, knowing where to begin your search for employment is important. Table 29-1 lists several sources for employment leads.

Social Media and Job Search

Social media broadly refers to a form of communication and networking. Social media is an extremely powerful tool when looking for employment opportunities and has become a fast and inexpensive *background check*. Employers search social media to verify facts on resumes, to check out knowledge and attitudes publicly expressed, and to evaluate communication skills. It helps employers gain a clearer idea of who you are and what you have done before talking with you. They can also pick up clues about your personality and how you might fit into their dental practice.

In general, the three major social media associated with job searches are LinkedIn, Facebook, and Twitter.

LinkedIn

LinkedIn is the largest professional network site in the world. Members connect with each other and directly with employers. Most employers prefer LinkedIn, and it is widely viewed as the most businesslike and professional of the social networks. Most importantly, your profile must be professional and up-to-date. Remove any photos or items that are politically divisive or could be considered offensive (https://www.linkedin.com).

Facebook

Facebook is the largest social networking Web site. Your Facebook wall must be either suitable for viewing by potential

TABLE 29-1
Employment Search

Type of Advertisement	Description
Social media	Employers search social media to find qualified applicants and often complete a search before inviting a job applicant in for an interview.
Newspaper advertisements	Dentists frequently place advertisements in the classified section in local newspapers that describe the available position and its requirements. The advertisement may contain a telephone number for you to call. More frequently, it will request that you send your resume to a post office box address or that you fax your resume to a specified number. Responses to newspaper advertisements give the employer an opportunity to screen prospective employees before scheduling interviews.
Employment agencies	Some agencies charge the employee a fee if they find him or her a position. Other agencies charge the employer the fee. The fees charged by most employment agencies are based on a percentage of the projected monthly or annual starting salary of the applicant.
Working interview	A working interview can be a good way to be certain if you have found the right position. On the basis of a resume and one interview, knowing whether the office is a good match for you and for the dentist can be difficult. In a working interview, you and the dentist have a chance to evaluate, first hand, the working relationship you will share. The dental assistant is paid for the day of the working interview.
Professional organizations	Local dental societies and dental-assisting organizations frequently serve as informal employment information centers. Professional journals also have a classified section of possible job opportunities.
Campus placement	Most formal dental-assisting programs offer a placement service with practicing dentists in the area. Dentists frequently contact local schools for new employees.
Sales representatives	When seeking employment, inform your local sales representative. They frequently know when a dentist is looking for a qualified dental assistant.

employers or sufficiently protected by your privacy settings (/social-networking/facebook-job-search/facebook-job-search.shtml).

Twitter

Twitter is a free social networking service that enables its users to send and read messages known as *tweets* (/social-networking/twitter-job search.shtml).

Seeking Employment

Whether you choose to pursue your job search through the use of social media or with a traditional method, you will go through stages. The following are the specific stages that are important in securing your new position.

Telephone Contact

If your first contact with a prospective employer is made by telephone, then identify yourself and explain your reason for calling. This first impression over the telephone is extremely important; if you do not make a good first impression, then you may not get a second chance to prove yourself in an interview. You may be asked to submit a completed application or a resume before being granted an interview.

BOX 29-2 Guidelines for a Cover Letter

- Prepare a one-page typed letter (never handwritten).
- Be brief, professional, and neat.
- Address the cover letter to a specific person.
- Identify the position for which you are applying.
- Request an interview.
- Give contact numbers where you can be reached.
- Thank the recipient for his or her consideration.

Cover Letter

A well-written cover letter serves to introduce you to a prospective employer and markets your skills and qualifications at the same time (Box 29-2). It also serves to create interest on the part of the reader to look at your resume. A variety of approaches and styles are available, but general guidelines should be followed (Figure 29-1).

Resume

A resume is a concise written statement that highlights your individual qualities and skills that would be valuable to a

1 **Your Contact Information**
Name
Address
City, State, Zip code
Phone number
Email address

2 **Date**

3 **Employer Contact Information**
Name
Address
City, State, Zip code

4 **Salutation**
Dear Dr. last name

5 **First Paragraph**
The first paragraph of your letter should include information on why you are writing. Mention the position you are applying for and where you found the job listing. Include the name of a mutual contact, if you have one.

6 **Middle Paragraph(s)**
The next section of your cover letter should describe what you have to offer the employer. Mention specifically how your qualifications match the job you are applying for. Remember, you are interpreting your resume, not repeating it.

7 **Final Paragraph**
Conclude your cover letter by thanking the employer for considering you for the position. Include information on how you will follow up.

8 **Complimentary Close**
Respectfully yours,

9 **Signature**
Handwritten signature (for a mailed letter)
Typed signature

1 Alicia Moore, CDA
121 Pleasant Drive
Any City, US 27740
(000) 555-1212
almoore@internet.com

2 Date, 20XX

3 Dr. Name
123 Cherry Lane
Any City, US 27740

Re: Clinical Assistant Position

4 Dear Dr. Name:

5 I am applying for the Clinical Assistant position advertised in the Any City newspaper.

6 I am a Certified Dental Assistant and a graduate of the Area Accredited School of Dental Assisting. My enclosed resume provides additional information about my experience and background in the dental field.

I would appreciate the opportunity to schedule an interview with you and your staff at your earliest convenience. I can also be reached on my cell phone at (000) 965-1255.

7 Thank you in advance for your consideration, and I look forward to hearing from you.

8 Sincerely,

9 *Alicia Moore*

Alicia Moore, CDA

FIGURE 29-1 Sample cover letter. (From Bird DL, Robinson DS: *Modern dental assisting,* ed 11, St. Louis, 2015, Saunders.)

prospective employer. A resume communicates a maximum amount of information through a minimum number of words (Figure 29-2). The primary purpose of a resume is to convince a prospective employer that you are an outstanding candidate for employment and that it would be worth his or her time to interview you in person.

The time and effort you devote to developing your own resume is a worthwhile investment in your future. Your resume should highlight your educational and professional accomplishments. There is no single correct way to write a resume; however, certain guidelines will assist you in preparing a good resume (Box 29-3).

BOX 29-3 Guidelines for Writing a Resume

Your resume should:
- Be 100% honest.
- Be easy to read with a lot of white space.
- Reflect your uniqueness.
- Stress your assets (avoid information that could screen you out).
- Focus on important information.
- Avoid containing personal pronouns (e.g., I, my, me).
- Stimulate the interest of the reader.
- Use language appropriate to the profession.

Alicia Moore, CDA
121 Pleasant Drive
Any City, US 27740
(000) 555-1212
almoore@internet.com

PROFESSIONAL OBJECTIVE:

Clinical Assistant with a pediatric or general dental practice.

PROFESSIONAL EXPERIENCE:

6/20XX to Present	**Clinical Assistant**, Dr. Janice Davison, New City, US Part-time employment (List your responsibilities and accomplishments here)
6/20XX to 9/20XX	**Coordinating Assistant**, Dr. Harold Randolph, Top City, US (List your responsibilities and accomplishments here)
1/20XX to 5/20XX	**Student Intern**, Dr. Janice Davison, New City, US (List your responsibilities and accomplishments here)

EDUCATION:

9/20XX to 6/20XX	Area Accredited School of Dental Assisting, Any City, US Graduated on Dean's List.
20XX to 20XX	Any City High School, Graduate City, US

CERTIFICATIONS:

Date, 20XX	Currently Certified Dental Assistant
Date, 20XX	Applied for Registered Dental Assistant
Date, 20XX	Treasurer of local Dental Assistants' Society, Any City, US

FIGURE 29-2 Sample resume.

Heading

The heading includes four items: full name (with credentials [CDA, RDA], if appropriate), complete address, home and cellular telephone numbers, and e-mail address. These items can be centered at the top of the page.

Professional Objective

A professional objective is a clear statement of the type of position you are seeking. However, it should not be too narrowly stated, which might limit your job opportunities.

Education

List your most recent to least recent education. If you have a college degree, then do not list your high school graduation. If you have taken special courses or have received honors that may be of interest to your potential employer, then you may want to make note of them in the education section.

Professional Experience

List your most recent to least recent work experiences. Provide the date (month and year only) of your employment, your position or title, the employer's name and location, and your responsibilities and accomplishments.

Note: If you are a recent graduate with minimal or no work experience, then you might wish to list your education first. If your strength is your experience, then list it first. Remember, the purpose of your resume is to make you shine!

Certifications

List your certification or registration, such as cardiopulmonary resuscitation (CPR) certification, and any other appropriate certification information. Emphasize any career-related affiliations, such as membership in the American Dental Assistants Association (ADAA).

It is not recommended that personal data be included in your resume. Under the federal regulations governed by the Equal Employment Opportunity Commission, employers may not ask questions regarding race, color, religion, gender, national origin, marital status, and child care arrangements unless they relate to bona fide occupational qualifications. However, you may be required to submit verification of citizenship or appropriate alien status.

References

Although a list of references is not required, if you choose to provided references, then be certain to contact those you list to get their permission before you provide their names. Your references should be individuals who can address your job-related skills.

Volunteer Experience

If you have done any volunteer work, then list it. Even if it does not pertain to dentistry, it will show that you are a caring individual. Do not list this category if it does not apply to you.

Awards and Scholarships

List any scholarships or awards you have received. Do not list this category if it does not apply to you.

See Procedure 29-1: Preparing a Professional Resume.

Job Application

Before the interview, you may be asked to complete an application form, which can serve as the initial basis of your conversation with the dentist or office manager. When completing this form, follow directions exactly and make certain that the information you provide is accurate, neat, and complete. Read the entire application before you begin filling in the answers. By doing this, you are less likely to make errors or to give information on the wrong line. Bringing a copy of your resume for reference as you fill out the application is also a good idea.

Interview

An interview can be an excellent experience, one in which you discuss your assets and accomplishments; or it can be an unpleasant experience, during which questions are asked of you, and the wrong answer could mean losing the job.

Controlling your nerves, projecting a positive image, and participating in the interview are your responsibility. Remember, not only will the dentist and staff members decide whether you are the assistant they are looking for, but you will also determine whether this job is right for you and whether you will be happy working in this office. Table 29-2 lists some tips that will help you do your best during your next interview.

Federal and state equal employment opportunity laws have a significant impact on the way employers may recruit and select employees. Employers may not discriminate on any legally recognized basis, including but not limited to race, age, color, sex, religion, creed, national origin, physical or mental disability, marital status, or veteran status. Box 29-4 lists the guidelines from the Equal Employment Opportunity Commission regarding questions that may and may not be legally asked during interviews.

Preparation

Rereading your resume before each interview will ensure that you present yourself as a well-organized person with a calm and

TABLE 29-2 Tips for a Good Interview

Be prepared	Make a list of all pertinent questions you would like to ask and points you would like to make.
Be honest	Do not be afraid to say, "I don't know." Then follow up by saying that you will find out.
Be prompt	Arrive approximately 15 minutes early. Never be late or too early. If for any reason you are delayed, then telephone and reschedule the interview.
Be aware	Do not divulge too much personal information. Questions about age, spouses, and children, among other personal information, are optional for you to answer. Keep the conversation about business.
Make eye contact	When you maintain eye contact, even during difficult questions, you display self-confidence.
Show enthusiasm	Be enthusiastic about your career potential, your interests, and your abilities. Remember, you must "sell" yourself. Be honest about your abilities.
Discuss salary if asked	Know the salary ranges in the area in which you are looking. Do not introduce salary negotiations; however, if asked what salary you are seeking, then answer without fear of rejection. Know your worth.
Be aware of body language	Pay attention to the way you nonverbally communicate. Sit upright, do not slouch or fidget, and avoid gestures and postures that show boredom or hostility.
Avoid multiple interviews	Do not arrange for more than one interview in the morning or afternoon.
Say "thank you"	Thank the interviewer at the end of the interview, and follow up with a thank-you note to help remind the interviewer about you and to indicate your continued interest.

BOX 29-4 What You May and May Not be Asked During an Interview*

What Applicants MAY NOT be Asked

- Age or date of birth
- Previous address
- Religion or race
- Mother's surname
- Marital status or maiden name
- Number or ages of children
- Who will care for children
- Spouse or parent's place of employment
- Parents' residence
- Whether you own or rent your residence
- Questions about your ability to speak a foreign language (unless job relevant)
- Questions about arrests
- Membership in social organizations
- Visible physical characteristics (e.g., scars, burns, missing limbs)
- Health status
- Psychologic well-being
- Past injuries or diseases
- Loans, financial obligations, wage attachments, or personal bankruptcies

What Applicants MAY Be Asked

- Reasons for termination of previous employment
- References
- Work schedules
- Previous work experience
- Job-related attitudes about previous assignments or present position
- Career interests
- Job duties
- Job training
- Education
- Qualifications for duties related to the position
- Verification of citizenship or appropriate alien status

*Guidelines from the Equal Employment Opportunity Commission, U.S. Department of Labor.

positive manner. It is also a means of helping you you recall facts, through association, that are not on the resume, but which that will probably come up in the interview.

Appearance

Your appearance is very important. In selecting your clothing, you want your appearance to reflect the fact that you are a neat, well-organized, and competent professional.

Do not wear your dental assisting uniform or scrubs to an interview. Wearing conservative business attire is best. Keep jewelry and makeup to a minimum.

Arrival

Plan to arrive 15 minutes before the scheduled time of the interview. If the interview is scheduled in a geographic area with which you are unfamiliar, it is advisable to make a "dry run" to find the office before the interview. In addition, make sure you arrive alone. Although you may think you need moral support, having a person accompany you would appear unprofessional.

Interviewing Professionally

The first 10 minutes of your interview are the most critical; during this time, both you and the interviewer will have formed first impressions. You may be nervous, but try to relax and be natural.

A smile; direct eye contact; the words, "Hello, I'm (first name and last name). It's a pleasure to meet you"; and a firm but gentle handshake are essential in creating a positive and professional first impression (Figure 29-3).

Many questions will be asked and answered on both sides. Try to answer all questions courteously, completely, and honestly. Be prepared for a variety of questions, and feel free to ask questions if it the time seems to be an appropriate time. Remember, that your attitude and motivation during the interview are important determining factors. You want to convey a positive attitude without overselling yourself.

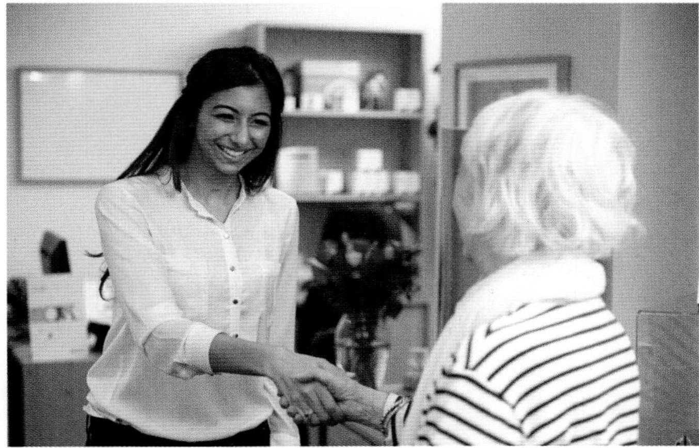

FIGURE 29-3 Your first impression is extremely important. (Copyright © iStock.com/monkeybusinessimages.)

Concluding the Interview

Let the prospective employer (or office manager) conclude the interview. If you think the interview has concluded, then you could say, "If you have no further questions, I would like to thank you for your time." Make the interviewer aware of your interest in the position and that you would like to be seriously considered for the position.

Make sure to extend your hand for a final handshake, and again, use direct eye contact before you say, "I look forward to hearing from you." Within the first week after the interview, you will have developed some intuition of how the interview went, and whether the office is the one in which you would like to pursue employment.

Follow-up Letter

A thank-you letter is an excellent way of following up with an employer after an interview. It serves to remind the employer of your interview, to accentuate your qualifications, to reaffirm your interest in the position, and to help you stand out in the interviewer's mind. The **follow-up letter** should be sent within 48 hours, should be addressed to the person with whom you interviewed, and should reaffirm your interest in the position in the practice. Make sure the letter is thoughtful and sincere (Figure 29-4).

Once you have landed the right position, it is also courteous to call or send a note to those offices with whom you have interviewed to let them know that you have found a position.

Salary Negotiations

Although salary and benefits are not the only factors to be considered when you are accepting a job, they are important issues that need to be clarified.

The interviewer may ask, "What do you expect in terms of salary?" If you have a definite and realistic idea, then by all means state it. Keep in mind that education, experience, and skills are important factors that should be considered in a fair and equitable salary and benefits package.

As you negotiate a compensation package with the dentist, you should realize the importance of the total dollar value when benefits are added to salary, the number of hours you will be working, and the working conditions.

Alicia Moore, CDA
121 Pleasant Drive
Any City, US 27740
(000) 555-1212
almoore@internet.com

Date, 20XX

Dr. Name and Staff
123 Cherry Lane
Any City, US 27740

Dear Dr. Name and Staff:

Thank you for taking time out of your busy schedule to interview me last Tuesday, October 25th. I enjoyed our conversation and am very enthusiastic about the possibility of working with you and your staff.

I know that my clinical and communication skills would be an asset to your practice. Please do not hesitate to call me should you have any other questions.

Again, thank you for your consideration. I look forward to hearing from you in hopes that you have reached a decision favorable to both of us.

Sincerely,

Alicia Moore

Alicia Moore, CDA

FIGURE 29-4 Sample follow-up letter. (From Bird DL, Robinson DS: *Modern dental assisting,* ed 11, St. Louis, 2015, Saunders.)

BOX 29-5 Exit Professionally: Tips for Terminating Employment

- Give adequate notice to your employer.
- Leave on a positive note. Do not vent anger and/or frustrations.
- Do not burn your bridges with angry remarks about others.
- Avoid new job-hunting activities during office hours.
- Do not slack off your duties during your last 2 weeks.
- When possible, find and train your replacement.

The negotiating discussion offers an excellent opportunity to ask about the frequency of reviews, salary increases, and opportunities to advance in the practice.

Job Termination

There may come a time when you will have to terminate employment. It should be ended in a professional manner (Box 29-5). If your practice has an employee handbook, follow the procedures for resigning your position. The employer should always learn—directly from you—of your intention to resign, not from another employee in the office.

The most common time frame for notifying your employer is 2 weeks. If asked, then help select and train your replacement. The time between giving notice and departing is a very important period of employment. Those employees who slack off in the final weeks should expect a less-than-positive recommendation. Commit yourself to leaving your job with honor and dignity. Remember, the last impression is the one that will always be remembered.

If your employment is terminated by your employer, then your departure should be handled in accordance with the terms of your employment agreement. Severance pay, which is the equivalent of salary for the notice period, is paid if your employer terminates your employment and is typically paid with the final paycheck.

Ethical Implications

The dental profession is a small community. Dentists socially and professionally interact with each other. They have formed connections through schools, dental societies, community and service organizations, and social activities.

Keeping good ties between you and former employers and coworkers is always a good idea. At some time in the future, these individuals can be valuable assets and can provide crucial help for future employment. During your career in the dental profession, you will find people who will enter and exit and enter your life again. Never allow angry words or unprofessional behavior burn the bridges behind you.

Your professional reputation can spread; therefore, always demonstrate ethical behavior at every job, from the first day to the last day.

Procedure 29-1

Preparing a Professional Resume

Goal

To prepare a resume to be used for seeking employment

Procedural Steps

1. Keep the resume to one page (see Figure 29-2).
2. Use standard letter size ($8\frac{1}{2} \times 11$) white or ivory rag paper.
3. Use common typefaces.
4. Use 1-inch margins on all sides.
5. Use a 12-point font size.
6. Ensure that the resume is neat and error free.
7. Keep the content concise and easy to read.

Chapter Exercises

Multiple Choice

Circle the letter next to the correct answer.

1. Dental assistants may be employed in which of the following areas?
   a. Private practice
   b. Teaching
   c. Dental sales
   d. All of the above
2. The purpose of a cover letter is to __________.
   a. introduce yourself to the prospective employer
   b. market your skills and qualifications
   c. create interest for reading your resume
   d. all of the above
3. Information about which of the following should NOT be included when writing a resume?
   a. Education
   b. Family
   c. Professional objective
   d. Professional experience
4. On a resume, your education should be listed __________.
   a. most recent to least recent
   b. top of the page
   c. least recent to most recent
   d. last item on the page
5. When should you arrive for an interview?
   a. 30 minutes early
   b. 15 minutes early
   c. Exactly on time
   d. Within the hour of the appointment
6. Which of the following is (are) NOT appropriate to wear on a job interview?
   a. Uniform
   b. Heavy makeup
   c. Scrubs
   d. All of the above
7. After an interview, you should __________.
   a. telephone the office and thank them once again
   b. send a thank-you letter
   c. fax an additional copy of your resume
   d. all of the above
8. When leaving a job, what is the usual minimum amount of notice that should be given to the employer?
   a. 24 hours
   b. 1 week
   c. 2 weeks
   d. 1 month
9. Which of the following social media sites is the largest for professional networking?
   a. Twitter
   b. Facebook
   c. LinkedIn
10. A resume communicates a minimum amount of information in a maximum amount of space.
    a. True
    b. False

Apply Your Knowledge

1. During a clinical internship in an orthodontic office, you decide that you would like to work in an orthodontic office after graduating from the dental-assisting program. You have an interview scheduled with Dr. Marcus, an orthodontist, and she is concerned about your lack of experience. What can you say to convince Dr. Marcus that you will make an excellent orthodontic assistant, despite your lack of experience?
2. Linda, a bubbly and experienced dental assistant, has finally had it with the inner-office politics and quarreling among the staff members. She decides that she is going to quit her job the next day and leave immediately after she tells her coworkers what she thinks of them. Then she is going to tell Dr. Elliott what she thinks of his management policies. Linda feels very satisfied with her plan. What danger do you see in this plan?
3. Trang Li has just graduated from a dental-assisting program and is very nervous about going for her first job interview. As a friend and classmate, how could you help her prepare?
4. An education in dental assisting can lead to a variety of career opportunities. Identify those areas in which a dental assistant can be employed, and think about which ones might interest you.

GLOSSARY

absorbed dose Amount of energy imparted by ionizing particles to unit mass of irradiated material at a place of interest (15)
abutment Tooth, root, or implant used for support and retention of a fixed or removable prosthesis (23)
act of commission Performance of an act that a "reasonable and prudent professional" would not perform (2)
act of omission Failure to perform an act that a "reasonable and prudent professional" would perform (2)
active learning Process during which the learner participates in teaching and learning activities (17)
acute infection Infection of short duration that is often severe (5)
acute myocardial infarction Occlusion or blockage of one or more arteries that supply the muscles of the heart, resulting in injury or necrosis of the heart muscle (heart attack) (13)
acute radiation exposure Large dose of radiation that is absorbed in a short period as in a nuclear accident (15)
aerosol 1. Suspension of materials in a gas or vapor 2. Substance dispensed as a constituent of a gas or vapor suspension (5)
air-powder polishing Use of a specially designed handpiece with a nozzle that delivers a high-pressure stream of warm water and sodium bicarbonate (Under high pressure, the combination of powder and water rapidly and efficiently removes stains.) (18)
ala of the nose Winglike tip on the outer side of each nostril (3)
ALARA principle Acronym for As Low As Reasonably Achievable (The ALARA principle pertains to radiation exposure encountered when taking x-ray images; it requires that every possible precaution be taken to limit radiation levels when exposing the patient or technician to radiation.) (15)
alcohol Transparent colorless liquid that is mobile and volatile (Alcohols are organic compounds formed from hydrocarbons by the substitution of hydroxyl radicals for the same number of hydrogen atoms.) (7)
alcohol-based hand rubs Waterless antiseptic agents that are alcohol-based products available in gels, foams, or rinses (6)
alginate Salt of alginic acid (e.g., sodium alginate), which, when mixed with water in accurate proportions, forms an irreversible hydrocolloid gel used for making impressions (22)
allergen Substance capable of producing an allergic response (Common allergens are pollens, dust, drugs, and food.) (13)
alloy Solution comprised of two metals dissolved in each other when in the liquid state (20)
alveolar socket Cavity or space within the alveolar process that surrounds the root of a tooth (3)
alveolitis Inflammation of a tooth socket after an extraction (26)
alveoloplasty Surgical shaping and smoothing of the margins of the tooth socket after the extraction of the tooth, generally in preparation for the placement of a prosthesis (26)
amalgam Alloy used for restoring teeth (Mercury is one of the constituents in amalgam.) (20)
amalgamator Mechanical device used to triturate the ingredients of dental amalgam into a mass (20)
analgesia Insensibility to pain without loss of consciousness; a state during which a painful stimulus is not perceived or interpreted as pain (Analgesia is usually induced by a drug.) (14)
anaphylaxis Allergic reaction characterized by sudden collapse, shock, or respiratory and circulatory failure from the presence of an allergen (13)
anatomic crown Portion of dentin covered by enamel (4)
anatomy Science of the form, structure, and parts of organisms (3)
anesthetics Drugs that generally or locally produce a loss of feeling or sensation (14)
angina pectoris Frequent symptom of cardiovascular disease (A severe viselike pain behind the sternum that sometimes radiates to the arms, neck, or mandible is characteristic of angina pectoris. Symptoms may also include a sense of constriction or pressure of the chest. Angina pectoris is caused by exertion or excitement and is relieved by rest.) (13)
angle of the mandible Lower posterior of the ramus (3)
anode Positive electrode in the x-ray tube (15)
anterior Toward the front surface (3)
anterior naris Nostril; plural, nares (3)
antianxiety Technique or drug used to prevent or relieve anxiety (14)
antigen Substance introduced into the body to stimulate the production of an antibody (13)
antiseptic Substance for killing microorganisms on the skin (7)
apex Tapered end of each root tip (4)
apical Pertaining to the end portion of the root (4)
apicoectomy Surgical procedure to remove the tip of a tooth root in endodontic therapy (25)
arch wires Contoured metal wires that provide force when guiding the teeth in movement for orthodontics (28)
articulator Dental laboratory device that simulates mandibular and temporomandibular joint movement when models of the dental arches are attached to it (23)
asepsis Condition of being without infection, of being free of pathogenic microorganisms (26)
asthma Respiratory disease often associated with allergies and characterized by sudden recurring attacks of labored breathing, chest constriction, and coughing (13)
attached gingivae Fibrous attachments of the gingival tissues to the teeth (3)
autoclave Instrument used for sterilization by means of moist heat under pressure (8)
automatic processing techniques Fast and efficient methods of processing during which the film is mechanically transferred

from the developer to the fixer, is washed, and is finally dried (16)

automix Mixing technique available for use with impression materials (Automix systems are designed by the manufacturers to complete the mixing process for the procedure. The unique automix system device provides a homogeneous mix with the appropriate amount of material without waste.) (22)

autonomy Childhood process of becoming independent (27)

auxiliaries Attachments located on the brackets and bands that hold arch wires and elastics (28)

avulsed Torn away or dislodged by force (27)

background radiation Particle emission arising from radioactive material other than the one directly under consideration (Background radiation can result from cosmic rays and natural radioactivity that is always present, and it may also exist because of radioactive substances in other parts of a building.) (15)

bacteria Small, unicellular microorganisms that morphologically vary in shape and size; spherical (cocci), rod-shaped (bacilli), spiral (spirochetes), or comma-shaped (vibrios) (5)

bacterial endocarditis Inflammation of the heart valves and lining of the heart as the result of a bacterial infection (5)

bands Stainless steel rings cemented to molars that hold the arch wire and auxiliaries for orthodontics (28)

bifurcation Division into two parts or branches, such as any two roots of a tooth (4)

bioburden Blood, saliva, and other bodily fluids (7)

biofilm Slime-producing bacterial communities that may also harbor fungi, algae, and protozoa; a complex, three dimensional arrangement of bacteria living together as a self-sufficient, secure, self-sustaining community that is resistant to conventional antibiotics and antimicrobial agents (Dental plaque is a biofilm; hence, the term *oral biofilm*.) (7, 17, 18)

biologic monitor Instrument that verifies sterilization by confirming that all spore-forming microorganisms have been destroyed (8)

bisecting angle technique Angle at which a periapical survey x-ray image is taken; horizontally angled so that the ray passes through the interproximal space as close to the center of the area being radiographed as possible and vertically angled so that the ray travels perpendicular to the bisection of the angle formed by the x-ray film and the long axes of the targeted tooth (16)

bite-wing image Radiographic image that includes the distal half of the crowns of the cuspids, both premolars, and often the first molars on both the maxillary and mandibular arches (16)

blood pressure Pressure of the blood that is applied against the walls of blood vessels within the arteries (11)

bloodborne diseases Viral diseases that are transmitted via contaminated blood and/or other bodily fluids (5)

Bloodborne Pathogens (BBP) Standard Most important standard of the Occupational Safety and Health Administration (OSHA) regarding infection control in dentistry (The BBP Standard is designed to protect employees against occupational exposure to bloodborne and disease-causing organisms.) 6)

bonding Technique that is used to adhere orthodontic attachments to the teeth (20)

brachial Related to the arm (brachium), as in brachial artery (11)

breach of contract Failure, without legal excuse, to perform an obligation or duty specified in a contract (2)

bridge Fixed prosthesis (23)

buccal Referring to structures closest to the inner cheek (3)

burs Rotary cutting instruments of steel or tungsten carbide and supplied with cutting heads of various shapes (19)

calculus Calcium and phosphate salts in saliva that become mineralized and adhere to tooth surfaces (17, 18)

canthus Fold of tissue at the corner of the eyelids (3)

career 1. Chosen pursuit; profession or occupation 2. General course or progression of one's working life or one's professional achievements (29)

carotid Related to either one of the two major arteries on each side of the neck that carries blood to the head (11)

carpal tunnel syndrome (CTS) Pain associated with continued flexion and extension of the wrist (9)

cassette Holder for extraoral films for exposure (16)

cathode Negative electrode in the x-ray tube (15)

cavity Area in a tooth caused by decay (21)

cavity classifications Standard classifications that describe the types and locations of decay or restorations (Carious lesions are classified according to the surfaces of the tooth on which they occur [e.g., lingual, buccal, occlusal], the type of surface [e.g., pit, fissure, smooth], and numeric grouping.) (12)

cells Basic units of vital tissue (3)

cements Materials that produce a mechanical interlocking effect of a direct restoration and the tooth (20)

cementoenamel junction Point at which the enamel of the crown and the cementum of the root of a tooth meet (The area above the cementoenamel junction corresponds to the anatomic crown of the tooth; the area apical to the junction constitutes the anatomic root of the tooth.) (4)

cementum Specialized, calcified connective tissue that covers the anatomic root of a tooth (4)

Centers for Disease Control and Prevention (CDC) Nonregulatory federal agency that issues recommendations on health and safety (6)

centric Having an object centered, such as maxillary teeth centered over mandibular teeth in correct relation (22)

cephalometric Extraoral radiograph exposed to show the bones and soft tissue areas of the facial profile (28)

cerebrovascular accident (CVA) Sudden loss of brain function caused by blockage or rupture of a blood vessel in the brain (A CVA is also called a stroke.) (13)

certified dental assistant (CDA) Person who successfully passes the Dental Assisting National Board Examination or State Board and remains current with continuing education requirements (2)

certified dental technician (CDT) Dental laboratory technician who passes the proper written examination (1)

cervical collar Leaded device that is positioned around the throat during radiographic procedures to protect the thyroid gland from exposure to radiation (15)

charge-coupled device (CCD) Solid-state image sensor used in intraoral digital imaging (16)

chemical label Identifies all hazardous ingredients and safety precautions for a product (A chemical label is required by the Hazard Communication Standard.) (6)

chemical vapor sterilization Process during which chemical vapors are created under heat and pressure for the sterilizing procedure (8)

chlorine dioxide Effective, rapid-acting environmental surface disinfectant or chemical sterilant (7)

chronic infection Infection of long duration (5)

chronic radiation exposure Exposure to small amounts of radiation that are repeatedly absorbed over a long period, the effects of which may not be observed until years after the original exposure (15)

civil law Category of law that deals with the relations of individuals, corporations, or other organizations (2)

clean areas Places where sterilized instruments, fresh disposable supplies, and prepared trays are stored (8)

clinical crown Portion of the tooth that is visible in the oral cavity (4, 18)

collimation Limiting the diameter of the x-ray beam to protect adjacent areas from exposure to radiation (15)

collimator Lead disc with an opening (rectangular or circular) designed to limit the dimension of a beam of radiation (15)

Commission on Dental Accreditation of the American Dental Association (CODA) Commission that accredits dental and dental assisting, dental hygiene, and dental laboratory educational programs (1)

composite resin Restorative material used for its esthetic purposes (The chemical makeup of composite resin includes an organic resin matrix, inorganic fillers, and a coupling agent.) (20)

contact point Area of the mesial or distal surface of a tooth that touches the adjacent tooth in the same arch (4)

contaminated area Place where contaminated items are brought for precleaning (8)

contract law Category of law that involves an agreement for services in exchange for payment (2)

contrast Differences in degrees of blackness on a radiograph (15)

control panel Master switch, indicator light, selector buttons, and exposure button (15)

control tooth Healthy tooth used as a standard to compare questionable teeth of similar size and structure during pulp vitality testing (25)

core Central part of or support for an indirect restoration (The core can be prepared from an existing amalgam restoration, a composite material, or reinforced glass ionomer cement.) (23)

cover letter Letter of introduction sent with other documents (e.g., resume) that provides more information to a prospective employer (29)

critical instruments Items used to penetrate soft tissue or bone (7)

cross-bite Tooth that is not properly aligned with its opposing tooth (27)

cross-contamination Direct transfer of an infection from one person to another or indirectly from one person to a second person via a fomite (5)

crown Portion of the tooth covered by enamel (23)

cumulative effects Exposure to radiation, resulting in a cumulative effect over a lifetime (When tissue is exposed to x-ray beams, some damage occurs. Although tissue can repair some damage, it does not return to its original state.) (15)

cumulative trauma disorder Condition caused by repetitive motion and overflexion and overextension of the wrist (9)

curing Act of polymerization (20)

cusp Major elevation on the masticatory surfaces of the canines and posterior teeth (4)

debridement Process of removing or cleaning out the pulpal canal (25)

demineralization Loss of minerals from the tooth; initial stage of tooth decay (17)

demographics Personal information about patients, such as address and work, as well as statistical characteristics of populations (11)

density Overall darkness or blackness of a radiograph (15)

dental assistant Oral health care professional trained to provide supportive procedures for the dentist and patients (1)

dental auxiliary Dental assistant, dental hygienist, and dental laboratory technician (2)

dental dam Thin, stretchable material that becomes a barrier when appropriately applied to selected teeth (When the dental dam is in place, only the selected teeth are visible through the dam. It is available in latex or nonlatex.) (10)

dental decay Infectious disease with progressive destruction of tooth substance, beginning on the external surface by demineralization of enamel or exposed cementum (17)

dental health care team Dentist, dental assistant, dental hygienist, and dental laboratory technician (The purpose of the dental health care team is to provide quality oral health care for the patients of the practice.) (1)

dental laboratory technician Professional who performs dental laboratory services, such as fabricating crowns, bridges, and dentures, as specified by the dentist's written prescription (1)

dental operatory Dental treatment room and control center of the clinical area (9)

dental public health Specialty that promotes oral health through organized community efforts (1)

dental sealant Resin-type material that is placed in the occlusal pits and fissures of teeth to prevent dental caries (18)

dental specialties Nine fields recognized by the American Dental Association (ADA): dental public health, endodontics, oral and maxillofacial radiology, oral and maxillofacial surgery, oral pathology, orthodontics, pediatric dentistry, periodontics, and prosthodontics (1)

dentin Portion of the tooth that lies between the enamel or cementum and the pulp (4)

dentinal fiber Fiber found in dentinal tubules (4)

dentinal tubules Microscopic canals found in dentin (4)

dentist Individual educated, trained, and licensed to treat diseases and injuries of the teeth and oral cavity and to construct and insert restorations of and for the teeth, jaws, and mouth (1)

diabetes Metabolic disorder characterized by high blood glucose levels and insufficient insulin (13)

diagnosis Identification or determination of the nature and cause of a disease or injury through an evaluation of a patient's history and examination (12)

diagnostic cast Stone or plaster model of dental structures for the purpose of study and treatment planning (22)

diagnostic quality image Image that has been properly placed, exposed, and processed (16)

diastolic Normal rhythmic relaxation and dilation of the heart chambers (11)

digital image Electronic representation of a radiographic, a film, or an x-ray image (16)

digital imaging Filmless method of capturing and displaying an image by using an image sensor, an electronic signal, and a computer to process and store the image (15)

digitizes Process of scanning a traditional film-based radiograph into a digital image (16)

direct pulp cap Application of a material to the exposed pulp to stimulate repair of the injured pulpal tissue (25)

direct supervision Level of supervision during which the dentist is physically present when the dental auxiliary performs a delegated function (2)

direct transmission Pathogens transferred by coming into direct contact with the infectious lesion or infected bodily fluids, including blood, saliva, semen, and vaginal secretions (5)

disclosing agents Coloring agents that make plaque visible when applied to teeth (17)

disinfection Process of destroying pathogenic organisms or rendering them inert (7)

distal Farther away from the trunk of the body; opposite of proximal (3)

doctor of dental surgery (DDS) Type of degree that some dental schools award to dentists upon graduation (1)

doctor of medical dentistry (DMD) Type of degree that some dental schools award to dentists upon graduation (1)

dose equivalence Product of absorbed dose and modifying factors, specifically, the quality factor, distribution factor, and any other necessary factors (15)

dry heat sterilizer Type of sterilization method for instruments that use dry heated air (8)

duration Time from induction to complete reversal of anesthesia (14)

edentulous Without teeth (23)

embrasure Triangular space in a gingival direction between the proximal surfaces of two adjoining teeth in contact (4)

emergency Unforeseen occurrence or a combination of circumstances that calls for immediate action or remedy; pressing necessity; exigency (13)

enamel 1. Hard, glistening tissue covering the anatomic crown of the tooth 2. Outermost layer or covering of the coronal portion of the tooth that overlies and protects the dentin (4)

enamel prisms Another term for enamel rods that make up the enamel structure (4)

endodontics Dental specialty that diagnoses and treats diseases of the pulp (1)

endodontist Dentist who practices endodontics, which focuses on the causes, diagnosis, prevention, and treatment of diseases of the dental pulp and their sequelae (25)

endogenous Developed from within the structure of the tooth (18)

endosteal Pertains to within the bone in a dental implant (23)

epilepsy Neurologic disorder that exhibits sudden, recurring seizures of motor, sensory, or psychic malfunctioning (13)

ergonomics Adaptation of the human body to the work environment (9)

esthetic dentistry Type of dentistry that improves the appearance of teeth by camouflaging defects and whitening teeth (21)

etching Process of preparing the tooth surface with the use of an acid product (18, 20)

ethics Moral standards of conduct; rules or principles that govern proper conduct (2)

evacuator Instrument used to remove saliva, blood, water, and debris during a dental procedure (10)

exfoliation Normal process of shedding the primary teeth (4)

exogenous Developed from external sources (18)

exothermic Characterized by the release of heat from a chemical reaction (20)

expanded function Specific intraoral function delegated to an auxiliary with the required advanced skill and training (9)

expanded function dental assistant (EFDA) Assistant who has received additional training and is legally permitted to provide certain intraoral patient care procedures beyond the duties traditionally performed by a dental assistant (1)

extraction Removal of a tooth from the oral cavity by means of elevators and/or forceps (26)

extrensic stain Stain within the structure of the tooth caused by external sources (e.g., amalgam stain) (18)

extrude To push or force out (22)

Facebook Popular free social networking Web site that allows registered users to create profiles, upload photos and videos, send messages, and keep in touch with other users (29)

Federation Dentaire Internationale (FDI) System Recognized method of dental charting used to identify and designate permanent and primary and deciduous teeth within the oral cavity (4)

film duplicating Process of copying a radiographic image (16)

filter Aluminum disc placed in the x-ray unit at the position indicator device (PID) to absorb less energetic (less penetrating) x-ray beams (15)

filtration Use of aluminum filters to remove long (less penetrating) wavelengths from a primary x-radiation beam (15)

fixed appliance Appliance that is cemented in place or attached by a bonding material (28)

fixed bridge Dental prosthesis with artificial teeth cemented in place and supported by attachment to natural teeth (23)

flange Part of a full or partial denture that extends from the teeth to the border of the denture (23)

fluoride Mineral that naturally occurs in food and water and is used for the prevention of tooth decay (Fluoride can be delivered through systemic and topical methods.) (17, 27)

fluoride varnish Concentrated topical fluoride within a resin or synthetic base that is applied to the teeth to prolong fluoride exposure (17)

fluorosis Form of enamel hypomineralization attributable to excessive ingestion of fluoride during the development of a tooth (17)

focusing cup Keeps electrons suspended in an electron cloud at the cathode (15)

follow-up letter Letter used to follow up with a potential employer after an interview (29)

force To cause a physical change through energy and strength (20)

forced air sterilizer Sterilizing instrument that circulates hot air throughout the chamber at high velocity, which permits the rapid transfer of heat energy from the air to the instruments, reducing the time needed for sterilization (A forced air sterilizer is also called a rapid heat transfer sterilizer.) (8)

fossae Pits, indentations, grooves, or depressions (4)

framework Metal skeleton of a removable partial denture (23)

Freeman, Robert Tanner First African-American student in the first dental class at Harvard University (1)

friction-grip Short and smooth shank that has no retention grooves (The friction-grip shank is held in the high-speed handpiece by the creation of friction that grips the entire shank.) (19)

frontal plane Vertical plane that divides the body into anterior (front) and posterior (back) portions (3)

F-speed film Currently the fastest-exposure dental x-ray film on the market (15)

fulcrum Finger rest within the mouth that is used when holding an instrument or handpiece for a specified time (18)

fungi Plants such as mushrooms, yeasts, and molds that lack chlorophyll, the substance that makes plants green (5)

galvanic Type of electrical current that takes place when two different or dissimilar metals come together (20)

general supervision Level of supervision during which the dental auxiliary performs delegated functions according to the instructions of the dentist, who is not necessarily physically present (2)

genetic changes Mutations that affect future generations (15)

gingival graft Surgical procedure during which tissue is removed from a donor site and attached (grafted) to another site (24)

gingival retraction Displacement of gingival tissue away from the tooth (23)

gingivectomy Surgical removal of diseased gingival tissue (24)

gingivitis Inflammation of gingival tissue (24)

gingivoplasty Surgical reshaping and contouring of gingival tissue (24)

glabella Smooth surface of the frontal bone and also the anatomic part directly above the root of the nose (3)

Globally Harmonized System (GHS) of Classification and Labeling of Chemicals International system of labeling and classifying chemicals that will be the same, regardless of where in the global market the chemical is manufactured or used (6)

glutaraldehyde Environmental Protection Agency (EPA)–registered high-level hospital disinfectant (7)

grasp Manner in which the dentist holds an instrument (9)

Gray-Rollins, Ida (1867-1953) First African-American woman in the United States to earn a dental degree (1)

gutta-percha Plastic type of filling material used in endodontics (25)

handpiece Electrical instrument used to hold rotary instruments (19)

hazard class Specific criteria for hazards that are developed to compare severity within a category (6)

Hazard Communication Standard (HCS) Occupational Safety & Health Administration (OSHA) standard regarding employees' "right to know" about hazardous chemicals in the workplace (6)

hazard statement Statement on a chemical label that indicates the specific hazard of a chemical (6)

hazardous waste Waste that poses a danger to humans or to the environment (6)

headgear External orthodontic appliance used to control growth and tooth movement (28)

hemisection Procedure during which the root and the crown are cut lengthwise and removed (25)

hepatitis A virus (HAV) Type of hepatitis that is spread from person to person via the oral-fecal route (HAV is the least serious form of viral hepatitis.) (5)

hepatitis B virus (HBV) Type of hepatitis that causes a very serious viral disease that may result in prolonged illness, liver cancer, cirrhosis of the liver, liver failure, and even death (HBV is a bloodborne disease that is transmitted by other bodily fluids including saliva.) (5)

hepatitis C virus (HCV) Type of hepatitis that is largely transmitted by blood transfusion or percutaneous inoculation, such as when intravenous drug users share needles (HCV progresses to chronic hepatitis in up to 50% of the patients acutely infected.) (5)

hepatitis D virus (HDV) Defective virus that cannot replicate itself without the presence of HBV (Infection with HDV may simultaneously occur as a co-infection with HBV or may occur in an HBV carrier.) (5)

Health Insurance Portability and Accountability Act (HIPAA) Federal regulations that ensure privacy regarding a patient's health care information (11)

HIV Human immunodeficiency virus; a bloodborne viral disease that attacks and weakens or destroys the immune system (5)

holding solution Used for instruments that cannot be immediately cleaned after the procedure (The holding solution prevents the drying of blood and debris on the instruments.) (8)

horizontal angulation Position of the tubehead and the direction of the central ray in a horizontal or side-to-side plane (16)

host Living cells that may be human, animal, plant, or bacteria in which viruses must live and replicate (5)

host susceptibility Ability of a host cell to resist the invasion of a virus (5)

hyperglycemia Abnormally high level of blood glucose (13)

hyperventilation Abnormally fast or deep breathing (13)

hypoglycemia Abnormally low level of blood glucose (13)

impaction Tooth that has not erupted (26)

implant Reproduction of a tooth and root placed into the bone to replace a tooth or bridge (23)

implied consent Patient's action that indicates consent for treatment (2)

impression Negative reproduction of an object from which a positive reproduction may be made (22)

indirect pulp cap Placement of dental material over a partially exposed pulp (25)

indirect supervision Level of supervision during which the legally qualified dental auxiliary performs delegated functions according to the instructions of the dentist, who is not necessarily physically present; also known as general supervision (2)

indirect transmission Indirect transfer of organisms to a susceptible person that can occur by handling contaminated instruments or by touching contaminated surfaces and then touching the face, eyes, or mouth (5)

induction Time from injection to effective anesthesia (14)

infectious disease Communicable disease (5)

infectious waste Term used to identify waste to be disposed of according to applicable federal, state, and local regulations (6)

inferior Below another part; closer to the feet (3)

informed consent Permission granted by a patient after being informed of the advantages, disadvantages, and alternatives of a procedure (2)

inlay Cast restoration designed for Class II cavity preparation (23)

innervation Distribution of an anesthetic agent to the nerves (3)

intrinsic stain Stain developed from within the structure of the tooth (18)

instrument Tool or appliance specifically designed for a technique or application in a dental procedure (19)

instrument processing Procedure required to prepare contaminated instruments for reuse on the next patient (8)

interdental aids Special devices recommended as aids for cleaning between teeth with large or open interdental spaces and under fixed bridges (17)

International Standards Organization (ISO) System Numbering system that assigns a two-digit number to each tooth (The first number is the quadrant; the second number is the tooth.) (4)

interview Formal meeting in person, especially one arranged for the assessment of the qualifications of an applicant (29)

iodophors Environmental Protection Agency (EPA)–registered intermediate-level hospital disinfectants with tuberculocidal action (7)

ionization Process during which electrons are removed from atoms, causing the harmful effects of radiation in humans (15)

irreversible hydrocolloid Material of choice when taking preliminary impressions (*hydro* means water, and colloid means a *gelatinous* substance) (22)

irreversible pulpitis Infectious condition in which the pulp is incapable of healing, requiring a root canal (25)

isolation Technique that protects a tooth against contamination from oral fluids during a surgical or restorative procedure, usually through the application of a dental dam or the use of cotton rolls (10)

Kells, C. Edmund (1856-1928) New Orleans dentist credited with employing the first dental assistant (1)

label elements (6) Labeling system used for chemical elements

latch-type Shank that has a small groove at the end that mechanically locks into the contra-angle attachment, which fits on the low-speed handpiece (19)

latent image Invisible image on the x-ray film after exposure but before processing (16)

latent infection Persistent infection with recurrent symptoms that "come and go" (5)

latent period Interval between exposure to ionizing radiation and the appearance of symptoms (15)

lateral Side or away from the midline (3)

lateral surface of the tongue Sides of the tongue (3)

leakage radiation Escape of radiation through the protective shielding of the x-ray unit tube head (Leakage radiation is detected at the sides, top, bottom, or back of the tube head; it does not include the useful beam.) (15)

legal 1. In compliance with the law 2. Not forbidden by law (2)

licensure License to practice in a specific state (2)

light-cured Technique to polymerize a dental material with a curing light (18)

lingual Surface of teeth closest to the tongue (3)

LinkedIn Business-oriented social networking service that is primarily used for professional networking (29)

luxate To dislocate, as a tooth from its socket (26)

malaligned Displaced out of line, such as teeth that are displaced from normal relation to line of the dental arch; maloccluded (10)

malocclusion Occlusion that is deviated from a Class I normal occlusion (28)

mandibular Lower jaw region (3)

manipulated Process of adapting an instrument to a procedure (19)

manual processing Procedure during which an exposed x-ray film is placed on a rack by hand and then inserted into processing chemicals, which causes the image to become visible on the film (16)

masticatory mucosa Oral mucosa that covers the hard palate, dorsum of the tongue, and gingiva (3)

matrix 1. Band that provides a temporary wall 2. Foundation that binds a substance together; continuous phases (organic polymer), during which particles of filler are dispersed in composite resin (21)

maxillary Upper jaw region (3)

maximum permissible dose (MPD) Amount of radiation to the whole body associated with minimal risk for injury (The MPD of whole-body radiation for persons occupationally exposed to radiation is 5000 millirem [mrem], or 5 rem, per year, which equals approximately 100 mrem per week.) (15)

medial Toward or nearer to the midline of the body (3)

medically compromised Individual who may be ill, in pain, or physically challenged (11)

mental protuberance Part of the mandible that forms the chin (3)

midsagittal plane Imaginary line that divides the patient's face into right and left sides (3)

mists Droplets of particles larger than those generated by the aerosol spray (Mists, such as those that result from coughing, can transmit a respiratory infection.) (5)

mixed dentition Complement of teeth in the jaws after the eruption of some of the permanent teeth but before all the primary teeth are absent (4)

mobility Loosening of a tooth in the alveolar socket attributable to the destruction of periodontal fibers (24)

model trimmer Machine used to trim stone or plaster models (22)

mucogingival junction Distinct line of color change in the tissue where the alveolar membrane meets with the attached gingivae (3)

mucous membrane Smooth tissue that lines the oral cavity and other canals and cavities of the body (3)

MyPlate Internet site (www.ChooseMyPlate.gov) designed to help consumers think about building a healthy plate and to offer more information to help consumers build a more healthy plate at mealtimes (17)

nasion Midpoint between the eyes just below the eyebrows (3)

necrotic Term used to describe a tooth that does not respond to sensory stimulus (25)

nitrous oxide–oxygen Combination of gas and oxygen used as an analgesic and sedative agent to ease a patient's anxiety (14)

noncritical instruments Items that come into contact with only intact skin (7)

nonvital Not living, as in oral tissue and tooth structure (25)

numbering systems Simplified means of identifying the teeth for charting and descriptive purposes (4)

object-film distance (OFD) Distance, usually expressed in centimeters or inches, between the object being radiographed and the cassette or film (15)

obturation Process of filling a root canal (25)

occlusal technique Used to examine large areas of the upper or lower jaw (16)

occupational exposure Any reasonably anticipated skin, eye, or mucous membrane contact or percutaneous injury with blood or any other potentially infectious materials (6)

Occupational Safety & Health Administration (OSHA) Federal agency charged with establishing guidelines and regulations regarding worker safety (OSHA guidelines include the storage and disposal of toxic chemicals and hazardous materials and the safety and proper use of clinical and office equipment.) (6)

onlay Cast restoration designed to cover the occlusal crown and proximal surfaces of posterior teeth (23)

operating zones Working positions of the dental team members; based on a "clock concept" (9)

operative dentistry Commonly used term to describe restorative and esthetic dentistry (21)

opportunistic infection Infection caused by normally nonpathogenic organisms and occurring in individuals whose resistance is decreased or compromised (5)

oral and maxillofacial radiology Dental specialty involved with the diagnosis of disease through various forms of imaging, including x-ray films (radiographs) (1)

oral and maxillofacial surgery (OMFS) Dental surgical specialty that diagnoses and treats conditions of the mouth, face, upper jaw (maxilla), and associated areas (1, 26)

oral biofilm Dense, nonmineralized complex mass of colonies in a gel-like matrix that adheres to the pellicle and hence to the teeth, calculus, and fixed and removable restorations (17)

oral pathology Dental specialty that diagnoses and treats diseases of the oral structures (1)

oral prophylaxis Complete removal of calculus, debris, stain, and plaque from the teeth (18)

organs Several types of tissues grouped together to perform a single function (e.g., heart, lungs, kidneys) (3)

orthodontics Specialty of dentistry designed to prevent, intercept, and correct skeletal and dental problems (1)

ortho-phthalaldehyde (OPA) Chemical used in high-level disinfection (7)

osseointegration Anchoring of an implant by the growth of bone (23)

ostectomy Surgery involving the removal of bone (24)

osteoplasty Surgical procedure during which bone is added, contoured, and reshaped (24)

palate Bone and soft tissue that close the space encompassed by the upper alveolar arch, extending posteriorly to the pharynx (3)

Palmer Notation System Method of charting in which each of the four quadrants is given its own tooth bracket made up of a vertical line and a horizontal line (4)

panoramic radiography Modality that delivers an image that provides a wide view of the upper and lower jaws (16)

paralleling technique Intraoral technique of exposing periapical films (16)

parenteral transmission Act of transmitting bloodborne pathogens through needlestick injuries, human bites, cuts, abrasions, or any break in the skin (5)

pathogen Disease-producing microorganism (5)

patient of record Individual who has been examined and diagnosed by the dentist and has had treatment planned (2)

patient record Document that is managed by the dentist for each patient in a dental practice (11)

pediatric dentistry Dental specialty involved with neonatal through adolescent patients and patients with special needs in these age groups (1)

percutaneous Through the skin, such as a needlestick, cut, or human bite (6)

periapical Apex and the surrounding area of a tooth (4)

periapical views Images that show the crown, root tip, and surrounding structures (16)

periodontal dressing Surgical dressing applied on a surgical site for protection, similar to a bandage (24)

periodontal flap surgery Incisional surgery performed when excisional surgery is not indicated (During periodontal flap surgery, the tissue is not removed but is pushed away from the underlying tooth roots and alveolar bone, similar to the flap of an envelope.) (24)

periodontal ligament System of collagenous connective tissue fibers that connect the root of a tooth to its alveolus (4)

periodontal pocket Deepening of the gingival sulcus beyond normal, resulting from periodontal disease (24)

periodontics Dental specialty involved with the diagnosis and treatment of diseases of the supporting tissue (1)

periodontist Dentist with advanced education in the specialty of periodontics—the art and science of examination, diagnosis, and treatment of diseases affecting the periodontium (24)

periodontitis Inflammatory disease of the supporting tissue of the teeth (24)

periodontium Structure that surrounds, supports, and is attached to a tooth (4, 24)

permanent dentition The 32 teeth of adulthood that replace or are added to the complement of deciduous teeth (4)

permucosal Contact with mucous membranes, such as the eyes or mouth (6)

personal protective equipment (PPE) Items that include protective clothing, masks, gloves, and eyewear to protect employees (6)

pestle Object that pounds or pulverizes a material (20)

philtrum Rectangular area from under the nose to the midline of the upper lip (3)

phosphor storage plates (PSPs) Thin flexible plates the size of conventional film that have been coated with phosphor crystals (This technology uses a reusable PSP as the image receptor.) (16)

photon Minute (tiny) bundle of pure energy that has no weight or mass (15)

physiology Study of the functions of the human body (3)

pictogram Graphic elements used on a hazard label to identify the specific hazard class and category (6)

pits and fissures Small pinpoint depressions located at the junction of developmental grooves and shallow grooves between the primary parts of the crown (Pits and fissures primarily occur on the occlusal surfaces of posterior teeth and on the lingual surfaces of the maxillary incisors.) (18)

plaque Soft deposit on teeth that consists of bacteria and bacterial by-products (17)

plaque control skillsinclude brushing, flossing, using interdental cleaning aids, and using antimicrobial solutions (17)

plaster Dental plaster of Paris (Plaster is used for pouring preliminary impressions and for making diagnostic models.) (22)

point of entry Specific location where the central beam is directed (16)

polyether Impression material that provides better mechanical properties than polysulfide and less dimensional change than silicone (22)

polymerization Bonding process of two or more monomers (20)

polysulfide Final impression material that has been used in dentistry for many years; also referred to as rubber base (Polysulfide is supplied as a two-paste system—the base and the catalyst.) (22)

pontic Artificial tooth that replaces a missing natural tooth within a bridge (23)

portal of entry Entrance that provides a pathogen the means of entering the body, which is necessary to cause an infection (5)

position indicator device (PID) Cone that directs the x-ray beam, has a round or rectangular shape, and is available in two lengths, short (8 inch) and long (16 inch) (15)

post Prefabricated pin that accurately fits within an endodontically treated tooth to provide added strength and stability to the final restoration (23)

posterior Toward the back (3)

postural hypotension Increased blood pressure that occurs when standing and may result in dizziness and fainting (13)

precleaning Removal of bioburden and other materials before disinfection or sterilization (7)

preparation Selected form given to a natural tooth when it is reduced by instrumentation to receive a prosthesis (e.g., an artificial crown or a retainer for a fixed or removable prosthesis) (21)

preventive dentistry Program of patient education, use of fluorides, application of dental sealants, proper nutrition, and plaque control to prevent dental disease (17)

primary dentition Teeth that erupt first and are replaced by the permanent teeth (This term is currently preferred over "deciduous.") (4)

primary radiation All radiation directly produced from the target in an x-ray tube (15)

process indicators Tapes, strips, or tabs with heat-sensitive chemicals that change color when exposed to a certain temperature (8)

process integrators Strips placed into packages that change colors when exposed to a combination of heat, temperature, and time (8)

professionalism Demonstration of specialized skills and knowledge in a manner that meets the standards of a profession (2)

prosthodontics Dental specialty that provides restoration and replacement of natural teeth (1)

provisional coverage Temporary protective crown or bridge that is cemented to a prepared tooth for a single crown or to abutment teeth for a bridge (23)

proximal Close to the trunk of the body (3)

pulp Central portion of teeth that is made up of blood vessels, nerves, and cellular elements, including odontoblasts, which forms the dentin (4)

pulpectomy Complete removal of a vital pulp from a tooth (25)

pulpotomy Removal of the coronal portion of a vital pulp from a tooth (25)

radiation monitoring Used to protect the operator by identifying occupational exposure to radiation (Both equipment and dental personnel can be monitored.) (15)

radiograph Image produced on conventional dental film (1, 16)

radiolucent Image on a radiograph that appears in ranges from shades of gray to black (15)

radiopaque Image on a radiograph that appears in ranges from shades of light gray to total white or clear (15)

rapport Sense of mutuality and understanding; harmony, accord, confidence, and respect underlying a relationship between two persons (27)

reciprocity System that allows individuals in one state to obtain a license in another state without retesting (2)

refractory periodontitis Progressive inflammatory destruction of the periodontal attachment that resists conventional mechanical treatment (24)

registered dental assistant (RDA) Dental assistant who has met the qualifications required by the state that issues the registration (2)

registered dental hygienist (RDH) Oral health care professional trained to remove deposits on the teeth, expose radiographs, place topical fluoride and dental sealants, and provide patients with oral health care instructions (1)

registration Act of completing forms with personal information (22)

regulated waste Infectious waste that requires special handling, neutralization, and disposal (6)

remineralization Replacement of minerals in the tooth structure (17)

removable appliance Appliance designed so that it can be removed and replaced by the patient (28)

res gestae (Latin, *things done*) Statements made by any person present at the time of an alleged negligent act that are admissible as evidence in a court of law (2)

respiration Act or process of inhaling and exhaling; breathing (11)

rests Metal projections designed to control the seating of a prosthesis as it is positioned in the mouth (23)

restorations Use of dental material to restore teeth to a functional permanent unit (21)

restorative dentistry Type of dentistry that restores teeth to their original structure by removing decay and restoring defects (21)

resume Brief account of one's professional or work experience and qualifications, often submitted with an employment application (29)

retainer 1. Device used to hold attachments and abutments of a removable prosthesis in place 2. Appliance used for maintaining the positions of the teeth and jaws after orthodontic treatment (23, 28)

retention Result of adhesion, mechanical locking, or both (20)

retrograde restoration Root end filling, which is completed when the apical seal is not adequate (25)

reversible pulpitis Form of pulpal inflammation in which the pulp may be salvageable (25)

Rickert, Jessica First Native-American woman dentist in the United States (1)

risk management Program designed to identify, contain, reduce, or eliminate the potential for harm to patients, visitors, and employees and potential financial loss to the facility if a compensable event occurs (2)

Roentgen, William Conrad Bavarian physicist (1845-1923) who discovered x-ray images, or radiographs, in 1895 (1)

root amputation Dental procedure during which one root is removed from a multiroot tooth (25)

root planing Procedure that smooths the surface of a tooth by removing abnormal toxic cementum or dentin that is rough, contaminated, or permeated with calculus (24)

rotary Part or device that rotates around an axis (19)

rubber-cup polishing Technique used to remove plaque and stains from the coronal surfaces of the teeth (18)

saddle 1. Part of a denture that fits the oral mucosa of the basal seat, restores the normal contours of the soft tissue of the edentulous mouth, and supports the artificial teeth 2. Portion of a denture that overlies the soft tissue, usually fabricated of resin or combinations of resins and metal (23)

safety data sheet (SDS) Form that provides health and safety information regarding materials that contain chemicals (6)

sagittal plane Any anteroposterior plane of the body parallel to the median sagittal plane (3)

scaling Removal of calcareous deposits from the teeth with the use of suitable instruments (24)

scanning Process immediately completed after radiographic exposure (16)

scatter radiation Form of secondary radiation that occurs when an x-ray beam has been deflected from its path by interaction with matter (15)

sealer Substance used to fill the space around silver or gutta-percha points in a pulp canal (25)

secondary radiation X-radiation that is created when the primary beam interacts with matter (15)

sedation Production of a sedative effect; act or process of calming (14)

semicritical instruments Items that come into contact with oral tissues but do not penetrate soft tissue or bone (7)

sensor-holding device Instrument that holds the image receptor in the patient's mouth during exposure (16)

separator Elastomeric ring or steel separating spring interproximally used to force the mesial and distal spaces of the tooth slightly apart (28)

septum 1. Dental dam material located between the holes of the punched dam 2. Tissue that divides the nasal cavity into two nasal fossae (3, 10)

sharps Pointed or cutting instruments, including needles, scalpel blades, orthodontic wires, and endodontic instruments, that are potentially infectious (6)

sign Indication of the existence of something; any objective evidence of a disease (13)

signal word Two words that are used on the safety data sheet: "Warning" for less severe hazard categories and "Danger" for more severe hazard categories (6)

silicone Compound of organic structural character in which all or some of the positions that could be occupied by carbon atoms are occupied by silicon (a plastic containing silicons) (22)

sodium fluoride (NaF) White, odorless powder used in 2% aqueous solution and topically applied to teeth as a caries-preventing agent; used as 33% NaF in kaolin and glycerin as a desensitizing agent for hypersensitive dentin; used as a caries-prophylactic substance (one part per million of NaF) in drinking water (17)

sodium hypochlorite Surface disinfectant commonly known as household bleach (7)

social media Online communications channels dedicated to community-based input, interaction, content sharing, and collaboration (29)

somatic changes Effects of radiation that cause illness and are responsible for poor health (e.g., cancer, leukemia, cataracts) but are not passed on to offspring (15)

source-film distance Distance from the focal spot of an x-ray tube to the radiographic film; also known as target-object distance (15)

space maintainer Fixed or removable appliance designed to preserve the space created by the premature loss of a tooth (27)

sphygmomanometer Instrument for measuring blood pressure in the arteries (11)

spore Form assumed by some bacteria that is resistant to heat, drying, and chemicals (Spores represent the most resistant form of life known.) (5)

stainless steel crown Preformed steel crown used for the restoration of badly decayed primary teeth and first permanent molars (27)

Standard Precautions Standard of care designed to protect health care providers from pathogens that can be spread by blood or any other bodily fluid, excretion, or secretion (Standard Precautions expand the concept of Universal Precautions.) (6)

stannous fluoride Type of topical fluoride that has been shown to be useful in treating dental hypersensitivity (17)

static air sterilizer Sterilizing instrument that circulates heat, similar to an oven (The heating coils of a static air sterilizer are on the bottom of the chamber, and the hot air rises inside through natural convection. Heat is transferred from the static [nonmoving] air to the instruments in approximately 1 to 2 hours.) (8)

sterilization Process that kills all microorganisms (8)

stethoscope Instrument that is used for listening to sounds produced within the body (11)

stone Abrading instrument or tool (22)

strain Distortion or change produced as a result of stress (20)

stress Internal reaction or resistance to an externally applied force (20)

subgingival Area below the gingivae (24)

subperiosteal Situated or occurring under the periosteum and on top of the bone (23)

subsupine Lying-down position in which the patient's head is lower than the feet (below the heart); used in emergency situations (9)

sulcus 1. Furrow, trench, or groove, as on the surface of the brain or in the folds of mucous membranes 2. Groove or depression on the surface of a tooth 3. Groove or depression surrounding the tooth (24)

superior Above another portion or closer to the head (3)

supine Lying-down position in which the patient's head, chest, and knees are at the same level (9)

supragingival Area above the gingivae (24)

surface barriers Fluid-resistant materials used to cover surfaces likely to become contaminated (7)

suture 1. Synarthrosis between two bones formed in a membrane, the uniting medium (which tends to disappear eventually) being a fibrous membrane continuous with the periosteum 2. Surgical stitch or seam 3. Material with which body structures are sewn, as after a surgical procedure or injury 4. To sew up a wound (26)

symptom Any morbid phenomenon or departure from normal in function, appearance, or sensation that is experienced by the patient and indicative of disease (13)

syncope Loss of consciousness caused by insufficient blood to the brain, also referred to as fainting (13)

synthetic phenol Environmental Protection Agency (EPA)–registered intermediate-level hospital disinfectant with broad-spectrum disinfecting action (7)

syringe Instrument consisting of a needle, barrel, and plunger that is used to inject liquid into a cavity or under the skin (14)

systemic fluoride Fluoride that is ingested and then circulated throughout the body (17)

systolic Rhythmic contraction of the heart, especially of the ventricles (11)

teledentistry Process of using electronic transfer of images and other information for consultation and/or insurance purposes in dentistry (16)

temperature Degree of heat or cold of a body or an environment (11)

thermometer Instrument for measuring temperature (11)

tipping Type of tooth movement in which the root of the tooth is facially or lingually tipped to correct the angle of the crown of the tooth (28)

tissue Aggregation of similarly specialized cells united in the performance of a particular function (3)

tooth whitening Noninvasive method of lightening the color of dark or discolored teeth; commonly known as vital bleaching (20)

topical fluorides Fluorides that are directly applied to teeth (17)

torque Twisting or turning force (19)

tort law Involvement in an act that brings harm to a person or damage to property (2)

toxic waste Waste that can have a poisonous effect (6)

trabeculae Thin plates of bone tissue arranged in an irregular pattern; found in spongy bone (3)

tragus Cartilaginous projection anterior to the external opening of the ear (3)

transosteal Insertion through the inferior border of the mandible and into the edentulous area (23)

transverse plane Imaginary plane that divides the body into superior (upper) and inferior (lower) portions; also known as the horizontal plane (3)

trays Receptacles or devices that hold or carry impression material to the oral cavity (22)

treatment plan In dentistry, a schedule of procedures and appointments designed to restore, step by step, the oral health of a patient (12)

trifurcation Area in which three roots divide (4)

trigeminal nerve Fifth cranial nerve that provides motor innervation to the muscles of mastication and sensory innervation to the face, jaws, and teeth (3)

trituration Process of mechanically mixing a material, as in using an amalgamator to mix an alloy and mercury to create dental amalgam (20)

tubehead Tightly sealed, heavy metal housing that contains the radiograph tube (15)

tuberculosis Infectious disease caused by *Mycobacterium tuberculosis* and characterized by the formation of tubercles in the tissue (Worldwide, tuberculosis is the leading cause of death from infectious diseases.) (5)

Twitter Online social networking service that enables users to send and read short 140-character messages called "tweets" (29)

ultrasonic cleaner Instrument that loosens and removes debris by sound waves traveling through a liquid (8)

ultrasonic scaler Device used for rapid calculus removal that operates on high-frequency sound waves (24)

unit Each component of the fixed bridge (23)

Universal National System Numbering system (1-32 for the permanent teeth and 1-20 for the primary teeth) that begins with the maxillary right and concludes at the mandibular right (4)

Universal Precautions Based on the concept that all human blood and certain bodily fluids (including saliva) are to be treated as if known to be infected with the bloodborne diseases hepatitis B, hepatitis C, or human immunodeficiency virus (HIV) infection (6)

vasoconstrictor Type of drug that constricts (narrows) blood vessels and used to prolong anesthetic action (14)

veneer Thin layer of composite resin or porcelain bonded or cemented to a prepared facial surface (21)

vertical angulation Angle measured within the vertical plane at which the central ray of the x-ray beam is projected, relative to a reference in the horizontal or occlusal plane (16)

vertical bite-wing radiograph Bite-wing film or receptor is placed in the mouth with the long portion of the film or receptor in a vertical direction (24)

virulence Strength of a pathogen's ability to cause disease; also known as pathogenicity (5)

viruses Ultramicroscopic infectious agents that contain either deoxyribonucleic acid (DNA) or ribonucleic acid (RNA) (5)

viscosity Physical property of fluids for resistance to flow (22)

vital bleaching Procedure during which a chemical oxidizing agent (sometimes in combination with light) is used to lighten tooth discolorations (21)

vital signs Clinical measurements used to evaluate a person's general physical condition (11)

wedge Wooden or plastic triangular device placed in the embrasure to provide the contour needed when restoring a Class II lesion (21)

white spot Earliest sign of demineralization (17)

zygomatic arch Arch formed by articulation of the temporal process of the zygomatic bone with the zygomatic process of the temporal bone (3)

INDEX

Page numbers followed by "*f*" indicate figures, "*t*" indicate tables, and "*b*" indicate boxes.

D

E